D1609503

Neuroglia

NEUROGLIA

Second Edition

Edited by

HELMUT KETTENMANN
BRUCE R. RANSOM

OXFORD
UNIVERSITY PRESS
2005

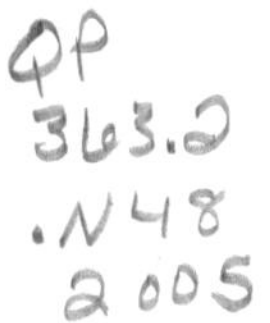

OXFORD
UNIVERSITY PRESS

Oxford New York
Auckland Bangkok Buenos Aires Cape Town Chennai
Dar es Salaam Delhi Hong Kong Istanbul Karachi Kolkata
Kuala Lumpur Madrid Melbourne Mexico City Mumbai Nairobi
São Paulo Shanghai Taipei Tokyo Toronto

Published by Oxford University Press, Inc.
198 Madison Avenue, New York, New York, 10016
www.oup.com

Library of Congress Cataloging-in-Publication Data
Neuroglia / edited by Helmut Kettenmann, Bruce R. Ransom.—2nd ed.
p. ; cm. Includes bibliographical references and index.
ISBN 0-19-515222-0 (cloth :)
1. Neuroglia. I. Kettenmann, Helmut. II. Ransom, Bruce R.
[DNLM: 1. Neuroglia—physiology.
2. Nervous System Diseases—physiopathology.
WL 102 N494555 2004] QP363.2.N48 2004 611′.0188—dc22 2004043482

Printing number: 9 8 7 6 5 4 3 2 1

Printed in the United States of America
on acid-free paper

To the memory of our friend
Richard K. Orkand (1936–2002),
a pioneer in glial research

Preface to the second edition

Almost 10 years have passed since the first edition of *Neuroglia* was published. *Neuroglia* was warmly received and we were pleased that it soon became a standard reference work in this field. The pace of glial research has continued to accelerate, however, and we could not ignore the obvious need for a fresh assessment and summary of this field.

The need for a comprehensive and contemporary book on glial cells has never been greater. All of the motivating factors mentioned in the preface to the first edition continue to operate, including the lack of glial coverage in general neuroscience textbooks. In fact, the practical impact of the second edition of *Neuroglia* may be greater than the first because it is offered at a time when a majority of neuroscientists would acknowledge that neuroglia are elemental to most, if not all, brain functions. This was certainly not the case when the first edition appeared.

This book is not simply an edited version of the first edition. We started with the proverbial "clean sheet" of paper in planning the second edition. Based on advice solicited from many of our colleagues, the book was entirely reorganized to more logically assemble current information about glial cells. We recruited many new contributors, reflecting the emergence of new topics and new experts in the field. Less than a fourth of the original chapters were retained, and most of these were revised so extensively that they are essentially new contributions themselves. Novel topics appearing in the second edition include: transmitter release by exocytosis from glia, glial derived stem cells, glia and synaptic transmission, glia and axon guidance, an entire section on mechanisms of glial injury, and several new chapters about the roles of glia in different diseases.

In many ways the second edition of *Neuroglia* was more challenging to conceive and produce than the first edition. With affordability in mind, we were committed to a second edition that was smaller than the first edition. We also wanted a greater degree of uniformity in terms of subject treatment than was true for the first edition. We struggled in the planning stages with how to condense topic areas without sacrificing crucial content. Accordingly, we urged authors to be concise, and we limited the number of citations and edited each chapter based on reviews provided by other contributors. But the universe of relevant knowledge about glial cells is much larger today and the need to include new topics while adhering to a strict page budget came at a price. Some "classic" topics covered in detail in the first edition such as glial anatomy and ion channel expression were significantly condensed, and the first edition of *Neuroglia* will remain useful for exactly that reason.

We predicted in the first edition preface that "As impressive as our gains in glial cell knowledge have been, the best is yet to come." The second edition of *Neuroglia* thoroughly documents our progress in understanding these cells and vindicates this statement, but we readily admit that this prediction remains true for the future. Not so long ago it was imagined that glia represented a functionally uniform cell population. This concept was discarded as we recognized that glia are a diverse and complex cell family whose only common feature is that they are not neurons. Situational plasticity and regional variability in these cells are emerging themes that promise to further enlarge their range of functions. But the path to the future always starts with a current and accessible base of information. We believe that the second edition of *Neuroglia* provides this important starting point.

Berlin, Germany H.K.
Seattle, Washington B.R.R.

Preface to the first edition

Nonneuronal cells, termed *neuroglia,* were recognized as independent elements of the nervous system nearly a century and a half ago by Virchow. These cells are present in primitive nervous systems and, undoubtedly driven by positive evolutionary pressures, have persisted in high density and acquired greater diversity in mammals. Knowledge about glial cells has accumulated at a phenomenal rate in the past 30 years, and has become relevant to all fields of neurobiology. With so much new information at hand, we felt that this was an important time to assemble the facts about these cells as we presently understand them.

Historically, glial cells were viewed as a type of central nervous system connective tissue whose main function was to provide support to the true functional cells of the brain, the neurons. This firmly entrenched concept remained virtually unquestioned for the better part of a century. But glial cells are neither connective tissue nor mere supportive cells. In contrast to early beliefs, glial cells are now recognized as intimate partners with neurons in virtually every function of the brain and as participants in the pathophysiology of the dysfunctional or diseased brain. These cells have been challenging to study, however, because their functions are not associated with easily recorded electrical signals, as is the case with neurons.

While books about the nervous system have grown in size and complexity, at-tempting to accommodate the frantic production of new neuroscience information, the incorporation of new facts about glia has not kept pace. One simply cannot learn about glial cells by turning to the typical neuroscience textbook (*From Neuron to Brain* by Nicholls, Martin, and Wallace, is a notable exception). This curious fact has also been a motivation for bringing together in the present volume a detailed summary of what is currently known about these cells. It will, we hope, also encourage better integration of the glial and neuronal information bases, which each suffer in the absence of the other. The brain cannot be understood as the functional sum of two isolated cellular compartments; it must, we think, be seen as a single entity containing neurons and glial cells working in seamless harmony with one another. Somehow, this essential message has gone too long undelivered.

Glial research is at a particularly exciting point in its evolution. Great advances in our knowledge about nervous system diseases have opened the door for thinking about the role of glial cells in the pathogenesis of these conditions and in their treatment. Therapies that would literally have been the stuff of science fiction only a decade ago are now in advanced stages of testing. Patients with Parkinson's disease who no longer respond to our best medicines, for example, have received brain tissue transplants, whose effectiveness may be enhanced by including glial cells as factories for the production of trophic substances. Glial transplants to refurbish areas of demyelination may also be possible in the near future. Our capacity to measure the brain's functional molecules and determine their cellular topography has revealed a baffling array of neurotransmitters, receptors, ion channels, adhesion molecules, and trophic factors associated with glial cells. These findings are stimulating and broadening the field of glial research. They provide critical insights into how neurons and glial cells might communicate with each other, and reveal an astonishing overlap between the features of the brain's two principal cell types that would have been heresy not long ago.

The many experts who wrote chapters for this volume contributed in other valuable ways as well. Before the writing began, they provided invaluable advice about what topics should be covered. In an unselfish manner, they adjusted the scope of their individual contributions so that they fit the context of the book as a whole. To enhance the quality and utility of the chapters, each underwent a stage of peer review and this was cheerfully provided by other authors. The editorial burden was significantly lightened by the satisfaction of dealing with this uniquely talented and energetically committed group of authors. They share our view of the importance of developing a compendium volume about glial cells and continuously reinforced our enthusiasm for the project as it moved forward. We acknowledge their essential partnership in the making of *Neuroglia* and thank them for their efforts.

One point should be made in concluding. As impressive as our gains in glial cell knowledge have been, the best is yet to come. Glial researchers have struggled with our own version of the Heisenberg uncertainty principle: how to study the role of glial cells in the multicellular actions of the nervous system without interfering with the very functions we wish to understand. Our initial efforts were a compromise. We retreated somewhat from the immense complexity of the intact nervous system in favor of simplified preparations that allowed more rigorous study. This reductionistic approach has produced a mountain of provocative information, as detailed here, but few definitive answers. Consequently, we have long lists of glial cell properties, while the list of proven functions is small. But starting with these demonstated properties, testable hypotheses of glial cell function can now be formulated with greatly improved precision, taking full advantage of new or refined research technologies. A rich yield of vital new insights into the functions of neuroglia should follow, and future editions of this book will survey those benefits.

Contents

Development

PART III DISEASE AND NEUROGLIAL CELLS

Mechanisms of Glial Injury

Recovery of Neural Function

Diseases

Contributors

FRANCESCA ALOISI
Laboratory of Organ and System Pathophysiology
Istituto Superiore di Sanità
Neurophysiology Unit
Rome
Italy

JACK ANTEL
Department of Neurology and Neurosurgery
McGill University, Montreal Neurology Institute
Montreal, Quebec
Canada

DOUGLAS ARNOLD
MR Spectroscopy Lab, McConnell Brain Imaging Centre
McGill University, Montreal Neurological Institute
Montreal, Quebec
Canada

RICHARD B. BANATI
University of Sydney
School of Medicine Radiation Sciences
Lindcombe, NSW
Australia

LAKSHMI BANGALORE
Department of Neurology
Yale University School of Medicine
New Haven, Connecticut

HANS-CHRISTIAN BAUER
Institut für Molekularbiologie
Österreichische Akademie der Wissenschaften
Salzburg
Austria

HANNELORE BAUER
Institute für Molekularbiologie
Österreichische Akademie der Wissenschaften
Salzburg
Austria

INGO BECHMANN
Institut für Anatomie
Charité, Humboldt Universität
Berlin
Germany

ETTY N. BENVENISTE
Department of Cell Biology
University of Alabama at Birmingham
Birmingham, Alabama

WILLIAM F. BLAKEMORE
Department of Clinical Veterinary Medicine
University of Cambridge
Cambridge
United Kingdom

INGOLF E. BLASIG
Forschungsinstitut für Molekulare Pharmakologie
Berlin
Germany

J. GORDON BOYD
Department of Anatomy and Cell Biology
Queen's University
Kingston, Ontario
Canada

NEVILLE BROOKES
Department of Pharmacology and Experimental Therapeutics
University of Maryland School of Medicine
Baltimore, Maryland

ARTHUR M. BUTT
Centre for Neuroscience Research
GKT Guy's Campus
London
United Kingdom

ANNACHIARA CAGNIN
Department of Neurology and Psychiatry
University of Padova
Padova
Italy

ANTHONY T. CAMPAGNONI
Department of Developmental Neuroscience
University of California, Los Angeles
School of Medicine
Los Angeles, California

JONATHAN A. COLES
INSERM, U 594
Grenoble
France

MARISA LUISA COTRINA
Division of Developmental Neurobiology
National Institute for Medical Research
London
United Kingdom

Rita M. Cowell
Department of Neurology
University of Michigan and Veterans Affairs Medical Center
Ann Arbor, Michigan

Martina Deckert
Abteilung für Neuropathologie
Universitätskliniken zu Köln
Köln
Germany

Joachim W. Deitmer
Abteilung für Allgemeine Zoologie
Universität Kaiserslautern
Kaiserslautern
Germany

Ulrich Dirnagl
Neurologische Klinik
Charité, Humboldt Universität
Berlin
Germany

Piet Eikelenboom
Department of Psychiatry
Valeriuskliniek
Amsterdam
The Netherlands

Lawrence F. Eng
Department of Pathology
Stanford University School of Medicine
Stanford, California and
Department of Veterans Affairs Medical Center
Palo Alto, California

Andreas Faissner
Zellmorphologie und molekulare Neurobiologie
Universität Bochum
Bochum
Germany

Christopher J. Feeney
Institute of Medical Science
University of Toronto
Toronto, Ontario
Canada

Robin J.M. Franklin
Department of Clinical Veterinary Medicine
University of Cambridge
Cambridge
United Kingdom

Mark P. Goldberg
Department of Neurology
Washington University School of Medicine
St. Louis, Missouri

James E. Goldman
Division of Neuropathology
Columbia University College of Physicians and Surgeons
New York, New York

Francisco González-Scarano
Department of Neurology
University of Pennsylvania
Philadelphia, Pennsylvania

Tessa Gordon
Department of Neuroscience
University Alberta Faculty of Medicine
Edmonton, Alberta
Canada

Bernd Hamprecht
Physiologisch-Chemisches Institut
Universität Tübingen
Tübingen
Germany

Reiner F. Haseloff
Forschungsinstitut für Molekulare Pharmakologie
Berlin
Germany

Jeroen J.M. Hoozemans
Departments of Pathology and Psychiatry
Vrije Universiteit
Amsterdam
The Netherlands

Lynn D. Hudson
National Institute of Neurological Disorders and Stroke
National Institutes of Health
Bethesda, Maryland

Lidija Ivic
Department of Neurology
Columbia College of Physicians and Surgeons
New York, New York

Kristján R. Jessen
Department of Anatomy
University College London
London
United Kingdom

Helmut Kettenmann
Zelluläre Neurowissenschaften
Max-Delbrück-Centrum für Molekulare Medizin
Berlin
Germany

Harold K. Kimelberg
Ordway Research Institute
Program for Nerve and Heart Cell Rescue
Albany, New York

ISABEL KLUSMAN
Scientific Coordinator
Brain Research Institute
Zürich
Switzerland

SHINICHI KOHSAKA
Department of Neurochemistry
National Institute of Neuroscience
Kodaira
Tokyo
Japan

DENNIS L. KOLSON
Departments of Neurology and Microbiology
University of Pennsylvania
Philadelphia, Pennsylvania

ARNOLD R. KRIEGSTEIN
Center for Neurobiology and Behavior
Columbia College of Physicians and Surgeons
New York, New York

YUEN LING LEE
Department of Pathology
Stanford University School of Medicine
Stanford, California
and
Department of Veterans Affairs Medical Center
Palo Alto, California

PIERRE J. MAGISTRETTI
Institut de Physiologie
Université de Lausanne
Lausanne
Switzerland

VERÓNICA MARTÍNEZ-CERDEÑO
Department of Neurology
Columbia College of Physicians and Surgeons
New York, New York

RUDOLF MARTINI
Universität Würzburg
Neurologie
Würzburg
Germany

JACOPO MELDOLESI
Department of Neurosciences
Vita-Salute University and Scientific Institute
San Raffaele
Milano
Italy

RHONA MIRSKY
Department of Anatomy and Developmental Biology
University College London
London
United Kingdom

ALEXANDER A. MONGIN
Division of Neurosurgery
Albany Medical College
Albany, New York

SEAN MURPHY
Medical School, QMC, Institute of Cell Signalling
University of Notingham
Nottingham
United Kingdom

KAZUYUKI NAKAJIMA
Neurobiology Laboratory
Soka University
Tokyo
Japan

KLAUS-ARMIN NAVE
Neurogenetik
MPI für Experimentelle Medizin
Göttingen
Germany

MAIKEN NEDERGAARD
Department of Cell Biology and Anatomy
New York Medical College
Valhalla, New York

JENNIFER K. NESS
Center for the Study of NS Injury, Department of Neurology
Washington University School of Medicine
St. Louis, Missouri

HARALD NEUMANN
Neuroimmunologie
European Neuroscience Institute Göttingen
Göttingen
Germany

ERIC A. NEWMAN
Department of Neuroscience
University of Minnesota
Minneapolis, Minnesota

ROBERT NITSCH
Institut für Anatomie
Charité, Humboldt Universität
Berlin
Germany

STEPHEN C. NOCTOR
Department of Neurology
Columbia College of Physicians and Surgeons
New York, New York

MICHELLE L. OLSEN
Department of Neurobiology and CIRC 545
University of Alabama at Birmingham
Birmingham, Alabama

Brian R. Pearce
Department of Pharmacology
University of London
School of Pharmacy
London
United Kingdom

Luc Pellerin
Institut de Physiology
Université de Lausanne
Switzerland

Josef Priller
Klinik und Poliklinik für Neurologie
Charité, Humboldt Universität
Berlin
Germany

Pasko Rakic
Department of Neurobiology
Yale University School of Medicine
New Haven, Connecticut

Bruce R. Ransom
Department of Neurology
University of Washington School of Medicine
Seattle, Washington

Andreas Reichenbach
Paul-Flechsig-Institut für Hirnforschung
Universität Leipzig
Leipzig
Germany

Bernhard Reuss
Zentrum für Anatomie, Neuroanatomie
Georg August Universität Göttingen
Göttingen
Germany

James W. Russell
Department of Neurology
University of Michigan and Veterans Affairs Medical Center
Ann Arbor, Michigan

Elena Ryzhova
Departments of Neurology and Microbiology
University of Pennsylvania
Philadelphia, Pennsylvania

Dirk Schlüter
Institut für Medizin Mikrobiologie und Hygiene
Universitätsklinikum Mannheim
Universität Heidelberg
Heidelberg
Germany

Martin E. Schwab
Institut für Hirnforschung
Universität Zürich
Zürich
Switzerland

Harald W. Sontheimer
Neurobiology Research Center
University of Alabama at Birmingham
Birmingham, Alabama

Christian Steinhäuser
Experimentelle Neurobiologie
Klinik für Neurochirurgie
Universität Bonn
Bonn
Germany

Wolfgang J. Streit
Department of Neuroscience
University of Florida COM
J. Hillis Miller Health Center
Gainesville, Florida

Peter K. Stys
Department of Neuroscience
University of Ottawa
Ottawa Hospital
Ottawa, Ontario
Canada

Olawale A.R. Sulaiman
Department of Surgery
Section of Neurosurgery
Health Sciences Centre
Winnipeg, Manitoba
Canada

Ueli Suter
Eidgenössische Technische Hochschule
Institute of Cell Biology
Zürich
Switzerland

Raymond A. Swanson
Department of Neurology
University of California, San Francisco
and
Veterans Affairs Medical Center
San Francisco, California

Klaus Unsicker
Abteilung Anatomie und Zellbiologie
Universität Heidelberg
Heidelberg
Germany

Robert Veerhuis
Departments of Pathology and Psychiatry
Vrije Universiteit
Academic Hospital
Amsterdam
The Netherlands

Stephan Verleysdonk
Physiologisch-Chemisches Institut
Universität Tübingen
Tübingen
Germany

ANDREA VOLTERRA
Institut de Biologie
Cellulaire et de Morphologie
Université de Lausanne
Lausanne
Suisse

STEPHEN G. WAXMAN
Department of Neurology
Yale University
New Haven, Connecticut

MICHAEL WELLER
Neurologische Klinik
Universität Tübingen
Tübingen
Germany

DUANE R. WESEMANN
School of Medicine Dean's Office
Department of Cell Biology
University of Alabama at Birmingham
Birmingham, Alabama

HEINRICH WIESINGER
Physiologisch-Chemisches Institut
Universität Tübingen
Tübingen
Germany

HARTWIG WOLBURG
Pathologisches Institut
Universität Tübingen
Tübingen
Germany

ZU-CHENG YE
Department of Neurology
University of Washington School of Medicine
Seattle, Washington

Neuroglia

1 The concept of neuroglia: a historical perspective

HELMUT KETTENMANN AND BRUCE R. RANSOM

Our intent in this chapter is to provide a historical perspective that highlights the early period of glial research. The scientific arguments and historical context were as important to us as the individual facts in trying to understand the emergence of the concept of neuroglia. One of the authors (H.K.) is German and has collected or has special access to a wide range of historical texts, most in German, permitting detailed study of some original material that has not been reviewed for decades. This was advantageous in unexpected ways. Many important nineteenth-century studies by early investigators of various nationalities were either directly published in German, such as the complete work of Gustav Retzius (Swedish), or were translated into German, including studies by Ranvier (French) and Golgi (Italian). Yet we are aware that there are more discoveries awaiting us in the historical literature recorded exclusively in Italian, Spanish, and French, particularly. We hope that this chapter will inspire individuals with unique access to documents in these languages to delve into them in an effort to bring greater clarity to the history of glial research. Several prior reviews touch on various aspects of the history of glial research (Deiters, 1865; Retzius, 1893; Lenhossék, 1895; Weigert, 1895; Robertson, 1897; Held, 1903; Penfield, 1932; Rand, 1953; Glees, 1955; Somjen, 1988; Jacobson, 1993).

It is worth considering momentarily the contentious issue of priority of discovery. The reason, of course, is that any historical work such as this cannot help but make pronouncements about the order in which scientific discoveries were made. In fact, scientists seem to have an appetite for such information, and we readily admit taking guilty pleasure in the practice. The process of assigning priority is imprecise, however, and we suggest keeping several points in mind as you read this account, or any historical account for that matter. First, the historical record itself is complicated and often incomplete. Historians inevitably view only portions of the relevant material, are influenced by their own presumptions and background, and are forced to depend, in many instances, on written accounts that are themselves derivative. Second, scientific papers from 100 or more years ago can be difficult to interpret because of ambiguous language and/or illustrations. Finally, there is the matter of defining what constitutes priority. In his enjoyable book *Foundations of Neuroscience*, Jacobson (1993) nicely states the problem: "Is priority established by the one who pronounced the original theory, or who gave the first inconclusive evidence, or who finally proved the theory? Or should priority be given to those who invented the techniques that made it possible to obtain the facts?" He does not provide an answer to this question, nor do we.

VIRCHOW COINS THE NAME

> Belief begins where science leaves off and ends where science begins.
>
> —*Rudolph Virchow*

Ironically, the concept of neuroglia may have been introduced prior to the actual discovery of the cells. In fact, as first used, the term *neuroglia* was more about interstitial substance than about cells. At a minimum, it can be said that Virchow's invention of the term *neuroglia* in 1856 predated clear histological recognition of the cells that we call neuroglia today.

Discovery is heavily influenced by the intellectual milieu. When the term *neuroglia* was coined, the *cell concept* was becoming established. Schleiden, and other botanists first developed the *cell theory* through the study of plants. An after-dinner conversation with Schleiden propelled Theodor Schwann (1810–1882) to search for and discover nucleated cells in animal tissues. This led Schwann to pronounce what Garrison (1929) calls "the most important generalization in the science of morphology, viz., the principle of structural similarity in animal and vegetable tissues." Other young scientists and students directed by Johannes Müller, the chairman of the department of physiology and anatomy at Berlin University, did pioneering work on the fundamental nature of tissues starting in the late

1830s. Along with Schleiden and Schwann, Jakob Henle, Rudolph Albert Kölliker, Robert Remak, and Rudolf Virchow studied various tissues and strengthened the concept that all tissues are built from cells. An error had crept into this theory, however. It was believed by the influential Schwann that cells developed from a matrix referred to as the *cytoblastema*. Virchow pointed out that this was tantamount to acceptance of *spontaneous generation*. One of Virchow's greatest contributions was his work supporting the concept that all cells derive from other cells ("Omnis cellula e cellula").

Rudolph Virchow (1821–1902) was a pathologist, and his main object of study was diseased tissue. He had abundant access to postmortem human tissue and was familiar with diseased brains. A prevailing theory, supported by Virchow, held that cells derived from ectoderm must directly contact cells of mesodermal origin. Moreover, he had published extensively on the topic of connective tissue, a mesodermal tissue that was a frequent site of inflammation. These ideas were in the air when *neuroglia* was first defined. Virchow, only 35 years old at the time, published an annotated two-volume collection of his papers in 1856 (Virchow, 1856). In a comment about his previous paper "Ueber das granulierte Ansehen der Wandung der Gehirnventrikel" (On the granulated appearance of the ventricular walls) (Virchow, 1846), he wrote: "In accordance with my studies, the ependyma does not only consist of an epithelium, but is a connective tissue layer covered by an epithelium. Despite the fact that it can be dissected from the surface, it does not form an isolated skin in the true sense of the word, but is a connective tissue originating from the brain and protruding on to the brain's surface. This connective substance forms a sort of cement (neuroglia) in the brain, spinal cord and higher sensory nerves, in which the nervous elements are embedded. Studied freshly, one finds a granulated, very rich substance with oval, fairly large nuclei, which was previously considered as a particular form of nerve tissue. These nuclei are contained in very soft and fragile cells, which can be observed in fresh objects, but more clearly after fixation."

In his book *Cellular Pathology*, Virchow elaborated further on neuroglia. This book, published in 1858, was based on a series of 20 lectures held between February and April 1858 in the Pathology Institute in Berlin. It has influenced a generation of scientists and also contains Virchow's first illustrations of neuroglia (Fig. 1.1). The historical importance of this book is that it introduces and provides support for the concept that diseases are a consequence of cellular changes. In the 13th lecture, held on April 3, 1858 Virchow states (Virchow, 1858; see also Virchow, 1978): "Hitherto, gentlemen, in considering the nervous system, I have only spoken of the really nervous parts of it. But if we would

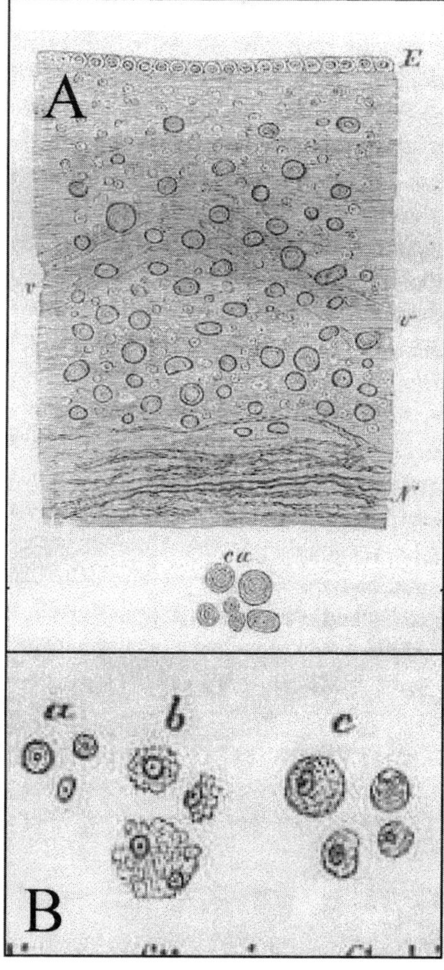

FIGURE 1.1 Virchow's illustration of neuroglia. *A.* Ependyma and neuroglia in the floor of the fourth ventricle. Between the ependyma and the nerve fibers is "the free portion of the neuroglia with numerous connective tissue corpuscles and nuclei." Numerous corpora amylacea are also visible, shown enlarged below the main illustration (*ca*). *E*: ependymal epithelium; *N*: nerve fibers; *v-w*: blood vessel. *B:* Elements of neuroglia from white matter of the human cerebral hemispheres. *a.* free nuclei with nucleoli; *b.* nuclei with partially destroyed cell bodies; *c*: complete cells. (From Virchow, 1858.)

study the nervous system in its real relations in the body, it is extremely important to have a knowledge of that substance also which lies between the proper nervous parts, holds them together and gives the whole its form in a greater or less degree" (p. 272). Further on he explains the term neuroglia:

"This peculiarity of the membrane (i.e., the layer immediately beneath the ependyma), namely, that it becomes continuous with the interstitial matter, the real cement, which binds the nervous elements together, and that in all its properties it constitutes a tissue different from the other forms of connective tissue, has induced me to give it a new name, that of *neuro-glia* (nerve-cement). The view that the substance in question belongs to the class of connective tissues has recently been admitted on nearly all sides, but with regard to the extent to which any isolated structures that occur in it are to be considered as belonging to this substance, opinions are divided" (1978, p. 277). In the end, however, he concludes: "where neuro-glia is met with, it also contains a certain number of cellular elements" (Virchow, 1978, p. 278). He referred to these cells variably as *connective tissue corpuscles* or *elements of the neuro-glia*, never as *neuro-glial cells*. He did not comment on the role of these cells or how they related to neuro-glia (i.e., brain interstitial substance).

We may conclude, therefore (although it is not emphasized in most historical accounts), that Virchow in 1856 used the term *neuro-glia* to refer to interstitial substance, not to the cellular elements within it. Time has blurred this distinction. What then is Virchow's interstitial substance or tissue in today's terms? It is undoubtedly the complex, space-filling processes of macroglial cells, especially astrocytes (Nedergaard et al., 2003). So, in retrospect, the meaning of Virchow's term *neuro-glia* morphed to accommodate the reality that neuroglial cells are the material between neurons. In other words, the two terms, *neuroglia* and *neuroglial cells*, soon became synonymous.

MÜLLER CELLS ARE THE FIRST WELL-DESCRIBED AND DEPICTED GLIAL CELLS

Virchow's published figures illustrating his "new" tissue (and the cells it contained) in *Cellular Pathology* are often considered the first images of glial cells. These illustrations show what are presumed to be "connective-tissue-corpuscles and nuclei" beneath ependymal cells in the floor of the fourth ventricle (Fig. 1.1). Historically, it has generally been accepted that these are the nuclei of astrocytes or oligodendrocytes but, given the location, it seems possible that some, maybe most, are the nuclei of small neurons. The influential neurohistologist Weigert summed up the evidence in 1895 and concluded that Virchow had described and illustrated neuroglial cells (see above). Jacobson (1993), however, provides an alternative view: "It is doubtful whether Virchow saw neuroglial cells in 1846 and there are no convincing pictures of them in Virchow's book, Die Cellularpathologie (1858), although he there discusses the theory of a neuroglial tissue." Given the vagaries of microscopy in this era, especially tissue fixation and staining, it is not possible to say with certainty what these objects were.

While most historians award Virchow exclusive credit for first recognizing glial cells, another pathologist published a picture of a glial cell in the same year, and his picture was vastly superior in clarity. Heinrich Müller (1820–1864) already noted in 1851 that the retina contains radial fibers (Müller, 1851), and in 1852 his colleague Kölliker termed these *Müller fibers* (Kölliker, 1852). In his detailed article Müller compares the retina in the fish (perch), amphibia (frog), bird (pigeon), and human. In his summary he states: "The presence of radial fibers is a common feature. In all cases, they extend from the inner surface of the retina to the inner granular layer where they show a swelling containing a nucleus; from there they continue to the outer layers." Müller had clearly recognized that these fibers are part of a cell with the soma in the inner granular layer. This is convincingly supported by his figures (Fig. 1.2*A*,*B*), which are, in fact, the first documentation of a glial cell (i.e., two years prior to Virchow's publication!). Still, one must credit Virchow for introducing the theory of a neuroglial tissue, even if "the theory led and the facts followed" (Jacobson, 1993). It is this theory or idea, more than anything else, that secures for Virchow his special place in the history of this field.

There is an interesting story about Virchow and Müller that influenced the discovery of the Müller cell. Müller was a senior assistant in the department of pathology at Würzburg with a research focus on cancer. He took over the chair of pathology as a deputy after the sudden death of Bernard Mohr, the previous chair holder, in 1848, and most of his colleagues in the faculty favored him as the next chair holder. At the same time that this nomination process was moving forward, Virchow was having political problems in Berlin because he was an active member in the 1848–1849 revolution. After the revolution failed, Virchow's career in Berlin seemed at an end. The faculty in Würzburg recognized their chance and offered the chair of pathology to Virchow, not to Müller. Virchow accepted the position (he returned to Berlin seven years later to become professor of pathology). Müller was so depressed by this unfortunate turn of events that he had to recover for half a year in a sanatorium. After his return, he decided to switch to comparative histology and joined Kölliker's department of anatomy and histology. There he began his thorough analysis of retinal histology.

While Müller's illustrations showed clearly the cell that bears his name, even judged by today's standards, soon thereafter (in 1859) utterly stunning pictures of these cells were published by Max Schultze (Fig. 1.2C). Schultze's illustrations seem almost modern in their detail and precision. He went on to have an illustrious career and is referred to by Garrison (1929) as "the master worker of histology." He succeeded the great Helmholtz in Bonn in 1859.

All these studies were done on unstained tissue. The cells were isolated by very carefully teasing the tissue apart with fine needles and thereby trying to isolate single cells or ensembles of a few cells. Of course, this was much easier in the retina than in the whole brain and explains why the first modern pictures of glial cells came from the retina.

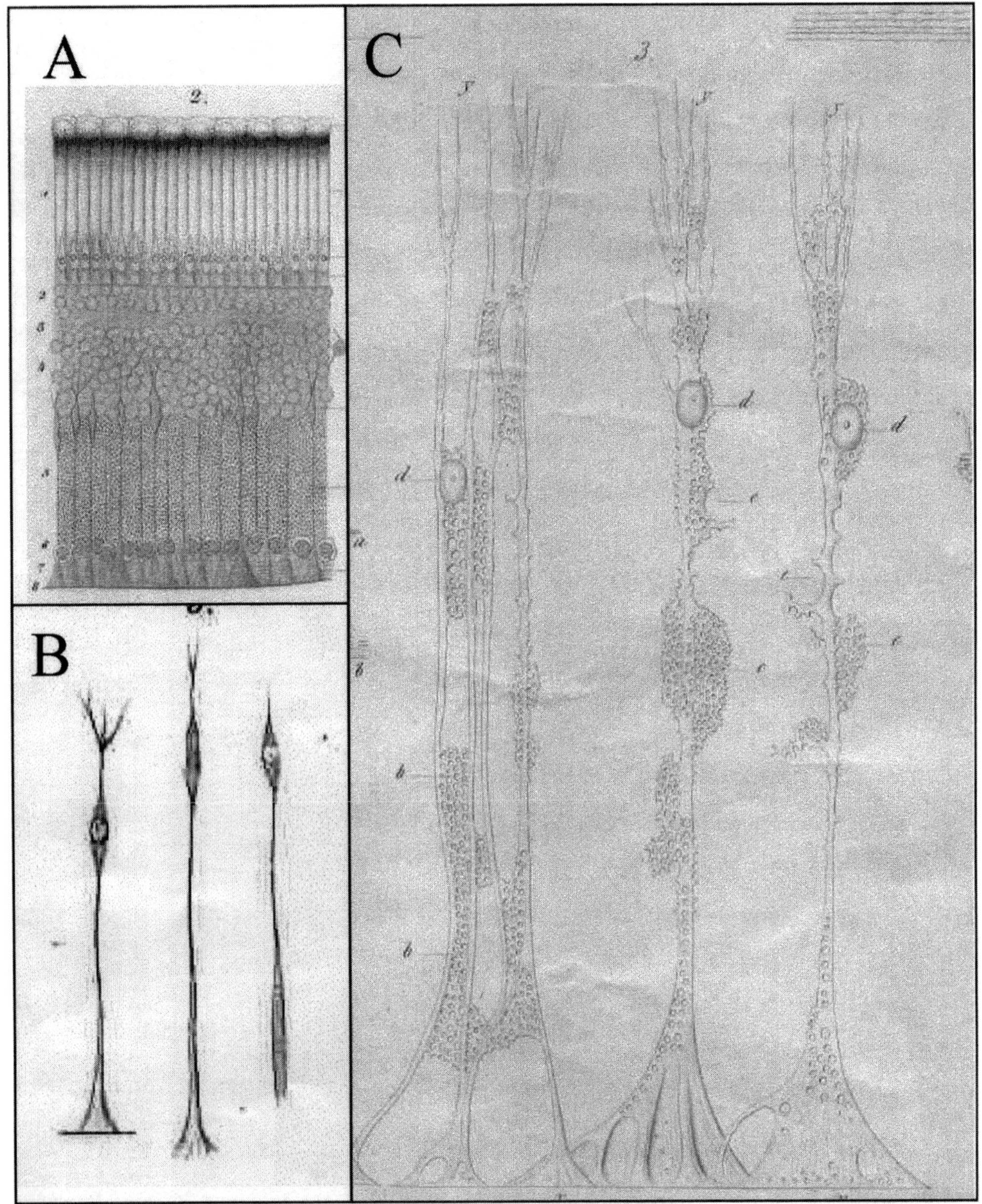

FIGURE 1.2 Retinal neuroglial cells. *A*. Cross section of frog retina. Note the radial (i.e., Müller) cells with their characteristic endfeet in the layer numbered "8." *B*. Isolated radial fibers from the frog retina. *C*. Müller fibers of the sheep retina. Brush-like processes extend from the Müller fiber in the outer granular layer (labeled *y*); *b*. very delicate network of fenestrated membranes similar to those in the ganglion cell layer; *c*. network in the molecular layer; *d*. nuclei shown as part of the Müller fibers; *e*. cavity in which the nuclei or the cells of the internal granular layer are located. *A* and *B* from Müller (1856). *C* from Schultze (1859).

STELLATE CELLS ARE FOUND IN WHITE AND GRAY MATTER

Otto Deiters (1834–1863) is considered the first to provide illustrations of a cell type that resembles our modern notion of an astrocyte (Cajal, 1909, 1911). In fact, in the chapter on neuroglia in his exhaustive neurohistology tome *Histology of the Nervous System* (1909), Santiago Ramon y Cajal (1852–1934) refers to Deiters as "the scholar who discovered them." As a consequence, authoritative textbooks (e.g., Ferguson, 1905; Cajal, 1909–1911) for many years used the term *Deiter's cell* synonymously with *astrocyte*. The story of Deiters' contribution is of interest, and we offer a small amendment to the historical record that strengthens his claims.

Deiters died at 29 of typhoid fever and left his crucial observations in the form of a draft manuscript. His friend Max Schultze (see above) finalized the manuscript and published it in 1865, two years after Deiters' death (Deiters, 1865). Deiters clearly described cells in white matter that were not neurons; he believed these were component parts of brain connective tissue, following the lead of Virchow. He described them as follows: "The shiny nucleus which lacks a nucleolus, is the origin of many fibers. They have a firm, but slender appearance and project in all directions . . . they are not only found in all forms of white matter, but also in grey matter" (Deiters, 1865). An apparent error in the labeling of his illustrations in 1865, never publicly corrected as far as we can tell, has led to questions about his observations (e.g., Somjen, 1988). Deiters illustrated two cells: as published, the one recognizable as a typical white matter fibrous astrocyte, using today's terminology, is *labeled* as located in gray matter (i.e., the hypoglossal nucleus). Unfortunately, the printer mixed up the legend and the picture. When one carefully reads the original text, it is clear that what Deiters saw in white matter was the cell in panel *A*, not the cell in panel *B*. Thus, the authenticity of his description rings true when one compares his picture (i.e., Fig. 1.3*A*) to modern images of dye-filled fibrous astrocytes (e.g., figure 9 in Butt and Ransom, 1993). The nature of the cell he illustrates in panel B (the cell from gray matter) is less certain, the confusion arising in part because of the admixture of neurons and neuroglia in this area. Deiters' posthumous 1865 publication is also famous for the exceptionally clear illustrations of axons having direct continuity with neuron cell bodies; this addressed the controversy of whether axons and neurons were connected.

Four years later, in 1869, Jakob Henle (1809–1885), together with his son-in-law Friedrich Merkel, published the first figure of a network of star-shaped cells in white matter (Fig. 1.3C). The stain he used was carmine red after fixation with chromic acid. Henle was an influential anatomist, and he opposed from the beginning Virchow's view that the brain contains connective tissue. Henle and Virchow knew each other from their time as students in Berlin, both completing a doctoral thesis in Müller's department. Virchow writes about Henle in his description of neuroglia in 1856: "Henle took efforts in his own interest to delay this insight (connective tissue in the brain). Moreover, he had the impudence to maintain, that I mixed up granules with nuclei and fine nerve fibers with connective tissue." While Henle's pictures enhanced the documentation of macroglia, his written interpretations were confusing and he argued against Virchow's concept of neuroglia.

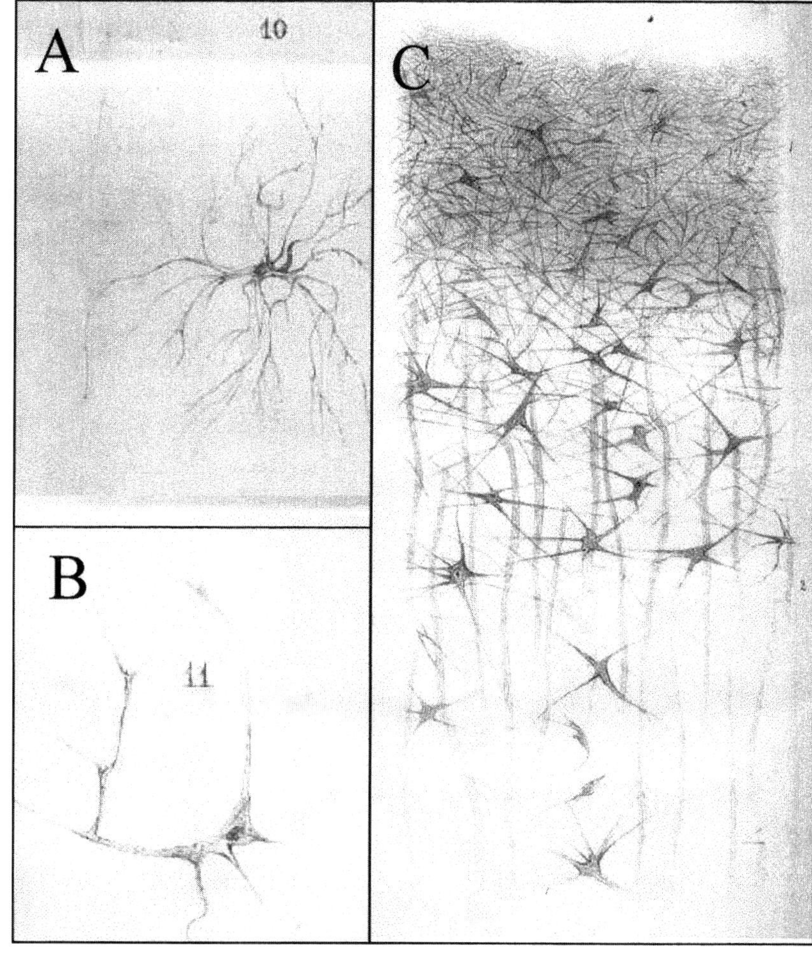

FIGURE 1.3 Deiters' illustrations of connective tissue cells. *A*. Connective tissue cell from white matter. *B*. Connective tissue cell from gray matter (hypoglossal nucleus). (From Deiters, 1865.) See text for details. *C*. Section from the spinal cord of the ox stained by carmine after chromic acid preparation. *1*. gray matter; *2*. white matter with exposed axons; multipolar connective tissue cells (magnification 400×). (From Henle and Merkel, 1869.)

GOLGI DESCRIBES CELLS WITH CHARACTERISTIC FEATURES OF ASTROCYTES AND OLIGODENDROCYTES

Camillo Golgi's (1843–1926) study of neuroglia began with papers in 1870 and 1871 using hematoxylin and carmine staining or no staining at all. Neither neurons nor neuroglia were stained completely by these techniques, but his publications suggested a diversity of glial cells in gray and white matter (Fig. 1.4). He also noted that blood vessels are contacted by glial cell processes (Fig. 1.4*B*). This passage is taken from his famous book *Contribuzione alla fina Anatomia degli organi centrali del sistema nervosos*, published in 1871: "Studying thin slices of treated cortical substance (osmium treated for 4 to 6 h) with addition of glycerin with the microscope, revealed numerous, roundish, oval or star-shaped cells, from which numerous, long, fine and never arborized prolongations originate. . . . Many (prolongations) extend to the vessel walls, including capillaries, vessels of medium size (particularly to those) and directly attach to the walls of the capillaries or to the lymphatic border of vessels with larger diameter. . . . The surround of the vessels is demarcated by a dense, regular network of fibers." That some of his cells contacted blood vessels is strong evidence that these represented astrocytes. In studying white matter, he may have recognized oligodendrocytes and specifically pointed out that processes of his white matter cells appeared to contact axons (Fig. 1.4*C*). His observation of cells aligned in a row, a characteristic feature of oligodendrocytes in white matter, is convincing: "In carmine-stained parallel slices, after carefully brushing and rinsing with water and watching them under the microscope in glycerin or water and glycerin, one can recognize the above mentioned cells in between the nerve fibers, which are

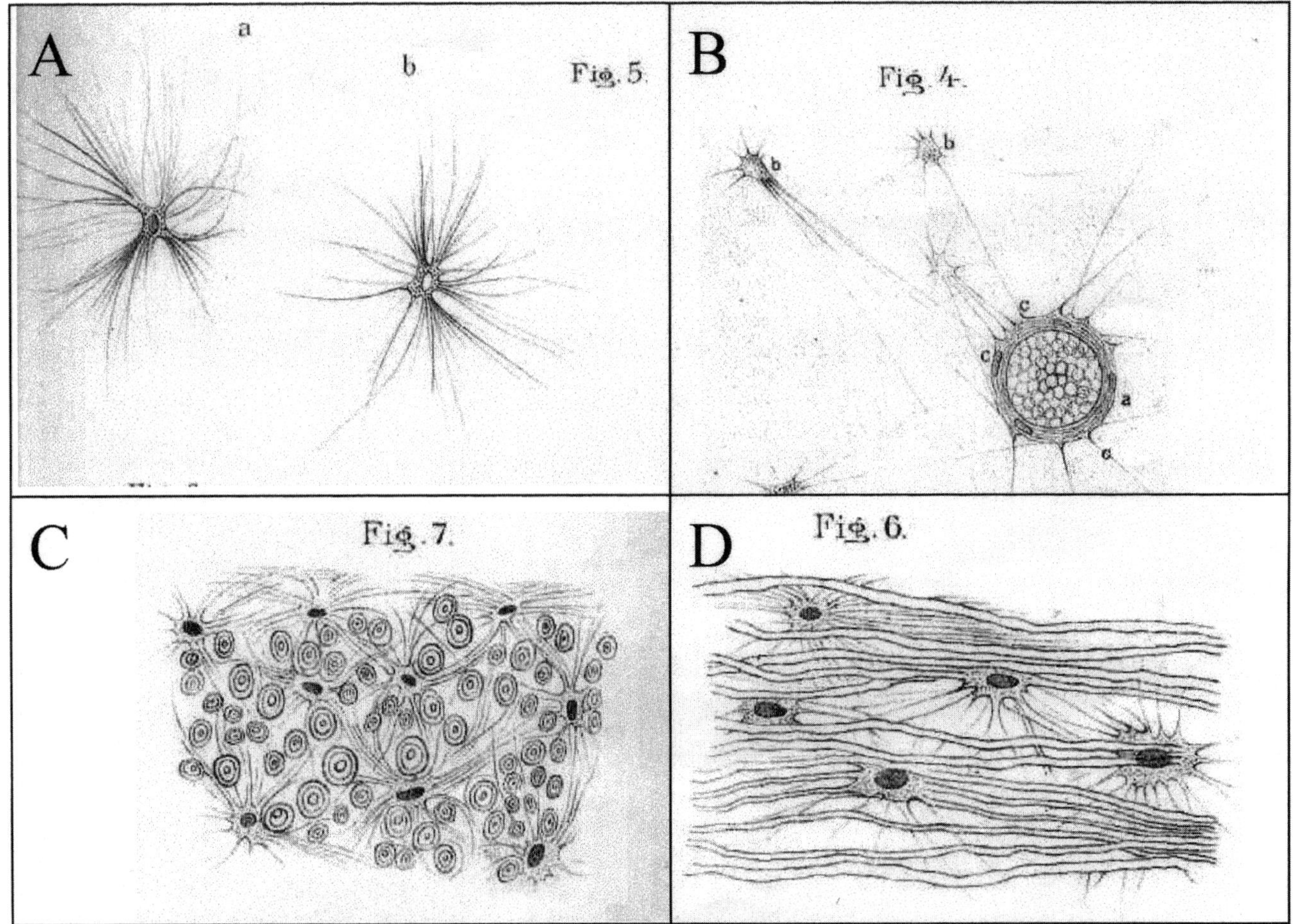

FIGURE 1.4 Neuroglial cells depicted in Golgi's early work. *A. a.* Neuroglial cell from the superficial layer of the cerebral cortex; *b.* neuroglial cell from the deeper cortical layer of the cerebrum from a 2-month-old child. The cell bodies and proximal processes contain fat droplets. *B.* Slice of the cerebral cortex hardened in osmium; *a.* blood vessel; *b.* neuroglial cells with multiple thread-like processes; *c.* processes from neuroglial cells terminating on the vessel wall. *C.* Section through deep white matter tracts. Between the axons and directly attached are several flattened neuroglial cells. Neuroglial processes project in all directions among the axons and attach to their ensheathments. *D.* Neuroglial cells in white matter. Longitudinal view of neuroglial cells showing their relationship to axons. All panels from Golgi (1894).

single or in groups or in rows of 3 to 4 or more; the thin processes are combined into bundles and run preferentially parallel with the nerve fibers and attach to them. Where these cells are numerous, they almost form an ensheathment of the fiber" (Fig. 1.4*C*,*D*).

Golgi's greatest contribution, some would argue, was his famous *reaziona nera*, or black reaction, that permitted entire neurons and glial cells to be stained (Fig. 1.5). While this method (potassium dichromate-silver) did not *distinguish* between neurons and neuroglia, it allowed them to be visualized better than ever before and in their entirety. Only later would specific stains for neuroglia appear (Cajal, 1913; Rio-Hortega, 1919). In the meantime, neuroglia were identified by a process of elimination. Reider (1906) quotes Carl Weigert (the German pathologist who introduced a specific stain for myelin) on this point: "one recognized neuroglia as the structure that one could not or would not call neuronal." Nevertheless, in the hands of workers like Golgi, Andriezen, and Cajal, the Golgi technique was a powerful tool that accelerated the understanding and classification of neuroglia. So impressive were the gains in knowledge that by 1909 Cajal could say (Cajal, 1995): "We have emphasized that two special elements, which are really abstractions derived from many examples, form all neural tissue: the neuron with its various processes and the glial cell."

In most of his beautiful drawings from hippocampus or cortex, Golgi depicts glial cells as a part of the tissue. One of his most intriguing pictures shows the glial populations of the cerebellum (Fig. 1.5). He recognized that the fibers in the molecular layer, originally discovered in 1857 by the German Karl Bergmann (1814–1865) (Bergmann, 1857), are processes of glial cells. For many years these cells were called *Golgi epithelial cells* for this reason (the term *Bergmann glia* has more recently become popular again).

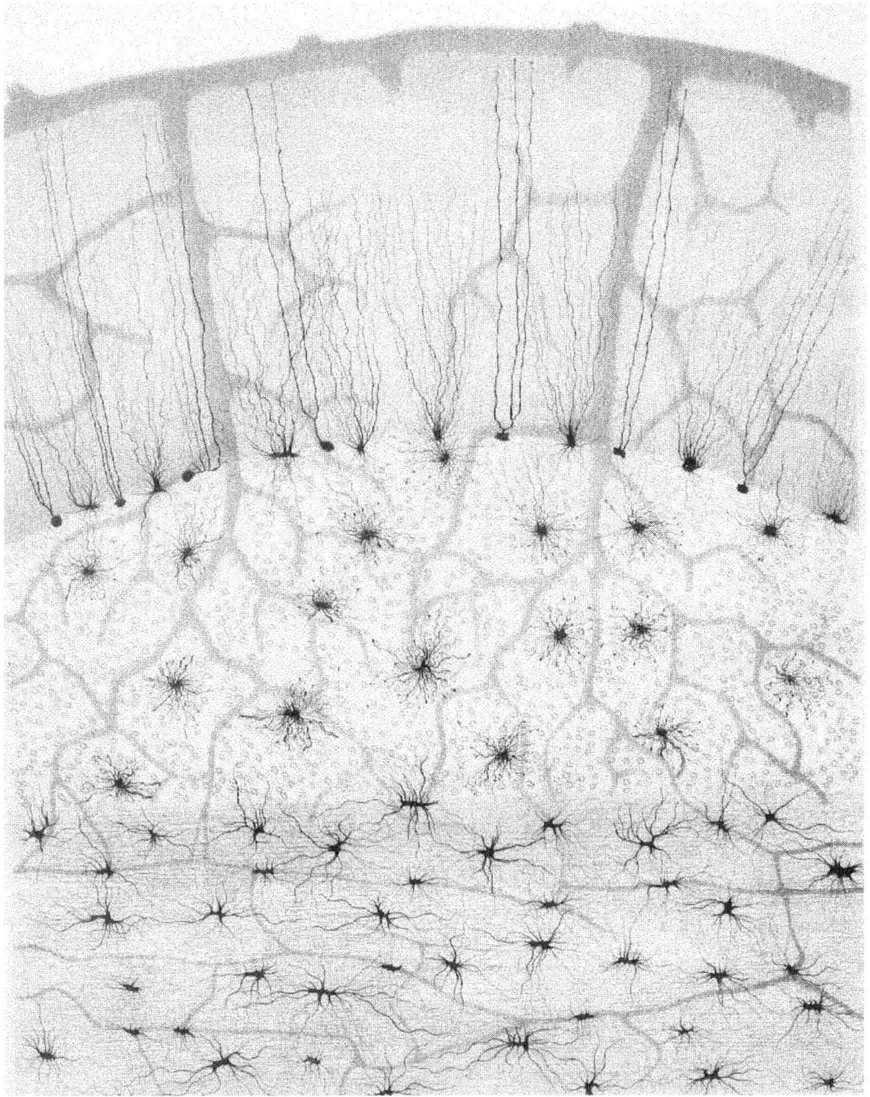

FIGURE 1.5 Vertical slice from the human cerebellum showing the glial cells in this structure, including the Golgi epithelial cells (also known as *Bergmann glial cells*). (From Golgi (1894).

A point of contention about glial fibers should be mentioned. Golgi's studies indicated that glial fibers existed as component parts of each glial cell. This was diametrically opposed to the view of Weigert (1895), supported by others including Ranvier (1883). Weigert contended that glial fibers were "neither branches of the cell nor identical in composition with the cytoplasm of the cell—they were therefore not cell branches but independent fibres" (Glees, 1955). In spite of this position, he seems to have believed that glial cells made the fibers and perhaps helped to maintain them. Cajal (1995) discussed this carefully and concluded that the results of the silver chromate staining method strongly favored Golgi's conclusion.

THE WORD *ASTROCYTE* IS INVENTED

In 1893 Michael von Lenhossek (1863–1937) from Würzburg introduced the term *astrocyte* to refer to star-shaped neuroglial cells. He wrote the first extensive review on glial cells in a textbook on the fine structure of the nervous system focusing on spinal cord. He states that what people had considered glial cells were a mixture of more than one cell type. He explained the need to use more specific terms in dealing with these cells (Leuhossek, 1893): "I would suggest that all supportive cells be named spongiocytes, and the most common form in vertebrates be named spider cells or astrocytes, and use the term neuroglia only cum grano salis (with a grain of salt), at least until we have a clearer view. . . . Astrocytes are the small elements, which form the supportive system of the spinal cord. They are star shaped and indeed no other comparison describes their form so clearly. While the term spider cell introduced by Jastrowitz has become popular and gives a proper impression of the cells, one should regard Gierke's note, namely that nobody has seen a spider with so many feet as these cells have processes." The cells he was describing are shown in Figure 1.6*A*.

The term *astrocyte* was used variably thereafter. Robertson did not use the term in his review of neuroglia in 1897 nor does Cajal in his general chapter on neuroglia in *Histology of the Nervous System* (1909–1911). Curiously, he employs the term regularly in later sections of these books. Andriezen (1893) and Koelliker (1889) divided glia (i.e. astrocytes, although they did not use this term) into two groups. Fibrous glia or *Langstrahler* (long projectors) had long processes and were found mainly in white matter, while protoplasmic astrocytes or *Kurzstrahler* (short projectors) either had only short processes or lacked obvious fibers and were more common in gray matter.

Because Virchow thought that neuroglia constituted connective tissue, it was assumed that these cells must arise from mesoderm. This idea died slowly. The failure of connective tissue stains, increasingly specific for mesoderm, to stain these cells was one line of evidence refuting the idea that they were mesodermal, but it left open the defense that negative results might only mean that neuroglial cells were a special type of connective tissue. Wilhelm His (1831–1904) studied early development and recognized that neuroblasts and spongioblasts, which formed radial glia, are both of ectodermal origin (His, 1889). Lenhossek (1893) showed that the radially aligned spongioblasts transformed into astrocytes (Fig. 1.6*B*) (later confirmed by Cajal [1913]). These findings were finally accepted as definitive proof that astrocytes were of ectodermal origin.

Another long-standing misimpression was that neuroglial cells formed a physical syncytium, often called the *neurospongium* (His, 1889). In retrospect, this mistake was mainly a consequence of limited microscopic resolution and misleading staining techniques. It was seriously questioned by many, including Lenhossek (Fig. 1.6) and Cajal, whose studies using the Golgi technique showed separate glial cells that transitioned from radial glial cells to typical astrocytes during development. The syncytium theory also came under attack when it became apparent that a normal glial cell could exist immediately adjacent to a glial cell showing marked pathological change; this did not make sense if the cells were continuous with one another. Unassailable evidence, however, was not provided until the 1950s, when the newly developed electron microscope showed that glial cells are always separated from each other by a thin layer of extracellular space.

THE SCHWANN CELL AND MYELIN

A comprehensive and insightful review of the history of myelin and the cells that produce it can be found in Jacobson's book (1993). This was an area of neuroscience that remained mired in controversy for more than a century. The questions being pondered, such as what cell makes myelin and how myelin forms on axons, simply could not be answered definitively until the invention of the electron microscope, a major technological leap of the mid-twentieth century. In other words, the history of this topic reveals the consequences of a persistent, unsolvable riddle: Contradictory theories flourished and became entrenched because no one point of view could gain the upper hand. The tale of myelin also teaches a humbling precept about scientific theories; theories most consistent with available evidence are not always destined to be right (for example, the highly plausible theory that myelin is secreted by axons).

Robert Remak (1815–1865) was the first to state that some nerve fibers in the peripheral nervous system had a distinct sheath and were thicker than fibers without this sheath (Fig. 1.7*A*,*B*) (1838). He called the fibers

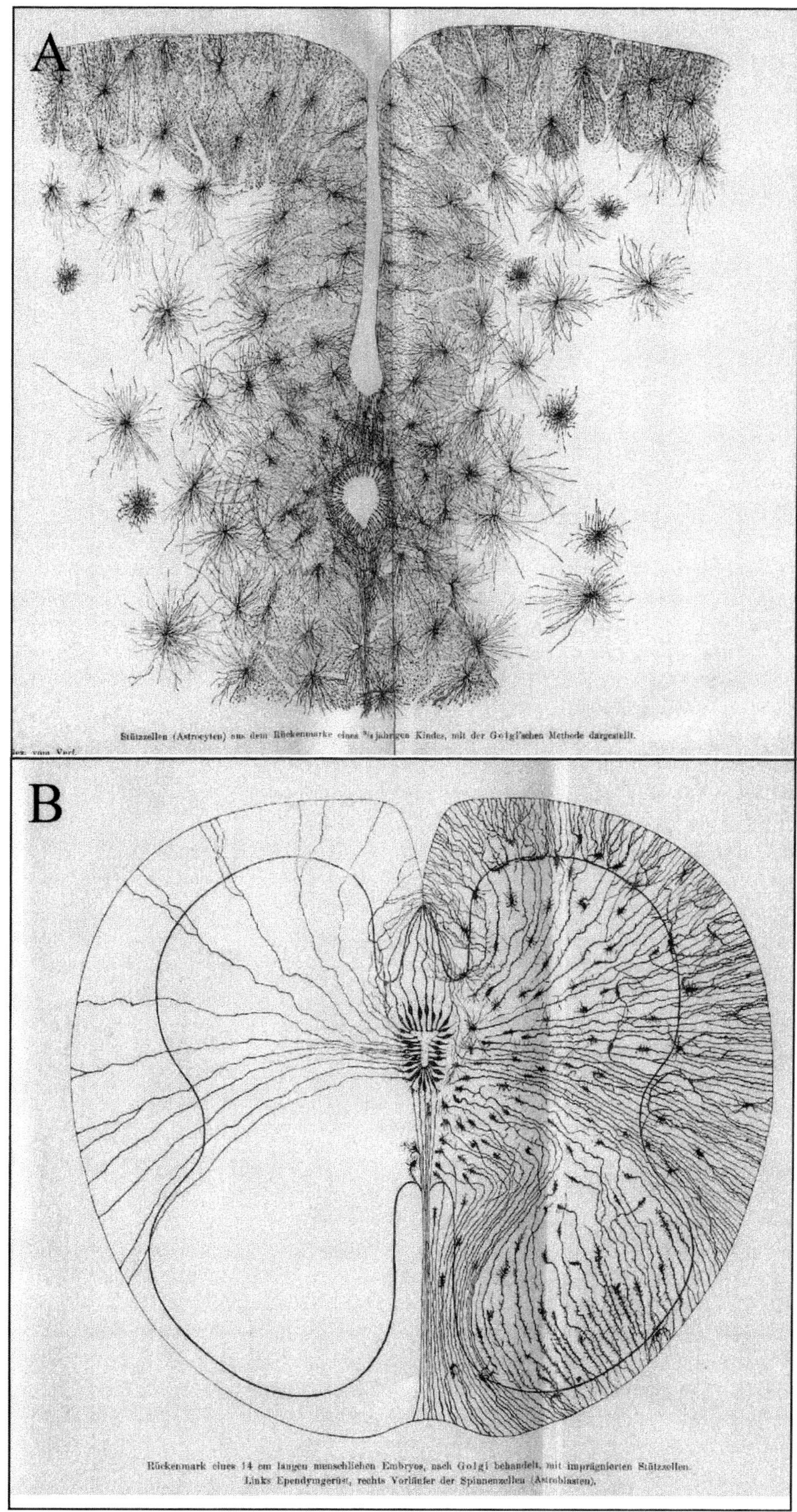

FIGURE 1.6 Astrocytes and radial glia in material prepared by Lenhossek in 1893. *A*: Supportive cells (i.e. astrocytes) from the spinal cord of a 9-month-old child; Golgi impregnation. *B*. Spinal cord of a 14 cm human embryo; Golgi impregnation of the supportive cells. *Left*: ependymal (i.e., radial glial) scaffold. *Right*: precursors of spider cells (astroblasts). (From Lenhossek, 1893.)

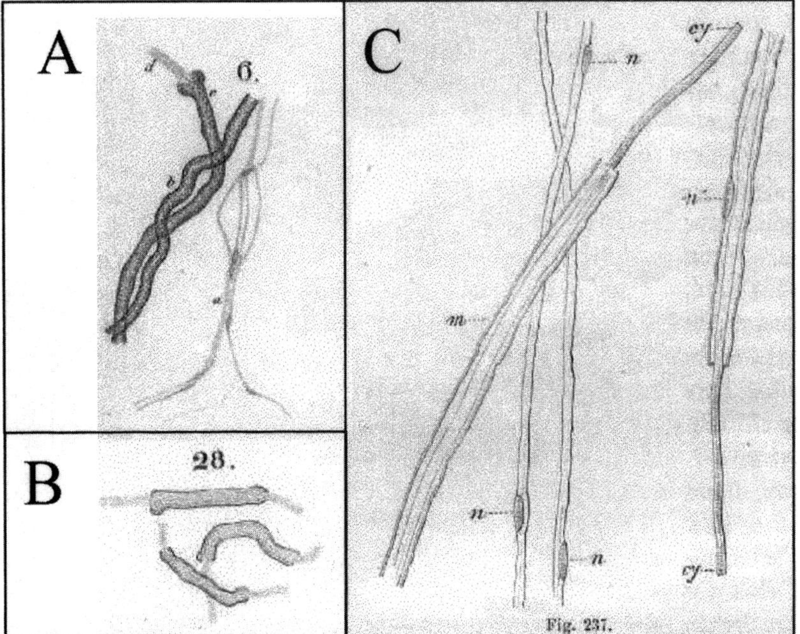

FIGURE 1.7 Illustrations of nerve fibers and their myelin sheaths. *A*. From the posterior root of the nervus alicujus lumbalis (magnification 200×). Organic fibers labeled *b* and *c*; primitive tubes labeled *a*. At *d*, the primitive fiber appears unsheathed. *B*. Fiber from rabbit cerebellum (magnification 110×). One can recognize the delicate sheath and the transparent fiber. *C*. Nerve fibers from the sciatic nerve of rabbit: *cy*: axon; *m*: myelin sheath; *n*: nuclei of the segments. *A* and *B* from Remak (1838). C from Ranvier (1875)

with sheaths *tubulus primitivus* (i.e., primitive tubes) and illustrated the nuclei associated with the sheaths. He called the nonmedullated fibers, that is, those without a sheath, *organic fibers*. His careful description of nonmedullated fibers in the sympathetic nervous system led to the practice of calling these *Remak fibers* (e.g., Cajal, [1995]). Schwann, in 1839, confirmed Remak's observation of medullated fibers with nuclei. He proposed that individual sheath nuclei were a remnant of an earlier stage when the nuclei formed a continuous chain of cells that coalesced to form the nerve fibers. Despite subsequent observations suggesting that axons grew independently of the sheath nuclei, Schwann's incorrect *cell-chain* or *catenary* theory held sway until the early twentieth century.

The medullary sheath came to be distinguished as a separate structure from a second sheath immediately external to it. This external covering was considered a "special investment of connective tissue, constituting the so-called sheath of Schwann" (Schultze, 1870). Although Schwann's name had gradually become attached to the external sheath, the term *Schwann cell* came much later. Illustrations in Ranvier's (1872) and Stricker's textbooks (1871) showed that Schwann sheaths contained or were associated with nuclei (Fig. 1.7C). To understand why the connection was not immediately made that the medullary sheath arose from a cell, one must recall that some scientists, like Jakob Henle, argued that the nervous system contained free nuclei. The term *Schwann cell* appears to have been first used by Louis-Antoine Ranvier (1835–1922) in 1871, but it may not have come into common usage until Cajal's treatise was published in 1909. It is not entirely clear why Schwann's name, and not Remak's, became associated with the sheath cells. Remak's clear illustration of the sheath with a nucleus in 1838 constitutes, at least technically, the first image of a glial cell.

Virchow enters the picture again in the story about peripheral glia. He introduced the term *myelin* in 1858 to refer to the fatty sheath surrounding some axons: "It is this substance, for which I have proposed the name of medullary matter (Markstoff), or *myeline*, that in extremely large quantity fills up the interval between the axis-cylinder and the sheath in primitive nerve-fibers" (Virchow, 1978). He, like many of his contemporaries, felt that myelin was secreted by the axon, not made by the Schwann cell. For example, in 1909 Cajal states: "Also, many writers, including ourselves, view myelin itself as nothing more than a secretory product of axons, rather than the contents of a cell that the axon passes through." This concept endured as long as it did, in part, because central nervous system (CNS) myelin appeared not to be associated with nuclei; in the apparent absence of a cell to make myelin, it seemed logical that the axon must make it. Ranvier was not the first to see interruptions in the myelin covering axons, but he was the first to realize that these interruptions were not artifacts. He correctly perceived that the axon was passing through a series of independent myelin segments and that each segment was associated with a single Schwann cell (Ranvier, 1872).

SPECULATIONS ON FUNCTION

In *Histology of the Nervous System*, Cajal (1995) summarized what was known about the functions of glia. He did not consider Schwann cells glia, and microglia and oligodendrocytes were not yet discovered, so his discussion was exclusively about astrocytes. He begins with these prescient remarks: "What is the function of glial cells in neural centers? The answer is still not known, and the problem is even more serious because it may remain unsolved for many years to come until physiologists find direct methods to attack it."

He first addressed the suggestion by Golgi and his students that glial cells carry important nutritional fluids from capillaries to neuronal cell bodies. This idea was spawned by Golgi's observation that most astrocytes contact capillaries with their processes. Cajal raised objections to this hypothesis: (*1*) Glial cells that surround neurons often lack processes that contact capillaries. He may have been referring, without realizing it, to perineuronal oligodendrocytes. However, he illustrates protoplasmic astrocytes from adult human gray matter with processes "never appearing to end near capillaries." In retrospect, limitations imposed by available staining methods and microscopes probably caused him to overestimate this population. (*2*) Amphibian and fish white matter does not contain glia. Subsequent studies have at least partially refuted this statement. Nevertheless, Cajal's disregard for this theory was echoed nearly 60 years later in Kuffler and Nicholl's review (1966). Only in the past 15 years has the nutritional theory of Golgi experienced an evidence-based renaissance (see Chapter 29, this volume).

Cajal carefully considered the *filling theory* of Weigert: "According to the celebrated neurologist, Weigert, glia serve an entirely passive role, filling spaces not occupied by neurons." Cajal strongly denigrated this notion based on careful reasoning. Despite his disdain, however, similar ideas have persisted and are sometimes encountered even today (Ransom et al., 2003).

The *isolation theory* developed by his brother, P. Ramon y Cajal, received strong support. The premise was that astrocytes act as physical insulation against the passage of neuronal impulses. "These processes are always arranged so as to prevent contact between either unmyelinated axons or dendrites, or between axons and dendrites, but only at points where these two different kinds of neuronal process should not lie immediately adjacent to one another" (Cajal, 1995). In white matter, he and others of this period intuitively assigned insulating function to myelin, which posed a nasty riddle: Why are there astrocytes in white matter? Cajal had no answer. Ironically, he failed to appreciate the glial origin of myelin and so was denied the key insight that makes the isolation theory credible today, at least in regard to the oligodendrocyte.

RIO-HORTEGA AND THE RECOGNITION OF OLIGODENDROGLIA AND MICROGLIA

Cajal introduced an improved staining technique for neuroglial cells (gold chloride-sublimate) in 1913 (Cajal, 1913). This stained astrocytes more completely than was previously possible and led him to recognize other nonnervous cells that were distinct from astrocytes. Although these other cells were poorly stained, they were clear enough to warrant naming, and he called them the *third element* of the CNS. Undoubtedly, others had seen such nonnervous cells, but previously they had only constituted a "group of cells with indefinite characteristics" variably described as "naked nuclei, round, indifferent, cuboidal or preameboid cells and apolar elements" (Rio-Hortega, 1932).

Cajal's understudy, Pio del Rio-Hortega (1882–1945), took up the problem of glial cells and developed his own stain (silver carbonate) that selectively stained the third element cells (Rio-Hortega, 1921). Two distinct cell populations emerged, which he named *oligodendroglia* (and later called *oligodendrocytes* to make the nomenclature consistent for the two forms of macroglia) and *microglia* (Fig. 1.8). Oligodendrocytes, so named because they exhibited fewer and smaller branches than astrocytes, were felt to be true classical neuroglial cells of ectodermal origin (Rio-Hortega, 1928). These findings put him painfully at odds with his mentor, Cajal, who could not reproduce Rio-Hortega's observations and therefore distrusted the existence of oligodendrocytes. This disagreement ruptured their close relationship.

William Ford Robertson (1867–1923), a Scotsman, probably stained third element cells earliest of all (Fig. 1.9). In experiments with platinous oxide he stained cells that had only a few short processes, none of which associated with blood vessels (Robertson, 1897, 1899). Robertson called these cells *mesoglia* to distinguish them from neuroglia and indicate his belief that they were derived from mesoderm. Penfield apparently looked at some of Robertson's histological preparations and felt that some of the stained cells were oligodendrocytes (Penfield, 1932). Robertson probably also stained microglial cells with his technique because he stated that "the mesoglia cells seem to have a phagocyte action in certain pathological conditions" (Fig. 1.9) (Robertson, 1900).

Rio-Hortega recognized that oligodendrocytes were most common in white matter. He considered the oligodendroglia to be a member of the macroglial or classical neuroglial family. Because these cells had a relationship to myelin sheaths that bore a striking resemblance to the relationship between Schwann cells and the myelin sheaths of peripheral fibers, he proposed that oligodendrocytes made and sustained CNS myelin (Fig. 1.8, left panel). While the idea that oligodendrocytes made myelin gained in popularity, it was not proven unequivocally until the electron microscope came on the scene.

Microglia were viewed by Rio-Hortega as distinct from all other neuroglial cells because his studies showed them to be of mesodermal origin and to have migratory and phagocytic capabilities (Fig. 1.8, right panel). Rio-Hortega sumed up his position on the mi-

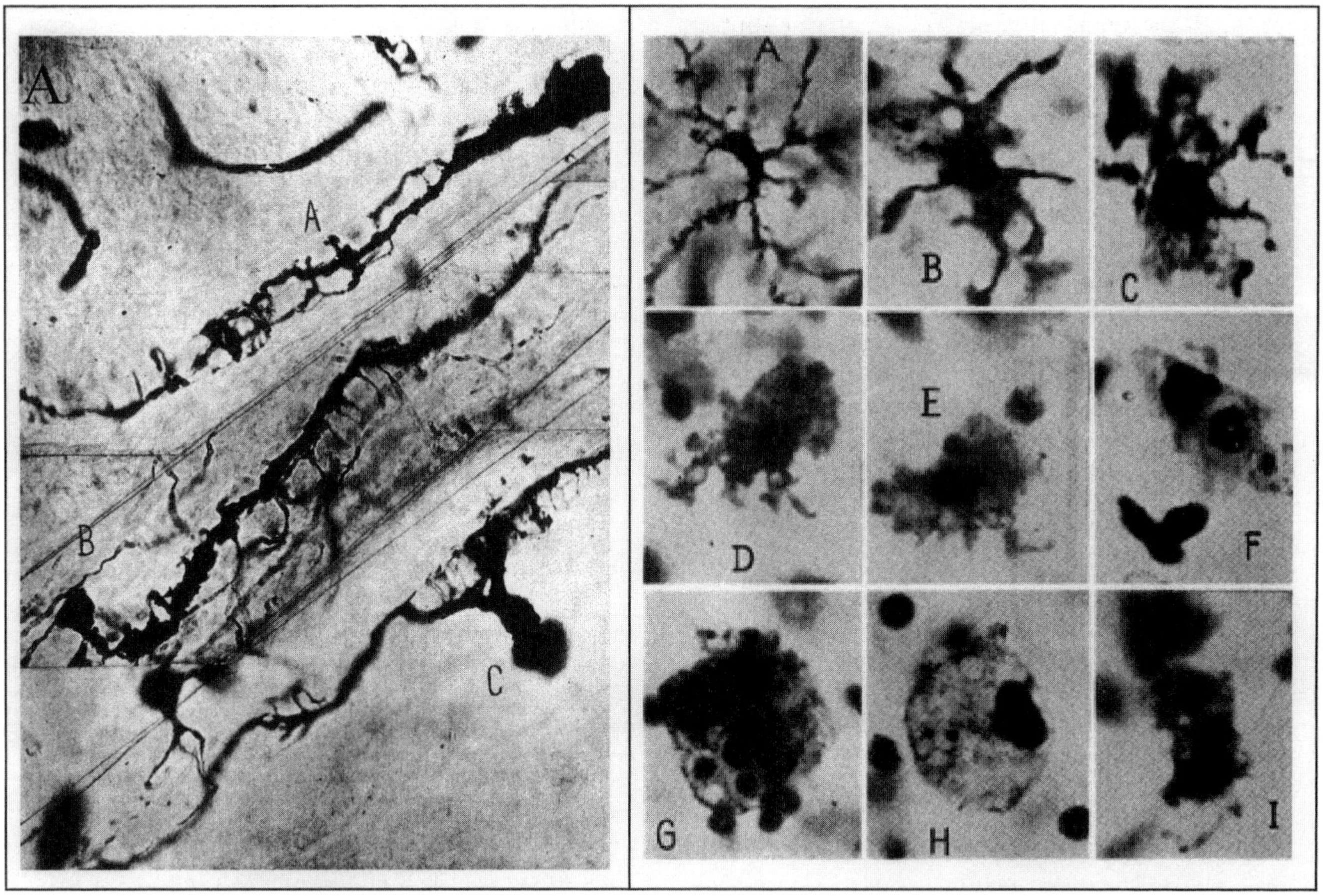

FIGURE 1.8 Early photomicrographs of oligodendrocytes and microglia. *Left panel*: interfascicular oligodendrocytes form a sheath about the myelin segments. *Right panels, A–I.* Evolution of microglial cells during phagocytic activity. *A.* Cell with thick, rough processes; *B.* cells with short processes and an enlarged cell body; *C.* hypertrophic cell with pseudopodia; *E.* ameboid form; *F.* cell with phagocytosed leukocyte; *G.* cell with numerous phagocytosed red cells; *H.* fat granule cell: *I.* cell in mitotic divisions. Left panel from Rio-Hortega (1928). *A-I* from Rio-Hortega (1932).

croglial cell as follows: "Since it is of different ancestry and its characteristics differ from those of the nerve cells (first element) and the neuroglial astrocytes (second element*), the microglia constitutes the *true* third element of the central nervous system" (Rio-Hortega, 1932). He acknowledged that microglia were the same cells, or closely related cells, as seen earlier by pathologists such as Nissl (1899; i.e., rod cells). In fact, Nissl and Alzheimer had argued that the glial cells seen under pathological conditions were of mesodermal origin.

Rio-Hortega's accomplishments in rigorously defining the final two members of the CNS glial family and in deducing their functions are impressive. Unfortunately, he is rarely accorded the credit he deserves for these accomplishments. He was the first to describe the two types of microglia: ameboid and ramified. He recognized that the ameboid form was mobile and phago-

*Rio-Hortega considered the oligodendroglia to be a member of the macroglial or classical neuroglial family.

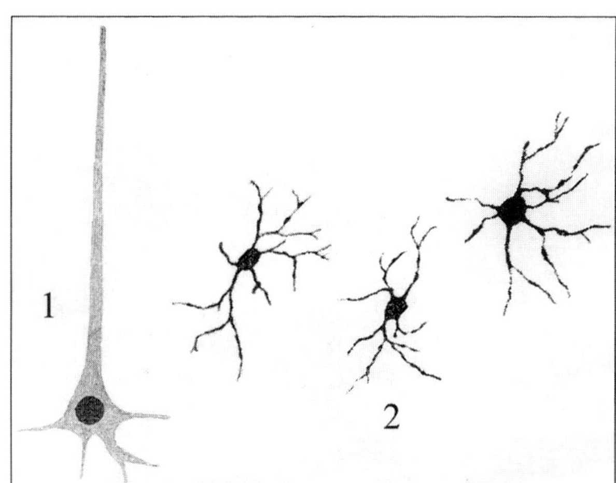

FIGURE 1.9. Illustration of cells stained with the platinum method of Robertson. Composite diagram showing (*1*) "large pyramidal nerve cell of cerebral cortex of sheep" and (*2*) "Three branching cells in cerebral cortex of dog." The cells labeled *2* were either microglia or oligodendrocytes. (From Robertson, (1899.)

cytic and was similar to a blood macrophage. In fact, he believed, as is believed today, that microglial cells originate from peripheral macrophages. He understood that the microglial cell can transform from its relatively inactive ramified form into the phagocytic ameboid form in response to a threat like infection. "In historical perspective we see that what Cajal is to the neuron, Rio-Hortega is to the neuroglia" (Jacobsen, 1993).

GLIAL CELLS RESPOND TO PATHOLOGY

Paralleling the development of knowledge about normal glial cells was the growing recognition that these same cells can alter their appearance in pathological states. In studying brains from deceased multiple sclerosis patients, Carl Frommann (1831–1892) noted that glial cells underwent changes in the demyelinated plaques (Frommann, 1864). He believed that the cells in the areas of fiber degeneration were glial cells that had undergone morphological changes. He stated that the cells became larger and had fewer processes compared to normal glia. It was also clear to him that glial cells were still present in the degenerated areas despite the fiber loss (Fig. 1.10*A*,*B*). He also claimed that some of the glial cells lacked a nucleus. In retrospect, it is likely that he observed activated microglia in these areas of fiber degeneration.

Franz Nissl (1860–1919) noted two new cell types that appeared in the pathological brain. One form was elongated and bipolar in shape, and he called such cells *Stäbchenzellen* (rod cells) (Fig. 1.10*D*). He described this cell type in brains of demented patients but found them also in animals. He originally described these cells as glial elements (Nissl, 1899) but later considered the possibility that they were of mesodermal origin (Nissl, 1904). A second cell type was found mainly in pathological tissue associated with disruption of the blood–brain barrier. These cells were round, without processes, and he termed them *Körnerzellen* (granule cells) or *Gitterzellen* (lattice cells) (Fig. 1.10*E*). Nissl speculated that they were infiltrating blood cells.

In 1910, Alois Alzheimer (1864–1915) published a book chapter summarizing the responses of neuroglia to different pathologies. It was clear to him and his contemporaries that any type of pathology is accompanied by a glial response. He described ameboid glial cells, or ameboid change, in response to both acute and

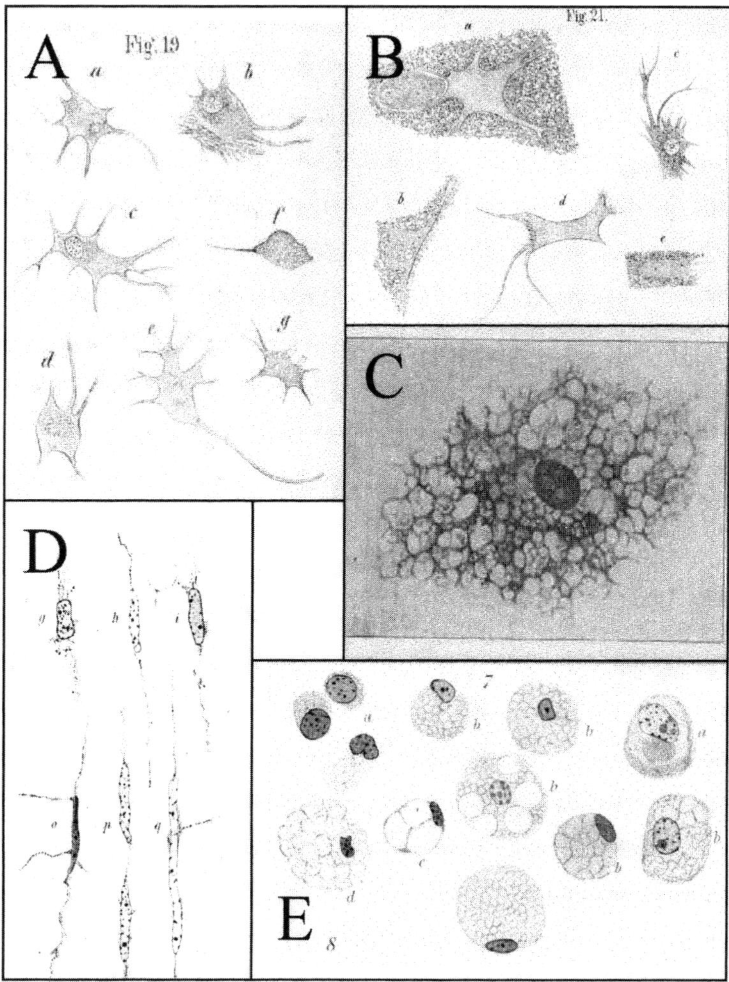

FIGURE 1.10 Neuroglial cells in pathological situations. *A*,*B*. Different types of glial cells found in multiple sclerosis plaques of human cortex. C. Glial cell close to a 14-day-old hemorrhage in human white matter. Axons pass through the network of the cell. *D*. Rod cells stained with toluidin blue. *E*. Gitter cells stained with toluidin blue. *A* and *B* from Frommann (1878). *C* from Alzheimer (1910). *D* and *E* from Alzheimer (1904).

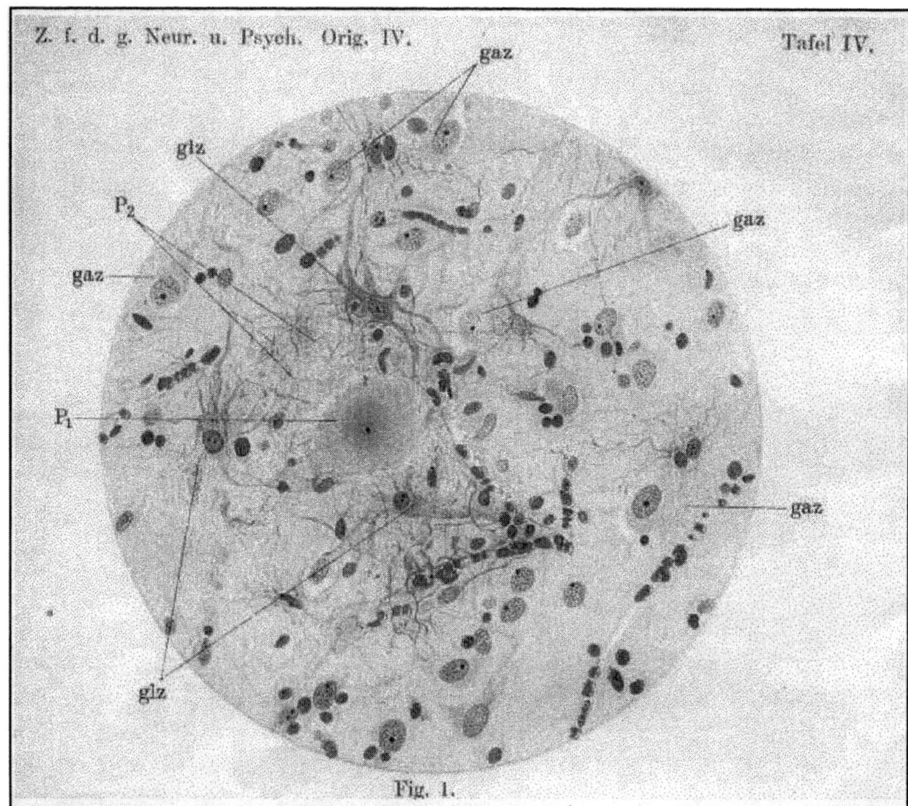

FIGURE 1.11 Relationship between (Alzheimer) plaque and glial cells; *gaz*: neuron; *glz*: glial cell; P_1: central part of the plaque; P_2: peripheral part of the plaque. (From Alzheimer, 1911.)

chronic diseases of the nervous system. The ameboid glial cell was believed to be a transformed astrocyte (swollen, with granular cytoplasm and fragmented processes) (Fig. 1.10C). Unfortunately, these cells were often, and easily, confused with Gitterzellen, as alluded to above. Alzheimer's discussion about these cells is a good example of how static microscopic images were used to draw conclusions about function. "The ameboid glial cells do not share the task of glia to provide structural support. They do not form fibers and networks, but they appear at areas of neuronal degeneration. They develop probably in response to a stimulus from the degradation products. Since we did not observe that they take up neuronal structures, we have to assume that they help to liquefy them. This we conclude from our observations on ganglion cells. Over time they grow in size and replace the ganglion cells which will completely disappear and they can be found everywhere in the (degenerating) tissue. This leads to the conclusion that they assimilate the products generated by the degradation of the ganglion cell and neuronal structures. After reaching the peak of their development, they undergo regressive changes while producing various granula and deteriorate rapidly. Their degradation products move to the lymphatic and perivascular space as fluid phase and are there taken up by mesodermal cells to be converted to lipoid matter. Thus, they clean the nervous tissue from waste, transform it to a substance harmless to ectodermal tissue and deliver it to the mesodermal tissue" (Alzheimer, 1910).

In addition to relating the occurrence of ameboid glia to neuronal degeneration, as in the case of acute postmortem change, Alzheimer realized that they could be present in chronic diseases such as epilepsy and syphilis. He also confirmed their presence in the disease that bears his name. His histopathological analysis of the first dementia patient illustrated activated glial cells surrounding the plaques (Fig. 1.11). His insights promoted glial cells to the status of important cellular elements in brain pathology. It was, however, Rio-Hortega who defined these pathological cell types and distinguished between astrocytes and microglia.

CONCLUSIONS

The early historical path to understanding neuroglia was circuitous. Penfield's general comment about the journey is telling: "Knowledge of the form and function of neuroglia is the result of progressive improvement in histological technique in the hands of careful workers. . . . Insight into the principles involved has been made difficult by numerous uncritical publications of men who, although doubtless sincere, are opportunists rather than cytologists" (Penfield, 1932). The essence of his sentiments continues to be valid today.

The history of discoveries about neuroglia highlights a major obstacle to rapid scientific progress. Scientists become so attached to their theories that contradictory evidence fails to modify their viewpoint. When conflicting data appear, new arguments are concocted to preserve the attacked notion. When evidence emerged that myelin was formed by cells, and not by axons, these contrary findings failed to convince the faithful committed to the older idea. It is provocative to ask ourselves what evidence would be necessary for us to abandon our own pet theories. Historians of our own era will, undoubtedly, have many examples to choose from to illustrate this point.

REFERENCES

Alzheimer, A. (1904) Histologische Studien zur Differenzial diagnose der progressiven Paralyse. In: Nissl, F., ed. *Histologische unsd histopathologische Arbeiten über die Grosshirnrinde mit besonderer Berücksichtigung der pathologischen Anatomie der Geisteskrankheiten*, Vol. 1. Jena: Gustav Fischer, pp. 18–314.

Alzheimer, A. (1910) Beiträge zur Kenntnis der pathologischen Neuroglia und ihrer Beziehungen zu den Abbauvorgängen im Nervengewebe. In: Nissl, F. and Alzheimer, A., eds. *Histologische unsd histopathologische Arbeiten über die Grosshirnrinde mit besonderer Berücksichtigung der pathologischen Anatomie der Geisteskrankheiten*, Vol. 3. Jena: Gustav Fischer, pp. 401–562.

Alzheimer, A. (1911) Über eigenartige Krankheitsfälle des späten Alters. *Z Neurol Psychiatrie* 4:356–385.

Andriezen, W.L. (1893) The neuroglia elements of the brain, *Br. Med. J.* 2:227–230.

Bergmann, K. (1857) Notiz über einige Strukturverhältnisse des Cerebellums und Rückenmarks. *Z. Med.* 8:360–363.

Butt, A.M. and Ransom, B.R. (1993) Morphology of astrocytes and oligodendrocytes during development in the intact optic nerve. *J. Comp. Neurol.* 338:141–158.

Cajal, S. Ramony (1995) *Histology of the Nervous System.* N. Swanson and L. Swanson, trans. New York: Oxford University Press.

Cajal, S. Ramon y (1909–1911) *Histologie de Systeme Nerveux de l'Homme et des Vertebres.* 2 vol. L. Azouloy, Trans. Paris: Maloine.

Cajal, S. Ramon y (1913) Contribucion al conocimiento de la neuroglia del cerebro humano. *Trab. Lab. Invest. Biol.* 11:255–315.

Deiters, O. (1865) *Untersuchungen über Gehirn und Rückenmark des Menschen und der Säugethiere.* Braunschweig: Vieweg.

Ferguson, J.S. (1905) *Normal Histology and Microscopical Anatomy.* New York: Appleton.

Frommann, C. (1864, 1877) *Untersuchung über die normale und pathologische Anatomie des Rückenmarks Teil I, II.* Jena.

Frommann, C. (1878) *Untersuchungen über die Gewebsveränderungen bei der Multiplen Sklerose des Gehirns.* Jena: Gustav Fischer.

Garrison, F.H. (1929) *History of Medicine*, 4th ed. Philadelphia: Saunders.

Glees, P. (1955) *Neuroglia Morphology and Function.* Oxford: Blackwell.

Golgi, C. (1871) Contribuzione alla fina Anatomia degli organi centrali del sistema nervosos. Bologna: Rivista clinica di Bologna

Golgi, C. (1894) *Untersuchungen über den feineren Bau des centralen und peripherischen Nervensystems.* Jena: Gustav Fischer.

Held, H. (1903) *Über den Bau der Neuroglia und über die Wand der Lymphgefässe in Haut und Schleimhaut.* Leipzig: Teubner.

Henle, J. and F. Merkel (1869) Ueber die sogenannte Bindesubstanz der Centralorgane des Nervensystems. Z. Med. 34:49–82.

His, W. (1889) Die Neuroblasten und deren Entstehung im embryonalen Mark. *Arch. Anat. Physiol.* 5:249–300.

Jacobson, M. (1993) *Foundations of Neuroscience.* New York: Plenum Press.

Kölliker, A. (1852) *Zur Anatomie und Physiologie der Retina, Verh. Physikal.-Med. Ges. Würzburg* 3:316–336.

Kölliker, A. (1889) *Handbuch der Gewebelehre des Menschen.* Leipzig: Wilhelm Engelmann.

Kuffler, S.W. and Nicholls, J.G. (1966). The physiology of neuroglial cells. *Ergeb. Physiol.* 57:1–90.

Lenhossék, M. von (1893) *Der feinere Bau des Nervensystems im Lichte neuester Forschung.* Berlin: Fischer's Medicinische Buchhandlung H. Kornfield.

Müller, H. (1856) Observations sur la structure de la rétine de certains animaux. Comptes Rendus de l'Académie der Sciences de Paris. 43:743–745.

Müller, H. (1851) Zur Histologie der Netzhaut, *Z. Wissenschaft. Zool.* 3:234–237.

Nedergaard, M., Ransom, B.R., Goldman, S.A. (2003) New roles for astrocytes: redefining the functional architecture of the brain. *TINS.* 26:523–530.

Nissl., F. (1899) Ueber einige Beziehungen zur Nervenzellenerkrankungen und gliosen Erscheinungen bei verschiedene Psychosen. *Arch. Psychiatrie.* 32:656–676.

Nissl, F. (1904) Die Histopathologie der paralytischen Rindenerkrankung. In: Nissl, F., ed. *Histologische unsd histopathologische Arbeiten über die Grosshirnrinde mit besonderer Berücksichtigung der pathologischen Anatomie der Geisteskrankheiten*, Vol. 1. Jena: Gustav Fischer, pp. 315–494.

Penfield, W. (1932) Neuroglia, normal and pathological. In: *Cytology and Cellular Pathology of the Nervous System*, Vol. 2. (W. Penfield, ed.) New York: Hafner, pp. 421–479.

Rand, C.W. (1953) The role of the astrocyte in the formation of cerebral scars with an introduction to Cajal's contribution to our knowledge of neuroglia. *Bull. Los Angeles Neurol. Soc.* 17:57–70.

Ransom, B., Goldman, S.A., and Nedergaard, M. (2003) New roles for astrocytes (stars at last). *TINS* 26:520–522.

Ranvier, L.-A. (1872) Recherche sur l'histologie et la physiologie des nerfs. *Arch. Physiol. Norm. Pathol.* 4:129–149.

Ranvier, L.A. (1875) Traité technique d'histologie, Figure from the German translation: *Technisches Lehrbuch der Histologie.* Leipzig: Vogel (published 1888).

Ranvier, L.-A. (1883) De la néuroglie. *Arch. de Physiol.* 3:177–185.

Remak, R. (1838) Observationes anatomicae et microscopicae de systematis nervosi structura, Dissertation, University of Berlin.

Retzius, G. (1893) Studien über Ependym und Neuroglia. *Biol. Untersuch.* 5:2–26.

Rieder, R. (1906) *Carl Weigert und seine Bedeutung fur die medizinische Wissenschaft unserer Zeit.* Berlin: Springer.

Rio-Hortega, P. del (1919) El tercer elemento de los centros nerviosos. *Bol. Soc. Esp. Biol.* 9:69–120.

Rio-Hortega, P. del (1921) Estudios sobre la neuroglia. La glia de escasas radiaciones oligodendroglia. *Bol. Soc. Esp. Biol.* 21:64–92.

Rio-Hortega, P. del (1928) Tercera aportacion al conocimiento morfologico e interpretacion functional de la oligodendroglia. *Mem. Real Soc. Esp. Hist. Nat.* 14:5–122.

Rio-Hortega, P. del (1932) Microglia. In: *Cytology and Cellular Pathology of the Nervous System*, Vol. II. (W. Penfield, ed.) New York: Hafner, pp. 483–534.

Robertson, W.F. (1897) The normal histology and pathology of the neuroglia. *J. Ment. Sci.* 43:733–752.

Robertson, W.F. (1899) On a new method of obtaining a black reaction in certain tissue elements of the central nervous system (platinum method). *Scot. Med. Surg. J.* 4:23.

Robertson, W.F. (1900) A microscopic demonstration of the normal and pathological histology of mesoglial cells. *J. Ment. Sci.* 46:733–752.

Schultze, M. (1859) Observationes de retinae structura penitiori. Published lecture at the University of Bonn

Schwann, T. (1839) *Mikroskopische Untersuchungen über die Übereinstimmung in der Struktur und dem Wachstum der Tiere und Pflanzen.* Berlin: Sander.

Somjen, G. (1988) Nervenkitt: Notes on the history of the concept of glia. *Glia* 1:2–9.

Stricker, S. (1871) *Handbuch der Lehre von den Geweben des Menschen und der Thiere.* Leipzig: Wilhelm Engelmann.

Virchow, R. (1978) *Cellular Pathology*, 2nd ed. Chance, F., trans. Birmingham, AL: Gryphon Editors.

Virchow, R. (1846) Über das granulierte ansehen der Wandungen der Gerhirnventrikel. *Allg. Z. Psychiatr.* 3:242–250.

Virchow, R. (1856) Gesammelte Abhandlungen zur wissenschaftlichen Medizin. Frankfurt: Verlag von Meidinger Sohn & Comp.

Virchow, R. (1858) Die Cellularpathologie in ihrer Begründung auf physiologische und pathologische Gewebelehre. Berlin: Verlag von August Hirschwald.

Weigert, K. (1895) *Beiträge zur Kenntnis der normalen menschlichen Neuroglia.* Frankfurt: Diesterweg.

I | PROPERTIES OF NEUROGLIAL CELLS

2 Astrocytes and ependymal glia

ANDREAS REICHENBACH AND HARTWIG WOLBURG

Macroglial cells, which comprise oligodendrocytes, astrocytes, and ependymoglial cells, may be classified according to the shapes and contacts of their cell processes (Reichenbach, 1989a) (Fig. 2.1). In contrast to oligodendrocytes, astroglial and ependymoglial cells are characterized by endfeet that contact a basal lamina around blood vessels and/or the pia mater or the vitreous body of the eye. Ependymoglial cells display a bipolar shape and additionally contact the ventricular surface (or the subretinal space). Astrocytes may be radially orientated (see the sections "Radial Astrocytes" and "Bergmann glia") but never contact the ventricular system.

MORPHOLOGY OF THE PECULIAR CELL TYPES

The morphology of astro- and ependymoglia is very diverse (Fig. 2.1). The soma of the cells may give rise to one or several *primary* or *stem* processes, from which secondary branches may origin. Much of this diversity is related to structural and functional interactions of a given cell with its microenvironment. Where macroglial cells form a *border sheath* against the ventricular space, pia, or blood vessels, they constitute epitheloid aggregates. This is observed in ependymocytes (Fig. 2.1, *X*), choroid plexus cells (Fig. 2.1, *XI*), and retinal pigment epithelial cells, (Fig. 2.5*A,E*) but also in marginal astrocytes (Fig. 2.1, *III*), perivascular astrocytes (Fig. 2.1, *VII*), and pecten glial cells (Fig. 2.5*A–C*). Typical astrocytes are more or less star-shaped (Fig. 2.1, *IV* and *VIII*), but this arrangement may be modified by adjacent neuronal cell bodies (e.g., Fig. 2.1, *V*) or axons (Fig. 2.1, *VI*) (see the sections "Radial Astrocytes," "Bergmann Glia," "Protoplasmic Astrocytes," "Fibrous Astrocytes," "Velate Astrocytes," and "Interlaminar Astrocytes"). The term *radial glia* should be restricted to bipolar ependymoglial cells that extend long processes throughout (most of) the thickness of the tissue. Early in embryonic development, the immature brain is spanned by a scaffold of fetal radial glial cells displaying wide morphological variability (Ramón y Cajal, 1911) (see Chapter 32, this volume). The persistent radial glia of the mature central nervous system (CNS) comprises tanycytes (in brain: Fig. 2.1, *I*) and Müller cells (in retina: Fig. 2.2) (see the sections "Tanycytes" and "Müller Cells").

It is noteworthy that fetal and even mature radial glial cells share many properties with neural stem cells, and in several instances they have been shown to generate neurons when they divide. The proliferative aspects of radial glia, as well as those of immature astrocytes / glioblasts (Fig. 2.1, *IX*), are beyond the topic of this chapter and are the subject of Chapter 6.

Tanycytes

Tanycytes (Fig. 2.1, *Ia* and *Ib*) (Leonhardt, 1980; Reichenbach and Robinson, 1995a) are the most common type of macroglia in the CNS of lower vertebrates. In adult mammals, they are restricted to brain regions where the tissue is rather thin, such as some periventricular organs, the stalk of the hypophysis, and the velum medullare, and to the raphe region of the spinal cord. In the periventricular organs of all vertebrates except sharks, the capillaries are fenestrated; in these regions, the tanycytes (and the choroid plexus cells (see the section "Ependymocytes, Choroid Plexus Cells, and Retinal Pigment Epithelial Cells") constitute a blood–cerebrospinal fluid barrier by expressing extensive tight junctions. Some of these tanycytes are specialized for the secretion of signaling molecules and of the material constituting Reissner's fiber.

Müller Cells

Müller cells (Reichenbach and Robinson, 1995a, 1995b; Reichenbach, 1999; Sarthy and Ripps, 2001) are the radial glia of the retina. In many vertebrates, including mammals with avascular retinae, they are the only macroglia. They contact virtually every neuronal and nonneuronal element of the retina. In the nuclear layers of the retina the Müller cell processes assume the shape of velate astrocytes (see the section "Velate Astrocytes), while in the plexiform (synaptic) layers the Müller cell processes resemble those of protoplasmic astrocytes (see the section "Protoplasmic Astrocytes"). Near the optic nerve head, the nerve fiber layer becomes very thick; there, the Müller cell processes are thin and smooth, like those of fibrous astrocytes (see

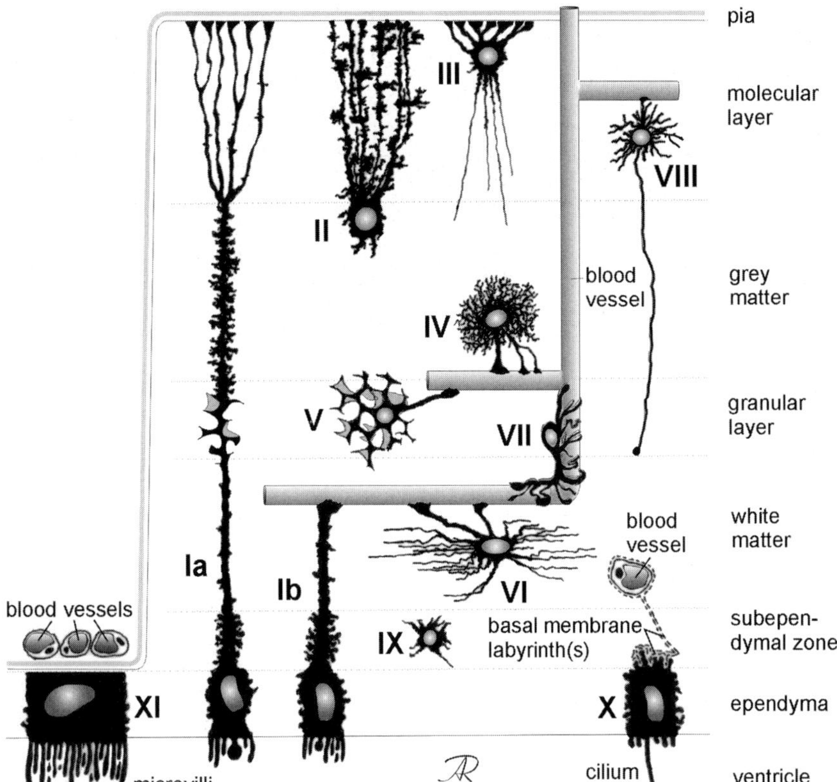

FIGURE 2.1 Semischematic survey of the main types of astroglial and ependymoglial cells and their localization in different layers/specialized regions of the central nervous system tissue. *I*: tanycyte (*a*: pial; *b*: vascular); *II*: radial astrocyte (Bergmann glial cell); *III*: marginal astrocyte; *IV*: protoplasmic astrocyte; *V*: velate astrocyte; *VI*: fibrous astrocyte; *VII*: perivascular astrocyte; *VIII*: interlaminar astrocyte; *IX*: immature astrocyte/glioblast; *X*: ependymocyte; *XI*: choroid plexus cell.

the section "Fibrous Astrocytes"). Müller cells occupy a variable volume fraction of the retinal tissue, ranging from about 3% (most lower vertebrates), to 5%–8% (mammals with vascularized retinae), to about 20% (mammals with avascular retinae). The volume of individual Müller cells may vary from 400 μm^3 (mouse) to >2000 μm^3 (rabbit, retinal periphery); their surface area ranges from 6000 to 12,000 μm^2. Müller cell densities per square millimeter of retinal surface area are 1550–2000 (frog, salamander), 5000–12,000 (most mammals), and >25,000 (fovea centralis of primates). Each Müller cell ensheaths and supports a columnar group of retinal neurons, the number of which ranges from 7 (tree shrew), about 16 (human, rabbit, and many herbivorous mammals), to about 30 (rodents and carnivores), up to 80 (frog) and to even more than 200 (deepsea teleosts). The size and shape of Müller cells depend on the animal species and, within a given retina, on retinal topography. Generally, in rod-dominant retinae (most fish and mammals), a Müller cell extends just one stem process from the soma to the inner limiting membrane, whereas in cone-dominant retinae (most reptiles and birds), the vitread stem processes of Müller cells are split into several branches (Fig. 2.2*E*). Notably, in species with native polyploidy (e.g., lungfish and salamander), not only the cell nucleus but the entire cell is huge; this advantage is being used for experiments on single cells.

Radial Astrocytes

Radial astrocytes (Fig. 2.1, *II*) (Stensaas and Stensaas, 1968; Miller and Luizzi, 1986) are common in the spinal cord and brain of lower vertebrates. As they cross white and gray matter, the properties of their cell processes may change from protoplasmic to fibrous (see the section "Protoplasmic Astrocytes" and "Fibrous Astrocytes"). Radial astrocytes with *velate* processes were also described (Pouwels, 1978). Some radial astrocytes are also found in the optic nerve of mammals (Fig. 2.4*C*).

FIGURE 2.2. Müller cells, the radial glia of the vertebrate retina. *A–D*. Müller cells in living unfixed sections (*A*) and whole mounts (*B–D*) of the midperipheral guinea pig retina, after uptake of the fluorescent dye MitoTracker; confocal microscopy. (courtesy of O. Uckermann, Leipzig.) Whereas the thick Müller cell endfeet form an almost complete *cobblestone panel* in the innermost retinal layers [interrupted only by the unstained ganglion cell somata (*asterisks*) and axon bundles, (*B*)], in the inner plexiform layer the vitread stem processes of Müller cells are separated from each other by the synaptic neuropile and constitute a rather regular framework (*C*). The somata of Müller cells are found within the inner nuclear layer (*D*); they appear irregularly shaped, as if indented by their neuronal neighbors. *E*, Survey of the shape of Müller cells in different vertebrate retinae. Most cells are drawn from Golgi-stained preparations; some are camera lucida drawings of dye-filled cells. As far as possible, all cells are shown at the same magnification. (Modified from Reichenbach, 1999, where the references can also be found.)

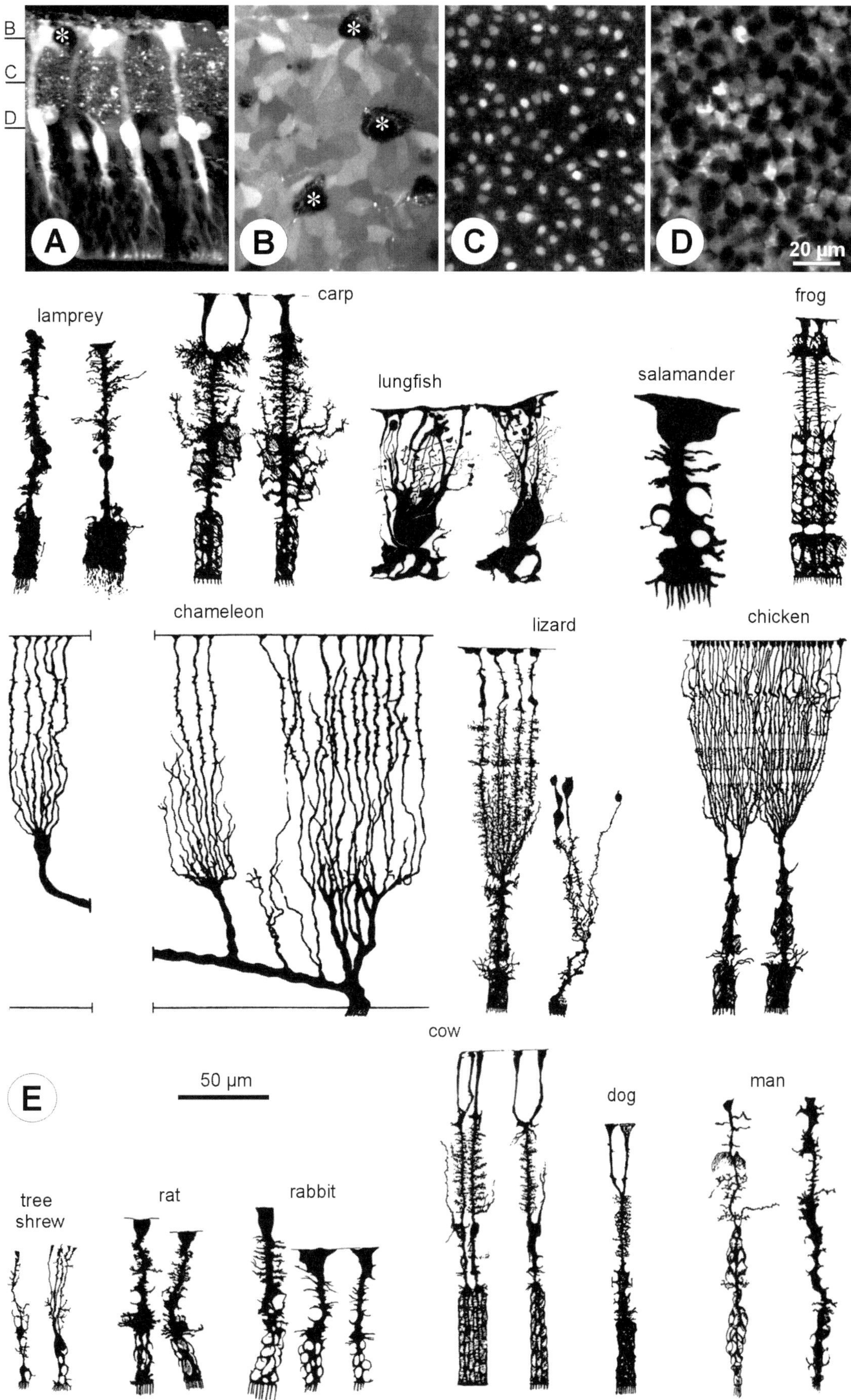
B
C
D
A
B
C
D
20 µm
lamprey
carp
lungfish
salamander
frog
chameleon
lizard
chicken
cow
E
50 µm
dog
man
tree shrew
rat
rabbit

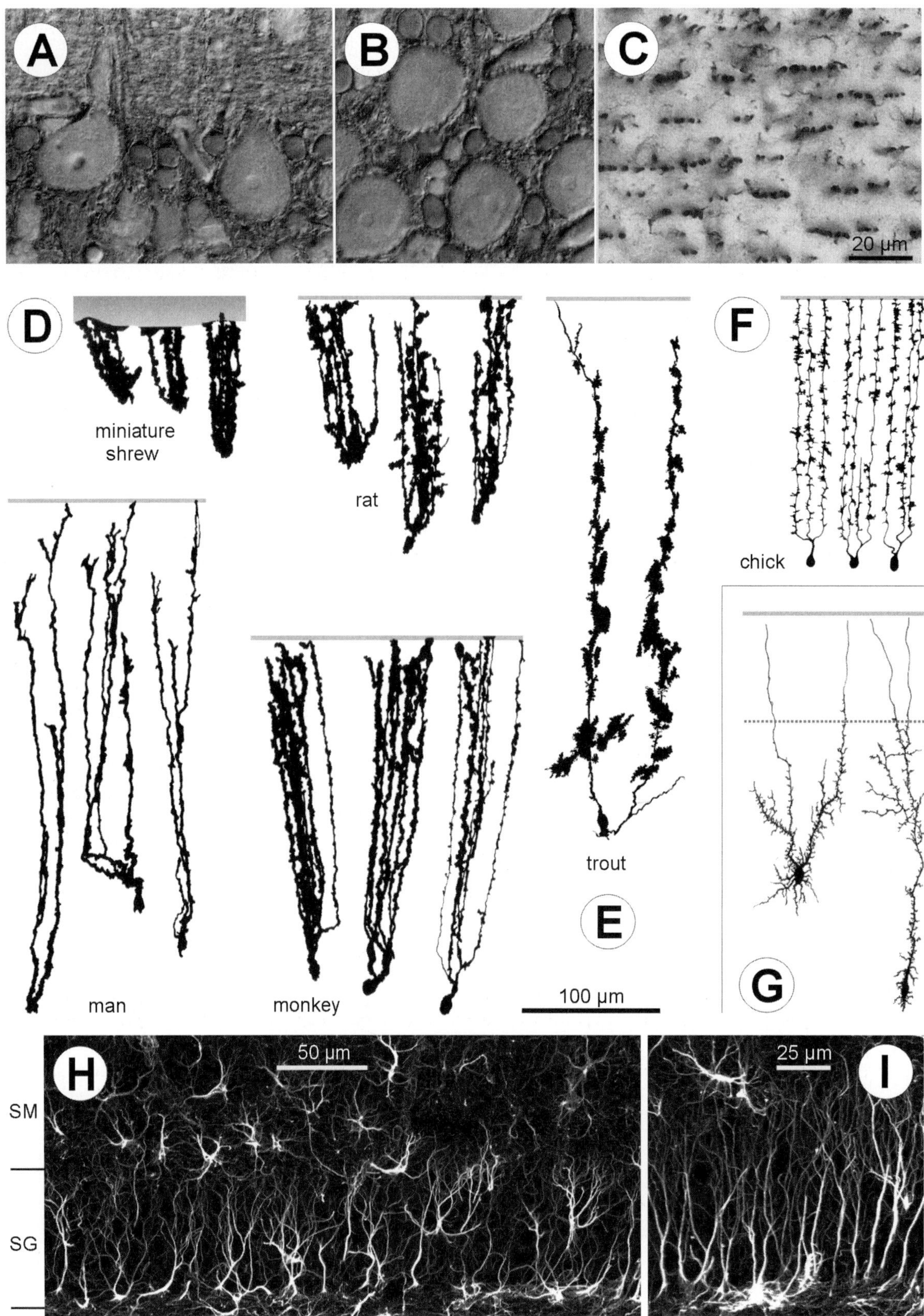
A
B
C
20 µm
D
miniature shrew
rat
trout
F
chick
man
monkey
E
100 µm
G
H
50 µm
SM
SG
25 µm
I

FIGURE 2.3. Bergmann glial cells, the radial astrocytes of the vertebrate cerebellum (*A–F*), radial astrocytes from turtle spinal cord (*G*), and radially oriented astrocytes from rat hippocampus (*H,I*). *A–C*. Bergmann glial cells of the adult rat cerebellum, immunocytochemistry. The glutamine synthetase–positive Bergmann glial cell somata (dark) surround and envelop the Purkinje cell somata (*A,B*), while their glial fibrillary acidic protein (GFAP)–positive stem processes run through the molecular layer where they form into rows or palisades (view from the cerebellar surface: *C*). *D–F*. Camera lucida drawings of Golgi-stained Bergmann glial cells in the cerebella of several different mammals including those of the human (*D*), the trout, *Salmo gairdneri* (*E*), and the chicken (*F*). *G*. Camera lucida drawings of Golgi-stained radial astrocytes in the spinal cord of the turtle. Note that the character of the processes changes from complex (protoplasmic) to smooth (fibrous) when they pass from gray to white matter (*dashed line*). (*A–C* modified from Reichenbach et al., 1995; *D* from Siegel et al., 1991; *E* from Pouwels, 1978; and *F* and *G* from Stensaas and Stensaas, (1968.) *H,I*. GFAP immunofluorescence of the dentate gyrus of the hippocampus of an adult rat; astroglial cell processes are radially aligned in the stratum granulare (*SG*), whereas typical star-shaped astrocytes are found in the stratum moleculare (*SM*). Original confocal microphotographs. (Courtesy of Gert Brückner, Leipzig.)

In the mammalian hippocampus, radially oriented astrocytes occur that do not abut the pia with their processes; rather, they are confined to the stratum granulare of the dentate gyrus (Kosaka and Hama, 1986) and to the stratum oriens of the CA1 region (Fig. 2.3*H*, *lower half*, 2.3*I*). They should be considered as a unique cell type, different from the radial astrocytes of lower vertrebrates.

Bergmann Glia

Bergmann glial cells, also termed *Golgi epithelial cells* (Fig. 2.3) (Palay and Chan-Palay, 1974), are the radial astrocytes of the cerebellum in all vertebrates. Their cell bodies reside in the layer of the Purkinje cell somata (Fig. 2.3*A,B*), and their processes (usually three to six per cell) cross the molecular layer, resembling those of the protoplasmic astrocytes (cf. the next section; Figs. 2.3*D–F*, 2.9*A*). The Bergmann glial cell processes form palisades parallel to the long axis of the folium (Fig. 2.3*C*). The many elaborate side branches (Figs. 2.8, 2.9) display complex interactions with the synapses on the Purkinje cell dendrites (see the section "Lamellar Neuron-Contact Processes, Glial Microdomains") (Fig. 2.9); they have a high surface-to-volume ratio of up to $>20\ \mu m^{-1}$ (Grosche et al., 1999, 2002). In rodent cerebellum, there are about eight Bergmann glial cells per Purkinje cell (i.e., about 8000 per square millimeter of cerebellar surface area). Each Bergmann glial cell ensheathes 2000–6000 Purkinje cell synapses (Reichenbach et al., 1995). Bergmann glial cells occupy about 15%–18% of the volume of the molecular layer; an average rodent Bergmann glial cell has a volume of about 3600 μm^3. The size and shape of Bergmann glial cells differ, depending on the animal species (Fig. 2.3). Generally, in small species (e.g., shrews) the Bergmann glial cell processes are short and densely covered with lateral appendages, while in large species (e.g., humans) they are much longer but show less dense lateral outgrowths (Siegel et al., 1991). Fañana's cells constitute a subtype of short Bergmann glial cells.

Protoplasmic Astrocytes

Protoplasmic astrocytes (Fig. 2.1, *IV*; Fig. 2.10*A–C*; Fig. 2.3*H*, *upper half*) (Wolff, 1968; Bushong et al., 2002; Chao et al., 2002) are found in the gray matter. Their numerous processes are spread more or less radially from the soma, and extend many fine, complex lamellar side branches (Wolff, 1968). These surface extensions occupy about 50% of the volume but as much as 80% of the surface area of the cell ($V_{cell} \sim 5500\ \mu m^3$; $S_{cell} \sim 80{,}000\ \mu m^2$: Chao et al., 2002), resulting in high surface-to-volume ratios of 10–20 μm^{-1}. Although the volume fraction of astroglia amounts to only 10%–20%, the astrocytic processes contact much of the available neuronal surfaces (Chao et al., 2002). At least one of the cell processes bears one or several perivascular endfeet such that the surfaces of CNS blood vessels are completely ensheathed by astroglial endfeet. The density of astrocytes in the cerebral cortex is high (layers III/IV: 4000–10,000 mm^{-3} in lissencephalic cortices of insectivores: Stolzenburg et al., 1989; 12,000–>30,000 mm^{-3} in rat gyrate cortex: Distler et al., 1991). The cortical glia-to-neuron index (largely determined by protoplasmic astrocytes) increases with the thickness of the tissue, from about 0.1 in shrew to about 5 in whale (see Reichenbach, 1989b). Every protoplasmic astrocyte establishes its own primarily exclusive territory (Bushong et al., 2002).

Fibrous Astrocytes

Fibrous astrocytes (Fig. 2.1, *VI*; Fig. 2.4) (Waxman, 1986; Schnitzer, 1988; Butt et al., 1994a, 1994b) are found in white matter tracts, in optic nerve, and in the nerve fiber layer of mammalian vascularized retinae. Their somata are often arranged in rows between the axon bundles (Fig. 2.4*G*). Their processes are comparatively smooth, and frequently oriented in parallel to the axons. Every fibrous astrocyte in murine optic nerve possesses several perivascular and/or subpial endfeet (Butt et al., 1994a, 1994b; see Fig. 2.4*C–E*). The processes of fibrous astrocytes extend multiple finger-like outgrowths into the perinodal space of adjacent axons (Figs. 2.4*F*, 2.4*I*). A density of about 200,000 fibrous astrocytes per cubic millimeter has been estimated for the anterior commissure of the mouse (Sturrock et al., 1977). The processes of fibrous astrocytes are generally longer (up to 300 μm) than those of protoplasmic astrocytes ($<50\ \mu m$), but their surface-to-volume ratio is significantly smaller (about 5 μm^{-1}).

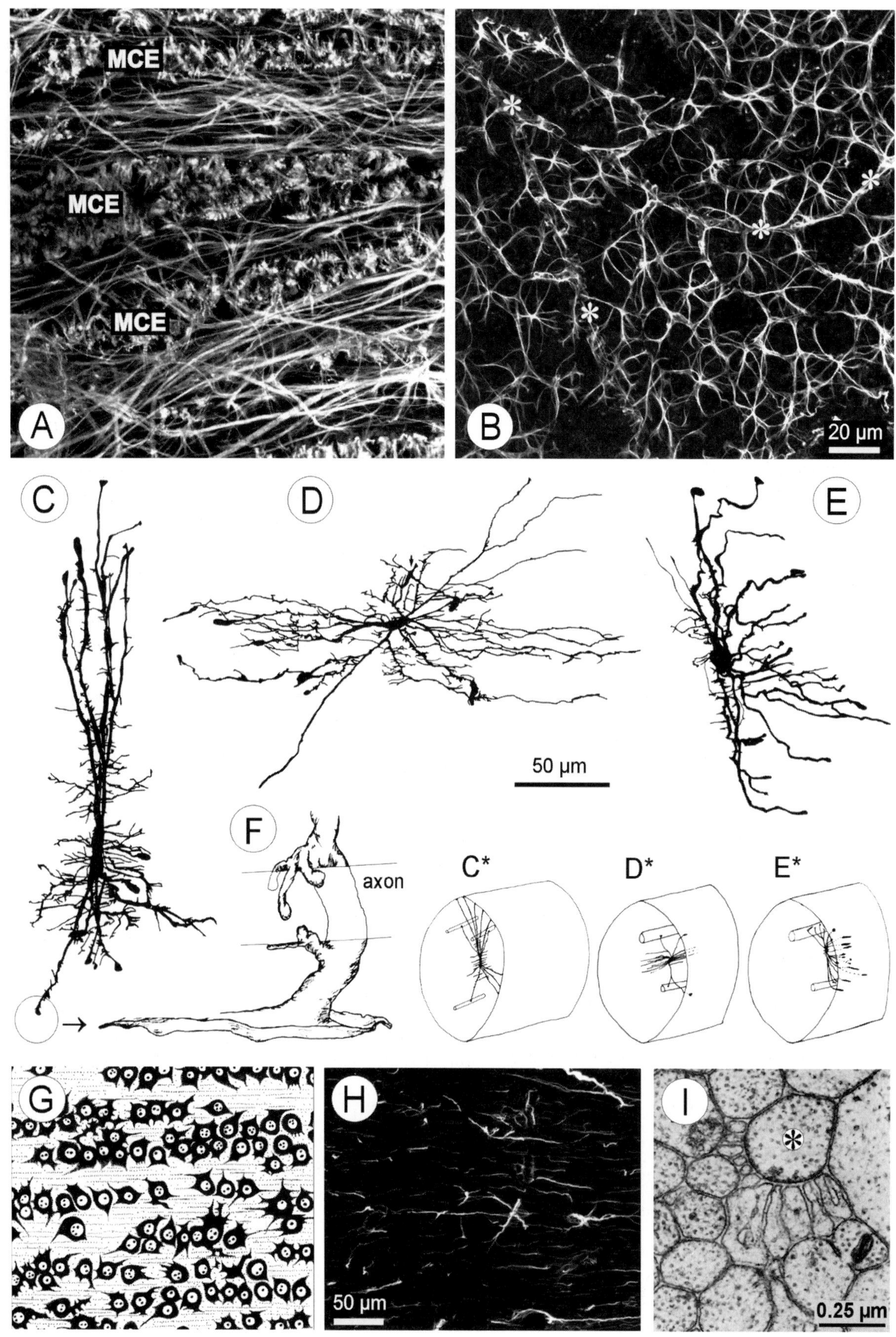
MCE
MCE
MCE
A
B
20 µm
C
D
E
50 µm
F
axon
C*
D*
E*
G
H
50 µm
I
0.25 µm

FIGURE 2.4. Fibrous astrocytes in the mammalian retina (*A, B, I*), optic nerve (*C–F*), spinal cord (*G*), and brain (*H*). *A,B*. Glial acidic fibrillary protein (GFAP)–labeled fibrous astrocytes in the flat-mounted murine retina, immunofluorescence. Close to the optic nerve (*A*), the astrocytic processes are aligned in parallel with the axon bundles that run between rows of Müller cell endfeet (*MCE*). In the retinal periphery (*B*) the cells are more or less star-shaped and form a regular pattern that is modified only by the contacts to retinal blood vessels (*asterisks*). (Courtesy of Bernd Biedermann, Leipzig.) *C–F*. Fibrous astrocytes from murine optic nerve. *C–E*. Camera lucida drawings of dye-injected cells show that the cell processes may be aligned radially (*C/C**), longitudinally (*D/D**), or randomly (*E/E**) but that all cells display several endfeet at the pia, the blood vessels, or both (*C*–E** give the orientation of the cells in the nerve). *F*. Artist's reconstruction of the finger-like perinodal processes of the cell shown in C, based upon electron microscopic serial sections of the dye-labeled cell. (Modified from Butt et al., 1994a, 1994b). *G*. Interfascicular rows of astrocytes and oligodendrocytes in the spinal cord of a newborn cat; silver carbonate stain. (Modified from Hortega, 1956.) *H*. GFAP-immunolabeled fibrous astrocytes in the murine optic chiasm. Original confocal microphotograph. (Courtesy of Gert Brückner, Leipzig.) *I*. Corona of finger-like astrocytic processes around a node-like specialization of an unmyelinated axon (*asterisk*) in the rat retinal nerve fiber layer. (Modified from Hildebrand and Waxman, 1983.)

Velate Astrocytes

Velate astrocytes (Fig. 2.1, V) were described in the granule layer of the cerebellum, where each of them surrounds several small neuronal granule cells with velate sheaths (rat: Chan-Palay and Palay, 1972; fish: Pouwels, 1978). Similar cells occur in the olfactory bulb (Valverde and Lopez-Mascaraque, 1991). This cell type develops at sites where many small, densely packed neurons occur. The surface-to-volume ratio of velate astrocytes is estimated to be very high (20–30 μm^{-1}).

Interlaminar Astrocytes

Interlaminar astrocytes (Fig. 2.1, *VIII*) (Colombo et al., 1995; Colombo, 2001) have been found in the supragranular layers of the cerebral cortex of higher primates including humans. They are similar to protoplasmic astrocytes but extend a long (up to 1.0 mm) process from the soma over at least two laminae, down to lamina IV, where it ends in a small bulb. Collectively these processes form a visible *palisade* that has been found to be severely disrupted in cases of Alzheimer's disease. It is speculated that interlaminar astrocytes may optimize the modular organization of the cortex.

Marginal Glia and Perivascular Astrocytes

Close to the pia mater, specialized astrocytes (Fig. 2.1, *III*) may form several layers of endfeet (Braak, 1975). Usually they extend several long, smooth processes into the neuropile, but their main function is thought to constitute a glial *limiting zone*.

In the human and rabbit retina, perivascular astrocytes (Fig. 2.1, VII), virtually devoid of neuron-contacting processes, form extensive endfoot contacts to blood vessels (see Schnitzer, 1988). They also seem to occur elsewhere in the brain, but their occurrence and possible function(s) (formation of a *glial barrier*?) have been poorly studied so far.

Ependymocytes, Choroid Plexus Cells, and Retinal Pigment Epithelial Cells

Ependymocytes, choroid plexus cells, and retinal pigment epithelial (RPE) cells (Leonhard, 1980; Reichenbach and Robinson; 1995a) line the ventricle (or the subretinal space). At their basal pole, mature ependymocytes (Fig. 2.1, *X*) contact remnants of embryonic blood vessels (so-called basement membrane labyrinths) (Leonhardt, 1980). On their other pole, they possess, in addition to microvilli, kinocilia to support the stream of the cerebrospinal fluid. The latter is secreted mainly by the choroid plexus cells (Fig. 2.1, *XI*), which requires a high permeability of the fenestrated plexus endothelial cells; thus, the blood–cerebrospinal fluid barrier is formed by the plexus epithelium.

Retinal pigment epithelial cells (Fig. 2.5*E*) line the subretinal space opposite the neuroretina. Their apical surface extends (*1*) long (5–7 μm), thin microvilli, maximizing the membrane area available for transepithelial transport, and (*2*) specially arranged shorter microvilli termed *photoreceptor sheaths*. The basal surface of the RPE cells contains numerous invaginations (Fig. 2.5*E*) to increase the surface area. Within the human macula, the RPE cells measure about 14 μm in diameter (12 μm in height), but they become wider (up to 60 μm in diameter) and flatter in the periphery. Like the choroid plexus cells, the RPE cells (*1*) are in close apposition to many blood vessels, (*2*) are specialized for transmembrane transport, and (*3*) form the blood–cerebrospinal (subretinal) fluid barrier by their tight junctions (Fig. 2.5*F*). However, RPE cells do not secrete fluid across their apical microvillous membrane but rather perform net fluid uptake from the subretinal space. This water resorption contributes to the attachment of the neuroretina to the RPE. Another specific feature of RPE cells is the presence of black (melanin) pigment granules, aimed at the avoidance of scattering light. By contrast, in some vertebrates adapted to dark environments (e.g., deep-sea fishes), the RPE cells may contain guanidin crystals in order to reflect light back to the photoreceptor cells. Melanin granula may also serve an important role as sinks for free radicals and excited oxygen species.

Pecten Glial Cells

The pecten oculi is a peculiar vascular structure of the avian eye, where it bulges from the optic nerve head into the vitreous body (Fig. 2.5*A*). It is composed of two types of cells, endothelial cells and specialized glial cells (Fig. 2.5*B–D*). The latter (like the RPE cells) originate in the outer leaflet of the optic cup; they contain pigment gran-

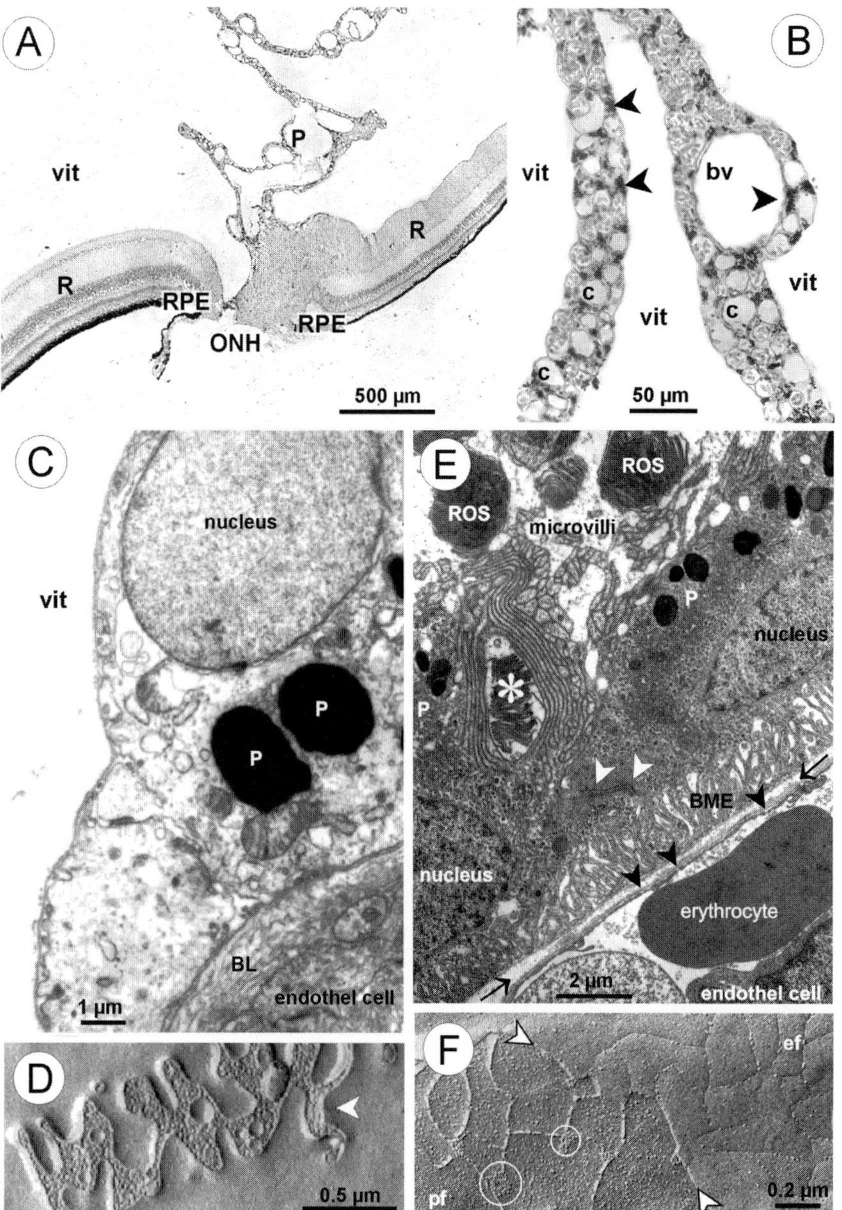

FIGURE 2.5. Specialized ependymoglia of the eye. *A*: Survey of the fundus of an avian (blue-and-yellow macaw) eye. Close to the optic nerve head (*ONH*), two peculiar forms of ependymoglia can be found: in the pecten (*P*), the pecten glial cells, and below the retina (*R*), the retinal pigment epithelial (*RPE*) cells. *B*. Higher magnification of an area of the pecten shown in *A*. Many capillaries (*c*) and larger blood vessels (*bv*) are embedded in a tissue that contains endothelial cells and pigmented pecten glial cells (*black arrowheads*) that contact the vitreous (*vit*). *C*. Electron microscopy of the chicken pecten; the pecten glial cells contain pigment granules (*P*) but do not form tight junctions (*D*, freeze fracture replica). *E*. The RPE cells (example from rabbit) contain pigment granula (*P*). Apically (i.e., toward the outer segments of the photoreceptor cells, *ROS*) they extend microvilli that may enclose the shed tips of ROS (*asterisk*) as the first step in phagocytosis. Basally, the cells face a basal lamina (Bruch's membrane, between the *arrows*) and display an enlarged surface area due to basal membrane enfoldings (*BME*). Since the capillaries of the underlying choroid possess a fenestrated endothelium (*black arrowheads*), the RPE cells form the blood–retina barrier by the expression of tight junctions (*white arrowheads*). *F*. Freeze-fracture replica of the tight junctions in the lateral membranes of chicken RPE cells; at the line between the white arrowheads, the fracture level changes from the protoplasmic (*pf*) to the external face (*ef*) of the cell membrane. In addition, gap junctions (*circled*) also occur between RPE cells. Original microphotographs.

ules (like RPE cells) but lose their tight junctions during differentiation (unlike RPE cells) such that the blood–retina barrier is maintained by the endothelial cells of the pecten. The pecten glial cells probably play important roles in the nutrition and detoxification of the avian retina.

IMMUNOCYTOCHEMICAL VISUALIZATION AND IDENTIFICATION OF ASTRO- AND EPENDYMOGLIAL CELLS

Astrocytic and ependymoglial cells can be visualized and even identified by immunocytochemical labeling of certain antigens that are, at least within the CNS, restricted to these cells. The immunoreactivities of certain cell types may change with differentiation or during pathological processes (Table 2.1). Furthermore, not all members of a cell population must express the same antigen; for instance, while it may be safely stated that every glial fibrillary acidic protein (GFAP)-immunopositive cell in brain is an astrocyte, there are many astrocytes that are not labeled by anti-GFAP antibodies. Moreover, some of the antigens (e.g., the intermediate filament proteins) allow mainly visualization of the stem processes (Fig. 2.6*A*) (delineating only 15% of the total astrocyte volume: Bushong et al., 2002), while antibodies directed to cytoplasmic proteins (such as glutamine synthetase and S-100β) may stain even fine cytoplasmic lamelles (Fig. 2.6*B*). By contrast, antibodies against membrane proteins may label (parts of) the cell surface (Fig. 2.6*C*). For a survey, see Table 2.1.

Ependymo- and astroglial cells have the capability to accumulate exogenously applied fluorescent dyes. Thus, such dyes can be used to monitor Ca^{2+} (Fig. 2.9*D*), glutathion, pH, and so on specifically in living glial cells and,

TABLE 2.1 *List of "Marker Antigens" Suitable to Visualize and/or to Identify the Various Types of Astro- and Ependymoglial Cells During Ontogenetic Development, in the Normal Mature Central Nervous System, and During Reactive Changes in Cases of Pathology*

Cell Type	*Antigen*	*Developing*	*Adult*	*Reactive*
Astroglia	GFAP	(+)	++	+++
	Vimentin	+++	−	++
	Nestin	++	−	++
	Cytokeratin [F,A]		++	
	Glutamine synthetase		++	
	iNOS		+	+++
	RC1/2 (antibodies)	++	−	
	RAN-2	+	++	
	BLBP*	++	−	
	S-100β	−	++	
	3CB2[C]			
	R-cadherin[C]	+	++	
Müller glia	GFAP [F]	−	−	+++
	Vimentin	+	++	+
	RAN-2		++	
	3CB2	++		
	nNOS/iNOS		+	+++
	CA		++	++
	S-100β		++	
	3CB2	++		
	B-cadherin[C]	+	++	
	F11*	++	++	
	Glutamine synthetase		++	
	CRALBP		++	
Bergmann glia	GFAP		++	
	Vimentin	++	+	
	Nestin	++		
	Glutamine synthetase		++	
	S-100β		++	
Ependymoglia	GFAP	(+)	++	
	Vimentin		++	
	Cytokeratin		+++	
	RAN-2		++	
Retinal pigment epithelium cells	Vimentin		++	
	CRALBP		+++	
	R-Cadherin[C]	++	−	
Pecten glia (only avian)	Vimentin	+	++	
	B-cadherin	+	++	
	Glutamin synthetase		++	
Choroid plexus epithelium	Cytokeratin		++	
	GFAP		−	++
	Vimentin		++	
	Neurofilament*		++	

Note: Whereas the list basically reflects the situation in mammals, many of the antigens can also be found in the particular cell types of other vertebrates. In cases when an antigen is found only in nonmammalian cells, it is labeled by a letter: F: fishes; A: amphibians; C: chicken. An asterisk indicates that the listed antigen (or antibody, respectively) labels not only selectively glial cells, but (in other regions of the central nervous system) also neurons. Antigens expressed in the cytoplasmic membranes such as ion channels, receptors, or adhesion molecules are excluded from the list since immunocytochemistry for these antigens usually results in "diffuse" labeling of the neuropile at the light microscopic level.

Abbreviations: BLBP: brain lipid-binding protein; CA: carbonic anhydrase; CRALBP: cellular retinaldehyde-binding protein; GFAP: glial fibrillary acidic protein; NOS: nitric oxide synthase (n, neuronal form, i, inducible form); RAN-2: rat neural antigen-2.

simultaneously, to study their morphology (Fig. 2.2*A–D*). Intracellular injections of fluorescent dyes can also be used to visualize individual glial cells (e.g., Fig. 2.4*D–F*). Finally, astroglial cells can be induced to express the green fluorescent protein (GFP) by coupling this gene to the GFAP promoter in transgenic mice (Fig. 2.9*A*).

ULTRASTRUCTURAL FEATURES

Cell Soma and Nucleus

The soma of astrocytes is usually rather poor in organelles compared to that of neurons. In most cases,

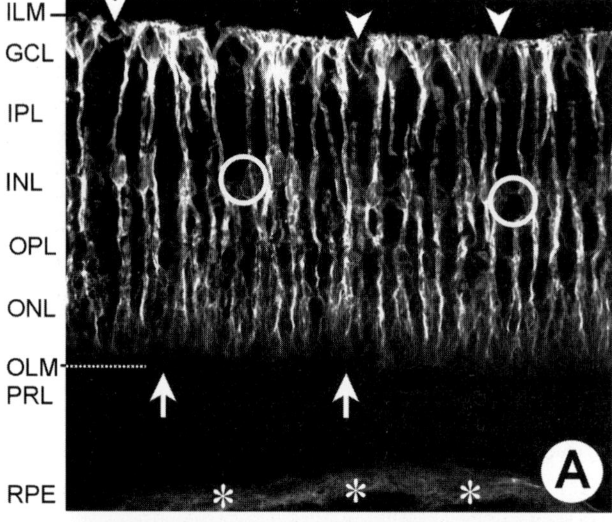

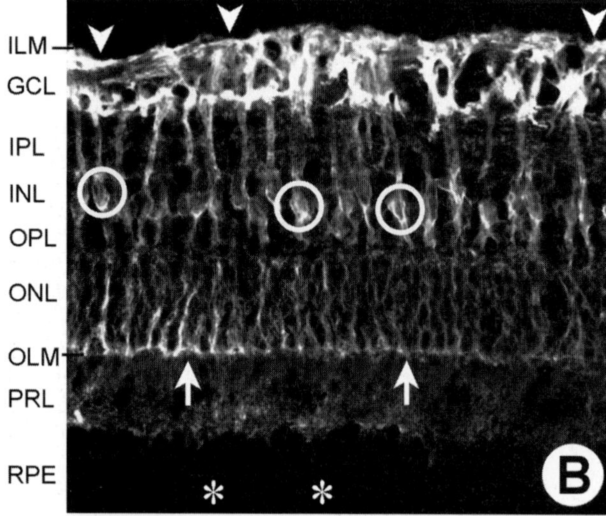

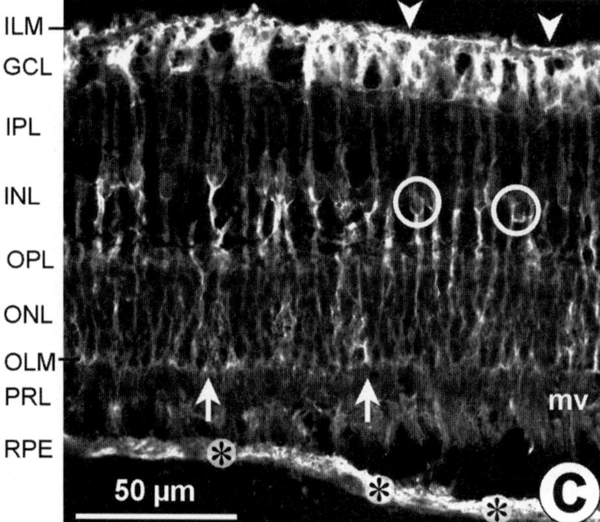

FIGURE 2.6. Immunocytochemical visualization of Müller cells in the adult guinea pig retina. *A*. Labeling of the intermediate filament protein, vimentin, demonstrates mainly the stem processes of the cells. The endfeet are not labeled throughout but only where they contain filament bundles; some appear empty (*arrowheads*). Likewise, neither the somata (*circles*) nor the sclerad ends of the cells (*arrows*) are labeled. Additional faint label is observed in the RPE (*asterisks*). *B*. Labeling of the cytoplasmic enzyme, glutamine synthetase, in addition reveals fine side branches in the plexiform layers (*IPL*, *OPL*), as well as the somata of the cells (*circles*). The cells are labeled throughout from the vitread endfeet (*arrowheads*) down to their sclerad ends (*arrows*). The RPE is not labeled (*asterisks*). *C*. Use of antibodies directed to the cellular retinaldehyde-binding protein (CRALBP) visualizes the membrane surface of the cells and thus reveals the most morphological details including the sclerad microvilli (mv). The RPE (including its microvilli) is also strongly labeled (*asterisks*). *ILM*: inner limiting membrane; *GCL*: ganglion cell layer; *IPL*: inner plexiform layer; *INL*: inner nuclear layer; *OPL*: outer plexiform layer; *ONL*: outer nuclear layer; *OLM*: outer limiting "membrane"; *PRL*: photoreceptor layer; *RPE*: retinal pigment epithelium. The RPE is artificially detached from the retina at some places. Original confocal images. (Courtesy of Ivona Goczalik and Mike Francke.)

characteristic bundles of intermediate filaments can be found. The somata of some ependymoglial cells contain melanin pigment granula (RPE cells, pecten glial cells, choroid epithelial cells: Fig. 2.5*C*,*E*). In many of these epitheloid glial cells, the lateral membranes of the somata are interconnected by zonulae adherentes and tight junctions, thus forming the blood–brain (or –retina) barrier (Wolburg and Lippoldt, 2002).

In astro- and ependymoglial cell nuclei, the nucleoplasm is rather evenly distributed (Fig. 2.5*C*,*E*) compared to that in oligodendrocytes and microglial cells. In many tanycytes, the cell nuclei are very irregularly shaped. The nuclei (and somata) of Müller cells seem to be (and may actually be) indented by neighboring neurons (cf. Fig. 2.2*D*).

Stem Processes

Stem processes arise directly from soma. Typically they contain bundles of intermediate filaments. Microtubuli are rarely found in astroglial cell processes; one of the few exceptions are the apical processes of Müller cells. The stem processes usually contain numerous mitochondria. An interesting exception are Müller cell processes in species with avascular retinae that contain mitochondria only at their apical pole (i.e., close to the choroid, which is the only source of oxygen supply).

Endfeet

Astrocytic endfeet cover all basal laminae within the CNS (along the blood vessels, the pia mater, and the vitreous body in the eye). They are often coupled to each other by gap junctions. In the case of tanycytes and Müller cells, the endfeet are densely filled with smooth endoplasmic reticulum. Bundles of intermediate filaments extend into the endfeet but fail to occupy the cytoplasm close to the basal lamina–contacting endfoot membrane. The endfeet are generally rich in mitochondria. The occurrence of caveolae, coated pits, and *Ω-vesicles* indicates an active material exchange with the compartment behind the basal lamina (i.e., blood plasma, vitreous body, or subarachnoidal fluid). A secretory function has been ascribed to the tanycytes of some circumventricular organs.

The most prominent and distinctive ultrastructural feature of endfoot membranes of all astroglial cells in higher vertebrates are the orthogonal arrays of intramembranous particles (OAPs) (Fig. 2.7). The OAPs accumulate in parts of the endfoot membrane that directly contact a basal lamina, whereas they are (almost) missing in neuropil-facing membranes. This polarity develops concomitantly with the maturation of the blood–brain barrier (BBB), is dependent on the perivascular extracellular matrix, and is lost in glial cell cultures and in astroglial tumors (Wolburg, 1995; Rascher-Eggstein et al., 2004). The particles seem to consist of the water channel protein, aquaporin-4 (AQP4) (Venero et al., 2001) and perhaps of other proteins such as the inwardly rectifying K^+ channel, Kir4.1 (Nagelhus et al., 1999) or the dystrophin-dystroglycan complex (Warth et al., 2004). OAP/AQP4 play an importent role in brain water homeostasis and in the maintenance of the BBB (Ke et al., 2001). It was recently shown that the Müller cell-specific member of the dystrophins, Dp71′, is crucial for the specific clustering of AQP4 and Kir4.1 in the endfoot membrane of the cells (Dalloz et al., 2003). At the opposite side, contact to mesenchymal cells and/or molecules (e.g., collagen, laminin, or agrin) is required to stimulate the insertion of Kir4.1 channels (Ishii et al., 1997) and the production of a basal lamina (Crawford 1983; Halfter, 1998).

Ventricular Contacts

Cell processes contacting the ventricular (or subretinal) space occur in all ependymoglial cells but never in astrocytes. They always display a large contact area provided by microvilli and abundant mitochondria, features that indicate high metabolic activity presumably

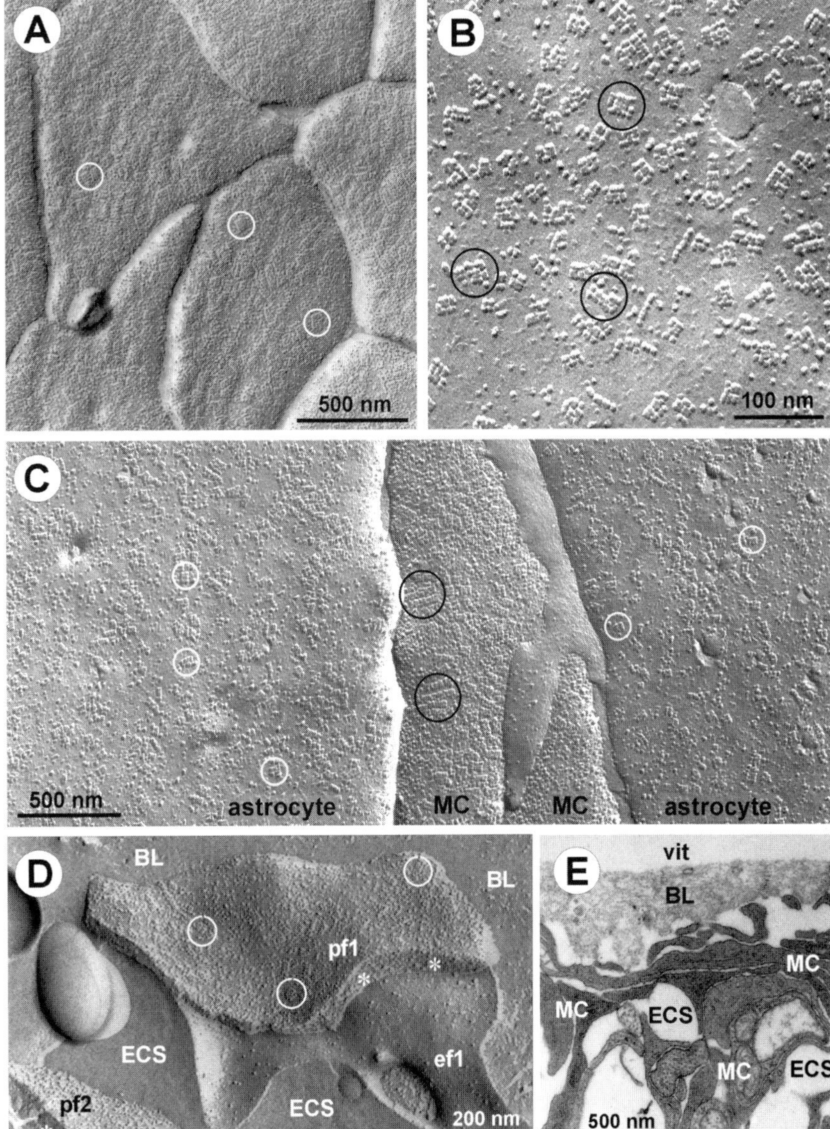

FIGURE 2.7. Freeze-fracture replicas of endfoot membranes of Müller cells and astrocytes. *A*. Müller cell endfeet of the adult pigeon retina. *B*. Subpial astrocytic endfoot membrane of the adult rat optic nerve at very high magnification. *C*. Inner surface of the adult rabbit retina; here (in the region of the *medullary rays*), endfeet of Müller cells (*MC*) and astrocytes are found in close proximity. Both Müller cell and astrocytic endfoot membranes display orthogonal arrays of particles (*OAPs*, encircled) but the size and distribution pattern of the OAPs differ between the two types of cells (as well as between animal species). *D,E*. Inner surface of the adult human retina (perifoveal region). In the central primate retina, the vitread basal lamina (*BL*) is extremely thick (up to several micrometers) and has a highly irregular surface toward the retina, where it interdigitates with the Müller cell endfeet (*MC* in *E*). As a further peculiarity, the Müller cell endfeet are subdivided into many small branchlets that may form several layers of very thin structures separated at some places by rather large extracellular spaces (*ECS*). A freeze-fracture replica of such a region is shown in *D*. The fracture level runs obliquely from the basal lamina (*top*) via a first vitread endfoot branchlet (*pf1*: protoplasmic face of the membrane adjacent to the basal lamina; asterisks: cytoplasm; *ef1*: external face of the membrane distant to the basal lamina) and an ECS to a second endfoot branchlet that is not in contact to the basal lamina (*pf2*: protoplasmic face of the membrane). Whereas OAPs are expressed in the endfoot membrane abutting the basal lamina, they are missing in the membrane of the second (distant) branchlet. *vit*: vitreous body. Original microphotographs.

related to active exchange of substances with the luminal fluid. The formation of microvilli seems to be triggered where glial cells abut large fluid compartments (Foos and Gloor, 1975; Anderson et al., 1983).

Neighboring glial ventricular contact processes (and adjacent neuronal cell processes, if present) are connected by apicolateral junctions (desmosomes). In regions without endothelial BBB (most circumventricular organs, RPE), ependymoglial cells form a cerebrospinal fluid–brain barrier by expressing tight junctions (cf. Fig. 2.5*E,F*). Apicolateral gap junctions occur between Müller cells in frogs but not in mammals. In homogeneous rabbit Müller cell cultures *in vitro*, however, gap and even tight junctions have been observed (Wolburg et al., 1990).

The apical processes of typical ependymocytes possess, depending on the species, 12 to 60 kinocilia. The cilia are 10 to 20 μm long and are of the $9 \times 2 + 2$ type. They beat rhythmically at a frequency of about 200 per minute and assist the rostro-caudad flow of cerebrospinal fluid.

Lamellar Neuron-Contact Processes; Glial Microdomains

The end branches of neuropilar astroglial cell processes are the site of glia-neuron interactions. These processes form flat or lamellar sheaths enclosing neuronal somata, synapses, or bundles of axonal internodes (Wolff, 1968; Chao et al., 2002) or finger-like extensions contacting the nodal membrane of myelinated axons (Fig. 2.4*F*). Such finger-like astroglial processes also contact node-like specializations of unmyelinated axons in the retinal nerve fiber layer and may originate from astrocytes (Hildebrand and Waxman, 1983) (Fig. 2.4*I*) and from Müller cells (Reichenbach et al., 1988). Such peripheral astroglial processes (PAPs) are poor in organelles (except actin filaments) but contain ezrin and radixin (Derouiche and Frotscher, 2001), two actin-binding proteins that link the cell membrane to the actin cytoskeleton and that may mediate the formation and stabilization of the very complex, thin side branches with their large surface-to-vol-

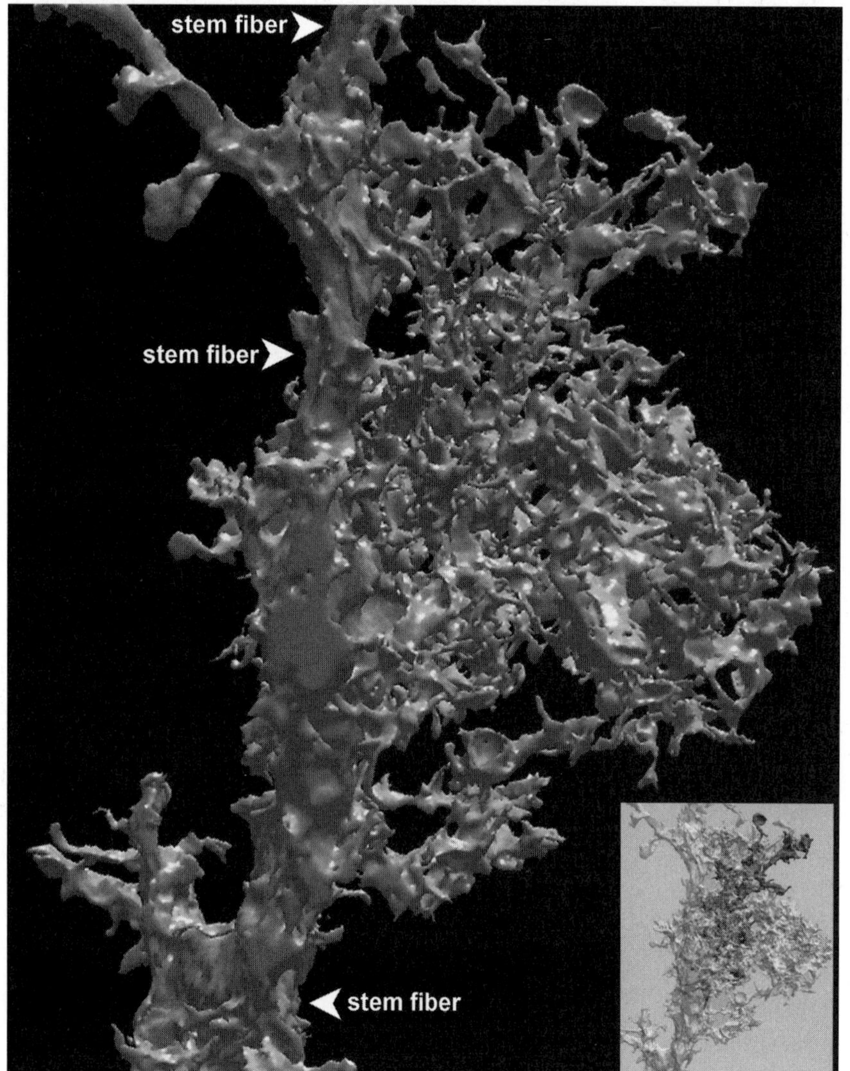

FIGURE 2.8. Three-dimensional reconstruction of part of a Bergmann glial cell process in the murine cerebellum. The living cell was dye-injected in a perfused cerebellar slice; then, after fixation and dye conversion, about 600 consecutive serial ultrathin sections were photographed in the electron microscope, and the images of the dye-labeled profiles were reconstructed by a computer program. The inset shows a substructure labeled in blue; this part was quantitatively analyzed (see Figure 2.9*B,C*). (Modified from Grosche et al., 1999.)

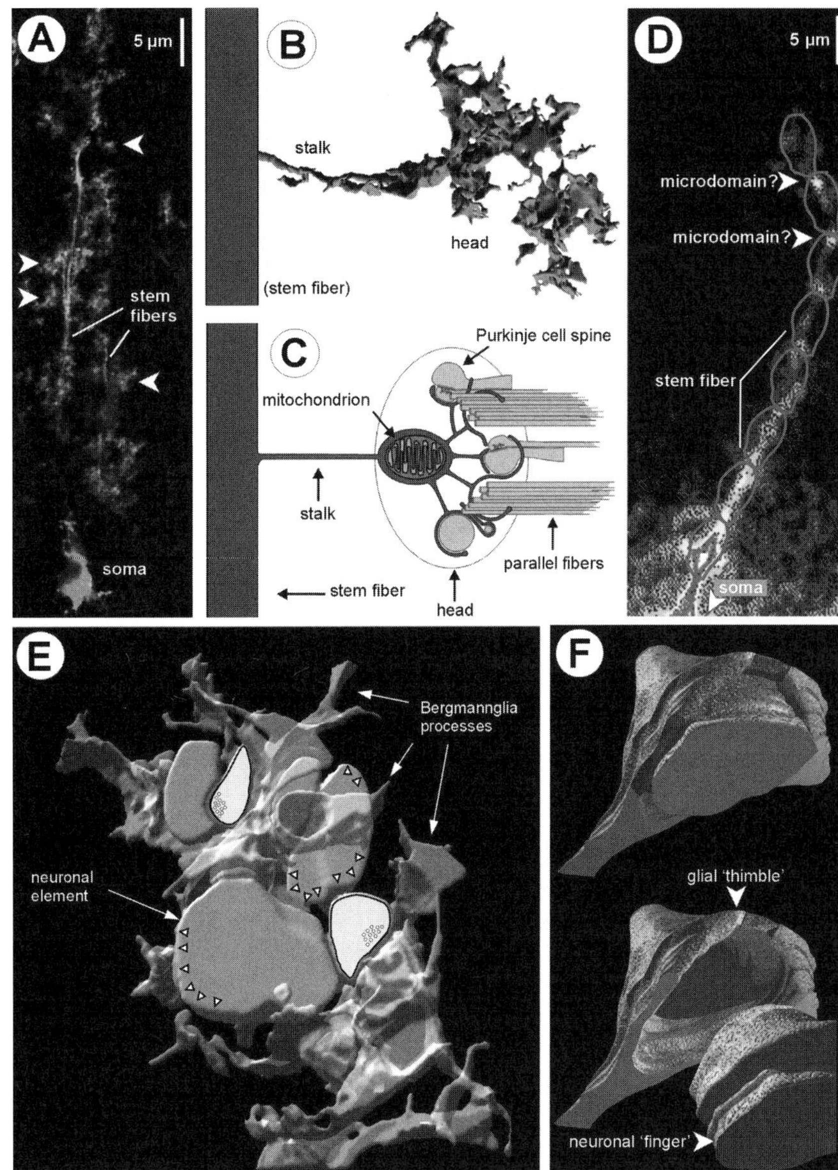

FIGURE 2.9. Microdomains of Bergmann glial cell processes in the murine cerebellum. *A*: Labeling of Bergmann glial cells in the murine cerebellum by green fluorescent protein (GFP) coupled to the glial fibrillary acidic protein (GFAP) promoter. Two typical cell processes are shown; they bear complex lateral appendages (*arrowheads*). Original confocal image. (courtesy of Gert Brückner, Leipzig, and Helmut Kettenmann, Berlin.) *B*. Glial microdomain as part of the three-dimensional reconstruction shown in Figure 2.8. *C*. Schematic drawing of such a glial microdomain and its relationships to the neuronal elements. *D*. Process of a murine Bergmann glial cell after injection of a Ca^{2+}-sensitive fluorescent dye and stimulation of the afferent parallel fibers. Ca^{2+} responses along the process are restricted to individual small compartments that may represent glial microdomains. *E*. Three-dimensional reconstruction of a group of neighboring cerebellar synapses together with the surrounding leaflets provided by the injected Bergmann glial cell. The arrowheads point to neuronal surfaces not covered by glial sheaths from the labeled cell. *F*. Three-dimensional reconstruction of a glial thimble and the neuronal "finger" covered by it; shown in apposition (*top*) and separated for better discrimination between the two compartments (*bottom*). [Modified from Grosche et al., 1999 (*B–D* and Grosche et al., 2002 (*E,F*).]

ume ratios (Figs. 2.8, 2.9). The ensheathing of neuronal elements by PAPs may vary considerably, even within the same area of the CNS (see Chao et al., 2002). There is an obvious tendency to ensheath the synapses; in rat neocortex, for example, about 56% of all synaptic perimeters are covered by astroglia, while astroglial membranes make up only 22% of all membranes in the neuropil (Landgrebe et al., cited in Chao et al., 2002). In particular, most (but not all: Ventura and Harris, 1999) synaptic clefts are "sealed" at their margins by glial lamellae (Figs. 2.9*E*, 2.10*G*). However, on synaptic glomeruli or *complex synapses*, glial coverage is very high (even multilamellar) but the glia does not penetrate the interior and, thus, cannot seal the individual synaptic clefts. As an extreme, there are astroglia-free neuropil compartments such as the *synaptic nests* in Rolando's substantia gelatinosa and in the cochlear nucleus.

In Bergmann glial cells, the existence of microdomains has been demonstrated (Grosche et al., 1999, 2002). These occur as *repetitive units* on the stem processes or as appendages of another microdomain. Each glial microdomain consists of a thin stalk and a cabbage-like, complex head structure that bears the lamellar perisynaptic sheaths for about five synapses (Fig. 2.9*B,C*). These microdomains may interact with "their" synapses, independent of each other and also of the stem process. Stimulation of the ensheathed synapses causes transient intracellular Ca^{2+} rises in individual microdomains (Grosche et al., 1999) (Fig. 2.9*D*). Furthermore, mathematical simulation reveals that even large depolarizations of the perisynaptic membranes are not conducted over the stalks toward neighboring microdomains or toward the stalk (Grosche et al., 2002). The energetic demands of the individual microdomain may be supported by its own mitochondria (Grosche et al., 1999, 2002). In every given volume unit of the molecular layer, at least two microdomains, originating from different Bergmann glial cells, interdigitate. This may fit with the observation that Purkinje cells express two functionally distinct, mutually independent populations of synaptic spines (Denk et al., 1995). In addition to the perisynaptic sheaths, the microdomains extend numerous *glial thimbles*, forming complete caps on small neuronal protrusions (Fig. 2.9*F*); the latter may represent dying or outgrowing synapses (see the following section).

ONTOGENESIS AND PHYSIOLOGICAL PLASTICITY

It is now clear that astroglial cell processes are by no means unchangeable, static structures. After the general shape and stem processes of an astroglial cell have been established in ontogenesis, the PAPs develop in (mutual) dependence on the developing neuronal cell processes and synapses (Waxman et al., 1983). The number and complexity of side branches then grow rapidly (Hanke and Reichenbach, 1987; Senitz et al., 1995; Grosche et al., 2002) and finally decline in the aged CNS (Senitz et al., 1995) (Fig. 2.10*A–C*).

The formation of PAPs may be triggered by the onset of neuronal activity, and their growing filopodia may be attracted (or repelled) by signals from active neurons. For such neuronal signals, K^+ ions (Reichelt et al., 1989) and neurotransmitters such as glutamate (Cornell-Bell et al., 1990; Ventura and Harris, 1999), γ-aminobutyric acid (GABA) (Matsutani and Yamamoto, 1997), and serotonin/noradrenaline (Paspalas and Papadopoulos, 1998) have been proposed as candidate molecules. Stimulation of protein kinase A induces the growth of short processes that extend flat, membranous sheaths from the glial growth cones (Althaus et al. 1990). The action of these mechanisms during ontogenesis may be modulated by the strength and/or pattern of neuronal activity, which, in turn, is triggered by sensory inputs and behavioral requirements. For instance, depending on whether rats are kept in an enriched (Sirevaag and Greenough, 1991)

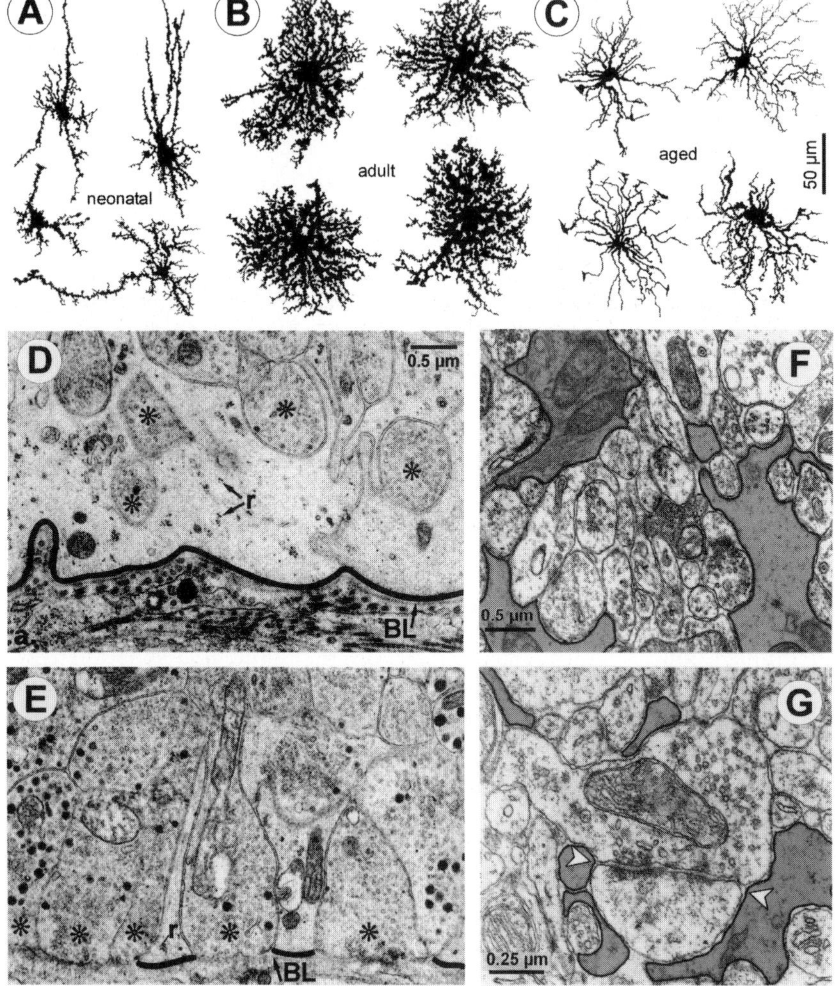

FIGURE 2.10 Development and plasticity of astroglial cell processes. *A–C*. Developmental changes of protoplasmic astrocytes in the human neocortex (area 11, layers III–V), Golgi impregnation. *A*. Four representative cells from neonatal brain; *B*. cells from normal adult brain (40 years old); *C*. cells from aged brain (72 years old). Whereas the number and complexitiy of the cell processes increase dramatically from birth to adulthood, in the aged brain the number and size of the side branches (but not of the stem processes) decrease. (Modified from Senitz et al., 1995.) *D,E*. The coverage of portal capillaries by glial endfeet is decreased when neurosecretion is induced by the activation of nicotinergic acetylcholine receptors. *D*. Under control conditions, much of the pericapillary basal lamina (*BL*) is covered by the endfeet of tanycytes, as identified by the presence of ribosomes (*r*) and the lack of neurosecretory vesicles in their cytoplasm; the endings of the neurosecretory axons (*asterisks*) do not contact the basal lamina. *E*. After stimulation, the glial coverage of the basal lamina is dramatically reduced (inked), and many vesicle-containing nerve endings establish direct access to the basal lamina. (Modified from Lichtensteiger et al., 1978.) *F,G*. After long-term potentiation (LTP), the perisynaptic astroglial coverage increases in dentate gyrus of adult rats. Whereas in the unstimulated neuropile many synapses are nearly devoid of astroglial contacts (*F*), 8 hours after LTP induction most of the synaptic clefts (*arrowheads*) and much of the pre- and postsynaptic elements are covered by glial sheaths (*G*). Glial profiles are labeled in grey. (Modified from Wenzel et al., 1991.)

or impoverished environment (Stewart et al., 1986), the complexity of their glial cell processes may differ significantly. Similar mechanisms seem to be maintained in the mature CNS, where they may modify the structure of glial cells even in the short term. In fact, morphological variations among perisynaptic glia at a fixed time point may largely reflect the plasticity of individual glial processes in response to the recent history of adjacent synaptic activity (Xu-Friedmann et al., 2001).

Hormonal or osmotic stimulation of neurons in the tubero-hypophyseal system evokes changes in the covering of blood vessels by tanycytic endfeet (Wittkowski, 1973; Lichtensteiger et al., 1978) (Fig. 2.10*D,E*) the ultrastructure of which changes with the physiological state (Rodríguez et al., 1979). These changes modify the neuro-humoral secretion (see Hatton, 1997). The structure of hypothalamic tanycytes differs between males and females, and the apical protrusions of tanycytes in females change their size and number with the oestrous cycle (Knowles and Anand-Kumar, 1969). Likewise, astrocytes may respond within less than one hour (Rohlmann et al., 1994) to changes of the activity of the ensheathed neuronal elements. The structure of PAPs may change due to long-term potentiation (Wenzel et al., 1991) (Fig. 2.10*F,G*), kindling (Hawrylak et al., 1998), stimulation of afferents (Güldner and Wolff, 1977), and altered estrogen levels (Klintsova et al., 1995). Such changes may involve not only an outgrowth of filopodia and lamellae but also retraction, autophagy, and lysosomal degradation of glial membranes (Landgrebe et al., cited in Chao et al., 2002). It is noteworthy that even minute changes in the size and/or shape of perisynaptic glial sheaths may cause dramatic changes of the efficacy of a given synapse (Oliet et al., 2001), as (*1*) changes in the extracellular volume modify the effective concentration and/or availability of neurotransmitters and (*2*) changes in the distance between the synaptic cleft and the perisynaptic glial membrane (and of the exposed surface area of the latter) modify the number of accessible glial uptake carriers, that is, the uptake rate and the effective concentration of transmitter molecules. The effective concentration of glial cell–derived neuroactive substances may be controlled by the same mechanisms. Similar morphological changes may modify the glial uptake/redistribution of neuronally released K^+ ions, modulating the extracellular K^+ concentration and, thereby, the neuronal excitability (cf. Chapters 26–28). Furthermore, the connexin-43-mediated gap junctional coupling among astrocytes is also rapidly modified by changes in neuronal activity (Rohlmann et al., 1994; Rouach et al., 2001). This changes the efficacy not only of individual synapses but also of large functional compartments of the neuropile (cf. Chapter 13).

In the normal adult rat cortex at any time, about 1% of all synapses are in the process of regression and remodeling (Wolff et al., 1995). Thus, *synaptic stripping* and phagocytosis of regressive synapses seem to be important functions of PAPs not only during ontogenesis (Missler et al., 1993) but also in adulthood (Wolff et al., 1995), which may be reflected by astrocytic profiles surrounding *empty presynaptic elements* and vacated postsynaptic densities (Adams and Jones, 1982) and by the glial thimbles (Grosche et al., 2002) (Fig. 2.9*F*). Furthermore, astroglia can not only remove "obsolete" synapses but also can contribute to the formation and maintenance of new synapses (Pfrieger and Barres, 1996), for instance, by providing cholesterol for neuronal lipoprotein synthesis (Mauch et al., 2001).

We want to leave the reader with the view that much of the morphological diversity of astrocytes and ependymoglial cells (Fig. 2.1) results from the different local microenvironments of a cell. Mesenchymal contact will induce the formation of endfeet with OAP-rich membranes, whereas contact with the cerebrospinal fluid will induce the outgrowth of microvilli and the formation of stabilizing cell-cell junctions. Where neuronal elements are contacted, the glial cells form delicate side branches that end in lamellar sheaths or finger-like branchlets. The number, size, and shape of these PAPs or microdomains are precisely adjusted to the requirements of the adjacent neuronal elements. This adjustment continues after ontogeny as a lifelong process of plasticity.

ACKNOWLEDGMENTS

The authors are greatly indepted to Bernd Biedermann, Gert Brückner, Ivona Goczalik, Heidrun Kuhrt, Jan Jandiev, Jens Grosche, Mike Francke, and Ortrud Uckermann for providing unpublished original microphotographs and/or help in compiling the Figures. Many thanks are due to T. Ivo Chao, Jorge A. Colombo, Menachim Hanani, and Joachim R. Wolff for intriguing discussions.

REFERENCES

Adams, J. and Jones, D.G. (1982) Synaptic remodelling and astrocytic hypertrophy in rat cerebral cortex from early to late adulthood. *Neurobiol. Aging* 3:179–186.

Althaus, H.H., Schwartz, P., Klüppner, S., Schröter, J., and Neuhoff, V. (1990) Protein kinases A and C are involved in oligodendroglial process formation. In: Jeserich, G., Althaus, H.H., and Waehneldt, T.V., eds. *Cellular and Molecular Biology of Myelination*. NATO ASI Series. Berlin: Springer-Verlag, pp. 247–253.

Anderson, D.H., Stern, W.H., Fisher, S.K., Erickson, P.A., and Borgula, G.A. (1983) Retinal detachment in the cat: the pigment epithelial-photoreceptor interface. *Invest. Ophthalmol. Vis. Sci.* 24:906–926.

Braak, E. (1975) On the fine structure of the external glial layer in the isocortex of man. *Cell Tissue Res* 157:367–390.

Bushong, E.A., Martone, M.E., Jones, Y.Z., and Ellisman, M.H. (2002) Protoplasmic astrocytes in CA1 stratum radiatum occupy separate anatomical domains. *J. Neurosci.* 22:183–192.

Butt, A.M., Colquhoun, K., Tutton, M., and Berry, M. (1994a)

Three-dimensional morphology of astrocytes and oligodendrocytes in the intact mouse optic nerve. *J. Neurocytol.* 23:469–485.

Butt, A.M., Duncan, A., and Berry, M. (1994b) Astrocyte associations with nodes of Ranvier: ultrastructural analysis of HRP-filled astrocytes in the mouse optic nerve. *J. Neurocytol.* 23:486–499.

Chan-Palay, V. and Palay, S.L. (1972) The form of velate astrocytes in the cerebellar cortex of monkey and rat: high-voltage electron microscopy of rapid-Golgi preparations. *Z. Anat. Entw.-Gesch.* 138:1–19.

Chao, T.I., Rickmann, M., and Wolff, J.R. (2002) The synapse-astrocyte boundary: anatomical basis for an integrative role of glia in synaptic transmission. In: Volterra, A., Magistretti, P., and Haydon, P., eds. *Tripartite Synapses: Synaptic Transmission with Glia.* Oxford · New York: Oxford University Press, pp. 3–23.

Colombo, J.A. (2001) A columnar-supporting mode of astroglial architecture in the cerebral cortex of adult primates? *Neurobiology* 9:1–16.

Colombo, J.A., Yáñez, A., Puissant, V., and Lipina, S. (1995) Long, interlaminar astroglial cell processes in the cortex of adult monkeys. *J. Neurosci. Res.* 40:551–556.

Cornell-Bell, A., Thomas, P.G., and Smith, S.J. (1990) The excitatory neurotransmitter glutamate causes filopodia formation in cultured hippocampal astrocytes. *Glia* 3:322–334.

Crawford, B.J. (1983) Some factors controlling cell polarity in chick retinal pigment epithelial cells in clonal culture. *Tissue Cell* 15:993–1005.

Dalloz, C., Sarig, R., Fort, P., Yaffe, D., Bordais, A., Pannicke, T., Grosche, J., Mornet, D., Reichenbach, A., Sahel, J., Nudel, U., and Rendon, A. (2003) Targeted inactivation of dystrophin gene product Dp71: phenotypic impact in mouse retina. *Human Molec. Genet.* 12:1543–1554.

Denk, W., Sugimori, M., and Llinas, R. (1995) Two types of calcium response limited to single spines in cerebellar Purkinje cells. *Proc. Natl. Acad. Sci. USA* 92:8279–8282.

Derouiche, A. and Frotscher, M. (2001) Peripheral astrocyte processes: monitoring by selective immunostaining for the actin-binding ERM proteins. *Glia* 36:330–341.

Distler, C., Dreher, Z., and Stone, J. (1991) Contact spacing among astrocytes in the central nervous system: an hypothesis of their structural role. *Glia* 4:484–494.

Foos, R.Y. and Gloor, B.P. (1975) Vitroretinal juncture: healing of experimental wounds. *Albrecht Graefes Arch. Klin. Exp. Ophthalmol.* 196:213–230.

Grosche, J., Kettenmann, H., and Reichenbach, A. (2002) Bergmann glial cells form distinct morphological structures to interact with cerebellar neurons. *J. Neurosci. Res.* 68:138–149.

Grosche, J., Matyash, V., Möller, T., Verkhratsky, A., Reichenbach, A., and Kettenmann, H. (1999) Microdomains for neuron-glia interaction: parallel fiber signaling to Bergmann glial cells. *Nature Neurosci.* 2:139–143.

Güldner, F.H. and Wolff, J.R. (1977) Perisynaptic reactions of astroglia in the visual cortex after optic nerve stimulation. In: Creutzfeldt, O., ed. *Afferent and Intrinsic Organization of Laminated Structures in the Brain.* Berlin: Springer-Verlag, pp. 343–347.

Halfter, W. (1998) Disruption of the retinal basal lamina during early embryonic development leads to retraction of vitreal endfeet, an increased number of ganglion cells, and aberrant axonal growth. *J. Comp. Neurol.* 397:89–104.

Hanke, S. and Reichenbach, A. (1987) Quantitative-morphometric aspects of Bergmann glial (Golgi epithelial) cell development in rats. A Golgi study. *Anat. Embryol.* 177:183–188.

Hatton, G.I. (1997) Function-related plasticity in hypothalamus. *Annu. Rev. Neurosci.* 20:375–397.

Hawrylak, N., Fleming, J.C., and Salm, A.K. (1998) Dehydration and rehydration selectively and reversibly alter glial fibrillary acidic protein immunoreactivity in the rat supraoptic nucleus and subjacent glia limitans. *Glia* 22:260–271.

Hildebrand, C. and Waxman, S.G. (1983) Regional node-like specializations in non-myelinated axons of rat retinal nerve fiber layer. *Brain Res.* 58:23–32.

Hortega, P. Del Rio. (1956) Variedas morfológicas de oligodendrocitos. *Arch. Histol. (B. Aires)* 6:239–291.

Ishii, M., Horio, Y., Tada, Y., Hibino, H., Inanobe, A., Ito, M., Yamada, M., Gotow, T., Uchiyama, Y., and Kurachi, Y. (1997) Expression and clustered distribution of an inwardly rectifying potassium channel, K_{AB}-2/Kir4.1, on mammalian retinal Müller cell membrane: their regulation by insulin and laminin signals. *J. Neurosci.* 17:7725–7735.

Ke, C., Poon, W.S., Ng, H.K., Pang, J.C., and Chan, Y. (2001) Heterogeneous responses of aquaporin-4 in oedema formation in a replicated severe traumatic brain injury model in rats. *Neurosci. Lett.* 301:21–24.

Klintsova, A., Levy, W.B., and Desmond, N.L. (1995) Astrocytic volume fluctuates in the hippocampal CA1 region across the estrous cycle. *Brain Res.* 690:269–274.

Knowles, F. and Anand Kumar, T.C. (1969) Structural changes, related to reproduction, in the hypothalamus and in the pars tuberalis of the rhesus monkey. *Phil. Trans. R. Soc. Lond. (Biol.) B* 256:357–375.

Kosaka, T. and Hama, K. (1986) Three-dimensional structure of astrocytes in the rat dentate gyrus. *J. Comp. Neurol.* 249:242–260.

Leonhardt, H. (1980) Ependym und circumventriculäre Organe. In: Oksche, A. (ed.). *Neuroglia I.* Volume 4, part 10 of *Handbuch der mikroskopischen Anatomie des Menschen.* Oksche, A. and Vollrath, L. (series eds.). Berlin, Heidelberg, New York: Springer, pp. 177–666.

Lichtensteiger, W., Richards, J.G., and Kopp, H.G. (1978) Changes in the distribution of non-neuronal elements in rat median eminence and in anterior pituitary hormone secretion after activation of tuberoinfundibular dopamine neurones by brain stimulation or nicotine. *Brain Res.* 157:73–88.

Matsutani, S. and Yamamoto, N. (1997) Neuronal regulation of astrocyte morphology in vitro is mediated by GABAergic signalling. *Glia* 20:1–9.

Mauch, D. H., Nägler, K., Schumacher, S., Göritz, C., Müller, E.-C., Otto, A., and Pfrieger, F.W. (2001) CNS synaptogenesis promoted by glia-derived cholesterol. *Science* 294:1354–1357.

Miller, R. H. and Liuzzi, F. (1986) Regional specialization of the radial glial cells of the adult frog spinal cord. *J. Neurocytol.* 15:187–196.

Missler, M., Wolff, A., Merker, H.-J., and Wolff, J.R. (1993) Pre- and postnatal development of the primary visual cortex of the common marmoset. II. Formation, remodelling, and elimination of synapses as overlapping processes. *J. Comp. Neurol.* 333:53–67.

Nagelhus, E.A., Horio, Y., Inanobe, A., Fujita, A., Haug, F.M., Nielsen, S., Kurachi, Y., and Ottersen, O.P. (1999) Immunogold evidence suggests that coupling of K^+ siphoning and water transport in rat retinal Müller cells is mediated by a coenrichment of Kir4.1 and AQP4 in specific membrane domains. *Glia* 26:47–54.

Oliet, S.H., Piet, R., and Poulain, D.A. (2001) Control of glutamate clearance and synaptic efficacy by glial coverage of neurons. *Science* 292:923–926.

Palay, S.L. and Chan-Palay, V. (1974) *Cerebellar Cortex, Cytology and Organization.* Stuttgart and New York: Springer-Verlag, pp. 288–311.

Paspalas, C.D. and Papadopoulos, G.C. (1998) Ultrastructural evidence for combined action of noradrenaline and vasoactive intestinal polypeptide upon neurons, astrocytes, and blood vessels of the rat cerebral cortex. *Brain Res. Bull.* 45:247–259.

Pfrieger, F.W. and Barres, B.A. (1996) New views on synapse-glia interactions. *Curr. Opin. Neurobiol* 6:615–621.

Pouwels, E. (1978) On the development of the cerebellum of the trout, *Salmo gairdneri. Anat. Embryol.* 3:67–83.

Ramón y Cajal, S. (1911) *Histologie du systéme nerveux de l'homme et des vertébrés*. Paris: Maloine.

Rascher-Eggstein, G., Liebner, S., and Wolburg, H. (2004) The blood–brain barrier in the human glioma. In: Sharma, H.S. and Westman, J., eds. *Blood–Spinal Cord and Brain Barriers in Health and Disease*. San Diego: Elsevier Science/Academic Press, pp. 567–576.

Reichelt, W., Dettmer, D., Brückner, G., Brust, P., Eberhardt, W., and Reichenbach, A. (1989) Potassium as a signal for both proliferation and differentiation of rabbit retinal (Müller) glia growing in cell culture. *Cell Signalling* 1:187–194.

Reichenbach, A. (1989a) Attempt to classify glial cells by means of their process specialization using the rabbit retinal Müller cell as an example of cytotopographic specialization of glial cells. *Glia* 2:250–259.

Reichenbach, A. (1989b) Glia:neuron index: review and hypothesis to account for different values in various mammals. *Glia* 2:71–77.

Reichenbach, A. (1999) *Neuroglia—das andere zelluläre Element im Nervensystem: Die Müllersche Gliazelle*. Wessobrunn: Socio Medico Verlag, pp. 1–216.

Reichenbach, A. and Robinson, S.R. (1995a) Ependymoglia and ependymoglia-like cells. In: Ransom, B.R. and Kettenmann, H., eds. *Neuroglial Cells*. Oxford: Oxford University Press, pp. 58–84.

Reichenbach, A. and Robinson, S.R. (1995b) Phylogenetic constraints on retinal organization and development: an Haeckelian perspective. *Prog. Retinal Res.* 15:139–171.

Reichenbach, A., Schippel, K., Schümann, R., and Hagen, E. (1988) Ultrastructure of rabbit nerve fibre layer—neuro-glial relationships, myelination, and nerve fiber spectrum. *J. Hirnforsch.* 29: 481–491.

Reichenbach, A., Siegel, A., Rickmann, M., Wolff, J.R., Noone, D., and Robinson, S.R. (1995) Distribution of Bergmann glial somata and processes: implications for function. *J. Brain. Res.* 36:509–517.

Rodríguez, E.M., Gonzalez, C.B., and Delannoy, L. (1979) Cellular organization of the lateral and postinfundibular regions of the median eminence in the rat. *Cell Tissue Res.* 201:377–408.

Rohlmann, A., Laskawi, R., Hofer, A., Dermietzel, R., and Wolff, J.R. (1994) Astrocytes as rapid sensors of peripheral axotomy in the facial nucleus of rats. *NeuroReport* 5:409–412.

Rouach, N., Glowinski, J., and Giaume, C. (2001) Activity-dependent neuronal control of gap-junctional communication in astrocytes. *J. Cell Biol.* 149:1513–1526.

Sarthy, V. and Ripps, H. (2001) *The Retinal Müller Cell. Structure and Function*. New York: Kluwer Academic/Plenum, pp. 1–278.

Schnitzer, J. (1988) Astrocytes in mammalian retina. *Progr. Retinal Res.* 7:209–231.

Senitz, D., Reichenbach, A., and Smith, T.G., Jr. (1995) Surface complexity of human neocortical astrocytic cells: changes with development, aging, and dementia. *J. Brain. Res.* 36:531–537.

Siegel, A., Reichenbach, A., Hanke, S., Senitz, D., Brauer, K., and Smith, T.G., Jr. (1991) Comparative morphometry of Bergmann glial (Golgi epithelial) cells. A Golgi study. *Anat. Embryol.* 183: 605–612.

Sirevaag, A.M. and Greenough, W.T. (1991) Plasticity of GFAP-immunoreactive astrocyte size and number in visual cortex of rats reared in complex environments. *Brain Res.* 540:273–278.

Stensaas, L.J. and Stensaas, S.S. (1968) Light microscopy of glial cells in turtles and birds. *Z. Zellforsch.* 91:315–340.

Stewart, M.G., Bourne, R.C., and Gabbott, P.L.A. (1986) Decreased levels of an astrocytic marker, glial fibrillary acidic protein, in the visual cortex of dark-reared rats: measurement by enzyme-linked immunosorbent assay. *Neurosci. Lett.* 63:147–152.

Stolzenburg, J.-U., Reichenbach, A., and Neumann, M. (1989) Size and density of glial and neuronal cells within the cerebral neocortex of various insectivorian species. *Glia* 2:78–84.

Sturrock, R.R., Smart, J.L., and Dobbing, J. (1977) Effect of undernutrition during the suckling period on the indisium griseum and rostrat part of the mouse anterior commissure. *Neuropathol. Appl. Neurobiol.* 3:369–375.

Valverde, F. and Lopez-Mascaraque, L. (1991) Neuroglial elements in the olfactory glomeruli of the hedgehog. *J. Comp. Neurol.* 307:658–674.

Venero, J.L., Vizuete, M.L., Machado, A., and Cano, J. (2001) Aquaporins in the central nervous system. *Prog. Neurobiol.* 63:321–336.

Ventura, R. and Harris, K.M. (1999) Three-dimensional relationships between hippocampal synapses and astrocytes. *J. Neurosci.* 19:6897–6906.

Warth, A. Kröger, S., and Wolburg, H. (2004) Redistribution of aquaporin-4 in human glioblastoma correlates with loss of agrin immunoreactivity from brain capillary basal laminae. *Acta Neuropathol.* 107:311–318.

Waxman, S.G. (1986) The astrocyte as a component of the node of Ranvier. *Trends Neurosci.* 9:250–253.

Waxman, S.G., Black, J.A., and Foster, R.E. (1983) Ontogenesis of the axolemma and axoglial relationships in myelinated fibers: electrophysiological and freeze-fracture correlates of membrane plasticity. *Int. Rev. Neurobiol.* 24:433–484.

Wenzel, J., Lammert, G., Meyer, U., and Krug, M. (1991) The influence of long-term potentiation on the spatial relationship between astrocyte processes and potentiated synapses in the dentate gyrus neuropil of rat brain. *Brain Res.* 560:122–131.

Wittkowski, W. (1973) Elektronenmikroskopische Untersuchungen zur funktionellen Morphologie des tubero-hypophysären Systems der Ratte. *Z. Zellforsch.* 139:101–148.

Wolburg, H. (1995) Orthogonal arrays of intramembranous particles. A review with special reference to astrocytes. *J. Brain Res.* 36:239–258.

Wolburg, H. and Lippoldt, A. (2002) Tight junctions of the blood–brain barrier: development, composition and regulation. *Vasc. Pharmacol.* 38:323–337.

Wolburg, H., Reichelt, W., Stolzenburg, J.-U., Richter, W., and Reichenbach, A. (1990) Rabbit retinal Müller cells in cell culture show gap and tight junctions which they do not express *in situ*. *Neurosci Lett.* 11:58–63.

Wolff, J. (1968) The role of astroglia in the brain tissue. In: Erbslöh, F. ed. Symposium on Neuroglia. Berlin: Springer-Verlag, *Acta Neuropathol., Suppl.* IV:33–39.

Wolff, J.R., Laskawi, R., Spatz, W.B., and Missler, M. (1995) Structural dynamics of synapses and synaptic components. *Behav. Brain Res.* 66:13–20.

Xu-Friedmann, M.A., Harris, K.M., and Regehr, W.G. (2001) Three-dimensional comparison of ultrastructural characteristics at depressing and facilitating synapses onto Purkinje cells. *J. Neurosci.* 21:6666–6672.

3 Structure and function of oligodendrocytes

ARTHUR M. BUTT

Oligodendrocytes are defined as the cells that produce the myelin sheaths that insulate central nervous system (CNS) axons. Rio-Hortega (1928) is credited with first identifying oligodendrocytes as process-bearing cells by metal impregnation and subdividing them into types I to IV, characterized by the number of their processes and the size of the fibres they contacted. He exhibited great insight when he suggested that oligodendrocytes make up the myelin sheath, but it was not until the advent of electron microscopy (EM) that the cellular connection between oligodendrocytes and myelin sheaths was finally demonstrated (Peters, 1964; Bunge, 1968; Hirano, 1968). Intracellular dye injection confirmed the conceptual picture developed from EM studies of an oligodendrocyte unit comprising the cell body and up to 30 radial processes that each terminate on and ensheath an axon to form one internodal myelin segment of variable thickness and length (Butt and Ransom, 1989). These morphological techniques have been superseded by immunohistochemical labelling of proteins that are characteristic of, or specific to, oligodendrocytes or myelin (Sternberger et al., 1978; Friedman et al., 1989).

This chapter deals with the morphology of oligodendrocytes, and is indebted to the chapter by Szuchet (1995) in the first edition of this book and to other authoritative book chapters and reviews that describe the topic more comprehensively (e.g. Bunge, 1968; Peters et al., 1991; Hildebrand et al., 1993). Modern studies show that oligodendrocyte polymorphism determines the function of axons within the unit, and that the growth of axons is inextricably linked to that of the myelin sheath. In addition to myelin-forming oligodendrocytes in CNS white matter, there are also many nonmyelinating *satellite oligodendrocytes* and *adult oligodendrocyte progenitors* (OPCs) in the adult CNS (Ludwin, 1979; Dawson et al., 2000). We know about the anatomy and ultrastructure of these cells, but their functions remain elusive. Key issues are how environmental, axonal, and genetic factors control the differentiation of oligodendrocyte phenotypes and how oligodendrocytes and myelin, in turn, determine axonal growth and integrity, as well as axolemmal specialization at nodes of Ranvier. This chapter will address these issues and integrate historical findings with modern concepts of the functions of oligodendrocytes. The chapter is divided into four main sections. The first reviews current findings on the morphology of oligodendrocytes and discusses them in the context of the classical work by Rio-Hortega. The second examines the functional significance of oligodendrocyte polymorphism, and the third deals with the environmental and axonal factors that are likely to control the differentiation of oligodendrocyte phenotypes. In the fourth section, recent findings on the functions of adult OPC are assessed.

See the list of abbreviations at the end of the chapter.

FROM RIO HORTEGA TO THE PRESENT DAY

Rio Hortega's Oligodendrocyte Phenotypes I to IV

Rio Hortega classified oligodendrocytes into types I–IV (Fig. 3.1) based on the characteristics of the number and orientation of their cellular processes, the shape and size of their somata, the size of the axons they were associated with, and their distributions within the CNS (Rio-Hortega, 1928; Penfield, 1932). Stensaas and Stensaas (1968) applied the same metal impregnation techniques to the toad spinal cord. They observed a range of morphologies between types I and II and between types III and IV, but there was less evidence of transitional forms between types I and II, on the one hand, and types III and IV, on the other, suggesting that there may not be a morphological continuum between types I and IV. This thesis has been amply confirmed by immunohistochemistry using the mouse monoclonal antibody Rip, which has the almost unique property of labeling entire units (Friedman et al., 1989; Berry et al., 1995; Butt et al., 1998). Type IV oligodendrocytes have also been identified in the chick spinal cord, where they are abundant, using the T4-O antibody (Anderson et al., 1999). Type I and II oligodendrocytes are indistinguishable and have four or more fine primary processes that branch repeatedly to myelinate 10–30 axons less than 2 μm in diameter (Fig. 3.1*A,B*). Type I oligodendrocytes can be found in the forebrain, cerebellum, and spinal cord, whereas type II oligodendrocytes are observed only in white matter. Type III oligodendrocytes have large cell bodies, often applied directly to an axon, with one or more thick primary processes that rarely branch and myelinate a small number of axons, usually less than five, with external sheath diameters ranging from 4 to 15 μm (Fig. 3.1*C,D*). Type III oligodendrocytes are localized in the cerebral and cerebellar peduncles, the medulla oblongata, and the spinal cord. Type IV units are similar to type III units but do not have processes and form a single long myelin sheath over a large-diameter fiber; they are restricted to tracts containing the largest diameter fibers and occur near the entrance of nerve roots into the CNS. The rarity of type IV oligodendrocytes in rodent brain may be related to the modest size of the largest diameter fibers compared to the chicken and larger mammals (Anderson et al., 1999). The myelin sheaths of type III and IV oligodendrocytes have a network of cytoplasmic interconnections or reticulations (Stensaas and Stensaas, 1968; Berry et al., 1995; Butt et al., 1998; Anderson et al., 1999), which are likely to correspond to the Schmidt-Lantermann incisures demonstrated at the EM level in fibers greater than 2 μm in diameter (Hildebrand et al., 1993).

Ultrastructure of Oligodendrocytes

Three-dimensional reconstructions of sequential electron micrographs of developing feline and rat spinal

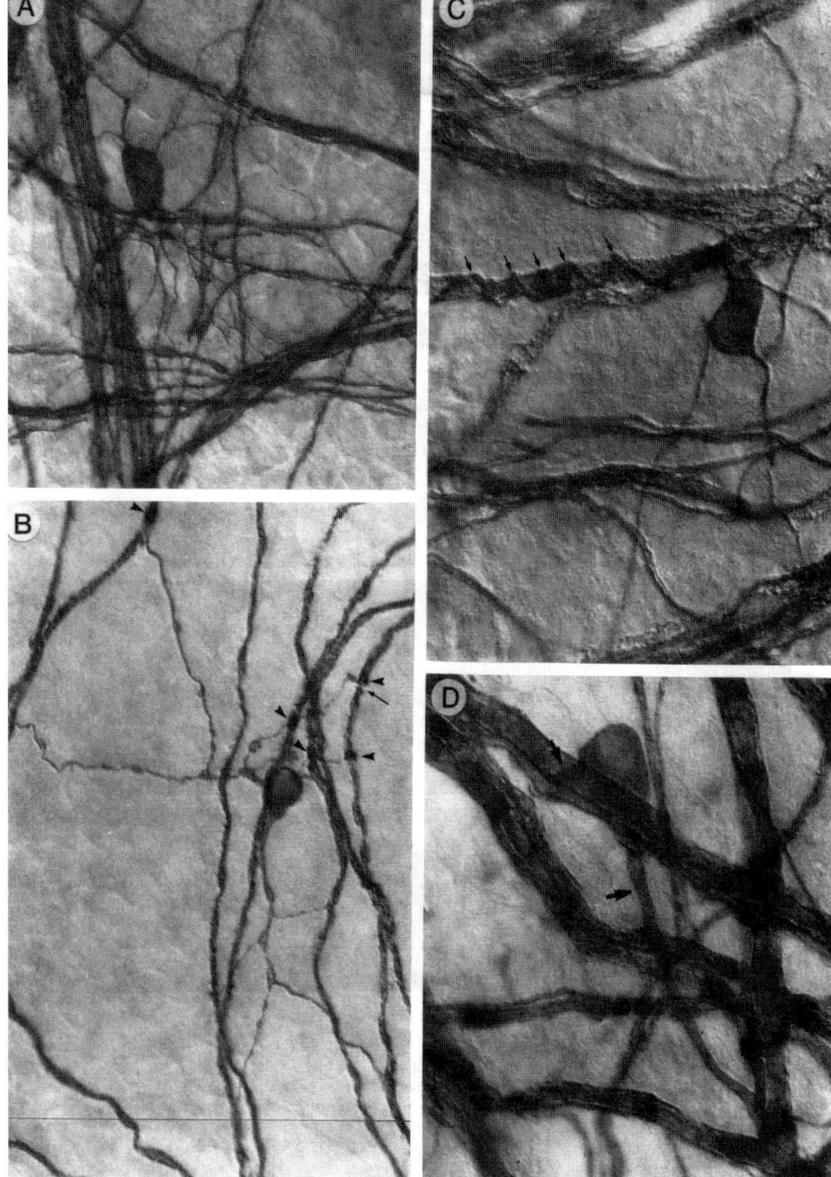

FIGURE 3.1 Immunolabeling of oligodendrocyte phenotypes with the Rip antibody in whole mounts of adult rat anterior medullary velum. *A,B*. Multipolar oligodendrocytes supporting numerous myelin sheaths for small-diameter axons. These correspond to Rio-Hortega's type I (*A*) and type II (*B*), which respectively have multiple branching processes supporting numerous radially oriented myelin sheaths, and less intricate processes supporting parallel myelin sheaths, but which are otherwise indistinguishable. *C,D*. Large type III oligodendrocytes with a small number of stout processes (*arrows* in *D*) that engage large-diameter axons. Both oligodendrocytes have a cell body directly applied to a large-diameter axon, a phenotypic characteristics of type IV oligodendrocytes. The oligodendrocyte in *C* also extends fine processes to numerous smaller-diameter axons, a feature of type I/II oligodendrocytes, whereas that in *D* has a single stout process extending to a large-diameter axon more characteristic of type III units. Arrowheads in *B* show Rip staining at points of engagement of oligodendrocyte processes with internodal myelin sheaths. This cell appears to extend processes to consecutive internodal myelin segments (*arrowheads*) on either side of a node (*arrow*). Spiraling of the outer cytoplasmic tongue process is clear in larger myelin sheaths (*arrows* in C). The number of axons engaged by each unit is inversely proportional to sheath diameter, but diameters vary within individual units (C). Magnification in A–D, ×1200. (From Berry et al., 1995, with permission.)

cord and corpus callosum by Hildebrand and colleagues (Remahl and Hildebrand, 1990a; Bjartmar et al., 1994) have identified two types of cell morphologies corresponding to Rio Hortega's types I/II (Fig. 3.2*A*,*B*) and III/IV (Fig. 3.2*C*,*D*). This was the first EM demonstration of the Schwann cell–like type IV oligodendrocyte (Remahl and Hildebrand, 1990a), and showed that the distribution of oligodendrocyte phenotypes is related to both fiber size and the developmental onset of myelination. Otherwise, no outstanding differences in the ultrastructure of oligodendrocytes from different areas of the CNS have been noted (Remahl and Hildebrand, 1990a; Peters et al., 1991; Bjartmar et al., 1994). In electron micrographs, oligodendrocyte cell bodies have a relatively small profile, with round nuclei and dense chromatin. The cytoplasm is usually scanty and opaque, rich in granular endoplasmic reticulum, ribosomes, and mitochondria. Mori and Leblond (1970) did describe three classes of oligodendrocyte in the corpus callosum of young rats on the basis of their fine structural appearances, namely, light, medium, and dark oligodendrocytes. Light oligodendrocytes are large cells with a pale nucleus that show rapid mitotic activity. Medium-shade oligodendrocytes, in comparison with the light cells, are smaller, with a more dense nucleus, and have reduced mitotic activity. Dark oligodendrocytes are the smallest cells with the most dense nucleus and are mitotically inactive. This classification reflects a maturation sequence of oligodendrocytes in which light cells represent the most immature form that develops into dark cells through an intermediate medium-shade type. These variants do not correspond to Rio Hortega's subtypes, and the cellular ultrastructural features of type I/II and type III/IV oligodendrocytes are not notably different (Remahl and Hildebrand, 1990a; Peters et al., 1991; Bjartmar et al., 1994).

Intracellular Injection of Dyes

Intracellular dye injection enables direct assessment of the number of axons myelinated by individual oligodendrocyte units and the length and diameter of the internodal myelin sheaths (Butt and Ransom, 1989, 1993; Ransom et al., 1991). Rat optic nerve type II oligodendrocytes have 5 to 30 parallel processes (Fig. 3.3*A*,*B*), which are the dye-filled internal and external tongue processes of the myelin sheath and are connected to the cell somata by a number of fine processes 15 to 30 μm in length (Butt and Ransom, 1989; Ransom et al., 1991). Type II oligodendrocytes have external sheath diameters in the range 0.2 to 4 μm, and internodal distances of individual myelin sheaths vary between 50 and 350 μm (Butt et al., 1994; Berry et al., 1995). Type III oligodendrocytes have been distinguished by intracellular dye injection in the adult rat anterior medullary velum (Berry et al., 1995). Figures

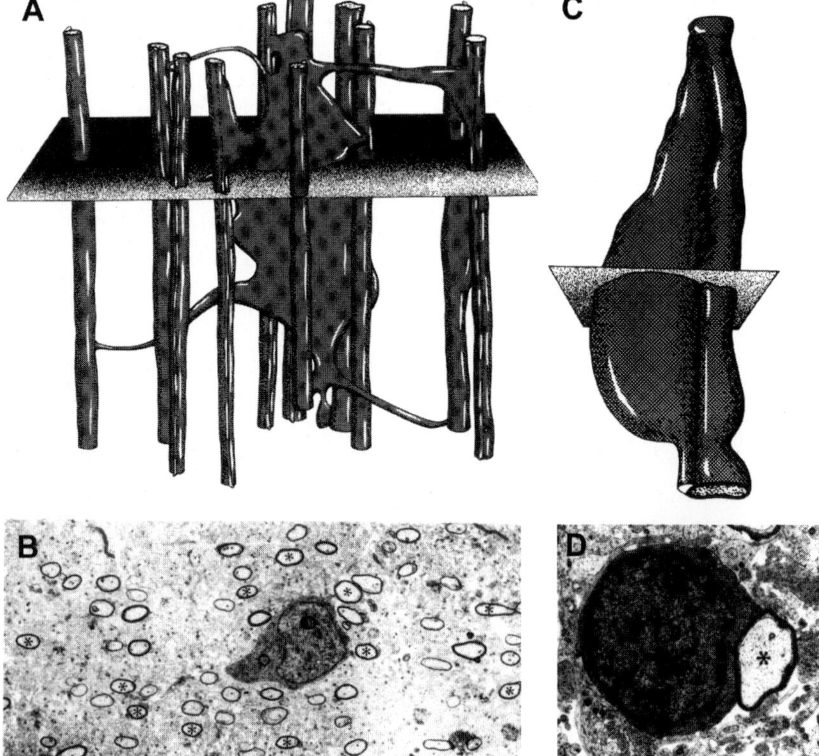

FIGURE 3.2 Electron micrographic reconstructions of oligodendrocytes from feline central nervous system. *A*,*B*. Type II oligodendrocyte from feline corpus callosum 21 days postnatally. The oligodendrocyte myelinates 11 nearby axons (*A*), indicated by asterisks in the electron micrograph (*B*), which corresponds to the plane marked in *A*. *C*,*D*. Type IV oligodendrocyte from feline spinal cord of a 47-day-old fetus. The oligodendrocyte is attached to a single axon that it myelinates (*C*), indicated by the asterisk in the electron micrograph (*D*). There are no ultrastructural distinguishing features between cell bodies and nuclei of type II and IV units (indicated by O in *B* and *D*). (From Remahl and Hildebrand, 1990a, with permission.)

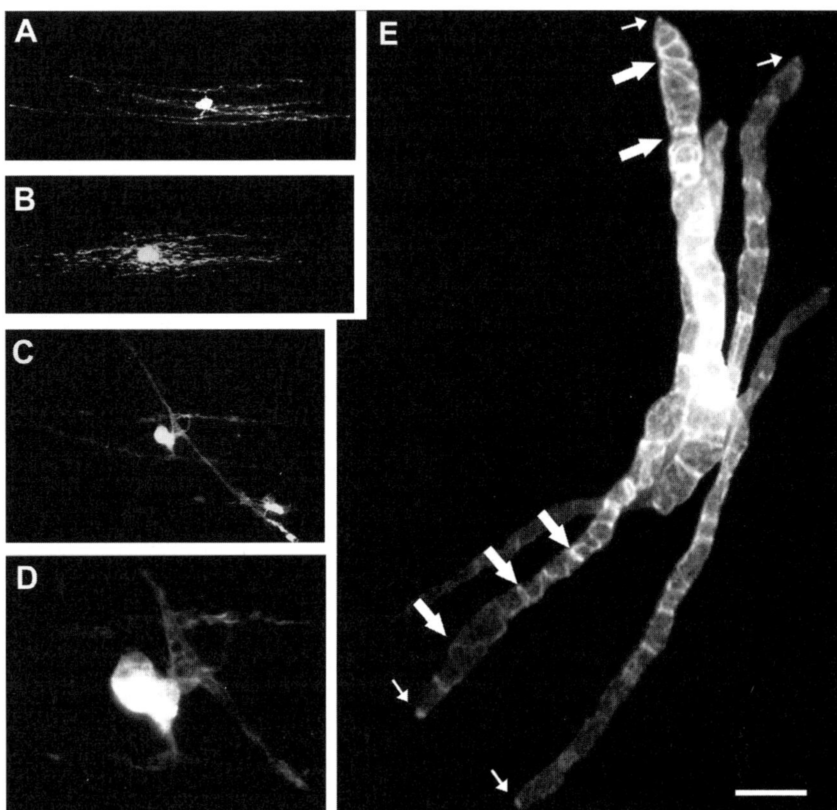

FIGURE 3.3 Confocal microscopy of oligodendrocytes intracellularly dye-filled with lysinated rhodamine dextran. *A,B*. Two type II oligodendrocytes from the adult rat optic nerve, with 10–30 parallel processes exclusively oriented along the long axis of the nerve. The processes are the dye-filled inner and outer tongue processes of the myelin sheaths and are connected to the cell body by tenuous processes. *A*. One unit myelinates 10 axons with uniform internodal lengths of 200 μm and external sheath diameters of approximately 1.5 μm. *B*. The second unit myelinates 20 or so axons, with internodal lengths varying in length from 50 to 200 μm and external sheath diameters of less than 0.5 μm. *C–E*. Two type III oligodendrocytes from the adult rat anterior medullary velum supporting four to five myelin sheaths of varying diameter and length. C. This unit has myelinated four axons (only three are clearly visible in the photomicrograph) of diameter 3–4 μm and internodal lengths of around 200 μm. *D*. A large oligodendrocyte unit myelinating five axons with external sheath diameters of 10–15 μm and internodal lengths of around 400 μm. Myelin sheaths are connected to the cell body by short, thick processes in type III units and have prominent reticulations C. Note the dye-filled paranodal loops (*small arrows* in *E*) and spirals of the cytoplasmic inner and outer tongue processes (*large arrows* in *E*). Scale bar is 40 μm in *A*, *B*, *C*, and *E* and 15 μm in *D*. [From Butt et al., 1994 (*A,B*), and Berry et al., 1995 (*C–E*), with permission.]

3.3*C* and 3.3*E* illustrate two type III oligodendrocyte units that myelinate four to five axons, with external sheath diameters ranging from 3 to 4 μm in one unit (Fig. 3.3C) and 10 to 15 μm in the second (Fig. 3.3*E*), and internodal lengths of around 400 μm. In both units, the sheaths display prominent dye-filled cytoplasmic tongues that spiral over the surface of the myelin sheaths up to the paranodal loops (Fig. 3.3*D*,*E*), contrary to published views of CNS myelin, where the outer cytoplasmic tongue is assumed to run linearly along the axon. Type I/II and III/IV phenotypes are defined by both the number and diameter of axons within the unit; type I/II oligodendrocytes myelinate six or more axons of diameter ≤2 μm, whereas type III/IV oligodendrocytes myelinate five or less axons of diameter ≥4 μm (Butt et al., 1998). Thus, small- and large-diameter axons in the adult CNS are myelinated by two discrete populations of oligodendrocyte phenotypes I/II and III/IV, whose distribution densities are determined by the spatial distribution of axons below and above a critical diameter of 2–4 μm. Thus, the optic nerve, corpus callosum, and corticospinal tracts contain small-diameter fibers (≤2 μm) and are populated only by type I/II oligodendrocytes, whereas the spinal cord fasciculi contain large-diameter axons (≥2 μm) and are populated by type III/IV oligodendrocytes.

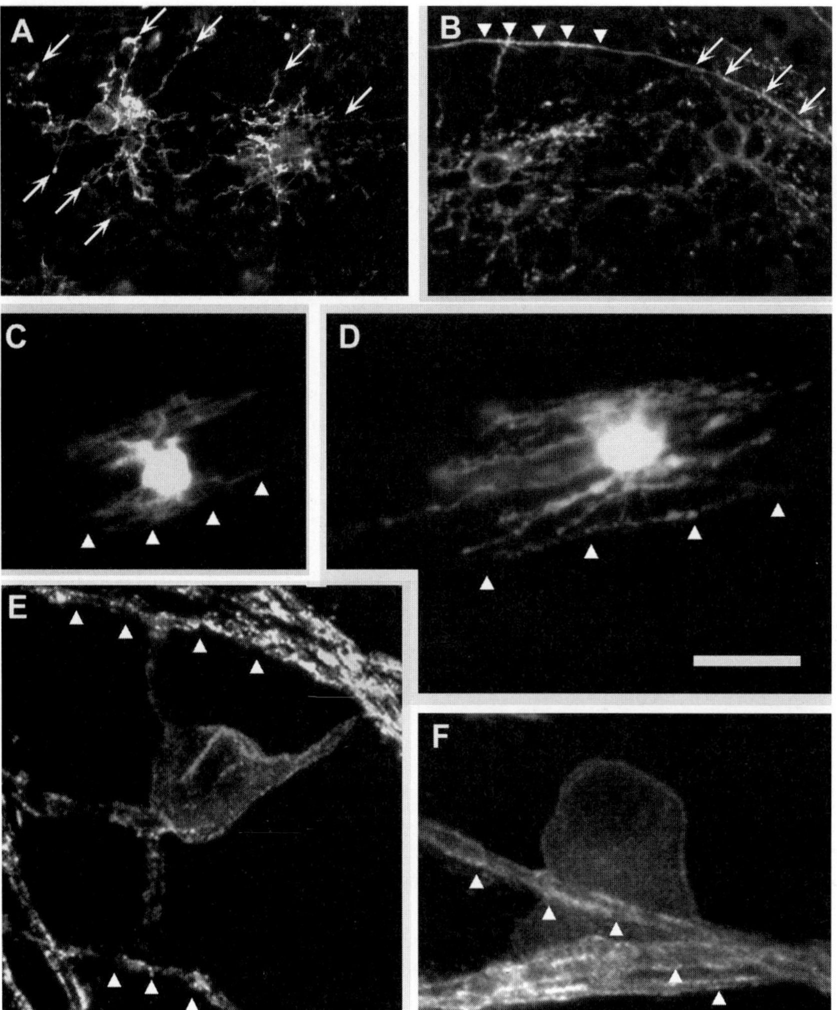

FIGURE 3.4 Axon-oligodendrocyte relations in developing oligodendrocyte units, resolved by double immunofluorescence labeling of the postnatal anterior medullary velum (*A,B,E,F*) and intracellular injection of Lucifer Yellow in the postnatal rat optic nerve (*C,D*). Vela are double immunofluorescence labeled with NG2, for oligodendrocyte progenitors (*A*), or with Rip, for oligodendrocytes (*B,E,F*), and NF-200 for axons *A*. Progenitors extend numerous radial processes that form multiple contacts with unmyelinated axons (*arrows*). *B*. Premyelinating oligodendrocytes have a starburst morphology and extend innumerable fine, branching processes. They contact axons via fine filipodia (*arrows*) and extend short initiator processes along axons prior to ensheathment (*arrowheads*). *C*. Transitional oligodendrocytes have commenced axonal ensheathment, recognized as linear process arrays (*arrowheads*), and initially extend both ensheathing and nonensheathing processes. *D–F*. Oligodendrocytes go through a remodeling phase during which they lose nonensheathing processes, and the number of sheaths per unit is established. Oligodendrocyte phenotypes II (*D*), III (*E*), and IV (*F*) are established early in unit development, and axons within the units are less than 2 μm in diameter (*arrowheads*). Bar in *D* represents 10 μm in *A*, *B*, *E*, and *F* and 20 μm in *C* and *D*. [From Butt and Ransom, 1993 (*C,D*), and Butt et al., 1997) (*B,E,F*), with permission.]

FUNCTIONAL IMPLICATIONS OF OLIGODENDROCYTE POLYMORPHISM

Biochemical Differences in Myelin Composition

Differences in myelin between large- and small-diameter CNS fibers have been noted with respect to structure, myelin turnover, and protein composition (reviewed by Hildebrand et al., 1993). Marchi staining, which is used to demonstrate degenerating myelin, also labels myelinoid bodies specifically in large-diameter myelinated fibers in normal spinal cord white matter (Hildebrand et al., 1993). There is also evidence that myelin basic protein (MBP) and proteolipid protein (PLP) are expressed more intensely in small- and large-diameter fibers, respectively (Hartman et al., 1982). In addition, phenotypic differences in the expression of carbonic anhydrase (CA)II and the S-isoform of myelin-associated glycoprotein (MAG) have been detected in the adult rat anterior medullary velum (reviewed by Butt and Berry, 2000). Two extreme variants are S-MAG$^-$/CAII$^+$ type I/II units and S-MAG$^+$/CAII$^-$ type III/IV units, which myelinate the smallest and largest diameter fibers, respectively. The different patterns of immunolabeling most likely reflect underlying biochemical differences and indicate that different types of myelin are found in different types of oligodendrocyte units, determined by the diameter of the axons in the unit.

Differences in Myelin Volume in Type I/II and Type III/IV Oligodendrocytes

There are direct relationships between fiber diameters and the number of myelin sheaths per oligodendrocyte unit, and between both the longitudinal (internodal lengths) and radial (number of lamellae) dimensions of the myelin sheaths (Hildebrand and Hahn, 1978; Ibrahim et al., 1995; Butt et al., 1998). The number of lamellae (*N*) determines the insulating properties of the sheath, whereas internodal myelin sheath length (*L*) determines the speed of conduction. Both *N* and *L* are directly and positively correlated with axon diameter (*D*), so thick axons conduct faster than slimmer ones.

Individual oligodendrocyte units support 1–50 myelin sheaths and have L values ranging from 50 to 1000 μm and values of N between 10 and 100, depending on D. Thus, each myelin sheath has dimensions of approximately $\pi \cdot D \cdot N \cdot L$. There is a clear demarcation between type I/II and type III/IV oligodendrocytes, which support myelin volumes of approximately 500 and 30,000 μm^3, respectively (Butt et al., 1998). In type IV units, where internodal lengths may attain 1000 μm, the volume of myelin supported is as great as 150,000 μm^3 (Remahl and Hildebrand, 1990a).

Oligodendrocyte Subtypes in Pathology

Oligodendrocyte polymorphism and differences in myelin biochemistry reflect the metabolic demand of the greater mass of myelin supported by type III/IV oligodendrocytes compared to type I/II oligodendrocytes. The large cell bodies and thick radial processes of type III/IV units and their prominent Schmidt-Lantermann incisures facilitate the distribution of myelin gene products. In addition, myelinoid bodies occur preferentially at large paranodes and reflect the greater myelin metabolism and turnover in type III/IV oligodendrocytes (Hildebrand et al., 1993). A number of studies indicate that type III/IV oligodendrocytes may be less susceptible to metabolic disruption and demyelination than type I/II oligodendrocytes. For example, in the *taiep* mutant rat, dysmyelination affects type I/II oligodendrocytes more severely than type III/IV oligodendrocytes (Song et al., 2001). Similarly, in two inherited metabolic disorders resulting in demyelination, Krabbe's disease and metachromatic leukodystrophy, late-myelinating tracts are more severely affected than early-myelinating tracts (Hildebrand et al., 1993).

DEVELOPMENT OF OLIGODENDROCYTE PHENOTYPES

Relation to Axon Diameter and the Age of Myelination

Since the dimensions of the axon and its myelin sheath determine the conduction properties of the axon, the question of what determines axon diameter and oligodendrocyte phenotype is of some importance. There are direct relationships between the age at which axons are myelinated, their final diameter in the adult, and the developmental divergence of oligodendrocyte phenotypes (Hildebrand et al., 1993). Thus, prospective large-diameter fibers ($\geq$4 μm) are myelinated early in development, by type III/IV oligodendrocytes that differentiate immediately prior to and after birth, whereas prospective small-diameter fibers ($\leq$2 μm) are myelinated later in development, by type I/II oligodendrocytes that differentiate in the first postnatal weeks. However, oligodendrocytes do not appear to be inherently programmed to myelinate axons of a specific size. Oligodendrocyte types I/II and III/IV appear to derive from common OPCs and premyelinating oligodendrocyte phenotypes (Fig. 3.4*A*,*B*) (Butt et al., 1997), and OPCs that normally develop into type I/II oligodendrocytes will remyelinate large-diameter fibers when transplanted into experimentally demyelinated spinal cord funiculi (Fanarraga et al., 1998). Oligodendrocytes initially contact and ensheath a large number of immature thin axons (Fig. 3.4*A*–*C*), and most of these processes are lost during myelination (Fig. 3.4*D*–*F*). Oligodendrocyte phenotypes II (Fig. 4.4*D*), III (Fig. 4.4*E*), and IV (Fig. 4.4*F*) are established during this remodeling phase, when axons within all units are of similar small diameters (<2 μm). This implies that oligodendrocyte phenotype is not determined by axon diameter at the onset of myelination. Indeed, axon growth depends on oligodendroglial contact and myelination (Collelo et al., 1994). The balance of evidence is that oligodendrocyte phenotype differentiation and axon and myelin growth are interdependent, controlled by local axo-glial interactions.

Axonal Control of Oligodendrocyte Phenotype Numbers

During development, oligodendrocyte phenotypes I/II and III/IV are defined by the number of axons within the unit and not by axon diameter. This implies that these are either inherent phenotypic characteristics of two separate oligodendrocyte lineages or they represent the divergence of a single lineage in response to the local environment. There is evidence for multiple oligodendroglial lineages in embryonic development (Spassky et al., 2000), but there is no evidence that they give rise to spatially and temporally separate oligodendrocyte phenotypes. It follows that axon-derived signals and environmental cues must differ qualitatively or quantitatively at different ages of myelination or between presumptive large- and small-diameter fibers.

The ratio of axons to oligodendrocytes is less than 5:1 in large-diameter fiber tracts and greater than 15:1 in small-diameter fiber tracts (Butt et al., 1994, 1998). How are the ratios of axons to oligodendrocytes established in small- and large-diameter fiber tracts? Barres and Raff (1999) have proposed a model by which the competition for limited axon-dependent survival factors precisely matches the final number of oligodendrocytes to the number and lengths of axons to be myelinated. Competition for extracellular and axonal factors may therefore be less for early-developing oligodendrocytes, which consequently myelinate a smaller number of axons per unit, compared with late-developing oligodendrocytes, when competition is greater. There are a number of possible growth factors that control oligodendrocyte numbers and differentiation, including platelet-derived growth factor-AA (PDGF-AA) and fibroblast growth factor-2 (FGF-2), while a strong candidate for the axon-derived survival signal is neuregulin (Barres et al., 1994; Barres and Raff, 1999; Butt and Berry, 2000). Possible mechanisms by which competition for these factors could control the developmental divergence of type III/IV and type I/II oligodendrocyte phenotypes are: (*1*) expression of axon-derived promoters of oligodendrocyte development is greater in presumptive large-diameter axons; (*2*) levels of axon-derived and extracellular factors decrease with age; or (*3*) the responsiveness to these factors is diminished in late-developing OPCs and oligodendrocytes. An important question is whether the levels of factors that control oligodendrocyte development, or their receptors, are developmentally regulated or differentially expressed in type I/II and type III/IV axon-oligodendrocyte units.

Oligodendrocyte Phenotype Maturation and Axon Growth Are Interdependent

It appears that differentiation of oligodendrocyte phenotypes, and therefore the composition, metabolism, and size of their myelin sheaths, are driven by axon-oligodendrocyte interactions via contact-mediated signals. The onset of axonal myelination is correlated with phenotypic changes in oligodendrocytes and axons, including the differential expression of myelin-related proteins (Sternberger et al., 1978), while axons thicken and there is induction of presumptive nodes of Ranvier (Rasband et al., 1999). Finally, there is interdependent maturation of axon-oligodendrocyte unit function and radial growth of the axon and its myelin sheath that, in the rat and cat, attain their adult dimensions late in development, many weeks after the commencement of myelination (Remahl and Hildebrand, 1990a, 1990b). A study in the rat optic nerve demonstrates that axon growth is substantially reduced in the absence of oligodendrocytes following X-irradiation (Collelo et al., 1994), which clearly points to local regulation of axon diameter by oligodendrocytes. This is possibly mediated in part by galactolipids (Popko, 2000), and there is evidence of a role for MAG as a myelin signal that modulates the calibre of myelinated axons (Yin et al., 1998). Long-term interactions between axons and their myelin sheaths are poorly understood, but transgenic mice show signs of axonal degeneration in the absence of the oligodendroglial protein PLP or the enzyme 2′,3′-cyclic nucleotide 3′-phosphodiesterase (CNP) (Griffiths et al., 1998; Lappe-Siefke et al., 2003). PLP is important for the fusion of the extracellular membranes of the myelin lamellae to form the intraperiod line, and axon degeneration may be secondary to myelin abnormalities observed in PLP knockout mice (Griffiths et al., 1998). However, in the Cnp1 knockout mouse, the ultrastructure and periodicity of myelin were unaffected, indicating that oligodendrocyte dysfunction alone, without demyelination, is sufficient to cause secondary axonal loss (Lappe-Siefke et al., 2003).

Oligodendrocytes and the Establishment of Nodes of Ranvier

Oligodendrocytes play an important role in sodium and potassium ion channel clustering and segregation in the nodal and juxtaparanodal axolemmal membranes, respectively (Kaplan et al., 1997; Rasband et al., 1999). The clustering of ion channels at presumptive nodes occurs at the same time as incipient internodal segments and axon-glial contacts at paranodal junctions are established, mediated in part via interactions between oligodendroglial neurofascin and the axonal paranodin/Caspr-contactin complex at the myelin attachment zone (Rasband et al., 1999; Charles et al., 2002; Poliak and Peles, 2003). The periodicity of nodes along axons is determined by axon diameter and myelin sheath internodal length (Ibrahim et al., 1995). However, it is far from clear how this is established early in the development of presumptive large- and small-diameter fibres. Induction of nodes does not depend on myelination, but is dependent on both oligodendroglial contact and diffusible factors from oligodendrocytes (Kaplan et al., 1997; Rasband et al., 1999). Both OPCs and premyelinating oligodendrocytes extend profuse filipodia that form multiple contacts with numerous axons (Fig. 3.4*A*,*B*), many of which are then lost (Fig. 3.4*C*,*D*), and so it seems unlikely that axonal contact alone could induce the relatively constant periodicity of nodes and spacing of oligodendrocytes along axons. As premyelinating oligodendrocytes engage axons, *initiator processes* extend along the axon and commence myelination (Fig. 3.4*B*,C), and nodal periodicity is established by the symmetrical growth of myelin sheaths along the axon from the connecting process. Nonmyelinating processes are lost, and the number of sheaths per oligodendrocyte unit and incipient internodal lengths are established during this remodeling phase (Fig. 3.4*D–F*). However, myelination of both presumptive large- and small-diameter axon tracts is asynchronous and multifocal, and axons are ensheathed intermittently along their length by both myelinating and premyelinating oligodendrocytes, with frequent heminodes and unmyelinated gaps that are myelinated by late-developing interstitial premyelinating oligodendrocytes (Butt et al., 1997). Despite this, internodal lengths and the periodicity of nodes of Ranvier are relatively constant along a given axon, depending on the diameter (Ibrahim et al., 1995), raising the question of how the spacing of oligodendrocytes along axons is determined.

Axon-Oligodendrocyte Recognition Signals

A number of recognition and adhesion events between axons and oligodendrocytes must be involved in the complex sequence of axon-oligodendrocyte interdependent maturation phases. Axon contact per se cannot be the factor determining whether an oligodendrocyte or its individual processes form myelin, since many processes that contact axons in OPCs and premyelinating oligodendrocytes do not form myelin and are subsequently lost (Fig. 3.4). The first step in axon myelination must therefore be a recognition event between oligodendrocyte processes and axons, or specific sites along axons, that are receptive for myelination. Oligodendrocyte phenotypic specification then occurs by remodeling, during which units compete for axons by axolemmal engagement/disengagement (Bjartmar et al., 1994), presumably mediated by contact-mediated recognition signals that must be qualitatively and/or quantitatively different for prospective large- and small-diameter axons. Axoglial Jagged/Notch signaling is likely to be important in controlling the onset of myelination, since axonal Jagged inhibits differentiation of OPCs, which express Notch, and both are developmentally downregulated in the optic nerve during myelination (Wang et al., 1998). Other possible axoglial signaling molecules have been identified by Brophy and colleagues from a subtractive cDNA library enriched for sequences that are upregulated at the onset of myelination (Collinson et al., 1998; Charles et al., 2002). For example, neurofascin is expressed by oligodendrocytes during the peak of myelination but declines after they have ensheathed their axons, indicating an early role for this cell adhesion molecule (CAM) in axoglial interactions (Collinson et al., 1998). Axonal receptors for neurofascin are part of the L1 CAM family, and binding of neurofascin to the paranodin/Caspr-contactin axonal complex may be most important in axo-glial interactions at the paranodal axoglial junction (Charles et al., 2002). Interactions between axonal contactin and oligodendroglial Notch receptors may also play an instructive role in oligodendrocyte development by promoting OPC differentiation and upregulation of myelin proteins (see Popko, 2003). Important unanswered questions are whether changes in the expression of axon-glial recognition molecules are differentially regulated in presumptive large- and small-diameter fibers, and whether their expression spatiotemporally correlates with myelination, which is multifocal and asynchronous.

ADULT NG2-GLIA: NONMYELINATING OLIGODENDROCYTES?

Relation to Oligodendrocyte Progenitors

A significant population of glia have been identified in the adult CNS by their expression of the NG2 chondroitin sulfate proteoglycan (Levine and Card, 1987). These cells have the antigenic phenotype of OPCs (Nishiyama et al., 1996) and are considered to be equivalent to adult OPCs identified in cultures of glial cells isolated from adult rat brain (Stallcup and Beasley, 1987). There is evidence that $NG2^+$ OPCs generate oligodendrocytes during development and following demyelination in the adult brain (Dawson et al., 2000), and it is reasonable to conclude that adult NG2-glia and oligodendrocytes are derived from a common $NG_2{}^+$ progenitor. However, it is not clear that all $NG_2{}^+$ cells in the adult or developing CNS are OPCs (Butt et al., 2002; Greenwood and Butt, 2003). Studies in transgenic mice support the concept that there are at least two populations of $NG_2{}^+$ cells in the developing brain (Mallon et al., 2002; Matthias et al., 2003), one that develops into myelinating oligodendrocytes and another that develops into nonmyelinating NG2-glia (Berry et al., 2002).

Adult NG2-Glia

Adult NG2-glia do not fit the conceptual picture of simple stem cells (Figs. 3.5 and 3.6). It has been proposed therefore that most, if not all, NG2-glia observed in adult gray matter (Fig. 3.5) and white matter (Fig. 3.6) are mature cells (Butt et al., 2002). The distribution of adult NG2-glia is clearly related to the neuronal layers of the cerebellum (Fig. 3.5*A*), and the process fields of individual NG2-glia traverse the Purkinje cell and granular cell layers (Fig. 3.5*B*). The density of NG2-glia in the molecular layer (Fig. 3.5*C*) is difficult to reconcile with their being a pool of adult OPCs sitting in the brain in order to regenerate oligodendrocytes throughout life, since oligodendrocytes do not develop in this area. NG2-glia form multiple contacts with neuronal cell bodies (Fig. 3.5*B*,*D*), shown by EM immunocytochemistry to contact synapses (Fig. 3.5*E–G*) (Bergles et al., 2000). NG2-glia have a similar complex morphology in white matter (Fig. 3.6*A*,*B*), where they extend processes along axons that EM immunocytochemistry has demonstrated contact nodes of Ranvier (Fig. 3.6C) (Butt et al., 1999). NG2-glia therefore have many morphological features of astrocytes (see Butt and Ransom, 1993), which also contact nodes of Ranvier and synapses, but they are not immunopositive for glial fibrillary acidic protein (GFAP) (Butt et al., 1999). However, in mice where expression of enhanced green fluorescent protein (EGFP) is driven by the GFAP promoter, $EGFP^+$ cells are colabeled by antibodies to AN2, the mouse homolog of NG2, and a subpopulation of these $EGFP(GFAP^+)/NG2^+$ cells also express the astroglial marker S-100β (Matthias et al., 2003). Furthermore, NG2-glia have some physiological properties of GFAP-negative *complex* astrocytes, which are distinguished from GFAP-positive *passive* astrocytes in electrophysiological studies on the basis of their ion currents, differential expression of glutamate receptors and transporters, and the extent of their intercellular

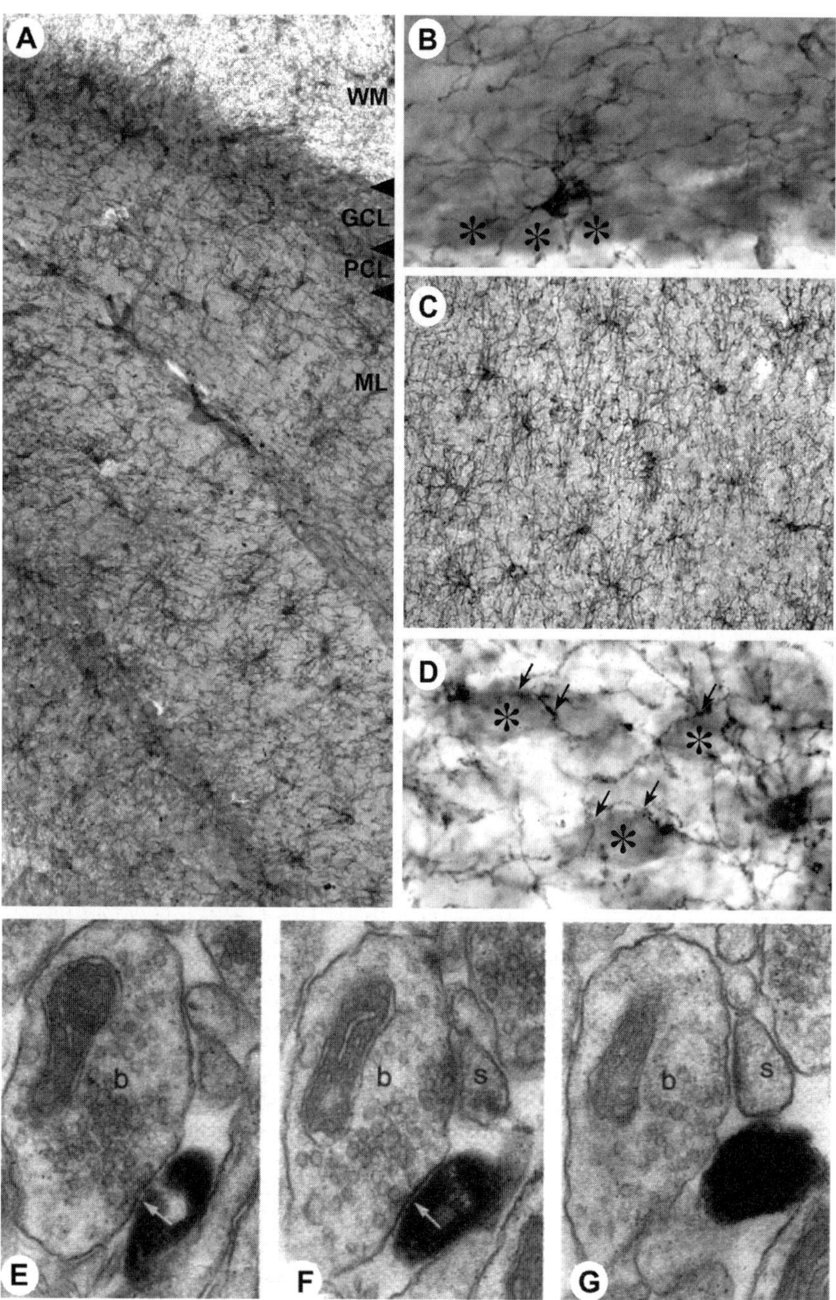

FIGURE 3.5 NG2-glia in gray matter of the adult rat brain. Immunolabeling with NG2, a marker for oligodendrocyte progenitor cells, is visualized in thick sections (50 μm), and neurons are counterstained with toluidine blue (*B*,*D*). *A*. NG2-glia have a stellate morphology, and their distribution in the cerebellum clearly demarcates the white matter (*WM*), granular cell layer (*GCL*), Purkinje cell layer (*PCL*), and molecular layer (*ML*). *B*. NG2-glia sited perineuronally and processes contacting and ensheathing Purkinje cells (*asterisks*). *C*. NG2-glia are numerous in the molecular layer, where there are no oligodendrocytes. *D*. NG2-glial cell forming multiple contacts (*arrows*) with granular cells of the dentate gyrus (*asterisks*). *E*,*F*. Serial electron micrographs illustrating the processes of an NG2-glial cell (*black*, peroxidase reaction) receives a synapse (*arrow*) from a bouton (*b*) that also gives a synapse to a dendritic spine (s) in rat hippocampus. Bar represents 100 μm in *A* and *C*, 20 μm in *B* and *D*, and 0.2 μm in *E–G* (*E–G* from Bergles et al., 2000, with permission.)

coupling (Lin and Bergles, 2002; Matthias et al., 2003; Schools et al., 2003). Adult NG2-glia therefore appear to have properties of both OPC and astrocytes, suggesting that there are either multiple populations of adult NG2-glia or a single population of multifunctional NG2-glia.

Injury Response of NG2-Glia

The stereotypic response of NG2-glia to almost any insult to the CNS is a reactive gliosis, irrespective of whether the insult is physical or excitotoxic injury, viral infection, chemical, X-irradiation, or immune-induced demyelination (reviewed by Levine et al., 2001). The balance of evidence is that NG2-glia are a highly reactive cell type, which responds rapidly to CNS injury by upregulation of NG2 expression, proliferation, and process outgrowth (Butt et al., 2002). Significantly, the NG2 chondroitin sulfate proteoglycan is a component of the glial scar matrix and is a potent inhibitor of axon regeneration in the CNS (Levine et al., 2001). NG2-glia are ideally situated to readily sense changes in neuronal activity via their perinodal and synaptic connections and their neurotransmitter receptors (Butt et al., 2002; Lin and Bergles, 2002). In addition, NG2-glia express receptors for PDGF-AA and FGF-2 (Nishiyama et al., 2002), and their activation induces an injury-like response (Butt et al., 2002).

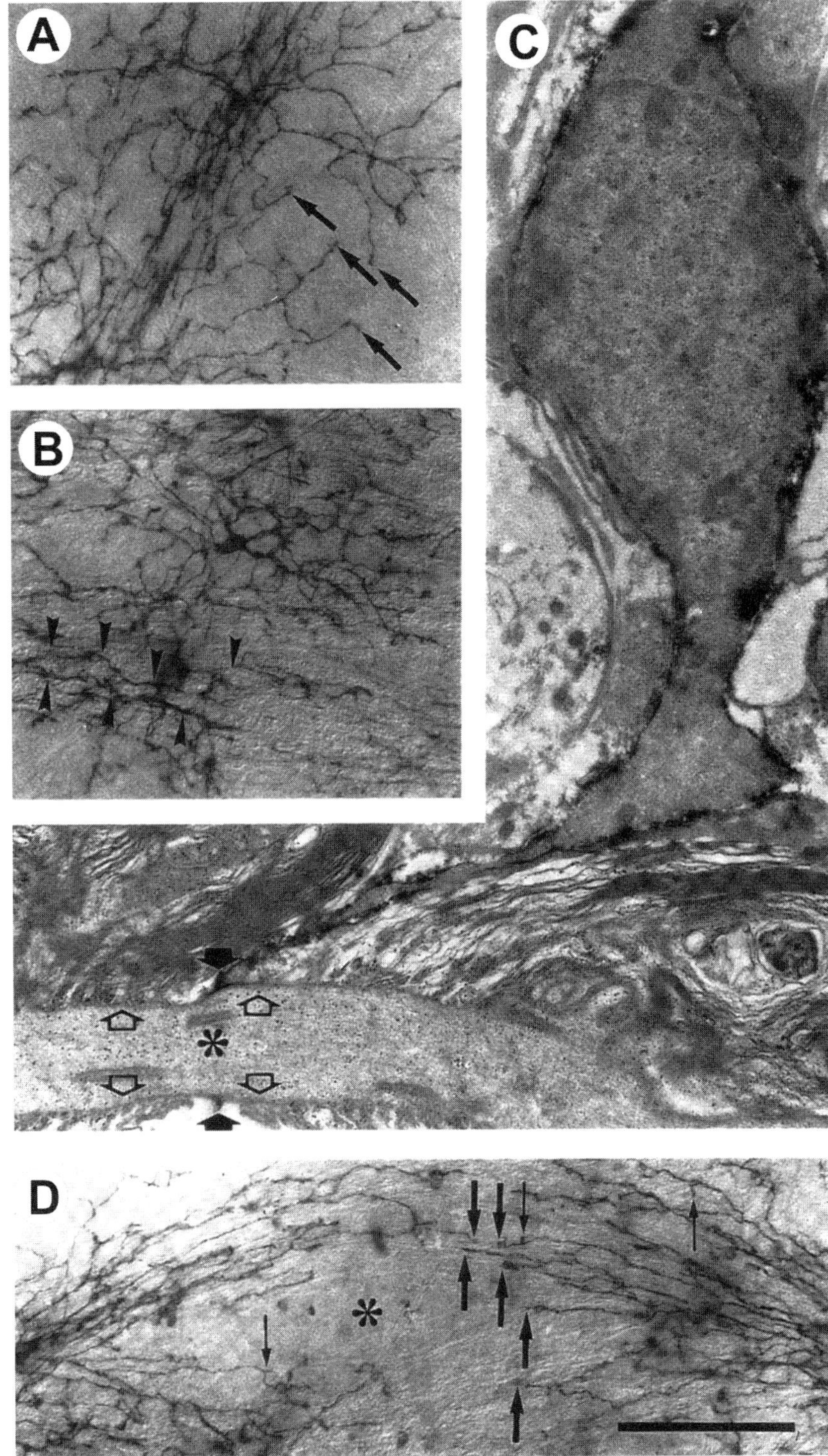

FIGURE 3.6 NG2-glia in white matter of the adult rat brain. *A,B,D*. Immunoperoxidase labeling in whole-mounted anterior medullary vela illustrates typical NG2-glia with small somata and multibranched varicose primary processes, which terminate on individual axons (*arrows* in *A*) and ramify in the long axis along axon bundles (*arrowheads* in *B*). *C*. Pre–embedding electron microscopic immunocytochemistry shows the surface labeling of the NG2 membrane-embedded chondroitin sulfate proteoglycan in a cell that sends a process (*filled arrows* in C) that wraps around the axolemma at a nearby node of Ranvier (*asterisk* in C), defined by the paranodal loops of the oligodendroglial myelin sheath (*open arrows* in C). *D*. The perinodal processes identified at the ultrastructural level are recognized at the light microscopic level as spines (*small arrows* in *D*) and free-ending processes (*large arrows* in *D*) that terminate on axons. NG2-glia processes appear to seek out axons, neglecting areas between axon bundles (*asterisk* in *D*), suggesting that they serve a specific perinodal function. Bar represents 80 μm in *A*, C, and *D* and 2.5 μm in C. (From Butt et al., 1999, and Butt and Berry, 2000, with permission.)

NG2-glia may therefore be specialized to monitor and respond rapidly to changes in neuronal activity and to help form the glial scar that localizes the site of injury and protects the surrounding neuropil from further damage. Butt and colleagues (2002) have termed NG2-glia *synantocytes*, from the Greek *synant* meaning "contact," to distinguish them from OPCs, which are undifferentiated, mitotic, and motile cells that develop into oligodendrocytes.

SUMMARY AND PERSPECTIVES

Rio-Hortega's thesis on oligodendrocyte heterogeneity is confirmed, although the significance of his findings is scarcely appreciated today. There are two oligodendrocyte subtypes in the brain and spinal cord, corresponding to Rio-Hortega's type I/II and III/IV, which are defined by the diameter of axons in the unit below and above 2–4 μm diameter, respectively. Type I/II oligodendrocytes myelinate a large number of small-diameter axons with thin myelin sheaths and short internodal lengths. Type III/IV oligodendrocytes are large cells that myelinate a small number of large-diameter axons with thick myelin sheaths and long internodal lengths. These phenotypic differences determine the conduction properties of axons within oligodendrocyte units. The numbers and distributions of oligodendrocyte phenotypes are related to the age of myelination, and are likely to be determined by the competition for axon-derived and environmental factors. The growth of axons and myelin sheaths is interdependent within oligodendrocyte unit phenotypes. Key issues are how environmental, axonal, and genetic factors control the differentiation of oligodendrocyte phenotypes and how oligodendrocytes and myelin, in turn, determine axonal growth and integrity, as well as the periodicity of nodes of Ranvier. Genetic techniques have began to provide insights into the factors controlling myelination and axo-glial interactions, but it is not clear that oligodendrocyte phenotypes I/II and III/IV obey the same rules of engagement. This is not trivial, because oligodendrocyte phenotypic heterogeneity determines axon growth and conduction properties, in addition to their susceptibility to demyelination and possibly degeneration. Nonmyelinating oligodendrocytes in the CNS are also of increasing interest, because they are important in the pathogenesis of degeneration/regeneration and demyelination/remyelination in the CNS. NG2-glia are a distinct class of glia that have the antigenic phenotype of OPCs and the morphological phenotype of astrocytes, with functional properties of both. An area of controversy is whether NG2-glia are adult OPCs, astrocytes or novel synantocytes, presumably with an oligodendrocyte lineage. Future studies should not neglect oligodendrocyte polymorphism if they are to answer these questions and determine how axo-glial interactions and environmental factors control oligodendrocyte genesis and myelinogenesis *in vivo*.

ACKNOWLEDGMENTS

I would like to thank all my coworkers past and present, with special thanks to Martin Berry, Merdol Ibrahim, Fraser Hornby, Sarah Kirvell, Paul Hubbard, and Alan Duncan.

ABBREVIATIONS

CAII	carbonic anhydrase II
CAM	cell adhesion molecule
CNS	central nervous system
CNP	2′,3′-cyclic nucleotide 3′-phosphodiesterase
EGFP	enhanced green fluorescent protein
EM	electron microscopy
GFAP	glial fibrillary acidic protein
MAG	myelin-associated glycoprotein
OPCs	oligodendrocyte progenitor cells
PDGF-AA	platelet-derived growth factor-AA
PLP	proteolipid protein

REFERENCES

Anderson, E.S., Bjartmar, C., Westermark, G., and Hildebrand, C. (1999) Molecular heterogeneity of oligodendrocytes in chicken white matter. *Glia* 27:15–21.

Barres, B.A and Raff, M.C. (1999) Control of oligodendrocyte number in the developing rat optic nerve. *Neuron* 12:935–942.

Bergles, D.E., Roberts, J.D.B., Somogyi, P., and Jahr, C.E. (2000) Glutamatergic synapses on oligodendrocyte precursor cells in the hippocampus. *Nature* 405:187–191.

Berry, M., Hubbard, P., and Butt, A.M. (2002) Cytology and lineage of NG2-positive glia. *J. Neurocytol.* 31:457–467.

Berry, M., Ibrahim, M., Carlile, J., Ruge, F., Duncan, A., and Butt, A.M. (1995) Axon glial relations in the anterior medullary velum of the adult rat. *J. Neurocytol.* 24:965–983.

Bjartmar, C., Hildebrand, C., and Loinder, K. (1994) Morphological heterogeneity of rat oligodendrocytes: electron microscopic studies on serial sections. *Glia* 11:235–244.

Bunge, R.P. (1968) Glial cells and the central myelin sheath. *Physiol. Rev.* 48:197–251.

Butt, A.M. and Berry, M. (2000) Oligodendrocytes and the control of myelination in vivo: new insights from the rat anterior medullary velum. *J. Neurosci. Res.* 59:477–488.

Butt, A.M., Colquhoun, K., and Berry, M. (1994) Confocal imaging of glial cells in the intact rat optic nerve. *Glia* 10:315–322.

Butt, A.M., Duncan, A., Hornby, M.F., Kirvell, S.L., Hunter, A., Levine, J.L., and Berry, M. (1999) Cells expressing the NG2 antigen contact nodes of Ranvier in adult CNS white matter. *Glia* 26:84–91.

Butt, A.M., Hubbard, P., Kiff, J., and Berry, M. (2002) Synantocytes: new functions for novel NG2 expressing glia. *J. Neurocytol.* 31:551–565.

Butt, A.M., Ibrahim, M., and Berry, M. (1997) The relationship between developing oligodendrocyte units and maturing axons during myelinogenesis in the anterior medullary velum of neonatal rats. *J. Neurocytol.* 26:327–338.

Butt, A.M., Ibrahim, M., and Berry, M. (1998) Axon-myelin sheath relations of oligodendrocyte unit phenotypes in the adult rat anterior medullary velum. *J. Neurocytol.* 27:259–269.

Butt, A.M. and Ransom, B.R. (1989) Visualization of oligodendrocytes and astrocytes in the intact rat optic nerve by intracellular injection of Lucifer yellow and horseradish peroxidase. *Glia* 2:470–475.

Butt, A.M. and Ransom, B.R. (1993) Morphology of astrocytes and oligodendrocytes during development in the intact rat optic nerve. *J. Comp. Neurol.* 338:141–158.

Charles, P., Tait, S., Faivre-Sarrailh, C., Barbin, G., Gunn-Moore, F., Denisenko-Nehrbass, N., Guennoc, A.-M., Girault, J.-A., Brophy, P.J., and Lubetzki, C. (2002) Neurofascin is a glial receptor for the paranodin/Caspr-contactin axonal complex at the axoglial junction. *Curr. Biol.* 12:217–220.

Colello, R.J., Pott, U., and Schwab, M.E. (1994) The role of oligodendrocytes and myelin on axon maturation in the developing rat retinofugal pathway. *J. Neurosci.* 14:2594–2605.

Collinson, J.M., Marshall, D., Gillespie, C.S., and Brophy, P.J. (1998) Transient expression of neurofascin by oligodendrocytes at the onset of myelinogenesis: implications for mechanisms of axon-glial interaction. *Glia* 23:11–23.

Dawson, R.L., Levien, J.M., and Reynolds, R. (2000) NG2-expressing cells in the central nervous system: are they oligodendrocyte progenitors? *J. Neurosci. Res.* 61:471–479.

Fanarraga, M.L., Griffiths, I.R., Zhao, M., and Duncan, I.D. (1998) Oligodendrocytes are not inherently programmed to myelinate a specific size of axon. *J. Comp. Neurol.* 399:94–100.

Friedman, B., Hockfield, S., Black, J.A., Woodruff, K.A., and Waxman, S.G. (1989) In situ demonstration of mature oligodendrocytes and their processes: an immunocytochemical study with a new monoclonal antibody, Rip. *Glia* 2:380–390.

Greenwood, K. and Butt, A.M. (2003) Evidence that perinatal and adult NG2-glia are not conventional oligodendrocyte progenitors and do not depend on axons for their survival. *Mol. Cell. Neurosci.* 23:544–558.

Griffiths, I.R., Klugman, M., Anderson, T.J., Thomson, C.E., Vouyiouklis, D.A., and Nave, H.-A. (1998) Current concepts of PLP and its role in the nervous system. *Science* 280:1610–1613.

Hartman, B.K., Agrawal, C.H., Agrawal, D., and Kalmbach, S. (1982) Development and maturation of central nervous system myelin: comparison of immunohistochemical localisation of proteolipid protein and basic protein in myelin and oligodendrocytes. *Proc. Natl. Acad. Sci. USA* 79:4217–4220.

Hildebrand, C. and Hahn, R. (1978) Relation between myelin sheath thickness and axon size in spinal cord white matter of some vertebrate species. *J. Neurol. Sci.* 38:421–434.

Hildebrand, C., Remahl, S., Persson, H. and Bjartmar, C. (1993) Myelinated nerve fibres in the CNS. *Prog. Neurobiol.* 40:319–384.

Hirano, A. (1968) A confirmation of oligodendroglial origin of myelin in the adult rat. *J. Cell Biol.* 38:637–640.

Ibrahim, M., Butt, A.M., and Berry, M. (1995) The relationship between myelin sheath diameter and internodal length in the anterior medullary velum of the rat. *J. Neurol. Sci.* 133:119–127.

Kaplan, M.R., Meyer-Franke, A., Lambert, S., Bennett, V., Duncan, I.D., Levinson, S.R., and Barres, B.A. (1997) Induction of sodium channel clustering by oligodendrocytes. *Nature* 386:724–728.

Lappe-Siefke, C., Goebbela, S., Gravel, M., Nicksch, E., Lee, J., Braun, P.E., Griffiths, I.R., and Nave, K.-A. (2003) Disruption of *Cnp1* uncouples oligodendroglial functions and axonal support and myelination. *Nature Genet.* 33:366–374.

Levine, J.M. and Card, J.P. (1987) Light and electron microscopic localization of a cell surface antigen (NG2) in the rat cerebellum: association with smooth protoplasmic astrocytes. *J. Neurosci.* 7:2711–2720.

Levine, J.M., Reynolds, R., and Fawcett, J.W. (2001) The oligodendrocyte precursor cell in health and disease. *Trends Neurosci.* 24:39–47.

Lin, S.-C. and Bergles, D.E. (2002) Physiological characteristics of NG2-expressing glial cells. *J. Neurocytol.* 31:537–549.

Ludwin, S.K. (1979) The perineuronal satellite oligodendrocyte. A role in remyelination. *Acta Neuropathol.* 47:49–53.

Mallon, B.S., Shick, H.E., Kidd, G.J., and Macklin, W.B. (2002) Proteolipid promoter activity distinguishes two populations of NG2-positive cells throughout neonatal cortical development. *J. Neurosci.* 22:876–885.

Matthias, K., Kirchhoff, F., Seifert, G., Huttmann, K., Matyash, M., Kettenmann, H., and Steinhauser, C. (2003) Segregated expression of AMP-type glutamate receptors and glutamate transporters defines distinct astrocyte populations in the mouse hippocampus. *J. Neurosci.* 23:1750–1758.

Mori, S. and Leblond, C.P. (1970) Electron microscopic identification of three classes of oligodendrocytes and a preliminary study of their proliferative activity in the corpus callosum of young rats. *J. Comp. Neurol.* 139:1–30.

Nishiyama, A., Lin, X.-L., Giese, N., Heldin, C.-H., and Stallcup, W.B. (1996) Co-localization of NG2 proteoglycan and PDGF α-receptor on O2A progenitor cells in the developing rat brain. *J. Neurosci. Res.* 43:299–314.

Nishiyama, A., Watanabe, M., Yang, Z., and Bu, J. (2002) Identity, distribution, and development of polydendrocytes: NG2-expressing glial cells. *J. Neurocytol.* 31:437–455.

Penfield, W. (1932) Neuroglia: normal and pathological. In: Penfield, W., ed. *Cytology and Cellular Pathology of the Nervous System*, Vol. 2. New York: Hoeber, pp. 423–479.

Peters, A. (1964) Observations on the connexions between myelin sheaths and glial cells in the optic nerves of young rats. *J. Anat.* 98:125–134.

Peters, A., Palay, S.L., and Webster, H. (1991) *The Fine Structure of the Nervous System: Neurons and their Supporting Cells*, 3rd ed. New York: Oxford University Press.

Poliak, S. and Peles, E. (2003) The local differentiation of axons at nodes of Ranvier. *Nat. Rev. Neurosci.* 4:968–980.

Popko, B. (2000) Myelin galactolipids: mediators of axon-glial interactions? *Glia* 29:149–153.

Popko, B. (2003) Notch signaling: a rheostat regulating oligodendrocyte differentiation? *Dev. Cell* 5:668–669.

Ransom, B.R., Butt, A.M., and Black, J. (1991) Ultrastructural identification of HRP-injected oligodendrocytes in the intact rat optic nerve. *Glia* 4:37–45.

Rasband, M.N., Peles, E., Trimmer, J.S., Levinson, S.R., Lux, S.E., and Shrager, P. (1999) Dependence of nodal sodium channel clustering on paranodal axoglial contact in developing CNS. *J. Neurosci.* 19:7516–7528.

Remahl, S. and Hildebrand, C. (1990a) Relation between axons and oligodendroglial cells during initial myelination. I. The glial unit. *J. Neurocytol.* 19:313–328.

Remahl, S. and Hildebrand, C. (1990b) Relation between axons and oligodendroglial cells during initial myelination. II. The individual axon. *J. Neurocytol.* 19:883–898.

Rio-Hortega P. (1928) Tercera apotación al conocimiento morfologica e interpretacion funcional de la oligodendroglia. *Mem. Real Soc. Esp. Hist. Nat. Madrid* 14:5–122.

Schools, G.P., Zhou, M., and Kimelberg, H.K. (2003) Electrophysiologically "complex" glial cells freshly isolated from the hippocampus are immunopositive for the chondroitin sulfate proteoglycan NG2. *J. Neurosci. Res.* 73:765–777.

Song, J., Goetz, B.D., Kirvell, S.L., Butt, A.M., and Duncan, I.D. (2001) Selective myelin defects in the anterior medullary velum of the *taiep* mutant rat. *Glia* 33:1–11.

Spassky, N., Olivier, C., Perez-Villegas, E., Goujet-Zalc, C., Martinez, S., Thomas, J., and Zalc, B. (2000) Single or multiple oligodendroglial lineages: a controversy. *Glia* 29:143–148.

Stallcup, W.B. and Beasley, L. (1987) Bipotential glial precursor cells of the optic nerve express the NG2 proteoglycan. *J. Neurosci.* 7:2737–2744.

Stensaas, L.J. and Stensaas, S.S. (1968) Astrocytic neuroglial cells, oligodendrocytes and microgliactyes in the spinal cord of the toad. I. Light microscopy. *Z. Zellforsch. Mikrosk. Anat.* 84:473–489.

Sternberger, N.H., Itoyama, Y., Kies, M.W., and Webster, H. de F. (1978) Myelin basic protein demonstrated immunocytochemically in oligodendroglia prior to myelin sheath formation. *Proc. Natl. Acad. Sci. USA* 75:2521–2524.

Szuchet, S. (1995) The morphology and ultrastructure of oligodendrocytes and their functional implications. In: Kettenmann, H. and Ransom, B.R., eds. *Neuroglia*. Oxford: Oxford University Press, pp. 23–43.

Wang, S.L., Sdrulla, A.D., diSibio, G., Bush, G., Nofziger, D., Hicks, C., Weinmaster, G., and Barres, B.A. (1998) Notch receptor activation inhibits oligodendrocyte differentiation. *Neuron* 21:63–75.

Yin, X., Crawford, T.O., Griffin, J.W., Tu, P., Lee, V.M., Li, C., Roder, J., and Trapp, B.D. (1998) Myelin-associated glycoprotein is a myelin signal that modulates the caliber of myelinated axons. *J. Neurosci.* 18:1953–1962.

4 Schwann cells and myelin

RUDOLF MARTINI

In the peripheral nervous system (PNS) there are different types of macroglial cells comprising perineuronal satellite cells of sensory and autonomic ganglia, the astrocyte-like glial cells of the enteric ganglia and plexus and the Schwann cells proper that are associated with axonal processes of peripheral nerves and spinal roots. The Schwann cells form the majority of the peripheral glial cells, and their origin, differentiation pathways, structural and molecular characteristics, and functional roles are best understood when compared to those of the other glial types of the peripheral nervous system.

Derived from the neural crest, two main populations develop during ontogeny, the myelinating (Fig. 4.1*A*,*B*) and the nonmyelinating Schwann cells (Fig. 4.1*B*). The latter usually collectively ensheath groups of small-caliber axons, whereas myelinating Schwann cells are always associated with one single axon of generally larger caliber. This differentiation in two groups is probably mediated by the axon. Of particular interest is the ability of Schwann cells to form myelin, a specialized structure that enables the rapid and saltatory conduction of action potentials. Recent studies not only have focused on the formation and maintenance of the internodal insulating myelin sheath, but also have disclosed the structural and molecular organization of another functionally important compartment involved in saltatory conduction, the node of Ranvier.

In addition to the myelinating and nonmyelinating Schwann cells, a third type of Schwann cells, the perisynaptic Schwann cell of the neuromuscular junction, has attracted interest due to its functional roles during neuromuscular transmission maintenance, and reinnervation of motor endplates. Besides these, there are terminal Schwann cell–like cells of the sensory system. However, their functional roles are less well understood than those of the perisynaptic Schwann cells.

This chapter will focus on the major structural characteristics of Schwann cells. Although treated in other chapters in more detail, molecular aspects will also be considered, especially where they help to clarify the cytoarchitecture of the highly organized axon–Schwann cell unit.

See the list of abbreviations at the end of the chapter.

EARLY DEVELOPMENT OF SCHWANN CELLS

Being predominantly derivatives of the neural crest (Le Douarin et al., 1991; Hagedorn et al., 1999; Paratore et al., 2002), embryonic Schwann cells travel along axon bundles during development (Billings-Gagliardi et al., 1974; Billings-Gagliardi, 1977). These cells are probably Schwann cell precursors, that is, prospective Schwann cells that still lack the ability to survive in the absence of axons (Jessen and Mirsky, 2002). In the rat, Schwann cell precursors have been identified up to embryonic days 14 and 15 and do not yet express significant levels of the glial marker S100, but show immunoreactivity for the low-affinity nerve growth factor (NGF) receptor p75 and for the cell adhesion molecules L1 and N-CAM (Martini, 1994; Dong et al., 1999) and, at a weaker level, for myelin protein 0 (P0), peripheral myelin protein 22 (PMP22), and proteolipid protein (PLP) (Mirsky and Jessen, 1999). Schwann cell precursors are not only the source for mature Schwann cells but also are pivotal cellular components for axon survival (Riethmacher et al., 1997). A role in guiding axons to their targets during development, as been proposed earlier (Noakes and Bennett, 1987), now appears less probable, since during development Schwann cell precursors follow rather than precede axons in the embryo (Billings-Gagliardi et al., 1974; Billings-Gagliardi, 1977; Sanes and Lichtman, 1999). In addition, Schwann cell precursors cannot survive when contact to axons is precluded (Jessen and Mirsky, 2002) and axons find their targets in the absence of Schwann cell precursors (Riethmacher et al., 1997).

Based on electron microscopic data (Peters and Muir, 1959; Cravioto, 1965; Billings-Gagliardi et al., 1974; Ziskind-Conhaim, 1988; Martini, 1994; Ciutat et al., 1996; Bentley and Lee, 2000), characteristic morphological features are that Schwann cell precursors are devoid of a basal lamina and intermingle with fasciculating axons extending processes between of the axon bundles (Fig. 4.2*A*,*B*). In addition, these cells are found at the margin of the prospective nerve or nerve fascicle and face the mesenchyme with their abaxonal surface (Fig. 4.2*A*).

When development proceeds, Schwann cell precursors start to form a basal lamina, proliferate, and col-

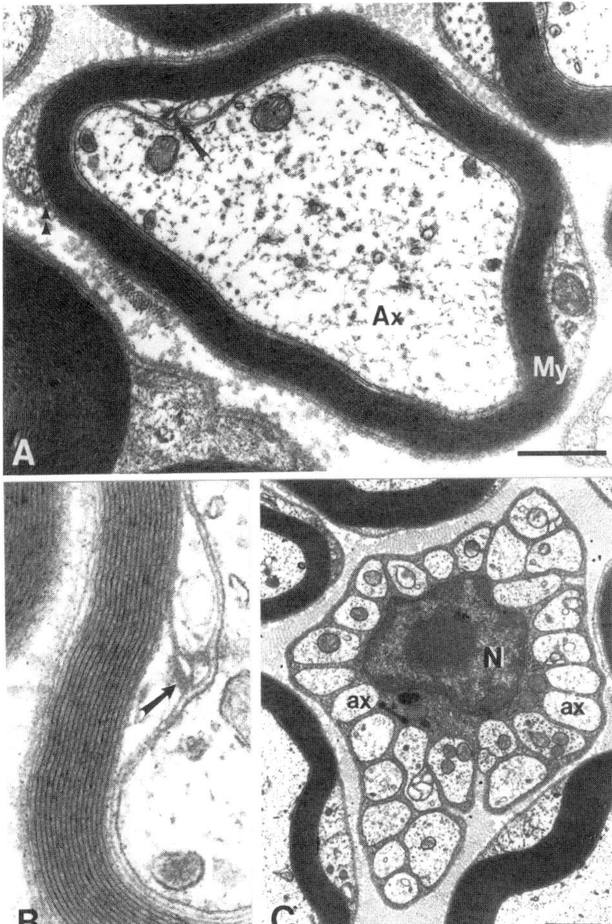

FIGURE 4.1 Two principle forms of Schwann cells are found in the peripheral nervous system: the myelinating (*A,B*) and the nonmyelinating Schwann cells (*C*). Plantar nerve of the adult mouse. *A*. Note the compacted myelin (*My*) that forms the bulk of the internodal segment. Inner (*arrow*) and outer mesaxon (*double arrowhead*) are indicated. *Ax*: axon. *B*. Higher magnification of *A* showing the inner mesaxon and its adherens-like junctions (*arrow*). Layers of compact myelin consist of major dense lines and intraperiod lines. *C*. Nonmyelinating Schwann cell cross-sectioned at the level of the nucleus (*N*). Note the rosette-like organization of the small-caliber axons (*ax*) and their ensheathment by slender Schwann cell processes. Bars: 0.5 μm (*A*), 0.25 μm (*B*), 1 μm (*C*).

lectively ensheath fasciculating axons forming so-called Schwann cell families, as initially described by Webster and colleagues (Fig. 4.2C) (Webster, 1971; Peters et al., 1991). Such glial cells probably reached the stage of *immature Schwann cells*, a term that characterizes the ability of the Schwann cells to survive independently of axons due to an autocrine survival mechanism (Lobsiger et al., 2000; Jessen and Mirsky, 2002). In the rat, all glial cells of the sciatic nerve are immature Schwann cells at embryonic day 17, whereas in the mouse, immature Schwann cells are already the main population in the nerve at embryonic day 15 (Dong et al., 1999; Jessen and Mirsky, 2002).

MATURATION AND ADULT STAGE

Ensheathment by Nonmyelinating Schwann Cells

Depending on still unknown axonal signals, immature Schwann cells develop in two directions. Those Schwann cells associated with larger-caliber axons eventually differentiate into the myelinating phenotype (see below). The Schwann cells remaining associated with small-caliber axons collectively ensheath them and eventually separate the individual axons from each other by slender processes (Fig. 4.1C). Thus, the axons are embedded in pocket-like structures. In the region of the Schwann cell nucleus, cross-cut axons are found

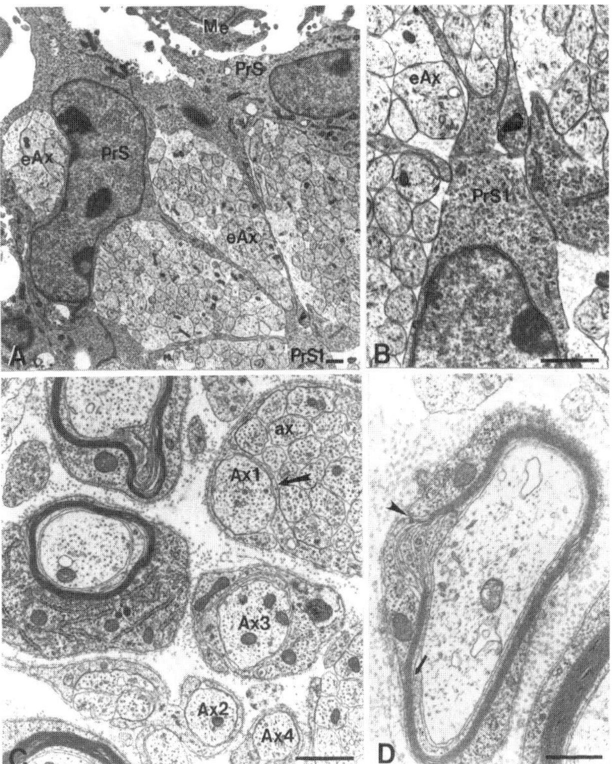

FIGURE 4.2 Developing peripheral nerve of the mouse. *A,B*. Sciatic nerve of a mouse at embryonic day 13. Schwann cell precursor cells (*PrS*) form a sheath-like structure around the embryonic axon bundles (*eAx*), and slender processes protrude between them (*A*). A Schwann cell precursor in a more central position of the nerve is also visible (*PrS1*) and is presented at a higher magnification in *B*. Basal laminae are not detectable around the Schwann cell precursor cells. Me: mesenchymal cell. *C,D*. Femoral nerve of the 4-day-old mouse. In *C*, two axons of larger caliber display a thin sheath of compacted myelin. The upper fiber shows a redundant myelin profile. An axon of larger caliber (*Ax1*) is positioned at the periphery of a bundle of prospective nonmyelinated axons (*ax*) and is separated from them by a process of the immature Schwann cell (*arrow*). Another axon (*Ax2*) is in a similar position. Ax3 and Ax4 have reached the promyelin stage. In *D*, the Schwann cell process has formed around six layers of compacted myelin. Note the stagged, noncompacted aspects reminiscent of a Schmidt-Lanterman incisure and the inner (*arrow*) and outer mesaxons (*arrowhead*). Bars: 1 μm (*A,B*), 1 μm (*C*), 0.5 μm (*D*).

at the periphery of the Schwann cell soma and show a rosette-like organization around the nucleus (Fig. 4.1C). In this position, the axons are often only partially covered by Schwann cell processes and are in direct apposition with the Schwann cell basal lamina. Mature nonmyelinating Schwann cells share a couple of cell surface molecules with immature Schwann cells that are not found on myelinating Schwann cells, such as the cell adhesion molecules L1, neural cell adhesion molecule (N-CAM) and the NGF receptor p75 (Martini, 1994; Jessen and Mirsky, 2002).

Although nonmyelinating Schwann cells are morphologically and molecularly distinct from myelinating Schwann cells, they can adopt a myelinating phenotype under experimental conditions. This has been impressively demonstrated by cross-anastomosis of sympathetic trunks and sciatic nerves. In this model, large-caliber axons growing into distal stumps of sympathetic trunks can initiate myelin formation in Schwann cells that were originally associated with small-caliber axons and displayed a nonmyelinating phenotype (Weinberg and Spencer, 1975; Aguayo et al., 1976a, 1976b).

Formation of the Myelin Internode

The increase in caliber of some axons that fasciculate within the confinements of immature Schwann cells leads to a separation of these prospective myelinated axons. They are positioned peripherally within the axon bundle and achieve a so-called 1:1 ratio with immature Schwann cells (Fig. 4.2C). Schwann cells at this stage are called *pro-myelinating*, since they precede proper myelin formation. At around this stage, many cell surface molecules related to immature or nonmyelinating Schwann cells are downregulated, whereas typical myelin molecules, such as P0, myelin-associated glycoprotein (MAG), PMP22, myelin basic protein (MBP) and periaxin are strongly upregulated at the pro-myelinating stage or shortly afterward (Martini, 1994; Jessen and Mirsky, 2002). In rodents, the generation of pro-myelinating Schwann cells occurs at around birth. However, myelin formation in the PNS is not a highly synchronized event. Axons with large calibers receive their myelin sheath earlier than smaller-caliber axons, so some pro-myelin stages can still be found in mice at approximately 3 weeks of age.

The pro-myelin stage is followed by spiral formation of one of the Schwann cell processes engulfing the axon (Fig. 4.2C). The apposition of Schwann cell membranes at the inner, axon-related site of the Schwann cell process is called *inner mesaxon*, whereas the contact of Schwann cell membranes at the endoneurial site is termed *outer mesaxon* (Fig. 4.1*B*, 4.2*D*). These cell contacts are characterized by the formation of epithelial (E)-cadherin-positive adherens (desmosome-like) junctions (Fig. 4.1*B*) (Fannon et al., 1995) and tight junctions (Scherer and Arroyo, 2002). In an elegant study, Richard P. Bunge and colleagues (Bunge et al., 1989) investigated the interesting question of which end of the Schwann cell—that is, the inner or outer one—turns around the axon during myelination. For this purpose, living rat Schwann cells cocultured with dorsal root ganglion neurons were video-recorded for up to 70 hours, followed by their investigation at the electron microscopic level (Fig. 4.3). These studies revealed that it is predominantly the inner, axon-related Schwann cell process that makes the turn around the axon and that the cell soma containing the nucleus is dragged behind at a much slower speed than the inner lip of the axon-related end of the Schwann cell process. This view is in line with older models stating that insertion of myelin components (e.g., radio-labeled lipids) (Peters et al., 1991) occurs along the entire extension of the developing spiral. Thus, relatively rapid turning of the inner lip of a relatively slowly moving Schwann cell body and the simultaneous overall insertion of myelin membrane components appear to be some of the characteristic events during myelin formation in the PNS.

In vivo studies revealed the myelinating process to be more complicated than just a spiral formation of the inner Schwann cell process around the axon. For instance, irregular forms with thin, redundant myelin loops are often observed in nerves of young rodents (Fig. 4.2C). In addition, the myelinating process in the internodal region near the Schwann cell nucleus turns at a higher speed around the axon than does the same process at the level of the Schwann cell edges, that is, near the prospective node of Ranvier. A comprehensive overview of the morphological events during myelin formation is summarized by Webster and colleagues (Webster, 1971; Peters et al., 1991).

A striking subcellular feature of myelinating glial cells is the compaction of the apposing membranes of the turning myelin spiral (Figs. 4.1*A*,*B*, 4.2*C*,*D*). In the case of the rodent Schwann cells, this starts after completion of several turns of the Schwann cell process around the axon. Two morphogenetic events occur nearly simultaneously, namely, (*1*) the narrowing of the spiraling cell surface membranes from approximately 12 nm to approximately 2 nm and (*2*) the "squeezing out" of cytoplasm. The collapsed cytoplasmatic sites of the Schwann cell membranes fuse and form a 3.5-nm-wide electron-dense band called the *major dense line*; the membrane leaflets facing the extracellular space of the spiral form the *intraperiod line*, which is double-stranded due to the 2-nm-wide gap separating the extracellular leaflets (Fig. 4.1*B*) (Peters et al., 1991).

The compaction of the Schwann cell membrane is a unique feature and therefore requires distinct molecular mechanisms that mediate this process. A pivotal molecular mediator for myelin compaction in the PNS is

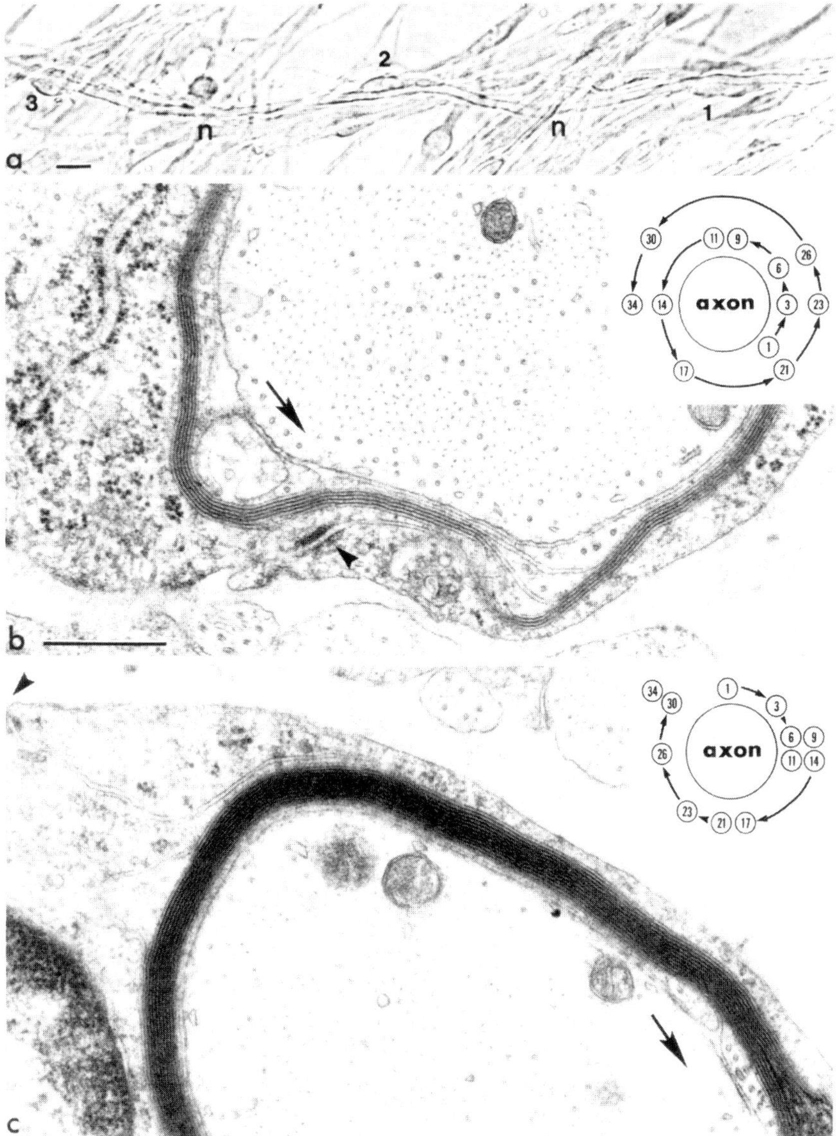

FIGURE 4.3 Light microscopic (*a*) and electron micrographs (*b,c*) of a profile of a myelinated nerve fiber grown *in vitro*. In *a*, three internodes (*1–3*) are visible. These internodes were investigated for 34 hours and nuclear movements were recorded. The insets in *b* and *c* show the position of the nuclei of internodes 1 (*b*) and 3 (*c*) at distinct time points. The electron micrographs show the direction of the inner lip of the myelinating Schwann cells (*arrows*). Note that movement of Schwann cell nuclei (insets) and of the corresponding inner lip (electron micrograph) are always in the same direction. Bars: 10 μm (*a*), 0.5 μm (*b,c*). (Courtesy of Dr. M. Bunge [Bunge et al., 1989] with copyright permission of The Rockefeller University Press.)

the cell adhesion molecule P0, also designated *myelin protein zero* (MPZ). It mediates homophilic adhesion leading to the close apposition of the extracellular aspects of the spiraling Schwann cell membrane forming the intraperiod line (reviewed in Martini and Schachner, 1997). This model received strong support from the determination of the three-dimensional structure of the extracellular domain of P0 by X-ray crystallography (Shapiro et al., 1996). The intracellular domain of P0 contains predominantly basic residues that have been suggested to interact with negatively charged phospholipids of the adjacent cytoplasmic parts of the Schwann cell membrane leading to the formation of the major dense line (Kirschner and Ganser, 1980; Lemke et al., 1988; Ding and Brunden, 1994). In addition, a role in signal transduction appears probable (Xu et al., 2001). Final proof that P0 mediates myelin development and compaction was provided by mice deficient in this molecule that show severe dysmyelination with disturbed myelin compaction (Giese et al., 1992; Martini et al., 1995).

Immature myelin sheaths are characterized by relatively expanded sites of still uncompacted myelin containing cytoplasm (Fig. 4.2*C,D*). During maturation, however, uncompacted myelin becomes restricted to distinct sites, such as the periaxonal collar (Fig. 4.1*B*), the outer Schwann cell loop (Fig. 4.1*B*), the paranodal loops (see below), and the Schmidt-Lanterman incisures. The last are cytoplasmic clefts that connect the periaxonal with the perinuclear (abaxonal) Schwann cell cytoplasm. In longitudinal sections of osmium tetroxide–fixed tissue, they can be identified by light microscopy as slim, bright lines obliquely transversing the myelin. In teased fiber preparations labeled for markers of noncompacted myelin [e.g., MAG, connexin 32 (Cx32)], Schmidt-Lanterman incisures appear as funnel-like profiles (Arroyo et al., 1999; Arroyo and Scherer, 2000; Scherer and Arroyo, 2002). Electron microscopy reveals that they consist of slender pockets of cytoplasm that form a helical funnel. Based on the observation that these cytoplasmic domains are Cx32-positive, it has been speculated that they form a rapid, radial cytoplasmic pathway for ions and small molecules between adaxonal and abaxonal Schwann cell cytoplasm (Scherer et al., 1995). Interestingly, recent immunohistochemical studies on teased fiber preparations revealed that Caspr1/paranodin and the voltage-gated K^+ channels Kv1.1 and 1.2 demarcate the axonal domain underlying the inner loop of the Schmidt-Lanterman incisures (Arroyo et al., 1999; Arroyo and Scherer, 2000; Scherer and Arroyo, 2002).

The Node of Ranvier

During the past few years, substantial progress in the understanding of the sophisticated molecular and cytological architecture of the node of Ranvier has been achieved (Arroyo et al., 1999; Arroyo and Scherer, 2000; Peles and Salzer, 2000; Arroyo, 2002; Poliak and Peles, 2003). The outer cytoplasmic aspect of the Schwann cells ends in the nodal region with microvilli-like protrusions that abut the nodal plasmalemma (Fig. 4.4*A,C,E*). These

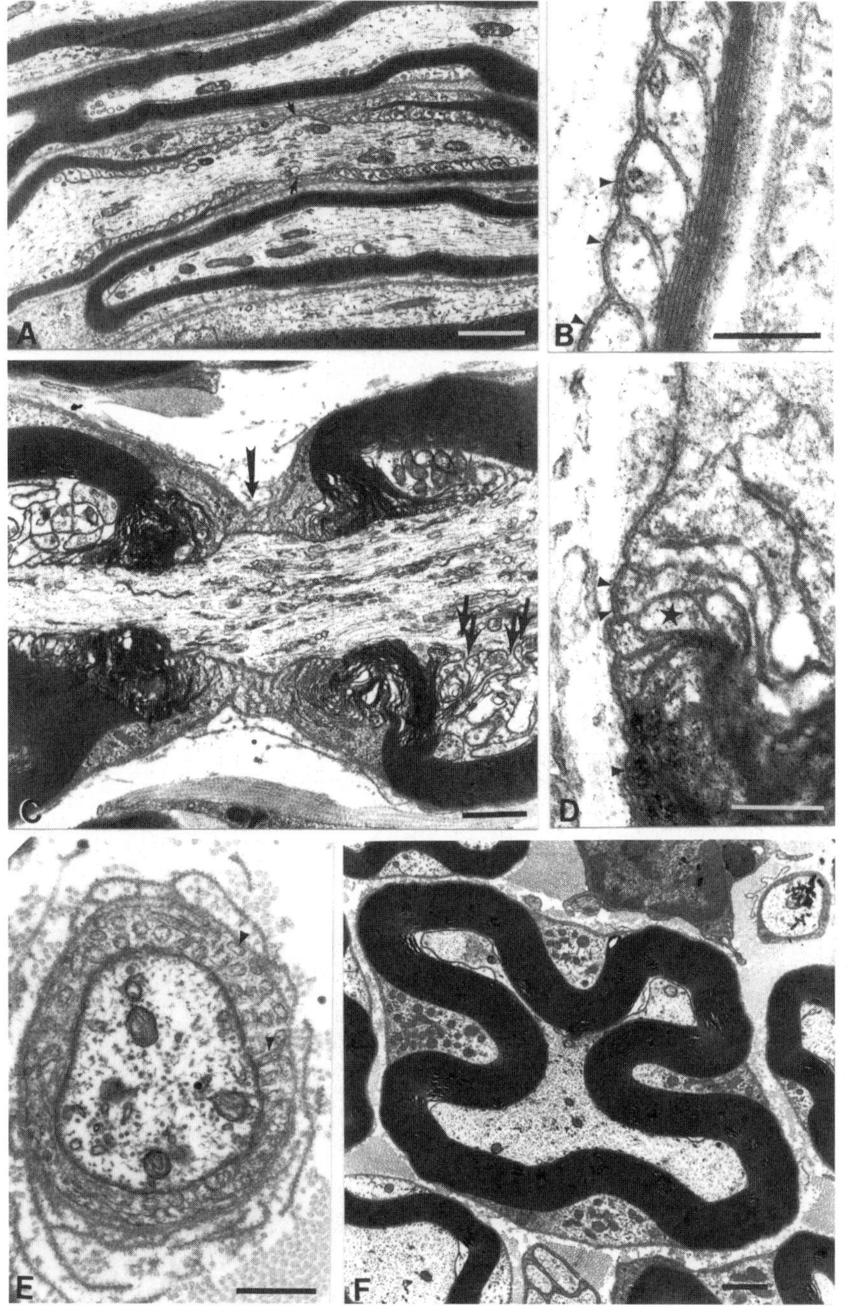

FIGURE 4.4 Nodal, paranodal, and juxtaparanodal aspects of the peripheral nerve of the adult mouse. *A,B*. Longitudinal section of the nodal region of a nerve fiber of small diameter. Small arrows in *A* indicate the node proper. The "regular" organization of the paranodal loops is characteristic, with each loop abutting the axolemma. Septate-like junctions are indicated by arrowheads (*B*). *C,D*. Longitudinal section of a nodal region of a larger-caliber nerve fiber. Note that magnifications are the same as in *A* and *B*. The arrow indicates the node proper. The organization of paranodal loops appears less regular, and some do not reach the axolemma (*asterisk* in *D*). Septate-like junctions are indicated by arrowheads. In *C*, the juxtaparanodal regions are conspicuous as typical of larger-caliber axons. Note the interdigitation between the inner Schwann cell loops and the protruding axolemma (*double arrows*). *E*. Cross section of a node of Ranvier. Nodal microvilli are indicated by arrowheads, and the typical electron-dense undercoating of the nodal axolemma is visible. *F*. Cross section of a juxtaparanodal region of a larger-caliber axon. Note the trefoil-like structure of the axon and the compact myelin sheath. Bars: 1 μm (*A,C,F*), 0.25 μm (*B,D*), 0.5 μm (*E*).

protrusions contain actin filaments (Trapp et al., 1989) and the typical microvilli-related cytoskeletal components ezrin, radixin, and moesin (ERM proteins) (Melendez-Vasquez et al., 2001; Scherer et al., 2001). The ERM proteins may bind to the actin filaments linking the cytoskeleton to integral membrane components, possibly adhesion molecules. It is assumed that ERM-linked adhesion molecules of the microvilli interact with cell surface molecules of the axolemma, possibly stabilizing these nodal cell surface components in their characteristic position (Bennett et al., 1997; Melendez-Vasquez et al., 2001; Scherer et al., 2001). In a recent in vitro study, Schwann cells have been shown to insert nodal microvilli compounds into growth cone-like structures. This process is mediated by Rho-stimulation and might increase the efficiency of node formation (Gatto et al., 2003). The nodal microvilli and the nodal axolemma are surrounded by an extracellular matrix consisting of tenascin-C and the proteoglycan NG2 (Arroyo et al., 1999; Arroyo and Scherer, 2000; Peles and Salzer, 2000; Martin et al., 2001).

The nodal axolemma is characterized by a typical electron-dense undercoating (Fig. 4.4*E*). In this region, cytoskeletal components, such as ankyrin-G and spectrin, are highly enriched and may organize the accumulation of the neuron-glia-related cell adhesion molecule (Nr-CAM) and neurofascin 186 and the typical clustering of the voltage-gated Na^+ channels (Fig. 4.5) (Bennett et al., 1997; Scherer and Arroyo, 2002). Therefore, it is plausible to assume that the electron-dense undercoating of the nodal axolemma is at least partially related to the accumulation of cytoskeletal elements. Other cytoskeletal components are neurotubules and neurofilaments. Characteristically, the latter components are at the low phosphorylation stage, as opposed to their internodal counterparts (Arroyo and Scherer, 2000). The low phosphorylation level may be related to the tapering of axon diameter at the nodal region (de Waegh et al., 1992).

Another distinct compartment of the nodal region consists of the paranodes. In longitudinal sections, myelin lamellae end as cytoplasmic pockets that abut the paranodal axolemma (Fig. 4.4*B,D*). Adaxonal myelin lamellae end farther from the node proper than the more abaxonal ones (Fig. 4.4*A*). Similar to the Schmidt-Lanterman incisures, they form a helix-shaped cytoplasmic band that connects the periaxonal with the abaxonal Schwann cell cytoplasm. Forming reflexive Cx32-positive gap junctions, both paranodal pockets and Schmidt-Lanterman incisures, may be used as rapid radial pathways between periaxonal and abaxonal cytoplasm (Balice-Gordon et al., 1998). Typical features of paranodal loops are adherens (desmosome-like) junctions that connect the paranodal pockets at their lateral sites. These junctions may be formed and stabilized by the Ca^{2+}-dependent adhesion molecule E-cadherin, which is expressed there (Fannon et al., 1995). Other subcellular components of the paranodal loops are microtubules that are helically oriented with respect to the longitudinal axis of the axon, so that they appear cross-cut in longitudinal nerve sections.

The paranodal pockets appear tightly associated with the paranodal axolemma. With conventional aldehyde fixation, the axolemma appears "scalopped" due to a slight protrusion of the convex axon–associated surfaces of the paranodal pockets into the axon surface

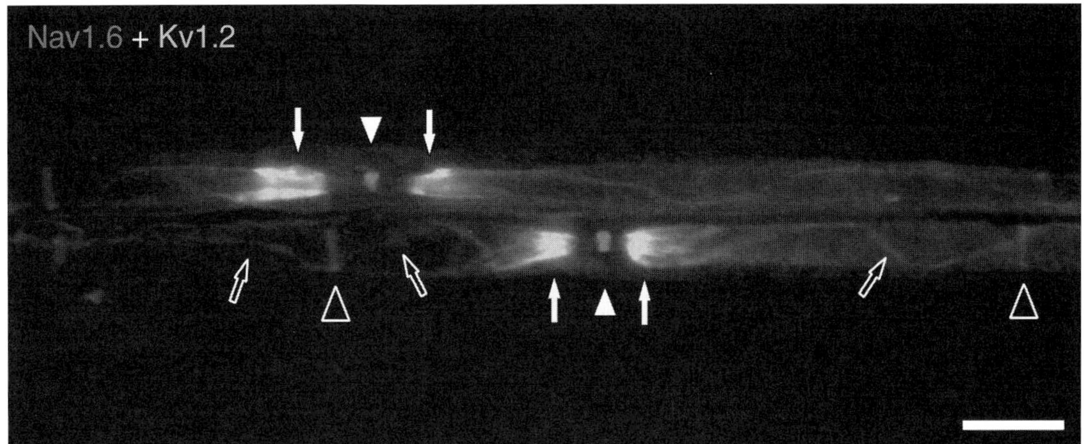

FIGURE 4.5 Two larger-caliber fibers isolated from the femoral nerve of the adult mouse and immunolabeled with antibodies to voltage-gated Na^+ (Nav 1.6) and K^+ channels (Kv 1.2). Note the nodal and juxtaparanodal position of Na^+ (*white arrowheads*) and K^+ channels (*white arrows*), respectively. Paranodal aspects appear as nonlabeled gaps between the Na^+ and K^+ channels. In addition to the juxtaparanodal accumulation, K^+ channels are weakly expressed at internodal aspects, such as the inner mesaxon (*black arrows*) and Schmidt-Lanterman incisures (*black arrowheads*). (Courtesy of Dr. Jochen Ulzheimer, Würzburg.) Bar: 10 μm.

(Fig. 4.4*B,D*). In addition, septate junctions form from the axonal surface and abut the paranodal Schwann cell membrane (Fig. 4.4*B,D*). Recent studies have focused on the molecular composition of these electron-dense bands and their putative functional roles. Two groups have independently identified a novel axonal component of these bands initially designated *contactin-associated protein* (*Caspr*) or *paranodin* (Einheber et al., 1997; Menegoz et al., 1997; Peles et al., 1997b). Due to the homology to the septate junction–related PDZ-related protein neurexin-IV in *Drosophila* (Peles et al., 1997a), the molecule has also been designated neurexin-Caspr-Paranodin (NCP1) (Bhat et al., 2001). The Caspr-contactin complex appears to trans-interact with neurofascin 155, an adhesive molecule of the immunoglobulin (Ig) superfamily (Tait et al., 2000; Charles et al., 2002). Possibly, the binding activity of neurofascin 155 is modulated by a novel, paranodal glial comopnent, CD9 (Ishibashi et al., 2004).

Depending on the size of the axon, there are in principle two different forms of paranodal regions (Phillips et al., 1972; Peters et al., 1991; Berthold, 1996) (compare Figs. 4.4*A* and 4.4*C*). In smaller-caliber fibers the cytoplasmic pockets approach the axon tangentially, and each pocket reaches the axolemma (Fig. 4.4*A,B*). They generally appear well organized. In larger-caliber fibers, the pockets approximate the axolemma in a steep and almost perpendicular fashion, and not all pockets reach the axolemma (Fig. 4.4*C,D*). They are usually smaller and often appear much more electron-dense than the pockets of the smaller-caliber axons. Due to these characteristics and to the fact that myelin structures of larger fibers are more prone to show fixation artifacts than small-caliber fibers, the paranodes of thick fibers often appear to be less organized structures than paranodes of the smaller fibers (Fig. 4.4*C*).

Another region of interest is the compartment near the paranodes, the juxtaparanodal region. From the morphological point of view, this compartment is particularly conspicuous in larger-caliber fibers (Fig. 4.4*C,F*). Due to the tapering of larger-caliber axons, the myelin sheath appears fluted, so that in cross sections the myelin sheath and the axon are cross-shaped or acquire the form of a trefoil (Fig. 4.4*F*). Here, the outer Schwann cell cytoplasm "fills" the grooves of the folded myelin and shows an accumulation of mitochondria. The axon–Schwann cell apposition often shows a complicated organization due to a profound interdigitation of inner Schwann cell loop and axolemma called the *axon-Schwann cell network* (Fig. 4.4*C*). In longitudinal sections, a striking asymmetry is often detectable in that the axon–Schwann cell network is much more conspicuous at the distal aspect of the nodal region than at the proximal one. In addition, axonal lysosomes containing acid phosphatase are found more frequently in the distal regions (Gatzinsky, 1996).

In the past, some authors included the juxtaparanodal region in the paranodal compartment (Berthold, 1996), but recent studies clearly demonstrate that the molecular characteristics of paranodal and juxtaparanodal sites are clearly distinct. For instance, Caspr 2, a molecule related to Caspr/NCP1, and the K^+ channel isoforms Kv1.1 and Kv 1.2 (Poliak et al., 1999) demarcate the juxtaparanodes (Fig. 4.5). During development, Caspr 2 and the K^+ channels are first expressed at the paranodal site and then shift to their final destination when Caspr is upregulated (Poliak et al., 2001). Transiently expressed axonal-surface glycoprotein 1 (TAG-1), a glycosylphosphatidylinositol-linked member of the Ig superfamily, has recently been localized at the juxtaparanodal region of developing and mature myelinated fibers. Its role at that position is still obscure, but the colocalization with voltage-gated K^+ channels suggests a participation in the distribution of the channels (Traka et al., 2002). From the physiological point of view, Kv1.1 and Kv 1.2 might buffer K^+ ions released by neuronal activity and might thus contribute to the maintenance of excitability of the nerve fiber under conditions of high activity.

The Schwann Cell Basal Lamina

As opposed to their myelinating counterparts in the central nervous system (CNS), the oligodendrocytes, Schwann cells typically form a basal lamina around their abaxonal cytoplasmic membrane (Figs. 4.1–4.4). Thus, the Schwann cell corresponds to a polarized cell with a highly specialized "apical," adaxonal compartment and a "basal" side represented by the abaxonal membrane that is separated from the mesenchymal endoneurial compartment by the basal lamina. In longitudinal sections, the Schwann cell basal lamina forms a continuous tube that even bridges the nodal gaps (Fig. 4.4*A,C,E*). The major Schwann cell basal lamina constituents are the extracellular matrix components laminin-2 (merosin), heparansulfate proteoglycans (e.g., perlecan, agrin), collagen type IV, and fibronectin (Chernousov and Carey, 2000). Since some of the extracellular matrix components of the basal lamina promote axonal growth, it is an important guidance structure under regenerative conditions (Martini, 1994; Stoll and Müller, 1999).

The role of the basal lamina in the process of myelination was initially investigated in the laboratory of Richard P. Bunge. In a sophisticated cell culture system, prevention of basal lamina secretion by omitting vitamin C in the medium blocked Schwann cell maturation and eventually myelin formation (Eldridge et al., 1987). Furthermore, addition of exogeneous basal lamina enabled the Schwann cells to form myelin in the absence of vitamin C (Eldridge et al., 1989). The interpretation of these findings was that Schwann cells need a solid scaffold, as provided by the basal lamina during the spiral formation of the adaxonal membrane. An additional hint that basal lamina formation is crucial for myelination is provided by the dysmyelinating phenotype of dystrophic mice, which are deficient in a major constituent of the Schwann cell basal lamina, laminin-2 (Matsumura et al., 1997).

Recent investigators consider the cell-substrate signaling mediated by the basal lamina component laminin 2 and the corresponding receptors of the abaxonal Schwann cell membrane as a pivotal prerequisite for Schwann cell differentiation. A recently established Schwann cell–related laminin receptor is the dystroglycan-dystrophin-related protein 2 (DRP2), which forms a complex with $\alpha\beta$-dystroglycan that interacts with laminin of the Schwann cell basal lamina (Sherman et al., 2001). Other Schwann cell–related laminin receptors are integrin heterodimers, such as $\alpha6/\beta1$ and $\alpha6/\beta4$ (Previtali et al., 2001). Function-blocking anti-$\beta1$ integrin antibodies prevent myelination *in vitro* (Fernandez-Valle et al., 1994). Furthermore, Schwann cell–specific gene inactivation of $\beta1$ leads to a severe dysmyelinating phenotype with impaired axonal sorting (Feltri et al., 2002). Although regulated similarly to myelin proteins (Einheber et al., 1993; Feltri et al., 1994), $\beta4$-integrin appears to be redundant during myelination, since absence of this component does not interfere with initial myelin formation *in vivo* or *in vitro* (Frei et al., 1999).

Relationship of Axon Diameter–Myelin Thickness and Axon Diameter–Internodal Length

An interesting question concerns the regulation of myelin thickness. A striking feature is the positive correlation between axonal caliber and myelin thickness. This is clearly reflected by the observation that the quotient between axon diameter and fiber diameter (taken at the outer aspect of the myelin sheath) is generally constant when axons of different diameters are compared (Friede and Beuche, 1985). A similarly constant ratio exists between internodal length and axon diameter in the adult nerve. Quantitative studies in various species revealed that a normal internode of a mature peripheral nerve is usually 100 times as long as the diameter of the corresponding axon (Friede and Beuche, 1985). However, developmental studies in nerves with a robust growth in length during maturation in the absence of Schwann cell proliferation modified this simple view, as shown in phrenic nerves in rabbits and several peripheral nerves in humans (Friede and Beuche, 1985; Schröder et al., 1988). In young rabbits, myelin sheaths are relatively thin for axon diameter followed by an increase in myelin thickness (Friede and Beuche, 1985). An extreme case is found in various peripheral nerves in humans, where radial growth of axons is finished at 5 years of age, whereas the corresponding myelin grows in thickness until the age of 17 years (Schröder et al., 1988). In rat tibial nerve branches supplying either the plantar or calf muscles, maximal axonal growth in diameter occurs between 3 weeks and 3 months. Here, the developmental change in relative myelin thickness is not uniform, since myelin sheaths of fibers of different caliber might behave in a slightly different way during development (Fraher et al., 1990).

PERISYNAPTIC (TERMINAL) SCHWANN CELLS OF THE NEUROMUSCULAR JUNCTION (TELOGLIA CELLS) AND SCHWANN-LIKE CELLS OF SENSORY CORPUSCLES

As described above, large-caliber axons usually induce myelination in adjacent Schwann cells. One exception is the perisynaptic Schwann cell at the neuromuscular junction. It forms an ensheathing structure around terminal axon branches and synaptic boutons and is covered by a basal lamina that fuses with that of the muscle fiber and with that of the motor endplate. Interestingly, the presynaptic membranes of the boutons are preserved from being ensheathed, whereas the axon terminals connecting the boutons are mostly entirely wrapped by the cells (Georgiou and Charlton, 1999).

Perisynaptic Schwann cells have many functions. During development, the cells contribute to the maturation and extension of the motor endplate as has been shown by immune ablation using an antibody against perisynaptic Schwann cells and complement (Herrera et al., 2000; Reddy et al., 2003). The same approach revealed that the cells stabilize the presynapse of the neuromuscular junction (Reddy et al., 2003). During normal function in the adult, the cells regulate the efficacy of synaptic transmission and neurotransmitter (acetylcholine) release by modulating perisynaptic Ca^{2+} concentration (Jahromi et al., 1992; Robitaille, 1998; Castonguay and Robitaille, 2001; Rochon et al., 2001). In this context, it is interesting that the perisynaptic cells show a Ca^{2+} response to presynaptic acetylcholine release by means of their muscarinic acetylcholine receptors (Rochon et al., 2001). Upon nerve injury, the perisynaptic Schwann cells upregulate growth associated protein-43 (GAP-43) and extend multiple processes along the muscle fiber that might guide regrowing motor axons toward their denervated endplates (Woolf et al., 1992; Love et al., 2003). Additionally, denervated perisynaptic Schwann cells upregulate the active form of the extracellular matrix component agrin and can induce aggregation of acetylcholine receptors at extrasynaptic sites of denervated muscle fibers (Yang et al., 2001).

Although they are associated with terminal axon branches that are not substantially smaller in diameter than myelin-competent axons, perisynaptic Schwann cells do not form myelin. The underlying mechanisms are not yet known, but it is possible that these cells are somehow inhibited from forming a myelin sheath. In addition, these cells are prevented from completely ensheathing the presynaptic membranes of the terminal boutons by the synaptic basal lamina–associated extracellular matrix component laminin 11 containing the synapse-specific laminin $\beta 2$ (Patton et al., 1988; Sanes and Lichtman, 1999). Although perisynaptic Schwann cells do not form myelin, they express typical myelin-related molecules, such as galactocerebroside, 2′,3′-cyclic nucleotide 3′-phosphodiesterase, MAG, and P0. Interestingly, the last two components show a distinct spatial expression pattern in that P0 is found on more extended aspects of the Schwann cell surface, whereas MAG, like myelinating Schwann cells, is confined to the adaxonal membrane (Fig. 4.6; Georgiou and Charlton, 1999). In addition, perisynaptic Schwann cells express cell adhesion molecules that are usually confined to nonmyelinating Schwann cells, such as L1 and N-CAM (Covault and Sanes, 1986; Sanes et al., 1986).

Schwann cell–like cells devoid of myelin and associated with terminal regions of myelinated axons are also found in the sensory part of the nervous system. One example is the multilamellar cells of the inner core of Pacinian corpuscles that express the Schwann cell marker S100. Similar to nonmyelinating Schwann cells, they constitutively express N-CAM, but L1 expression is confined to developmental stages (Nolte et al., 1989). Thus, these cells might share molecular features of both myelinating (L1 negativity in adulthood) and nonmyelinating Schwann cells (maintenance of N-CAM positivity). The lamellar cells of Meissner's corpuscles also express S100 and transiently the low-affinity NGF receptor p75, possibly reminiscent of the downregulation of p75 in myelinating Schwann cells (Albuerne et al., 2000).

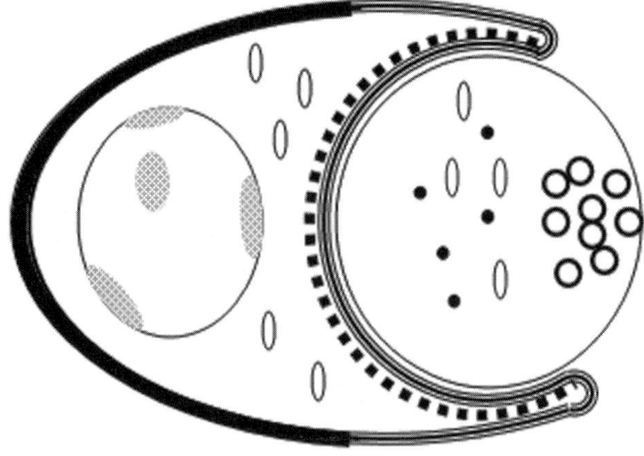

FIGURE 4.6 Schematic representation of a perisynaptic Schwann cell at the neuromuscular junction. Distribution of myelin-associated glycoprotein (*broken line*) and of myelin protein 0 (*triple line*) is indicated. (Adapted from (Georgiou and Charlton, 1999.)

SUMMARY AND PERSPECTIVES

Schwann cells are the major glial cells of the PNS. Dependent on still unknown axonal cues, two principal phenotypes develop, the myelinating and nonmyelinating Schwann cells. The myelinating Schwann cells have a pivotal role in the saltatory propagation of action potentials. The node of Ranvier is the myelin-related compartment responsible for the generation of the action potential. Both nodal and paranodal axolemmas, as well as the corresponding Schwann cell domains, are highly specialized due to a presumably intimate cell-cell communication between axon and myelinating glia that eventually leads to the functionally important clustering of Na^+ and K^+ channels at the nodal and juxtaparanodal sites, respectively. The internode consists of compacted myelin, a membrane specialization that is unique to the nervous system. It is interrupted by the Schmidt-Lanterman incisures that might direct the position of internodal K^+ channels and functionally connects the perinuclear and adaxonal Schwann cell cytoplasm. Another example of an intimate communication between axons and myelinating Schwann cells is the relatively constant ratio between axon diameter, myelin thickness, and internodal length. Both the myelinating and nonmyelinating Schwann cells are surrounded by a basal lamina that not only forms the demarcation to the mesenchymal environment within the nerve, but also appears to be essential for the differentiation of the cells. In addition to the two major Schwann cell groups, less conspicuous cells, such as synaptic terminal Schwann cells, might have important functions during formation of the cytoarchitecture of the neuromuscular junction and during neuromuscular transmission. Thus, Schwann cells are essential determinants of the functional integrity of the peripheral part of the axon, and it is not surprising that disorders primarily affecting the Schwann cells have serious consequences for axon structure, nodal organization, and axon survival. Therefore, knowledge of the basic biology of Schwann cells is not only helpful in understanding peripheral nerve development and function, but is also instrumental in comprehending the features of glia-related neurological disorders of the PNS. Moreover, the still unknown axonal cues initiating myelination and determining myelin thickness and Schwann cell extension along the axon are of outstanding interest for future studies.

ACKNOWLEDGMENTS

The author is grateful to Dr. Mary Bunge (Miami) and The Rockefeller University Press for permission for reproduction of Figure 4.3. Many thanks also to all the colleagues at my laboratory, especially Dr. Jochen Ulzheimer, Heinrich Blazyca, and Carolin Kiesel, for their patient assistance in generating the figures. The author is grateful to Dr. Claudia Sommer for reading the manuscript and to Dr. Jochen Ulzheimer for providing Figure 4.5.

ABBREVIATIONS

Caspr	contactin-associated protein
CNS	central nervous system
Cx32	connexin 32 (kDa)
DRP2	dystroglycan-dystrophin-related protein 2
E-cadherin	epithelial cadherin
ERM proteins	ezrin, radixin, moesin proteins
GAP-43	growth-associated protein-43
Ig	immunoglobulin
MAG	myelin-associated glycoprotein
MBP	myelin basic protein
N-CAM	neural cell adhesion molecule
NCP1	Neurexin-caspr-paranodin 1
NGF	nerve growth factor
Nr-CAM	neuron-glia-related cell adhesion molecule
P0	(myelin) protein 0 (zero)
PDZ	postsynaptic density protein 95, *Drosophila* discs large tumor suppressor, zonula occludens-1
PLP	proteolipid protein
PMP22	peripheral myelin protein 22 (kDa)
PNS	peripheral nervous system
TAG-1	transiently expressed axonal-surface glycoprotein 1

REFERENCES

Aguayo, A.J., Charron, L., and Bray, G.M. (1976a) Potential of Schwann cells from unmyelinated nerves to produce myelin: a quantitative ultrastructural and radiographic study. *J. Neurocytol.* 5:565–573.

Aguayo, A.J., Epps, J., Charron, L., and Bray, G.M. (1976b) Multipotentiality of Schwann cells in cross-anastomosed and grafted myelinated and unmyelinated nerves: quantitative microscopy and radioautography. *Brain Res.* 104:1–20.

Albuerne, M., De Lavallina, J., Esteban, I., Naves, F.J., Silos-Santiago, I., and Vega, J.A. (2000) Development of Meissner-like and Pacinian sensory corpuscles in the mouse demonstrated with specific markers for corpuscular constituents. *Anat. Rec.* 258:235–242.

Arroyo, E.J. and Scherer, S.S. (2000) On the molecular architecture of myelinated fibers. *Histochem. Cell Biol.* 113:1–18.

Arroyo, E.J., Xu, Y.-T., Zhou, L., Messing, A., Peles, E., Chiu, S.Y., and Scherer, S.S. (1999) Myelinating Schwann cells determine the internodal localization of Kv1.1, Kv1.2, Kvβ2, and Caspr. *J. Neurocytol.* 28:333–347.

Balice-Gordon, R.J., Bone, L.J., and Scherer, S.S. (1998) Functional gap junctions in the Schwann cell myelin sheath. *J. Cell Biol.* 142:1095–1104.

Bennett, V., Lambert, S., Davis, J.Q., and Zhang, X. (1997) Molecular architecture of the specialized axonal membrane at the node of Ranvier. *Soc. Gen. Physiol. Series* 52:107–120.

Bentley, C.A. and Lee, K.F. (2000) p75 is important for axon growth and Schwann cell migration during development. *J. Neurosci.* 20:7706–77015.

Berthold, C.H. (1996) Development of nodes of Ranvier in feline nerves: an ultrastructural presentation. *Microsc. Res. Technique* 34:399–421.

Bhat, M.A., Rios, J.C., Lu, Y., Garcia-Fresco, G.P., Ching, W. St Martin, M., Li, J., Einheber, S., Chesler, M., Rosenbluth, J., Salzer, J.L., and Bellen, H.J. (2001) Axon-glia interactions and the domain organization of myelinated axons requires neurexin IV/Caspr/Paranodin. *Neuron* 30:369–383.

Billings-Gagliardi, S. (1977) Mode of locomotion of Schwann cells migrating in vivo. *Am. J. Anat.* 150:73–88.

Billings-Gagliardi, S., Webster, H.D., and O'Connel, M.F. (1974) In vivo and electron microscopic observations on Schwann cells in developing tadpole nerve fibers. *Am. J. Anat.* 141:375–392.

Bunge, R.P., Bunge, M.B., and Bates, M. (1989) Movements of the Schwann cell nucleus implicate progression of the inner (axon-related) Schwann cell process during myelination. *J. Cell Biol.* 109:273–284.

Castonguay, A. and Robitaille, R. (2001) Differential regulation of transmitter release by presynaptic and glial Ca^{2+} internal stores at the neuromuscular synapse. *J. Neurosci.* 21:1911–1922.

Charles, P., Tait, S., Faivre-Sarrailh, C., Barbin, G., Gunn-Moore, F., Denisenko-Nehrbass, N., Guennoc, A.M., Girault, J.A., Brophy, P.J., and Lubetzki, C. (2002) Neurofascin is a glial receptor for the paranodin/Caspr-contactin axonal complex at the axoglial junction. *Curr. Biol.* 12:317–320.

Chernousov, M.A. and Carey, D.J. (2000) Schwann cell extracellular matrix molecules and their receptors. *Histol. Histopathol.*, 15:593–601.

Ciutat, D., Caldero, J., Oppenheim, R.W., and Esquerda, J.E. (1996) Schwann cell apoptosis during normal development and after axonal degeneration induced by neurotoxins in the chick embryo. *J. Neurosci.* 16:3979–3990.

Covault, J. and Sanes, J.R. (1986) Distribution of N-CAM in synaptic and extrasynaptic portions of developing and adult skeletal muscle. *J. Cell Biol.*102:716–730.

Cravioto, H. (1965) The role of Schwann cells in the development of human peripheral nerves. An electron microscopic study. *J. Ultrastructure Res.* 12:634–651.

de Waegh, S.M., Lee, V.M.Y., and Brady, S.T. (1992) Local modulation of neurofilament phosphorylation, axonal caliber, and slow axonal transport by myelinating Schwann cells. *Cell* 68:451–463.

Ding, Y. and Brunden, K.R. (1994) The cytoplasmic domain of myelin glycoprotein P0 interacts with negatively charged phospholipid bilayers. *J. Biol. Chem.* 269:10764–10770.

Dong, Z., Sinanan, A., Parkinson, D., Parmantier, E., Mirsky, R., and Jessen, K.R. (1999) Schwann cell development in embryonic mouse nerves. *J. Neurosci. Res.* 56:334–348.

Einheber, S., Milner, T.A., Giancotti, F., and Salzer, J.L. (1993) Axonal regulation of Schwann cell integrin expression suggests a role for alpha6 beta4 in myelination. *J. Cell Biol.* 123:1223–1236.

Einheber, S., Zanazzi, G., Ching, W., Scherer, S., Milner, T.A., Peles, E., and Salzer, J.L. (1997) The axonal membrane protein Caspr, a homologue of neurexin IV, is a component of the septate-like paranodal junctions that assemble during myelination. *J. Cell Biol.* 139:1495–1506.

Eldridge, C.F., Bunge, M.B., and Bunge, R.P. (1989) Differentiation of axon-related Schwann cells in vitro: II. Control of myelin formation by basal lamina. *J. Neurosci.* 9:625–638.

Eldridge, C.F., Bunge, M.B., Bunge, R.P., and Wood, P.M. (1987) Differentiation of axon-related Schwann cells in vitro. I. Ascorbic acid regulates basal lamina assembly and myelin formation. *J. Cell Biol.,* 105:1023–1034.

Fannon, A.M., Sherman, D.L., Ilynia, G., Brophy, P., Friedrich, V.L., and Colman, D.R. (1995) Novel E-cadherin-mediated adhesion in peripheral nerve: Schwann cell architecture is stabilized by autotypic adherens junctions. *J. Cell Biol.* 129:189–202.

Feltri, M.L., Graus Porta, D., Previtali, S.C., Nodari, A., Migliavacca, B., Cassetti, A., Littlewood-Evans, A., Reichardt, L.F., Messing, A., Quattrini, A., Mueller, U., and Wrabetz, L. (2002) Conditional disruption of beta 1 integrin in Schwann cells impedes interactions with axons. *J. Cell Biol.* 156:199–209.

Feltri, L., Scherer, S.S., Nemni, R., Kamholz, J., Vogelbacker, H., Scott, M.O., Canal, N., Quaranta, V., and Wrabetz, L. (1994) $\beta 4$ integrin expression in myelinating Schwann cells is polarized, developmentally regulated and axonally dependent. *Development* 120:1287–1301.

Fernandez-Valle, C., Gwynn, L., Wood, P.W., Carbonetto, S., and Bunge, M.B. (1994) Anti-$\beta 1$ integrin antibody inhibits Schwann cell myelination. *J. Neurobiol.* 25:1207–1226.

Fraher, J.P., O'Leary, D., Moran, M.A., Cole, M., King, R.H., and Thomas, P.K. (1990) Relative growth and maturation of axon size and myelin thickness in the tibial nerve of the rat. 1. Normal animals. *Acta Neuropathol.* 79:364–374.

Frei, R., Dowling, J., Carenini, S., Fuchs, E., and Martini, R. (1999) Myelin formation by Schwann cells in the absence of $\beta 4$ integrin. *Glia* 27:269–274.

Friede, R.L. and Beuche, W. (1985) A new approach toward analyzing peripheral nerve fiber populations. I. Variance in sheath thickness corresponds to different geometric proportions of the internodes. *J. Neuropathol. Exp. Neurol.* 44:60–72.

Gatto, C.L., Walker, B.J., Lambert, S. (2003) Local ERM activation and dynamic growth cones at Schwann cell tips implicated in efficient formation of nodes of Ranvier. *J. Cell Biol.* 162:489–498.

Gatzinsky, K.P. (1996) Node-paranode regions as local degradative centres in alpha-motor axons. *Microsc. Res. Technique* 34:492–506.

Georgiou, J. and Charlton, M.P. (1999) Non-myelin-forming perisynaptic Schwann cells express protein zero and myelin-associated glycoprotein. *Glia* 27:101–109.

Giese, K.P., Martini, R., Lemke, G., Soriano, P., and Schachner, M. (1992) Mouse P0 gene disruption leads to hypomyelination, abnormal expression of recognition molecules, and degeneration of myelin and axons. *Cell* 71:565–576.

Hagedorn, L., Suter, U., and Sommer, L. (1999) P0 and PMP22 mark a multipotent neural crest-derived cell type that displays community effects in response to TGF-β family factors. *Development* 126:3781–3794.

Herrera, A.A., Qiang, H., and Ko, C.P. (2000) The role of perisynaptic Schwann cells in development of neuromuscular junctions in the frog (*Xenopus laevis*). *J. Neurobiol.* 45:237–254.

Ishibashi, T., Ding, L., Ikenaka, K., Inoue, Y., Miyado, K., Mekada, E., and Baba, H. (2004) Tetraspanin protein CD9 is a novel paranodal component regulating paranodal junctional formation. *J. Neurosci.* 24:96–102.

Jahromi, B.S., Robitaille, R., and Charlton, M.P. (1992) Transmitter release increases intracellular calcium in perisynaptic Schwann cells in situ. *Neuron* 8:1069–1077.

Jessen, K.R. and Mirsky, R. (2002) Signals that determine Schwann cell identity. *J. Anat.* 200:367–376.

Kirschner, D.A. and Ganser, A.L. (1980) Compact myelin exists in the absence of basic protein in the shiverer mutant mouse. *Nature* 283:207–210.

Le Douarin, N., Dulac, C., Dupin, E., and Cameron-Curry, P. (1991) Glia cell lineages in the neural crest. *Glia* 4:175–184.

Lemke, G., Lamar, E., and Patterson, J. (1988) Isolation and analysis of the gene encoding peripheral myelin protein zero. *Neuron* 1:73–83.

Lobsiger, C.S., Schweitzer, B., Taylor, V., and Suter, U. (2000) Platelet-derived growth factor-BB supports the survival of cultured rat Schwann cell precursors in synergy with neurotrophin-3. *Glia* 30:290–300.

Love, F.M., Son, Y.J., Thompson, W.J. (2003) Activity alters muscle reinnervation and terminal sprouting by reducing the number of Schwann cell pathways that grow to link synaptic sites. *J. Neurobiol.* 54:566–576.

Martin, S., Levine, A.K., Chen, Z.J., Ughrin, Y., and Levine, J.M. (2001) Deposition of the NG2 proteoglycan at nodes of Ranvier in the peripheral nervous system. *J. Neurosci.* 21:8119–8128.

Martini, R. (1994) Expression and functional roles of neural cell surface molecules and extracellular matrix components during development and regeneration of peripheral nerves. *J. Neurocytol.* 23:1–28.

Martini, R., Mohajeri, M.H., Kasper, S., Giese, K.P., and Schachner, M. (1995) Mice doubly deficient in the genes for P0 and myelin basic protein show that both proteins contribute to the formation of the major dense line in peripheral nerve myelin. *J. Neurosci.* 15:4488–4495.

Martini, R. and Schachner, M. (1997) Molecular bases of myelin formation as revealed by investigations on mice deficient in glial cell surface molecules. *Glia* 19:298–310.

Matsumura, K., Yamada, H., Saito, F., Sunada, Y., and Shimizu, T. (1997) Peripheral nerve involvement in merosin-deficient congenital muscular dystrophy and dy mouse. *Neuromusc. Disord.* 7:7–12.

Melendez-Vasquez, C.V., Rios, J.C., Zanazzi, G., Lambert, S., Bretscher, A., and Salzer, J.L. (2001) Nodes of Ranvier form in association with ezrin-radixin-moesin (ERM)-positive Schwann cell processes. *Proc. Natl. Acad. Sci. USA* 98:1235–1240.

Menegoz, M., Gaspar, P., Le Bert, M., Galvez, T., Burgaya, F., Palfrey, C., Ezan, P., Arnos, F., and Girault, J.A. (1997) Paranodin, a glycoprotein of neuronal paranodal membranes. *Neuron* 19: 319–331.

Mirsky, R. and Jessen, K.R. (1999) The neurobiology of Schwann cells. *Brain Pathol.* 9:293–311.

Noakes, P.G. and Bennett, M.R. (1987) Growth of axons into developing muscles of the chick forelimb is preceded by cells that stain with Schwann cell antibodies. *J. Comp. Neurol.* 259:330–347.

Nolte, C., Schachner, M., and Martini, R. (1989) Immunocytochemical localization of the neural cell adhesion molecules L1, N-CAM, and J1 in Pacinian corpuscles of the mouse during development, in the adult and during regeneration. *J. Neurocytol.* 18:795–808.

Paratore, C., Hagedorn, L., Floris, J., Hari, L., Kleber, M., Suter, U., and Sommer, L. (2002) Cell-intrinsic and cell-extrinsic cues regulating lineage decisions in multipotent neural crest-derived progenitor cells. *Int. J. Dev. Biol.* 46:193–200.

Patton, B.L., Chiu, A.Y., and Sanes, J.R. (1988) Synaptic laminin prevents glial entry into the synaptic cleft. *Nature* 393:698–701.

Peles, E., Joho, K., Plowman, G., and Schlessinger, J. (1997a) Close similarity between *Drosophila* neurexin IV and mammalian Caspr protein suggests a conserved mechanism for cellular interactions. *Cell* 88:745–746.

Peles, E., Nativ, M., Lustig, M., Grumet, M., Schilling, J., Martinez, R., Plowman, G.D., and Schlessinger, J. (1997b) Identification of a novel contactin-associated transmembrane receptor with multiple domains implicated in protein-protein interactions. *EMBO J.* 16:978–988.

Peles, E. and Salzer, J.L. (2000) Molecular domains of myelinated axons. *Curr. Opin. Neurobiol.* 10:558–565.

Peters, A. and Muir, A.R. (1959) The relationship between axons and Schwann cells during development of peripheral nerves in the rat. *Q. J. Exp. Physiol.* 44:117–130.

Peters, A., Palay, S.L., and Webster, H.D. (1991) *The Fine Structure of the Nervous System*. New York and Oxford: Oxford University Press, pp. 222–232.

Phillips, D.D., Hibbs, R.G., Ellison, J.P., and Shapiro, H. (1972) An electron microscopic study of central and peripheral nodes of Ranvier. *J. Anat.* 111:229–238.

Poliak, S., Gollan, L., Martinez, R., Custer, A., Einheber, S., Salzer, J.L., Trimmer, J.S., Shrager, P., and Peles, E. (1999) Caspr2, a new member of the neurexin superfamily, is localized at juxtaparanodes of myelinated axons and assoziates with K^+ channels. *Neuron* 24:1037–1047.

Poliak, S., Gollan, L., Salomon, D., Berglund, E.O., Ohara, R., Ranscht, B., and Peles, E. (2001) Localization of Caspr2 in myelinated nerves depends on axon-glia interactions and the generation of barriers along the axon. *J. Neurosci.* 21:7568–7575.

Poliak, S., and Peles, E. (2003) The local differentiation of myelinated axons at nodes of Ranvier. Nat. Rev. Neurosci. 4:968–980.

Previtali, S.C., Feltri, M.L., Archelos, J.J., Quattrini, A., Wrabetz, L., and Hartung, H. (2001) Role of integrins in the peripheral nervous system. *Prog. Neurobiol.* 64:35–49.

Reddy, L.V., Koirala, S., Sugiura, Y., Herrera, A.A., and Ko, C.P. (2003) Glial cells maintain synaptic structure and function and promote development of the neuromuscular junction in vivo. *Neuron* 40:563–580.

Riethmacher, D., Sonnenberg-Rietmacher, E., Brinkmann, V., Yamaai, T., Lewin, R.G., and Birchmeier, C. (1997) Severe neuropathies in mice with targeted mutations in the ErbB3 receptor. *Nature* 389:725–730.

Robitaille, R. (1998) Modulation of synaptic efficacy and synaptic depression by glial cells at the frog neuromuscular junction. *Neuron* 21:847–855.

Rochon, D., Rousse, I., and Robitaille, R. (2001) Synapse-glia interactions at the mammalian neuromuscular junction. *J. Neurosci.* 21:3819–3829.

Sanes, J.R. and Lichtman, J.W. (1999) Development of the vertebrate neuromuscular junction. *Annu. Rev. Neurosci.* 22:389–442.

Sanes, J.R., Schachner, M., and Covault, J. (1986) Expression of several adhesive macromolecules (NCAM, L1, J1, NILE, uvomorulin, laminin, fibronectin and heparan sulfate proteoglycan) in embryonic, adult, and denervated adult skeletal muscles. *J. Cell Biol.* 102:420–431.

Scherer, S.S. and Arroyo, E.J. (2002) Recent progress on the molecular organization of myelinated axons. *J. Peripheral Nerv. Syst.* 7:1–12.

Scherer, S.S., Deschênes, S.M., Xu, Y.T., Grinspan, J.B., Fischbeck, K.H., and Paul, D.L. (1995) Connexin32 is a myelin-related protein in the PNS and CNS. *J. Neurosci.* 15:8281–8294.

Scherer, S.S., Xu, T., Crino, P., Arroyo, E.J., and Gutmann, D.H. (2001) Ezrin, radixin, and moesin are components of Schwann cell microvilli. *J. Neurosci. Res.* 65:150–164.

Schröder, J.M., Bohl, J., and Bardeleben, U. v. (1988) Changes of the ratio between myelin thickness and axon diameter in human developing sural, femoral, ulnar, facial, and trochlear nerves. *Acta Neuropathol.* 76:471–483.

Shapiro, L., Doyle, J.P., Hensley, P., Colman, D.R., and Hendrickson, W.A. (1996) Crystal structure of the extracellular domain from P0, the major structural protein of peripheral nerve myelin. *Neuron* 17:435–449.

Sherman, D.L., Fabrizi, C., Gillespie, C.S., and Brophy, P.J. (2001) Specific disruption of a Schwann cell dystrophin-related protein complex in a demyelinating neuropathy. *Neuron* 30:677–687.

Stoll, G. and Müller, H.W. (1999) Nerve injury, axonal degeneration and neural regeneration: basic insights. *Brain Pathol.* 9:313–325.

Tait, S., Gunn-Moore, F., Collinson, J.M., Huang, J., Lubetzki, C., Pedraza, L., Sherman, D.L., Colman, D.R., and Brophy, P.J. (2000) An oligodendrocyte adhesion molecule at the site of assembly of the paranodal axo-glial junction. *J. Cell Biol.* 150:657–666.

Traka, M., Dupree, J.L., Popko, B., and Karagogeos, D. (2002) The neuronal adhesion protein TAG-1 is expressed by Schwann cells and oligodendrocytes and is localized to the juxtaparanodal region of myelinated fibers. *J. Neurosci.* 22:3016–3024.

Trapp, B.D., Andrews, S.B., Wong, A., O'Connell, M., and Griffin, J.W. (1989) Co-localization of the myelin-associated glycoprotein and the microfilament components, F-actin and spectrin, in Schwann cells of myelinated nerve fibres. *J. Neurocytol.* 18:47–60.

Webster, H.D. (1971) The geometry of peripheral myelin sheaths during their formation and growth in rat sciatic nerves. *J. Cell Biol.* 48:348–367.

Weinberg, H.J. and Spencer, P.S. (1975) Studies on the control of myelinogenesis. I. Myelination of regenerating axons after entry into a foreign unmyelinated nerve. *J. Neurocytol.* 4:395–418.

Woolf, C.J., Reynolds, M.L., Chong, M.S., Emson, P., Irwin, N., and Benowitz, L.I. (1992) Denervation of the motor endplate results in the rapid expression by terminal Schwann cells of the growth-associated protein GAP-43. *J. Neurosci.* 12:3999–4010.

Xu, W., Shy, M., Kamholz, J., Elferink, L., Xu, G., Lilien, J., and Balsamo, J. (2001) Mutations in the cytoplasmic domain of P0 reveal a role for PKC-mediated phosphorylation in adhesion and myelination. *J. Cell Biol.* 155:439–445.

Yang, J.F., Cao, G., Koirala, S., Reddy, L.V., and Ko, C.P. (2001) Schwann cells express active agrin and enhance aggregation of acetylcholine receptors on muscle fibers. *J. Neurosci.* 21:9572–9584.

Ziskind-Conhaim, L. (1988) Physiological and morphological changes in developing peripheral nerves of rat embryos. *Dev. Brain Res.* 42:15–28.

5 Microglial cells

WOLFGANG J. STREIT

Microglial cell numbers are thought to make up 5% to 20% of the entire central nervous system (CNS) glial cell population. As a conservative estimate, assuming that microglia represent 10% of the total glial cell pool and knowing that there are at least 10 times as many glial cells as there are neurons in the CNS, it is apparent that there are at least as many microglia as there are neurons. This simple calculation is astonishing only insofar as some scientists questioned the very existence of microglial cells as recently as 15 years ago.

Research on microglia has grown significantly during the past two decades. This trend can be attributed largely to the development of reliable histological methods for identifying the cells in CNS tissue sections using light microscopy. Most of these methods, which are described in this chapter, can also be carried to the electron microscopic level, allowing verification of microglial identity through direct comparison of the presence of a specific marker with ultrastructural morphology. Before the advent of microglia-specific markers, electron microscopy was almost always needed for positive identification using solely morphological criteria. Modern neurobiology now has available an assortment of reliable light microscopic techniques that enable identification of microglial cells by neuroscientists from all backgrounds.

Regarding the terminology used in this chapter, it is important to point out that microglial cells in the adult CNS can assume at least three clearly identifiable states: (*1*) resting (ramified) microglia, as in the normal and nonpathological CNS; (*2*) activated (reactive) microglia, which occur in pathological states but are nonphagocytic; and (*3*) phagocytic microglia that appear as rounded brain macrophages. For more detailed descriptions of these microglial states the reader is referred elsewhere (Streit et al., 1988; Morioka et al., 1992; Chapter 35, this volume).

HISTORICAL PERSPECTIVE

Following early descriptions of neuroglia by Virchow in the mid-nineteenth century, other contemporary pathologists and psychiatrists, including Nissl and Alzheimer, commented on the possibility that the developing CNS was populated by cells of nonneuroectodermal origin. Speculation abounded as to the source of these invading cells, but with increasing consistency attention was being focused on the possibility that mesodermally derived cells were the invaders. Ultimately this led to the formulation by Cajal of *el tercer elemento*, the third element of the CNS, referring to a group of cells that was morphologically distinct from both the first and second elements (neurons and astrocytic neuroglia). Cajal's third element, defined by him in strictly morphological terms, received further classification into oligodendrocytes and microglia by del Rio-Hortega, the Spanish neuroanatomist, who provided the first systematic investigation on microglial cells (del Rio-Hortega, 1932). Del Rio-Hortega's detailed cytological observations, which remain quite relevant even today, gave rise to a long-standing controversy over the origin of microglia that dominated microglial research into the 1990s.

In recent history, the debate over microglial ontogeny has been succeeded by another fervent discussion, this one focusing on the functional significance of activated microglial cells, that is, whether activation of microglial cells is a beneficial or harmful process. The significance of this discussion pertains primarily to the issue of bystander damage, a phenomenon that is thought to be important in both acute and chronic CNS injury and disease. For example, regarding the pathogenesis of Alzheimer's disease, many scientists believe that microglial activation represents a type of chronic glial inflammation that is triggered by the presence of beta-amyloid proteins and causes neurodegenerative changes, such as neurofibrillary tangles, through production of neurotoxic molecules (Akiyama et al., 2000; Chapter 45, this volume).

ORIGIN AND LINEAGE OF MICROGLIA

Two related issues were at the heart of a long-standing debate over the origin of microglia: (*1*) Are microglia derived from mesoderm or from neuroectoderm? (*2*) When and how do microglia populate the CNS? As discussed recently (Streit, 2001), both issues have now been resolved and it is clear that (*1*) microglia are of the myelomonocytic lineage and therefore are derived from hemangioblastic mesoderm, and (*2*) microglia become part of the CNS parenchyma early during embryonic development at about the time neurulation has been completed. Microglial precursor cells are an integral component of the CNS during embryonic and postnatal development. Cells that are most aptly described as *fetal macrophages* (Takahashi et al., 1989) populate the developing neuroectoderm as early as embryonic day 8 in rodents (Alliot et al., 1999). These fetal macrophages can be visualized using lectin histochemical markers that also label microglia (Sorokin et al., 1992), and they are therefore considered the earliest detectable microglial precursor cells. Importantly, fetal macrophages can be found in the primitive neuroectoderm before it becomes vascularized (Fig. 5.1), which eliminates the possibility that bloodborne monocytes serve as direct microglial precursors. It is most likely that fetal macrophages are a common precursor for both microglia and blood monocytes, as well as for other tissue macrophages. As the embryonic CNS develops toward the perinatal stage and various neural cell types mature and differentiate, fetal macrophages also metamorphose from rounded cells to more differentiated embryonic microglia with short processes. These process-bearing embryonic microglia are at an intermediate stage of differentiation and have not yet matured to the fully ramified morphology that is characteristic of adult microglia.

As CNS development reaches the perinatal stage (which begins at about embryonic day 20 in rodents), a unique constellation of so-called ameboid microglial cells becomes apparent (Ling and Wong, 1993). Ameboid microglia aggregate as clusters of rounded cells at specific anatomical locations, most prominently in the supraventricular corpus callosum (Ling and Wong, 1993; Hurley et al., 1999). Ameboid microglia undergo mitosis in the postnatal CNS, and the prominent supraventricular clusters of proliferating cells were recognized by early microglial researchers, who termed them *fountains of microglia* (del Rio-Hortega, 1932). Contemporary neurobiologists might be inclined to apply the term *microglial progenitor cells* instead of *ameboid microglia* to emphasize their status as immature precursor cells. Microglial progenitor cells in the corpus callosum persist through the first 2 postnatal weeks, and during that time the cells migrate into the overlying cerebral cortex, differentiating into fully ramified microglia. This perinatal burst of microgliogenesis occurs to facilitate microglial colonization of the forebrain, which undergoes its most expansive growth during the postnatal period (Fig. 5.1).

During adult life there is little replacement of microglia from exogenous sources, such as the bone marrow, as shown in studies using bone marrow chimeras (Lassmann et al., 1993). Microglia have the greatest mitotic potential of all mature parenchymal cells in the CNS, and they are therefore capable of self-renewal. Microglial mitosis in the normal CNS occurs at a low rate, indicating slow but continuous turnover. A small fraction of microglial cells may undergo replacement by bone marrow–derived cells by way of perivascular cells. The latter are mononuclear phagocytes that reside in the Virchow-Robin (perivascular) spaces surrounding medium-sized and small cerebral vessels. Perivascular cells, which are replaced continuously by bone marrow–derived progenitors, may on occasion penetrate the perivascular basement membrane, enter the parenchyma, and differentiate into process-bearing microglia. Studies using bone marrow chimeras and localization of major histocompatibility antigens support this idea (Hickey and Kimura, 1988; Streit et al., 1989).

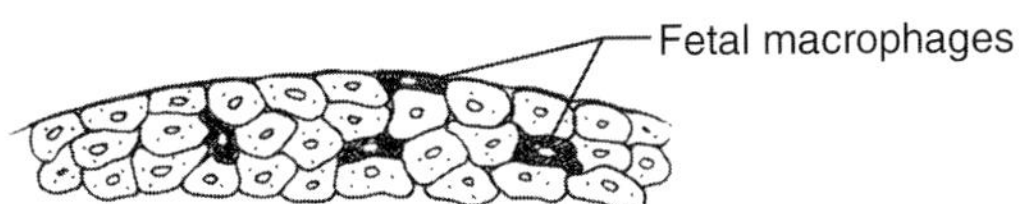

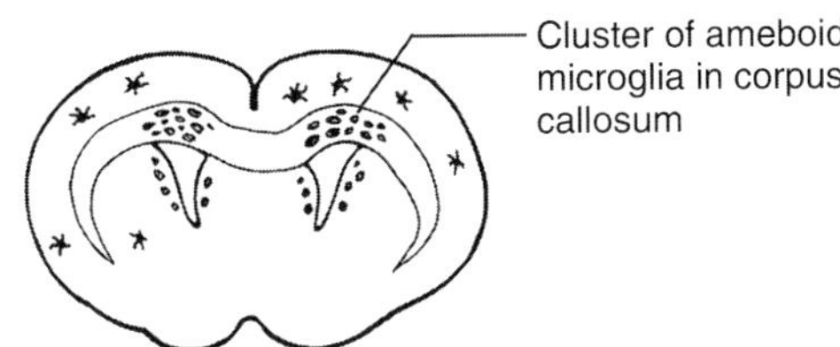

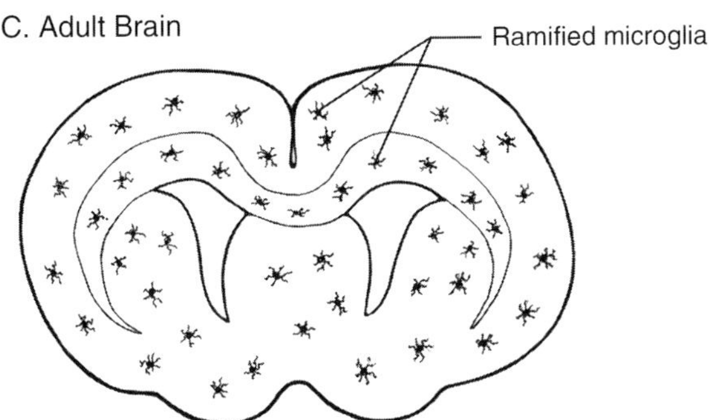

FIGURE 5.1 Summary of microglial ontogeny during three developmental stages. *A.* Fetal macrophages are found in the developing neurectoderm as early as embryonic day 8 in rodents. *B.* In the perinatal brain, clusters of dividing ameboid microglia are found in the supraventricular corpus callosum. The cells migrate from the clusters into the cerebral cortex and differentiate into ramified microglia. *C.* Ramified microglia colonize throughout the adult brain.

METHODS FOR STAINING MICROGLIA

Silver Carbonate Method

The first selective stain for microglia was the weak silver carbonate method developed by del Rio-Hortega (1919). Despite its capriciousness, this method remained the only useful histochemical procedure for at least 50 years. As with many other histochemical techniques involving metallic silver impregnations, Hortega's weak silver carbonate method for microglia has very specific fixation requirements, which do not, however, guarantee reproducible results in every preparation. The results obtained are quite variable in terms of numbers of microglia stained, and vary also with the animal species used. For unknown reasons, the method seems to work reliably only in rabbit brain. While it can be carried to the electron microscopic level, its usefulness is limited due to poor structural preservation and the deposition of metallic precipitates that obscure much of the cellular detail.

Enzyme Histochemical Methods

Thiamine pyrophosphatase (TPPase) and nucleoside diphosphatase (NDPase) are the most reliable and specific enzyme histochemical methods for staining resting microglial cells in a variety of species. These methods have been used successfully to localize microglia at both the light and electron microsocpic levels (Murabe and Sano, 1981; Schnitzer, 1989). Thiamine pyrophosphatase activity, originally described to be localized to the Golgi apparatus in a variety of cell types, including neurons, was later found to be associated specifically with the plasma membrane of microglial cells and with blood vessels in the CNS (Murabe and Sano, 1981).

Nonspecific esterase (NSE) is an enzyme used to identify microglia in mixed brain cultures (Sawada et al., 1990). However, NSE staining is of little use for detecting resting microglial cells in tissue sections. Actively proliferating, reactive microglial cells in the hypoglossal nucleus after peripheral nerve transection do not show any staining for this enzyme (Schelper and Adrian, 1980). However, NSE can be found in microglia-derived and other brain macrophages that are prevalent in stab wounds. Thus, NSE enzyme histochemistry supports the view that microglia *in vitro* are, in fact, microglia that have transformed into brain macrophages as a consequence of having been placed into cell culture.

Activated and/or phagocytic microglia in cell culture or in the pathological brain show increased activities for a number of other enzymes that are absent from resting microglial cells. These include acid phosphatase, 5′-nucleotidase, and oxidoreductase. Other studies have shown the presence of nitric oxide synthase, cyclooxygenase, lysosomal proteinases, plasminogen activator, lysozyme, purine nucleoside phosphorylase, and elastase (Castellano et al., 1990; Nakajima et al., 1992; Banati et al., 1993; Walsh et al., 2000). It is worth noting that some of these enzymatic activities are also found in other glial cells types and are therefore not always useful as selective histochemical markers for microglial cells.

Immunohistochemical Detection of Microglia

The microglial plasma membrane is complex, containing a large variety of receptor and adhesion molecules in addition to enzymatic activities. Due to this large repertoire of surface antigens, numerous antibodies are now available to facilitate immunohistochemical staining of microglia. Interestingly, many of these monoclonal antibodies were not produced with the intention of specifically marking microglia, but were meant to target differentiation antigens found on cells of the immune system, such as macrophages, thymocytes, and lymphocytes. Following initial failures to demonstrate the presence of monocytic and lymphoid antigens on human microglia (Oehmichen et al., 1979), it was found that a mouse macrophage–specific antigen could be localized on resting microglia with a monoclonal antibody designated F4/80 (Hume et al., 1983; Perry et al., 1985). These investigators also succeeded in showing the presence of Fc and complement receptors on resting mouse microglia using antibodies 2.4G2 and Mac-1, respectively. Analogously, ramified microglia in rat brain can be demonstrated reliably using the OX-42 antibody against the CD11b antigen, also known as the *CR3 complement receptor* (Graeber et al., 1988). It is important to note that these receptors are also found on macrophages in nonneural tissues, and their presence on microglia underscores the phagocytic potential of these cells, as well as their close relationship to the myelomonocytic cell lineage. Cross-reactivity of macrophage-specific antibodies with microglia and blood monocytes has been taken as evidence that microglia are derived from monocytes. However, a direct lineage relationship between monocytes and microglia is not likely since both microglia and monocytes are fully differentiated cell types that may arise from a common precursor cell, as discussed above.

A distinction between microglia and "other brain macrophages" has also been made using flow cytometric analyses, which have shown that "other CNS macrophages" are phenotypically distinct (CD11b/c+ and CD45 hi) from parenchymal microglia (CD11b/c+ and CD45 low) (Ford et al., 1995).

In the human brain, microglia can also be localized using antibodies against macrophage surface receptors (Akiyama and McGeer, 1990). In addition to the expression of Fc and complement receptors, other cell adhesion molecules are expressed constitutively on resting microglia in normal brain. Belonging to the integrin superfamily of adhesion molecules, these include typical lymphocytic antigens, such as lymphocyte function antigen, CD4 antigen, as well as leukocyte common antigen (Perry and Gordon, 1987; Akiyama and

McGeer, 1990). Species differences between the mouse, rat, and human in the constitutive expression of these molecules on resting microglia have been observed. These are likely due to both antibody specificities, as well as to variations in tissue processing techniques. B-lymphocyte antigens are detectable on human microglial cells using monoclonal antibodies LN-1 and LN-3, the latter recognizing human leukocyte antigen–([HLA]-DR) antigens (Miles and Chou, 1988; Dickson and Mattiace, 1989). While the LN-1 antibody may label both astrocytes and microglia, depending on fixation and tissue processing techniques, antibody LN-3 has an exclusive specificity for microglia in both normal and pathological human brain. Figures 5.4 through 5.6 provide examples of LN-3 staining of microglia in human brain. Importantly, staining with LN-3 is fixation-sensitive, and optimal preparations require lightly fixed tissues (Streit and Sparks, 1997).

It is apparent that the microglial surface membrane bears molecules usually associated with white blood cells. Consistent with this is the localization of antigens of the major histocompatibility complex (MHC) on microglia. While it was once thought that MHC antigens were entirely absent from brain, supporting the notion of the brain as an immunologically privileged organ, it is now well documented that MHC antigens are expressed in normal brain and that the principal parenchymal cell type expressing MHC antigens is the microglial cell (Hayes et al., 1987; Streit et al., 1989). The constitutive expression of MHC antigens in normal brain also includes endothelial cells and perivascular cells, and there are considerable species differences in the levels of constitutive MHC antigen expression on these various cell types. Major histocompatibility complex antigen expression on microglia is increased dramatically under pathological conditions, but also with aging in the normal brain (Streit and Sparks, 1997; Finch et al., 2002).

To date, a truly specific marker for microglia, that is, one that does not cross-react with other macrophages, has not been generated. All antibodies and lectins that react with resting microglial cells also label activated microglia and microglia-derived brain macrophages, as well as peripheral macrophages. Conversely, not all antibodies that react with brain or other macrophages label resting microglia, suggesting that the antigenic repertoire of resting microglia is smaller than that of activated microglia and brain macrophages, and/or that the level of expression of certain antigens in resting cells is below the detection limit of the immunohistochemical procedure (Table 5.1).

Immunohistochemical localization of ramified microglia has been achieved through the use of phosphotyrosine antibodies (Griffith et al., 2000). This procedure detects the products of an enzymatic reaction carried out by tyrosine kinase. There are important functional implications for this observation, since it is known that tyrosine kinases are often associated with

TABLE 5.1 In Vivo *States of Microglial Biology and Associated Phenotypic Characteristics*

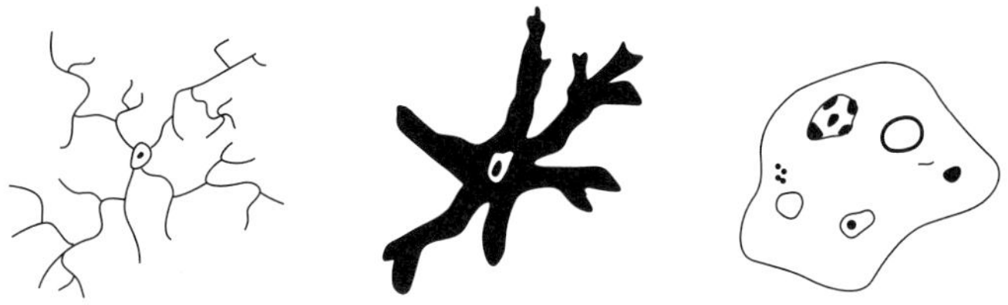

	Resting	*Activated*	*Phagocytic*
Proliferation	−/+	+	+
Griffonia simplicifolia			
B_4-isolectin	+	+	+
Vimentin	−	+	+
Macrophage markers			
(ED1, ED2, OX-41)	−	−/+	−/+
CR3 complement receptor (OX-42)	+	+	+
MHC class I antigen (OX-18)	−	+	+
MHC class II antigen (OX-6)	−/+	+	+
CD4 antigen (W3/25)	−/+	+	+
CD8 antigen (OX-8)	−	−/+	+
Leukocyte common antigen (OX-1)	−	+	+

Antibody designations in parentheses are specific for rat.
Symbols: − absent; −/+ weak; + strong.
MHC: major histocompatibility complex.

cell surface receptors, which are plentiful on the microglial membrane. Various other immunohistochemical methods aimed at detecting somewhat unconventional antigens, such as vaults, ferritin, and lipocortin-1, have also been described (Kaneko et al., 1989; Chugani et al., 1991; McKanna, 1993). Vaults, which are multiarched ribonucleoprotein particles of unknown function, appear to be enriched in microglia during ontogeny but mostly disappear in adult cells. Ferritin, on the other hand, is a well-known iron-storage protein, and its detection in microglia suggests their active participation in iron metabolism, as in the case of blood monocytes and other tissue macrophages. Lipocortin-1 is a Ca^{2+}-binding protein that is thought to function as an anti-inflammatory or immunosuppressive molecule.

In summary, remarkable progress has been made in the development of immunohistochemical procedures that are useful for the detection and identification of microglia. Given the great variety of receptor molecules known to cover the microglial cell surface, it is likely that more antibodies will be developed in the future, and these will undoubtedly be important for the continued study of microglial cell functions.

Lectin Histochemical Detection of Microglia

During the course of investigations examining the distribution of complex carbohydrates in nervous tissue with lectin histochemistry, it was noted that the B_4-isolectin derived from *Griffonia simplicifolia* resulted in the selective visualization of a population of rat glial cells that were identified tentatively as microglia (Streit et al., 1985). This observation was confirmed soon thereafter in human tissue where it was shown that the lectin from *Ricinus communis* could be used as a histochemical marker for microglia (Mannoji et al., 1986). Both lectins have similar sugar-binding characteristics in recognizing anomeric forms of galactose, with *G. simplicifolia* binding to α-D-galactose and *R. communis* recognizing β-D-galactose residues. An additional β-D-galactose binding lectin derived from mistletoe has been shown to preferentially stain human over rat microglia (Suzuki et al., 1988), emphasizing the subtle difference in glycocalyx composition between rodent and human microglial cells, being one of anomeric configuration. The galactose sugar residues occur as terminal sugars in the oligosaccharide side chains of nervous system glycoproteins that are embedded in the microglial plasma membrane, as revealed by electron microscopy (Streit and Kreutzberg, 1987). Interestingly, the lectin from *Lycopersicum esculentum* (tomato), which has an affinity for poly-*N*-acetyl lactosamine residues, can also be used for staining rat microglia (Acarin et al., 1994), indicating the diversity of carbohydrate domains present on the microglial cell surface. The specific nature and function of lectin-binding glycoproteins on microglial cells has not yet been resolved; however, it is likely that the carbohydrate domains of many of the surface receptors, described in the preceding section, account in large part for lectin binding. Lectin staining is perhaps the quickest and most resilient method for visualizing microglia in tissue sections since the carbohydrate epitopes, unlike most proteins, are largely unaffected by cross-linking through aldehyde-based fixation and tissue processing techniques.

Other Methods for Labeling Microglia

Among all the mature parenchymal cell types in the mature CNS, microglia are the cells with the greatest potential for mitosis. Their ability to divide and proliferate makes them susceptible to labeling with ^3H-thymidine and other markers of dividing cells, such as 5-bromo-2′-deoxyuridine or proliferating cell nuclear antigen. Microglial cell division is usually triggered by perturbations in CNS homeostasis, such as neuronal injury, but there is also evidence that microglial cell division occurs normally in the rodent brain, albeit at a low rate (Korr et al., 1983). Microglia may also be labeled directly or indirectly using various dyes and tracer substances. Following intraperitoneal injection of the fluorescent dye rhodamine isothiocyanate (RhIC), labeled ameboid microglia were observed in the corpus callosum. Subsequently, the ameboid cells were observed to transform into RhIC-labeled, ramified microglial cells (Leong and Ling, 1992), confirming earlier observations using colloidal carbon introduced in the form of India ink. An indirect method for labeling microglia makes use of their ability to phagocytose dead or dying neurons. Following injection of the appropriate tracer substance into axons, the tracer is retrogradely transported toward the parent neuron cell bodies. If the injected nerve is also axotomized, in many instances this will cause degeneration of the parent neurons, followed by removal of dead neurons by local microglia that phagocytose not only the neuronal debris but also the tracer substance and thus become labeled.

Such experiments have been successfully carried out in various sytems, including the visual system, resulting in the labeling of retinal microglia with the carbocyanine dye DiI (Thanos, 1991); the dorsal motor nucleus of the vagus, where the neural tracer fluorogold was used (Rinaman et al., 1991); and the rat facial nucleus, where fluorogold was used in conjunction with toxic ricin to induce motor neuron degeneration (Streit and Graeber, 1993). Interestingly, direct injection of fluorogold into the brain does not label ramified microglial cells, but if the cells are maintained in culture, where they undergo macrophage transformation, they do take up fluorogold rather avidly (Pennell and Streit, 1998).

MICROGLIA AND RELATED CELL TYPES

Definitions

Microglial cells, because they can change their morphology and appearance in certain pathological and developmental states, have been given various descriptive names and attributes, such as *rod cells, gitter cells, globoid cells*, and *ameboid cells*, to name a few. Even though these terms accurately reflect the cells' changed appearance, the descriptive terminology has somewhat obscured the true identity of the cells associated with the term *microglia*. In the normal adult brain, resting microglia can be defined in terms of both morphology and phenotype. They are highly branched (ramified) glial cells with a small amount of perinuclear cytoplasm and a small, dense, heterochromatic nucleus (Figs. 5.2, 5.3). They can be distinguished easily from other glial cells by their surface immunophenotype. That is, they are the only glial cell type that constitutively expresses the CR3 complement receptor (recognized by monoclonal antibody OX-42 in the rat) and binds lectins with a specificity for galactose residues. Furthermore, at the ultrastructural level, microglia are recognizable as true parenchymal constituents of the CNS because they are located outside of the vascular basement membrane. At the same time, they may be considered part of the perivascular glia limitans, since microglial cytoplasmic processes are found incorporated intermingled with the layer of astrocytic foot processes (Lassmann et al., 1991).

The observation that microglia are frequently found in the vicinity of blood vessels has resulted in the use of the term *perivascular microglia*, which is yet another descriptive term referring to parenchymal microglial cells, as defined above, that happen to be located near a cerebral blood vessel (Fig. 5.4). Perivascular microglia are not to be confused with the so-called *perivascular cells*, which, unlike microglia, are not part of the CNS parenchyma since they are separated from it by a perivascular basement membrane. Perivascular cells are components of the vascular wall and are located in the perivascular spaces. They fit the morphological definition of a pericyte (Mato et al., 1986; Graeber and Streit, 1990). Perivascular cells are phagocytic and may express MHC antigens (Mato et al., 1986; Streit et al., 1989), which has made it difficult in certain pathological situations to distinguish between perivascular cells and perivascular microglia. In the normal brain, these two cell types are readily distinguished by their morphology and surface immunophenotype. Perivascular cells are seen only in association with blood vessels. They are not ramified but have an elongate shape, and they can be specifically labeled in the rat with an antibody designated as ED2 (Graeber et al., 1989). Thus, at least two clearly definable and indigenous sources

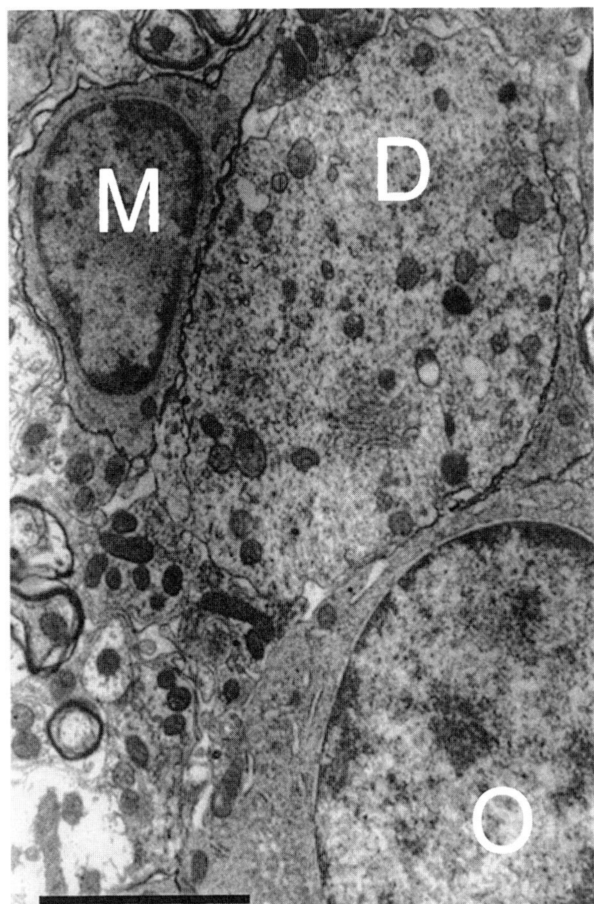

FIGURE 5.3 This electron micrograph shows a microglial cell (*M*), an oligodendrocyte (O), and a large dendrite (*D*). Both cell types have a heterochromatic nucleus that is larger in the oligodendrocyte. Bar = 2 μm.

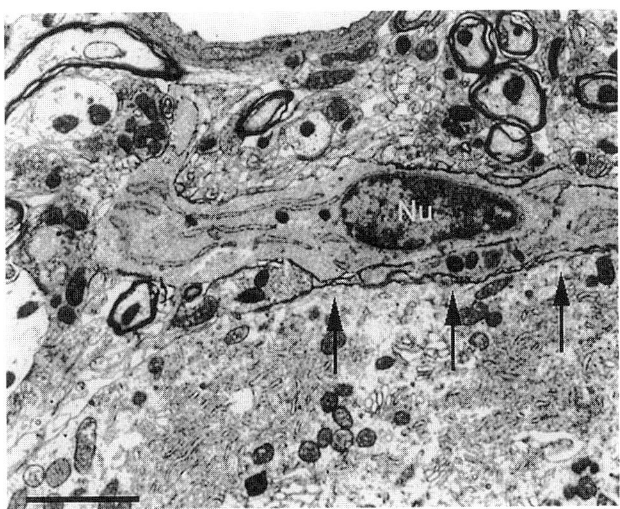

FIGURE 5.2 Ultrastructural appearance of a perineuronal microglial cell in the rat brain. The cell has a heterochromatic nucleus (*Nu*) and prominent cisternae of rough endoplasmic reticulum. Its plasma membrane, which is accentuated by lectin staining, is directly apposed to the neuronal plasma membrane (*arrows*). Bar = 2 μm.

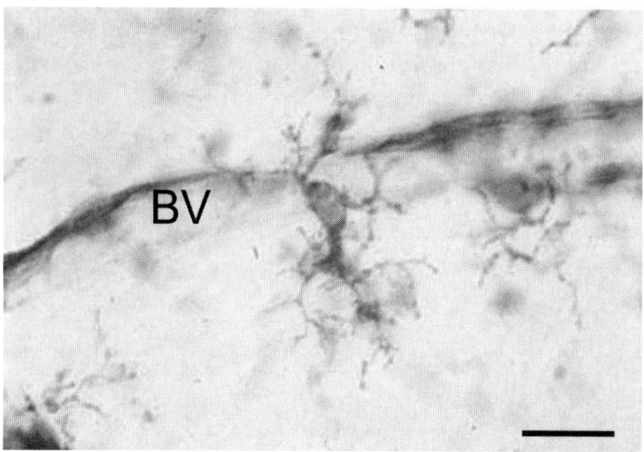

FIGURE 5.4 Ramified resting microglial cell in a perivascular position. The blood vessel (*BV*) is seen coursing horizontally. LN-3 immunohistochemistry in the nonpathological brain of a 68-year-old individual. Bar = 20 μm.

of brain macrophages are present in normal brain: microglia and perivascular cells. The term *brain macrophage* is generic and encompasses all phagocytic cells in the CNS, including blood-derived monocytes, which may enter the CNS following development of a lesion that disrupts the blood brain barrier.

Factors Affecting Distribution, Morphology, and Phenotype of Microglia

Microglia are distributed ubiquitously throughout the normal CNS, with regional differences having been reported in mouse brain (Lawson et al., 1990). According to these authors, the highest microglial densities are encountered in the hippocampal formation, the olfactory telencephalon, portions of the basal ganglia, and the substantia nigra. A total number of 3.5×10^6 microglia is estimated to reside in the adult mouse brain (Lawson et al., 1990), although that estimate is probably too conservative. Individual microglial cells typically occupy a distinct territory; that is, neighboring cells do not contact each other with their cytoplasmic processes.

The morphology and branching patterns of microglial cells show heterogeneity between different brain regions, which is perhaps most remarkable when comparing cells in gray and white matter. While microglia in gray matter tend to be profusely ramified, with processes extending in all directions, cells in the white matter often align their cytoplasmic extensions in parallel, but also at right angles to nerve fiber bundles. Thus, the cell shape of microglia adapts to the geometry of the brain region they populate. The microglial immunophenotype is heterogeneous and appears to be influenced by the chemical composition of the microenvironment. For example, MHC class II-positive, as well as CD4-positive, microglia are localized preferentially in white matter of normal brain (Hayes et al., 1987; Perry and Gordon, 1987; Streit et al., 1989). Brain regions lacking a blood–brain barrier, such as the circumventricular organs, do show microglia and microglia-like cells, such as the Kolmer cells of the choroid plexus, with a different phenotype, suggesting that components of the serum exert an influence on microglial phenotype. This suggestion is supported further by *in vivo* studies showing profound changes in microglial phenotype after brain lesioning, such as by forebrain ischemia and kainic acid injections that compromise the blood–brain barrier. Similar changes in microglial immunophenotype also occur when the cells are maintained *in vitro* using serum-containing culture medium.

Microglia in Cell Culture

Although the maintenance of microglia/brain macrophages in cell culture was used and described in the 1930s, possibly even earlier, the procedure did not gain widespread popularity until the 1980s. The technique described by Giulian and Baker (1986) is now widely used with numerous modifications. When culturing microglial cells, perhaps more so than with any other neural cell type, it is apparent that microglia *in vitro* are quite different from microglia *in vivo*. The preparation of primary mixed brain cultures, from which microglia are isolated, causes the generation of large amounts of tissue debris. This, together with a high serum content of the growth media, promotes rapid transformation of microglial cells into brain macrophages. Isolated microglia plated onto plastic culture dishes take on a rounded cell shape resembling that of immature ameboid microglial precursor cells, and it was once widely accepted that cultured microglia are the same as ameboid microglia. Since isolated microglia *in vitro* are essentially brain macrophages, it is important to distinguish this advanced functional (phagocytic) state from the precursor state that defines ameboid microglial cells in the developing CNS. Brain macrophages, like cultured microglia, secrete a variety of cytokines and growth factors, whereas ameboid microglial progenitor cells do not (Hurley et al., 1999).

Another important consideration with regard to cultured microglial cells concerns the issue of microglial activation. Microglia are activated *in vitro* by exposure to potent immunostimulatory agents, such as lipopolysaccharide (LPS) and/or interferon-gamma, which means that cells already transformed into brain macrophages by the culturing process itself become superactivated when exposed to LPS. This *in vitro* stimulation produces a different kind of activated microglia than that seen *in vivo* when resting microglia are activated by neuronal injury. Microglia *in vivo* progress to become brain macrophages only if debris from degenerating cells needs to be phagocytosed; in the absence of cell death, activated microglia *in vivo* do not become brain macrophages. Accordingly, cultured microglia/brain macrophages, before LPS stimulation, are already at an activation state that is equivalent to what is perceived as maximal microglial activation *in vivo*, that is, the brain macrophage stage. Clearly, it is important not to equate microglial activation *in vitro* with microglial activation *in vivo*. Techniques for inducing microglial ramification *in vitro*, including the use of organotypic or slice cultures, coculturing microglia with astrocytes or exposing them to astrocyte-conditioned medium, or treating them with ramifying agents such as vitamin E and thapsigargin (Sievers et al., 1994; Tanaka and Maeda, 1996; Kloss et al., 1997; Heppner et al., 1998; Czapiga and Colton, 1999; Eder 1999; Yagi et al., 1999; Bouscein et al., 2000; Mertsch et al., 2001), may allow researchers to study ramified microglia more effectively. It remains to be seen, however, whether ramified microglia *in vitro* show the same gene expression patterns as ramified microglia *in vivo* and can therefore be considered identical.

Microglia activated *in vitro* with LPS or other immunostimulants can produce neurotoxic molecules, such as nitric oxide, glutamate, reactive oxygen and nitrogen species, and proinflammatory cytokines. These observations have fostered the idea that microglia are potentially harmful, and that activated microglia may be responsible for exacerbating damage in the injured or diseased CNS by producing neurotoxic compounds that cause neurodegeneration secondarily. This idea is difficult to prove *in vivo*, where, in fact, most observations support the notion that microglial activation is a result of neuronal damage rather than its cause. The secondary injury concept also clashes with studies showing that cultured microglial cells can produce neurotrophic factors and other neuroprotective substances (for review see Nakajima and Kohsaka, 2002). Microglia *in vitro* behave much like other tissue macrophages in a dish, and as such are capable of the full repertoire of immune functions, including phagocytosis, antigen presentation, and cellular cytotoxicity. Importantly, though, this type of immunological activity does not necessarily reflect what occurs in the normal or injured CNS, where inhibitory influences and cell-cell interactions may dampen immune responses and inflammation.

MICROGLIA IN THE NORMAL ADULT AND AGING BRAIN

Microglia are ubiquitous in the CNS, where they are spaced evenly in a network-like fashion throughout the brain and spinal cord. However, microglia are not known to form connections with each other normally, and it appears that each cell occupies its own individual plot of three-dimensional space, which is approximately 50,000 μm^3 in volume. In the normal uninjured CNS the cells are referred to as *resting* microglia to distinguish them from the *activated* or *reactive* microglia that are encountered after brain injury. Resting microglia have a characteristic cell shape marked by finely branched, ramified cell processes that extend in all directions (Fig. 5.5). This ramified cell morphology reflects the cells' recognized function as *sensors* on the lookout for biochemical or bioelectric changes in their microenvironment that may signal ongoing brain pathology (Kreutzberg, 1996).

It would be correct to say that a major functional role of microglia in the normal CNS is that of a sentry. This role, of course, is clearly analogous to the roles served by cells of the immune system, such as macrophages and lymphocytes, in the rest of the body. The concept of microglia as *the brain's immune system* thus reconciles the discrepancy between the absence of leukocytes in the brain and the brain's ability to defend itself against infections, injury, and disease. With microglia, evolution has found a way to achieve compatibility between the destructive power of the immune system and the relative vulnerability of the CNS to injury and disease. Functionally speaking, one might therefore view microglia as a hybrid cell type that combines characteristics of a neural cell with some of the attributes of macrophages and lymphocytes.

In line with the role of microglia as sensors of pathology, their cell surface is covered with an abundance of receptor molecules that range from ion channels to immunological recognition molecules to neurotransmitter receptors. In many instances, receptor molecules have been identified in cultured microglia but not in mi-

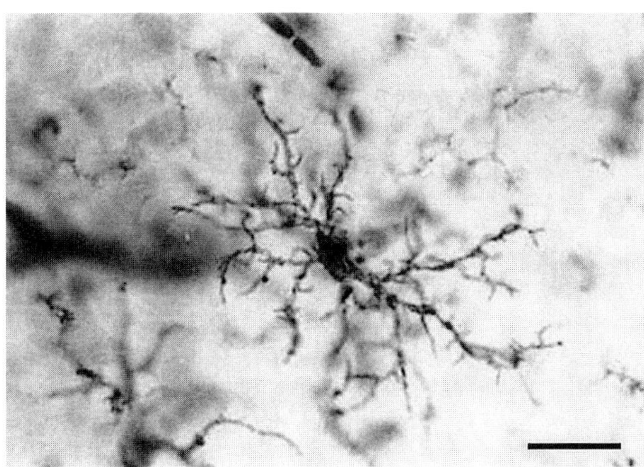

FIGURE 5.5 Ramified resting microglial cell in the nonpathological brain of a 64-year-old human visualized with monoclonal antibody LN-3. Note the extensive branching of cytoplasmic processes. Bar = 20 μm.

croglia within brain tissue sections. This is because some receptors, especially cytokine receptors and their ligands, are present in such small amounts in healthy tissues that they cannot be detected reliably *in vivo*. Low levels of many cytokines and their receptors in the normal CNS may contribute to an immunologically quiescent CNS microenvironment thought to be sustained, in part, by inhibitory influences. Accordingly, the functional roles of most cytokines/chemokines and their respective receptors in the normal CNS are largely unknown. However, immediately following acute brain injury, many of the cytokines and cytokine receptor proteins are present in increased amounts, as they are needed to regulate postinjury inflammatory and repair processes. Microglia, which are both sources and targets of numerous cytokines and chemokines, thus play an integral role in the cellular mechanisms that regulate postinjury events.

For the normal CNS, one chemokine, termed *fractalkine* (CX3CL1), is of some interest because both it and its receptor (CX3CR1) are expressed constitutively in relatively large amounts (Harrison et al., 1998; Nishiyori et al., 1998). Fractalkine, which is present in both membrane-bound and secreted forms in neurons of the CNS, is bound by the fractalkine receptor, which is present on microglial cells. The distinct separation in cellular localization of CX3CL1 and CX3CR1 suggests a role for fractalkine in mediating neuron-microglia interactions normally, as well as after injury. It is currently thought that high levels of fractalkine in uninjured CNS neurons function in a constitutively inhibitory fashion to help maintain microglia in their resting state. Constitutive inhibition of microglia in the normal CNS is thought to be mediated by other neuronal molecules as well. Recently, the CD200 molecule, which is found in neurons, has been implicated in suppressing microglial activation through interactions with the CD200 receptor, which is thought to be present on microglia (Hoek et al. 2000).

The examples of fractalkine and CD200 as neuronal molecules that regulate microglial cell activity and activation provide not only an illustration of how biochemical signaling may occur between neurons and microglia, but also make clear the necessity for neuron-microglia signaling to occur constantly within the CNS. Structural observations of perineuronal microglial satellite cells in the normal CNS support these molecular studies. Perineuronal microglial satellites are microglia that are located near CNS neurons in such a way that the glial processes are partially wrapped around the neuronal somata (Palacios, 1990; Figs. 5.2, 5.3). There is close physical proximity between microglial satellites and neurons, a spatial arrangement that is ideal for facilitating specific cell-cell interactions involving the targeted exchange of minute quantities of signaling molecules. Since not all neurons have perineuronal microglial satellites, it is likely that those neurons with satellite microglia may have attracted the cells for a reason. Neurons with perineuronal microglial satellites may require increased trophic support from microglia owing to increased metabolic stress or increased physiological activity. In addition to providing trophic support, perineuronal microglial satellites may be involved in the remodeling of synaptic contacts on these neurons. Microglia have long been known to engage in synaptic remodeling, a phenomenon first reported more than 35 years ago (Blinzinger and Kreutzberg, 1968). However, this potentially important role of microglia in synaptic plasticity has received very little attention to date, and the molecular mechanisms that underlie this function are far from clear. Microglia are well equipped to participate in synaptic remodeling since they generate a number of enzymes, including matrix metalloproteinase, elastase, and plasminogen activator. They also produce extracellular matrix molecules, such as laminin, thrombospondin, and keratan sulfate, as well as neurotrophic factors. Research into the possible role of microglia in synaptic plasticity may be important for better understanding the physiological functions of microglia, not only in the normal CNS but also in neurodegenerative diseases, where the loss of synaptic connections is thought to be the major correlate to diminished cognitive function.

Microglia in the normally aging brain undergo changes that have been interpreted to represent progressive microglial activation (Perry et al., 1993; Streit and Sparks, 1997; Finch et al., 2002). Most conspicuous is the cells' increased immunoreactivity for MHC antigens and the formation of microglial rod cells and clusters (Fig. 5.6). This is a curious phenomenon since age-dependent microglial activation occurs in the absence of the usual triggers of acute microglial activation, such as neuronal injury or death (Finch et al., 2002). What exactly happens to microglial cells with aging is largely unknown, but clearly two cellular characteristics are affected: cell morphology and cell surface antigen expression. Microglial morphology and immunophenotype are also changed in activated microglia after acute injury, but these changes are transient and with time the cells revert back to their normal resting morphology and phenotype. In contrast, microglial changes that occur with aging are progressive. This raises the question of whether such aging-related microglial activation should be classified as microglial activation at all. It may be more accurate to consider age-related microglial activation a process that is perhaps closer to cellular senescence (Flanary and Streit, 2004; Streit et al., 2004). Microglial senescence is currently an understudied subject, and much remains to be done in this area since senescence could provide important and novel perspectives for understanding the aging process as well as aging-related neurodegenerative disorders.

SUMMARY AND PERSPECTIVES

Microglial cells have moved into the mainstream of neuroscience research, and their importance for maintaining tissue homeostasis in the normal, and particularly in the injured, CNS is increasingly being understood. The concept of microglia as the brain's immune system has become a widely accepted idea and, indeed, a very useful one because it emphasizes the unique structure of the brain in immunological terms. The brain's immune system is essential for maintaining the organ's viability and functionality, and any impairment in its function could have detrimental consequences. Evidence is beginning to emerge that the brain's immune system is subject to aging-related deterioration and that microglial cell function may wane over the lifetime of an organism (Streit, 2002). If dysfunction of microglia can be shown to occur with advancing age, it could form the basis for a new perspective on aging-related neurodegenerative diseases such as Alzheimer's disease. Similar to impairment in systemic immune function that can produce some of the most devastating diseases, a specific impairment of the brain's immune system could have destructive effects on mental abilities such as cognition and memory. In sum, microglia have come a long way in a relatively short period of time: from barely being on the radar screen of neuroscience 20 years ago to taking center stage in theories regarding the pathogenesis of neurodegenerative disease today. With new knowledge on microglia accumulating rapidly, one can look forward to a day when treatment of microglia becomes the treatment of choice for brain dysfunction.

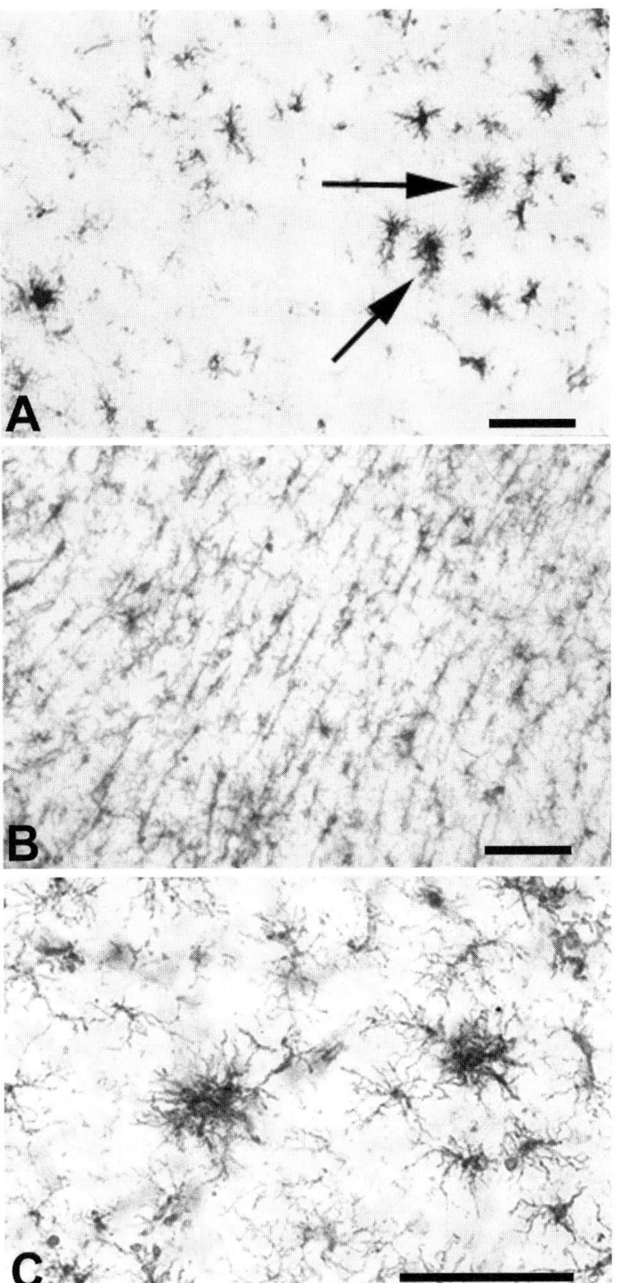

FIGURE 5.6 Resting and apparently activated microglia stained with LN-3 in nonpathological human brain. Panel *A* shows that activated microglia stain more strongly than resting ones and have a bushy appearance in a 41-year-old individual (*arrows*). Panel *B* shows microglial rod cells in the cerebral cortex of a 94-year-old individual. Panel *C* shows very large, bushy microglia in the 94-year-old, possibly representing two or more cells that have fused to form a microglial cluster. Bar = 100 μm.

ACKNOWLEDGMENTS

I thank Dr. Larry Sparks for providing samples of nonpathological human brain that were processed for LN-3 staining. I also thank David Peace for help with the artwork in Figure 5.1 and Amanda Kuhns for digital processing of micrographs and the manuscript.

REFERENCES

Acarin, L., Vela, J.M., Gonzalez, B., and Castellano, B. (1994) Demonstration of poly-*N*-acetyl lactosamine residues in ameboid and ramified microglial cells in rat brain by tomato lectin binding. *J. Histochem. Cytochem.* 42:1033–1041.

Akiyama, H., Barger, S., Barnum, S., Bradt, B., Bauer, J., Cole, G.M., Cooper, N.R., Eikelenboom, P., Emmerling, M., Fiebich, B.L., Finch, C.E., Frautschy, S., Griffin, W.S.T., Hampel, H., Hull, M., Landreth, G., Lue, L.F., Mrak, R., Mackenzie, M., O'Banion, K., Pachter, J., Pasinetti, G., Plata-Salaman, C., Rogers, J., Rydel, R., Shen, Y., Streit, W., Strohmeyer, R., Tooyoma, I., Van Muiswinkel, F.L., Veerhuis, R., Walker, D., Webster, S., Wegrzyniak, B., Wenk, G., and Wyss-Coray, A. (2000) Inflammation and Alzheimer's disease. *Neurobiol. Aging* 21:383–421.

Akiyama, H. and McGeer, P.L. (1990) Brain microglia constitutively express β-2 integrins. *J. Neuroimmunol.* 30:81–93.

Alliot, F., Godin, I., and Pessac, B. (1999) Microglia derive from progenitors, originating from the yolk sac, and which proliferate in the brain. *Brain Res.* 117:145–152.

Banati, R.B., Gehrmann, J., Schubert, P., and Kreutzberg, G.W. (1993) Cytotoxicity of microglia. *Glia* 7:111–118.

Blinzinger, K. and Kreutzberg, G. (1968) Displacement of synaptic terminals from regenerating motoneurons by microglial cells. Z. *Zellforsch* 85:145–157.

Boucsein, C., Kettenmann, H., and Nolte, C. (2000) Electrophysiological properties of microglial cells in normal and pathologic rat brain slices. *Eur. J. Neurosci.* 12:2049–2058.

Castellano, B., Gonzales, B., Finsen, B.R., and Zimmer, J. (1990) Histochemical demonstration of purine nucleoside phosphorylase (PNPase) in microglial and astroglial cells of adult rat brain. *J. Histochem. Cytochem.* 38:1535–1539.

Chugani, D.C., Kedersha, N.L., and Rome, L.H. (1991) Vault immunofluorescence in the brain: new insights regarding the origin of microglia. *J. Neurosci.* 11:256–268.

Czapiga, M. and Colton, C.A. (1999) Function of microglia in organotypic slice cultures. *J. Neurosci. Res.* 56:644–651.

del Rio-Hortega, P. (1919) Notas tecnicas. Coloración rápida de tejidos normales y patológicos con carbonato de plata amoniacal. *Trab. Lab. Invest. Biol. Univ. Madrid* 17:229–235.

del Rio-Hortega, P. (1932) Microglia. In: Penfield, W., ed. *Cytology and Cellular Pathology of the Nervous System, Vol. II.* New York: Hoeber, pp. 481–534.

Dickson, D.W. and Mattiace, L.A. (1989) Astrocytes and microglia in human brain share an epitope recognized by a B-lymphocyte-specific monoclonal antibody (LN-1). *Am. J. Pathol.* 135:135–147.

Eder, C., Schilling, T., Heinemann, U., Haas, D., Hailer, N., and Nitsch, R. (1999) Morphological, immunophenotypical and electrophysiological properties of resting microglia in vitro. *Eur. J. Neurosci.* 11:4251–4261.

Finch, C.E., Morgan, T.E., Rozovsky, I., Xie, Z., Weindruch, R., and Prolla, T. (2002) Microglia and aging in the brain. In: Streit, W.J., ed. *Microglia in the Regenerating and Degenerating Central Nervous System.* New York: Springer, pp. 275–305.

Flanary, B.E. and Streit, W.J. (2004) Progressive telomere shortening occurs in cultured rat microglia, but not astrocytes. *Glia* 45:75–88.

Ford, A.L., Goodsall, A.L., Hickey, W.F., and Sedgwick, J.D. (1995) Normal adult ramified microglia separated from other central nervous system macrophages by flow cytometric sorting. Phenotypic differences defined and direct ex vivo antigen presentation to myelin basic protein-reactive CD4+ T cells compared. *Journal of Immunology* 154:4309–4321.

Giulian, D. and Baker, T.J. (1986) Characterization of ameboid microglia isolated from developing mammalian brain. *J. Neurosci.* 6:2163–2178.

Graeber, M.B. and Streit, W.J. (1990) Perivascular microglia defined. *Trends Neurosci.* 13:366.

Graeber, M.B., Streit, W.J., and Kreutzberg, G.W. (1988) Axotomy of the rat facial nerve leads to increased CR3 complement receptor expression by activated microglial cells. *J. Neurosci. Res.* 21:18–24.

Graeber, M.B., Streit, W.J., and Kreutzberg, G.W. (1989) Identity of ED2-positive perivascular cells in rat brain. *J. Neurosci. Res.* 22:103–106.

Griffith, R., Soria, J., and Wood, J.G. (2000) Regulation of microglial tyrosine phosphorylation in response to neuronal injury. *Exp. Neurol.* 161:297–305.

Harrison, J.K., Jiang, Y., Chen, S., Xia, Y., Maciejewski, D., McNamara, R.K., Streit, W.J., Salafranca, M.N., Adhikari, S., Thompson, D.A., Botti, P., Bacon, K.B., and Feng, L. (1998) Role for neuronally-derived fractalkine in mediating interactions between neurons and CX3CR1-expressing microglia. *Proc. Natl. Acad. Sci. USA* 95:10896–10901.

Hayes, G.M., Woodroofe, M.N., and Cuzner, M.L. (1987) Microglia are the major cell type expressing MHC class II in human white matter. *J. Neurol. Sci.* 80:25–37.

Heppner, F.L., Roth, K., Nitsch, R., and Hailer, N.P. (1998) Vitamin E induces ramification and downregulation of adhesion molecules in cultured microglial cells. *Glia* 22:180–188.

Hickey, W.F. and Kimura, H. (1988) Perivascular microglial cells of the CNS are bone marrow-derived and present antigen in vivo. *Science* 239:290–292.

Hoek, R.M., Ruuls, S.R., Murphy, C.A.,Wright, G.J., Goddard, R., Zurawski, S.M., Blom, B., Homola, M.E., Streit, W.J., Brown, M.H., Barclay, A.N., and Sedgwick, J.D. (2000) Down-regulation of the macrophage lineage through interaction with OX2 (CD200). *Science* 290:1768–1771.

Hume, D.A., Perry, V.H., and Gordon, S. (1983) Immunohistochemical localization of a macrophage-specific antigen in developing mouse retina: phagocytosis of dying neurons and differentiation of microglial cells to form a regular array in the plexiform layers. *J. Cell Biol.* 97:253–247.

Hurley, S.D., Walter, S.A., Semple-Rowland, S.L., and Streit, W.J. (1999) Cytokine transcripts expressed by microglia in vitro are not expressed by ameboid microglia of the developing rat central nervous system. *Glia* 25:304–309.

Kaneko, Y., Kitamoto, T., Tateishi, J., and Yamaguchi, K. (1989) Ferritin immunohistochemistry as a marker for microglia. *Acta Neuropathol.* 79:129–136.

Kloss, C.U., Kreutzberg, G.W., and Raivich, G. (1997) Proliferation of ramified microglia on an astrocyte monolayer: characterization of stimulatory and inhibitory cytokines. *J. Neurosci. Res.* 49:248–254.

Korr, H., Schilling, W.-D., Schultze, B., and Maurer, W. (1983) Autoradiographic studies of glial proliferation in different areas of the brain of the 14-day-old rat. *Cell Tissue Kinetics* 16:393–413.

Kreutzberg, G.W. (1996) Microglia: a sensor for pathological events in the CNS. *Trends Neurosci.* 19:312–318.

Lassmann, H., Schmied, M., Vass, K., and Hickey, W.F. (1993) Bone marrow derived elements and resident microglia in brain inflammation. *Glia* 7:19–24.

Lassmann, H., Zimprich, F., Vass, K., and Hickey, W.F. (1991) Microglial cells are a component of the perivascular glia limitans. *J. Neurosci. Res.* 28:236–243.

Lawson, L.J., Perry, V.H., Dri, P., and Gordon, S. (1990) Heterogeneity in the distribution and morphology of microglia in the normal adult mouse brain. *Neuroscience* 39:151–170.

Leong, S.K. and Ling, E.A. (1992) Amoeboid and ramified microglia: their interrelationship and response to brain injury. *Glia* 6:39–47.

Ling, E.A. and Wong, W.C. (1993) The origin and nature of ramified and amoeboid microglia: a historical review and current concepts. *Glia* 7:9–18.

Mannoji, H., Yeger, H., and Becker, L.E. (1986) A specific histochemical marker (lectin *Ricinus communis* agglutinin-1) for normal human microglia, and application to routine histopathology. *Acta Neuropathol.* 71:341–343.

Mato, M., Ookawara, S., and Saito-Taki, T. (1986) Serological determinants of fluorescent granular perithelial cells along small cerebral blood vessels in rodent. *Acta Neuropathol.* 72:117–123.

McKanna, J.A. (1993) Lipocortin 1 immunoreactivity identifies microglia in adult rat brain. *J. Neurosci. Res.* 36:491–500.

Mertsch, K., Hanisch, U.K., Kettenmann, H., and Schnitzer, J. (2001) Characterization of microglial cells and their response to stimulation in an organotypic retinal culture system. *J. Comp. Neurol.* 431:217–227.

Miles, J.M. and Chou, S.M. (1988) A new immunoperoxidase marker for microglia in paraffin section. *J. Neuropathol. Exp. Neurol.* 47:579–587.

Morioka, T., Baba, T., Black, K.L., and Streit, W.J. (1992) Response of microglial cells to experimental rat glioma. *Glia* 6:75–79.

Murabe, Y. and Sano, Y. (1981) Thiaminepyrophosphatase activity in the plasma membrane of microglia. *Histochemistry* 71:45–52.

Nakajima, K. and Kohsaka, S. (2002) Neuroprotective roles of microglia in the central nervous system. In: Streit, W.J., ed. *Microglia in the Regenerating and Degenerating Central Nervous System.* New York: Springer Verlag, pp. 188–208.

Nakajima, K., Shimojo, M., Hamanoue, M., Ishiura, S., Sugita, H., and Kohsaka, S. (1992) Identification of elastase as a secretory protease from cultured rat microglia. *J. Neurochem.* 58:1401–1408.

Nishiyori, A., Minami, M., Ohtani, Y., Takami, S., Yamamoto, J., Kawaguchi, N., Kume, T., Akaike, A., and Satoh, M. (1998) Localization of fractalkine and CX_3CR1 mRNAs in rat brain: does fractalkine play a role in signaling from neuron to microglia? *FEBS Lett.* 429:167–172.

Oehmichen, M., Wiethölter, H., and Greaves, M.F. (1979) Immunological analysis of human microglia: lack of monocytic and lymphoid differentiation antigens. *J. Neuropathol. Exp. Neurol.* 38:99–103.

Palacios, G. (1990) A double immunocytochemical and histochemical technique for demonstration of cholinergic neurons and microglial cells in basal forebrain and neostriatum of the rat. *Neurosci. Lett.* 115:13–18.

Pennell, N.A. and Streit, W.J. (1998) Tracing of fluoro-gold-prelabeled microglia injected into the adult rat brain, *Glia* 23:84–88.

Perry, V.H. and Gordon, S. 1987. Modulation of CD4 antigen on macrophages and microglia in rat brain. *J. Exp. Med.* 166:1138–1143.

Perry, V.H., Hume, D.A., and Gordon, S. (1985) Immunohistochemical localization of macrophages and microglia in the adult and developing mouse brain. *Neuroscience* 15:313–326.

Perry, V.H., Matyszak, M.K., and Fearn, S. 1993. Altered antigen expression of microglia in the aged rodent brain. *Glia* 7:60–67.

Rinaman, L., Milligan, C.E., and Levitt, P. (1991) Persistence of fluoro-gold following degeneration of labeled motoneurons is due to phagocytosis by microglia and macrophages. *Neuroscience* 44:765–776.

Sawada, M., Suzumura, A., Yamamoto, H., and Marunouchi, T. (1990) Activation and proliferation of the isolated microglia by colony stimulating factor-1 and possible involvement of protein kinase C. *Brain Res.* 509:119–124.

Schelper, R.L. and Adrian, E.K. (1980) Non-specific esterase activity in reactive cells in injured nervous tissue labeled with ^{3}H-thymidine or ^{125}iododeoxyuridine injected before injury. *J. Comp. Neurol.* 194:829–844.

Schnitzer, J. (1989) Enzyme-histochemical demonstration of microglial cells in the adult and postnatal rabbit retina. *J. Comp. Neurol.* 282:249–263.

Sievers, J., Parwaresch, R., and Wottge, H.U. (1994) Blood monocytes and spleen macrophages differentiate into microglia-like cells on monolayers of astrocytes: morphology. *Glia* 12:245–258.

Sorokin, S.P., Hoyt, R.F., Jr., Blunt, D.G., and McNelly, N.A. (1992) Macrophage development: II. Early ontogeny of macrophage populations in brain, liver, and lungs of rat embryos as revealed by a lectin marker. *Anat. Rec.* 232:527–550.

Streit, W.J. (2001) Microglia and macrophages in the developing CNS. *Neurotoxicology* 22:619–624.

Streit, W.J. (2002) Microglia as neuroprotective: immunocompetent cells of the CNS. *Glia* 40:133–139.

Streit, W.J. and Graeber, M.B. (1993) Heterogeneity of microglial and perivascular cell populations—Insights gained from the facial nucleus paradigm. *Glia* 7:68–74.

Streit, W.J., Graeber, M.B., and Kreutzberg, G.W. (1988) Functional plasticity of microglia: a review. *Glia* 1:301–307.

Streit, W.J., Graeber, M.B., and Kreutzberg, G.W. (1989) Expression of Ia antigens on perivascular and microglial cells after sublethal and lethal neuronal injury. *Exp. Neurol.* 105:115–126.

Streit, W.J. and Kreutzberg, G.W. (1987) Lectin binding by resting and reactive microglia. *J. Neurocytol.* 16:249–260.

Streit, W.J., Schulte, B.A., Balentine, J.D., and Spicer, S.S. (1985) Histochemical localization of galactose containing glycoconjugates in sensory neurons and their processes in the central and peripheral nervous system of the rat. *J. Histochem. Cytochem.* 33:1042–1052.

Streit, W.J. and Sparks, D.L. (1997) Activation of microglia in the brains of humans with heart disease and hypercholesterolemic rabbits. *J. Mol. Med.* 75:130–138.

Streit, W.J., Sammons, N.W., Kuhns, A.J., and Sparks, D.L. (2004) Dystrophic microglia in the aging human brain. *Glia* 45:208–212.

Suzuki, H., Franz, H, Yamamoto, T., Iwasaki, Y., and Konno, H. (1988) Identification of the normal microglial population in human and rodent nervous tissue using lectin-histochemistry. *Neuropathol. Appl. Neurobiol.* 14:221–227.

Takahashi, K., Yamamura, F., and Naito, M. (1989) Differentiation, maturation, and proliferation of macrophages in the mouse yolk sac: a light-microscopic, enzyme-cytochemical, immunohistochemical, and ultrastructural study. *J. Leukocyte Biol.* 45:87–96.

Tanaka, J. and Maeda, N. (1996) Microglial ramification requires nondiffusible factors derived from astrocytes. *Exp. Neurol.* 137: 367–375.

Thanos, S. (1991) Specific transcellular carbocyanin-labelling of rat retinal microglia during injury-induced neuronal degeneration. *Neurosci. Lett.* 127:108–112.

Walsh, D.T., Perry, V.H., and Minghetti, L. (2000) Cyclooxygenase-2 is highly expressed in microglial-like cells in a murine model of prion disease. *Glia* 29:392–396.

Yagi, R., Tanaka, S., and Koike, T. (1999) Thapsigargin induces microglial transformation from amoeboid to ramified type in vitro. *Glia* 29:49–52.

6 Lineages of astrocytes and oligodendrocytes

JAMES E. GOLDMAN

CENTRAL NERVOUS SYSTEM GLIAL LINEAGES

Any model of glial development must account for the wide variety of glial cells that populate the central nervous system (CNS). As described in this volume, those include astrocytes of many and diverse forms, oligodendrocytes of assorted varieties, ependymal cells, choroid plexus epithelial cells, tanycytes and other subependymal glia, and a heterogeneous collection of immature glial cells that continue to populate the nervous system throughout adulthood. Constructed from both observations *in vivo* and studies of cultured cells, current development schemes show a linear sequence of stages reflecting progressive fate restrictions and progressive acquisitions of mature characteristics. This chapter will review these schemes and point out gaps in our understanding.

Patterns of Glial Development in Different Regions of the Central Nervous System: Is Glial Development Identical Everywhere in the Brain?

It is unlikely that the details of glial development are identical in every region of the CNS. Development needs to be placed in an appropriate anatomical context, because different types of glia need to be generated at different times in different regions and because the anatomy of different regions varies (the white matter of the spinal cord is at its periphery, while the white matter of the hemispheres is more centrally located, for example). There seem to be several general rules, however: (*1*) glia, along with neurons, originate from VZ cells in the embryonic CNS; (*2*) the immature cells that give rise to oligodendrocytes are located mainly in ventral regions of the neuraxis, although migratory routes to their final destinations are different in different regions (there are a few exceptions to this ventral rule, as noted below); (*3*) astrocytes have at least two different origins—one from radial glial cells and the other from migratory cells that populate the subventricular zone (SVZ); (*4*) some radial glia share a common origin with neurons, and in fact, give rise to certain classes of neurons; (*5*) a series of soluble and cell surface molecules regulate gliogenesis; (*6*) these molecules induce different combinations of transcription factors that specify glial or neuronal fate or progressively restrict the fate of immature cells.

The idea that glia and neurons share common origins is obvious, but when the lineages diverge has been controversial. It appears that there are different common progenitors in different regions: motor neuron/oligodendrocyte in spinal cord, radial glia/projection neuron in cortex and cerebellum, astrocyte/oligodendrocyte/interneuron in forebrain and cerebellum and perhaps in cord as well. Thus, one should be cautious in transplanting a lineage scheme in its entirety from one region of the CNS to another.

Glial Development in the Forebrain

Some astrocytes arise from radial glia

The ventricular zone (VZ) is a pseudostratified epithelium composed of the earliest neuroectodermal cells. At about the time when cortical neurons begin to develop (around E11 in mouse), elongated, radially oriented cells appear in the VZ that have many characteristics in common with astrocytes, such as the GLAST type of glutamate transporter, glycogen granules, brain lipid binding protein (BLBP), and glial fibrillary acidic protein (GFAP) (Malatesta et al., 2003). The historical term for these cells is *radial glia*. Radial glia span the width of the neural tube from ventricular to pial surface and are found in all regions of the developing CNS. In the cerebral cortex, radial glia give rise to neurons, primarily projection neurons (Malatesta et al., 2000, 2003; Noctor et al., 2001), with perhaps some interneurons as well (Fig. 6.1). At a later time, after neuronal migration has ceased, some of the radial glial cells transform into astrocytes (Fig. 6.2). We do not know, however, what proportion of astrocytes are generated in this way or if those astrocytes have different properties from those generated from SVZ cells (see below). The generation of astrocytes from radial glia likely oc-

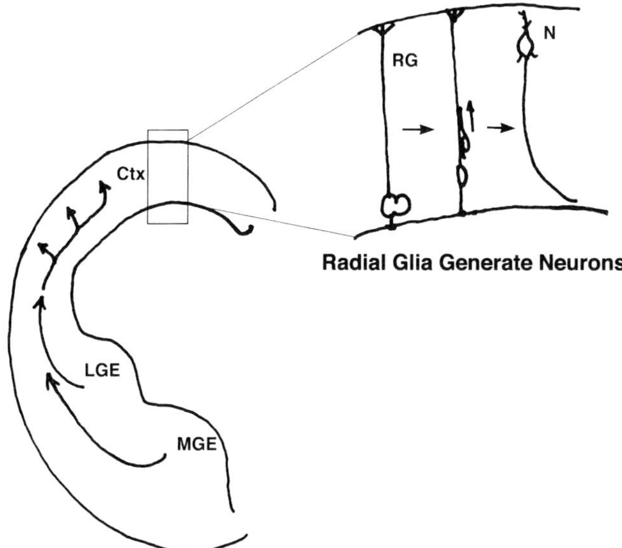

FIGURE 6.1 During embryonic development, immature cells from the ventral forebrain migrate tangentially through the intermediate zone and into the cortex. There they develop into inhibitory interneurons and oligodendrocytes. The diagram also shows generation of cortical projection neurons from radial glia in the dorsal telencephalon. Radial glia then go on to generate astrocytes (see Figure 6.2). MGE, medial ganglionic eminence; LGE, lateral ganglionic eminence; RG, radial glial cell; N, neuron. (Adapted from Anderson et al., 2001 and Noctor et al., 2001.)

curs in all areas of the CNS, although this transformation has been visualized directly only in forebrain (Voigt, 1989; Gaiano et al., 2000). Thus, astrocytes and some neurons share a common progenitor, a lineage that has been most clearly shown in the neocortex but also observed in the developing chick optic tectum (Galileo et al., 1990; Gray and Sanes, 1992).

What regulates astrocyte versus neuronal differentiation from VZ cells? Members of the Notch family of transmembrane receptors and their ligands, jagged and delta, play an important role: Notch 1, when constitutively expressed in an activated form in VZ cells of the E9.5 mouse CNS, strongly promotes an astrocyte fate (Gaiano et al., 2000) instead of the normal neuronal and astrocyte fates. Similarly, expressing Notch 1 in cells of the embryonic retina strongly promotes differentiation of Müller glial cells, apparently at the expense of rod photoreceptors (Furukawa et al., 2000). Thus, as in invertebrates, Notch activation appears to promote a glial fate while inhibiting a neuronal fate. It is not yet clear what downstream signaling systems of Notch are activated either to repress neurogenesis or to promote astrogenesis.

There is no direct evidence, however, that oligodendrocytes of the cortex or subcortical white matter arise directly from cortical radial glial cells. Indeed, oligodendrocytes in the forebrain appear to emerge from immature cells that are generated ventrally and migrate dorsally into the cortex (see below).

Oligodendrocytes as well as some astrocytes arise from immature cells in ventral regions of the neural axis

As noted above, some astrocytes arise from VZ cells via radial glia intermediates. Other astrocytes, along with oligodendrocytes, arise from immature cells that emigrate in the perinatal period from the SVZ into the brain to colonize both gray and white matter (Levison

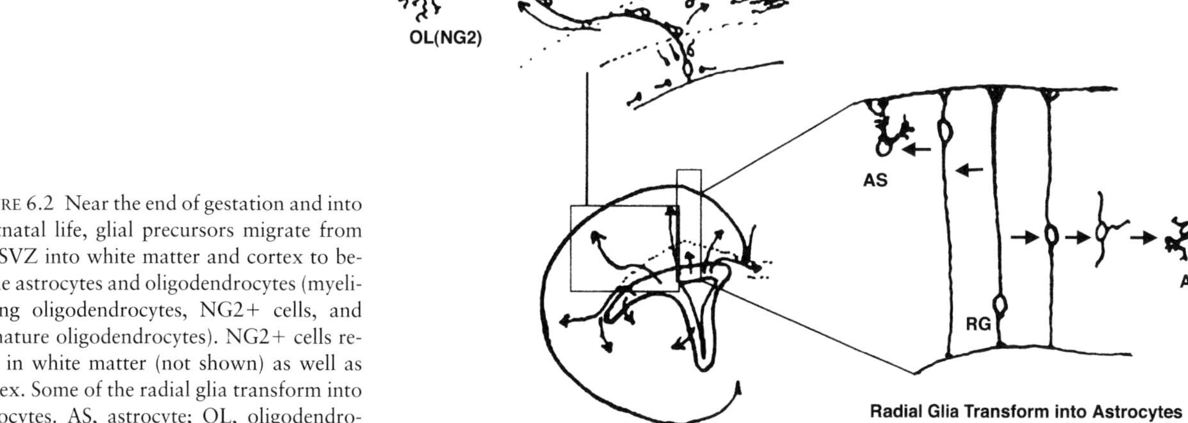

FIGURE 6.2 Near the end of gestation and into postnatal life, glial precursors migrate from the SVZ into white matter and cortex to become astrocytes and oligodendrocytes (myelinating oligodendrocytes, NG2+ cells, and immature oligodendrocytes). NG2+ cells reside in white matter (not shown) as well as cortex. Some of the radial glia transform into astrocytes. AS, astrocyte; OL, oligodendrocyte; OL(NG2), NG2+ glia; RG, radial glia.

and Goldman, 1993; reviewed in Marshall et al., 2003). To consider the lineage of glia that arise from SVZ cells, we need to consider three interrelated issues: the ventral origin of oligodendrocytes, the ventral origin of cortical interneurons, and the genesis of the SVZ itself.

The earliest appearance of cells that express early oligodendrocyte markers occurs in the ventral forebrain, around the third ventricle. Progenitors expressing DM-20, an alternatively spliced product from the *plp* gene, are first seen in the ventral forebrain around E9.5 in mouse (Timset et al., 1995). Progenitors expressing PDGFRα also first arise in the ventral forebrain, around E12–13 (Pringle and Richardson, 1993). DM-20 and PDGFRα+ do not appear to be expressed in the same cells, however. The lineage relationship between the PDGFRα+ cells and the DM-20+ cells is not completely clear, and it is possible that these two cell classes give rise to different classes of oligodendrocytes (Richardson et al., 2000; Spassky et al., 2000). The DM-20+ cells do not depend upon signaling through the PDGFRα, however, consistent with the idea of two separate oligodendrocyte precursor types (Spassky et al., 2001). Alternatively, it is possible that the markers belong to cells in the same lineage but are just not expressed simultaneously.

Oligodendrocyte precursors migrate extensively in a ventral-to-dorsal direction. During the late embryonic period in mice, cells expressing DM-20 are progressively observed in more lateral and dorsal locations. Furthermore, transplantation experiments to produce chick-quail or chick-mouse chimeras clearly show the migration of oligodendrocyte precursors from the anterior entopeduncular area to colonize both ventral and dorsal telencephalon (Olivier et al., 2001). PDGFRα+ cells also appear in more and more dorsal locations, first in the intermediate zone and then in the neocortex (Tekki-Kessaris et al., 2001). These and other observations imply that there is a ventral-to-dorsal migration of progenitors, some of which express PDGFRα or DM-20. This migratory population is a heterogeneous one, however. Many of the GABAergic cortical interneurons arise from cells initially located in the ventral forebrain, specifically in the lateral or medial ganglionic eminences (LGE, MGE) (Anderson et al., 1997, 2001). These immature cells migrate dorsally through the intermediate zone to reach the neocortex, a migratory path tangential to the cortical surface and one that is similar to that of early oligodendrocyte precursors (Fig. 6.1). Later in embryonic development, the ventral cells take a more medial migratory course, in a path close to the ventricular surface, to form the large SVZ at the dorsolateral angle of the lateral ventricle in perinatal life (Marshall and Goldman, 2002). The SVZ cells do not express early markers for oligodendrocytes or astrocytes within the SVZ. They begin to express early glial antigens like PDGFRα, NG2, and zebrinII after they exit from the SVZ (Pringle and Richardson, 1993; Staugaitis et al., 2001).

This dorsolateral SVZ gives rise to astrocytes and oligodendrocytes of the cortex, white matter, and striatum, as well as to interneurons of the olfactory bulb (Levison and Goldman, 1993; Luskin, 1993; Luskin and McDermott, 1994) (Figs. 6.2 and 6.3).

The ventral origins of some interneurons, oligodendrocytes, and some astrocytes raise the question of whether glia and interneurons might arise from common progenitors. This question is difficult to answer now, although cells isolated from the embryonic LGE and placed in culture will generate clones composed of neurons and oligodendrocytes (He et al., 2001) but, interestingly, not astrocytes, at least under those particular conditions. In the neonatal period, forebrain SVZ cells placed in culture give rise to clones containing neurons and glia, but under these conditions the glia are both astrocytes and oligodendrocytes (Levison and Goldman, 1997). Thus, at least some of the immature cells from these regions have the potential to differentiate into both neurons and glia; whether they actually do *in vivo* is not known.

Glia lineages *in vivo* have been studied using replication-deficient retroviruses, an approach that can determine lineage relationships by defining the set of cells

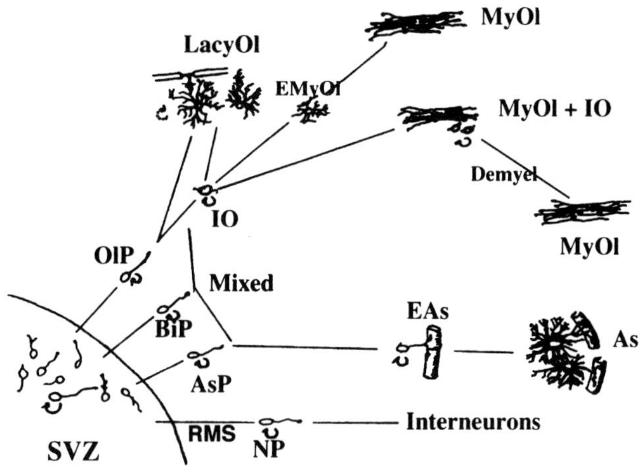

FIGURE 6.3 Lineage relationships among the progenitors of the forebrain SVZ—these migrate from the SVZ into white matter and gray matter to become glia and along the rostral migratory stream (RMS) to become interneurons in the olfactory bulb. Oligodendrocytes do not differentiate synchronously—some remain immature and cycling in the adult CNS. These are induced to develop into myelinating oligodendrocytes during demyelination/remyelination. The diagram is based upon in vivo retroviral analyses and in vitro clonal studies. SVZ, subventricular zone; OlP, oligodendrocyte precursor; AsP, astrocyte precursor; BiP, bipotential precursor, likely a glial restricted progenitor (GRP, Rao et al., 1998); RMS, rostral migratory stream; NP, neuronal precursor; IO, immature oligodendrocyte; EMyOl, early myelinating oligodendrocyte; MyOl, myelinating oligodendrocyte; Lacy Ol, NG2+ cells; EAS, early astrocyte (shown here contacting a blood vessel); As, astrocyte.

that arise from the viral infection of a single dividing progenitor. In some cases, both neurons and glia arise from the same progenitor. For example, single progenitors in the embryonic retina give rise to neurons and Müller glia (Turner and Cepko, 1987). The developmental potential of retinal cells becomes restricted over time, however, and in the late embryonic and early postnatal periods, dividing progenitors give rise largely to Müller glia and photoreceptor cells. Obviously, the descendants of a given progenitor depend in large part on the time when the retrovirus is introduced and the location in which it is placed. Individual progenitors in the embryonic neocortex and the striatum can generate both astrocytes and neurons (Halliday and Cepko, 1992; Walsh and Cepko, 1993), possibly through radial glial intermediates (see above). But other retroviral fate studies have concluded that embryonic CNS cells give rise largely or entirely to one cell type—neurons, astrocytes, or oligodendrocytes (Luskin et al., 1988, 1993; Grove et al., 1993; Price and Thurlow, 1988).

In the application of retroviruses to gliogenesis, most studies find that retroviral-labeled cells accumulate in groups or clusters, which are in most cases homogeneous—either astrocytic or oligodendrocytic. However, a small proportion of clusters, about 15%, are mixed, either containing astrocytes and oligodendrocytes or, more rarely, neurons and glia (Luskin et al., 1988; Price and Thurlow, 1988; Grove et al., 1993; Levison and Goldman, 1993; Luskin et al., 1993; Luskin and McDermott, 1994; Parnevales, 1999). Most, if not all, of these clusters are clonal, at least if the titer of injected retrovirus is low and clusters are spatially distinct (Zerlin et al., in press). Thus, a clonal cluster is formed from a single progenitor that migrates to a particular place, stops migrating, but continues to proliferate. The presence of mixed astrocyte-oligodendrocyte clusters tells us that a small proportion of the gliogenic SVZ cells are not specified to either of the lineages until they have stopped migrating.

The clonal analysis becomes more complex due to spatial dispersion of members of a single clone. Immature glia continue to divide as they migrate, but the two progeny of a dividing cell may not necessarily continue to migrate together, and therefore would not necessarily end up in the same cluster. Indeed, direct visualization of migrating glia shows that cells cease migrating before they divide and recommence migration after they divide, the two progeny moving off in different directions.

Glial development in the optic nerve

Studies of optic nerve development have heavily influenced thinking about glial lineages. In this structure, both astrocytes and oligodendrocytes are generated at around the end of gestation and during the first week or two of life in rodents. These two glial types appear to originate from separate progenitors (Skoff and Knapp, 1991). The oligodendrocytes originate as precursors in the SVZ at the base of the third ventricle and migrate into and along the nerve (migration and developmental stages are reviewed in Miller, 2002). These immature oligodendrocytes, if removed from the neonatal optic nerve, however, display plasticity in that they can develop into either oligodendrocytes or astrocytes, depending upon the culture conditions (Raff et al., 1983). These progenitors, termed *O-2A* (*oligodendrocyte-type 2 astrocyte*) cells, will differentiate into oligodendrocytes in serum-free media but can be induced to differentiate along an astrocytic pathway, yielding *type 2 astrocytes*, by serum, or interleukin-6 (IL-6)/leukemia inhibitor factor (LIF)/ciliary neuronotrophic factor (CNTF) family members (see below). The bipotential nature of these cells reveals that the environment of the developing optic nerve promotes their differentiation into oligodendrocytes and/or inhibits their differentiation into astrocytes. The pattern of immature glia differentiating largely into oligodendrocytes in a region of white matter also seems to be followed elsewhere in the forebrain, since the large majority of SVZ cells that settle in subcortical white matter in the neonatal period differentiate into oligodendrocytes (Levison et al., 1993).

Optic nerve astrocytes appear to be intrinsic to the nerve and likely arise from radial glial cells, which are derived in turn from the initial optic nerve neuroepithelium. The conversion of the precursors into astrocytes goes through a stage during which they express the vimentin type of intermediate filament and the gangliosides recognized by the monoclonal antibody, A2B5, but do not express either GFAP or S-100β, markers of more mature astrocytes in rodents (Mi and Barres, 1999). *In vivo* the vimentin-positive cells will eventually also express GFAP. In culture, the astrocyte progenitors can be induced to express GFAP by CNTF or LIF.

Glial Development in the Cerebellum

The cerebellum contains oligodendrocytes as well as a variety of astrocyte forms, including the fibrous astrocytes of white matter, velate astrocytes of the internal granule cell layer, and Bergmann glia, which send radially directed processes from the cell bodies in the Purkinje cell layer up to the pial surface (Palay and Chan-Palay, 1972).

Early morphological and ^{3}H-thymidine studies suggested that some Bergmann glia are generated from other Bergmann glia (since they incorporate thymidine) and/or from some progenitor of an unknown type (Basco et al., 1977; Choi and Lapham, 1980). It is likely that some Bergmann glia as well as other astrocytes

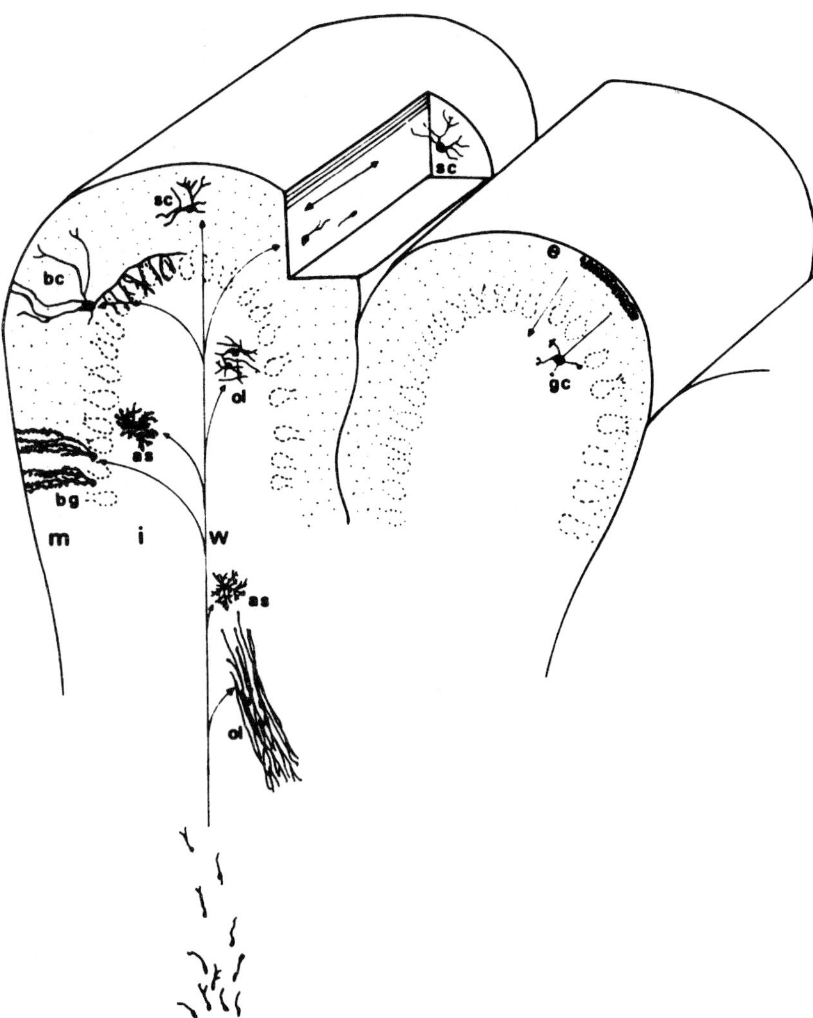

FIGURE 6.4 During late gestation and into postnatal life, glial and neuronal precursors generated at the base of the cerebellum migrate through white matter into cortex and differentiate into oligodendrocytes, several astrocyte forms (including Bergmann glia), and interneurons. as, astrocyte; bc, basket cell; bg, Bergmann glia; e, external granule layer; gc, granule cell; i, internal granule layer; m, molecular layer; ol, oligodendrocyte; pro, progenitor; sc, stellate cell; w, white matter. (From Zhang and Goldman, 1996.)

arise from embryonic radial glia of the cerebellum. Some astrocytes, including Bergmann glia, share a common lineage with Purkinje cells, as determined by retroviral tracing in chick (Lin and Cepko, 1999).

During the perinatal period, glial progenitors arise in the base of the cerebellum, just dorsal to the fourth ventricle, and migrate through the white matter in a largely radial direction (Miyake et al., 1995; Zhang and Goldman, 1996). These migratory progenitors give rise to astrocytes of all types and to oligodendrocytes, as well as to interneurons (Fig. 6.4). At least some of these progenitors in the white matter begin to differentiate as they migrate, since they express astrocyte characteristics, such as GLAST, and oligodendrocyte markers, such as NG2 (Milosevic and Goldman, 2002).

Gliogenesis in the Spinal Cord

In the spinal cord, oligodendrocyte development is strongly linked to dorsoventral patterning. A series of domains, as defined by the expression of transcription factors, partition the ventral neuroepithelium of the embryonic cord (for review see Rowitch et al., 2002). Cells within the motor neuron progenitor domain (pMN), defined by the expression of the basic helix-loop-helix (bHLH) factor *olig2*, first give rise to motorneurons and then, after neurogenesis, produce oligodendrocytes (Fig. 6.5). Oligodendrocytes are generated from the ventral cord for at least two reasons. First, both motorneurons and oligodendrocytes require the presence of Sonic hedgehog (Shh), produced ventrally by the notochord and floorplate. Second, the differentiation of oligodendrocytes from precursors located more dorsally appears to be actively inhibited by signals from the dorsal cord (Wada et al., 2000).

How is the switch from neuronal to oligodendrocyte fate regulated? Current models envision a changing constellation of transcription factors accompanying this change in fate. Immature cells of the pMN domain initially express *olig2* as well as the proneuronal gene, *neurogenin-2*, but the latter decreases at the end of neurogenesis (Zhou et al. 2000), at which time *olig2*+ cells

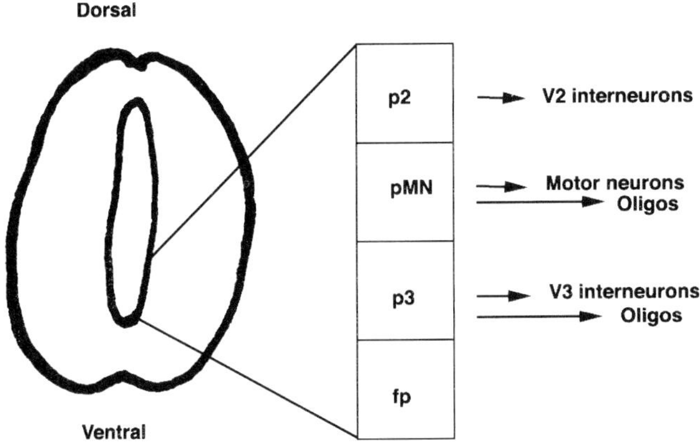

FIGURE 6.5 Oligodendrocytes in the spinal cord originate from ventral ventricular zone, specifically the pMN domain, which generates motor neurons at first, then oligodendrocytes. The p3 domain may also give rise to oligodendrocytes (not shown—see Fu et al., 2002). (Adapted from Rowitch et al., 2002.)

begin to express the early oligodendrocyte marker, *PDGFRα*, and eventually the homeobox transcription factor, *Nkx2.2*. However, it is likely that oligodendrocytes also originate from the more ventral p3 domain of the cord neuroepithelium (Fu et al., 2002). The cells in the p3 domain are initially *Nkx2.2+*, *olig2−*, and *PDGFRα−* but eventually express early oligodendrocyte markers. Whether these closely proximate regions generate oligodendrocytes with equivalent characteristics is not yet known.

Where do cord astrocytes come from? Evidence to date suggests that astrocytes and oligodendrocytes arise from separate progenitors in separate VZ domains. Pringle et al. (2003) find that the expressions of *olig2* (in the PMN domain) does not overlap with the expression of fibroblast growth factor receptor type 3 (*Fgfr3*), which has a far more widespread localization in dorsal as well as ventral neuroepithelium. The expression of molecular markers argues for separate astrocyte and oligodendrocyte lineages in the cord, at least by around E13–14 in mouse. *Fgfr3+* cells, which do not represent oligodendrocyte precursors and apparently not neuronal precursors either, likely correspond to very early astrocyte precursors. Other evidence for a separation of astrocyte from oligodendrocyte lineages includes the observation that oligodendrocytes in cord require Shh for their development (Orentas et al., 1999), whereas astrocytes do not (Pringle et al., 2003), and astrocytes can be generated from dorsal neuroepithelium, whereas oligodendrocytes cannot (Pringle et al., 1998). However, in *olig1/olig2* double knockout (−/−) mice, in which oligodendrocytes do not develop, fate mapping studies show astrocytes arising from cells that had originated in the domain where *olig2* would have been normally expressed (Zhou and Anderson, 2002). This observation raises the possibility that the Olig factors normally repress astrocyte differentiation in a population that develops into oligodendrocytes and neurons. Neither *olig1* nor *olig2* appears to be expressed in astrocytes in the normal spinal cord, consistent with the idea that these genes inhibit astrocyte development (Lu et al., 2000; Zhou et al., 2000). However, developing astrocytes in other regions of the CNS do express *olig2* (Marshall and Goldman, unpublished observations).

How astrocytes arise in cord, then, is not fully understood. By analogy to the radial glial–astrocyte transformation in the forebrain (see above), it seems likely that at least some of the cord astrocytes arise from VZ cells via radial glia.

The above considerations argue for a common lineage of oligodendrocytes with some neurons and a separate lineage for astrocytes in the cord. Nevertheless, Rao et al. (1998) have isolated a progenitor from embryonic spinal cord that appears to be restricted to glial lineages, able to generate both astrocytes and oligodendrocytes in culture, but not neurons. These cells bind the monoclonal antibody A2B5. They can be isolated from both dorsal and ventral regions of the cord. These observations do not appear to coincide with observations *in vivo*, as noted above. There are at least two ways to harmonize these findings. First, one can argue that development is highly regulated in spatial and temporal patterns, and thus that immature cells are prevented from assuming all of their potential fates. Removing progenitors from their normal environment relieves fate restrictions to some degree and allows progression through lineages not otherwise taken. Second, one could argue that there are indeed three lineages for oligodendrocytes (which might in fact give rise to different oligodendrocyte populations): one in common with motorneurons, one from the p3 domain, and the other in common with astrocytes, although there is no definitive evidence for the latter *in vivo*, at least in the cord.

Astrocyte and Oligodendrocyte Development in the Adult Central Nervous System

Astrocytes and oligodendrocytes are generated in the adult CNS, although at a low rate. Early studies used ^{3}H-thymidine to estimate glial turnover in the adult rodent brain, concluding that both glial types continue to be generated. It appears that the number of oligodendrocytes increases slowly, while the number of astrocytes remains approximately constant (Hommes and Leblond, 1967; Korr et al., 1973; Paterson, 1983). A similar conclusion was drawn from retroviral labeling, which showed an increase in the size of oligodendrocyte clonal clusters, but not astrocyte clusters, over time (Levison et al., 1999).

New glia may arise either from the proliferation of mature astrocytes and oligodendrocytes or from the differentiation of progenitors. The bulk of evidence strongly favors the latter possibility. Although astrocytes and oligodendrocytes will divide in pathological states (Norton, 1999), there is little evidence that mature glia divide in the unperturbed brain. A variety of immature glial cells, however, populate the adult CNS. Thymidine labeling studies (see above) all described proliferating cells that did not have characteristics of mature astrocytes or oligodendrocytes, based on nuclear morphology and ultrastructural characteristics. It was difficult at the time to place all of these cells into specific lineages, however; the more recent use of antigenic markers has begun to sort out the nature of these progenitors. The thymidine studies estimated that cycling cells constituted a small but significant proportion of the total cell number. For example, proliferating cells in the adult rodent white matter make up as much as 2% of the total (Paterson, 1983).

One approach to studying immature cells has been to isolate them on the basis of antigenic characteristics. Thus, cells that bind the A2B5 monoclonal antibody and proliferate in culture have been isolated from the adult CNS (Wolswijk and Noble, 1989). These progenitors cycle more slowly *in vitro* than their A2B5+ counterparts taken from the neonatal brain, but can be induced to cycle as rapidly as the neonatal cells with platelet-derived growth factor (PDGF) and basic fibroblast growth factor (bFGF) (Wolswijk and Noble, 1992), consistent with a model in which cycle times depend upon the availability/local concentrations of specific growth factors. The A2B5+ progenitors from adult brain will differentiate in culture into more mature oligodendrocytes or into astrocytes (A2B5+/GFAP+) as a function of culture conditions.

Populations isolated directly from adult CNS (Gensert and Goldman, 2001) and enriched for immature cells are heterogeneous, expressing various combinations of markers, including A2B5, O4, and vimentin, although not mature markers such as GFAP, O1, or myelin basic protein (MBP). In culture, these cells can generate oligodendrocytes and astrocytes, although the majority appear to be O4+ oligodendrocyte progenitors. Whether astrocytes are generated from O4+ cells seems less likely, although Armstrong et al. (1992) isolated the rare cell from adult human white matter that became both O4+ and GFAP+ in culture.

The Nature and Lineages of NG2-Expressing Cells in the Adult Central Nervous System

Glia expressing the NG2 chondroitin sulfate proteoglycan were first found in the cerebellum, where they display a lacy shape with many delicate processes; similar cells reside in the forebrain (reviewed in Levine et al., 2001). While the NG2 marker is found on oligodendrocytes during their early development (Nishiyama et al., 1996), the NG2+ glia in the adult brain do not myelinate. Furthermore, they do not ensheath blood vessels or the pial surface. Their classification has been controversial, and it is not clear whether NG2 marks a single type of glial cell or multiple types. Some authors believe that these cells represent a type of glial precursor cell in the adult brain (Levine et al., 2001) Many of the NG2+ cells contact nodes of Ranvier in white matter and synapses in gray matter (Butt et al., 1999; Bergles et al. 2000), suggesting that they play roles in saltatory conduction along axons and synaptic regulation, and also suggesting that at least some of the NG2+ cells constitute a stable glial population in the brain (Butt et al., 2002). In terms of lineage, it is likely that the NG2+ population is related to oligodendrocytes rather than astrocytes. In retroviral studies *in vivo* the NG2+ cells either form their own clonal clusters or are part of clusters of myelinating oligodendrocytes (Levison et al., 1999). Why and how the oligodendrocyte lineage diverges to generate myelinating oligodendrocytes and NG2+ cells is not understood.

$NG2^+$ cells in the adult optic nerve and the molecular layer of the adult cerebellum have far lower labeling index than NG2+ cells in the developing CNS (Levine et al., 1993; Shi et al., 1998). However, a higher bromodeoxyuridine (BrdU) labeling index has been reported for NG2+ cells in the rat CNS after a series of BrdU pulses (Alonso, 2000). Retroviral labeling of dividing cells in adult rat white matter *in situ* results in reporter gene expression in NG2− cells as well as NG2+ cells (J. Mason, unpublished results). The former appear relatively simple in morphology, while the latter display many thin, lacy processes. To make matters more complex, there is a population of NG2+/vimentin+ cells in the adult rat spinal cord (Horner et al., 2000). These appear to be relatively simple cells that assume a radial orientation and do not look at all like the lacy cells in the brain. Furthermore, in rodents under some pathological conditions, and in humans, the NG2 proteoglycan is expressed by microglia/macrophages and endothelial cells (Pouly et al., 1999; Bu et al., 2001; Pouly et al., 2001). Thus, cells expressing NG2 may differ in different regions of the adult CNS; NG2 is likely not to be a specific marker for a specific oligodendrocyte progenitor cell; and while some NG2+ cells do indeed divide in the adult CNS, they are not the only proliferative cell population.

There Are Cycling Cells in the Adult Central Nervous System That Have Astrocytic Properties

The adult CNS contains cells that possess *stem-like* properties, at least in culture, generating *neurospheres* containing oligodendrocytes, astrocytes, and neurons, as noted initially by Reynolds and Weiss (1992) and Richards et al. (1992). Among this potentially multipotent population are cycling cells that express astrocyte qualities, including GFAP (Doetsch et al., 1999; Laywell et al., 2000; Seri et al., 2001; Fabel et al., 2003). Such cells give rise to neurons in the adult CNS—specifically, astrocytic cells in the residual forebrain SVZ generate olfactory interneurons (Doetsch et al., 1999), while astrocytic cells in the subgranular zone of the hippocampus generate dentate granule cells (Fabel et al., 2003). The adult spinal cord also contains cycling cells that express GFAP or S-100β (Horner et al., 2000), but their fate has not been followed. The astrocytic character neither implies that these immature cells have all of the characteristics of mature astrocytes nor implies that all astrocytes are potential stem cells. The astrocytic nature of such cells has, however, engendered discussions as to the nature of "astrocyteness" and even as to the nature of a "glial" cell. The origin of such cells is not entirely clear, but they may turn out to be direct descendants of VZ cells or of radial glia, which, as noted above, possess many of the characteristics of astrocytes and generate neurons and astrocytes during development.

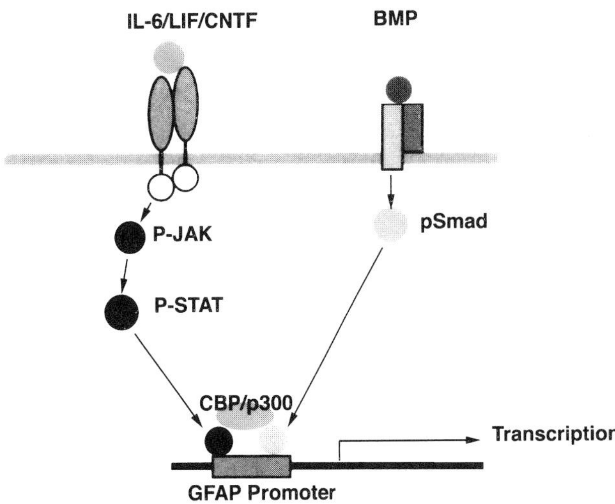

FIGURE 6.6 Members of the IL-6 and BMP families induce astrocyte genes through Jak/Stat and Smad activation pathways.

Astrocyte and Oligodendrocyte Development Is Regulated by Different Classes of Molecules and Different Intracellular Pathways

For astrocytes, attention has focused on the IL-6/LIF family of cytokines and the LIF receptor/gp130 pair, the TGFβ transforming growth factor family, particularly bone morphogenetic proteins (BMPs) and BMP receptors, and the Notch and Notch ligand pairs. For oligodendrocytes, attention has focused on shh pathways, on transcription factors such as the Olig genes, and, later in oligodendrocyte differentiation, or a series of growth factors, including PDGF, bFGF, insulin-like growth factor, type 1 (IGF1), neuregulins, and thyroid hormone. The signals that determine early fate designation are likely to interact to regulate glial cell choices or neuronal-glial choices.

Signaling pathways that regulate astrocyte development

The interleukin-6 (IL-6) family of proteins includes ciliary neuronotrophic factor (CNTF), leukemia inhibitory factor (LIF), cardiotropin 1 (CT1), and oncostatin M (OSM). All of these stimulate astrocytic differentiation, usually defined as the induction of *GFAP*, in cells cultured from the embryonic CNS or from the neonatal optic nerve (Hughes et al., 1988; Gard et al., 1995; Johe et al., 1996; Bonni et al., 1997; Yanigisawa et al., 1999; Ochiai et al., 2001). These ligands signal through the LIF receptor/gp130 complex (Nakashima et al., 1999a), to activate the Janus kinase (JAK)-signal transducers and activators of transcription (STAT) intracellular signaling pathway (Bonni et al., 1997; Kahn et al., 1997) (Fig. 6.6). This pathway is linked to *GFAP* regulation, since phosphorylated JAK then phosphorylates STAT3, a transcription factor, which then binds to the CBP/p300 complex to bind to and activate the S3BE sequence in the *GFAP* promoter (Yanagisawa et al., 2001) Interleukin 6 family members act synergistically with the extracellular matrix of mesenchymal cells (Lillien and Raff, 1990; Mayer et al., 1994) in inducing GFAP expression. As noted above, astrocytes have extensive interactions with basal laminae of blood vessels and the pial surface of the brain. In fact, cerebral endothelial cells do express LIF (Mi et al., 2001). Such an interaction might help induce astrocyte differentiation, a mechanism that could appropriately match the number of astrocytes with vessels (Zerlin and Goldman, 1997).

However, bear in mind that astrocyte differentiation must involve the induction of many genes other than *GFAP*. Indeed, some of the GFAP-negative progenitors that migrate through the forebrain and cerebellum express astrocyte markers such as the glutamate transporter, GLAST (Milosovic and Goldman, 2001, 2002), or zebrin II (Staugaitis et al., 2001) prior to contacting basal laminae. Thus, early stages of astrocyte development may begin prior to mesenchymal interactions.

The TGFβ family of proteins, particularly BMP2 and BMP7, promote astrocyte development from cells of the embryonic telencephalon (Gross et al., 1996). These ligands bind to BMP receptors to active Smad transcription factors. The BMPs can act synergistically with IL-6 family members (Nakashima et al., 1999c), inducing a complex that has both Smad and STAT3 (Nakashima et al., 1999b) (Fig. 6.6). In addition to inducing astrocyte differentiation, BMP2 may be reponsible for inhibiting neuronal differentiation—that is, controlling a switch from one fate to the other or promoting astrocyte development at the expense of neurogenesis. In favor of this idea is that BMP2 upregulates Id1, Id3, and

Hes-5 in embryonic brain cells in culture (Nakashima et al., 2001). The inhibitor of differentiation genes (Id genes) play important roles in repressing specific differentiation pathways, in this case neurogenic pathways. These two Ids and Hes-5, which lies in the Notch signaling pathway, inhibit the expression of the neurogenic bHLH genes, *mash1* and *neurogenin.*

The activation of Notch, by its interaction with Notch ligands on adjacent cells, promotes the development of radial glia and astrocytes. Thus, constitutive expression of an activated Notch by cells in the E9.5 mouse forebrain directed cells toward a radial glial fate, cells which in the postnatal brain then developed into astrocytes (Gaiano et al., 2000). Similarly, expression of Notch in the P0 retinal progenitors directed cells toward a Müller glial fate, and away from a photoreceptor fate (Furukawa et al., 2000).

Clearly, progenitors are subjected to a large variety of signals, and the interactions among these signals result in fate decisions. For example, when neurogenin 1 was overexpressed in embryonic neural cells, it not only promoted neurogenesis but also inhibited the cells from differentiating into astrocytes, even when stimulated by LIF (Sun et al., 2001). If neurogenin 1 competes with STATs for binding to the CBP/p300 complex, then one can think of a model of fate determination in which the relative levels of transcription factors are the critical variables (Sun et al., 2001). Consistent with this idea is the finding that the mouse double knockout of neurogenin 2 and Mash 1 did not contain large numbers of astrocytes at the expense of neurons (Nieto et al., 2001).

Another astrogenic pathway may function through cyclic adenosine monophosphate (cAMP), since the induction of cAMP in embryonic forebrain cells induces an astrocytic fate (McManus et al., 1999). How cAMP interacts with the pathways described above is not yet clear. It is well known to increase the transcription of *GFAP* in astrocytes (Shafit-Zagardo et al., 1988; Masood et al., 1993), possibly via the cyclic AMP response element (CRE) sequence in the GFAP promoter (Besnard et al., 1991; Masood et al., 1993).

Signaling Pathways That Regulate Oligodendrocyte Development

A great deal more is known about the regulation of oligodendrocyte development than about astrocyte development. For details concerning the various factors that regulate oligodendrocyte progenitor proliferation, differentiation, and survival, the reader is referred to excellent and comprehensive reviews (Hudson, 2001; Richardson, 2001; Miller, 2002). As noted above, many if not all of the oligodendrocytes in the cord and forebrain originate from progenitors in ventral regions. Sonic hedgehog (shh), which plays a major role in establishing dorsal-ventral polarity in the developing neural tube and is required for the differentiation of spinal motor neurons, also plays a major role in oligodendrocyte development. Thus, inhibiting shh prevents the development of oligodendrocytes in the cord (Orentas et al., 1999). In the forebrain, *shh* is expressed in the ventral hypothalamus (see Nery et al., 2001; Tekki-Kessaris et al., 2001) and olfactory bulb (Spassky et al., 2001). Furthermore, deleting the *Nkx2.1* homeobox gene deletes the ventral hypothalamic *shh* focus and delays oligodendrocyte development in the telencephalon (Nery et al., 2001; Tekki-Kessaris et al., 2001). Oligodendrocytes will eventually develop, however, suggesting that there may be other sources of shh or other hedgehog family members. In fact, *shh* is expressed in the embryonic ventral thalamus, amygdala, and olfactory bulb, but it is not known how these sources influence oligodendrocyte development. Oligodendrocytes will arise in cell cultures from either dorsal or ventral telencephalon of wild-type or *Nkx2.1* (−/−) mice (Nery et al., 2001; Tekki-Kessaris et al., 2001), although the development is delayed. The presence of oligodendrocyte development in these cultures may reflect the activity of shh congeners in the CNS, since blocking all hedgehog-like signaling in cultures prevents all oligodendrocyte development (Tekki-Kessaris et al., 2001). Furthermore, placing cells in culture may in some way activate *shh* or related genes. As a further indication of the shh requirement for oligodendrocyte development, oligodendrocytes in the chick metencephalon are generated at multiple points, ventral, lateral, and dorsal (Davies and Miller, 2001), and each of these points lies in close proximity to a source of shh. The pathways through which shh specifies oligodendrocyte fate are not well understood. The homeobox gene *gsh2* lies downstream of *shh* (Corbin et al., 2000); *olig 1* and *olig 2* also depend on shh signaling (Lu et al., 2000); and the transcription factors *Gli1-3* are also linked to shh signaling (Ruiz i Altaba, 1998).

Several of the factors noted above to promote astrocyte differentiation also appear to inhibit oligodendrocyte development, suggesting that these molecules control fate-switching mechanisms. For example, BMPs inhibit oligodendrocyte development in embryonic or perinatal progenitors (Mabie et al., 1997; Mehler et al., 2000). The BMP antagonist, noggin, overcomes the inhibition of oligodendrocyte differentiation, at least *in vitro*, suggesting that a balance between BMP-derived activation and inhibition is an important regulator of astrocyte versus oligodendrocyte fate. Note that BMPs can also inhibit neuronal development (see above). Thus, BMPs have different effects on different progenitors at different times (see Mehler et al., 2000).

Oligodendrocyte precursors develop through a series of stages. The earliest stages are characterized by a highly migratory pheonotype and by the expression polysialylated neural cell adhesion molecule (PSA-NCAM) and of gangliosides that react with the A2B5 monoclonal antibody. Note that neither of these markers is specific for the oligodendrocyte lineage, however. In the forebrain, as oligodendrocyte precursors exit the SVZ, they acquire the PDGFRα and NG2. In these early stages, PDGF-A plays a major role in regulating oligodendrocyte progenitor numbers, both by promoting proliferation and by inhibiting cell death, phenomena easily observed in cell culture (reviewed in Richardson, 2001, and Miller, 2002). The value of PDGF-A in oligodendrocyte development *in vivo* has been demonstrated with murine PDGF-A knockouts, which show a severe decrease in oligodendrocytes and hypomyelination (Fruttiger et al., 1999), and with a PDGF-A overexpressor, which initially creates more than the normal number of oligodendrocytes (Calver et al., 1998). Some oligodendrocytes do develop in the PDGF-A knockout, however, probably being generated from the DM-20 population, which does not require PDGFRα signaling (see above).

In addition to PDGF, bFGF also acts as a major mitogen for progenitors, at least in tissue culture, where the combination of these two growth factors can keep oligodendrocyte progenitors in an immature, cycling state (Bogler et al., 1990). Other factors play roles in oligodendrocyte development and survival, among them insulin-like growth factor, type 1 (IGF1) and tri-iodothyronine (T3) (Barres et al., 1993). The interaction of differentiating oligodendrocytes with axons provides survival signals to the progenitors (Barres and Raff, 1994), likely to be mediated through the interaction of axonal β-neuregulin-1 with epidermal growth factor receptor, type B (erbB) on oligodendrocyte progenitors. For example, spinal cord explants from mice deficient in β-neuregulin-1 do not myelinate, but will display myelination after the addition of neuregulin (Vartanian et al., 1999). Whether the absence of neuregulin prevents progenitors from differentiating or surviving is not yet clear, although *in vitro*, β-neuregulin-1 strongly promotes survival (Canoll et al., 1996).

Progenitors stop migrating at about the stage of O4 expression, but as noted above, they remain proliferative for some time. The number of divisions oligodendrocyte progenitors go through at this stage can be roughly estimated by the size of oligodendrocyte clonal clusters, defined by retroviral labeling. Grove et al. (1993) and our laboratory (Zerlin et al., in press) have observed clusters of myelinating oligodendrocytes as large as 24 cells. This size requires five divisions. Given that a certain proportion of glial cells die during development, a cluster this large might require even more divisions. As noted above, it appears that most oligodendrocyte progenitors either go on to myelinate axons or die, but a few survive into adulthood as immature cells, which contribute to a slow turnover of myelin and which will rapidly turn into myelinating oligodendrocytes during a demyelinating insult.

CONCLUSIONS AND PERSPECTIVES

Among the fascinating questions left to be answered are the following:

1. A detailed understanding of molecular mechanisms of fate specification

   What are the downstream effectors of *shh*? What are the molecular mechanisms of glial fate induction?

   What role(s) do local environmental signals play in determining glial cell fate (e.g., interactions between blood vessels and astrocytes, between astrocytes and oligodendrocytes, or between axons and oligodendrocytes)?

2. Coordination of glial and neuronal development

   How is the development of astrocytes coordinated with the development of neurons, including dendritic growth and synapse formation?

   How is the development of astrocytes coordinated with the growth of blood vessels?

   How is the development of oligodendrocytes coordinated with myelination—what are the signals to begin myelination? Why does myelination occur asynchronously throughout the CNS?

3. Glial heterogeneity

   How is the molecular and morphological heterogeneity of glia generated? In what ways are glia functionally heterogeneous?

4. A better understanding of the nature of glial progenitors in the adult CNS

   How can we characterize this heterogeneous population? What is the developmental potential(s) of these cells? Why is their development normally restricted?

   How might adult progenitors be treated to induce differentiation and aid in repair in neurological diseases?

ACKNOWLEDGMENTS

Work in the author's laboratory has been supported by NIH Grant NS17125 and by the National Multiple Sclerosis Society. I am particularly grateful to Christine Marshall, Peter Canoll, Jeff Mason, Bernard Zalc, and Ben Barres for their helpful discussions on this chapter.

REFERENCES

Alonso, G. (2000) Prolonged corticosterone treatment of adult rats inhibits the proliferation of oligodendrocyte progenitors present throughout white and gray matter regions of the brain. *Glia* 31:219–231.

Anderson, S.A., Eisenstat, D.D., Shi, L., and Rubenstein, J.L.R. (1997) Interneuron migration from basal forebrain to neocortex: dependence on *Dlx* genes. *Science* 278:474–476.

Anderson, S.A., Marin, O., Horn, C., Jennings, K., and Rubenstein,

J.L.R. (2001) Distinct cortical migrations from the medial and lateral ganglionic eminences. *Development* 128:353–363.

Armstrong, R.C., Dorn, H.H., Kufta, C.V., Friedman, E., and Dubois-Dalcq, M.E. (1992) Pre-oligodendrocytes from adult human CNS. *J. Neurosci.* 12:1538–1547.

Barres, B.A. and Raff, M.C. (1994) Control of oligodendrocyte number in the developing rat optic nerve. *Neuron* 12:935–942.

Barres, B.A., Schmid, R., Sendnter, M., and Raff, M.C. (1993) Multiple extracellular signals are required for long-term oligodendrocyte survival. *Development* 118:283–295.

Basco, E., Hajos, F., and Fulop, Z. (1977) Proliferation of Bergmann-glia in the developing rat cerebellum. *Anat. Embryol.* (Berl) 151: 219–222.

Bergles, D.E., Roberts, J.D., Somogyi, P., and Jahr, C.E. (2000) Glutamatergic synapses on oligodendrocyte precursor cells in the hippocampus. *Nature* 405:187–191.

Besnard, F., Brenner, M., Nakatani, Y., Chao, R., Purohit, H.J., and Freese, E. (1991) Multiple interacting sites regulate astrocyte-specific transcription of the human gene for glial fibrillary acidic protein. *J. Biol. Chem.* 266:18877–18883.

Bogler, O., Wren, D., Barnett, S.C., Land, H., and Noble, M. (1990) Cooperation between two growth factors promotes extended self-renewal and inhibits differentiation of oligodendrocyte-type-2 astrocyte (O-2A) progenitor cells. *Proc. Natl. Acad. Sci. USA* 87: 6368–6372.

Bonni, A., Sun, Y., Nadal-Vicens, M., Bhatt, A., Frank, D.A., Rozovsky, I., Stahl, N., Yancopoulos, G.D., and Greenberg, M.E. (1997) Regulation of gliogenesis in the central nervous system by the JAK-STAT signaling pathway. *Science* 278:477–483.

Bu, J., Akhtar, N., and Nishiyama, A. (2001) Transient expression of the NG2 proteoglycan by a subpopulation of activated macrophages in an excitotoxic hippocampal lesion. *Glia* 34:296–310.

Butt, A.M., Duncan, A., Hornby, M.F., Kirvall, S.L., Hunter, A., Levine, J., and Berry, M. (1999) Cells expressing the NG2 antigen contact nodes of Ranvier in adult CNS white matter. *Glia* 26:84–91.

Butt, A.M., Kiff, J., Hubbard, P., and Berry, M. (2002) Synantocytes: new functions for novel NG2 expressing glia. *J. Neurocytol.* 31:551–565.

Calver, A.R., Hall, A.C., Yu, W.-P., Walsh, F.S., Heath, J.K., Betsholtz, C., and Richardson, W.D. (1998) Oligodendrocyte population dynamics and the role of PDGF in vivo. *Neuron* 20:869–882.

Canoll, P.D., Musacchio, J.M., Hardy, R., Reynolds, R., Marchionni, M.A., and Salzer, J.L. (1996) GGF/neuregulin is a neuronal signal that promotes the proliferation and survival and inhibits the differentiation of oligodendrocyte progenitors. *Neuron.* 17:229–243.

Choi, B., and Lapham, L. (1980) Evolution of Bergmann glia in developing human fetal cerebellum: a Golgi, electron microscopic and immunofluorescent study. *Brain Res.* 190:369–383.

Corbin, J.G., Gaiano, N., Machold, R.P., Langston, A., and Fishell, G. (2000) *GSH2* homeodomain gene controls multiple aspects of telencephalic development. *Development* 127:5007–5020.

Davies, J.E., and Miller, R.H. (2001) Local sonic hedgehog signaling regulates oligodendrocyte precursor appearance in multiple ventricular zone domains in the chick metencephalon. *Dev. Biol.* 233:513–525.

Doetsch, F., Caille, I., Lim, D.A., Garcia-Verdugo, J.M., and Alvarez-Buylla, A. (1999) Subventricular zone astrocytes are neural stem cells in the adult mammalian brain. *Cell* 97:730–716.

Fabel, K., Todas, H., Fabel, K., and Palmer, T. (2003) Copernican stem cells: regulatory constellations in adult hippocampal neurogenesis. *J. Cell. Biochem.* 88:41–50.

Fruttiger, M., Karlsson, L., Hall, A.C., Abramsson, A., Calver, A.R., Bostrom, H., Willetts, K., Bertold, C.-H., Betsholtz, C., and Richardson, W.D. (1999) Defective oligodendrocyte development and severe hypomyelination in PDGF-A knockout mice. *Development* 126:457–467.

Fu, H., Qi, Y., Tan, M., Cai, J., Takebayashi, H., Nakafuku, M., Richardson, W., and Qiu, M. (2002) Dual origin of spinal oligodendrocyte progenitors and evidence for the cooperative role of Olig2 and Nkx2.2 in the control of oligodendrocyte differentiation. *Development* 129:681–693.

Furukawa, T., Mukherjee, S., Bao, Z.-Z., Morrow, E.M., and Cepko, C.L. (2000) *rax*, *Hes1*, and *notch1* promote the formation of Müller glia by postnatal retinal progenitor cells. *Neuron* 26:383–394.

Gaiano, N., Nye, J.S., and Fishell, G. (2000) Radial glial identity is promoted by Notch1 signaling in the murine forebrain. *Neuron* 26:395–404.

Galileo, D.S., Gray, G.C., Owens, G.C., Majors, J., and Sanes, J.R. (1990) Neurons and glia arise from a common progenitor in chicken optic tectum: demonstration with two retroviruses and cell-type-specific antibodies. *Proc. Natl. Acad. Sci. USA* 87:458–462.

Gard, A.L., Williams, W.C., and Burrell, M.R. (1995) Oligodendroblasts distinguished from O-2A glial progenitors by surface phenotype (O4+/GalC−) and response to cytokines using signal transducer LIFR. *Dev. Biol.* 167:596–608.

Gensert, J.M. and Goldman, J.E. (2001) Heterogeneity of cycling glial progenitors in the adult mammalian neocortex and white matter. *J Neurobiol.* 48:75–86.

Gray, G.E. and Sanes, J.R. (1992) Lineage of radial glia in the chicken optic tectum. *Development* 114:271–283.

Gross, R.E., Mehler, M.F., Mabie, P.C., Zang, Z., Santschi, L., and Kessler, J.A. (1996) Bone morphogenetic proteins promote astroglial lineage commitment by mammalian subventricular zone progenitor cells. *Neuron* 17:595–606.

Grove, E.A., Williams, B.P., Da-Qing, L., Hajihosseini, M., Friedrich, A. and Price, J. (1993) Multiple restricted lineages in the embryonic rat cerebral cortex. *Development* 117:553–561.

Halliday, A.L., and Cepko, C.L. (1992) Generation and migration of cells in the developing striatum. *Neuron* 9:15–26.

He, W., Ingraham, C., Rising, L., Goderie, S., and Temple, S. (2001) Multipotent stem cells from the mouse basal forebrain contribute GABAergic neurons and oligodendrocytes to the cerebral cortex during embryogenesis. *J. Neurosci.* 21:8854–8862.

Hommes, O.R. and Leblond, C.P. (1967) Mitotic division of neuroglia in the normal adult rat. *J. Comp. Neurol.* 129:269–278.

Horner, P.J., Power, A.E., Kempermann, G., Kuhn, H.G., Palmer, T.D., Winkler, J., Thal, L.J., and Gage, F.H. (2000) Proliferation and differentiation of progenitor cells throughout the intact rat spinal cord. *J. Neurosci.* 20:2218–2228.

Hudson, L.D. (2001) Control of gene expression by oligodendrocytes. In: Jessen, K.R. and Richardson, W.D., eds. *Glial Cell Development*, 2nd ed. Oxford: Oxford University Press, pp. 209–221.

Hughes, S.M., Lillien, L.E., Raff, M.C., Rohrer, H., and Sendtner, M. (1988) Ciliary neurotrophic factor induces type-2 astrocyte differentiation in culture. *Nature* 335:70–73.

Johe, K.K., Hazel, T.G., Müller, T., et al. (1996) Single factors direct the differentiation of stem cells from fetal and adult central nervous system *Genes Dev.* 10:3129–3140.

Kahn, M.A., Huang, C.J., Caruso, A., et al. (1997) Ciliary neurotrophic factor activates JAK/Stat signal transduction cascade and induces transcriptional expression of glial fibrillary acidic protein in glial cells. *J. Neurochem.* 68:1413–1423.

Korr, H., Schultze, B., and Maurer, W. (1973) Autoradiographic investigations of glial proliferation in the brain of adult mice. *J. Comp. Neurol.* 150:169–176.

Laywell, E.D., Rakic, P., Kukekov, V.G., Holland, E., and Steindler, D.A. (2000) Identification of a multipotent astrocytic stem cell in the immature and adult mouse brain. *Proc. Natl. Acad. Sci. USA* 97:13883–13888.

Levine, J.M., Reynolds, R., and Fawcett, J.W. (2001) The oligodendrocyte precursor cell in health and disease. *Trends Neurosci.* 24:39–47.

Levine, J.M., Stincone, F., and Lee, Y.-S. (1993) Development and differentiation of glial precursor cells in the rat cerebellum. *Glia* 7:307–321.

Levison, S.W., Chuang, C., Abramson, B.J., and Goldman, J.E. (1993) The migrational patterns and developmental factors of glial precursors in the rat subventricular zone are temporally regulated. *Development* 119:611–622.

Levison, S.W. and Goldman, J.E. (1993) Both oligodendrocytes and astrocytes develop from progenitors in the subventricular zone of postnatal rat forebrain. *Neuron* 10:201–212.

Levison, S.W. and Goldman, J.E. (1997) Multipotential progenitors co-exist with lineage restricted precursors in the mammalian postnatal subventricular zone. *J. Neurosci. Res.* 48:83–94.

Levison, S.W., Young, G.M., and Goldman, J.E. (1999) Cycling cells in the adult rat neocortex produce oligodendrocytes. *J. Neurosci. Res.* 57:435–446.

Lillien, L.E. and Raff, M.C. (1990) Differentiation signals in the CNS: type-2 astrocyte development in vitro as a model system. *Neuron* 5:111–119.

Lin, J.C. and Cepko, C.L. (1999) Biphasic dispersion of clones containing Purkinje cells and glia in the developing chick cerebellum. *Dev. Biol.* 211:177–197.

Lu, Q.R., Yuk, D., Alberta, J.A., Zhu, A.Z. Pawlitzky, I., Chan, J., McMahon, A.P., Stiles, C.D., and Rowitch, D.H. (2000) Sonic hedgehog-related oligodendrocyte lineage genes encoding bHLH proteins in the mammalian central nervous system. *Neuron* 25:317–329.

Luskin, M. (1993) Restricted proliferation and migration of postnatally generated neurons derived from the forebrain subventricular zone. *Neuron* 11:173–189.

Luskin, M.B. and McDermott, K. (1994) Divergent lineages for oligodendrocytes and astrocytes originating in the neonatal forebrain subventricular zone. *Glia* 11:211–226.

Luskin, M.B., Parnavelas, J.G., and Barfield, J.A. (1993) Neurons, astrocytes, and oligodendrocytes of the rat cerebral cortex originate from separate progenitor cells: an ultrastructural analysis of clonally related cells. *J. Neurosci.* 13:1730–1750.

Luskin, M.B., Pearlman, A.L., and Sanes. J.R. (1988) Cell lineage in the cerebral cortex of the mouse studied in vivo and in vitro with a recombinant retrovirus. *Neuron* 1:635–647.

Mabie, P.C., Mehler, M.F., Marmur, R., Papavasiliou, A., Song, Q., and Kessler, J.A. (1997) Bone morphogenetic proteins induce astroglial differentiation of oligodendroglial-astroglial progenitor cells. *J. Neurosci.* 17:4112–4120.

Malatesta, P., Hack, M.A., Hartfuss, E., Kettenmann, H., Klinkert, W., Kirchoff, F., and Gotz, M. (2003) Neuronal or glial progeny: regional differences in radial glial fate. *Neuron* 37:751–764.

Malatesta, P., Hartfuss, E., and Gotz, M. (2000) Isolation of radial glial cells by fluorescent-activated cell sorting reveals a neuronal lineage. *Development* 127:5253–5263.

Marshall, C.A.G., and Goldman, J.E. (2002) Subpallial Dlx2-expressing cells give rise to astrocytes and oligodendrocytes in the cerebral cortex and white matter. *J. Neurosci.* 22:9821–9830.

Marshall, C.A.G.., Suzuki, S.O., and Goldman, J.E. (2003) Gliogenic and neurogenic progenitors of the subventricular zone: who are they, where did they come from, and where are they going? *Glia* 43:52–61.

Masood, K., Besnard, F., Su, Y., and Brenner, M. (1993) Analysis of a segment of the human glial fibrillary acidic protein gene that directs astrocyte-specific transcription. *J. Neurochem.* 61:160–166.

Mayer, M., Bhakoo, K., and Noble, M. (1994) Ciliary neuronotrophic factor and leukemia inhibitory factor promote the generation, maturation and survival of oligodendrocytes in vitro. *Development* 120:143–153.

McManus, M.F., Chen, L.-C., Vallejo, I., and Vallejo, M. (1999) Astroglial differentiation of cortical precursor cells triggered by activation of the cAMP-dependent signaling pathway. *J. Neurosci.* 19:9004–9015.

Mehler, M.F., Mabie, P.C., Zhu, G., Gokhan, S., and Kessler, J.A. (2000) Developmental changes in progenitor cell responsiveness to bone morphogenetic proteins differentially modulate progressive CNS lineage fate. *Dev. Neurosci.* 22:74–85.

Mi, H. and Barres, B.A. (1999) Purification and characterization of astrocyte precursor cells in the developing rat optic nerve. *J. Neurosci.* 19:1049–1061.

Mi, H.M., Haeberle, H., and Barres, B.A. (2001) Induction of astrocyte differentiation by endothelial cells. *J. Neurosci.* 21:1538–1547.

Miller, R.H. (2002) Regulation of oligodendrocyte development in the vertebrate CNS. *Prog. Neurobiol.* 67:451–467.

Milosovic, A. and Goldman, J.E. (2002) Progenitors in the postnatal cerebellar white matter are antigenically heterogeneous. *J. Comp. Neurol.* 452:192–203.

Miyake, T., Fujiwara, T., Fukunaga, T., Takemura, K., and Kitamura, T. (1995) Glial cell lineage *in vivo* in the mouse cerebellum. *Dev. Growth Differ.* 37:273–285.

Nakashima, K., Takizawa, T., Ochiai, W., Yanigisawa, M., Hisatsune, T., Hakafuku, M., Miyazono, K., Kishimoto, T., Kageyama, R., and Taga, T. (2001) BMP2-mediated alteration in the developmental pathway of fetal mouse brain cells from neurogenesis to astrocytogenesis. *Proc. Natl. Acad. Sci. USA* 98:5868–5873.

Nakashima, K., Wiese, S., Yanagisawa, M., Arakawa, H., Kimura, N., Hisatsune, T., Yoshida, K., Kikshimoto, T., Sendtner, M., and Taga, T. (1999a) Developmental requirement of gp130 signaling in neuronal survival and astrocyte differentiation. *J. Neurosci.* 19:5429–5434.

Nakashima, K., Yanagisawa, M., Arakawa, H., Kimura, N., Hisatsune, T., Kawabata, M., Miyazono, K., and Taga, T. (1999b) Synergistic signaling in fetal brain by STAT3-Smad1 complex bridged by p300. *Science* 284:479–482.

Nakashima, K., Yanagisawa, M., Arakawa, H., and Taga, T. (1999c) Astrocyte differentiation mediated by LIF in cooperation with BMP2. *FEBS Lett.* 457:43–46.

Nery, S., Wichterle, H., and Fishell, G. (2001) Sonic hedgehog contributes to oligodendrocyte specification in the mammalian forebrain. *Development* 128:527–540.

Nieto, M., Schuurmans, C., Britz, O., and Guillemot, F. (2001) Neural bHLH genes control the neuronal versus glial fate decision in cortical progenitors. *Neuron* 29:401–413.

Nishiyama, A., Lin, X.-H., Giese, N., Heldin, C.-H., and Stallcup, W.B. (1996) Co-localization of NG2 proteoglycan and PDGF α-receptor on O2A progenitor cells in the developing rat brain. *J. Neurosci. Res.* 43:299–314.

Noctor, S.C., Flint, A.C., Weissman, T.A.l., Dammerman, R.S., and Kriegstein, A.R. (2001) Neurons derived from radial glial cells establish radial units in neocortex. *Nature* 409:714–720.

Norton, W.T. (1999) Cell reactions following acute brain injury: a review. *Neurochem. Res.* 24:213–218.

Ochiai, W., Yanagisawa, M., Takizawa, T., Hakashima, K., and Taga, T. (2001) Astrocyte differentiation of fetal neuroepithelial cells involving cardiotrophin-1-induced activation of STAT3. *Cytokine* 14:264–271.

Olivier, C., Cobos, I., Villegas, E.M.P., Spassky, N., Zalc, B., Martinex, S., and Thomas, J.-L. (2001) Monofocal origin of telencephalic oligodendrocytes in the anterior entopeduncular area of the chick embryo. *Development* 128:1757–1769.

Orentas, D.M., Hayes, J., Dyer, K., and Miller, R.H. (1999) Sonic hedgehog signaling is required during the appearance of spinal cord oligodendrocyte precursors. *Development* 126:2419–2429.

Palay, S., and Chan-Palay, V. (1972) *Cerebellar Cortex: Cytology and Organization.* New York: Springer-Verlag.

Parnevales, J.G. (1999) Glial cell lineages in the rat cerebral cortex. *Exp. Neurol.* 156:418–429.

Paterson, J.A. (1983) Dividing and newly produced cells in the corpus callosum of adult mouse cerebrum as detected by light microscopic radioautography. *Anat. Anz. (Jena)* 153:149–168.

Pouly, S., Becher, B., Blain, M., and Antel, J.P. (1999) Expression of a homologue of rat NG2 on human microglia. *Glia* 27:259–268.

Pouly, S., Prat, A., Blain, M., Olivier, A., and Antel, J. (2001) NG2 immunoreactivity on human brain endothelial cells. *Acta Neuropathol (Berl).* 102:313–320.

Price, J. and Thurlow, L. (1988) Cell lineage in the rat cerebral cortex: a study using retroviral-mediated gene transfer. *Development* 104:473–482.

Pringle, N.P., Guthrie, S., Lumsden, A., and Richardson, W.D. (1998) Dorsal spinal cord neuroepithelium generates astrocytes but not oligodendrocytes. *Neuron* 20:883–893.

Pringle, N.P. and Richardson, W.D. (1993) A singularity of PDGF alpha receptor expression in the dorsoventral axis of the neural tube may define the origin of the oligodendrocyte lineage. *Development* 117:525–533.

Pringle, N.P., Yu, W.-P., Howell, M., Colvin, J., Ornitz, D.M., and Richardson, W.D. (2003) Fgfr3 expression by astrocytes and their precursors: evidence that astrocytes and oligodendrocytes originate in distinct neuroepithelial domains. *Development* 130:93–102.

Raff, M.C., Miller, R.H., and Noble, M. (1983) A glial progenitor cell that develops in vitro into an astrocyte or an oligodendrocyte depending on culture medium. *Nature* 303:390–396.

Rao, M.S., Noble, M., and Mayer-Proschel, M. (1998) A tripotential glial precursor cells is present in the developing spinal cord. *Proc. Natl. Acad. Sci. USA* 95:3996–4001.

Reynolds, B.A. and Weiss, S. (1992) Generation of neurons and astrocytes from isolated cells of the adult mammalian central nervous system. *Science* 255:1707–1710.

Richards, L.J., Kilpatrick, T.J, and Bartlett, P.F. (1992) De novo generation of neuronal cells from the adult mouse brain. *Proc. Natl. Acad. Sci. USA* 89:8591–8595.

Richardson, W.D. (2001) Oligodendrocyte development. In: Jessen, K.R. and Richardson, W.D., eds. Glial Cell Development, 2nd ed. Oxford: Oxford University Press, pp. 21–54.

Richardson, W.D., Smith, H.K., Sun, T., Pringle, N.P., Hall, A., and Woodruff, R. (2000) Oligodendrocyte lineage and the motor neuron connection. *Glia* 29:136–142.

Rowitch, D.H., Lu, R.Q., Kessaris, N., and Richardson, W.D. (2002) An "oligarchy" rules neural development. *Trends Neurosci.* 25: 417–422.

Ruiz i Altaba AR (1998) Combinatorial Gli gene function in floor plate and neuronal inductions by Sonic hedgehog. *Development* 125:2203–2212.

Seri, B., Garcia-Verdugo, J.M., McEwen, B.S., and Alvarez-Buylla, A. (2001) Astrocytes give rise to new neurons in the adult mammalian hippocampus. *J. Neurosci.* 21:7153–7161.

Shafit-Zagardo, B., Iwaki, A.K., and Goldman, J.E. (1988) Astrocytes regulate GFAP mRNA levels by cAMP and protein kinase C dependent mechanisms. *Glia* 1:346–354.

Shi, J., Marinovich, A., and Barres, B.A. (1998) Purification and characterization of adult oligodendrocyte precursor cells from the rat optic nerve. *J. Neurosci.* 18:4627–4636.

Skoff, R.P. and Knapp, P.E. (1991) Division of astroblasts and oligodendroblasts in postnatal rodent brain: evidence for separate astrocyte and oligodendrocyte lineages. *Glia* 4:165–174.

Spassky, N., Heydon, K., Mangatal, A., Jankovski, A., Olivier, C., Queraud-Lesaux, F., Goujet-Zalc, C., Thomas, J.L., and Zalc, B. (2001) Sonic hedgehog–dependent emergence of oligodendrocytes in the telencephalon: evidence for a source of oligodendrocytes in the olfactory bulb that is independent of PDGFRalpha signaling. *Development* 128:4993–5004.

Spassky, N., Olivier, C., Perez-Villegas, E., Goujet-Zalc, C., Martinex, S., Thomas, J., and Zalc, B. (2000) Single or multiple oligodendrocyte lineages: a controversy. *Glia* 29:143–148.

Staugaitis, S.M., Zerlin, M., Levine, J.M., Hawkes, R., and Goldman, J.E. (2001) Aldolase C/Zebrin II expression in neonatal rat forebrain reveals cellular heterogeneity within the subventricular zone and early astrocyte differentiation. *J. Neurosci.* 21:6195–6205.

Sun, Y., Nadal-Vicens, M., Misono, S., Lin, M.Z., Zubiaga, A., Hua, X., Fan, G., and Greenberg, M.E. (2001) Neurogenin promotes neurogenesis and inhibits glial differentiation by independent mechanisms. *Cell* 104:365–376.

Tekki-Kessaris, N., Woodruff, R., Hall, A.C., Garfield, W., Kimura, S., Stiles C., and Richardson, W.D. (2001) Hedgehog-dependent oligodendrocyte specification in the telencephalon. *Development* 128:2545–2554.

Timsit, S., Martinez, S., Allinquant, B., Peyron, F., Puelles, L., and Zalc, B. (1995) Oligodendrocytes originate in a restricted zone of the embryonic ventral neural tube defined by DM-20 mRNA expression. *J. Neurosci.* 15:1012–1024.

Turner, D. and Cepko, C. (1987) Cell lineage in the rat retina: a common progenitor for neurons and glia persists late in development. *Nature (Lond)* 328:131–136.

Vartanian, T., Fischbach, G., and Miller, R. (1999) Failure of spinal cord oligodendrocyte development in mice lacking β-neuregulin-1. *Proc. Soc. Natl. Acad. Sci. USA* 96:731–735.

Voigt, T. (1989) Development of glial cells in the cerebral wall of ferrets: direct tracing of their transformation from radial glia into astrocytes. *J. Comp. Neurol.* 289:74–88.

Wada, T., Kagawa, T., Ivanova, A., Zalc, B., Shirasaki, R., Murakami, F., Iemura, S., Ueno, N., and Ikenaka, K. (2000) Dorsal spinal cord inhibits oligodendrocyte development. *Dev Biol.* 227:42–55.

Walsh, C. and Cepko, C.L. (1993) Clonal dispersion in proliferating layers of developing cerebral cortex. *Nature* 362:632–635.

Wolswijk, G. and Noble, M. (1989) Identification of an adult-specific glial progenitor cell. *Development* 105:387–400.

Yanagisawa, M., Nakashima, K., and Taga, T. (1999) STAT3-mediated astrocyte differentiation from mouse fetal neuroepithelial cells by mouse oncostatin M. *Neurosci. Lett.* 269:169–172.

Yanagisawa, M., Nakashima, K., Takizawa, T., Ochiai, W., Arakawa, H., and Taga, T. (2001) Signaling crosstalk underlying synergistic induction of astrocyte differentiation by BMPs and IL-6 family of cytokines. *FEBS Lett.* 489:139–143.

Zerlin, M. and Goldman, J.E. (1997) Interactions between glial progenitors and blood vessels during early postnatal corticogenesis: blood vessel contact represents an early stage of astrocyte differentiation. *J. Comp. Neurol.* 387:537–546.

Zhang, L. and Goldman, J.E. (1996) Developmental fates and migratory pathways of dividing progenitors in the postnatal rat cerebellum. *J. Comp. Neurol.* 370:536–550.

Zhou, Q. and Anderson, D.J. (2002) The bHLH transcription factors Olig2 and Olig1 couple neuronal and glial subtype specification. *Cell* 109:61–73.

Zhou, Q., Wang, S., and Anderson, D.J. (2000) Identification of a novel family of oligodendrocyte specific basic helix-loop-helix transcription factors. *Neuron* 25:331–343.

Zerlin, M., Milosevic, A., and Goldman, J.E. (2004) Glial progenitors of the neonatal subventricular zone differentiate asynchronously, leading to spatial dispersion of glial clones and to the persistence of immature glia in the adult mammalian CNS., *Dev. Biol.*, in press.

7 The Schwann cell lineage

KRISTJÁN R. JESSEN AND RHONA MIRSKY

OUTLINE OF SCHWANN CELL DEVELOPMENT

The two types of Schwann cells found in peripheral nerve trunks, myelinating and nonmyelinating cells, differ radically in structure, function, and molecular properties. These cells develop from a common pool of apparently homogeneous cells, immature Schwann cells, in a process that starts in rodents at around birth, that is, after about 3 weeks of embryonic development. Immature Schwann cells originate in embryonic nerves from Schwann cell precursors that, in turn, arise from neural crest cells. Therefore, three major developmental transitions lie between migrating neural crest cells and mature Schwann cells (Figs. 7.1, 7.2). Since crest cells can generate several cell types, including neurons and melanocytes, in addition to Schwann cell precursors, and since immature Schwann cells will become either myelinating or nonmyelinating cells, the first and last of these transitions involve a fate choice. The second transition, in contrast, represents lineage progression, rather than lineage choice, since it is very likely that Schwann cell precursors in normal nerves are fated only to become Schwann cells or die by programmed cell death.

It is believed that the fate of individual immature Schwann cells is randomly determined by which axons the cell becomes associated with during complex rearrangements between axons and Schwann cells in perinatal nerves. During this poorly understood process, some cells come to envelop single large-diameter axons (referred to as the *1:1 relationship* between axon and Schwann cell) and progress to myelinate, while other cells remain associated with more than one smaller-diameter axon and develop as nonmyelinating cells (Fig. 7.2). Remarkably, the axon–Schwann cell signaling that instructs those cells associated with the large-diameter axons to myelinate is unknown, as are the signals that control the development of nonmyelinating cells. Similarly, the extracellular signals that cause crest cells to choose the Schwann cell lineage are unclear.

While we do not have definitive information on the key extracellular signals that control the choice points in the lineage, more is known about signals that are important for the progression of the lineage in embryonic nerves. *In vivo* studies and cell culture experiments have implicated two factors, endothelin and, in particular, β-neuregulin-1 (neuregulin-1), in the control of this phase of Schwann cell development. A number of transcription factors that are important in this system have also been identified. Sox-10 is essential for the establishment of the Schwann cell lineage, Krox-20 is required for myelination, and Oct-6 (SCIP) is involved in timing the onset of myelination (Britsch et al., 2001; Topilko and Meijer, 2001).

Most of the embryonic phase of Schwann cell differentiation is compatible with ongoing cell division since Schwann cell precursors and immature Schwann cells are rapidly proliferating cells, and it is not until the last transition, when immature cells form myelinating and nonmyelinating cells, that cell division stops (Mirsky and Jessen, 2001). This last step of Schwann cell development is strikingly reversible. Even mature Schwann cells in adult nerves can readily reenter the cell cycle, abandon their morphological and molecular differentiation, and readopt a phenotype that is quite similar to that of immature Schwann cells in perinatal nerves. This process is typically triggered in nerve segments distal to an injury leading to axonal death, and is in this case referred to as *Wallerian degeneration*. Essentially the same dedifferentiation process takes place if Schwann cells are isolated from nerves and placed in neuron-free cultures. Dedifferentiated Schwann cells can easily redifferentiate again. This is seen, for instance, during nerve regeneration, presumably because this process allows Schwann cells to reestablish contact with axonal differentiation signals (Scherer, 1997; Scherer and Salzer, 2001).

Ready reversibility, as described here for the last major transition in the lineage, is also seen in the first transition, since Schwann cell precursors can be reprogrammed by exposure to signaling molecules to generate other cell types including neurons *in vitro* (Jessen and Mirsky, 2003). On the other hand, reversal of immature Schwann cells to form Schwann cell precursors has not yet been described.

THE USE OF MARKERS TO IDENTIFY DISTINCT STAGES OF EMBRYONIC SCHWANN CELL DEVELOPMENT

Studies on postnatal Schwann cell development and myelination have greatly benefited from the availability of molecular differentiation markers that can be used to pinpoint the developmental stage of Schwann

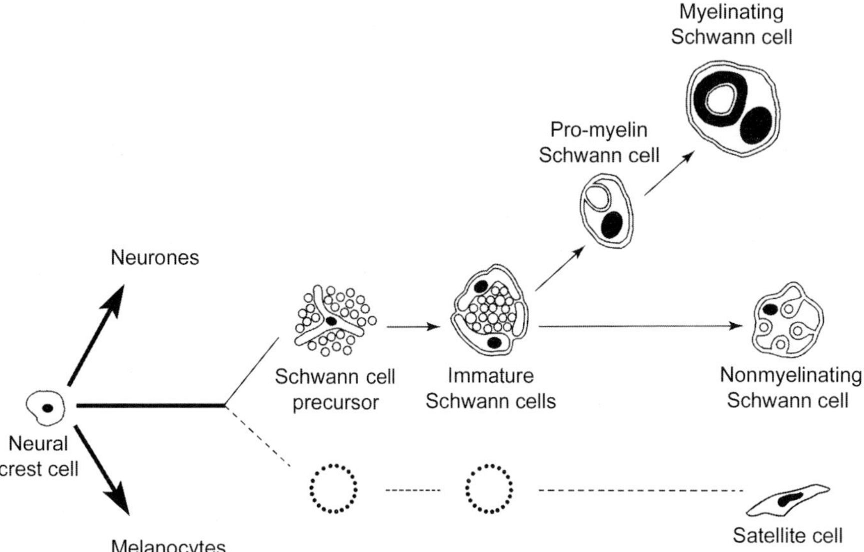

FIGURE 7.1 The Schwann and satellite cell lineages in rat and mouse. *Upper line*: There are three main transitions in the Schwann cell lineage: (*1*) The formation of Schwann cell precursors from undifferentiated migrating neural crest cells, (*2*) the precursor–Schwann cell transition, and (*3*) the formation of mature myelinating and nonmyelinating Schwann cells. The phenotypic changes that characterize each developmental step are summarized in Figure 7.3. The reversibility of postnatal Schwann cell development is indicated by stippled arrows. *Lower line*: The formation of satellite cells in sensory ganglia. These cells are also derived from the neural crest. They are flattened and located around neuronal cell bodies. They differ from Schwann cells in expression of the transcription factor Erm (Lobsiger et al., 2002) and in their ability to survive in the absence of neuregulin-1 (Garratt et al., 2000) Whether they go through a precursor stage similar to that of Schwann cells has not been determined. Similar cells exist in sympathetic and parasympathetic ganglia.

cells in normal and damaged nerves. The absence of comparable markers for the embryonic phase of Schwann cell development has made careful analysis of early Schwann cell development much more difficult. Many more markers have been established for use in studies on early neurons, including neuron-specific tubulin (β3-tubulin; TUJ1), neurofilament and peripherin in addition to early markers of distinct neuronal lineages. With these tools, it has been possible to determine and separate early and late stages of embryonic development of peripheral neurons. In contrast, investigators working on glia have had to resort to using antigens that appear relatively late in embryonic Schwann cell development, in particular glial fibrillary acidic protein (GFAP) and S100, to detect early events such as the initiation of glial differentiation in neural crest cells.

Currently, however, a set of markers is beginning to be established for examining glial development in embryonic nerves of rodents (Fig. 7.3) (Jessen and Mirsky, 2003). These markers fall into four groups: (*1*) those that are present throughout on crest cells and embryonic peripheral nervous system (PNS) glia exemplified by the transcription factor Sox-10; (*2*) those that are expressed by crest cells and precursors but not, or at much lower levels, by immature Schwann cells, such as the transcription factor AP2α; (*3*) those present in Schwann cell precursors and Schwann cells but not on early-migrating crest cells, such as brain fatty acid binding protein (BFABP) and protein zero (P0); and (*4*) molecules that are expressed by immature Schwann cells but are absent or present at very low levels in precursors and crest cells, such as GFAP and S100. Markers in the last two groups should be particularly useful for studying the two main lineage transitions in embryonic nerves.

In addition to these markers, it is now possible to use characteristic response patterns to survival factors as a way to discriminate between different stages of the lineage. Differences in survival responses are particularly striking between migrating crest cells and Schwann cell precursors (Woodhoo et al., 2004).

THE ORIGIN OF GLIAL CELLS FROM THE NEURAL CREST

The neural crest is a transient population of cells that migrates from the dorsal aspect of the neural plate as it curves and closes to form the neural tube. In the trunk region the crest cells give rise to several cell types, including dorsal root sensory and autonomic neurons, melanocytes, and satellite glial cells of sensory and sympathetic ganglia, in addition to Schwann cells (Le Douarin and Kalcheim, 1999; Anderson, 2000; Knecht and Bronner-Fraser, 2002). It is likely that some crest cells have already entered these lineages at the onset of crest migration, while other cells choose lineages later, during migration or at their destination, such as developing skin, condensing ganglia, or emerging nerves. It is now recognized that even though a cell has taken the first differentiation steps along a lineage, that is, has entered the lineage, as detected, for instance, by the expression of early differentiation markers, the cell may, at least initially, retain alternative developmental

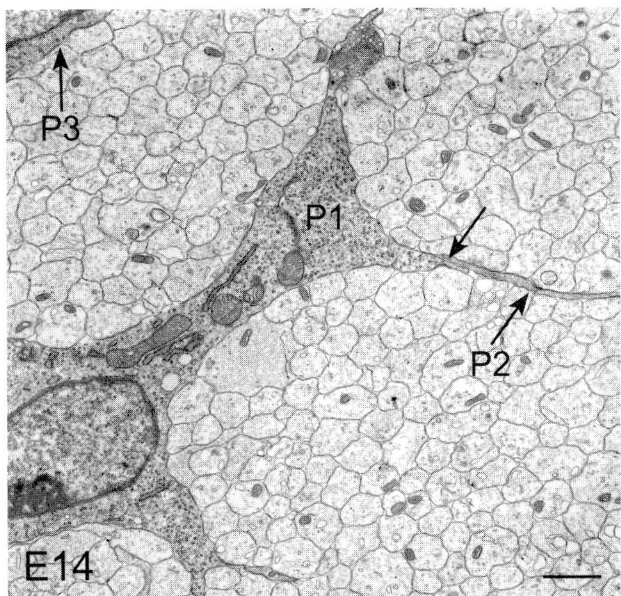

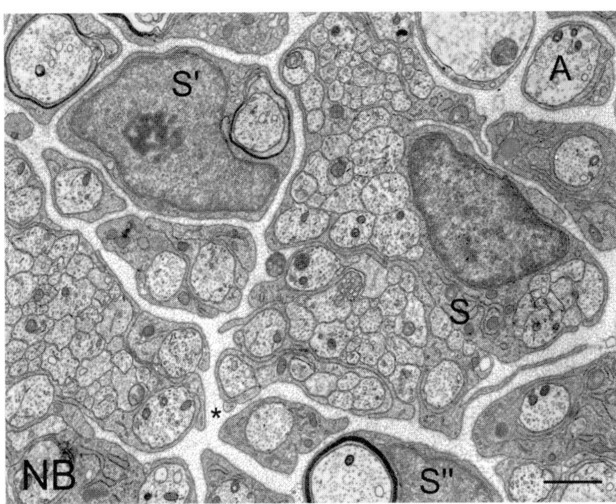

FIGURE 7.2 The appearance of early cells in the Schwann cell lineage. *Upper panel*: Parts of three Schwann cell precursors (P1–3) can be seen in this hind-limb nerve of a rat embryo at E14. Most of the nucleus of P1 is visible (*left*). The cells ramify and form close contacts (*arrow*) with each other and are either embedded between axons inside the nerve, as shown here, or found in close apposition to axons at the surface of the nerve. Because connective tissue spaces, extracellular matrix, and blood vessels are essentially absent, these nerves are more compact than older ones. The axons also have a smaller and more uniform diameter than those seen in mature nerves. Bar: 1 μm. *Lower panel*: Schwann cells in the sciatic nerve of a newborn rat at the same magnification (*NB*). Immature Schwann cells (e.g., S) communally envelop a group of axons of various diameters. As the first step toward myelination, some axons (e.g., A) have segregated to form a 1:1 relationship with a Schwann cell (the pro-myelin stage). Other cells (e.g., *S'*) are at a very early stage of myelination, while the cell S" has already formed a thin myelin sheath. Note that in contrast to the compact arrangement seen in the E14 nerve, perinatal nerves contain considerable collagen (e.g., *asterisk*) and extracellular space. Bar: 1 μm. (Both micrographs courtesy of Aman Kumar.)

Neural crest cells	Schwann cell precursors	Immature Schwann cells
Sox10 ErbB3 P75 L1	Sox10 ErbB3 P75 L1	Sox10 ErbB3 P75 L1
AP-2α N-cad*	AP-2α N-cad*	
	B-FABP Po Dhh CD9* GAP-43* PMP22* PLP*	B-FABP Po Dhh CD9* GAP-43* PMP22* PLP*
		S100 GFAP Oct-6** O4**
Associate with ECM	Associate with axons	Associate with axons
Neuregulin survival signalling is ECM dependent	Neuregulin survival signaling is ECM independent	Neuregulin survival signalling is ECM independent
		Autocrine survival circuits

FIGURE 7.3 Markers of embryonic Schwann cell development. Neural crest cells, Schwann cell precursors, and Schwann cells are characterized by molecular markers, as indicated in the gray boxes. The text below the boxes summarizes some important differences in cellular properties between the three developmental stages. Additional differences relate to the mitogenic response to fibroblast growth factor (FGF), since in rat cells FGF2 is a mitogen for rat Schwann cells but not for precursors. Also, precursors are highly motile *in vitro*, in comparison to Schwann cells (Jessen et al., 1994; Dong et al., 1995). *ECM*: extracellular matrix.

potentials that can be revealed by removing it from the normal environment and exposing it to alternative signals (Tosh and Slack, 2002). In spite of such plasticity, the signals that control initial lineage choices are of great interest, as they determine cell fate, if not developmental potential, during normal development. Three main systems have been implicated in the establishment of the Schwann cell lineage from the neural crest: Delta/Notch signaling, neuregulin-1 signaling, and the transcription factor Sox-10.

Notch activation suppresses neurogenesis in neural crest cultures. In experiments employing clonal analysis, Notch activation also promotes glial differentiation, as judged by an increase in the number of clones expressing the Schwann cell marker GFAP (Morrison et al., 2000; Wakamatsu et al., 2000). It is not clear whether Notch signaling triggers glial differentiation directly in these experiments or whether Notch activation allows other gliogenic signals to act more effectively. For instance, the Notch-mediated suppression of neuronal differentiation is likely to prolong the period during which crest cells are available to respond to constructive gliogenic signals present in the culture medium. Notch activation has recently been implicated in the promotion of gliogenesis in the central nervous system (CNS) (Wang and Barres, 2000).

Neuregulin-1 also inhibits neurogenesis in crest cultures, and it has been suggested that both neuregulin-1 and Delta/Notch signaling could provide a mechanism whereby early neurons block neuronal development in neighboring cells, thereby preventing excessive neurogenesis within condensing ganglia (Shah et al., 1994; Morrison et al., 2000). Although exposure to neuregulin-1 promotes gliogenesis relative to neurogenesis in crest cultures due to suppression of neuronal development, clonal analysis shows that equally many clones generate glia in the presence and absence of neuregulin-1 (Shah et al., 1994). In agreement with this, satellite glial cells within dorsal root ganglia (DRGs) develop apparently normally in mice in which neuregulin-1 has been inactivated (although Schwann cell precursors in nerve trunks are severely depleted; see the section "Neuregulins and Schwann Cell Development"). The role of neuregulin-1 in the initiation of glial development from neural crest cells therefore remains unclear.

The transcription factor Sox-10 is expressed in migrating crest cells and persists in the Schwann cell lineage while it is downregulated in early neurons. It is essential for the generation of both Schwann cell precursors and glial cells within DRGs, since these cells are missing in mice in which Sox-10 has been inactivated and in Dominant megacolon (Dom) mice that have a spontaneous inactivating mutation in the Sox-10 gene (Britsch et al., 2001). The DRG neurons are generated in normal numbers in these mice, although they die later, perhaps due in part to the absence of glial cells and glial-derived trophic support. Sox-10 mutants also have defects in the enteric nervous system of the gut and abnormal pigmentation. In the absence of Sox-10, crest cells do not maintain expression of the neuregulin-1 receptor ErbB3. Since neuregulin-1 signaling is important for the survival and proliferation of Schwann cell precursors (see the section "Neuregulins and Schwann Cell Development") the loss of ErbB3 could contribute to the elimination of these cells in Sox-10 mutants. It is equally possible that Sox-10 is needed for the process that allows migrating crest cells to become early glia and that entry to the glial lineage is therefore blocked in Sox-10 mutants (Britsch et al., 2001).

SCHWANN CELL PRECURSORS

Schwann cell precursors are the glial cells found in limb nerves of embryo day (E) 14/15 rats (E12/13 mice). They represent the earliest well-defined stage of PNS glial development and the cell from which the immature Schwann cell, characterized in numerous studies on perinatal nerves, is derived (Jessen et al., 1994; Dong et al., 1995; Jessen and Mirsky, 1999).

Schwann cell precursors are first seen at the edge of early embryonic nerves but soon spread throughout the nerves, communally enveloping large numbers of axons with sheet-like processes (Fig. 7.2). Peripheral nerves at this stage are compact structures that contain essentially no connective tissue and are not vascularized. Between E15 and E17, connective tissue spaces and vessels appear within nerves; concomitantly, Schwann cell precursors progress to generate Schwann cells. Therefore, while the large majority of cells in E14/15 rat nerves (E12/13 in mouse) are Schwann cell precursors, essentially all the glial cells in E17/18 rat (E15/16 in mouse) nerves are Schwann cells. It is likely that the precursor/Schwann cell transition takes place somewhat earlier in more proximal nerves.

One of the most striking phenotypic differences between Schwann cell precursors and immature Schwann cells concerns survival regulation. Schwann cells can maintain their own survival by autocrine survival circuits, but this mechanism is absent from Schwann cell precursors (Meier et al., 1999). Instead, the precursors appear to rely entirely on axon-associated survival signals, in particular neuregulin-1. Another difference noted in early studies was that Schwann cell precursors expressed very low levels of the S100 protein in comparison to Schwann cells. More recent studies have defined a number of phenotypic differences between Schwann cell precursors and immature Schwann cells, on the one hand, and between Schwann cell precursors and the neural crest, on the other (Fig. 7.3) (Mirsky and Jessen, 2001; Jessen and Mirsky, 2003). Thus Schwann cell precursors are specified glial cells that represent the first stage in the process that transforms some migrating neural crest cells eventually into the myelinating and nonmyelinating Schwann cells found in postnatal nerves.

Unlike immature Schwann cells, which have two developmental options, Schwann cell precursors are likely to be unifated, namely, destined only to become Schwann cells (or die) during normal development. This does not have to mean that Schwann cell precursors are irreversibly committed to a glial fate. In fact, there is clear evidence in both avians and rodents that $P0^+$ Schwann cell precursors or $P0^+$ nonneuronal cells from sensory ganglia can be reprogrammed to generate glial-melanocytic precursors or melanocytes, neurons, and other crest derivatives after prolonged culture in complex media (Sherman et al., 1993; Hagedorn et al., 1999; Dupin et al., 2003). It remains an interesting additional possibility that early nerves might, apart from Schwann cell precursors, also contain a distinct population of multipotent crest-like cells that in culture can be diverted to nonglial lineages. It was suggested that absence of P0 expression distinguishes these cells from Schwann cell precursors and that they amount to ≈15% of the total number of cells dissociated from E14 rat nerves (Morrison et al., 2000).

NEUREGULINS AND SCHWANN CELL DEVELOPMENT

Neuregulin-1 is involved in all stages of Schwann cell development from the neural crest to adult cells and is the most important known external regulator of the lineage. Two of the three other members of the neuregulin gene family, neuregulins-2 and -3, are expressed in the nervous system, but their function in nerve development is unknown (Adlkofer and Lai, 2000). Glial growth factor (GGF), later identified as the type II isoform of neuregulin-1, was one of the earliest identified Schwann cell mitogens, and neuregulin-1 is now considered to be the major axonally derived Schwann cell mitogen (Lemke, 2001).

The embryonic nerves of mice in which neuregulin-1 or its receptors ErbB2 or ErbB3 have been genetically inactivated are essentially devoid of Schwann cell precursors. Sympathetic ganglia also fail to form properly, probably due to impaired ventral migration of neural crest cells. On the other hand, DRG neurons initially develop normally and their associated satellite glial cells appear unaffected. These striking results suggest a crucial role for neuregulin-1 in the development of the PNS, and in particular in the development of the peripheral glial lineage (Garratt et al., 2000). The normal development of DRG satellite cells in the mutants indicates that neuregulin-1 is not required *in vivo* for the development of at least one branch of this lineage, a conclusion supported by studies showing that cultured neural crest cells give rise to GFAP-positive glia in the absence or presence of added neuregulin-1 (Shah et al., 1994). The paucity of precursors in neuregulin mutants is therefore unlikely to reflect a need for neuregulin-1 in the process of glial differentiation from crest cells.

A likely reason for the lack of Schwann cell precursors in early nerves of these mutant mice relates to the function of neuronally derived neuregulin-1 as a survival factor for Schwann cell precursors and early Schwann cells both *in vivo* and *in vitro* (Dong et al., 1995; Winseck et al., 2002). In mice lacking isoform III of neuregulin-1, the major isoform in peripheral nerves, precursors initially populate the nerves at E11, presumably using other neuregulin isoforms for survival, but by E14, a stage when precursors are converting rapidly to Schwann cells, cell numbers are severely depleted (Wolpowitz et al., 2000). Taken together, these findings strongly support the idea that a major function of neuregulin-1 *in vivo* is to ensure the survival of Schwann cell precursors.

Although the evidence is not unequivocal, reduced migration of glia from DRGs into nerves may also play a part, since an important reason for the failure to develop sympathetic ganglia in ErbB3-deficient mice is thought to be impaired migration of neural crest cells in the ventromedial pathway (Garratt et al., 2000; Mirsky and Jessen, 2001).

The experiments using mutant mice described above highlight the importance of neuregulin-1, isoform I Neudifferentiation factor, acetylcholine receptor inducing activity (NDF, ARIA), isoform II (GGF) and, in particular, isoform III stromal cell-derived factor, cysteine-rich domains (SDF, CRD-NRG-1) in Schwann cell development (Garratt et al., 2000; Lemke, 2001). In these mutants, Schwann cell precursors in peripheral nerve trunks are most severely depleted in animals with inactivation of the neuregulin-1 gene, and therefore all three isoforms, or of the neuregulin receptors ErbB2 or ErbB3. In mice with selective inactivation of isoform III, the initial phenotype is milder, although at later stages Schwann cell precursor numbers are severely depleted and Schwann cells are essentially absent from the distal portions of the nerves (see above) (Wolpowitz et al., 2000). In contrast, in mice lacking isoforms I and II, Schwann cell development in peripheral nerves is normal (Garratt et al., 2000), highlighting the importance of isoform III, which is mostly expressed as a transmembrane protein (Wang et al., 2001; Leimeroth et al., 2002).

In addition to its prominent role at the embryonic stages of Schwann cell development, neuregulin-1 is important for events that take place in older nerves.

As mentioned above, neuregulin-1 is likely to be the major axon-associated mitogen for immature Schwann cells in perinatal nerves. Axonal neuregulin-1 is also likely to act, in concert with autocrine signals, to support the survival of these cells (see the section "Schwann Cell Survival Signals"). There is evidence that neuregulin-1 is involved in the control of myelin thickness since selective inactivation of the neuregulin receptor ErbB3 in myelinating Schwann cells *in vivo* results in the formation of thinner myelin sheaths (Garratt et al., 2000). Other studies, carried out *in vitro*, indicate that neuregulin-1 signaling might delay the onset of myelination (see the section "Myelination") and promote demyelination under traumatic or pathological conditions (Scherer and Salzer, 2001).

Neuregulin-1 activates a variety of intracellular signaling pathways in precursors and Schwann cells. It induces phosphorylation and dimerization of its receptors ErbB2 and ErbB3, events that are potentiated by the transmembrane glycoprotein CD44. Downstream pathways that may be activated, depending on the conditions under which neuregulin is applied, include the phosphoinositide (PI) 3 kinase, mitogen-activated protein kinase (MAPK/extracellular signal-regulated kinase [ERK]), protein kinase A (PKA), p38 MAPK pathways and c-Jun-N-terminal kinase pathways (Adlkofer and Lai, 2000; Jessen and Mirsky, 2003).

Activation of the PI3 kinase pathway is crucial to proliferative and survival responses since inhibition of PI3 kinase prevents both axonally induced and neuregulin-1-induced DNA synthesis and survival, whereas inhibition of the MAPK pathway has no effect on DNA synthesis. Inhibition of MAPK induces significant cell death (in some studies, but not all), while in Schwann cell precursors inhibition of either of these pathways completely inhibits survival in neuregulin-1 (Meier et al., 1999; Maurel and Salzer, 2000; Li et al., 2001; Mirsky and Jessen, 2001; Jessen and Mirsky, 2003).

Elevation of intracellular cyclic adenosine monophosphate (cAMP) levels and PKA activation have profound effects on both proliferation and differentiation *in vitro* (see the sections "Cell Culture Studies on Schwann Cell Proliferation and Differentiation" and "Myelination"). Neuregulin-1 induces a delayed rise in intracellular cAMP levels, PKA activation and cAMP response element binding protein (CREB) phosphorylation. This may account for its ability to stimulate proliferation in the absence of cAMP-elevating agents, although both forskolin and insulin-like growth factors (IGF) potentiate the response (Conlon et al., 2001; Mirsky and Jessen, 2001).

Both neuregulin-1 and autocrine-mediated survival of Schwann cells (see the section "Schwann Cell Survival Signals") depend on the activity of Ets transcription factors, several of which are expressed by Schwann cells (Parkinson et al., 2002a).

REGULATION OF THE PRECURSOR–SCHWANN CELL TRANSITION

Schwann cell generation from precursors *in vivo* involves coordinated changes in antigenic profile, survival regulation, response to mitogens, motility and cell-cell interactions (see Fig. 7.3; see also the section "Schwann Cell Precursors"). This transition can also be accomplished *in vitro* by culture of precursors in the absence of neurons in chemically defined medium containing neuregulin-1 for 4 days (E14 + 4 = E18). When cells cultured under these conditions are dissociated and replated, over 80% of cells have a Schwann cell phenotype with respect to antigenic profile, mitogenic response, and the presence of autocrine survival loops (see the section "Schwann Cell Survival Signals"; Dong et al., 1995). This means that neuregulin-1 supports not only precursor survival but also lineage progression and Schwann cell generation.

In vivo it is likely that multiple signals control the rate of Schwann cell generation. Endothelin, acting through the endothelin B receptor, is likely to be one of these signals. Endothelins 1–3 support precursor survival *in vitro*, and endothelin and its receptors are present in embryonic nerves. Endothelins, unlike neuregulin-1, do not promote DNA synthesis in precursors, and lineage progression is also affected differently by these two factors. Schwann cells are generated very slowly in endothelin alone, while the rate of Schwann cell generation in neuregulin-1 and endothelin is intermediate between the rates seen in neuregulin-1 and endothelin alone. This suggests that neuregulin actively promotes the generation of Schwann cells, whereas endothelin slows the process. *In vivo* experiments using the *spotting lethal* rat, in which endothelin B receptors are nonfunctional, confirm this proposition, since Schwann cells are generated ahead of schedule, as expected, if in normal nerves activation of endothelin B receptors exerts a brake on the rate of lineage progression (Brennan et al., 2000).

To date, only one transcription factor, AP2α, has been implicated in the control of Schwann cell generation from precursors. It is sharply downregulated at the precursor–Schwann cell transition *in vivo* in both rats and mice. Furthermore, enforced expression of AP2α in precursors *in vitro* delays the conversion to Schwann cells, suggesting that the downregulation seen *in vivo* may help to control the rate at which conversion occurs (Jessen and Mirsky, 2003). Both Schwann cell precursors and Schwann cells express the helix-loop-helix (HLH) genes Ids 1–4, but their expression is not regulated in a simple way and there is at present no evidence that they are involved in controlling the precursor–Schwann cell transition (but see the section "Myelination").

SCHWANN CELL SURVIVAL SIGNALS

Both axon-associated neuregulin-1 and autocrine Schwann cell signals appear to play a role in promoting the survival of immature Schwann cells in perinatal nerves (Fig. 7.4). Neonatal sciatic nerve transection

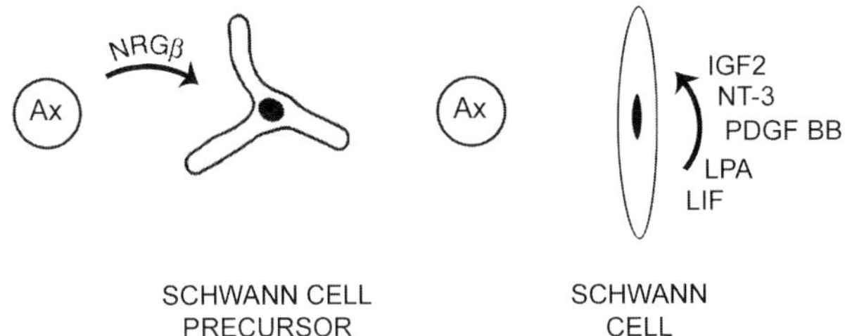

FIGURE 7.4 Survival regulation in the Schwann cell lineage. Both axon-derived and autocrine signals regulate survival of cells in the Schwann cell lineage. Schwann cell precursors rely exclusively on axonal signals, principally neuregulin-1, for survival, but as development proceeds and precursors generate Schwann cells, there is a shift to the establishment of autocrine loops, the main components of which are likely to include insulin-like growth factor-2 (*IGF-2*), platelet-derived growth factor-BB (*PDGF-BB*), and neurotrophin 3 (*NT3*), leukemia inhibitory factor (*LIF*), and lysophosphatidic acid (*LPA*)-like activity. *NRGβ*: neuregulin *β*.

results in the death of all teloglia at the neuromuscular junction (Trachtenburg and Thompson, 1996). Although most Schwann cells survive, there is also increased Schwann cell death within the nerve, indicating a partial dependence on axonal signals for full survival (Scherer and Salzer, 2001). This death is probably caused by loss of axon-associated neuregulin-1 as axons degenerate after transection, an idea supported by the fact that exogenous neuregulin-1 rescues both Schwann cells and teloglia from death. After the first postnatal week, nerve transection no longer results in immediate cell death, although death is seen in regenerating adult nerves at 3 weeks after crush at a time when there is a requirement to match the number of axons and Schwann cells (Scherer and Salzer, 2001; Jessen and Mirsky, 2003).

The ability of adult Schwann cells to survive in the absence of axons for several months after injury is crucial for nerve regeneration because Schwann cells provide both adhesive substrates and trophic factors that promote axon regrowth. It is likely that Schwann cell survival in the absence of axons is due in large part to the existence of autocrine Schwann cell circuits that enable Schwann cells to support their own survival. This represents a fundamental difference between Schwann cells and precursors, which are wholly dependent on axonal neuregulin for survival (see the sections "Schwann Cell Precursors" and "Neuregulins and Schwann Cell Development"). Conditioned medium from densely plated Schwann cells that supports Schwann cell survival will not support precursor survival and is not mitogenic for either precursors or Schwann cells. Major components of the autocrine loop have been identified as IGF-2 plus platelet-derived growth factor BB (PDGF-BB) and neurotrophin 3 (NT3) combined, leukemia inhibitory factor (LIF), and a lysophosphatidic acid (LPA)-like activity, while laminin acts with these components to promote longer-term survival (Jessen and Mirsky, 2003).

Both IGF and LPA signal via PI3 kinase and Akt, in the case of IGF leading to inhibition of c-Jun terminal kinases and caspase-mediated apoptosis (Cheng et al., 2000; Weiner et al., 2001). Unlike neuregulin-1 and autocrine survival factors, LPA-induced survival does not require the activity of Ets transcription factors (see above and the section "Neuregulins and Schwann Cell Development"; Parkinson et al., 2002a).

There is evidence that nerves contain factors that actively promote cell death. Two such factors, nerve growth factor (NGF) and transforming growth factor (TGF) *β*, have been identified (Soilu-Hanninen et al., 1999; Parkinson et al., 2001). Nerve growth factor promotes cell death in cultured Schwann cells, and there is less cell death in nerves of p75 neurotrophin receptor (NTR)-deficient mice than in normal mice after neonatal nerve transection or in regenerating adult nerves at 3 weeks after crush. Furthermore, cultured expanded Schwann cells from these mice survive better than normal Schwann cells when deprived of serum and growth factors (Soilu-Hanninen et al., 1999; Jessen and Mirsky, 2002). Several Schwann cell proteins interact directly with p75NTR. These include the anti-apoptotic receptor-interacting protein (RIP)-2, acting to prevent cell death via activation of NF*κ*B, and the pro-apoptotic TNF receptor-associated factor (TRAF), which activates the c-Jun-N-terminal kinase pathway. Receptor-interacting protein-2 is expressed by freshly isolated cultured Schwann cells, which are not killed by NGF, but is lost from Schwann cells on prolonged culture, when they become susceptible to NGF-induced cell death, possibly induced by TRAF (Khursigara et al., 2001).

The TGF*β*s, like NGF, can induce apoptotic cell death in neonatal Schwann cells after nerve transection *in vivo* and also in freshly isolated cultured Schwann cells (Parkinson et al., 2001). *In vitro* TGF*β*-induced death can be blocked by the combined presence of neuregulin-1 and the IGF-2, PDGF-BB, NT3 autocrine survival signal. Transforming growth factor-β_1 signals via c-Jun-N-terminal kinase and phosphorylation of c-Jun. By postnatal day 4, myelinating Schwann cells are resistant to cell death, and in these cells TGF*β* fails to phosphorylate c-Jun and does not induce apoptosis (Grinspan et al., 1996; Parkinson et al., 2001).

The actions of TGF*β* on Schwann cells are strikingly context dependent. In addition to killing cells, as seen *in vivo* or in primary cultures in defined medium (above), TGF*β* can act as a Schwann cell mitogen in the presence of serum and cAMP-elevating agents. Furthermore, in neuron-Schwann cell cocultures TGF*β* blocks myelination, and in pure Schwann cell cultures TGF*β* suppresses the induction of myelin-related genes by cAMP (see the following two sections).

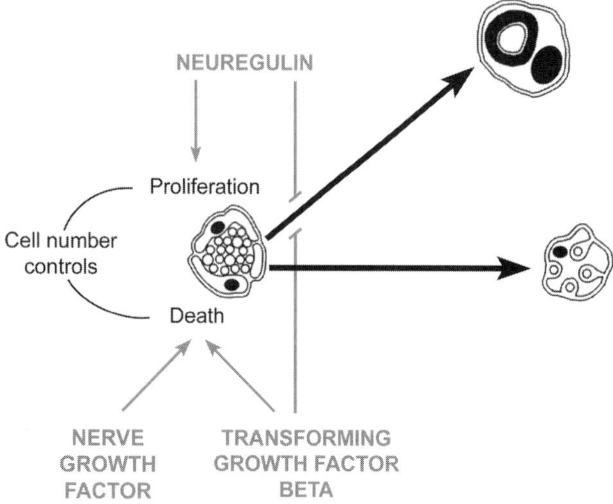

FIGURE 7.5 Schwann cell numbers in developing nerves are regulated by proliferation and cell death. A model of how transforming growth factor beta, nerve growth factor, and neuregulin-1 might cooperate in the perinatal period of Schwann cell development to ensure correct Schwann cell numbers.

As outlined above, the population of immature Schwann cells in perinatal nerves is exposed to death signals (NGF and TGFβ), survival signals (neuregulin-1 and autocrine signals), and mitogens (principally neuregulin-1). It is likely that this complex signaling provides a mechanism for matching the number of Schwann cells and axons. Two of these signals, TGFβ and neuregulin-1, can also suppress myelination (see above and the section "Myelination") and could therefore take part in timing the duration of this premyelination phase of Schwann cell development (Fig. 7.5).

CELL CULTURE STUDIES ON SCHWANN CELL PROLIFERATION AND DIFFERENTIATION

Besides neuregulin (see the section "Neuregulins and Schwann All Development"), other growth factors present in neurons induce Schwann cell DNA synthesis. These factors may therefore take part in regulating proliferation *in vivo* (Mirsky and Jessen, 2001). Two *in vitro* models have been used extensively to study proliferation and myelin-related differentiation in Schwann cells. The first model uses cocultures of DRG neurons and Schwann cells to study proliferation and myelination, both of which can occur in defined media. In particular, it has been used to establish neuregulin-1 as the principal axonal mitogen and the importance of the basal lamina in myelination (Bunge, 1993; see the section "Neuregulin and Schwann Cell Development"). Axon-induced proliferation and myelination occur sequentially in these cultures, and the effects of antibodies, added growth factors, genetically engineered constructs, or intracellular pathway inhibitors on both of these processes have been investigated. The other model uses elevation of intracellular cAMP levels in purified cultures of Schwann cells, grown in media with or without identified growth factors or serum, to mimic the effects of axon-induced proliferation and differentiation. In this model, elevation of cAMP levels in the absence of growth factors (see below) strongly stimulates expression of myelin-related proteins, including P0, peripheral myelin protein (PMP22), periaxin and galactocerebroside, without inducing DNA synthesis, thus mimicking events that occur when myelination is induced by axons. When cAMP levels are elevated in the presence of growth factors or serum, cell division is stimulated, and elevation of proteins such as P0 in the population as a whole is greatly reduced (reviewed in Mirsky and Jessen, 2001; Jessen and Mirsky, 2003). Results using these two models largely complement one another.

Studies on the regulation of Schwann cell DNA synthesis in serum-purified rat Schwann cell cultures have identified growth factors, including fibroblast growth factor (FGF)-1 and -2, PDGF-BB, TGFβs, and Reg-2, that act as mitogens in the presence or absence of serum, provided that cAMP levels are elevated (Livesey et al., 1997; Mirsky and Jessen, 2001). Insulin-like growth factors or high levels of insulin, presumably acting via type 1 IGF receptors, potentiate the effects of most if not all Schwann cell mitogens, acting in Schwann cells and other cells as progression factors, and to increase cell size in the G1 phase of the cell cycle (Conlon et al., 2001; Kim et al., 2001). None of these factors stimulate significant DNA synthesis when used alone in the absence of cAMP elevation. In contrast, neuregulin-1 and hepatocyte growth factor (HGF) both stimulate Schwann cell proliferation in the absence of other factors, although DNA synthesis in neuregulin-1 is potentiated by both cAMP elevation and IGFs, while HGF-induced DNA synthesis is inhibited by cAMP elevation (Kim et al., 2000; Mirsky and Jessen, 2001).

Early studies suggested that cAMP promoted Schwann cell proliferation by increasing the expression of receptors for mitogenic growth factors on the cells (Weinmaster and Lemke, 1990). Recent studies have confirmed this observation but indicate that other mechanisms that act at earlier stages in the process are involved. Using the interaction between cAMP and PDGF-BB as a model, they show that PDGF acts upstream of cAMP in the G1 phase of the cell cycle as a competence factor. The primary effect of cAMP is to induce sustained elevation of the G1 phase–specific protein cyclin-D1, which is transiently elevated when PDGF is applied alone, thus allowing progression through G1. Ectopic expression of cyclin-D1 alleviates the requirement for cAMP elevation, while the tumor suppressor neurofibromin antagonizes cAMP accumulation and expression of cyclin-D1 (Kim et al., 2000,

2001). Cyclic AMP may interact with other Schwann cell mitogens in similar ways. Studies on Schwann cells and thyroid follicular cells suggest that activation of the p70 ribosomal S6 kinase (p70s6k) is also required for cAMP-dependent proliferation since inhibition of this kinase with rapamycin lowers cAMP-induced DNA synthesis in both cell types. In thyroid cells two separate cAMP-activated pathways converge to activate p70s6k, one of which is PKA dependent while the other is PI3 kinase dependent, PKA independent (Cass and Meinkoth, 2000).

Schwann cell proliferation in the early postnatal period of nerve development proceeds normally in cyclin-D1 or -D2 null mice. In contrast, in cyclin-D1 null mice, there is little proliferation after nerve transection or in serum-purified cultures of cyclin-D1 null Schwann cells in response to PDGF/forskolin or neuregulin-1. Thus, cyclin-D1 is required for proliferation in the absence of axons, either in transected adult nerves or in neonatal cell cultures, whereas it is not necessary for axonally driven proliferation in development (Kim et al., 2000; Atanasoski et al., 2001).

Interestingly, retroviral inhibition of cAMP-dependent PKA does not inhibit proliferation in neuron–Schwann cell cocultures, although it blocks proliferation in purified Schwann cell cultures driven by cAMP-elevating agents and growth factors. This suggests that neuron-dependent proliferation in development may not involve PKA-dependent pathways (Howe and McCarthy, 2000).

- Upregulation of myelin-associated proteins, e.g., P0, periaxin, and MBP.
- Downregulation of protein markers of immature Schwann cells, e.g., p75 and L1.
- Withdrawal from the cell cycle.
- Resistance to TGFβ-mediated killing.
- Membrane synthesis and wrapping movements.

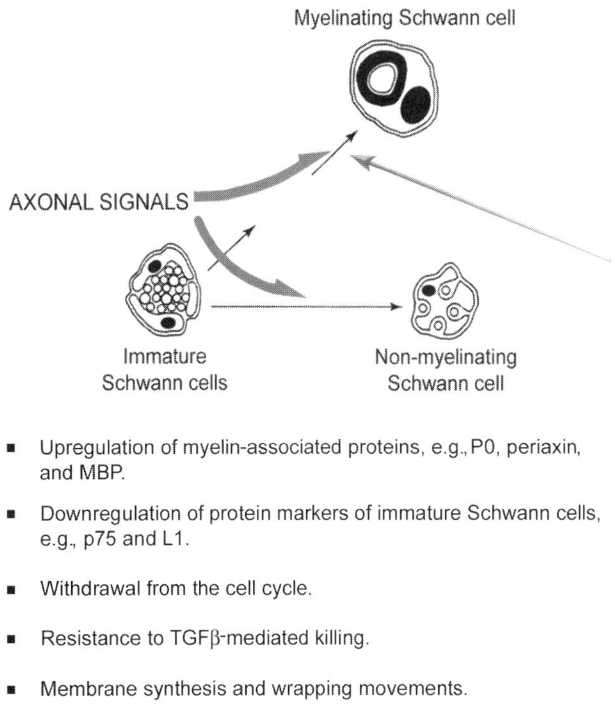

FIGURE 7.6 Activation of the myelin program. Axonal signals (*curved gray arrows*) drive the differentiation of both myelinating and non-myelinating Schwann cells (*black arrows*). Some of the major changes associated with myelination (*straight gray arrow*) are indicated by the bullet points below the diagram, all of which are discussed in greater detail in the text and in Figure 7.7.

MYELINATION

Schwann cell myelination is a remarkable example of cell-cell interaction in which an intimate association of a Schwann cell with a large-diameter axon induces a radical change in the immature Schwann cell phenotype, leading to the formation and elaboration of the myelin sheath and reciprocal changes in axonal ion channels and cytoskeleton that enable saltatory conduction along large nerves (Figs. 7.6, 7.7). At present, the identity of the axonal signal(s) and Schwann cell receptors that induce myelination is unknown.

Despite this, several other key steps in the process have been identified. The importance of the basal lamina in enabling myelination is well established and will not be covered in here (for reviews see Bunge, 1993; Chernousev and Carey, 2000; Previtali et al., 2001). More recently, the role of three key transcription factors in controlling myelination has been revealed. The importance of the transcription factor Sox-10 in early development of the glial lineage has been discussed (see the section "The Origin of Glial Cells from the Neural Crest"), but it also participates in later lineage events (see below). Two transcription factors, the POU domain protein Oct-6 (SCIP, Tst-1) and the zinc-finger protein Krox-20 (Egr-2), are essential for normal myelination *in vivo* (Scherer, 1997; Jaegle and Meijer, 1998; Mirsky and Jessen, 1999; Topilko and Meijer, 2001).

In Oct-6 null mice myelination is severely delayed, while in Krox-20 null mice it does not occur. In both of these mice Schwann cells are arrested either temporarily (Oct-6) or permanently (Krox-20) at the pro-myelinating stage, wrapping up to one and a half times round the large axons (Topilko and Meijer, 2001). In humans, Krox-20 (Egr-2) mutations are associated with Charcot-Marie-Tooth, Dejerrine-Sottas, and hereditary sensory and motor neuropathies, underlining the pivotal role of this transcription factor in controlling myelination (Kamholz et al., 2000).

Krox-20 is expressed selectively in cells that are destined to myelinate (Zorick et al., 1999; Topilko and Meijer, 2001; Parkinson et al., 2003, 2004). In contrast, Oct-6 can be detected in late precursors/early Schwann cells from about E13 (mouse), E15 (rat) on (Jessen and Mirsky, 2003). Although it is expressed most highly in pro-myelinating Schwann cells, it is seen in essentially all Schwann cells in perinatal nerves but is downregulated in mature nerves (Topilko and Meijer, 2001). Schwann cells of Oct-6 null mice fail to express Krox-20 at the appropriate time, but do so at the time when they eventually myelinate after a developmental delay of about 2 weeks (Topilko and Meijer, 2001). In this case, a related POU-domain transcrip-

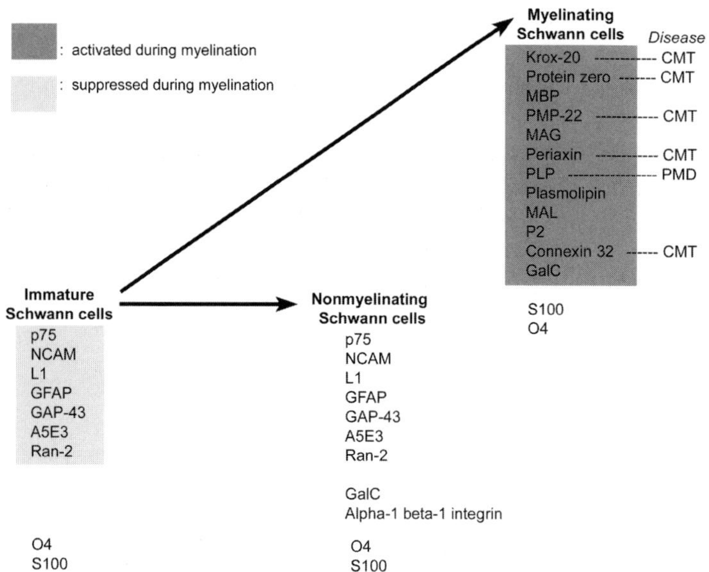

FIGURE 7.7 The main changes in protein and lipid expression that take place as the population of immature Schwann cells diverges to generate myelinating and nonmyelinating cells during development. Myelination involves a combination of downregulation and upregulation of key molecules, most of which are associated with formation of the myelin sheath. *Dark gray box*: molecules that are strongly upregulated on myelination. *Light gray box*: molecules associated with immature Schwann cells that are downregulated when cells myelinate. The generation of mature nonmyelinating cells from immature cells involves far fewer molecular changes, and most of the molecules typical of immature Schwann cells are also expressed by nonmyelinating cells, as indicated. Galactocerebroside (*GalC*) is expressed by both myelinating and nonmyelinating Schwann cells but not by immature cells, while $\alpha 1\beta 1$ integrin is upregulated specifically on nonmyelinating cells as they mature. 04 antigen and S100 are expressed by all Schwann cells in peripheral nerves, although 04 is downregulated in the absence of axons. Hereditary demyelinating neuropathies that result from abnormal expression of some of the myelin-associated proteins are indicated. *CMT*: Charcot-Marie-Tooth neuropathy; *GFAP*: glial fibrillary acid protein; *NCAM*: neural cell adhesion molecule; *PMD*: Pelizaeus-Merzbacher disease.

tion factor, Brn-2, can partially substitute for the missing Oct-6 in initiating myelination. It is intriguing that even in the combined absence of Brn-2 and Oct-6, myelination is not permanently blocked and a large number of fibers eventually myelinate (Jaegle et al., 2003). In contrast, in Krox-20 null mice, Oct-6 is expressed on schedule, and expression is maintained at higher than normal levels in the early postnatal period, suggesting that *in vivo* Krox-20 may downregulate Oct-6 (Topilko and Meijer, 2001; Ghazvini et al., 2002). It may also regulate cell death and proliferation since Schwann cells in these nerves have elevated DNA synthesis and death rates (Zorick et al., 1999; and see below). Krox-20 mRNA and protein levels are axonally regulated. They fall sharply on nerve transection and are reinduced on axonal regeneration and myelination, and in cultured Schwann cells by cAMP elevation (Zorick et al., 1999; Topilko and Meijer, 2001). Oct-6 is also reexpressed as Schwann cells remyelinate regenerating nerves and on cAMP elevation in cultured Schwann cells (Topilko and Meijer, 2001). Gene array technology has been used to show that enforced expression of Krox-20 in cultured Schwann cells is sufficient to induce a large and diverse set of genes, including those involved in myelin protein and lipid synthesis (Nagarajan et al., 2001). This and other studies indicate that Krox-20 organizes a widespread set of phenotypic changes associated with the transition from immature proliferating cells to quiescent myelinating cells, including a block of neuregulin-1-induced proliferation; activation of periaxin, P0, and myelin basic protein (MBP); downregulation of L1 protein; and inhibition of TGFβ-induced cell death (Nagarajan et al., 2001; Jessen and Mirsky, 2002; Parkinson et al., 2002b, 2004). There is evidence that the underlying mechanisms relate to the capacity of Krox-20 to inactivate the c-Jun-N-terminal kinase pathway. Not only is activation of this pathway required for both Schwann cell proliferation and death, but it also functions to inhibit myelin differentiation. The ability of Krox-20 to suppress c-Jun-N-terminal kinase activity therefore gives Krox-20 integrated control over myelination, proliferation, and death (Parkinson et al., 2004; D.B. Parkinson, A. Bhaskaran, R. Mirsky, and K.R. Jessen, unpublished). Krox-20 also induces P0 and periaxin expression and inhibits DNA synthesis and death in an unrelated cell type, NIH 3T3 cells, behavior reminiscent of master regulatory genes such as the bHLH factors or peroxisome proliferator-activated receptor (PPAR) γ (Jessen and Mirsky, 2002).

The promoter regions of *Oct-6* and *Krox-20* contain Schwann cell specific enhancer (SCE) elements that are controlled by axonally regulated transcription factors. The *Oct-6* SCE, present within a 4.3 kb sequence 12 kb downstream of the transcription initiation site, is sufficient to drive temporally and spatially correct expression of the gene developmentally and during regeneration (Mandemakers et al., 2000; Ghazvini et al., 2002). The *Krox-20* gene contains two separate elements, the immature Schwann cell element (ISE), situated upstream of the transcription start site, and the myelinating Schwann cell element (MSE), which is within a 1.3 kb sequence situated 35 kb downstream of the *Krox-20* open reading frame. The MSE is active from E18.5 on in myelinating Schwann cells, contains multiple Oct-6 binding sites, and requires Oct-6 for activation, while the ISE is active in immature Schwann cells from E15.5 on, but not in actively myelinating cells (Ghislain et al., 2002).

Sox-10 can function synergistically with Oct-6 to promote gene expression and can modulate Pax-3 and Krox-20 activity *in vitro* (Kuhlbrodt et al., 1998). It positively regulates the P0 promoter and functions synergistically with Krox-20 to activate the gap junction connexin32 (Cx32) promoter (Peirano et al., 2000; Bondurand et al., 2001). Connexin 32 is expressed in myelinating Schwann cells, and mutations in the Krox-20/Sox-10 binding region of the human Cx32 promoter are among the more than 80 mutations that result in X-linked Charcot-Marie-Tooth neuropathy. Furthermore, mutated forms of Sox-10 or Krox-20, identified in patients with other forms of Charcot-Marie-Tooth neuropathy, fail to transactivate the Cx32 promoter (Bondurand et al., 2001).

Recent experiments indicate that the transcription factor NFκB plays a role in myelination (Nickols et al., 2003). Like Oct-6, NFκB is highly expressed in premyelinating Schwann cells in sciatic nerves and is downregulated in adult nerves. In myelinating neuron–Schwann cell cocultures NFκB is activated prior to Oct-6 upregulation, and inhibition of NFκB activity prevents upregulation of Oct-6 and myelination. Proper alignment of Schwann cells along axons is disturbed, and myelination is severely reduced when Schwann cells null for the p65 subunit of NFκB are cocultured with DRG neurons, suggesting that NFκB is required for Schwann cells to enter the pro-myelinating stage (Nickols et al., 2003). Roles for HLH factors in regulating myelination have been suggested but not proved. These include the bHLH factor Mash-2, expressed in a subset of myelinating Schwann cells, and the inhibitory Id HLH factors, Ids 1 and 3. Ids 1 and 3 repress myelin gene promoter activity and are more highly expressed in mature nerves than perinatal ones (Thatikunta et al., 1999; Kury et al., 2002).

Cell culture studies suggest the importance of cAMP pathways in myelination (Mirsky and Jessen, 2001). Retroviral inhibition of PKA prevents myelination in neuron–Schwann cell cocultures (Howe and McCarthy, 2000), and as mentioned earlier, numerous studies indicate that elevation of Schwann cell intracellular cAMP levels, particularly under nonproliferating conditions in the absence of growth factors such as FGF, partially mimics the axonal signal by strongly upregulating expression of Oct-6, Krox-20, and myelin proteins and lipids (see the section "Cell Culture Studies on Schwann Cell Proliferation and Differentiation"; Mirsky and Jessen, 2001). Among growth factors, IGFs promote cAMP-induced P0 induction in purified Schwann cell cultures and myelination in cocultures (Cheng et al., 1999; Mirsky and Jessen, 2001). Similarly, brain-derived neurotrophic factor (BDNF) enhances myelination in cocultures, while inhibition of BDNF signaling in these cultures and in regenerating nerves retards myelination (Chan et al., 2001). Another growth factor, glial-derived neurotrophic factor (GDNF), induces Schwann cell proliferation and promotes myelination of small-diameter axons that would normally not myelinate when it is administered exogenously to adult rats (Hoke et al., 2003). It is argued that the direct effect of GDNF is to increase the size and axon diameter of the smaller neurons and, that its effects on proliferation and myelination of Schwann cells are indirect.

The steroid hormone progesterone increases the rate of myelination both *in vivo* and *in vitro*, and upregulates P0 and PMP22 mRNA (Magnaghi et al., 2001). Coculture studies have suggested that progesterone synthesized by Schwann cells may also activate neuronal target genes (Chan et al., 2000). In cocultures between Schwann cells and neurons, TGFβs and neuregulins inhibit myelination. Both of these factors also suppress P0 expression in purified Schwann cells under certain culture conditions. It is therefore possible that *in vivo* they take part in regulating the time of onset of myelination (Mirsky and Jessen, 2001).

NEURAL ACTIVITY

Several studies indicate that neural activity may regulate the development of immature Schwann cells (Fields and Stevens, 2000; Colomar and Amedee, 2001). Electrical stimulation of neurons in DRG–Schwann cell cocultures results in neuronal calcium elevation. This leads to delayed calcium elevation in neurite-associated Schwann cells, caused by nonsynaptic release of adenosine triphosphate (ATP) from neurons acting via P2 receptors (Fields and Stevens, 2000). Cell division is inhibited in response to ATP, and Schwann cell differentiation, measured by expression of 04 antigen and myelination, is delayed. The reduced proliferation is likely caused by inhibition of adenylate cyclase activity induced by activation of P2Y receptors, though P2X7 and P2U receptors are also present on primary Schwann cells or immortalized cells, respectively (Fields and Stevens, 2000; Colomar and Amedee, 2001). In normal nerve development, cessation of proliferation occurs just prior to myelination and takes place well after 04 antigen is expressed, so it is not clear how signaling via ATP will integrate with other signals to generate the coordinated pattern of Schwann cell maturation, proliferation, and myelination that occurs *in vivo*.

Complicated patterns of neural activity also lower neuronal but not Schwann cell expression of N-cadherin and L1 in these cocultures (Itoh et al., 1997; Fields and Stevens, 2000). Reduced L1 induced by low-impulse activity lowers myelination to one-third of the normal level and, in a short-term assay, adhesion of Schwann cells to neurites. The involvement of L1 in axon–Schwann cell interactions is supported by other studies. Antibodies to L1 prevent myelination in the coculture system by disrupting correct alignment along the axon, and decreased axonal L1 expression leads to defasciculation of nerve bundles both *in vivo* and *in vitro* (Wood et al., 1990; Honig et al., 2002). Nevertheless, no major disturbance of development of either myelinated or unmyelinated fibres has been described in L1 null mice, although in older mice disturbances occur in axon–Schwann cell interactions in sensory fibers (Haney et al., 1999).

THE EXTRACELLULAR MATRIX AND THE CYTOSKELETON IN SCHWANN CELL DEVELOPMENT

New research on the extracellular matrix and interactions with the Schwann cell membrane and cytoskeletal components during development has pinpointed the importance of direct interactions between the major Schwann cell basal lamina protein laminin 2 ($\alpha2$, $\beta1$, $\gamma1$) and its three major receptors in maintaining normal Schwann cell function in peripheral nerves (see below). Two of these receptors, namely, integrin $\alpha6\beta1$ and $\alpha\beta$dystroglycan, appear to be more crucial than the $\alpha6\beta4$ receptor, which is highly expressed in myelinating Schwann cells (Previtali et al., 2001; Brophy, 2002; Rambukkana et al., 2002).

Use of a P0-Cre transgene to excise $\beta1$ integrin from a floxed allele between E13.5 and 14.5 in mice has revealed a role for integrin $\beta1$ in subsequent phases of nerve development. In these mice, Schwann cells proliferate and survive normally but show severely abnormal relationships with axons (Feltri et al., 2002). In many instances, axons fail to segregate properly and never achieve the 1:1 ratio with Schwann cells that is required for myelination. In the minority of nerve fibers in which myelination does occur, it is developmentally delayed. Because aspects of the phenotype strongly resemble the pathology seen in the spinal roots of the *dy/dy* mouse, which lacks functional laminin 2, it is suggested that the main extracellular partner for the $\beta1$ integrin in Schwann cells in normal development is likely to be laminin 2, acting via the $\alpha6\beta1$ receptor, which is highly expressed in embryonic Schwann cells. Lack of $\beta1$ integrin would then lead to a failure to link the basal lamina to the Schwann cell cytoskeleton, a process necessary for Schwann cell polarization and proper axonal ensheathment (Feltri et al., 2002; Previtali et al., 2002).

There is considerable evidence that interactions between integrins and the actin cytoskeleton are important in Schwann cells. Integrin $\beta1$ interacts with and phosphorylates focal adhesion kinase and associates with the actin-linked protein paxillin in differentiating Schwann cells in DRG-neuron cocultures (Chen et al., 2000). Lysophosphatidic acid causes focal adhesion assembly of paxillin and vinculin, acting via Rho, the rearrangement of the actin cytoskeleton into wreath-like structures, and the induction of N-cadherin/catenin-mediated cell contacts (Weiner et al., 2001). In culture, N-cadherin mediates the axon-aligned process growth of Schwann cells and contacts between Schwann cells, a role consistent with its distribution *in vivo* (Wanner and Wood, 2002). Paxillin also interacts with the tumor suppressor cytoskeletal protein Schwannomin (Fernandez-Vallé et al., 2002). The actin-binding protein dystonin may also be involved in Schwann cell myelination. Schwann cells from mice with dystonin mutations fail to attach normally to laminin and show abnormal myelination (Bernier et al., 1998).

Binding of laminin to dystroglycan promotes basal lamina formation (Tsiper and Yurchenko, 2002). In Schwann cells, basal lamina formation occurs just prior to myelination *in vivo* (Bunge, 1993; Masaki et al., 2002). In Schwann cells, α-dystroglycan binds to transmembrane β-dystroglycan, which in turn binds to the dystrophin-related-protein (DRP) 116, which lacks an actin-binding domain, or to utrophin, which has one (Sherman et al., 2001). In myelinating Schwann cells, dystroglycan also binds to an additional form of dystrophin, DRP2. In turn, this binds to the cytoskeletal PSD-95/DLg-A/ZO-1 (PDZ) domain protein periaxin, with which it forms morphologically discrete membrane-associated complexes in myelinating Schwann cells (Sherman et al., 2001). Mutations in periaxin result in Charcot-Marie-Tooth neuropathy type 4F in humans and severe sensory neuropathy in mice, emphasizing the importance of these complexes in myelin stability (Williams and Brophy, 2002). Phenolic-glycolipid-1 of *Mycobacterium leprae*, the infective agent in leprosy, interacts specifically with the G domain of the laminin-$\alpha2$ domain. This blocks the laminin2-α-dystroglycan interaction and allows entry of the bacterium into non-myelinating Schwann cells in DRG-neuron cocultures while inducing demyelination in myelinating cells (Rambukkana et al., 2002).

There is also evidence that two integrins, α4 and α5, are required for survival and proliferation, respectively, in the early stages of the Schwann cell lineage. Early glial cells in DRG and nerves initially develop normally in mice lacking α4 integrin, but later their survival is severely compromised both *in vivo* and *in vitro*, while in mice lacking α5 integrin, proliferation of early glial cells is inhibited (Haack and Hynes, 2001).

DEVELOPMENTAL SIGNALS FROM SCHWANN CELLS TO OTHER COMPONENTS OF THE NERVE

Schwann cell precursors and Schwann cells are an important source of developmental signals in embryonic and neonatal nerves (Jessen and Mirsky, 1999) (Fig. 7.8). It is likely that they provide trophic factors for embryonic DRG and motor neurons, as well as signals that regulate axonal architecture and Na-channel clustering (Jessen and Mirsky, 1999). Schwann cells also generate autocrine survival factors and release chemokines such as interleukin-6 (IL-6), LIF, and monocyte-chemoattractant protein (MCP)-1 that attract macrophages into damaged nerves (Tofaris et al., 2002). In addition, they secrete the signaling molecule Dhh, which controls the proper formation of the connective tissue sheaths of the nerve, in particular the perineurial sheaths that surround nerve fascicles (Parmantier et al., 1999).

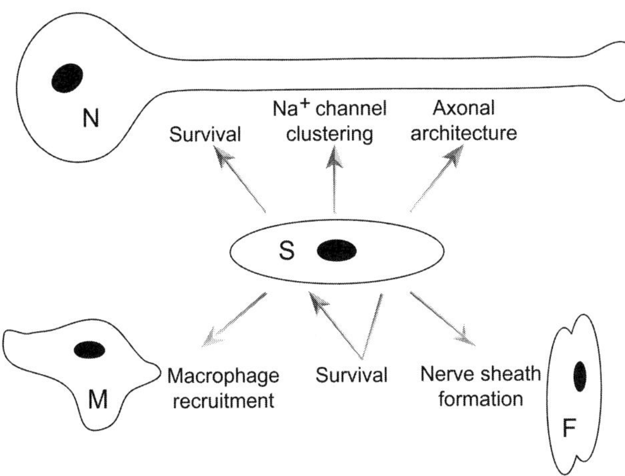

FIGURE 7.8 A summary of signaling from developing Schwann cells during nerve development. Signals from developing Schwann cells and their precursors (*S*) regulate numerous events in nerve development. They secrete Desert hedgehog to signal correct formation of the perineurium from fibroblastic cells, and after injury chemotactic signals that attract macrophages to the nerve. They provide autocrine signals that enable Schwann cell survival in the absence of axons. Developing Schwann cells are also likely to supply trophic factors that support the survival of embryonic sensory and thoracic motor neurons, and provide signals that control sodium channel clustering in myelinating axons and other aspects of axonal architecture, including axonal diameter. F: fibroblast; M: macrophage; N: neuron.

Some of the diverse roles that cells of the Schwann cell lineage play in building and maintaining peripheral nerves are shown in Figure 7.8. It should be emphasized, however, that mutual interplay between all the cellular components—neurons, Schwann cells, and fibroblasts—is required for normal nerve development and function.

ACKNOWLEDGMENTS

We would like to thank the Wellcome Trust for supporting some of the work described in this chapter and Mrs. Debbie Bartram for editorial assistance.

REFERENCES

Adlkofer, K., and Lai, C. (2000) Role of neuregulins in glial cell development. *Glia* 29:104–111.

Anderson, D.J. (2000) Genes, lineages and the neural crest: a speculative review. *Philos. Trans. R. Soc. Lond. B Biol. Sci.* 355:953–964.

Atanasoski, S., Shumas, S., Dickson, C., Scherer, S.S., and Suter, U. (2001) Differential cyclin D1 requirements of proliferating Schwann cells during development and after injury. *Mol. Cell. Neurosci.* 18:581–592.

Bernier, G., De Repentigny, Y., Mathieu, M., David, S., and Kothary, R. (1998) Dystonin is an essential component of the Schwann cell cytoskeleton at the time of myelination. *Development* 125:2135–2148.

Bitgood, M.J., Shen, L., and McMahon, A.P. (1996) Sertoli cell signaling by Desert hedgehog regulates the male germline. *Curr. Biol.* 6:298–304.

Bondurand, N., Girard, M., Pingault, V., Lemort, N., Dubourg, O., and Goossens, M. (2001) Human connexin 32, a gap junction protein altered in the X-linked form of Charcot-Marie-Tooth disease, is directly regulated by the transcription factor SOX10. *Hum. Mol. Genet.* 10:2783–2795.

Brennan, A., Dean, C.H., Zhang, A.L., Cass, D.T., Mirsky, R., and Jessen, K.R. (2000) Endothelins control the timing of Schwann cell generation *in vitro* and *in vivo*. *Dev. Biol.* 227:545–557.

Britsch, S., Goerich, D.E., Riethmacher, D., Peirano, R.I., Rossner, M., Nave, K.A., Birchmeier, C., and Wegner, M. (2001) The transcription factor Sox10 is a key regulator of peripheral glial development. *Genes Dev.* 15:66–78.

Brophy, P.J. (2002) Microbiology. Subversion of Schwann cells and the leper's bell. *Science* 296:862–863.

Bunge, R.P. (1993) Expanding roles for the Schwann cell: ensheathment, myelination, trophism and regeneration. *Curr. Opin. Neurobiol.* 3:805–809.

Cass, L.A. and Meinkoth, J.L. (2000) Ras signaling through PI3K confers hormone-independent proliferation that is compatible with differentiation. *Oncogene* 19:924–932.

Chan, J.R., Cosgaya, J.M., Wu, Y.J., and Shooter, E. M. (2001) Neurotrophins are key mediators of the myelination program in the peripheral nervous system. *Proc. Natl. Acad. Sci. USA* 98:14661–14668.

Chan, J.R., Rodriguez-Waitkus, P.M., Ng, B.K., Liang, P., and Glaser, M. (2000) Progesterone synthesized by Schwann cells during myelin formation regulates neuronal gene expression. *Mol. Biol. Cell* 11:2283–2295.

Chen, L.M., Bailey, D., and Fernandez-Vallé, C. (2000) Association of beta 1 integrin with focal adhesion kinase and paxillin in differentiating Schwann cells. *J. Neurosci.* 20:3776–3784.

Cheng, H.L., Russell, J.W., and Feldman, E.L. (1999) IGF-I promotes peripheral nervous system myelination. *Ann. NY Acad. Sci.* 883:124–130.

Cheng, H.L., Steinway, M., Delaney, C.L., Franke, T.F., and Feldman, E.L. (2000) IGF-I promotes Schwann cell motility and survival via activation of Akt. *Mol. Cell. Endocrinol.* 170:211–215.

Chernousov, M.A. and Carey, D.J. (2000) Schwann cell extracellu lar matrix molecules and their receptors. *Histol. Histopathol.* 15:593–601.

Colomar, A, and Amedee, T. (2001) ATP stimulation of P2X(7) receptors activates three different ionic conductances on cultured mouse Schwann cells. *Eur. J. Neurosci.* 14:927–936.

Conlon, I.J., Dunn, G.A., Mudge, A.W., and Raff, M.C. (2001) Extracellular control of cell size. *Nature Cell Biol.* 3:918–921.

Dong, Z., Brennan, A., Liu, N., Yarden, Y., Lefkowitz, G., Mirsky, R., and Jessen, K.R. (1995) NDF is a neuron-glia signal and regulates survival, proliferation, and maturation of rat Schwann cell precursors. *Neuron* 15:585–596.

Dupin, E., Real, C., Glavieux-Pardanaud, C., Vaigot, P., and Le Douarin, N.M. (2003) Reversal of developmental restrictions in neural crest cell lineages: transition from Schwann cells to glial-melanocytic precursors in vitro. *Proc. Natl. Acad. Sci. USA* 100: 5229–5233.

Feltri, M.L., Graus Porta, D., Previtali, S.C., Nodari, A., Migliavacca, B., Cassetti, A., Littlewood-Evans, A., Reichardt, L.F., Messing, A., Quattrini, A., Mueller, U., and Wrabetz, L. (2002) Conditional disruption of beta 1 integrin in Schwann cells impedes interactions with axons. *J. Cell Biol.* 156:199–209.

Fernandez-Vallé, C., Tang, Y., Ricard, J., Rodenas-Ruano, A., Taylor, A., Hackler, E., Biggerstaff, J., and Iacovelli, J. (2002) Paxillin binds schwannomin and regulates its density-dependent localization and effect on cell morphology. *Nat. Genet.* 31:354–362.

Fields, R.D. and Stevens, B. (2000) ATP: an extracellular signaling molecule between neurons and glia. *Trends Neurosci.* 23:625–633.

Garratt, A.N., Britsch, S., and Birchmeier, C. (2000) Neuregulin, a factor with many functions in the life of a Schwann cell. *BioEssays* 22:987–996.

Ghazvini, M., Mandemakers, W., Jaegle, M., Piirsoo, M., Driegen, S., Koutsourakis, M., Smit, X., Grosveld, F., and Meijer, D. (2002) A cell type–specific allele of the POU gene *Oct-6* reveals Schwann cell autonomous function in nerve development and regeneration. *EMBO J.* 21:4612–4620.

Ghislain, J., Desmarquet-Trin-Dinh, C., Jaegle, M., Meijer, D., Charnay, P., and Frain, M. (2002) Characterisation of cis-acting sequences reveals a biphasic, axon-dependent regulation of Krox20 during Schwann cell development. *Development* 129:155–166.

Grinspan, J.B., Marchionni, M.A., Reeves, M., Coulaloglou, M., and Scherer, S.S. (1996) Axonal interactions regulate Schwann cell apoptosis in developing peripheral nerve: neuregulin receptors and the role of neuregulins. *J. Neurosci.* 16:6107–6118.

Haack, H. and Hynes, R.O. (2001) Integrin receptors are required for cell survival and proliferation during development of the peripheral glial lineage. *Dev. Biol.* 233:38–55.

Hagedorn, L., Suter, U., and Sommer, L. (1999) P0 and PMP22 mark a multipotent neural crest–derived cell type that displays community effects in response to TGF-beta family factors. *Development* 126:3781–3794.

Haney, C.A., Sahenk, Z., Li, C., Lemmon, V.P., Roder, J., and Trapp, B.D. (1999) Heterophilic binding of L1 on unmyelinated sensory axons mediates Schwann cell adhesion and is required for axonal survival. *J. Cell Biol.* 146:1173–1184.

Hoke, A., Ho, T., Crawford, T.O., LeBel, C., Hilt, D., and Griffin, J.W. (2003) Glial cell line–derived neurotrophic factor alters axon Schwann cell units and promotes myelination in unmyelinated nerve fibers. *J. Neurosci.* 23:561–567.

Honig, M.G., Camilli, S.J., and Xue, Q.S. (2002) Effects of L1 blockade on sensory axon outgrowth and pathfinding in the chick hindlimb. *Dev. Biol.* 243:137–154.

Howe, D.G. and McCarthy, K.D. (2000) Retroviral inhibition of cAMP-dependent protein kinase inhibits myelination but not Schwann cell mitosis stimulated by interaction with neurons. *J. Neurosci.* 20:3513–3521.

Itoh, K., Ozaki, M., Stevens, B., and Fields, R.D. (1997) Activity-dependent regulation of N-cadherin in DRG neurons: differential regulation of N-cadherin, NCAM, and L1 by distinct patterns of action potentials. *J. Neurobiol.* 33:735–748.

Jaegle, M., Ghazvini, M., Mandemakers, W., Piirsoo, M., Driegen, S., Levavasseur, F., Raghoenath, S., Grosveld, F., and Meijer, D. (2003) The POU proteins *Brn-2* and *Oct-6* share important functions in Schwann cell development. *Genes Dev.* 17:1380–1391.

Jaegle, M. and Meijer, D. (1998) Role of *Oct-6* in Schwann cell differentiation. *Microsc. Res. Tech.* 41:372–378.

Jessen, K.R., Brennan, A., Morgan, L., Mirsky, R., Kent, A., Hashimoto, Y., and Gavrilovic, J. (1994) The Schwann cell precursor and its fate: a study of cell death and differentiation during gliogenesis in rat embryonic nerves. *Neuron* 12:509–527.

Jessen, K.R. and Mirsky, R. (1999) Schwann cells and their precursors emerge as major regulators of nerve development. *Trends Neurosci.* 22:402–410.

Jessen, K.R. and Mirsky, R. (2002) Signals that determine Schwann cell identity. *J. Anat.* 200:367–376.

Jessen, K.R. and Mirsky, R. (2003) Embryonic Schwann cell development and the initiation of myelination. In: Lazzarini, R.A., ed. *Biology and Disorders*, Volume 1, Chapter 13. Elsevier Inc., San Diego, pp. 329–370.

Kamholz, J., Menichella, D., Jani, A., Garbern, J., Lewis, R.A., Krajewski, K.M., Lilien, J., Scherer, S.S., and Shy, M.E. (2000) Charcot-Marie-Tooth disease type 1: molecular pathogenesis to gene therapy. *Brain* 123:222–233.

Khursigara, G., Bertin, J., Yano, H., Moffett, H., DiStefano, P.S., and Chao, M.V. (2001) A prosurvival function for the p75 receptor death domain mediated via the caspase recruitment domain receptor-interacting protein 2. *J. Neurosci.* 21:5854–5863.

Kim, H.A., Pomeroy, S.L., Whoriskey, W., Pawlitzky, I., Benowitz, L.I., Sicinski, P., Stiles, C.D., and Roberts, T.M. (2000) A developmentally regulated switch directs regenerative growth of Schwann cells through cyclin D1. *Neuron* 26:405–416.

Kim, H.A., Ratner, N., Roberts, T.M., and Stiles, C.D. (2001) Schwann cell proliferative responses to cAMP and Nf1 are mediated by cyclin D1. *J. Neurosci.* 21:1110–1116.

Knecht, A.K. and Bronner-Fraser, M. (2002) Induction of the neural crest: a multigene process. *Nat. Rev. Genet.* 3:453–461.

Kuhlbrodt, K., Herbarth, B., Sock, E., Enderich, J., Hermans-Borgmeyer, I., and Wegner, M. (1998) Cooperative function of POU proteins and SOX proteins in glial cells. *J. Biol. Chem.* 273: 16050–16057.

Kury, P., Greiner-Petter, R., Cornely, C., Jurgens, T., and Muller, H.W. (2002) Mammalian achaete scute homolog 2 is expressed in the adult sciatic nerve and regulates the expression of Krox24, Mob-1, CXCR4, and p57kip2 in Schwann cells. *J. Neurosci.* 22:7586–7595.

Le Douarin, N.M., and Kalcheim, C. (1999) *The Neural Crest.* Cambridge, UK: Cambridge University Press.

Leimeroth, R., Lobsiger, C., Lüssi, A., Taylor, V., Suter, U., and Sommer, L. (2002) Membrane-bound neuregulin1 type III actively promotes Schwann cell differentiation of multipotent progenitor cells. *Dev. Biol.* 246:245–258.

Lemke, G. (2001) Glial control of neuronal development. *Annu. Rev. Neurosci.* 24:87–105.

Li, Y., Tennekoon, G.I., Birnbaum, M., Marchionni, M.A., and Rutkowski, J.L. (2001) Neuregulin signaling through a PI3K/Akt/Bad pathway in Schwann cell survival. *Mol. Cell. Neurosci.* 17:761–767.

Livesey, F.J., O'Brien, J.A., Li, M., Smith, A.G., Murphy, L.J., and Hunt, S.P. (1997) A Schwann cell mitogen accompanying regeneration of motor neurons. *Nature* 390:614–618.

Lobsiger, C.S., Taylor, V., and Suter, U. (2002) The early life of a Schwann cell. *Biol. Chem.* 383:245–253.

Magnaghi, V., Cavarretta, I., Galbiati, M., Martini, L., and Melcangi, R.C. (2001) Neuroactive steroids and peripheral myelin proteins. *Brain Res. Brain Res. Rev.* 37:360–371.

Mandemakers, W., Zwart, R., Jaegle, M., Walbeehm, E., Visser, P., Grosveld, F., and Meijer, D. (2000) A distal Schwann cell–specific enhancer mediates axonal regulation of the Oct-6 transcription factor during peripheral nerve development and regeneration. *EMBO J.* 19:2992–3003.

Masaki, T., Matsumura, K., Hirata, A., Yamada, H., Hase, A., Arai, K., Shimizu, T., Yorifuji, H., Motoyoshi, K., and Kamakura, K. (2002) Expression of dystroglycan and the laminin-alpha 2 chain in the rat peripheral nerve during development. *Exp. Neurol.* 174:109–117.

Maurel, P., and Salzer, J.L. (2000) Axonal regulation of Schwann cell proliferation and survival and the initial events of myelination requires PI 3-kinase activity. *J. Neurosci.* 20:4635–4645.

Meier, C., Parmantier, E., Brennan, A., Mirsky, R., and Jessen, K.R. (1999) Developing Schwann cells acquire the ability to survive without axons by establishing an autocrine circuit involving IGF, NT-3 and PDGF-BB. *J. Neurosci.* 19:3847–3859.

Mirsky, R. and Jessen, K.R. (1999) The neurobiology of Schwann cells. *Brain Pathol.* 9:293–311.

Mirsky, R. and Jessen, K.R. (2001) Embryonic and early postnatal development of Schwann cells. In: Jessen, K.R. and Richardson, W.D., eds. *Glial Cell Development: Basic Principles and Clinical Relevance*, 2nd ed. Oxford, U: Oxford University Press, pp. 1–20.

Morrison, S.J., Perez, S.E., Qiao, Z., Verdi, J.M., Hicks, C., Weinmaster, G., and Anderson, D.J. (2000) Transient Notch activation initiates an irreversible switch from neurogenesis to gliogenesis by neural crest stem cells. *Cell* 101:499–510.

Nagarajan, R., Svaren, J., Le, N., Araki, T., Watson, M., and Milbrandt, J. (2001) *EGR2* mutations in inherited neuropathies dominant-negatively inhibit myelin gene expression. *Neuron* 30: 355–368.

Nickols, J.C., Valentine, W., Kanwal, S., and Carter, B.D. (2003) Activation of the transcription factor NF-kappaB in Schwann cells is required for peripheral myelin formation. *Nat. Neurosci.* 6:161–167.

Parkinson, D.B., Bhaskaran, A., Droggiti, A., Dickinson, S., D'Antonio, M., Mirsky, R., and Jessen, K.R. (2004) Krox-20 inhibits Jun-NH_2-terminal kinase/c-Jun to control Schwann cell death. *J. Cell Biol.* 164, 3, 385–394.

Parkinson, D.B., Dickinson, S., Bhaskaran, A., Kinsella, M.T., Brophy, P.J., Sherman, D.L., Sharghi-Namini, S., Duran Alonso, M.B., Jessen, K.R., and Mirsky, R. (2002b) Krox 20 activates a set of complex changes in Schwann cells that characterize myelination. *Glia* (Supp 1):S69.

Parkinson, D.B., Dickinson, S., Bhaskaran, A., Kinsella, M.T., Brophy, P.J., Sherman, D.L., Sharghi-Namini, S., Duran Alonso, M.B., Mirsky, R., and Jessen, K.R. (2003) Regulation of the myelin gene periaxin provides evidence for Krox-20 independent myelin-related signalling in Schwann cells. *Mol. Cell. Neurosci.* 23:13–27.

Parkinson, D.B., Dong, Z., Bunting, H., Whitfield, J., Meier, C., Marie, H., Mirsky, R., and Jessen, K.R. (2001) Transforming growth factor β (TGFβ) mediates Schwann cell death in vitro and in vivo: examination of c-Jun activation, interactions with survival signals, and the relationship of TGFβ mediated death to Schwann cell differentiation. *J. Neurosci.* 21:8572–8585.

Parkinson, D.B., Langner, K., Namini, S.S., Jessen, K.R., and Mirsky, R. (2002a) β-Neuregulin and autocrine mediated survival of Schwann cells requires activity of Ets family transcription factors. *Mol. Cell. Neurosci.* 20:154–167.

Parmantier, E., Lynn, B., Lawson, D., Turmaine, M., Sharghi Namini, S., Chakrabarti, L., McMahon, A.P., Jessen, K.R., and Mirsky, R. (1999). Schwann cell-derived Desert Hedgehog controls the development of peripheral nerve sheaths. *Neuron* 23:713–724.

Peirano, R.I., Goerich, D.E., Riethmacher, D., and Wegner, M. (2000) Protein zero gene expression is regulated by the glial transcription factor Sox10. *Mol. Cell. Biol.* 20:3198–3209.

Previtali, S.C., Feltri, M.L., Archelos, J.J., Quattrini, A., Wrabetz, L., and Hartung, H. (2001) Role of integrins in the peripheral nervous system. *Prog. Neurobiol.* 64:35–49.

Previtali, S., Nodari, A., Dina, G., Messing, A., Quattrini, A., Wrabetz, L., and Feltri, M.L. (2002) Cell-type specific knockouts in the study of glia-basement membrane interactions. *Glia* supplement I, S7.

Rambukkana, A., Zanazzi, G., Tapinos, N., and Salzer, J.L. (2002) Contact-dependent demyelination by *Mycobacterium leprae* in the absence of immune cells. *Science* 296:927–931.

Scherer, S.S. (1997) The biology and pathobiology of Schwann cells. *Curr. Opin. Neurol.* 10:386–397.

Scherer, S.S. and Salzer, J.L. (2001) Axon-Schwann cell interactions during peripheral nerve degeneration and regeneration. In: Jessen, K.L. and Richardson, W.D., eds. *Glial Cell Development: Basic Principles and Clinical Relevance*, 2nd ed. Oxford, UK: Oxford University Press, pp. 299–330.

Shah, N.M., Marchionni, M.A., Isaacs, I., Stroobant, P., and Anderson, D.J. (1994) Glial growth factor restricts mammalian neural crest stem cells to a glial fate. *Cell* 77:349–360.

Sherman, D.L., Fabrizi, C., Gillespie, C.S., and Brophy, P.J. (2001) Specific disruption of a Schwann cell dystrophin-related protein complex in a demyelinating neuropathy. *Neuron* 30:677–687.

Sherman, L., Stocker, K.M., Morrison, R., and Ciment, G. (1993) Basic fibroblast growth factor (bFGF) acts intracellularly to cause the transdifferentiation of avian neural crest–derived Schwann cell precursors into melanocytes. *Development* 118:1313–1326.

Soilu-Hanninen, M., Ekert, P., Bucci, T., Syroid, D., Bartlett, P.F., and Kilpatrick, T.J. (1999) Nerve growth factor signaling through p75 induces apoptosis in Schwann cells via a Bcl-2-independent pathway. *J. Neurosci.* 19:4828–4838.

Thatikunta, P., Qin, W., Christy, B.A., Tennekoon, G.I., and Rutkowski, J.L. (1999) Reciprocal Id expression and myelin gene regulation in Schwann cells. *Mol. Cell. Neurosci.* 14:519–528.

Tofaris, G.K., Patterson, P.H., Jessen, K.R., and Mirsky, R. (2002) Denervated Schwann cells attract macrophages by secretion of leukemia inhibitory factor (LIF) and monocyte chemoattractant protein-1 in a process regulated by interleukin-6 and LIF. *J. Neurosci.* 22:6696–6703.

Topilko, P. and Meijer, D. (2001) Transcription factors that control Schwann cell development and myelination. In: Jessen, K.R. and Richardson, W.D., eds. *Glial Cell Development: Basic Principles and Clinical Relevance*, 2nd ed. Oxford, UK: Oxford University Press, pp. 223–244.

Tosh, D. and Slack, J.M. (2002) How cells change their phenotype. *Nature Rev. Mol. Cell Biol.* 3:187–194.

Trachtenberg, J.T., and Thompson, W.J. (1996) Schwann cell apoptosis at developing neuromuscular junctions is regulated by glial growth factor. *Nature* 379:174–177.

Tsiper, M.V. and Yurchenco, P.D. (2002) Laminin assembles into separate basement membrane and fibrillar matrices in Schwann cells. *J. Cell Sci.* 115:1005–1015.

Wakamatsu, Y., Maynard, T.M., and Weston, J.A. (2000) Fate determination of neural crest cells by NOTCH-mediated lateral inhibition and asymmetrical cell division during gangliogenesis. *Development* 127:2811–2821.

Wang, J.Y., Miller, S.J., and Falls, D.L. (2001) The N-terminal region of neuregulin isoforms determines the accumulation of cell surface and released neuregulin ectodomain. *J. Biol. Chem.* 276:2841–2851.

Wang, S. and Barres, B.A. (2000) Up a notch: instructing gliogenesis. *Neuron* 27:197–200.

Wanner, I.B. and Wood, P.M. (2002) N-cadherin mediates axon-aligned process growth and cell-cell interaction in rat Schwann cells. *J. Neurosci.* 22:4066–4079.

Weiner, J.A., Fukushima, N., Contos, J.J., Scherer, S.S., and Chun, J. (2001) Regulation of Schwann cell morphology and adhesion by receptor-mediated lysophosphatidic acid signaling. *J. Neurosci.* 21:7069–7078.

Weinmaster, G. and Lemke, G. (1990) Cell-specific cyclic AMP–mediated induction of the PDGF receptor. *EMBO J.* 9:915–920.

White, P.M., Morrison, S.J., Orimoto, K., Kubu, C.J., Verdi, J.M., and Anderson, D.J. (2001) Neural crest stem cells undergo cell-intrinsic developmental changes in sensitivity to instructive differentiation signals. *Neuron* 29:57–71.

Williams, A.C. and Brophy, P.J. (2002) The function of the *Periaxin* gene during nerve repair in a model of CMT4F. *J. Anat.* 200:323–330.

Winseck, A.K., Calderó, J., Ciutat, D., Prevette, D., Scott, S.A., Wang, G., Esquerda, J.E., and Oppenheim, R.W. (2002) *In vivo* analysis of Schwann cell programmed cell death in the embryonic chick: regulation by axons and glial growth factor. *J. Neurosci.* 22:4509–4521.

Wolpowitz, D., Mason, T.B., Dietrich, P., Mendelsohn, M., Talmage, D.A., and Role, L.W. (2000) Cysteine-rich domain isoforms of the neuregulin-1 gene are required for maintenance of peripheral synapses. *Neuron* 25:79–91.

Wood, P.M., Schachner, M., and Bunge, R.P. (1990) Inhibition of Schwann cell myelination in vitro by antibody to the L1 adhesion molecule. *J. Neurosci.* 10:3635–3645.

Woodhoo, A., Dean, C.H., Droggiti, A., Mirsky, R., and Jessen, K.R. (2004) The trunk neural crest and its early glial derivatives: a study of survival responses, developmental schedules and autocrine mechanisms. *Mol. Cell. Neurosci.* 25, 30–41.

Zorick, T.S., Syroid, D.E., Brown, A., Gridley, T., and Lemke, G. (1999) Krox-20 controls SCIP expression, cell cycle exit and susceptibility to apoptosis in developing myelinating Schwann cells. *Development* 126:1397–1406.

8 The role of neurogenic astroglial cells in the developing and adult central nervous system

STEPHEN C. NOCTOR, LIDIJA IVIC,
VERÓNICA MARTÍNEZ-CERDEÑO, AND ARNOLD R. KRIEGSTEIN

The brain is comprised of neurons and glia that perform distinct functions, but the lineage relationships between some types of glial cells and neurons are not as divergent as was once thought. Recent evidence indicates that some glial cells function *in vivo* as neural precursor cells. This has been most clearly demonstrated in the telencephalon, where it has been shown that radial glial cells in the neocortical ventricular zone (VZ) generate neurons during embryonic development (Malatesta et al., 2000; Miyata et al., 2001; Noctor et al., 2001; Tamamaki et al., 2001), and that astrocytes generate neurons in the subventricular zone (SVZ, Doetsch et al., 1999) and dentate gyrus (Seri et al., 2001) of postnatal animals. Radial glial cells and astrocytes share several key identifying features that indicate glial phenotype such as electron-lucent cytoplasm, glycogen granule storage, and blood vessel encapsulation (Choi and Lapham, 1978). The known transformation of radial glial cells into astrocytes (Choi and Lapham, 1978; Schmechel and Rakic, 1979; Voigt, 1989), together with the new appreciation of the neurogenic role of radial glial cells and astrocytes, indicates that cells in the astroglial lineage play crucial roles in neurogenesis.

The central nervous system (CNS) is derived from the neuroepithelium, which at the earliest stages of development consists of a thin monolayer of epithelial cells, the neural plate. As the neuroepithelial cells continue to divide, the neural plate thickens and the neuroepithelium becomes a pseudostratified structure. The neural groove forms within the neural plate and closes dorsally to form the neural tube, thus creating a lumen, which becomes the ventricular system. The apical pole (ventricular endfoot) of the neuroepithelial cells maintains contact with the lumen, or ventricular system, while the basal pole maintains contact with the basal lamina, or pial surface. Throughout neurogenesis VZ precursor cells maintain these apical and basal relationships (Levitt and Rakic, 1980).

The neuroepithelial cells of the neural tube constitute a population of proliferative precursor cells that ultimately give rise to all of the neurons and macroglia in the CNS. Just before the onset of neurogenesis, radial glial cells emerge in the neuroepithelium. The radial glia may be generated by dividing neuroepithelial cells or, alternatively, through the transformation of neuroepithelial cells. Radial glial cells can be distinguished from neuroepithelial cells on the basis of several criteria. For example, neuroepithelial cells do not express the astroglial markers such as brain lipid-binding protein (BLBP), tenascin C, or the glutamate transporter GLAST that are expressed by radial glial cells during neurogenesis (Malatesta et al., 2003). Tight junctions that are found between the apical (ventricular) surfaces of neuroepithelial cells disappear at the onset of neurogenesis, and may be functionally replaced by gap junctions in amphibians (Decker and Friend, 1974) and by adherens junctions in mammals (Aaku-Saraste et al., 1996). Furthermore, ultrastructural analysis has revealed that radial glial endfeet possess glycogen storage granules (Choi and Lapham, 1978). As radial glia replace neuroepithelial cells in the proliferative VZ, they also acquire defining morphological features, such as multiple branching endfeet at the pial surface and frequent contact with blood vessels that enter the developing cortex during early stages of cortical development (Bauer et al., 1992).

At the onset of neurogenesis, cortical neurons migrate out of the proliferative zones to the cortical plate in the well-described inside-out fashion. At nearly the same time, the SVZ forms at the outer margin of the VZ (Boulder Committee, 1970; Bayer and Altman, 1991; Zecevic, 1993). The SVZ contains a second population of proliferative cells that can be distinguished from VZ precursor cells because they do not undergo interkinetic nuclear migration, and they divide away from the ventricular surface (Takahashi et al., 1995b; Noctor et al., 2004). The SVZ precursor cells are derived from precursor cells in the VZ and are mitotically active throughout the remaining period of neurogenesis (Takahashi et al., 1995b; Noctor et al., 2004). The SVZ reaches a maximum size postnatally when it is thought to produce glial cells (Privat, 1975). However, the SVZ is also the site of postnatal neurogenesis (Luskin, 1993; Doetsch et al., 1999), and recent evidence indicates that some upper-layer neurons may be generated in the SVZ prenatally as well (Tarabykin, 2001; Letinic et al., 2002; Noctor et al., 2004).

HISTORICAL PERSPECTIVE

Our understanding of the key events during corticogenesis has developed over the past 100 years, starting with the work of the classical neuroanatomists in the late nineteenth century. In the 1880s scientists began to study the developing nervous system, paying particular attention to the proliferative zones surrounding the ventricular system. Golgi (1886) first used his impregnation technique on embryonic chick spinal cord and described cylindrical neuroepithelial cells lining the central canal that possessed radial fibers extending out to the periphery of the spinal cord and terminating in the pia and on blood vessels. Magini (1888) applied Golgi's technique to the developing mammalian cerebral cortex, and described bipolar *neuroglial* cells with soma in the neuroepithelium and thin radial fibers extending through the cortical mantle. Magini also described varicosities located along the radial fibers of the neuroglia, and he argued that these swellings represented neuroblasts migrating along radial fibers out of the VZ (Magini, 1888). Wilhelm His combined histological staining methods with Golgi's technique and described two populations of cells in the VZ: mitotic cells at the ventricular surface that he termed *germinal cells* and long, thin bipolar *spongioblasts*. His also described short bipolar cells migrating toward the forming gray matter of the neocortex that he called *neuroblasts*. Based on these findings, His proposed that neocortical neurons were generated at the ventricular surface by the dividing germinal cells, and that the immature neurons, or neuroblasts, then migrated out to the forming gray matter of the cerebral cortex along the radially arranged fibers of the spongioblast cells (His, 1889). Sauer (1935) concluded that the dividing germinal cells and radial spongioblast cells that had been described by His "are not two separate types of cells, but are the interkinetic and mitotic stages of the same cell." Later use of thymidine analogs confirmed interkinetic nuclear migration of cortical precursor cells (Sauer, 1959), and also confirmed that the VZ was a site of cortical neurogenesis (Sidman et al., 1959; Angevine and Sidman, 1961; Rakic, 1974; Miller and Nowakowski, 1988). Thymidine analog studies also revealed the inside-out gradient of cortical laminar genesis that confirmed earlier hypotheses that the formation of the cortical laminae "progresses from deep to superficial with small pyramidal cells developing last" (Ramón y Cajal, 1911). Finally, Rakic performed a series of detailed ultrastructural analyses to determine that radial glial cells play a crucial role in guiding the radial migration of cortical neurons (Rakic, 1978; see Chapter 31). Although cortical neurogenesis in the VZ had been described very early in the history of neuroscience research, the exact identity of the neural precursor cell(s) remained elusive.

RADIAL GLIA CELLS AS NEURONAL PRECURSOR CELLS IN NEOCORTICAL DEVELOPMENT

Prevailing opinion has often held that neuronal and glial lineages are distinct by the time neurogenesis begins in the CNS proliferative zones. Indeed, Levitt and Rakic's studies of the early 1980s described two populations of cells within the macaque VZ, one negative for glial fibrillary acidic protein (GFAP), and the other GFAP positive, and thought to represent separate neuronal and glial lineages, respectively (Levitt et al., 1981). However, studies in other species demonstrated commonalities between radial glial cells and neural precursors and gave hints that perhaps the distinction did not exist across all species. For example, antibodies that identify neural precursor cells such as anti-nestin (Hockfield and McKay, 1985) also label radial glial cells (Frederiksen and McKay, 1988), indicating a functional overlap between neural precursors and radial glial cells. Misson et al. (1988) provided more evidence of a close relationship by demonstrating that radial glia are mitotically active during neurogenesis and exhibit the same characteristic interkinetic nuclear movements as neural precursors. Alvarez-Buylla et al. (1990) examined neurogenesis in songbird and described an overlap of thymidine analog labeling with the location of vimentin-positive *radial cells* in the VZ. They speculated that these cells might be neural precursors. Lineage studies using replication-incompetent retroviruses in chick and rodent telencephalon reported clones containing single radial glial cells and multiple neurons indicating that, at a minimum, radial glia and neurons are lineally related (Gray and Sanes, 1992; Halliday and Cepko, 1992). Recent studies have since confirmed that rodent radial glial cells act as neural precursor cells (Malatesta et al., 2000; Miyata et al., 2001; Noctor et al., 2001; Tamamaki et al., 2001; Noctor et al., 2002; Noctor et al., 2004).

The Majority of Mitotically Active Cortical Ventricular Zone Cells Have Radial Glial Morphology

The evidence demonstrating that radial glial cells are neural precursors has been obtained both *in vitro* and *in vivo* using several techniques, including those that allow identification and study of labeled cells in live tissue. The traditional method for identifying radial glial cells has been based on their characteristic bipolar morphology and contact with both the ventricular and pial surfaces. Researchers have taken advantage of this morphological feature to label radial glia by applying dye to either the pial or ventricular surfaces. For example, delivery of 1,1′-dioctadecyl-3,3,3′,3′,-tetramethylindocarbocyanine perchlorate (DiI) to the ventricular surface using DiI-coated microbeads randomly labels all cells in contact with the ventricular surface and has demonstrated that 85% of the cells in the VZ have radial glial morphology (Noctor et al., 2002). Whole-cell patch-clamp recordings have been used to simultaneously label and measure the membrane properties of randomly chosen cells in contact with the ventricular surface. These experiments have demonstrated that cells with the characteristic morphological features of radial glial cells have the physiological properties of precursor cells (LoTurco and Kriegstein, 1991; Noctor et al., 2002). Similarly, the application of DiI or fluorescent microbeads to the pial surface of developing neocortex labels mitotically active VZ cells with distinct radial glial morphology (Malatesta et al., 2000; Miyata et al., 2001; Götz et al., 2002) and has demonstrated that these cells constitute more than 90% of mitotically active cells in the VZ (Noctor et al., 2002).

Radial Glial Cells Generate Neurons *in Vitro*

In vitro assays have demonstrated that isolated radial glial cells can generate neurons in culture. In one study, radial glial cells were labeled by painting fluorescent dyes on the pial surface. Fluorescence-activated cell (FAC) sorting of the fluorescent radial glial cells followed by single-cell cultures demonstrated that radial glial cells remained mitotically active and generated neurons in culture (Malatesta et al., 2000). Similarly, DiI-labeled radial glial were shown to divide and generate neurons in slice culture assays (Miyata et al., 2001; Tamamaki et al., 2001). Rodent radial glial cells do not express the astrocytic protein GFAP during embryonic development, but the GFAP promoter is present and active. Thus, radial glial cells can be isolated and FAC-sorted from transgenic mice with GFAP promoter–driven expression of green fluorescent protein (GFP). Such cells can generate neurons when plated in single-cell cultures (Malatesta et al., 2000).

Radial glial cells have also been identified as the predominant mitotically active cell type in the VZ of embryonic cortical explants (Noctor et al., 2002). In this system, developing neocortex retains much of its natural environment, with minimal disruption to the processes and connections of cells such as radial glia. Fluorescent microbeads applied to the pial surface of cortical explants are taken up by the pial endfeet of radial glial cells. Through pulse labeling with bromodeoxyuridine (BrdU), it was determined that more than 90% of the mitotic VZ cells contained the microbeads that had been deposited on the pial surface, thus identifying the mitotic cells as radial glial cells.

Radial glial cells can also be labeled through *in utero* injections of retroviruses (Gray and Sanes, 1992; Halliday and Cepko, 1992; Noctor et al., 2001). Retrovirally labeled radial glial cells identified in slice cultures during late stages of rodent neurogenesis were monitored through time-lapse microscopy, and were directly observed to undergo interkinetic nuclear migration and to generate neurons (Noctor et al., 2001; Noctor et al., 2004; see Fig. 8.1).

Radial Glial Cells Generate Neurons *in Vivo*

Evidence that radial glial cells are neural precursors has also been obtained *in vivo*. A short pulse of the thymidine analog BrdU during rodent neurogenesis labels mitotic neural precursor cells in S-phase, and the vast majority of S-phase-labeled VZ cells express the rodent radial glial markers vimentin or RC2 in both fixed slices and dissociated cells (Noctor et al., 2002). Furthermore, it has been shown that radial glial cells express a phosphorylated form of vimentin (4A4) during mitosis (Kamei et al., 1998), allowing quantification of the percentage of cycling VZ cells that express the radial glial marker vimentin. Nearly all of the mitotic figures at the ventricular surface during neurogenesis express 4A4, indicating that radial glial cells represent the predominant neural precursor cell in the rodent and human neocortical VZ (Noctor et al., 2002; Weissman et al., 2003; see Fig. 8.2*a*).

Vimentin is not a promiscuous marker and is not present in all classes of rodent neural precursor cells. For example, dividing neural precursor cells found in the external granular layer (EGL) of the postnatal rat cerebellum do not express vimentin (Kamei et al., 1998; Noctor et al., 2002). Neural precursor cells present in this layer generate granule neurons that then migrate along the radial fibers of the Bergmann glial cells to the internal granular layer (Levitt and Rakic, 1980). Interestingly, while the EGL neural precursors are vimentin negative, Bergmann glial cells are mitotically active during this period and stain positive for 4A4 (Noctor et al., 2002).

The vast majority of dividing cells in the neocortical VZ, either in S-phase or in M-phase, express radial glial markers. This, together with the observation that ra-

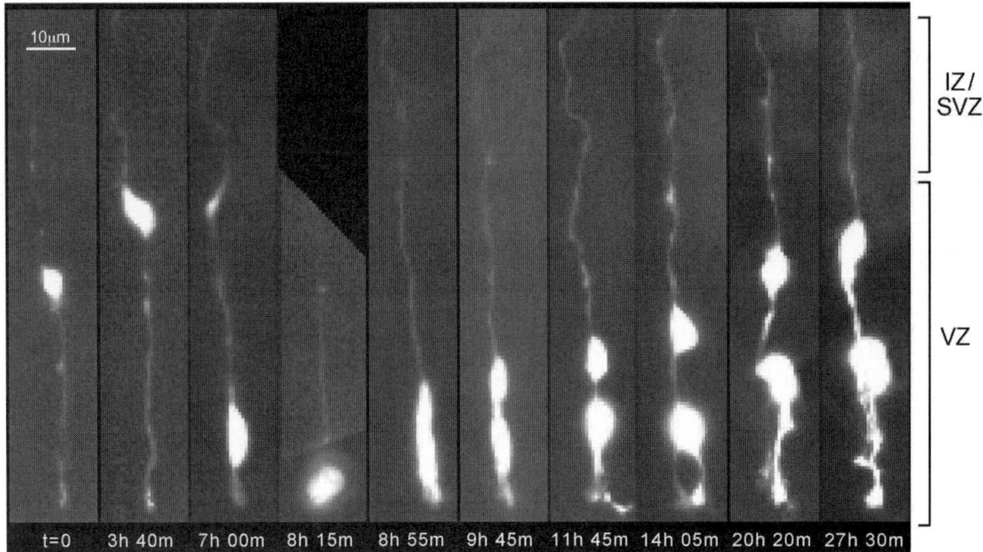

FIGURE 8.1 Time-lapse video microscopy of radial glial cell division. A single radial glial cell labeled *in utero* with green fluorescent protein–expressing retrovirus viewed in slice culture 24 hours post-infection ($t = 0$). The radial glial cell has an endfoot contacting the ventricular surface and a radial process extending to the pia. The radial glial soma descends to the ventricular surface, divides, and translocates to the top of the VZ, while its daughter cell begins migration to the cortical plate. Times indicated at bottom. *CP*: cortical plate; *IZ*: intermediate zone; *SVZ*: subventricular zone; *VZ*: ventricular zone.

dial glial cells are the only mitotic cells in radial clones consisting of neurons and radial glia (see Fig. 8.3), confirms that radial glia generate neurons *in vivo* and, furthermore, that this cell class may represent the predominant neural precursor within the VZ of developing neocortex.

Radial Glial Cells Retain Their Pial Fibers During Division

In addition to generating neurons, radial glial cells guide neuronal migration, as originally described by Rakic (1978). Both *in vivo* and *in vitro*, evidence has

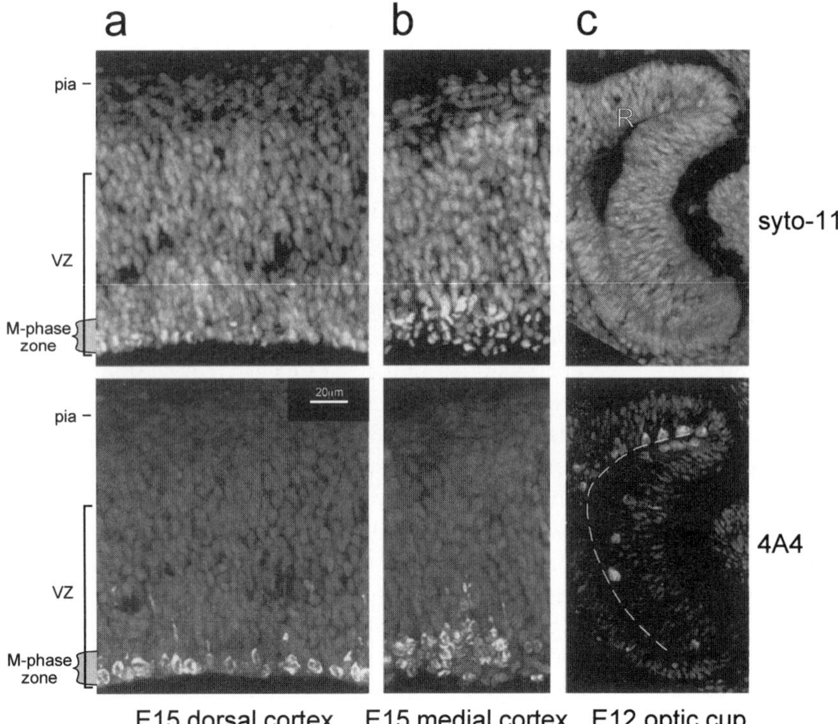

FIGURE 8.2 M-phase cells in the VZ express the radial glial marker phosphorylated vimentin (*4A4*). Confocal sections in the coronal plane from E15 rat cortex demonstrate that M-phase cells identified by the pattern of Syto-11 labeling (*top panels*) are costained with the 4A4 antibody (*bottom panels*) in *a* dorsolateral neocortex and *b* medial wall of cortex. *c*. 4A4-positive cells are also located at the apical surface of the optic cup in E12 rat. *R*: developing retina; *VZ*: ventricular zone.

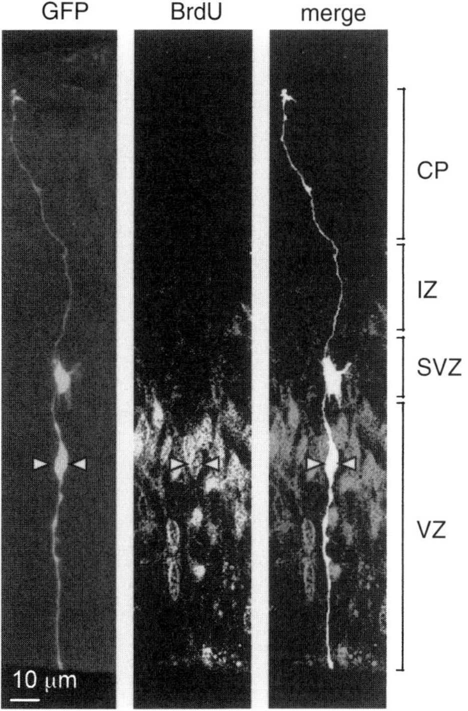

FIGURE 8.3 Radial clones in embryonic neocortex contain mitotic radial glial cells and neurons. *Left panel*: retroviral labeling reveals radial clones consisting of radial glia (*arrowheads*) and daughter cells located on the radial glial fiber. *Middle panel*: single injections of the thymidine analog bromodeoxyuridine 30 to 48 hours after retroviral infection label S-phase cells and show that radial glia are the only mitotically active cells in the radial clones (*right panel*). *CP*: cortical plate; *GFP*: green fluorescent protein; *IZ*: intermediate zone; *SVZ*: subventricular zone; *VZ*: ventricular zone.

demonstrated that daughter neurons migrate along the pial fibers of parent radial glial cells out of the VZ, and many of these cells maintain an association with the parental fiber as they migrate to the cortical plate (Noctor et al., 2001). But what happens to the migrating daughter neurons during subsequent divisions of the mother radial glial cells? It has long been assumed that neural precursor cells round up at the ventricular surface when they divide, retracting the basal process that contacts the pial surface. However, recent observations have shown that dividing radial glial cells in neocortex also maintain their long pial fiber during division (Miyata et al., 2001; Noctor et al., 2001; Tamamaki et al., 2001; Götz et al., 2002; Noctor et al., 2004). Evidence obtained from several species indicates that daughter neurons may inherit the pial fiber of the parent radial glial cell, and daughter neurons then translocate to the cortical plate within the pial fiber (Morest, 1970; Miyata et al., 2001; Tamamaki et al., 2001). However, evidence obtained from the rat at late stages of neurogenesis suggests that radial glial cells keep the pial fiber after division, while daughter neurons migrate to the cortex via glial-guided locomotion (Noctor et al., 2001; Hatanaka and Murakami, 2002; Tabata and Nakajima, 2003; Noctor et al., 2004). These contrasting findings may be due to species differences or perhaps to different modes of neuronal migration during early versus later stages of cortical neurogenesis (Nadarajah and Parnavelas, 2002). Alternatively, different classes of cortical neurons may use different mechanisms to migrate to the cortical plate. Nonetheless, recent evidence has revealed that the migration of cortically derived neurons is more complex than once thought. It has recently been shown that most, if not all, cortical neurons pause during their migration while in the SVZ or intermediate zone, and assume a multipolar morphology (Bai et al., 2003; Tabata and Nakajima, 2003; Noctor et al., 2004). During the multipolar phase, these neurons do not contact either the pial or ventricular surfaces, and after a day or more, they assume a bipolar morphology and resume radial migration towards the cortical plate (Noctor et al., 2004).

Are There Distinct Subsets of Radial Glial Cells?

The radial glial cell class may be comprised of several subsets. Indeed, it has been shown that several subsets of radial glial cells can be distinguished on the basis of antigen and/or transcription factor expression (Hartfuss et al., 2001). Furthermore, proliferative VZ cells express different markers during early, middle, and late stages of neocortical development (Malatesta et al., 2003). For example, in some mammals radial glial cells express the astroglial intermediate filament marker vimentin throughout neurogenesis, but after neurogenesis radial glia downregulate vimentin expression while upregulating expression of the mature astrocyte marker GFAP (Schmechel and Rakic, 1979; Voigt, 1989). Similarly, proliferative neuroepithelial cells do not express radial glial markers such as GLAST or tenascin C, while these markers are expressed by radial glia during neurogenesis and by transformed astrocytes in postnatal animals (Malatesta et al., 2003). Subsets of radial glial cells can also be distinguished by the specific functions performed by these cells. For example, expression of the radial glial marker BLBP is induced only in radial glial cells that support migrating neurons (Feng and Heintz, 1995).

In the mouse it has been determined that cortical neurogenesis occurs over approximately 11 cell cycles (Takahashi et al., 1995a). But it is not known whether all radial glial cells contribute to each of the 11 neurogenic cell cycles or rather have shorter proliferative periods that encompass only portions of neurogenesis. The different subsets of radial glia that have been described may represent distinct classes of radial glial cells that perform different functions and perhaps generate different cell types. Alternatively, radial glial cells may express specific markers during distinct stages and while performing distinct functions, but do so asynchronously throughout cortical neurogenesis. There may also be significant differences between radial glial cells located in different regions of the CNS. For example, recent evidence using fate-mapping analysis suggests that radial glial cells from the ventral telencephalon do not generate neurons, unlike radial glial cells located in the dorsal telencephalon that generate the majority of the principal neurons (Malatesta et al., 2003). This difference may reflect distinct subclasses of radial glial cells in the dorsal and ventral telencephalon, or perhaps different mechanisms of neurogenesis such as through an intermediate precursor cell generated by a radial glial cell. Recently, it has been shown that neurons in the dorsal telencephalon are generated both directly through asymmetric neurogenic divisions of radial glial cells, and indirectly through terminal symmetric divisions of intermediate progenitor cells that are generated by radial glia (Noctor et al., 2004). It may thus be possible that neurogenesis in the ventral telencephalon may occur predominantly through the division of intermediate progenitor cells, and these may not have been labeled by the fate-mapping technique.

What Types of Neurons Do Radial Glial Cells Generate?

The cerebral cortex is a six-layered structure composed of two broad classes of neurons: pyramidal and nonpyramidal. Pyramidal neurons are the neocortical projection neurons that send axons to other brain regions and communicate via the excitatory neurotransmitter glutamate. Nonpyramidal cells, or interneurons, are a diverse class of mostly inhibitory neurons that are organized into local circuits and use γ-aminobutyric acid (GABA) as a neurotransmitter. The lineage of neocortical cells has been investigated through the use of replication-incompetent retroviruses that label dividing neural precursor cells at the ventricular surface. The retroviral lineage studies examined the location and identity of clonal cells in mature cortex after embryonic labeling. Price and Thurlow (1988) suggested that both pyramidal and nonpyramidal neurons derive from the same progenitor, and that there is a wide tangential spread of clonally related neurons within a given cortical layer. Similarly, Walsh and Cepko (1988, 1992) reported clones consisting of morphologically diverse types of neurons, and even some clones that had both neurons and glia. However, studies combining retroviral infections with ultrastructural (Luskin et al., 1993) or immunohistochemical (Mione et al., 1994) analyses indicated that clones consist of only one cell type, and in particular noted that pyramidal neurons and interneurons derive from separate precursors. Most lineage analyses have supported the view that clones are either purely neuronal or purely glial (Grove et al., 1993; Luskin et al., 1993; Mione et al., 1994). The use of retroviral libraries that include more than 100 constructs that were identified through PCR amplification determined that clonal cells can be dispersed widely across cortex (Walsh and Cepko, 1992; Reid et al., 1995). In addition, while clustered clones were mostly uniform in cell type, the widespread clones consisted of variable cell types. The discovery that GABAergic interneurons are generated in the ganglionic eminences, particularly the medial ganglionic eminence, and migrate tangentially into the developing neocortex may partially explain some but not all of the tangential spread of clonal cells in the neocortex (de Carlos et al., 1996; Anderson et al., 1997; Tamamaki et al., 1997; Wichterle et al., 2001).

More recent retroviral lineage studies have found that radially organized clones are composed exclusively of pyramidal neurons, or glial cells, or a mix of pyramidal neurons and astrocytes, while the widely dispersed clusters usually consist of nonpyramidal cells (Mione et al., 1997). Chimeric mouse studies have indicated the existence of separate progenitors for radially oriented pyramidal neurons and tangentially dispersed GABAergic neurons (Tan et al., 1998). Furthermore, use of Cre recombinase has demonstrated that principal neurons and astrocytes derive from Emx1-positive precursors, while the majority of GABA-positive cells lie outside of this lineage (Gorski et al., 2002). Together these data indicate that radial glial cells generate glutamatergic principal neurons in the neocortical VZ, while the majority of GABAergic interneurons are generated in the ganglionic eminence and migrate tangentially into the cortex (for review see Parnavelas, 2000). However, there may be significant species differences. For example, recent evidence in human indicates that a substantial proportion of neocortical interneurons are derived from the neocortical VZ/SVZ, while a smaller percentage derive from the ganglionic eminence (Letinic et al., 2002).

Postneurogenesis Fate of Radial Glial Cells

After cortical neurogenesis is complete in the VZ, radial glial cells transform into astrocytes (Choi and Lapham, 1978; Schmechel and Rakic, 1979; Voigt, 1989; Noctor et al., 2004). During early stages of transformation, radial glial cells lose their attachment to the ventricular surface while retaining their pial attachment, and the nuclei translocate within the pial fiber toward the pial surface. This mass exodus of VZ cells contributes to the considerable thinning of the VZ that occurs during the end stages of neurogenesis. The translocation of astroglial cells occurs not only in the dorsolateral neocortex, but also in the medial wall of the telencephalon that gives rise to the hippocampal formation and in the developing cerebellum. The translocation and transformation of these cells is accompanied by a decrease in the expression of the radial glial marker vimentin and by a concomitant increase in the expression of the mature astrocyte marker GFAP (Voigt, 1989).

NEUROGENIC GLIA IN OTHER CENTRAL NERVOUS SYSTEM REGIONS

The Role of Astroglia in Other Central Nervous System Regions

Radial glial cells line the ventricular system throughout the developing CNS. However, their role as neural precursor cells has been confirmed only in the dorsal neocortex and in the spinal cord (Malatesta et al., 2003). Nevertheless, translocation and transformation of radial glial cells into astrocytes has been documented for several CNS areas including the neocortex, hippocampus, and cerebellum (see Cameron and Rakic, 1991). Postnatal neurogenesis by GFAP-positive astrocytes has been demonstrated in two of these areas, the forebrain SVZ (Doetsch et al., 1999) and the dentate gyrus of the hippocampus (Seri et al., 2001). The cerebellar EGL is also the site of postnatal neurogenesis, but the neural precursor cells have not yet been identified. The EGL precursors may represent a distinct class of neural precursor cells since they are not vimentin positive (Kamei et al., 1998; Noctor et al., 2002). However, the postnatal cerebellum contains a population of mitotically active, vimentin-positive Bergmann glial cells. The Bergmann glial cells derive from transformed radial glial cells and share important characteristics with neocortical radial glial cells. These include multiple branching endfeet at the pial surface (Ramón y Cajal, 1890; Rakic, 1971), labeling with the same antibody markers (Schmechel and Rakic, 1979; Voigt, 1989; Yuasa, 1996; Kamei et al., 1998), and guidance of neuronal migration (Rakic, 1971; Levitt and Rakic, 1980). In addition, both cell types are mitotically active during neurogenesis (Basco et al., 1977) and do not retract their pial fibers during division, a feature that could allow for the uninterrupted guidance of migrating neurons (Basco et al., 1977; Noctor et al., 2002). Dividing Bergmann glia are thought to generate other Bergmann glial cells, but in light of recent findings regarding neurogenic glia in the postnatal brain, this issue should be revisited.

Astroglial cells called *Müller glia* are also present in the developing and adult retina. The Müller glial cell is the predominant glial cell type in the retina, and it stains positive for vimentin (Pixley and de Vellis, 1984), 4A4 (Fig. 8.2*c*), and GFAP (Bignami, 1984). Lineage data show that retinal neurons and Müller glial cells are closely related, and that clones labeled during eye development consist of several neurons and one Müller glial cell (Turner and Cepko, 1987). Furthermore, recent evidence obtained from postnatal chick indicates that under conditions of stress or injury, Müller glia can dedifferentiate, proliferate, and generate retinal neurons (Fischer and Reh, 2001). The neurogenic capacity of Müller glia has not been demonstrated during development, nor has it been shown in mammals. Nevertheless, the lineage relationships between Müller glia and retinal neurons in addition to their potential for generating neurons point to similarities between cortical radial glial cells and Müller glia in the retina. Furthermore, the ability of Müller glia to generate neurons in response to injury indicates that the retina may serve as an ideal system for elucidating conditions that promote neurogenesis after injury.

NEUROGENIC GLIA IN NONMAMMALIAN VERTEBRATES

The Role of Radial Glia in the Formation of the Avian Central Nervous System

Nonmammalian vertebrate species differ from mammalian species in that extensive neurogenesis persists postnatally. Neurogenesis continues throughout adulthood in songbirds, and both projection neurons and interneurons are generated within the avian telencephalon (Alvarez-Buylla et al., 1990). Coincident with postnatal neurogenesis in the songbird, radial glial cells persist in the VZ, where neurogenesis occurs. Nottebohm and colleagues conclusively determined the neuronal identity of postnatally generated cells through ultrastructural and electrophysiological analysis of tritiated, thymidine-labeled cells (Goldman and Nottebohm, 1983; Paton and Nottebohm, 1984). Alvarez-Buylla et al. (1990) found that radial glial cell bodies were located in the neurogenic regions of the songbird forebrain and that radial glial cells incorporated thymidine analogs. Noting the colocalization of mitotic radial glial cells with the site of neurogenesis, they proposed that radial glial cells might in fact be the neural progenitors in songbirds.

Early studies using a recombinant retrovirus to study cell lineage in the chicken optic tectum revealed that individual clones contained different types of neurons (Gray et al., 1988), and also that both neurons and glia derive from a common progenitor cell (Galileo et al., 1990). Gray and Sanes (1992) examined clonal relationships during embryonic development in the chick, and determined that individual clones consisted of neurons and usually one radial glial cell. They found that the number of labeled radial glial cells declines after the main period of neurogenesis and that transitional forms of radial glia begin to appear, suggesting that some radial glial cells in the optic tectum transform into astrocytes. Based on their findings, Gray and Sanes

(1992) also proposed that radial glial cells are neural precursor cells.

SUMMARY

Neurogenic Astroglial Cells

Recent findings have elucidated a more complex role for astroglial cells in the development of CNS structures across many species. Mitotically active radial glial cells line the ventricular system throughout the developing CNS and have been shown to generate neocortical neurons in rodents (Malatesta et al., 2000; Miyata et al., 2001; Noctor et al., 2001; Tamamaki et al., 2001). Precursor cells in the VZ can divide symmetrically or asymmetrically, and evidence indicates that both types of divisions coexist throughout the entire period of cortical neurogenesis (Caviness et al., 1995; Kornack and Rakic, 1995; Noctor et al., 2004). However, it is thought that a preponderance of symmetric proliferative divisions increases the number of neural progenitors during early stages of cortical development, while asymmetric neurogenic divisions generate many of the principal excitatory neurons during later stages (see Fig. 8.4).

Localization of fate-determining factors including Notch, Numb, and Numb-like during cell division plays a role in daughter cell fate (Chenn and McConnell, 1995; Zhong et al., 1997; Gaiano et al., 2000), but the mechanisms that control how and when radial glial cells divide symmetrically or asymmetrically have yet to be determined. After neurogenesis is complete, vimentin-positive radial glial cells transform into GFAP-positive astrocytes in several developing CNS structures (Cameron and Rakic, 1991).

It has recently been shown directly that some neurogenic radial glial cells translocate and transform into

a Early-stage symmetric proliferation

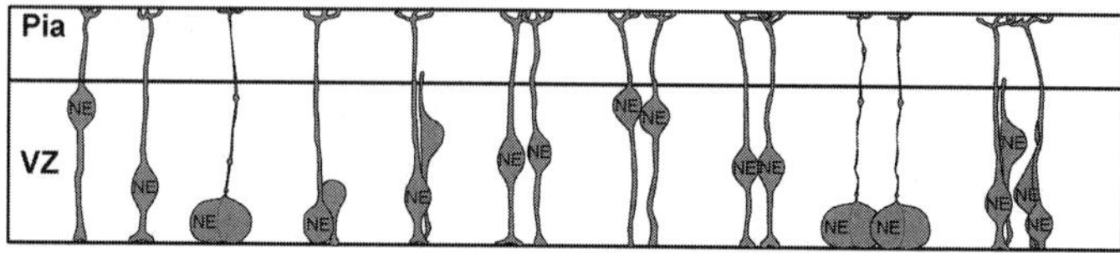

b Mid-stage asymmetric neurogenesis

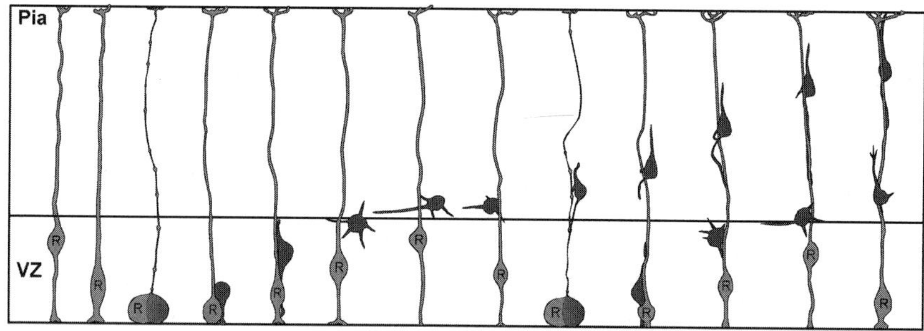

c End-stage astroglial transformation

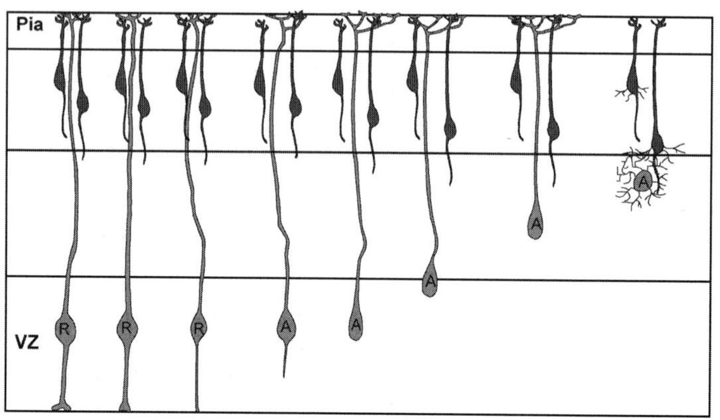

FIGURE 8.4 Schematic representation of the patterns of precursor cell divisions during the development of cortical structures. *a.* Neuroepithelial cells undergo symmetric proliferative divisions during the earliest stages of cortical development, increasing the number of progenitor cells for neuronal production. *b.* During the middle stages of cortical development, radial glial cells divide asymmetrically to generate principal excitatory neurons that migrate radially along radial glial fibers to the cortical plate. *c.* At the end of neurogenesis, some radial glial cells translocate toward the overlying cortical structures and transform into astrocytes. *VZ*: ventricular zone.

astrocytes after neurogenesis (Noctor et al., 2004). Astrocytes are known to remain mitotically active in the postnatal brain and serve as neural precursor cells in some regions of the adult brain (Doetsch et al., 1999; Seri et al., 2001). In addition, astrocytes are found in regions that have suffered brain trauma. However, future studies will have to determine if embryonic radial glial cells are lineally related to neurogenic astrocytes found in the adult CNS, and whether other CNS regions harbor postnatal neurogenic astrocytes under normal conditions or after trauma.

Defining Neural Precursor Cells: Are Radial Glial Cells Stem Cells?

Neuroepithelial cells in the neural tube are pluripotent, and ultimately give rise to the many subtypes of neurons and glia that populate mature cerebral cortex. During later stages of cortical development, radial glial precursor cells are more restricted in their potential (Frantz and McConnell, 1996) but may retain the ability to generate astrocytes in addition to neurons. Definitions of stem cells vary, but all include the stipulation that a stem cell must have the capacity to self-regenerate and to produce more than one type of cell. Both *in vitro* and *in vivo* studies have demonstrated that precursor cells in the embryonic VZs can divide to generate both a daughter neuron and a self-replenished precursor cell (Malatesta et al., 2000; Miyata et al., 2001; Noctor et al., 2001; Shen et al., 2002; Noctor et al., 2004). Recent data has shown that neurogenic radial glial cells also generate intermediate progenitor cells, and that the final radial glial division generates a translocating astrocyte (Noctor et al,. 2004). The embryonic generation of neurons intermediate progenitor cells, and astrocytes indicates that at least some radial glia possess the capacity to generate multiple cell types and thus may be classified as a form of neuronal "stem cell", albeit one with limited potential. However, future studies that examine the lineage relationships between embryonic radial glia and neurogenic astrocytes in the adult SVZ, dentate gyrus, and cortex should clarify the full potential of astroglial cells.

REFERENCES

Aaku-Saraste, E., Hellwig, A., and Huttner, W.B. (1996) Loss of occludin and functional tight junctions, but not ZO-1, during neural tube closure—remodeling of the neuroepithelium prior to neurogenesis. *Dev. Biol.* 180(2):664–679.

Alvarez-Buylla, A., Garcia-Verdugo, J.M., and Tramontin, A.D. (2001) A unified hypothesis on the lineage of neural stem cells. *Nat. Rev. Neurosci.* 2(4):287–293.

Alvarez-Buylla, A., Theelen, M., and Nottebohm, F. (1990) Proliferation "hot spots" in adult avian ventricular zone reveal radial cell division. *Neuron* 5(1):101–109.

Anderson, S.A., Eisenstat, D.D., Shi, L., and Rubenstein, J. (1997) Interneuron migration from basal forebrain to neocortex: dependence on dlx genes. *Science* 278(5337):474–476.

Angevine, J.B.J., and Sidman, R.L. (1961) Autoradiographic study of cell migration during histogenesis of cerebral cortex in the mouse. *Nature* 192:766–768.

Bai, J., Ramos, R.L., Ackman, J.B., Thomas, A.M., Lee, R.V., and LoTurco, J.J. (2003) RNAi reveals doublecortin is required for radial migration in rat neocortex. *Nat. Neurosci.* 6(12):1277–1283.

Basco, E., Hajos, F., and Fulop, Z. (1977) Proliferation of Bergmann-glia in the developing rat cerebellum. *Anat. Embryol. (Berl.)* 151(2):219–222.

Bauer, H.C., Steiner, M., and Bauer, H. (1992) Embryonic development of the CNS microvasculature in the mouse: new insights into the structural mechanisms of early angiogenesis. *Exs* 61: 64–68.

Bayer, S.A. and Altman, J. (1991) *Neocortical Development*. New York: Raven Press.

Bignami, A. (1984) Glial fibrillary acidic (GFA) protein in Muller glia. Immunofluorescence study of the goldfish retina. *Brain Res.* 300(1):175–178.

Boulder Committee. (1970) Embryonic vertebrate central nervous system: revised terminology. *Anat. Rec.* 166(2):257–261.

Cameron, R.S. and Rakic, P. (1991) Glial cell lineage in the cerebral cortex: a review and synthesis. *Glia* 4(2):124–137.

Caviness, V., Jr., Takahashi, T., and Nowakowski, R.S. (1995) Numbers, time and neocortical neuronogenesis: a general developmental and evolutionary model. *Trends Neurosci.* 18(9):379–383.

Chenn, A. and McConnell, S.K. (1995) Cleavage orientation and the asymmetric inheritance of Notch1 immunoreactivity in mammalian neurogenesis. *Cell* 82(4):631–641.

Choi, B.H. and Lapham, L.W. (1978) Radial glia in the human fetal cerebrum: a combined Golgi, immunofluorescent and electron microscopic study. *Brain Res.* 148(2):295–311.

de Carlos, J.A., Lopez-Mascaraque, L., and Valverde, F. (1996) Dynamics of cell migration from the lateral ganglionic eminence in the rat. *J. Neurosci.* 16(19):6146–6156.

Decker, R.S. and Friend, D.S. (1974) Assembly of gap junctions during amphibian neurulation. *J. Cell Biol.* 62(1):32–47.

Doetsch, F., Caille, I., Lim, D.A., Garcia-Verdugo, J.M., and Alvarez-Buylla, A. (1999) Subventricular zone astrocytes are neural stem cells in the adult mammalian brain. *Cell* 97(6):703–716.

Feng, L. and Heintz, N. (1995) Differentiating neurons activate transcription of the brain lipid-binding protein gene in radial glia through a novel regulatory element. *Development* 121(6):1719–1730.

Fischer, A.J. and Reh, T.A. (2001) Muller glia are a potential source of neural regeneration in the postnatal chicken retina. *Nat. Neurosci.* 4(3):247–252.

Frantz, G.D. and McConnell, S.K. (1996) Restriction of late cerebral cortical progenitors to an upper-layer fate. *Neuron* 17:55–61.

Frederiksen, K. and McKay, R.D. (1988) Proliferation and differentiation of rat neuroepithelial precursor cells in vivo. *J. Neurosci.* 8(4):1144–1151.

Gaiano, N., Nye, J.S., and Fishell, G. (2000) Radial glial identity is promoted by Notch1 signaling in the murine forebrain. *Neuron* 26(2):395–404.

Galileo, D.S., Gray, G.E., Owens, G.C., Majors, J., and Sanes, J.R. (1990) Neurons and glia arise from a common progenitor in chicken optic tectum: demonstration with two retroviruses and cell type-specific antibodies. *Proc. Natl. Acad. Sci. USA* 87(1): 458–462.

Goldman, S.A. and Nottebohm, F. (1983) Neuronal production, migration, and differentiation in a vocal control nucleus of the adult female canary brain. *Proc. Natl. Acad. Sci. USA* 80(8):2390–2394.

Golgi, C. (1886) *Sulla fina anatomia degli organi centrali del sistema nervoso*. Milano: Hoepli.

Gorski, J.A., Talley, T., Qiu, M., Puelles, L., Rubenstein, J.L., and Jones, K.R. (2002) Cortical excitatory neurons and glia, but not GABAergic neurons, are produced in the Emx1-expressing lineage. *J. Neurosci.* 22(15):6309–6314.

Götz, M., Hartfuss, E., and Malatesta, P. (2002) Radial glial cells as neuronal precursors: a new perspective on the correlation of morphology and lineage restriction in the developing cerebral cortex of mice. *Brain Res. Bull.* 57(6):777–788.

Gray, G.E., Glover, J.C., Majors, J., and Sanes, J.R. (1988) Radial arrangement of clonally related cells in the chicken optic tectum: lineage analysis with a recombinant retrovirus. *Proc. Natl. Acad. Sci. USA* 85(19):7356–7360.

Gray, G.E. and Sanes, J.R. (1992) Lineage of radial glia in the chicken optic tectum. *Development* 114(1):271–283.

Grove, E.A., Williams, B.P., Li, D.Q., Hajihosseini, M., Friedrich, A., and Price, J. (1993) Multiple restricted lineages in the embryonic rat cerebral cortex. *Development* 117(2):553–561.

Halliday, A.L. and Cepko, C.L. (1992) Generation and migration of cells in the developing striatum. *Neuron* 9(1):15–26.

Hartfuss, E., Galli, R., Heins, N., and Götz, M. (2001) Characterization of CNS precursor subtypes and radial glia. *Dev. Biol.* 229(1):15–30.

Hatanaka, Y. and Murakami, F. (2002) In vitro analysis of the origin, migratory behavior, and maturation of cortical pyramidal cells. *J. Comp. Neurol.* 454(1):1–14.

His, W. (1889) Die Neuroblasten und deren Entstehung im embryonalen Mark. *Abh. Kgl. Ges. Wissensch. Math. Phys. Kl.* 15: 311–372.

Hockfield, S. and McKay, R.D. (1985) Identification of major cell classes in the developing mammalian nervous system. *J. Neurosci.* 5(12):3310–3328.

Kamei, Y., Inagaki, N., Nishizawa, M., Tsutsumi, O., Taketani, Y., and Inagaki, M. (1998) Visualization of mitotic radial glial lineage cells in the developing rat brain by Cdc2 kinase-phosphorylated vimentin. *Glia* 23(3):191–199.

Kornack, D.R. and Rakic, P. (1995) Radial and horizontal deployment of clonally related cells in the primate neocortex: relationship to distinct mitotic lineages. *Neuron* 15(2):311–321.

Letinic, K., Zoncu, R., and Rakic, P. (2002) Origin of GABAergic neurons in the human neocortex. *Nature* 417(6889):645–649.

Levitt, P., Cooper, M.L., and Rakic, P. (1981) Coexistence of neuronal and glial precursor cells in the cerebral ventricular zone of the fetal monkey: an ultrastructural immunoperoxidase analysis. *J. Neurosci.* 1(1):27–39.

Levitt, P. and Rakic, P. (1980) Immunoperoxidase localization of glial fibrillary acidic protein in radial glial cells and astrocytes of the developing rhesus monkey brain. *J. Comp. Neurol.* 193(3): 815–840.

LoTurco, J.J. and Kriegstein, A.R. (1991) Clusters of coupled neuroblasts in embryonic neocortex. *Science* 252(5005):563–566.

Luskin, M.B. (1993) Restricted proliferation and migration of postnatally generated neurons derived from the forebrain subventricular zone. *Neuron* 11(1):173–189.

Luskin, M. B., Parnavelas, J.G., and Barfield, J.A. (1993) Neurons, astrocytes, and oligodendrocytes of the rat cerebral cortex originate from separate progenitor cells: an ultrastructural analysis of clonally related cells. *J. Neurosci.* 13(4):1730–1750.

Magini, G. (1888) Nouvelles recherches histologiques sur le cerveau du foetus. *Arch. Ital. Biol.* 10:384–387.

Malatesta, P., Hack, M.A., Hartfuss, E., Kettenmann, H., Klinkert, W., Kirchhoff F., and Götz, M. (2003) Neuronal or glial progeny. Regional differences in radial glia fate. *Neuron* 37(5): 751–764.

Malatesta, P., Hartfuss, E., and Götz, M. (2000) Isolation of radial glial cells by fluorescent-activated cell sorting reveals a neuronal lineage. *Development* 127(24):5253–5263.

Miller, M.W. and Nowakowski, R.S. (1988) Use of bromodeoxyuridine-immunohistochemistry to examine the proliferation, migration, and time of origin of cells in the central nervous system. *Brain Res.* 457:44–52.

Mione, M.C., Cavanagh, J.F.R., Harris, B., and Parnavelas, J.G. (1997) Cell fate specification and symmetrical/asymmetrical divisions in the developing cerebral cortex. *J. Neurosci.* 17(6): 2018–2029.

Mione, M.C., Danevic, C., Boardman, P., Harris, B., and Parnavelas, J.G. (1994) Lineage analysis reveals neurotransmitter (GABA or glutamate) but not calcium-binding protein homogeneity in clonally related cortical neurons. *J. Neurosci.* 14(1):107–123.

Misson, J.P., Edwards, M.A., Yamamoto, M., and Caviness, V.S., Jr. (1988) Mitotic cycling of radial glial cells of the fetal murine cerebral wall: a combined autoradiographic and immunohistochemical study. *Brain Res.* 466(2):183–190.

Miyata, T., Kawaguchi, A., Okano, H., and Ogawa, M. (2001) Asymmetric inheritance of radial glial fibers by cortical neurons. *Neuron* 31(5):727–741.

Morest, D.K. (1970) A study of neurogenesis in the forebrain of opossum pouch young. *Z. Anat. Entwicklungs.* 130:265–305.

Nadarajah, B. and Parnavelas, J.G. (2002) Modes of neuronal migration in the developing cerebral cortex. *Nat. Rev. Neurosci.* 3(6):423–432.

Noctor, S.C., Flint, A.C., Weissman, T.A., Dammerman, R.S., and Kriegstein, A.R. (2001) Neurons derived from radial glial cells establish radial units in neocortex. *Nature* 409:714–720.

Noctor, S.C., Flint, A.C., Weissman, T.A., Wong, W.S., Clinton, B.K., and Kriegstein, A.R. (2002) Dividing precursor cells of the embryonic cortical ventricular zone have morphological and molecular characteristics of radial glia. *J. Neurosci.* 22(8):3161–3173.

Noctor, S.C., Martínez-Cerdeño, V., Ivic, L., and Kriegstein, A.R. (2004) Cortical neurons arise in symmetric and asymmetric division zones and migrate through specific phases. *Nat. Neurosci.* 7(2):136–144.

Nowakowski, R.S. and Rakic, P. (1979) The mode of migration of neurons to the hippocampus: a Golgi and electron microscopic analysis in foetal rhesus monkey. *J. Neurocytol.* 8(6):697–718.

Parnavelas, J.G. (2000) The origin and migration of cortical neurones: new vistas. *Trends Neurosci.* 23(3):126–131.

Paton, J.A. and Nottebohm, F.N. (1984) Neurons generated in the adult brain are recruited into functional circuits. *Science* 225(4666):1046–1048.

Pixley, S.K. and de Vellis, J. (1984) Transition between immature radial glia and mature astrocytes studied with a monoclonal antibody to vimentin. *Brain Res.* 317(2):201–209.

Price, J. and Thurlow, L. (1988) Cell lineage in the rat cerebral cortex: a study using retroviral-mediated gene transfer. *Development* 104(3):473–482.

Privat, A. (1975) Postnatal gliogenesis in the mammalian brain. *Int. Rev. Cytol.* 40:281–323.

Rakic, P. (1971) Neuron-glia relationship during granule cell migration in developing cerebellar cortex. A Golgi and electronmicroscopic study in *Macacus rhesus*. *J. Comp. Neurol.* 141(3):283–312.

Rakic, P. (1974) Neurons in rhesus monkey visual cortex: systematic relation between time of origin and eventual disposition. *Science* 183(123):425–427.

Rakic, P. (1978) Neuronal migration and contact guidance in the primate telencephalon. *Postgrad. Med. J.* 1:25–40.

Rakic, P. (2004) Radial glial cells: scaffolding for cortical development and evolution. In: Kettenmann, H., and Ransom, B.R., eds. *Neuroglia*. New York: Oxford University Press.

Ramón y Cajal, S. (1890) Sur les fibres nerveuses de la couche granuleuse du cervelet et sur l'évolution des éléments cerebelleux. *Int. Mschr. Anat. Physiol.* 7:12–30.

Ramón y Cajal, S. (1911) *Histologie du système nerveux de l'homme et des vertébrés*. Paris: Maloine.

Reid, C.B., Liang, I., and Walsh, C. (1995) Systematic widespread clonal organization in cerebral cortex. *Neuron* 15(2):299–310.

Rickmann, M., Amaral, D.G., and Cowan, W.M. (1987) Organization of radial glial cells during the development of the rat dentate gyrus. *J. Comp. Neurol.* 264(4):449–479.

Sauer, F.C. (1935) Mitosis in the neural tube. *J. Comp. Neurol.* 62(2): 377–405.

Sauer, M.E. (1959) Radioautographic study of the location of newly synthesized deoxyribonucleic acid in the neural tube of the chick embryo. *Anat. Rec.* 133:456.

Schmechel, D.E. and Rakic, P. (1979) A Golgi study of radial glial cells in developing monkey telencephalon: morphogenesis and transformation into astrocytes. *Anat. Embryol.* 156(2):115–152.

Seri, B., Garcia-Verdugo, J.M., McEwen, B.S., and Alvarez-Buylla, A. (2001) Astrocytes give rise to new neurons in the adult mammalian hippocampus. *J. Neurosci.* 21(18):7153–7160.

Shen, Q., Zhong, W., Jan, Y.N., and Temple, S. (2002) Asymmetric Numb distribution is critical for asymmetric cell division of mouse cerebral cortical stem cells and neuroblasts. *Development* 129(20): 4843–4853.

Sidman, R.L., Miale, I.L., and Feder, N. (1959) Cell proliferation and migration in the primitive ependymal zone: an autoradiographic study of histogenesis in the nervous system. *Exp. Neurol.* 1:322–333.

Smart, I.H. (1982) Radial unit analysis of hippocampal histogenesis in the mouse. *J. Anat.* 135(4):763–793.

Tabata, H. and Nakajima, K. (2003) Multipolar migration: the third mode of radial neuronal migration in the developing cerebral cortex. *J. Neurosci.* 23(31):9996–10001.

Takahashi, T., Nowakowski, R.S., and Caviness, V., Jr. (1995a) The cell cycle of the pseudostratified ventricular epithelium of the embryonic murine cerebral wall. *J. Neurosci.* 15(9):6046–6057.

Takahashi, T., Nowakowski, R.S., and Caviness, V., Jr. (1995b) Early ontogeny of the secondary proliferative population of the embryonic murine cerebral wall. *J. Neurosci.* 15(9):6058–6068.

Tamamaki, N., Fujimori, K.E., and Takauji, R. (1997) Origin and route of tangentially migrating neurons in the developing neocortical intermediate zone. *J. Neurosci.* 17(21):8313–8323.

Tamamaki, N., Nakamura, K., Okamoto, K., and Kaneko, T. (2001) Radial glia is a progenitor of neocortical neurons in the developing cerebral cortex. *Neurosci. Res.* 41(1):51–60.

Tan, S.S., Kalloniatis, M., Sturm, K., Tam, P.P., Reese, B.E., and Faulkner-Jones, B. (1998) Separate progenitors for radial and tangential cell dispersion during development of the cerebral neocortex. *Neuron* 21(2):295–304.

Tarabykin, V., Stoykova, A., Usman, N., and Gruss, P. (2001) Cortical upper layer neurons derive from the subventricular zone as indicated by *Svet1* gene expression. *Development* 128:1983–1993.

Turner, D.L. and Cepko, C.L. (1987) A common progenitor for neurons and glia persists in rat retina late in development. *Nature* 328(6126):131–136.

Voigt, T. (1989) Development of glial cells in the cerebral wall of ferrets: direct tracing of their transformation from radial glia into astrocytes. *J. Comp. Neurol.* 289(1):74–88.

Walsh, C. and Cepko, C.L. (1988) Clonally related cortical cells show several migration patterns. *Science* 241(4871):1342–1345.

Walsh, C. and Cepko, C.L. (1992) Widespread dispersion of neuronal clones across functional regions of the cerebral cortex. *Science* 255(5043):434–440.

Weissman, T., Noctor, S.C., Clinton, B.K., Honig, L.S., and Kriegstein, A.R. (2003) Neurogenic radial glial cells in reptile, rodent and human: from mitosis to migration. *Cereb. Cortex* 13(6):550–559.

Wichterle, H., Turnbull, D.H., Nery, S., Fishell, G., and Alvarez-Buylla, A. (2001) In utero fate mapping reveals distinct migratory pathways and fates of neurons born in the mammalian basal forebrain. *Development* 128(19):3759–3771.

Yuasa, S. (1996) Bergmann glial development in the mouse cerebellum as revealed by tenascin expression. *Anat. Embryol. (Berl.)* 194(3):223–234.

Zecevic, N. (1993) Cellular composition of the telencephalic wall in human embryos. *Early Hum. Dev.* 32(2–3):131–149.

Zhong, W., Jiang, M.M., Weinmaster, G., Jan, L.Y., and Jan, Y.N. (1997) Differential expression of mammalian Numb, Numblike and Notch1 suggests distinct roles during mouse cortical neurogenesis. *Development* 124(10):1887–1897.

9 Voltage-activated ion channels in glial cells

MICHELLE L. OLSEN AND HARALD W. SONTHEIMER

In 1984, Ritchie and colleagues used patch-clamp recordings to directly demonstrate the expression of voltage-gated Na^+ and K^+ channels in cultured Schwann cells (Chiu et al., 1984) and astrocytes (Bevan et al., 1985). This discovery was surprising and served as catalyst for a thorough examination of the biophysics of glial cells. Numerous laboratories have now provided unequivocal evidence that glial cells contain a large variety of voltage-gated channels that are also commonly found in neurons. However, unlike their neuronal counterparts, these channels do not appear to be engaged in generating short-duration transient electrical signals, but are most likely involved in other fundamental cell biological functions.

SODIUM CHANNELS

Voltage-gated Na^+ channels generate and propagate electrical impulses. Mammalian Na^+ channels comprise a gene family with nine cloned, pore-forming α subunits named $Na_V1.1–1.9$ (Goldin et al., 2000). While Na^+ channels differ significantly with regard to their tissue-specific expression of biophysical and pharmacological properties, most members of this family show some degree of sensitivity to the pufferfish toxin, tetrodotoxin (TTX), and the related marine guanidinium toxin, saxitoxin (STX). The first evidence that Na^+ channels may be expressed by nonneuronal cells came from STX binding studies in axon-free distal nerve stumps of rabbit sciatic nerves undergoing Wallerian degeneration (Ritchie and Rang, 1983). This surprising finding prompted a search for Na^+ channels in isolated glial cells and indeed revealed the presence of TTX/STX-sensitive voltage-activated Na^+ channels on cultured Schwann cells (Chiu et al., 1984) and astrocytes (Bevan et al. 1984).

Numerous laboratories have since used patch-clamp electrophysiology to also demonstrate the expression of Na^+ channels in essentially all cultured macroglial cell types (for review see Sontheimer et al., 1996; Verkhratsky and Steinhauser, 2000). Some of these studies revealed a surprising degree of biophysical and pharmacological diversity. For example, Schwann cell Na^+ currents showed all the hallmarks of Na^+ currents recorded in the nerve they ensheath, with the exception of a positively shifted current-voltage curve (Bevan et al., 1984). This biophysical difference suggested that larger depolarizations are required to activate Schwann cell Na^+ channels than neuronal Na^+ channels. Studies on cultured astrocytes in hippocampus (Sontheimer et al., 1992b), spinal cord (Sontheimer and Waxman, 1992), and optic nerve (Barres et al., 1990a) showed two Na^+ current types that differed in their sensitivity to TTX and their steady-state inactivation parameters. These two current types segregated to two morphologically distinct subtypes of astrocytes. Specifically, flat, protoplasmic astrocytes, refered to as *Type 1* in optic nerve and pancake cells in spinal cord, showed Na^+ channels that were TTX-resistant (TTX-R) and had steady-state inactivation curves that were 20 mV more negative than those in typical neurons (Sontheimer and Waxman, 1992) (Fig. 9.1). Fibrous process-bearing astrocytes, called *Type 2* in optic nerve, showed TTX-sensitive (TTX-S) currents with biophysical features reminiscent of those of most neurons. O2A progenitor cells, by comparison, always showed the most "neuronal" Na^+ channels, with typical high sensitivity for TTX and steady-state inactivation curves reminiscent of those of most cultured neurons (Barres et al., 1989b).

Several laboratories have now succeeded in demonstrating Na^+ channel expression in glial cells in acute tissue preparations, dismissing any concerns that these channels may be aberrantly expressed only in cultured cells. For example, astrocytes in whole mount retinas showed voltage-activated Na^+ channels (Clark and Mobbs, 1994), as did a subpopulation of astrocytes in hippocampus (Bordey and Sontheimer, 1997), cortex (Bordey and Sontheimer, 2000), and spinal cord (Chvátal et al., 1995). Mouse cortical astrocytes similarly showed small Na^+ currents *in situ* (Steinhäuser et al.,

See the list of abbreviations at the end of the chapter.

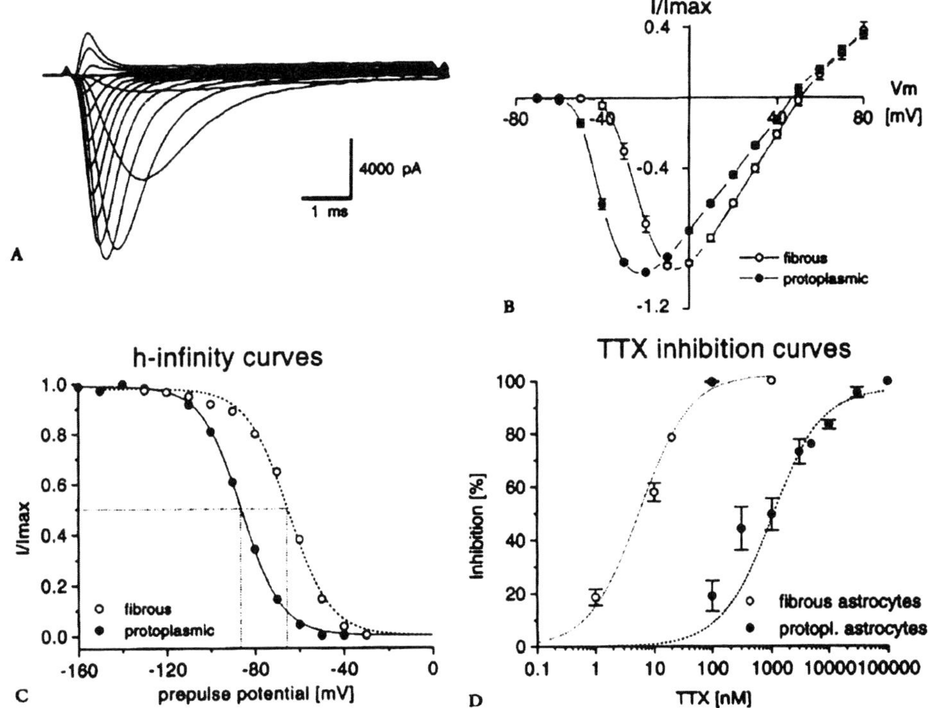

FIGURE 9.1 Astrocyte subtypes express Na^+ currents with different tetrodotoxin (TTX) sensitivity, activation, and inactivation curves. *A*. Na^+ currents expressed by astrocytes are fast, transient currents. Time to peak at 20°C is $<800\ \mu s$, and current kinetics show overall resemblance of Na^+ currents in excitable cells. *B*. Na^+ currents recorded in stellate and protoplasmic spinal cord astrocytes differ in their current-voltage (*I–V*) curves in that the peak activation threshold of the curve is 16 mV more positive than in protoplasmic cells. *C*. Steady-state current inactivation differs similarly and shows a 20 mV positive shift in fibrous astrocytes. Data in *C* and *D* were normalized means from at least 20 recordings each, and the data were fit to Boltzmann equations. *D*. The two astrocyte subtypes differ in their sensitivity to TTX. Na^+ currents in fibrous astrocytes are highly TTX-sensitive (K_d = 5.7 nM), whereas protoplasmic astrocytes are comparatively TTX-resisitant (K_d = 1000 nM). Data displayed were obtained from 39 cells, and means were fitted to Langmuir binding isotherms (dotted and dashed lines). (From Sontheimer et al., 1992a, and Sontheimer and Waxman, 1992, with permission.)

1994), as did Schwann cells that were still associated with sciatic nerves (Chiu and Schwarz, 1987). In the corpus callosum slice, immature O2A progenitor cells showed the same small TTX-S Na^+ currents observed for cultured O2A cells (Berger et al., 1991). Interestingly, some differences became apparent when tissue culture studies were compared to *in situ* recordings. Neither the TTX-R Na^+ currents that characterize protoplasmic astrocytes in rat optic nerve, spinal cord, and hippocampus nor the Na^+ currents with very negative steady-state inactivation curves have yet been identified *in situ*. To date, only retinal astrocytes have been shown to express TTX-R currents *in situ* (Clark and Mobbs, 1994). Moreover, *in situ,* Na^+ channels appear to be expressed only in a subpopulation of cells.

Our detailed biophysical understanding of Na^+ channels in glial cells by far eclipses our knowledge of the molecular biology of these proteins (see Table 9.1). Single-cell polymerase chain reaction (PCR) experiments have demonstrated transcripts for the $rNa_v1.1–1.3$ in cultured spinal cord astrocytes (Black et al., 1994b), but only $rNa_v1.2$ channels were detected immunohistochemically in tissue slices (Black et al., 1994a). In addition, spinal cord astrocytes contain transcripts for rH1, a TTX-R Na^+ channel typically restricted to the heart muscle (Black et al., 1998). By immunostaining, rH1 channels were restricted to the flat (pancake) cells that have TTX-R currents (Sontheimer and Waxman, 1992), suggesting that the TTX-R current in this subpopulation of astrocytes may be mediated by rH1 channels. Polymerase chain reaction studies demonstrated $rNa_v1.1–1.3$ transcripts in rat optic nerve astrocytes (Oh et al., 1994b), and one study demonstrated expression of $Na_v1.6$ in astrocytes, Schwann cells, and neurons (Schaller et al., 1995). $Na_v1.2$ and 1.3 are expressed in cultured Schwann cells (Oh et al., 1994a), and a partial clone of a novel Na^+ channel was isolated from rabbit Schwann cells that contained both conserved and novel sequences (Belcher et al., 1995). Whether this gene gives rise to Na^+ channels with altered properties in Schwann cells is not known. At the protein level, the use of subtype-specific antibodies con-

TABLE 9.1 *Molecularly Identified Ion Channels in Glial Cells*

Channel and Subunit	*Preparation*	*Detection Method*	*Reference*
Na^+ channel			
rNav1.1–1.3	Cultured spinal cord astrocytes	PCR	Black et al. (1994b)
rNav1.1	Spinal cord astrocytes (tissue)	Immunohistochemistry	Black et al. (1994a)
rNav1.1–1.3	Cultured astrocytes	Immunocytochemistry	Black et al. (1995)
rNav1.1–1.3	Rat optic nerve astrocytes	PCR	Oh et al. (1994b)
Nav1.6	Astrocytes, Schwann cells, and neurons	PCR	Schaller et al. (1995)
Nav1.2, 1.3	Cultured Schwann cells	PCR	Oh et al. (1994a)
rNa_x	Astrocytes (glial-specific Na^+ channel)	Cloning	Gautron et al. (1992)
rH1	Spinal cord pancake astrocytes	PCR	Black et al. (1995)
Ca^{2+} channels			
L-type	Reactive astrocytes following injury	Immunostaining	Westenbroek et al. (1998)
α1D, α2 and β3	Müller cells	RT-PCR	Puro et al. (1996a)
K^+ channels			
$K_{ir}4.1$	Mouse Müller cells	Knockout mouse	Kofuji et al. (2000)
$K_{ir}4.1$	Müller cells	Immunogold EM	Nagelhus et al. (1999)
$K_{ir}4.1$	Adult rat CNS gray matter astrocytes	Immunohistochemistry	Pooalasundaram et al. (1999)
$K_{ir}4.1$	White matter astrocytes	Immunohistochemistry	Li et al. (2001)
$K_{ir}2.1$	Müller cells	Immunohistohemistry	Kofuji et al. (2002)
$K_{ir}2.1$, 2.2, 2.4, 3.1, 3.2, 4.1 and 6.1	Retina and primary cultured Müller cells	RT-PCRRaap et al. (2002)	
K_{ir} 6.1	Hippocampal, cortical, and cerebellar astrocytes, tanycytes, Bergmann glial cells	Immunohistochemistry	Thomzig et al. (2001)
Kv1.1, 1.2, 1.5, 2.1 3.1b and 3.1	Schwann cells	Immunoblotting	Sobko et al. (1998)
Kv1.1 and 1.5	Schwann cells	Immunostaining	Mi et al. (1995)
Kv1.2, 1.4, 1.5 and 1.6	Cultured oligodendrocyte progenitor cells	Immunoblotting	Chittajallu et al. (2002)
Kv1.1, 1.2, 1.5 and 1.6	Cultured spinal cord astrocytes	Immunoblotting	MacFarlane and Sontheimer (2000b)
Kv1.4	Cultured Schwann cells from sciatic nerve	Immunoblotting	Sobko et al. (1998)
Kv1.4	Oligodendrocytes and progenitor cells	RT-PCR	Attali et al. (1997)
BK	Mylinating Schwann cells in sciatic nerve	Immunostaining	Mi et al. (1999)
BK	Brain and spinal cord astrocytes	Immunostaining	Price et al. (2002)
Cl^- channels			
ClC2 and ClC3	Cultured cortical astrocytes	PCR	Stegen et al. (2000)
BR1-VDAC	Bovine brain	Cloning	Dermietzel et al. (1994)
ClC2	Astrocytes	Immunohistochemistry	Sik et al. (2000)

EM: electron microscopy; RT-PCR; reverse transcriptase–polymerase chain reaction.

firms PCR data supporting variable levels of expression of $Na_v1.1$–1.3 in cultured astrocytes (Black et al., 1995). The molecular identity of Na^+ channels in O2A progenitor cells is largely unknown. One of the earliest efforts to clone glial-specific Na^+ channels isolated a seemingly astrocyte-specific Na^+ channel gene candidate named NaG (now rNa_x) (Gautron et al., 1992). However, efforts to show functional NaG channels have thus far been unsuccessful.

Several studies have examined potential interactions between astrocytes and neurons, or between Schwann cells and axons, and have demonstrated that such interactions can modulate the expression and/or function of Na^+ channels on glial membranes. These studies provide preliminary evidence for channel regulation by contact, secreted substances, or second messenger signaling pathways. Rat optic nerve astrocytes that were deprived of neuronal influences by either nerve transection or ablation of the retina showed a loss of Na^+ channels (Minturn et al., 1992), suggestive of a trophic role for axons on Na^+ channel expression. Yet spinal cord astrocytes cultured in the presence of dorsal root ganglion (DRG) neurons or DRG-conditioned medium show a decrease in Na^+ channels. This suggests a suppressant role of an unknown factor secreted by DRG neurons (Thio et al., 1993). In hippocampus, the percentage of astrocytes that express Na^+ channels increases as a function of postnatal development (Bordey and Sontheimer, 1997), whereas in mouse hippocampal slices the opposite is the case (Kressin et al., 1995). Again, the reason for this discrepancy is unclear.

The density of Na^+ channels in Schwann cells changes markedly, depending on the myelination state of the cell (Chiu, 1993). Cells that do not ensheath axons with myelin are rich in Na^+ channels, whereas those that have significant myelin investment do not express Na^+ channels. It appears that Schwann cell Na^+ channels are suppressed by axonal contact, similar to that demonstrated for spinal cord astrocytes. Interestingly, a large literature now supports the notion that Schwann cells regulate the expression and localization of Na^+ channels in axons, a topic discussed in Chapter 21.

Na^+ channel β subunits contain several phosphorylation sites (Catterall et al., 1990), and functional modulation of glial Na^+ channels via kinases has been demonstrated. In cultured spinal cord astrocytes, exposure of cells to protein kinase C (PKC) activators led to enhanced TTX-R Na^+ currents, while it reduced the magnitude of TTX-S Na^+ currents (Thio and Sontheimer, 1993). In cultured Schwann cells, exposure to glial-derived growth factor and/or forskolin enhanced Na^+ channels (Wilson and Chiu, 1993).

The role or functional importance of Na^+ channels in glial cells is a complete enigma. These channels are expressed at very low density (<0.1 channel/μm^2) and, at least in astrocytes, the high K^+ conductance essentially clamps the cells at the resting potential, making activation of Na^+ channels by depolarization very unlikely. A number of ideas concerning Na^+ channel function in glial cells have been proposed; however, none has firm support by experimental evidence. Ritchie and colleagues proposed the *channel transfer hypothesis*, by which Schwann cells and possibly astrocytes synthesize Na^+ channel protein for the primary purpose of donating it to adjacent axons (Gray and Ritchie, 1985). While this theory is intriguing, the transfer of membrane proteins from glial cells to neurons has not yet been demonstrated. Moreover, the cloning of Na^+ channel β subunits from Schwann cells provided evidence for molecularly distinct Na^+ channels in Schwann cells (Belcher et al., 1995). In cultured spinal cord astrocytes, it has been suggested that the unique biophysical properties of Na^+ channels may provide for a potential influx of Na^+ through the few Na^+ channels that are open in resting cells (Sontheimer et al., 1994). Over a voltage range near the resting potential, steady-state inactivation and activation curves for Na^+ channels overlap, suggesting a small degree of channel activation in resting cells. These small *window* currents may provide a pathway for Na^+ to enter and fuel the astrocytes Na^+/K^+-ATPase (Sontheimer et al., 1994) that requires intracellular Na^+ to operate. This notion, while attractive, has been called into question by a study that measured intracellular Na^+ dynamics and suggests that this modus operandi occurs only following Na^+ channel inactivation (Rose et al., 1997).

A third idea concerning the function of Na^+ channels derives from the cancer literature. Na^+ channel activity appears to play a significant role in determining the morphological development of MAT-LyLu prostate cancer cells in such a way as to enhance their metastatic potential (Fraser et al., 1999). The recent finding that some glial-derived tumor cells express Na^+ channels in high density (Labrakakis et al., 1997) suggests that Na^+ channels may be equally involved in some aspect of the unique biology of these highly invasive tumor cells. Furthermore, glial progenitor cells, which are highly migratory, express similarly high densities of Na^+ channels (Barres et al., 1989b). Clearly, this interesting idea warrants further examination.

The field of Na^+ channel biology in glia has made major inroads in describing their presence, but has failed to identify both the proteins that mediate these currents and the function they play. In the authors' opinion, the failure to assign a function to these channels has greatly reduced recent interest in the further study of Na^+ channel biology in glia cells, a void that needs to be filled.

CALCIUM CHANNELS

Voltage-activated Ca^{2+} channels are abundantly expressed in excitable cells and are designed to mediate Ca^{2+} entry in response to transient membrane depolarization. Like Na^+ channels, Ca^{2+} channels are composed of a pore-forming α subunit that can associate with additional accessory subunits ($\alpha 2$, β, γ, δ). The initial characterization of voltage-activated Ca^{2+} channels distinguished two biophysically and pharmacologically distinct groups of Ca^{2+} channels: (*1*) high voltage-activated (HVA) Ca^{2+} channels, which require relatively large cell depolarizations (threshold of approx. −30 mV) and (*2*) low voltage activated (LVA) Ca^{2+} channels that require only modest cell depolarizations (threshold of approx. −60 mV). The HVA channels include those designated pharmacologically as L (*long-lasting*), N (*neuron*), P (*Purkinje*), Q, and R types of Ca^{2+} channels. These show distinct pharmacology that includes sensitivity to certain animal venom toxins including agatoxin and conotoxins. By comparison, T (*transient*)-type Ca^{2+} channels are the only LVA channels and are abundantly expressed in muscle. They are sensitive to a number of class IV antiarrhythmic drugs including nifedipine and verapamil.

Ca^{2+} is an important intracellular messenger, and its cytoplasmic concentration is well regulated. Ca^{2+} channels have been shown to comprise one important pathway for Ca^{2+} entry into cells and hence to regulate intracellular Ca^{2+}. Many investigators have examined the intracellular Ca^{2+} dynamics in glial cells using Ca^{2+}-sensitive indicator dyes. Particularly in astrocytes, propagating Ca^{2+} waves have been described as unique intraglial signals (see Chapter 17). Some of these studies provide pharmacological evidence for an important role of Ca^{2+} influx through Ca^{2+} channels in the propagation of these glial Ca^{2+} waves.

Our current knowledge of Ca^{2+} channels in glial cells stems almost exclusively from biophysical studies; the molecular identity of glial Ca^{2+} channels remains largely uninvestigated (see Table 9.1). The first evidence that glial cells express voltage-gated Ca^{2+} channels came from recordings in cultured rat cortical astrocytes (MacVicar, 1984). Current clamp recordings, in the presence of Ba^{2+} as charge carrier, demonstrated large voltage transients in response to current injection (Fig. 9.2). These transients were reminiscent of Ca^{2+} *spikes* in some neurons. These spikes were inhibited by Mn^{2+} or Cd^{2+}, suggesting that they were mediated by voltage-gated Ca^{2+} channels. Two subsequent studies revealed that the ability to record Ca^{2+} currents required exposure of astrocytes to agents that raise intracellular cyclic adenosine monophosphate (cAMP) levels such as dibutyryl cAMP (MacVicar and Tse, 1988), forskolin, or vasoactive intestinal peptide (Barres et al., 1989a). In rat optic nerve astrocytes, both L-type and T-type Ca^{2+} currents could be identified under these conditions (Fig. 9.2*B,C*). Even then, Ca^{2+} currents were relatively small in amplitude (25–200 pA), at least one to two orders of magnitude smaller than Na^+ or K^+ currents. In most untreated primary astrocyte cultures, however, voltage-activated Ca^{2+} channels remained undetectable.

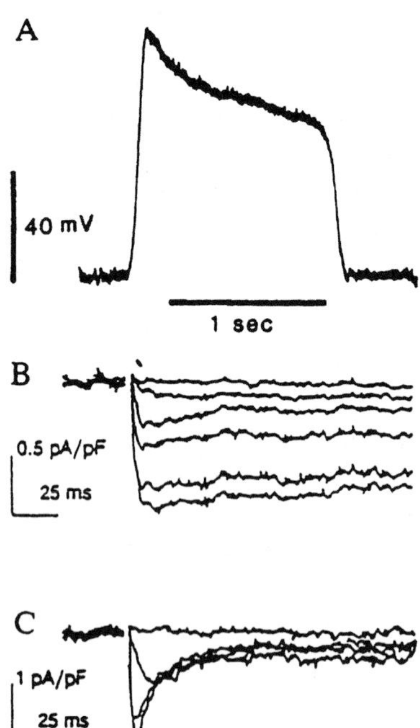

FIGURE 9.2 *(A)* Spontaneous Ca^{2+} action potential in rat astrocyte (in Ba^{2+} Locke solution). (From MacVicar, 1984, with permission. Copyright 1984, American Association for the Advancement of Science.) *B,C*. L-type and T-type Ca^{2+} currents in type 1 rat optic nerve astrocytes in response to families of depolarizing steps between -60 and $+25$ mV and between -60 and -5 mV, respectively. (From Barres et al., 1990a, with permission from Elsevier.)

Barres et al. (1989a) showed that certain batches of serum were able to induce Ca^{2+} channel expression in a limited number of cells, and Corvalan et al. (1990) demonstrated that coculture of rat cortical astrocytes with DRG neurons induced both L- and T-type Ca^{2+} currents in astrocytes that were not expressed in the absence of neurons. This neuronal regulation of glial Ca^{2+} channel expression is reminiscent of that previously described for Na^+ channels (as discussed in the previous section). Interestingly, a similar dependence on the presence of neuronal factors or agents that alter cAMP levels has been described for Schwann cells (Beaudu-Lange et al., 1998). These studies, while intriguing, raise significant concerns as to the usefulness of tissue-cultured cells for study and have motivated a detailed examination of astrocytic Ca^{2+} channels in rat brain slice preparations.

In mouse hippocampal slices, subpopulations of presumably immature astrocytes or progenitor cells showed both L- and T-type Ca^{2+} channels (Akopian et al., 1996). Similarly, studies of immature O2A lineage cells showed expression of L- and T-type Ca^{2+} channels in cultured O2A cells (Verkhratsky et al., 1990) and progenitor cells in slices of corpus callosum (Berger et al., 1992). In the retina, a developmental decrease in the expression of LVA channels occurs with highest expression at P2–P5 (Bringmann et al., 2000b). Hence, not only the context in which the cells are found but probably their lineage relationship and developmental stage also appear to influence the expression of Ca^{2+} channels. This notion is also supported by a study examining reactive astrocytes *in vivo* with Ca^{2+} channel–specific antibodies (Westenbroek et al., 1998). Here, staining for L-type channels was upregulated in reactive astrocytes following brain injury. It has frequently been noted that reactive astrocytes may recapitulate some earlier developmental phenotype.

To complicate matters further, it appears that Ca^{2+} channels in glial cells are regulated not only at the transcriptional level but also at the functional/activity level. For example, in retinal (Müller) glial cells, arachidonic acid reversibly depressed both LVA and HVA currents (Bringmann et al., 2001).

Ca^{2+} channels appear to be absent from oligodendrocytes and Schwann cells unless cocultured with DRGs. The failure to demonstrate Ca^{2+} channels in myelinating cells *in vivo* may be technical. Due to space clamp issues, patch-clamp recordings cannot identify small currents arising from distal processes on either of these cell types, even if they were present. At present, a molecular identification of glial Ca^{2+} channels has been attempted only in the retina. It showed the presence of transcripts for α1D, α2, and α3 subunits in Müller cells by reverse transcription–polymerase chain reaction (RT-PCR) (Puro et al., 1996a).

As with Na^+ channels, the function of astrocytic Ca^{2+} channels is an enigma. However, HVA Ca^{2+} channels are activated at potentials that could conceivably be reached under physiological conditions. Increases in extracellular K^+ and the subsequent depolarization may cause the activation of Ca^{2+} channels, leading to channel-mediated Ca^{2+} influx. In isolated astrocytes, the removal of Ca^{2+} abolishes a significant component of high K^+-induced Ca^{2+} influx (Duffy and MacVicar, 1994) that is sensitive to Ca^{2+} channel blockers. Therefore, at least under some circumstances, Ca^{2+} channels can contribute to the intracellular Ca^{2+} dynamics of astrocytes. Of note, such interactions may occur in microdomains far out in distal processes, similar to those demonstrated for Bergmann glial cells (Grosche et al., 1999).

POTASSIUM CHANNELS

Voltage-activated potassium channels are the most numerous and diverse family of the voltage-dependent channels. To date there are at least 50 different genes, cloned from mammals, that code for voltage-activated potassium channels (Coetzee et al., 1999). To add to their diversity, these channels often form heteromultimers, and different splicing isoforms allow single genes to give rise to distinctly different channel proteins with different properties. Based on the macroscopic currents that arise from channel activation, voltage-activated potassium channels have long been divided into several families: the inward rectifier potassium channel (K_{ir}), the delayed rectifier potassium channels (K_D), the rapidly inactivating A-type potassium channels (K_A), and the calcium-activated potassium channels (K_{Ca}).

Electrophysiological studies have demonstrated each of these K^+ channels in central and peripheral glial cells. Unfortunately, as with Na^+ and Ca^{2+} channels, the assignment of molecular identity to whole-cell currents is poorly developed (for a summary of molecularly identified K^+ channels in glia, see Table 9.1). Instead, glial potassium channel types have been identified and cataloged largely on the basis of biophysical and pharmacological properties that include single-channel conductance, voltage dependence, whole-cell current profiles, and pharmacological inhibition or activation. We will briefly summarize the key features, channel distribution, preliminary molecular identification, and putative roles for each of the four macroscopically distinct K^+ channel classes: K_{ir}, K_D, K_A, and K_{Ca}.

INWARD RECTIFIER POTASSIUM CHANNELS

Inward rectifier potassium channels (K_{ir}) are a particularly prominent feature of differentiated glial cells and are thought to be responsible for the negative resting membrane potential (RMP) typical of many glial cells. When K_{ir} channels were first identified, they were termed *anomalous rectifiers* because of their unusual current-voltage profile. Unlike all other voltage-gated K^+ currents, K_{ir} currents are largest at hyperpolarized potentials and decrease with membrane depolarization. The channels that mediate these currents are not voltage-dependent in the classical sense. Instead, the inward rectification of K_{ir} channels is achieved by intracellular polyamines and/or Mg^{2+}, which block the pore at depolarized potentials. At relatively negative potentials (around the RMP for most glial cells, -80 mV), the block is released and K^+ ions flow into the cell. Additionally, rectification is regulated by extracellular K^+ ($[K^+]_o$) that is, extracellular potassium. These channels show a large open probability near or negative of the potassium equilibrium potential (E_k), thus conferring a *K^+ leak* conductance to glial cells. Indeed, K_{ir} channels are thought to be the main contributor to the negative RMP that is typical of most glial cells.

Numerous studies have described macroscopic K_{ir} currents in essentially all glial cell types. The majority of these studies suggest that glial K_{ir} currents are weakly rectifying. A molecular identification of the underlying K_{ir} channels has just begun. Biophysical studies have demonstrated some heterogeneity with regard to channel properties, including unitary conductance, activation and inactivation parameters, and voltage dependence. However, all currents identified show two fundamental properties that are shared by all glial K_{ir} channels: (*1*) dependence on extracellular K^+, whereby the inward current increases with increasing $[K^+]_o$ concentrations (current proportional to the square root of $[K^+]_o$) (Fig. 9.3*A*) and (*2*) inhibition of channel activity by extracellular applications of Ba^{2+} or Cs^{2+} at micro- and millimolar concentrations (Fig. 9.3*C*,*D*).

K_{ir} currents in glia were first described in cultured rat astrocytes in the early 1980s (Bevan and Raff 1985;

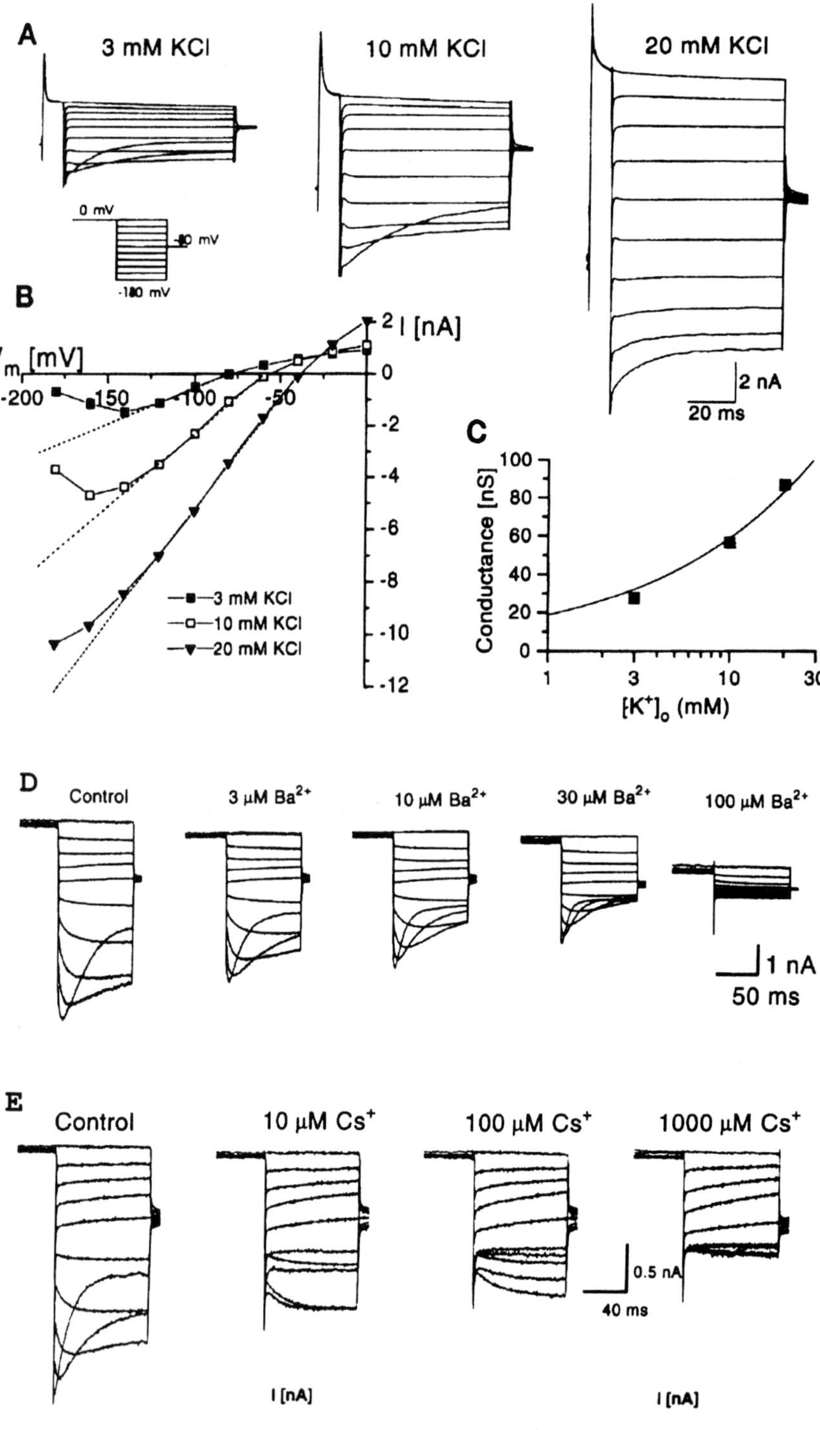

FIGURE 9.3 Whole-cell recordings from cultured spinal cord astrocytes. *A*. K_{ir} conductance depends on $[K^+]_o$. K^+ dependence of K_{ir} was studied by recording currents in response to families of voltage steps (*A*, *inset*) in 3, 10, and 20 mM extracellular K^+. Current amplitude depends critically on $[K^+]_o$ and increases with increasing $[K^+]_o$. Inactivation at negative potentials was reduced in elevated $[K^+]_o$. *B*. Peak currents from the experiments in *A* were plotted as a function of applied potential and yielded the current-voltage (*I–V*) curves under the three ionic gradients. *I–V* curves were shifted toward more positive potentials, and conductances increased. *C*. Slope conductances were determined by linear fit to the inward current component of the *I–V* curves (- - - in *B*) and were plotted as a function of $[K^+]_o$. The resulting data could be well fitted to a square-roots function of the form $f(x) = A * \mathrm{sqrt}(x)$. *D*. Ba^{2+} block of K_{ir} currents examined by external application of solutions containing 3, 10, 30, and 300 μM BaCl. *E*. $[Cs^+]_o$ block of K_{ir} currents is voltage-dependent. Currents were recorded in the presence of 10, 100, and 1000 μM Cs^+; increasing Cs^+ concentrations resulted in suppression of K_{ir} currents. (From Ransom et al., 1995, with permission.)

Bevan et al., 1985), and soon thereafter in dissociated salamander Müller cells (astrocyte-like cells in the retina) (Newman, 1985). Prior to the cloning of the first K_{ir} channel in 1993 (Kubo et al., 1993), biophysical evidence described K_{ir} currents in cultured mouse brain and spinal cord oligodendrocytes (Sontheimer and Kettenmann, 1988), adult human oligodendrocytes (McLarnon and Kim, 1989), astrocytes from rat spinal cord (Sontheimer et al., 1992a), and astrocytes from hippocampus (Tse et al., 1992). Subsequent studies examined K_{ir} channels in acute brain slices and showed prominent expression of weakly rectifying K_{ir} currents in astrocytes and oligodendrocytes from the rat (Sontheimer and Waxman, 1993) and mouse hippocampus (Steinhauser et al., 1992). Inward rectifier currents were observed in freshly isolated Schwann cells (Chiu, 1991). Here, channel density was affected by myelination status as well as the proliferative state of the cell. Additionally, K_{ir} currents were described in acutely dissociated retinal Müller cells (Newman, 1985). In general, these *in situ* studies agreed well with previous *in vitro* studies, and collectively suggest that K_{ir} channels contribute to the cells resting potential and possibly contribute to K^+ uptake (buffering) under conditions when $[K^+]_o$ is elevated.

Cloning of K_{ir} channels provided the tools to identify molecularly the proteins that give rise to glial K_{ir} currents, and several groups have examined channel expression by PCR, by Western blot, or by immunohistochemistry with channel-specific antibodies. $K_{ir}4.1$ is the most well-characterized subunit in glial cells. Recombinant expression of $K_{ir}4.1$ in HEK cells gives rise to weakly rectifying K_{ir} currents that are nearly indistinguishable from K_{ir} currents in astrocytes (Li et al., 2001) or Müller cells (Ishii et al., 1997). These studies directed immediate attention to $K_{ir}4.1$ as the major glial K_{ir} channel candidate. Subsequent immunogold electron microscopic studies colocalized $K_{ir}4.1$ and aquaporin-4 in rat Müller cells (Nagelhus et al., 1999), and immunohistochemical studies identified $K_{ir}4.1$ as an abundant astrocytic K_{ir} protein throughout the adult rat central nervous system (CNS) (Poopalasundaram et al., 2000). Some controversy remains as to whether $K_{ir}4.1$ is expressed only in gray matter astrocytes (Poopalasundaram et al., 2000) or is also expressed in white matter astrocytes (Li et al., 2001). The most conclusive evidence that $K_{ir}4.1$ is an important glial K_{ir} channel protein came from the examination of a transgenic mouse harboring a homozygotic deletion of the $K_{ir}4.1$ gene. Kofuji and colleagues (2000) elegantly demonstrated that Müller cells in the $K_{ir}4.1-/-$ knockout mouse have a 10-fold increase in input resistance, suggesting a low resting K^+ permeability. Moreover, these knockout mice had very depolarized membrane potentials (-13.2 ± 2.9 mV) compared to control littermates (-85.2 ± 0.7 mV). Importantly, the slow PIII response, a component of the light-evoked electroretinogram, believed to be caused by glial potassium currents (Newman, 2003), was selectively absent from the retinas of the $K_{ir}4.1-/-$ mice. Thus, at least in Müller cells of the retina, $K_{ir}4.1$ is essential for setting the resting potential of glial cells and mediating K^+ buffering in response to light stimuli.

Several other K_{ir} channel subunits have been identified in glial cells, yet their relative contribution to resting potential or K^+ fluxes remains to be demonstrated. For example, RT-PCR studies from both retina and primary cultured Müller cells show the presence of transcripts for $K_{ir}2.1$, $K_{ir}2.2$, $K_{ir}2.4$, $K_{ir}3.1$, $K_{ir}3.2$, $K_{ir}4.1$, and $K_{ir}6.1$ (Raap et al., 2002). $K_{ir}6.1$ is expressed in hippocampal, cortical, and cerebellar astrocytes, as well as in tanycytes and Bergmann glial cells (Thomzig et al., 2001). Some of these channels would be expected to give rise to strongly rectifying K_{ir} currents, which have not been observed in these cells. However, it is possible that these subunits form heterodimeric channels with altered properties. Clearly, further molecular studies, preferentially using targeted knockouts and/or antisense techniques, will be required to determine the relative importance of these K_{ir} channel genes.

Interestingly, a consistent observation from *in vitro* and *in situ* studies has been the developmental expression profile of K_{ir} channels. K_{ir} channel activity appears to be selectively associated with a more mature or differentiated, possibly postmitotic cell phenotype. Specifically, in many glial preparations, the expression of K_{ir} first appears postnatally, around P8–P12. Concomitant with increased K_{ir} channel expression, the cell's RMP becomes gradually more negative. For example, in astrocytes in the rat hippocampal slice, K_{ir} currents increase dramatically between P5 and P20, at which time K_{ir} becomes the dominant conductance (Sontheimer et al., 1989). This developmental expression pattern is maintained *in vitro* as cultured spinal cord astrocytes begin to express K_{ir} channels only after 7–10 days in culture (Sontheimer et al., 1992a; MacFarlane and Sontheimer, 2000a). Similarly, in rabbit Müller cells, K_{ir} channel activity increases substantially after P7 (Bringmann et al., 1999a), and channel expression correlates positively with the cell's RMP; the higher the K_{ir} expression, the more negative the RMP. The correlation between cell differentiation and K_{ir} expression is even more pronounced in cells of the oligodendrocyte lineage. Here, A2B5 and O4 antigen-positive glial precursor cells do not express any K_{ir} channels, yet these channels are expressed as cells differentiate into mature oligodendrocytes (Sontheimer et al., 1989). Again, the developmental appearance of K_{ir} channels correlates with increasingly negative RMPs.

If K_{ir} channels were selectively expressed in postmitotic glial cells, one might expect their expression and/or activity to be lost when cells reenter the cell cycle. This can indeed be demonstrated following the induction of gliotic cell division. Acute injury to spinal cord astrocytes in culture leads to an acute loss of K_{ir} currents (MacFarlane and Sontheimer, 1997). Additionally, retinal diseases that present with glial proliferation show a similar loss of K_{ir} channel activity, resulting in glial cells with more depolarized RMP and reduced resting K^+ conductance (Francke et al., 1997). In culture, pharmacological inhibition of K_{ir} channels causes an increase in spinal cord astrocyte proliferation; conversely, arrest of actively proliferating astrocytes leads to a premature increase in K_{ir} channel expression (MacFarlane and Sontheimer, 2000a). Hence, one may surmise that K_{ir} channel expression is essential for cells to exit the cell cycle and differentiate. The best evidence that this may indeed be the case again comes from the $K_{ir}4.1-/-$ mice (Kofuji et al., 2000; Neusch et al., 2001). In addition to a loss of resting K^+ conductance, these mice exhibited severe motor impairment that can be attributed to defects in oligodendrocyte differentiation and myelination. Peripheral myelination by Schwann cells may similarly require functional K_{ir} channels, as *in situ*, K_{ir} currents can only be recorded from Schwann cells with visible myelin (Wilson and Chiu, 1990). Taken together, these studies provide compelling evidence that K_{ir} channel activity correlates with cell development. However, the causal link between K_{ir} expression/function and cell maturation or differentiation remains unclear.

Buffering of extracellular K^+ remains the oldest and most frequently discussed hypothesis implicating K^+ channels (Orkand et al., 1966). By all accounts, K_{ir} channels appear to be perfectly suited to the task of taking up extracellular K^+; they are open at rest, and their conductance increases with increasing $[K^+]_o$. Moreover, in glial cells, K_{ir} channels show the polarized distribution that one would expect from a channel type that serves in K^+ redistribution. Specifically, in brain, $K_{ir}4.1$ is enriched in the processes of astrocytes that surround blood vessels (Higashi et al., 2001). In Müller cells, $K_{ir}2.1$ preferentially localizes to the plasma membrane that is in direct contact with neurons, ideally situated to take up potassium after neuronal discharge (Kofuji et al., 2002).

Neuronal activity may regulate glial K_{ir} channel activity. For example, K_{ir} currents in spinal cord astrocytes decrease as extracellular sodium concentrations decrease even slightly (Ransom et al., 1996), as would be the case under conditions of enhanced neuronal excitation. Two β-adrenergic receptor agonists, isoproterenol and epinephrine, significantly reduce K_{ir} currents through the action of adenylate cyclase (Roy and Sontheimer, 1995). Importantly, γ-amino-3-hydroxy-5-methyl-isoazolepropionic acid (AMPA) receptor activation in response to glutamate release causes a transient inhibition of K_{ir} currents in hippocampal astrocytes (Schroder et al., 2002), while in Müller cells, *N*-methyl-D-aspartate (NMDA) receptor activation inhibits K_{ir} currents (Puro et al., 1996b). Each of these examples exemplifies real possibilities whereby neuronal activity may regulate the K_{ir} channel activity of astrocytes and hence may indirectly modulate the composition of the extracellular space. Alternatively, controlling glial K_{ir} channel activity may modulate neuronal responses. Pharmacological blockade of K_{ir} channels with Cs^{2+} altered the epileptform neuronal discharge in hippocampal brain slices (Bordey and Sontheimer, 1997).

OUTWARDLY RECTIFYING POTASSIUM CHANNELS

Outwardly rectifying potassium channels constitute a second family of diverse voltage-activated channels abundantly expressed in glial cells. Collectively, these channels are activated by membrane depolarization.

The outwardly rectifying potassium channels consist of at least 15 subfamilies (for review see Coetzee et al., 1999). This section will focus on a subset of this superfamily. The Kv family of voltage-gated channels is composed of both delayed rectifier (K_D)-type potassium channels and fast-inactivating or transient (K_A) A-type potassium channels. Distantly related to these, yet still in the same superfamily of channels, are the calcium-activated potassium (K_{Ca}) channels, which are activated by intracellular Ca^{2+} concentrations as well as membrane depolarization. Multiple homologs and isoforms have been identified, leading to an exceptionally large and surprisingly diverse family of channels.

Traditionally, these three channel types, K_D, K_A and K_{Ca}, were distinguished on the basis of pharmacological and biophysical characteristics. The activation threshold for these channels as well as unitary conductance, channel kinetics, activation and inactivation, and permeation properties vary tremendously between channel types. Most outwardly rectifying potassium channels are sensitive to varying concentrations of the potassium channel blockers, tetraethylammonium (TEA), 4-aminopyridine (4-AP), or both. Moreover, the majority of these channels are sensitive to one or multiple naturally occurring toxins derived from plants, snake venoms, and scorpion venoms. However, there are very few examples of subunit-specific blockers (for a review on voltage-sensitive K^+ channel pharmacology, see Kaczorowski and Garcia, 1999). Each of these three types of outwardly rectifying potassium channels has been identified in glial cells, and these findings will be discussed below.

DELAYED RECTIFIER POTASSIUM CHANNELS

Delayed rectifier potassium (K_D) channels are responsible for repolarization of action potentials and for controlling the release of neurotransmitters in excitable cells. Generally, K_D channels are not open at the resting membrane potential. The typical activation threshold is -40 mV, and characteristically, these channels inactivate minimally with sustained depolarization.

K_D channels have been described in essentially all glial cells. As with K_{ir} channels, the initial identity of specific subtypes in glia has been primarily through biophysical characteristics. Ritchie and colleagues were the first to describe delayed rectifier-type currents in glial cells (Chiu et al., 1984). At the time, they reported it as surprising that Schwann cells, which "lack[ed] excitability," did indeed possess voltage-gated potassium channels similar to those found in neurons. This current was activated by depolarization and blocked by extracellular application of 4-AP and internal application of CsCl (CsCl in the pipette solution is also frequently used to block K^+ channels). Similar findings

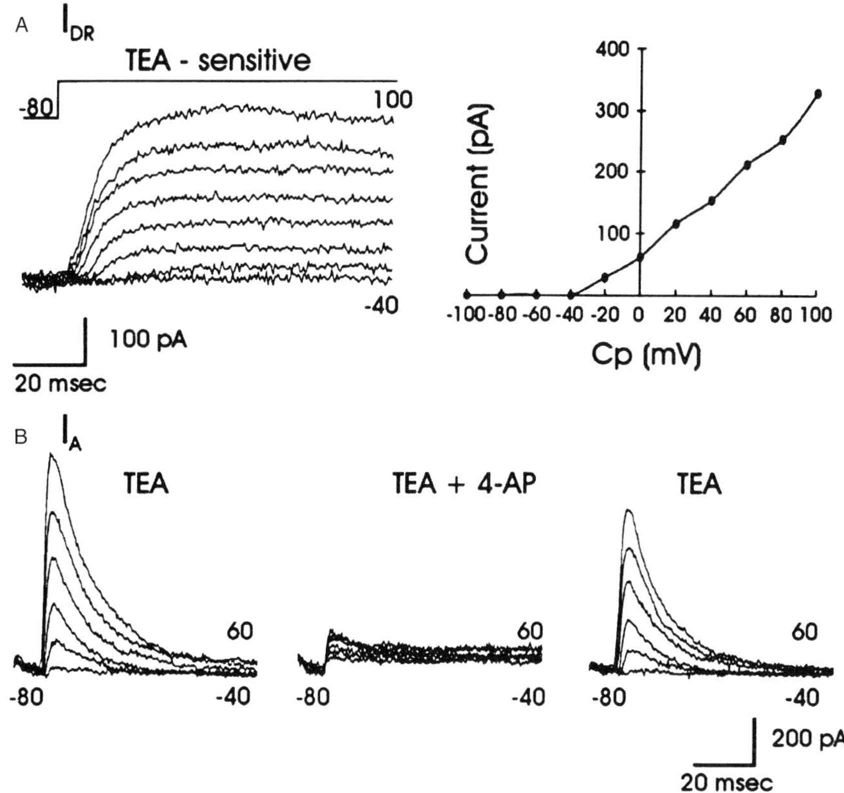

FIGURE 9.4 Whole-cell voltage clamp recordings from acutely isolated hippocampal astrocytes demonstrating the presence of K_D currents (I_{DR}) and K_A currents (I_{KA}). *A*. Membrane potential was stepped from −40 mV to 100 mV from a holding potential of −80 mV in external solutions with or without tetraethylammonium (TEA, 40 mM). The outward current that was blocked by TEA (I_{DR}) is illustrated in the left panel, and the current-voltage (*I–V*) relationship of the peak outward current is plotted. There was no significant inactivation of the current over this time frame. The current had a threshold for turn-on of −40 mV. *B*. In the presence of external TEA to block I_{DR}, a rapidly inactivating outward current (I_A) was still observed. I_A turned on with a much faster time course than I_{DR} and inactivated almost completely over a time course in which I_{DR} exhibited no decrement. I_A was totally blocked by by external 4-aminopyridine (4-AP) in a reversible manner. (From Tse et al. Copyright 1992, with permission by the Society for Neuroscience.)

were soon confirmed in nearly every glial cell type and preparation (Fig. 9.4*A*). *In vitro*, delayed rectifier potassium channels were described in rat astrocytes (Bevan and Raff, 1985), cultured rabbit Schwann cells (Konishi, 1989), mouse A2B5 and O4-positive oligodendrocytes precursor cells (Sontheimer et al., 1989), cultured and acutely isolated O2A progenitor cells (Barres et al., 1990b) and acutely isolated mammalian Müller cells from 22 species (Chao et al., 1997). Similar currents were reported in astrocytes from rat hippocampal slices (Sontheimer and Waxman, 1993) and Schwann cells from organotypic cultures of dorsal root ganglion (Amedee et al., 1991). Single-channel conductance varies between cell types and suggests that more than one subunit gives rise to the currents that were observed.

Cloning of K_D channels provided the tools needed to identify molecularly the currents electrophysiologists had been characterizing for more than four decades. As biophysical evidence had suggested, many glial cell types possess more than one K_D channel subtype. For example, in mouse Schwann cells, both cloning and immunoblotting revealed expression of the delayed rectifier channels Kv1.1, Kv1.2, Kv1.5, Kv2.1, Kv3.1b, and Kv3.2 (Sobko et al., 1998). Channel localization in Schwann cells appears to be quite specialized. Kv1.5 is found in the Schwann cell membrane at the node of Ranvier, whereas Kv1.1 is located intracellularly (Mi et al., 1995). Cultured oligodendrocyte progenitor cells express Kv1.2, Kv1.4, Kv1.5, and Kv1.6 (Chittajallu et al., 2002), while cultured astrocytes have been shown to express Kv1.1, Kv1.2, Kv1.6, and Kv1.5 (MacFarlane and Sontheimer, 2000b). The physiological significance of the diversity of subtype expression in glial cells is still unclear.

Although K_D channels appear to be expressed throughout the cell lineage, there is mounting evidence for an upregulation of channel expression as cells enter the cell cycle and are downregulation of channel expression as cells exit the cell cycle and differentiate. For example, in spinal cord astrocytes, antisense oligonucleotide knockdown of Kv1.5 inhibits cell proliferation by 50% (MacFarlane and Sontheimer, 2000b). Arrest of the cell cycle at various stages indicates that although there are no changes in the overall channel expression level, there is a decrease in the amount of tyrosine-phosphorylated Kv1.5. Moreover, activated Src appears to enhance cell proliferation, while a Src inhibitor decreases cell proliferation. Another study demonstrates that K_D channels are downregulated in the soma of Schwann cells as proliferation slows and myelination proceeds (Sobko et al., 1998), and blockers of K_D channels inhibited cell proliferation. Yet another study finds that oligodendrocyte progenitor cell proliferation and differentiation is inhibited by TEA (Ghiani et al., 1999). Moreover, when cultured oligodendrocyte progenitors are induced to enter the cell cycle there is a marked upregulation of the delayed rectifier channels Kv1.3 and Kv1.5 (Chittajallu et al., 2002) Furthermore, immunocytochemical staining of cells acutely isolated from slices demonstrates a concomitant downregulation of these two channel subunits as progenitor cells progress along their cell lineage to mature oligodendrocytes. In contrast to K_{ir} channels, K_D channel expression correlates positively with a more depolarized membrane potential.

Several studies have reported that K_D channel activity can be modulated by tyrosine kinases. Sobko and colleagues demonstrated that mouse Schwann cell K_D currents were sensitive to two broad-spectrum tyrosine kinase inhibitors, genistein and herbimycin (Peretz et al., 1999). In good agreement with this study, spinal cord astrocyte K_D currents were potentiated when active Src was included in the pipette and were inhibited by a Src-specific inhibitor, PP2 (MacFarlane and Sontheimer, 2000b).

RAPIDLY INACTIVATING A-TYPE POTASSIUM CHANNELS

In response to membrane depolarization, rapidly inactivating potassium (K_A) channels undergo a conformational change that allows ion permeation. An additional conformational change then takes place that leads to a nonconducting state or channel inactivation. When originally characterized, the currents mediated by K_A channels inactivated rapidly; thus, the terms *fast-inactivating* or *transient K^+ current* were used to describe them (Connor and Stevens, 1971). In excitable cells, these channels are responsible for regulating the interspike interval (Hille, 2001). Since the initial studies that first described K_A type currents, the rate and extent of inactivation have been shown to vary. The clear biophysical distinction that had previously been thought to exist between the currents mediated by both K_A and K_D channel subunit types regarding their inactivation has become blurred. A delayed rectifier-type channel behaves as a transient-type channel if expressed with the proper β subunit (Heinemann et al., 1994). Indeed, the Kv channel family is not composed of subunits that give rise to classical K_A- and K_D-like currents, but to currents that exhibit a continuum of inactivation ranging from no inactivation to very transient currents.

Like K_D channels, K_A channels are typically not open at the resting membrane potential. They activate transiently at membrane potentials of approximately -40 mV after a sustained hyperpolarization. The biophysical protocol introduced by Conner and Stevens remains a reliable means to isolate A-type currents biophysically (Connor and Stevens 1971). Additionally, K_A channels can be isolated pharmacologically, as they are less sensitive to TEA and more sensitive to 4-AP than other members in the same superfamily (Fig. 9.4B).

Many of the same studies that identified K_D channel currents in glia also identified I_A (current mediated by K_A) (Newman, 1985). For example, these fast or transient currents were detected in rat and human cultured mammalian Schwann cells (Konishi, 1989), mouse A2B5 and O4-positive oligodendrocyte precursor cells (Sontheimer et al., 1989), cultured acutely isolated O2A progenitor cells (Barres et al., 1990b), rat spinal cord astrocytes (MacFarlane and Sontheimer, 2000a) and Müller cells of the rabbit retina (Chao et al., 1994). These types of currents were also found *in situ* in organotypic slice cultures from Schwann cells (Amedee et al., 1991) and in rat hippocampal slices (Bordey and Sontheimer, 1997).

K_A channels appear to be expressed in glial cells as abundantly as other voltage-gated potassium channels, yet only one channel subunit, Kv1.4, has been identified molecularly. Western blotting detected Kv1.4 from cultured Schwann cells of the mouse sciatic nerve (Sobko et al., 1998). In this study Kv1.4 was shown to form heteromultimers with the K_D channel subunit Kv1.5. In contrast to the K_D channel subunit expression in these cells, which declined during postnatal development, Kv1.4 expression remained relatively constant. Reverse transcriptase–polymerase chain reaction revealed expression of Kv1.4 in oligodendrocytes and progenitor cells (Attali et al., 1997). It is possible that other members of the Kv channel subfamily interact with β subunits or form different combinations through heteromultimerization to give rise to transient currents.

The modulation and regulation of currents mediated by K_A channels have not been extensively studied in glial cells. Tyrosine kinases have been shown to change the amplitude of transient currents as well as modulate the gating properties (Peretz et al., 1999). In freshly isolated Müller cells, varying the $[Ca^{2+}]_o$ (extracellular Ca^{2+}) shifted the activation and inactivation curves, slowed the activation and inaction kinetics, and increased the peak amplitude of I_A (Bringmann et al., 1999b). The role that K_A channels play in glial cell biology is unclear.

CALCIUM-ACTIVATED POTASSIUM CHANNELS

Ca^{2+}-activated potassium (K_{Ca}) channels differ from other voltage-activated potassium channels in that their activation is controlled by two physiological processes: intracellular Ca^{2+} concentration and membrane voltage. Calcium binding is required for channel activation under normal physiological conditions.

Three channel types (BK, IK, and SK) can be distinguished by their biophysical properties and have differential sensitivities to specific toxins. BK channels have large unitary conductance (>100 pS), are sensitive to $[Ca^{2+}]$ in the low micromolar range, show a relatively steep voltage dependence, and are blocked by iberiotoxin, charybdotoxin, and micromolar concentrations of TEA. IK channels have an intermediate conductance (30–70 pS), are minimally voltage-dependent, and are found sparingly in the nervous system (Sah and Faber, 2002). SK channels have a relatively small single-channel conductance (5–20 pS), are sensitive to 200–400 nanomolar concentrations of $[Ca^{2+}]_i$, are also minimally voltage-dependent, and are relatively insensitive to TEA but blocked by the bee venom toxin, apamin.

The first description of K_{Ca} channels in glia was presented by Newman and colleagues (Newman, 1985). They described an outward Ca^{2+}-activated potassium current in enzymatically dissociated Müller cells that was blocked by TEA and Cd^{2+}. They questioned the physiological relevance of this channel. At normal membrane potentials, it remained closed unless there was a large increase in $[K^+]_o$ that might depolarize the membrane potential enough for the channel to open.

Similar to the other voltage-activated potassium channels described thus far, expression of K_{Ca} channels has been demonstrated in many glial cell types by either channel activity (Fig. 9.5) or protein expression. For example, early studies revealed currents mediated by both SK (Quandt and MacVicar, 1986) and BK channels (Nowak et al., 1987) in cultured rat and mouse cortical astrocytes, respectively. Both types of channels were observed in cultured striatal astrocytes (Bychkov et al., 2001). An apamin-sensitive current was detected in $A2B5^+/O4+$ O2A progenitor cells (Sontheimer et al., 1989). Immunocytochemistry has revealed that BK channels are enriched in the outer membrane of myelinating Schwannn cells at the node of Ranvier of the sciatic nerve (Mi et al., 1999). Channel expression was also detected in rat astrocytes from the brain and spinal cord at perivascular endfeet (Price et al., 2002). It was suggested that activation of these channels, possibly by local increases in $[Ca^{2+}]_i$, may allow these channels to efflux K^+ and therefore aid in K^+ homeostasis.

Reichenbach's group has extensively studied K_{Ca} channels in mammalian Müller cells and, more specifically, their role in cell differentiation. They have shown that BK channel expression decreases dramatically during development (Bringmann et al., 1999a). They described a decrease in the open probability (P_{open}) of the channel from P2 ($P_{open} = 0.69$) to P14 ($P_{open} = 0.06$). These investigators attribute this decrease in channel activity to an increasingly hyperpolarized membrane

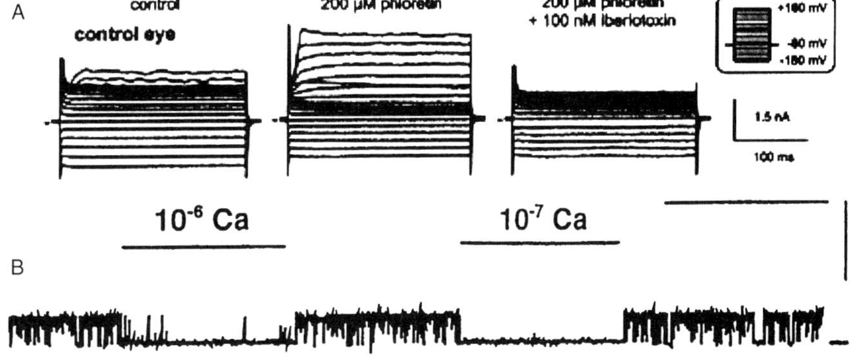

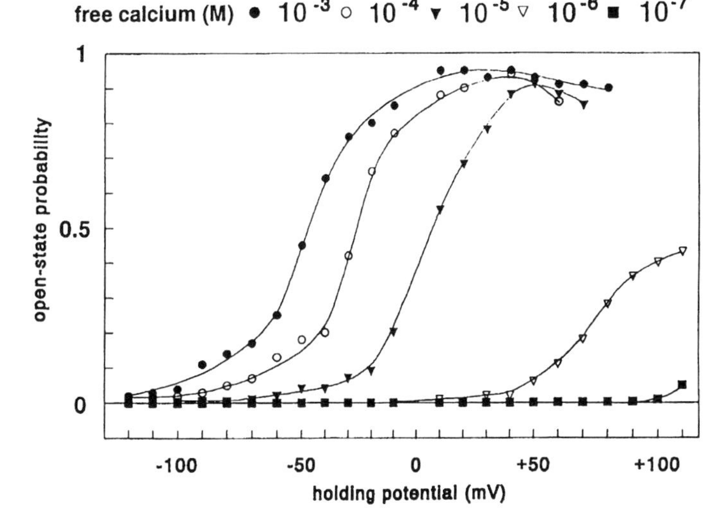

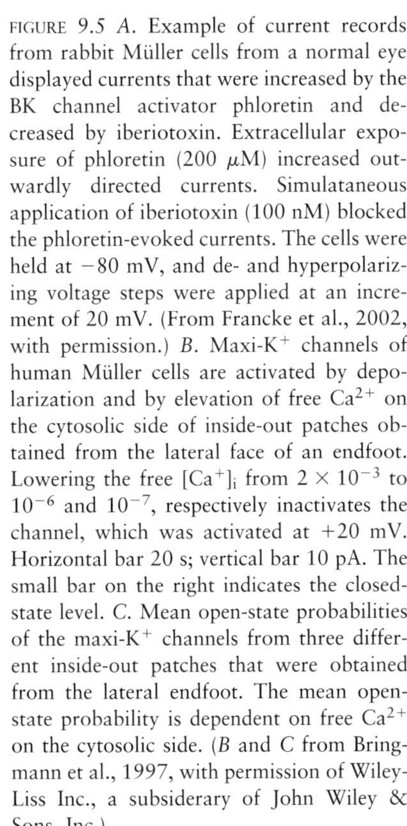

FIGURE 9.5 *A*. Example of current records from rabbit Müller cells from a normal eye displayed currents that were increased by the BK channel activator phloretin and decreased by iberiotoxin. Extracellular exposure of phloretin (200 μM) increased outwardly directed currents. Simulataneous application of iberiotoxin (100 nM) blocked the phloretin-evoked currents. The cells were held at -80 mV, and de- and hyperpolarizing voltage steps were applied at an increment of 20 mV. (From Francke et al., 2002, with permission.) *B*. Maxi-K^+ channels of human Müller cells are activated by depolarization and by elevation of free Ca^{2+} on the cytosolic side of inside-out patches obtained from the lateral face of an endfoot. Lowering the free $[Ca^+]_i$ from 2×10^{-3} to 10^{-6} and 10^{-7}, respectively inactivates the channel, which was activated at +20 mV. Horizontal bar 20 s; vertical bar 10 pA. The small bar on the right indicates the closed-state level. *C*. Mean open-state probabilities of the maxi-K^+ channels from three different inside-out patches that were obtained from the lateral endfoot. The mean open-state probability is dependent on free Ca^{2+} on the cytosolic side. (*B* and *C* from Bringmann et al., 1997, with permission of Wiley-Liss Inc., a subsiderary of John Wiley & Sons, Inc.)

potential that is characteristic of more differentiated cells. Supporting the notion that BK channel activity is more prominent in dividing cells, they have found enhanced expression of BK currents in gliotic cells following injury of the retina (Bringmann et al., 2000a). Blockade of BK channels decreases the rate of DNA synthesis, possibly by increasing mitogen-induced increases in $[Ca^{2+}]_i$ (Kodal et al., 2000) in Müller cells. Furthermore, activation of P2Y receptors, by exposing Müller cells to extracellular adenosine triphosphate (ATP), increased DNA synthesis. This increase was dependent on increased $[Ca^{2+}]_i$ and blocked by iberiotoxin (Moll et al., 2002). Indeed, increased K_{Ca} channel activity in immature cells is not confined to Müller cells. As stated above, K_{Ca} channels were described in oligodendrocyte precursor cells but not in mature oligodendrocytes in culture (Sontheimer et al., 1989). Transformed astrocytes, which are also highly proliferative, express BK channels (Ransom et al., 2001).

In addition to Ca^{2+}, K_{Ca} channel activity is also modulated by neurotransmitters, nucleotides, hormones, ATP, protein kinase A (PKA), PKC, lipids, and G-proteins. Only a few studies have examined modulation of Ca^{2+} activated potassium channels in glial cells. For example, the open probability of BK channels increases when PKA is activated by exposure to dibutyryl-cAMP, and channel activity can be inhibited by activation of PKC. Additionally, a protein kinase inhibitor, staurosporine, also enhances channel activity (Schopf et al., 1999). Müller cell maxi-K^+ or BK channels are modulated by raising intracellular pH and Mg^{2+} ions (Hille, 2001). Moreover, these authors demonstrated that channel phosphorylation in the presence of Mg-ATP enhanced channel sensitivity to both Ca^{2+} and voltage. Clearly, the most important regulator of BK channels is intracellular Ca^{2+}. Ca^{2+} is a fundamental and universal second messenger, and Ca^{2+} signaling has been demonstrated to be involved in cell proliferation, differentiation, secretion, excitation, migration, and apoptosis (Bootman et al., 2002). Indeed, Ca^{2+} signaling, including the propagation of Ca^{2+} waves between cells, has been extensively studied in glial cells (for review see (Verkhratsky et al., 1998). Therefore, it is possible that cell-to-cell signaling or communication between glial cells may, in turn, activate BK channels. As mentioned above, the synergy between membrane depolarization and local or global increases in intracellular Ca^{2+} enhances the probability of channel opening.

CHLORIDE AND ANION CHANNELS

Cl^- is the major anion in all physiological saline environments, and essentially all living cells express a combination of transporters and ion channels to move Cl^- across cell membranes. In the brain, changes in osmolarity or water content occur primarily in the context of disease, brain edema being the primary example. However, it has been proposed that buffering of K^+ by glial cells may also be associated with Cl^- fluxes (for discussion see Walz, 2000). This Cl^- flux may be mediated by Cl^- channels under physiological conditions.

Cloned mammalian Cl^- channels can be grouped into four molecular superfamilies: the cystic fibrosis transmembrane conductance regulator (CFTR) channels, Ca^{2+}-activated Cl^- channels, voltage-dependent anion-selective channels (VDACs), and voltage-gated chloride channels (ClCs) (Jentsch et al., 1999). Only a few representatives of these channel families have been unequivocally identified in glial cells (see Table 9.1). The majority of our knowledge regarding Cl^- channel expression in glial cells stems from biophysical recordings. Using patch-clamp recordings, Ritchie and colleagues (Gray and Ritchie, 1986) recorded outwardly rectifying 4,4′-diisothiocyanato-stilbene-2,2′-disulfonic acid (DIDS)-sensitive currents from cultured astrocytes that persisted when extracellular Cl^- was replaced with acetate but disappeared when Cl^- was replaced by glu-

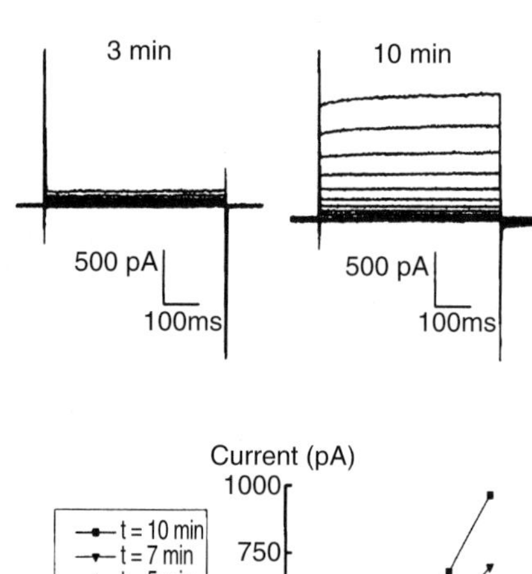

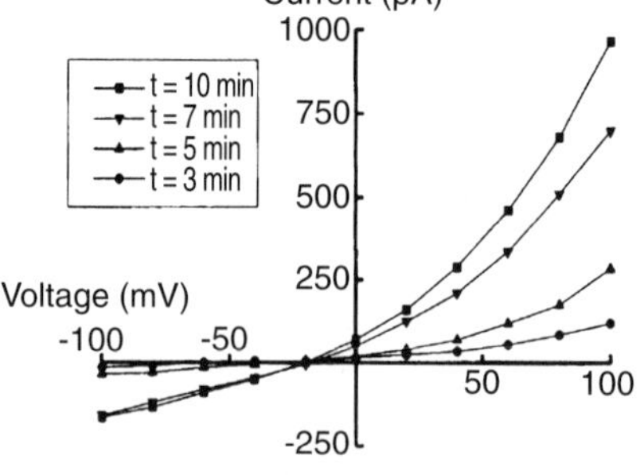

FIGURE 9.6 Cytochalasins activate Cl^- currents in cultured cortical astrocytes. Whole-cell Cl^- currents were elicited in flat polygonal cells when dialyzed with 5 μM cytochalasin B (n = 6), cytochalasin D (n = 4), and dihydrocytochalasin B (n = 3). Average peak current amplitude for all cytochalasin-treated cells was 420 ± 108 pA (n = 13), comparable to the peak amplitude of Cl^- currents in each morphological transformation. The mean zero-current potential for all cells was −28.4 ± 0.9 mV. Some Cl^- current was usually evident 3 minutes after going whole-cell and became maximal 10–20 minutes after the start of the recordings. The cell in this figure expressed peak current 10 minutes after the start of the experiment with 5 μM cytochalasin B. (From Lascola and Kraig Copyright 1996, with permission, by the Society for Neuroscience.)

conate. This indicated the presence of outwardly rectifying Cl^- currents in astrocytes. Surprisingly, however, astrocytes do not show a significant resting Cl^- conductance (Walz, 2002). Indeed, only cell swelling or changes in the morphology of the cells activates these otherwise silent Cl^- channels. This was elegantly demonstrated by Lascola and Kraig (Lascola et al., 1998) (Fig. 9.6) when they showed that changes in the cell's cytoskeleton were both necessary and sufficient to activate outwardly rectifying Cl^- channels in astrocytes. Rounding up cells by brief exposure to trypsin or by exposure to serum-free Ringer's solution, as well as swelling cells by exposure to hypo-osmotic solution, both induced the same outwardly rectifying Cl^- currents. These studies strongly suggest that glial Cl^- channels are intrinsically connected to the cell's cytoskeleton, which may participate in channel activation. The cytoskeleton does not appear to be the only point of regulation of these channels. MacVicar and colleagues showed that hypotonic challenge activates Cl^- currents in cortical astrocytes and that the development of currents is dependent on the activation of mitogen-activated protein kinases (Crépel et al., 1998).

In addition to these outwardly rectifying Cl^- channels that require strong membrane depolarization or changes in cell shape for their activation, glial cells also express inwardly rectifying Cl^- currents under certain conditions. For example, Ferroni and colleagues treated astrocytes for 2 weeks with dibutyryl cyclic adenosine monophosphate (dBcAMP), a drug frequently used to round up cells (Ferroni et al., 1997). Under these conditions they were able to record Cl^- currents. These channels were of small conductance (3–6 pS) and were inhibited by Cd^{2+}. Cl^- currents with similar conductance had previously been demonstrated in mouse cerebral astrocytes (Nowak et al., 1987). Currents were potentiated by hyperpolarization and showed a $Cl^- = Br^- = I^- > F^- >$ cyclamate $>$ gluconate permeability sequence. External application of the putative Cl^- channel blockers DIDS or 4-acetamido-4′-isothiocyanato-2,2′-stilbene disulfonic acid (SITS) did not affect these currents, but anthracene-9-carboxylic acid and Cd^{2+} or Zn^{2+} inhibited it. These features are consistent with those of recombinant ClC-2 channels expressed in oocytes (Furukawa et al., 1998). Analogous to outwardly rectifying Cl^- channels in astrocytes, ClC-2 expressed in oocytes is activated upon actin cytoskeleton disruption (Ahmed et al., 2000). Polymerase chain reaction studies have demonstrated the presence of ClC-2 and ClC-3 transcripts in cultured cortical astrocytes (Stegen et al., 2000), and BR1-VDAC, a member of the VDAC family, has been cloned from bovine brain and shown to constitute a porin in astrocytes (Dermietzel et al., 1994).

The presence of ClC-2 in astrocytes is further supported by immunohistochemical studies that demonstrate the expression of ClC-2 in astrocytes *in vivo*. These channels appear to show a laminar distribution that coincides with that of GABAergic axon terminals (Sik et al., 2000). Based on these findings, the authors suggest that astrocytes may participate in GABAergic transmission by delivering Cl^- ions to layers with intense GABAergic transmission.

Several studies have reported on the expression of swelling-activated Cl^- channels in glia and glioma cells (Jackson and Madsen, 1997) that largely contradict the reported properties for cloned Cl^- channels. These elusive channels, dubbed $I_{CLswell}$ in other cell types, show $I > Cl$ permeability, are blocked by tamoxifen and DIDS, and may require intracellular ATP to be activated (Bond et al., 1999). These channels probably mediate the release of osmotically active anions, possibly including organic osmolites such as taurine (Jackson and Strange, 1993). It is thus possible that the same channel population engages in Cl^- and osmolite secretion.

Astrocytes and Schwann cells do not show significant resting Cl^- conductance, whereas oligodendrocytes do. In addition, astrocytes actively accumulate intracellular Cl^- such that the equilibrium potential for Cl^- in these cells is positive (~ -40 mV) to the resting membrane potential (~ -80 mV) (Kettenmann, 1987). This explains why activation of γ-aminobutyric acid (GABA) receptors, which are ligand-gated Cl^- channels, depolarize astrocytes (Kettenmann et al., 1987), whereas the typical neuronal response is hyperpolarizing. Embryonic neurons also show intracellular Cl^- accumulation that disappears upon cell differentiation (Andersen et al., 1980). This change in the Cl^- gradient across neuronal membranes appears to be influenced by astrocytes (Li et al., 1998).

Opening of Cl^- channels in astrocytes leads to Cl^- efflux. Hence Cl^- channels may play important roles in cell shape and cell volume changes associated with cell proliferation or cell migration. The best evidence for such a role comes from studies of glioma cells that express a high resting Cl^- conductance (Ransom et al., 2001), which is at least partially mediated by CLC-2 channels (Olsen et al., 2003). Inhibition of these channels retards glioma cell migration and invasion (Ransom et al., 2001).

A significant body of work supports the notion that cell swelling induced by hypotonicity or elevated K^+ activates Cl^- channels that are normally silent. Indeed, numerous neurological conditions have been reported to present with edema and show marked swelling of astrocytes (Kimelberg, 1995). At least *in vitro*, astrocytes respond to hypotonic swelling with a characteristic regulatory volume decrease (RVD) (Pasantes-Morales et al., 1994). This process is still not entirely understood but clearly involves the extrusion of osmotically active anions, Cl^- and taurin among them, to aid the secretion of water and may regulate the cell volume back to a normal value (Pasantes-Morales, 1996). As alluded to before, the molecular identity of the channel(s) involved in this process is unknown.

SUMMARY

Following the exciting discovery of voltage-activated ion channels in glial cells, a very significant effort has been made to validate their expression *in situ* and *in vivo*. Through the collective effort of numerous laboratories, the notion that these channels were a culture artifact has now been dismissed, and this represents a significant achievement. These studies have also uncovered evidence that glial membrane properties are not static and that glial cells respond to signals in their native microenvironment. Tantalizing findings suggest that they may be much more engaged in shaping neuronal responses than had previously been thought.

ACKNOWLEDGMENTS

The authors wish to acknowledge the diligent work in many laboratories that has contributed to our current understanding of ion channels in glial cells. Space limitations and a limit on the number of references prevented us from discussing and citing many important studies. Our objective was to distill common themes, and we apologize to those who feel that their valuable contributions are not represented. We wish to thank those investigators who allowed us to reproduce figures from their published work. We also wish to acknowledge the valuable input provided by Kimberly Parkerson. The authors are grateful for the continued supported by grants from the National Institutes of Health (RO1 NS-31234, RO1 NS-36692, and PO1-HD38760).

ABBREVIATIONS

4-AP	4-aminopyridine
ATP	adenosine triphosphate
BK	large-conductance K_{Ca} channel
$[Ca^{2+}]_i$	intracellular Ca^{2+}
$[Ca^{2+}]_o$	extracellular Ca^{2+}
cAMP	cyclic adenosine monophosphate
CFTR	cystic fibrosis transmembrane conductance regulator
ClC	voltage-gated chloride channel
CNS	central nervous system
dBcAMP	dibutyryl cyclic adenosine monophosphate
DIDS	4,4′-diisothiocyanato-stilbene-2,2′-disulfonic acid
DRG	dorsal root ganglion
E_K	potassium equilibrium potential
GABA	γ-aminobutyric acid
HVA	high voltage-activated
I_A	current mediated by K_A
IK	intermediate-conductance K_{Ca} channel
$[K^+]_o$	extracellular potassium
K_A	rapidly inactivating A-type potassium channel
K_{Ca}	calcium-activated potassium channel
K_D	delayed rectifier potassium channel
K_{ir}	inwardly rectifying potassium channel
Kv	voltage-dependent potassium channel
LVA	low voltage-activated
Na_v	voltage-gated sodium channel
NMDA	*N*-methyl-D-aspartate
PCR	polymerase chain reaction
pg322 AMPA	α-amino-3-hydroxy-5-methyl-isoxazolepropionic acid
PKA	protein kinase A
PKC	protein kinase C
RMP	resting membrane potential
RT-PCR	reverse transcriptase–polymerase chain reaction
RVD	regulatory volume decrease
SK	small-conductance K_{Ca} channel
SITS	4-acetamido-4′ isothiocyanato-2,2′-stilbenedisulfonic acid
STX	saxitoxin
TEA	tetraethylammonium
TTX	tetrodotoxin
TTX-R	tetrodotoxin-resistant
TTX-S	tetrodotoxin-sensitive
VDAC	voltage-dependent anion-selective channel

REFERENCES

Ahmed, N., Ramjeesingh, M., Wong, S., Varga, A., Garami, E., and Bear, C.E. (2000) Chloride channel activity of ClC-2 is modified by the actin cytoskeleton. *Biochem. J.* 352:3–794.

Akopian, G., Kressin, K., Derouiche, A., and Steinhauser, C. (1996) Identified glial cells in the early postnatal mouse hippocampus display different types of Ca^{2+} currents. *Glia* 17:181–194.

Amedee, T., Ellie, E., Dupouy, B., and Vincent, J.D. (1991) Voltage-dependent calcium and potassium channels in Schwann cells cultured from dorsal root ganglia of the mouse. *J. Physiol.* (*Lond.*) 441:35–56.

Andersen, P., Dingledine, R., Gjerstad, L., Langmoen, I.A., and

Laursen, A.M. (1980) Two different responses of hippocampal pyramidal cells to application of gamma-aminobutyric acid. *J. Physiol.* 305:279–296.

Attali, B., Wang, N., Kolot, A., Sobko, A., Cherepanov, V., and Soliven, B. (1997) Characterization of delayed rectifier Kv channels in oligodendrocytes and progenitor cells. *J. Neurosci.* 17:8234–8245.

Barres, B.A., Chun, L.L.Y., and Corey, D.P. (1989a) Calcium current in cortical astrocytes: induction by cAMP and neurotransmitters and permissive effect of serum factors. *J. Neurosci.* 9: 3169–3175.

Barres, B.A., Chun, L.L.Y., and Corey, D.P. (1989b) Glial and neuronal forms of the voltage-dependent sodium channel: characteristics and cell type distribution. *Neuron* 2:1375–1388.

Barres, B.A., Koroshetz, W.J., Chun, L L.Y., and Corey, D.P. (1990a) Ion channel expression by white matter glia: the type-1 astrocyte. *Neuron* 5:527–544.

Barres, B.A., Koroshetz, W.J., Swartz, K.J., Chun, L.L.Y., and Corey, D.P. (1990b) Ion channel expression by white matter glia: the O2A glial progenitor cell. *Neuron* 4:507–524.

Beaudu-Lange, C., Despeyroux, S., Marcaggi, P., Coles, J.A., and Amedee, T. (1998) Functional Ca^{2+} and Na^{+} channels on mouse Schwann cells cultured in serum-free medium: regulation by a diffusible factor from neurons and by cAMP. *Eur. J. Neurosci.* 10: 1796–1809.

Belcher, S.M., Zerillo, C.A., Levenson, R., Ritchie, J.M., and Howe, J.R. (1995) Cloning of a sodium channel α subunit from rabbit Schwann cells. *PNAS* 92:11034–11038.

Berger, T., Schnitzer, J., and Kettenmann, H. (1991) Developmental changes in the membrane current pattern, K^{+} buffer capacity, and morphology of glial cells in the corpus callosum slice. *J. Neurosci.* 11:3008–3024.

Berger, T., Schnitzer, J., Orkand, P.M., and Kettenmann, H. (1992) Sodium and calcium currents in glial cells of the mouse corpus callosum slice. *Eur. J. Neurosci.* 4:1271–1284.

Bevan, S., Chiu, S.Y., Gray, P.T.A., and Ritchie, J.M. (1984) Sodium channels in rat cultured astrocytes. *J. Physiol. (Lond.)* 361:18P.

Bevan, S., Chiu, S.Y., Gray, P.T.A., and Ritchie, J.M. (1985) The presence of voltage-gated sodium, potassium and chloride channels in rat cultured astrocytes. *Proc. R. Soc. Lond. B Biol. Sci.* B225:299–313.

Bevan, S. and Raff, M. (1985) Voltage-dependent potassium currents in cultured astrocytes. *Nature* 315:229–232.

Black, J.A., Dib-Hajj, S., Cohen, S., Hinson, A.W., and Waxman, S.G. (1998) Glial cells have heart: rH1 Na^{+} channel mRNA and protein in spinal cord astrocytes. *Glia* 23:200–208.

Black, J.A., Westenbroek, R., Minturn, J.E., Ransom, B.R., Catterall, W.A., and Waxman, S.G. (1995) Isoform-specific expression of sodium channels in astrocytes in vitro: immunocytochemical observations. *Glia* 14:133–144.

Black, J.A., Westenbroek, R., Ransom, B.R., Catterall, W.A., and Waxman, S.G. (1994a) Type II sodium channels in spinal cord astrocytes in situ: immunocytochemical observations. *Glia* 12: 219–227.

Black, J.A., Yokoyama, S., Waxman, S.G., Oh, Y., Zur, K.B., Sontheimer, H., Higashida, H., and Ransom, B.R. (1994b) Sodium channel mRNAs in cultured spinal cord astrocytes: in situ hybridization in identified cell types. *Mol. Brain. Res.* 23:235–245.

Bond, T., Basavappa, S., Christensen, M., and Strange, K. (1999) ATP dependence of the ICl, swell channel varies with rate of cell swelling. Evidence for two modes of channel activation. *J. Gen. Physiol.* 113:441–456.

Bootman, M.D., Berridge, M.J., and Roderick, H.L. (2002) Calcium signalling: more messengers, more channels, more complexity. *Curr. Biol.* 12:R563–R565.

Bordey, A. and Sontheimer, H. (1997) Postnatal development of ionic currents in rat hippocampal astrocytes in situ. *J. Neurophysiol.* 78:461–477.

Bordey, A. and Sontheimer, H. (2000) Ion channel expression by astrocytes in situ: comparison of different CNS regions. *Glia* 30: 27–38.

Bringmann, A., Faude, F,. Reichenbachx, A. (1997) Mammalian retinal glial (Müller) cells express large-conductance Ca^{2+}-activated K^{+} channels that are modulated by Mg^{2+} and pH and activated by protein kinase A. *Glia* 19:311–323.

Bringmann, A., Biedermann, B., and Reichenbach, A. (1999a) Expression of potassium channels during postnatal differentiation of rabbit Müller glial cells. *Eur. J. Neurosci.* 11:2883–2896.

Bringmann, A., Francke, M., Pannicke, T., Biedermann, B., Kodal, H., Faude, F., Reichelt, W., and Reichenbach, A. (2000a) Role of glial K^{+} channels in ontogeny and gliosis: a hypothesis based upon studies on Müller cells. *Glia* 29:35–44.

Bringmann, A., Schopf, S., Faude, F., and Reichenbach, A. (2001) Arachidonic acid-induced inhibition of Ca^{2+} channel currents in retinal glial (Müller) cells. *Graefes Arch. Clin. Exp. Ophthalmol.* 239:859–864.

Bringmann, A., Schopf, S., Faude, F., Skatchkov, S.N., Enzmann, V., and Reichenbach, A. (1999b) The activity of a transient potassium current in retinal glial (Müller) cells depends on extracellular calcium. *J. Hirnforsch.* 39:539–550.

Bringmann, A., Schopf, S., and Reichenbach, A. (2000b) Developmental regulation of calcium channel-mediated currents in retinal glial (Müller) cells. *J. Neurophysiol.* 84:2975–2983.

Bychkov, R., Glowinski, J., and Giaume, C. (2001) Sequential and opposite regulation of two outward K(+) currents by ET-1 in cultured striatal astrocytes. *Am. J. Physiol. Cell Physiol.* 281:C1373–C1384.

Catterall, W.A., Nunoki, K., Lai, Y., De, J.K., Thomsen, W., and Rossie, S. (1990) Structure and modulation of voltage-sensitive sodium and calcium channels. *Adv. Second Messenger Phosphoprotein Res.* 24:30–35.

Chao, T.I., Grosche, J., Friedrich, K.J., Biedermann, B., Francke, M., Pannicke, T., Reichelt, W., Wulst, M., Mühle, C., Pritz-Hohmeier, S., Kuhrt, H., Faude, F., Drommer, W., Kasper, M., Buse, E., and Reichenbach, A. (1997) Comparative studies on mammalian Müller (retinal glial) cells. *J. Neurocytol.* 26:439–454.

Chao, T.I., Henke, A., Reichelt, W., Eberhardt, W., Reinhardt-Maelicke, S., and Reichenbach, A. (1994) Three distinct types of voltage-dependent K^{+} channels are expressed by Müller (glial) cells of the rabbit retina. *Pflügers Arch.* 426:51–60.

Chittajallu, R., Chen, Y., Wang, H., Yuan, X., Ghiani, C.A., Heckman, T., McBain, C.J., and Gallo, V. (2002) Regulation of Kv1 subunit expression in oligodendrocyte progenitor cells and their role in G1/S phase progression of the cell cycle. *Proc. Natl. Acad. Sci. USA* 99:2350–2355.

Chiu, S.Y. (1991) Functions and distribution of voltage-gated sodium and potassium channels in mammalian Schwann cells. *Glia* 4:541–558.

Chiu, S.Y. (1993) Differential expression of sodium channels in acutely isolated myelinating and non-myelinating Schwann cells of rabbits. *J. Physiol.* 470:485–499.

Chiu, S.Y., Schrager, P., and Ritchie, J.M. (1984) Neuronal-type Na^{+} and K^{+} channels in rabbit cultured Schwann cells. *Nature* 311:156–157.

Chiu, S.Y. and Schwarz, W. (1987) Sodium and potassium currents in acutely demyelinated internodes of rabbit sciatic nerves. *J. Physiol. (Lond.)* 391:631–649.

Chvátal, A., Pastor, A., Mauch, M., Syková, E., and Kettenmann, H. (1995) Distinct populations of identified glial cells in the developing rat spinal cord slice: ion channel properties and cell morphology. *Eur. J. Neurosci.* 7:129–142.

Clark, B.A. and Mobbs, P. (1994) Voltage-gated currents in rabbit retinal astrocytes. *Eur. J. Neurosci.* 6:1406–1414.

Coetzee, W.A., Amarillo, Y., Chiu, J., Chow, A., Lau, D., McCormack, T., Moreno, H., Nadal, M.S., Ozaita, A., Pountney, D.,

Saganich, M., Vega-Saenz, D.M., and Rudy, B. (1999) Molecular diversity of K+ channels. *Ann. NY Acad. Sci.* 868:233–285.

Connor, J.A. and Stevens, C.F. (1971) Voltage clamp studies of a transient outward membrane current in gastropod neural somata. *J. Physiol.* 213:21–30.

Corvalan, V., Cole, R., deVellis, J., and Hagiwara, S. (1990) Neuronal modulation of calcium channel activity in cultured rat astrocytes. *PNAS* 87:4345–4348.

Crépel, V., Panenka, W., Kelly, M.E.M., and MacVicar, B.A. (1998) Mitogen-activated protein and tyrosine kinases in the activation of astrocyte volume-activated chloride current. *J. Neurosci.* 18:1196–1206.

Dermietzel, R., Hwang, T.-K., Buettner, R., Hofer, A., Dotzler, E., Kremer, M., Deutzmann, R., Thinnes, F.P., Fishman, G.I., Spray, D.C., and Siemen, D. (1994) Cloning and *in situ* localization of a brain-derived porin that constitutes a large-conductance anion channel in astrocytic plasma membranes. *PNAS* 91:499–503.

Duffy, S. and MacVicar, B.A. Potassium-dependent calcium influx in acutely isolated hippocampal astrocytes. *Neuroscience* 61:51–61.

Ferroni, S., Marchini, C., Nobile, M., and Rapisarda, C. (1997) Characterization of an inwardly rectifying chloride conductance expressed by cultured rat cortical astrocytes. *Glia* 21:217–227.

Francke, M., Pannicke, T., Biedermann, B., Faude, F., Wiedemann, P., Reichenbach, A., and Reichelt, W. (1997) Loss of inwardly rectifying potassium currents by human retinal glial cells in diseases of the eye. *Glia* 20:210–218.

Francke, M., Weick, M., Pannicke, T., Uckermann, O., Grosche, J., Groczalik, I., Milenkovic, I., Uhlmann, S., Faude, F., Wiedemann, P., Reichenbach, A., Bringmann, A. (2002) Upregulation of extracellular ATP-induced Müller cell responses in adipase model of proliferative vitreoretinopathy. *Invest. Ophthalmol. Vis. Sci.* 43:870–81.

Fraser, S.P., Ding, Y., Liu, A., Foster, C.S., and Djamgoz, M.B. (1999) Tetrodotoxin suppresses morphological enhancement of the metastatic MAT-LyLu rat prostate cancer cell line. *Cell Tissue Res.* 295:505–512.

Furukawa, T., Ogura, T., Katayama, Y., and Hiraoka, M. (1998) Characteristics of rabbit ClC-2 current expressed in Xenopus oocytes and its contribution to volume regulation. *Am. J. Physiol.* 274:C500-12.

Gautron, S., Dossantos, G., Pintohenrique, D., Koulakoff, A., Gros, F., and Berwald-Netter, Y. (1992) The glial voltage-gated sodium channel—cell-specific and tissue-specific messenger RNA expression. *PNAS* 89:7272–7276.

Ghiani, C.A., Yuan, X.Q., Eisen, A.M., Knutson, P.L., DePinho, R.A., McBain, C.J., and Gallo, V. (1999) Voltage-activated K^+ channels and membrane depolarization regulate accumulation of the cyclin-dependent kinase inhibitors $p277^{Kip1}$ and $p21^{CIP1}$ in glial progenitor cells. *J. Neurosci.* 19:5380–5392.

Goldin, A.L., Barchi, R.L., Caldwell, J.H., Hofmann, F., Howe, J.R., Hunter, J.C., Kallen, R.G., Mandel, G., Meisler, M.H., Netter, Y.B., Noda, M., Tamkun, M.M., Waxman, S.G., Wood, J.N., and Catterall, W.A. (2000) Nomenclature of voltage-gated sodium channels. *Neuron* 28:365–368.

Gray, P.T.A. and Ritchie, J.M. (1985) Ion channels in Schwann and glial cells. *TINS* 8:411–415.

Gray, P.T.A. and Ritchie, J.M. (1986) A voltage-gated chloride conductance in rat cultured astrocytes. *Proc. R. Soc. Lond. B Biol. Sci.* 228:267–288.

Grosche, J., Matyash, V., Moller, T., Verkhratsky, A., Reichenbach, A., and Kettenmann, H. (1999) Microdomains for neuron-glia interaction: parallel fiber signaling to Bergmann glial cells. *Nat. Neurosci.* 2:139–143.

Heinemann, S., Rettig, J., Scott, V., Parcej, D.N., Lorra, C., Dolly, J., and Pongs, O. (1994) The inactivation behaviour of voltage-gated K-channels may be determined by association of alpha- and beta-subunits. *J. Physiol.* (*Paris*) 88:173–180.

Higashi, K., Fujita, A., Inanobe, A., Tanemoto, M., Doi, K., Kubo, T., and Kurachi, Y. (2001) An inwardly rectifying K(+) channel, Kir4.1, expressed in astrocytes surrounds synapses and blood vessels in brain. *Am. J. Physiol. Cell Physiol.* 281:C922–C931.

Hille, B. (2001) *Ionic Channels of Excitable Membranes*. Sunderland, MA: Sinauer.

Ishii, M., Horio, Y., Tada, Y., Hibino, H., Inanobe, A., Ito, M., Yamada, M., Gotow, T., Uchiyama, Y., and Kurachi, Y. (1997) Expression and clustered distribution of an inwardly rectifying potassium channel, KAB-2/Kir4.1, on mammalian retinal Müller cell membrane: their regulation by insulin and laminin signals. *J. Neurosci.* 17:7725–7735.

Jackson, P.S. and Madsen, J.R. (1997) Identification of the volume-sensitive organic osmolyte anion channel in human glial cells. *Pediatr. Neurosurg.* 27:286–291.

Jackson, P.S. and Strange, K. (1993) Volume-sensitive anion channels mediate swelling-activated inositol and taurine efflux. *Am. J. Physiol.* 265:C1489–500.

Jentsch, T.J., Friedrich, T., Schriever, A., and Yamada, H. (1999) The CLC chloride channel family. *Pflügers Arch.* 437:783–795.

Kaczorowski, G.J. and Garcia, M.L. (1999) Pharmacology of voltage-gated and calcium-activated potassium channels. *Curr. Opin. Chem. Biol.* 3:448–458.

Kettenmann, H. (1987) K^+ and Cl^- uptake by cultured oligodendrocytes. *Can. J. Physiol. Pharmacol.* 65:1033–1037.

Kettenmann, H., Backus, K.H., and Schachner, M. (1987) Gamma-aminobutyric acid opens Cl-channels in cultured astrocytes. *Brain Res.* 404:1–9.

Kimelberg, H.K. (1995) Current concepts of brain edema. *J. Neurosurg.* 83:1051–1059.

Kodal, H., Weick, M., Moll, V., Biedermann, B., Reichenbach, A., and Bringmann, A. (2000) Involvement of calcium-activated potassium channels in the regulation of DNA synthesis in cultured Müller glial cells. *Invest. Ophthalmol. Vis. Sci.* 41:4262–4267.

Kofuji, P., Biedermann, B., Siddharthan, V., Raap, M., Iandiev, I., Milenkovic, I., Thomzig, A., Veh, R.W., Bringmann, A., and Reichenbach, A. (2002) Kir potassium channel subunit expression in retinal glial cells: implications for spatial potassium buffering. *Glia* 39:292–303.

Kofuji, P., Ceelen, P., Zahs, K.R., Surbeck, L.W., Lester, H.A., and Newman, E.A. (2000) Genetic inactivation of an inwardly rectifying potassium channel (Kir4.1 subunit) in mice: phenotypic impact in retina. *J. Neurosci.* 20:5733–5740.

Konishi, T. (1989) Voltage-dependent potassium channels in cultured mammalian Schwann cells. *Brain Res.* 499:273–280.

Kressin, K., Kuprijanova, E., Jabs, R., Seifert, G., and Steinhäuser, C. (1995) Developmental regulation of Na^+ and K^+ conductances in glial cells of mouse hippocampal brain slices. *Glia* 15:173–187.

Kubo, Y., Baldwin, T.J., Jan, Y.N., and Jan, L.Y. (1993) Primary structure and functional expression of a mouse inward rectifier potassium channel [see comments]. *Nature* 362:127–133.

Labrakakis, C., Patt, S., Weydt, P., Cervos-Navarro, J., Meyer, R., and Kettenmann, H. (1997) Action potential-generating cells in human glioblastomas. *J. Neuropathol. Exp. Neurol.* 56:243–254.

Lascola, C.D., Kraig, R.P. (1996) Whole-cell chloride currents in rat astrocytes accompany changes in cell morphology. *J. Neuro. Sci.* 16:2532–2545.

Lascola, C.D., Nelson, D.J., and Kraig, R.P. (1998) Cytoskeletal actin gates a Cl^- channel in neocortical astrocytes. *J. Neurosci.* 18: 1679–1692.

Li, L., Head, V., and Timpe, L.C. (2001) Identification of an inward rectifier potassium channel gene expressed in mouse cortical astrocytes. *Glia* 33:57–71.

Li, Y.X., Schaffner, A.E., Walton, M.K., and Barker, J.L. (1998) Astrocytes regulate developmental changes in the chloride ion gradient of embryonic rat ventral spinal cord neurons in culture. *J. Physiol.* 509:847–858.

MacFarlane, S.N. and Sontheimer, H. (1997) Electrophysiological changes that accompany reactive gliosis *in vitro*. *J. Neurosci.* 17:7316–7329.

MacFarlane, S.N. and Sontheimer, H. (2000a) Changes in ion channel expression accompany cell cycle progression of spinal cord astrocytes. *Glia* 30:39–48.

MacFarlane, S.N. and Sontheimer, H. (2000b) Modulation of kv1.5 currents by src tyrosine phosphorylation: potential role in the differentiation of astrocytes. *J. Neurosci.* 20:5245–5253.

MacVicar, B.A. (1984) Voltage-dependent calcium channels in glial cells. *Science* 226:1345–1347.

MacVicar, B.A. and Tse, F.W.Y. (1988) Norepinephrine and cyclic adenosine 3′:5′-cyclic monophosphate enhance a nifedipine-sensitive calcium current in cultured rat astrocytes. *Glia* 1:359–365.

McLarnon, J.G. and Kim, S.U. (1989) Existence of inward potassium currents in adult human oligodendrocytes. *Neurosci. Lett.* 101:107–112.

Mi, H., Deerinck, T.J., Ellisman, M.H., and Schwarz, T.L. (1995) Differential distribution of closely related potassium channels in rat Schwann cells. *J. Neurosci.* 15:3761–3774.

Mi, H., Harris-Warrick, R.M., Deerinck, T.J., Inman, I., Ellisman, M.H., and Schwarz, T.L. (1999) Identification and localization of Ca(2+)-activated K+ channels in rat sciatic nerve. *Glia* 26: 166–175.

Minturn, J.E., Sontheimer, H., Black, J.A., Ransom, B.R., and Waxman, S.G. (1992) Sodium channel expression in optic nerve astrocytes chronically deprived of axonal contact. *Glia* 6:19–29.

Moll, V., Weick, M., Milenkovic, I., Kodal, H., Reichenbach, A., and Bringmann, A. (2002) P2Y receptor-mediated stimulation of Müller glial DNA synthesis. *Invest. Ophthalmol. Vis. Sci.* 43:766–773.

Nagelhus, E.A., Horio, Y., Inanobe, A., Fujita, A., Haug, F.M., Nielsen, S., Kurachi, Y., and Ottersen, O.P. (1999) Immunogold evidence suggests that coupling of K^+ siphoning and water transport in rat retinal Müller cells is mediated by a coenrichment of Kir4.1 and AQP4 in specific membrane domains. *Glia* 26:47–54.

Neusch, C., Rozengurt, N., Jacobs, R.E., Lester, H.A., and Kofuji, P. (2001) Kir4.1 potassium channel subunit is crucial for oligodendrocyte development and in vivo myelination. *J. Neurosci.* 21:5429–5438.

Newman, E.A. (1985) Voltage dependent calcium and potassium channels in retinal glial cells. *Nature* 317:809–811.

Newman, E.A. (2003) Müller cells in retinal pigment epithelium. In: Albert, D.M. and Jakobiec, F.A., eds. *Principles and Practice of Opthalmology*. Philidelphia: Saunders, pp. 1763–1785.

Nowak, L., Ascher, P., and Berwald-Netter, Y. (1987) Ionic channels in mouse astrocytes in culture. *J. Neurosci.* 7:101–109.

Oh, Y., Black, J.A., and Waxman, S.G. (1994a) Rat brain Na^+ channel mRNAs in non-excitable Schwann cells. *FEBS Lett.* 350: 342–346.

Oh, Y., Black, J.A., and Waxman, S.G. (1994b) The expression of rat brain voltage-sensitive Na^+ channel mRNAs in astrocytes. *Brain Res. Mol.* 57–65.

Olsen, M.L., Schade, S., Lyons, S.A., Amaral, M.D., Sontheimer, H. (2003) Expression of voltage-gated Cl^- channels in human glioma cells. *J. Neurosci.* 23:5572–5582.

Orkand, R.K., Nicholls, J.G., and Kuffler, S.W. (1966) Effect of nerve impulses on the membrane potential of glial cells in the central nervous system of amphibia. *J. Neurophysiol.* 29:788–806.

Pasantes-Morales, H. (1996) Volume regulation in brain cells: cellular and molecular mechanisms. *Metab. Brain Dis.* 11:187–204.

Pasantes-Morales, H., Murray, R.A., Lilja, L., and Moran, J. (1994) Regulatory volume decrease in cultured astrocytes. I. Potassium- and chloride-activated permeability. *Am. J. Physiol.* 266:C165–71.

Peretz, A., Sobko, A., and Attali, B. (1999) Tyrosine kinases modulate K^+ channel gating in mouse Schwann cells. *J. Physiol.* 519: 373–384.

Poopalasundaram, S., Knott, C., Shamotienko, O.G., Foran, P.G., Dolly, J.O., Ghiani, C.A., Gallo, V., and Wilkin, G.P. (2000) Glial heterogeneity in expression of the inwardly rectifying K^+ channel, Kir4.1, in adult rat CNS. *Glia* 30:362–372.

Price, D.L., Ludwig, J.W., Mi, H., Schwarz, T.L., and Ellisman, M.H. (2002) Distribution of rSlo Ca(2+)-activated K(+) channels in rat astrocyte perivascular endfeet. *Brain Res.* 956:183–193.

Puro, D.G., Hwang, J.J., Kwon, O.J., and Chin, H.M. (1996a) Characterization of an L-type calcium channel expressed by human retinal Müller (glial) cells. *Mol. Brain Res.* 37:41–48.

Puro, D.G., Yuan, J.P., and Sucher, N.J. (1996b) Activation of NMDA receptor-channels in human retinal Müller glial cells inhibits inward-rectifying potassium currents. *Vis. Neurosci.* 13:319–326.

Quandt, F.N. and MacVicar, B.A. (1986) Calcium activated potassium channels in cultured astrocytes. *Neuroscience* 19:29–41.

Raap, M., Biedermann, B., Braun, P., Milenkovic, I., Skatchkov, S.N., Bringmann, A., and Reichenbach, A. (2002) Diversity of Kir channel subunit mRNA expressed by retinal glial cells of the guinea-pig. *NeuroReport* 13:1037–1040.

Ransom, C.B. and Sontheimer H. (2001) BK channels in human glioma cells. *J. Neurophysiol.* 85:790–803.

Ransom, C.B., O'Neal, J.T., and Sontheimer, H. (2001) Volume-activated chloride currents contribute to the resting conductance and invasive migration of human glioma cells. *J. Neurosci.* 21:7674–7683.

Ransom, C.B. and Sontheimer, H. (1995) Biophysical and pharmacological characterization of inwardly rectifying K^+ currents in rat spinal cord astrocytes. *J. Neurophysiol.* 73:333–345.

Ransom, C.B., Sontheimer, H., and Janigro, D. (1996) Astrocytic inwardly rectifying potassium currents are dependent on external sodium ions. *J. Neurophysiol.* 76:626–630.

Ritchie, J.M. and Rang, H.P. (1983) Extraneuronal saxitoxin binding sites in rabbit myelinated nerve. *PNAS* 80:2803–2807.

Rose, C.R., Ransom, B.R., and Waxman, S.G. (1997) Pharmacological characterization of Na^+ influx via voltage-gated Na^+ channels in spinal cord astrocytes. *J. Neurophysiol.* 78:3249–3258.

Roy, M.-L. and Sontheimer, H. (1995) β-Adrenergic modulation of glial inwardly rectifying potassium channels. *J. Neurochem.* 64:1576–1584.

Sah, P. and Faber, E.S. (2002) Channels underlying neuronal calcium-activated potassium currents. *Prog. Neurobiol.* 66:345–353.

Schaller, K.L., Krzemien, D.M., Yarowsky, P.J., Krueger, B.K., and Caldwell, J.H. (1995) A novel, abundant sodium channel expressed in neurons and glia. *J. Neurosci.* 15:3231–3242.

Schopf, S., Bringmann, A., and Reichenbach, A. (1999) Protein kinases A and C are opponents in modulating glial Ca^{2+}-activated K^+ channels. *NeuroReport*. 10:1323–1327.

Schroder, W., Seifert, G., Huttmann, K., Hinterkeuser, S., and Steinhauser, C. (2002) AMPA receptor-mediated modulation of inward rectifier K(+) channels in astrocytes of mouse hippocampus. *Mol. Cell Neurosci.* 19:447–458.

Sik, A., Smith, R.L., and Freund, T.F. (2000) Distribution of chloride channel-2-immunoreactive neuronal and astrocytic processes in the hippocampus. *Neuroscience* 101:51–65.

Sobko, A., Peretz, A., Shirihai, O., Etkin, S., Cherepanova, V., Dagan, D., and Attali, B. (1998) Heteromultimeric delayed-rectifier K^+ channels in Schwann cells: developmental expression and role in cell proliferation. *J. Neurosci.* 18:10398–10408.

Sontheimer, H., Black, J.A., Ransom, B.R., and Waxman, S.G. (1992a) Ion channels in spinal cord astrocytes in vitro: I. Transient expression of high levels of Na^+ and K^+ channels. *J. Neurophysiol.* 68:985–1000.

Sontheimer, H., Black, J.A., and Waxman, S.G. (1996) Voltage-gated Na^+ channels in glia: properties and possible functions. *TINS* 19:325–331.

Sontheimer, H., Fernandez-Marques, E., Ullrich, N., Pappas, C.A., and Waxman, S.G. (1994) Astrocyte Na^+ channels are required for maintenance of Na^+/K^+-ATPase activity. *J. Neurosci.* 14: 2464–2475.

Sontheimer, H. and Kettenmann, H. (1988) Heterogeneity of potassium currents in cultured oligodendrocytes. *Glia* 1:415–420.

Sontheimer, H., Ransom, B.R., and Waxman, S.G. (1992b) Different Na^+ currents from P0 and P7-derived hippocampal astrocyes in vitro: evidence for a switch in Na^+ channel expression in vivo. *Brain Res.* 597:24–29.

Sontheimer, H., Trotter, J., Schachner, M., and Kettenmann, H. (1989) Channel expression correlates with differentiation stage during development of oligodendrocytes from their precursor cells in culture. *Neuron* 2:1135–1145.

Sontheimer, H. and Waxman, S.G. (1992) Ion channels in spinal cord astrocytes in vitro: II. Biophysical and pharmacological analysis of two Na+ current types. *J. Neurophysiol.* 68:1001–1011.

Sontheimer, H. and Waxman, S.G. (1993) Expression of voltage-activated ion channels by astrocytes and oligodendrocytes in the hippocampal slice. *J. Neurophysiol.* 70:1863–1873.

Stegen, C., Matskevich, I., Wagner, C.A., Paulmichl, M., Lang, F., and Broer, S. (2000) Swelling-induced taurine release without chloride channel activity in *Xenopus laevis* oocytes expressing anion channels and transporters. *Biochim. Biophys Acta* 1467:91–100.

Steinhauser, C., Berger, T., Frotscher, M., and Kettenmann, H. (1992) Heterogeneity in the membrane current pattern of identified glial cells in the hippocampal slice. *Eur. J. Neurosci.* 4:472–484.

Steinhäuser, C., Kressin, K., Kuprijanova, E., Weber, M., and Seifert, G. (1994) Properties of voltage-activated Na^+ and K^+ currents in mouse hippocampal glial cells in situ and after acute isolation from tissue slices. *Pflügers Arch.* 428:610–620.

Thio, C.L. and Sontheimer, H. (1993) Differential modulation of TTX-sensitive and TTX-resistant Na^+ channels in spinal cord astrocytes following activation of PKC. *J. Neurosci.* 13:4889–4897.

Thio, C.L., Waxman, S.G., and Sontheimer, H. (1993) Ion channels in spinal cord astrocytes in vitro: III. Modulation of channel expression by co-culture with neurons and neuron-conditioned medium. *J. Neurophysiol.* 69:819–831.

Thomzig, A., Wenzel, M., Karschin, C., Eaton, M.J., Skatchkov, S.N., Karschin, A., and Veh, R.W. (2001) Kir6.1 is the principal pore-forming subunit of astrocyte but not neuronal plasma membrane K-ATP channels. *Mol. Cell Neurosci.* 18:671–690.

Tse, F.W., Fraser, D.D., Duffy, S., and MacVicar, B.A. (1992) Voltage-activated K+ currents in acutely isolated hippocampal astrocytes. *J. Neurosci.* 12:1781–1788.

Verkhratsky, A.N., Orkand, R.K., and Kettenmann, H. (1998) Glial calcium: homeostasis and signaling function. *Physiol. Rev.* 78:99–141.

Verkhratsky, A.N. and Steinhauser, C. (2000) Ion channels in glial cells. *Brain Res. Brain Res. Rev.* 32:380–412.

Verkhratsky, A.N., Trotter, J., and Kettenmann, H. (1990) Cultured glial precursor cells from mouse cortex express two types of calcium currents. *Neurosci. Lett.* 112:194–198.

Walz, W. (2000) Role of astrocytes in the clearance of excess extracellular potassium. *Neurochem. Int.* 36:291–300.

Walz, W. (2002) Chloride/anion channels in glial cell membranes. *Glia* 40:1–10.

Westenbroek, R.E., Bausch, S.B., Lin, R.C.S., Franck, J.E., Noebels, J.L., and Catterall, W.A. (1998) Upregulation of L-type Ca^{2+} channels in reactive astrocytes after brain injury, hypomyelination, and ischemia. *J. Neurosci.* 18:2321–2334.

Wilson, G.F. and Chiu, S.Y. (1990) Ion channels in axon and Schwann cell membranes at paranodes of mammalian myelinated fibers studied with patch-clamp. *J. Neurosci.* 10:3263–3274.

Wilson, G.F. and Chiu, S.Y. (1993) Mitogenic factors regulate ion channels in Schwann cells cultured from newborn rat sciatic nerve. *J. Physiol. (Lond.)* 470:501–520.

10 Receptors for neurotransmitters and hormones

HELMUT KETTENMANN AND CHRISTIAN STEINHÄUSER

Until about 20 years ago, the expression of neurotransmitter receptors in the nervous system was considered an exclusive property of neurons. Astrocytes were viewed as electrically silent elements that would not participate in the information processing of the central nervous system (CNS). The complete lack of synaptic structures onto or from glial cells supported this assumption. This view was challenged by a series of studies in cell culture demonstrating that astrocytes, oligodendrocytes, and Schwann cells had the potential to express transmitter receptors. In the culture dish, the astrocyte seemed to be the most versatile glial cell type in that almost all receptors for important transmitter systems were expresssed. Two exceptions remained: *N*-methyl-D-aspartate (NMDA) and glycine receptors. In the early 1990s the studies were extended to acute brain slices, and it became evident that astrocytes and, to a lesser extent, oligodendrocytes expressed functional receptors in this more intact preparation. Interestingly, the two receptor types lacking in culture, namely, NMDA and glycine, were now found to be functionally expressed by glial cells from defined regions of the CNS. Very recently, microglial cells also joined the club of transmitter receptor expressing cells. In the following sections, we will describe the receptor repertoire expressed by the different types of glial cells.

ASTROCYTES

Ionotropic Glutamate Receptors

A wealth of information is available describing properties of ionotropic glutamate receptors (iGluRs) in astrocytes both in cell culture and *in situ* (recently reviewed by Seifert and Steinhäuser, 2001). About 20 years ago, two groups provided the first evidence that not only neurons but also astrocytes express functional iGluRs (Bowman and Kimelberg, 1984; Kettenmann et al., 1984). Cultured astrocytes express both α-amino-3-hydroxy-5-methyl-γ-isoxazolepropionate (AMPA) (assembled from subunits GluR1–GluR4) and kainate receptors (GluR5–GluR7, KA1, KA2). Functional AMPA receptors have been described in astrocytes *in situ* in various brain regions, including cortex, hippocampus, cerebellum, nucleus ruber, and retina. In the hippocampus, two types of astrocytes were shown to coexist, with one type expressing and the other lacking AMPA receptors (Matthias et al., 2003). While in most brain regions astrocyte AMPA receptors display low Ca^{2+} permeability, Bergmann glial cells in the cerebellum lack the GluR2 subunit and hence allow passage of divalent cations (Müller et al., 1992). The physiological relevance of this subunit combination has been nicely demonstrated by experimentally inducing the expression of GluR2 in Bergmann glial cells, which results in a significant neuronal rearrangement (Iino et al., 2001). The pharmacological properties and single-channel conductances of astroglial AMPA receptors mimic those of their neuronal counterparts. In the hippocampus, astroglial receptors possess intermediate Ca^{2+} permeability and are assembled primarily from the subunits GluR1, GluR2, and GluR4. Receptor activation leads to a reversible block of outward- and inward-rectifying K^+ channels. This effect is mediated by intracellular accumulation of Na^+, which blocks the channels from inside and might be relevant for regulation of astroglial proliferation and extracellular K^+ homeostasis (Schröder et al., 2002) (Fig. 10.1). Early in postnatal development, astrocytes coexpress AMPA receptors with variable Ca^{2+} permeability, while later in development only receptors with low Ca^{2+} permeability are expressed due to the presence of GluR2 in the receptor complex. In addition, changes in receptor splicing occur within the first 3 postnatal weeks: In contrast to hippocampal neurons, the portion of flip splice variants (primarily GluR2 flip) increases in the astrocytes, resulting in prolonged receptor opening (Seifert et al., 2003). Joint stimulation of AMPA and metabotropic glutamate receptors in hippocampal and neocortical astrocytes triggers Ca^{2+} oscillations and mediates glutamate release (Bezzi et al., 1998). AMPA receptor activity seems to be important for the generation of correlated astrocytic network activity (Aguado et al., 2002). Interestingly, non-NMDA receptor activation in astrocytes recently was shown to trigger ATP release from these cells, which in turn caused homo- and heterosynaptic suppression in CA1 neurons of the hippocampus (Zhang et al., 2003) (Fig. 10.1). Astroglial AMPA receptors have also been investigated in the diseased CNS (reviewed by Seifert and Steinhäuser, 2001; Steinhäuser and Seifert, 2002). For example, molecular and functional changes occur in epilepsy, and these alterations have been proposed to contribute to the generation and spread of seizure activity in human temporal lobe epilepsy (Seifert et al., 2004). In addition, significant changes in iGluR expression are observed in the ischemic brain, and excessive activation of AMPA receptors leads to astrocyte injury.

Although antibody staining and *in situ* hybridization demonstrated widespread distribution of kainate receptors in brain, clear evidence for functional expression of these receptors in astrocytes is lacking. Apparently, no such receptors are functionally expressed by hippocampal astrocytes. A modulation of kainate and quisqualate responses by concanavalin A has been observed in cultured cerebellar and cortical astrocytes, but the low level of potentiation suggested an effect on AMPA receptors. At the transcript level, GluR6 but not GluR5 was detected in cultured cortical and hippocampal astrocytes, and in contrast to neurons, GluR6 was only partially edited at the Q/R site. Transcripts of all five kainate receptor subunits, GluR5–7, KA1, and KA2 have been found in adult bovine white matter astrocytes *in situ*. Antibodies against GluR5–7, GluR6,7 and KA2 confirmed the expression of kainate receptor protein (García-Barcina and Matute, 1996), but functional receptors have yet to be identified.

The presence of NR1 protein in astroglial processes in cortex and amygdala indicates that glial cells can also express NMDA receptor. Bergmann glial cells express mRNAs for NR2B, and a physiological study in acute brain slices reported NMDA-induced membrane currents in Bergmann glial cells. However, these responses displayed unusual properties (e.g., no Mg^{2+} and glycine sensitivity), and indirect effects cannot be excluded. Evidence for the presence of functional NMDA receptors *in situ* comes from cortical astrocytes. In these cells, astroglial NMDA responses were observed that resembled NMDA response in neurons, including sensitivity to extracellular Mg^{2+} and blockade by MK-801 (Schipke et al., 2001b). Moreover, a recent report demonstrated the activation of functional NMDA receptors in hippocampal astrocytes after ischemia *in vivo* due to upregulation of the NR2B subunit (Krebs et al., 2003). Investigations on cultured Müller cells suggested an involvement of NMDA receptors, presumably NR1, in the regulation of proliferation. Taken together, these studies demonstrate that astrocytes are capable of expressing NMDA receptors.

Metabotropic Glutamate Receptors

The metabotropic glutamate receptor (mGluR) family couples to G-proteins and can be classified into three groups: Group I comprises mGluR1 and mGluR5, and their activation leads to stimulation of phospholipase C (PLC), increase in inositol 1,4,5-triphosphate (IP_3), and release of Ca^{2+} from internal stores, while group II (mGluR2, mGluR3) and group III (mGluR4, mGluR6–8) receptors couple to adenylate cyclase. Metabotropic glutamate receptors 3 and 5 are the predominant subtypes expressed by astrocytes and have been described in cultured cells as well as *in situ*, including human hippocampus (reviewed by Winder and Conn, 1996; Porter and McCarthy, 1997; Condorelli et al., 1999). Metabotropic glutamate receptor 1 has been reported in hippocampal astrocytes and in the spinal cord. Accordingly, activation of these receptors led to an increase in intracellular Ca^{2+} and inhibition of cyclic adenosine monophosphate (cAMP) accumulation, although G-protein (Gs)-coupled cAMP stimulation has also been reported. Stimulation of astroglial mGluRs leads to intracellular Ca^{2+} oscillations and Ca^{2+} wave propagation within the astrocyte network, activates Ca^{2+}-dependent K^+ channels, and induces ATP release as well as prostaglandin-mediated glutamate release from astrocytes that activates glial and neuronal receptors (Chen et al., 1997; Pasti et al., 1997; Bezzi et al., 1998; Sul et al., 2004). These responses are likely to occur under physiological conditions because astroglial mGluR activation and subsequent Ca^{2+} responses could be evoked by electrical stimulation of fibre tracts, causing neuronal glutamate release in acute brain slices. Activation of mGluRs induced other astrocyte responses, including swelling, ac-

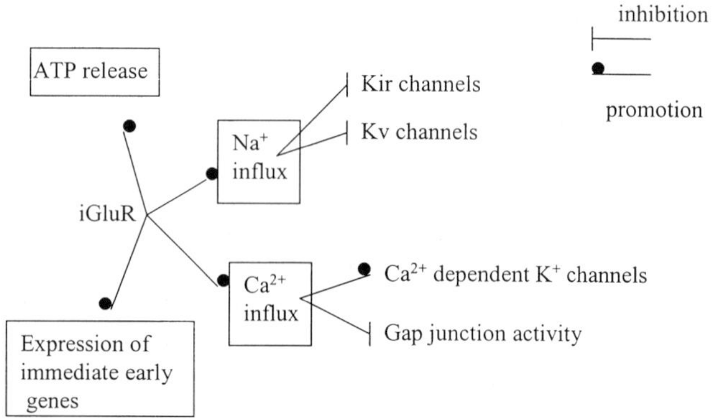

FIGURE 10.1 The figure illustrates the multiple actions triggered by ionotropic glutamate receptor activation in astrocytes. ATP: adenosine triphosphate.

tivation of phospholipase D (PLD) and glutamine synthetase, release of arachidonic acid, cAMP-dependent block of K^+ currents, modulation of proliferation, and regulation of the expression of the glutamate transporter, GLAST. Together, these findings suggest that mGluRs play a pervasive role in modulating astrocyte function and intercellular communication in the CNS.

Expression of mGluR can change under pathophysiological conditions. Metabotropic glutamate receptor 1 on astrocytes have been implicated in the pathophysiology of spinal cord injury (Agrawal et al., 1998). Upregulation of astroglial mGluR1 and mGluR5 was observed in amyotrophic lateral sclerosis in human spinal cord (Aronica et al., 2001). In epilepsy, reactive astrocytes of the hippocampus persistently upregulate mGluR3, mGluR5, and mGluR8 protein (reviewed by Steinhäuser and Seifert, 2002). Electron microscopic inspection of hippocampal tissue from temporal lobe epilepsy patients revealed the expression of mGluR2/3, mGluR4, and mGluR8 in astrocytes, suggesting involvement of these receptors in gliosis. Frequent activation of mGluR5 during seizures enhanced IP_3 hydrolysis in astrocytes and increased $[Ca^{2+}]_i$(intracellular Ca^{2+}). Because group I mGluRs induce glial Ca^{2+} oscillations, induce Ca^{2+} wave propagation, and influence neuronal excitability (see above), their upregulation, as observed in epilepsy, might indicate astroglial involvement in seizure generation or spread. A protective role of mGluRs has been suggested in Alzheimer's disease since stimulation of the receptors accelerates processing of amyloid precursor protein (APP) into nonamyloidogenic APPs (Lee et al., 1996).

Gamma-Aminobutyric Acid$_A$ Receptors

Ionotropic γ-aminobutyric acid$_A$ (GABA$_A$) receptors are expressed by astrocytes both in culture and *in situ* (reviewed by Verkhratsky and Steinhäuser, 2000). *In situ*, functional GABA$_A$ receptors have been demonstrated in Bergmann glial cells, astrocytes of the spinal cord, optic nerve, retina, hippocampus, and pituitary gland. As in neurons astrocytic GABA$_A$ receptors form Cl^- channels with a conductance of about 30 pS. In contrast to mature neurons, GABA$_A$ receptor activation leads to a large depolarization in astrocytes studied in culture (Kettenmann et al., 1984). The Cl^- reversal potential can be as positive as -40 mV, indicating that GABA can lead to a substantial depolarization from the normal resting membrane potential of about -80 mV. In astrocytes of the pituitary gland, postsynaptic potentials were activated by neuronally released GABA (Mudrick-Donnon et al., 1993). Besides opening Cl^- channels, GABA$_A$ receptor activation in astrocytes triggers a long-lasting blockade of K^+ conductances, thereby augmenting depolarization (e.g., in Bergmann glial cells and astrocytes of the spinal cord and hippocampus; Müller et al., 1994; Pastor et al., 1995; Bekar et al., 1999) and activating voltage-gated Ca^{2+} channels with subsequent cytosolic Ca^{2+} increase (in freshly isolated astrocytes from hippocampus; Fraser et al., 1995).

The GABA$_A$ receptor has a complex pharmacology. As in neurons, barbiturates and steroids enhance the astrocytic GABA response. There is a difference between the responses in neurons and cultured astrocytes: While normal benzodiazepines like diazepam enhance the GABA response in both neurons and cultured astrocytes, the inverse benzodiazepine agonist, dimeth-oxyethylcarbolinie carboxylate (DMCM), enhances the response in astrocytes opposite to its action in neurons. In contrast, Bergmann glial cells studied in cerebellar slices showed GABA responses that were benzodiazepine-insensitive. Immunocytochemistry revealed that these cells do not express the γ subunits responsible for benzodiazepine binding at the GABA receptor complex; they express instead the δ subunit (Müller et al., 1994). In freshly isolated astrocytes from the hippocampus, the benzodiazepine sensitivity was as described in neurons (Fraser et al., 1995). This indicates that GABA$_A$ receptor subunit composition is heterogeneous in astrocytes, resulting in different populations of astrocytes with respect to their GABA$_A$ receptor profile.

In Bergmann glial cells, GABA$_A$ receptors were prominently expressed in immature cells but were downregulated in the mature cerebellum. In addition, an uneven distribution was reported in these cells: Immunolabeling preferentially identified receptors along the processes. There is evidence from both cell culture and *in situ* studies that GABA$_A$ receptor activation promotes differentiation of astrocytes. In culture, GABA triggers formation of processes and leads to a more complex morphological shape of the astrocytes. A similar effect has been observed in the hypothalamus *in situ*: Gamma-aminobutyric acid released from neurons activated astroglial GABA$_A$ receptors and induced differentiation (Mong et al., 2002). This finding is contrary to the observation in culture that GABA triggers thymidine incorporation and, presumably, proliferation (Fig. 10.2).

Gamma-Aminobutyric Acid$_B$ Receptors

There is evidence from culture studies that astrocytes express metabotropic GABA$_B$ receptors (see the review by Fraser et al., 1994). In culture, GABA$_B$ receptor activity controls the release of endozepine, an endogeneous ligand of benzodiazepine receptors (Patte et al., 1999). In hippocampal slices GABA release from inhibitory neurons triggers Ca^{2+}, signaling through activation of $GABA_B$ receptors (Kang et al., 1998). Activation of $GABA_B$ receptors in these astrocytes has an impact on neuronal function by potentiating inhibitory postsynaptic currents in pyramidal neurons. Thus, in the hippocampus, astrocytic $GABA_B$ receptors are part of a functional circuit involving inhibitory neurons, astrocytes, and pyramidal neurons.

Purinergic Receptors

Astrocytes can express a large number of purinergic receptors linked to different effector mechanisms, as summarized by Ciccarelli et al. (2001) and James and Butt (2002). The presence of adenosine receptors *in situ* has been established in the hippocampus and in acutely isolated cortical astrocytes. In both preparations, the activation of adenosine receptors led to the accumulation of intracellular Ca^{2+} via release from cytoplasmic stores (Porter and McCarthy, 1995; Pilitsis and Kimelberg, 1998). All three types of adenosine receptors (A_1, A_2, A_3) can be expressed by astrocytes. A_2 receptor activation increased the internal cAMP concentration and stimulated astroglial proliferation (G_S-coupled). In contrast, activation of A_1 (G_i-coupled) and A_3 receptors (G_i- and G_q-coupled) had opposite effects, namely, inhibition of proliferation (Fig. 10.2). A_1 receptor activation also stimulated the production of neurotrophic factors [nerve growth factor (NGF), S100β, transforming growth factor β (TGFβ)] (Ciccarelli et al., 1999) and enhanced mGluR5-induced intracellular Ca^{2+} responses (Cormier et al., 2001). Receptor subtypes can have opposing actions: While A_1 receptor stimulation inhibited purine release, A_2 receptor activation stimulated this release *in situ*. A_3 receptor stimulation also leads to apoptosis and induces reorganization of the astroglial cytoskeleton (Abbracchio et al., 1997; Di Iorio et al., 2002). Thus, adenosine is a receptor system that triggers a complex response in astrocytes that can lead either to proliferation or to apoptosis, depending on the expression levels of A_1 and A_3 receptors, respectively. A_{2a} receptor signaling is linked to an important function of astrocytes, namely, the control of glutamate levels in the extracellular space. Activating A_{2a} receptors inhibited glutamate transporter (GLT-1)-mediated glutamate uptake and facilitated glutamate release (Nishizaki et al., 2002) (Fig. 10.2). Thus, astrocyte A_{2a} receptor activation leads to an increase in extracellular glutamate levels. As demonstrated in culture, stimulation of A_{2a} receptors inhibited the release of nitric oxide (NO), while A_{2b} receptor activation induced synthesis and release of interleukin-6 (IL-6).

Both types of adenosine triphosphate (ATP) receptors, P2X and P2Y, have been identified in astrocytes. In cell culture, activation of P2X receptors leads to the opening of a cationic conductance. Such responses have not been observed in astrocytes *in situ* despite positive immunolabeling for various P2X subunits (Kukley et al., 2001). Only in Müller cells of the human retina have $P2X_7$-induced currents been recorded, and this property seems to be species-specific (Pannicke et al., 2000). In these cells, $P2X_7$ receptor activation triggered Ca^{2+}-activated K^+ (BK) channels possibly linked to $P2X_7$-dependent regulation of proliferation. In addition, the activation of $P2X_7$ receptors was found to induce expression of monocyte chemoattractant protein-1 (Panenka et al., 2001), indicating that purinergic receptors control chemokine synthesis.

P2Y receptors are widely expressed in astrocytes in culture and *in situ*. P2Y-mediated signaling has been identified in Bergmann glial cells in acute slices of cere-

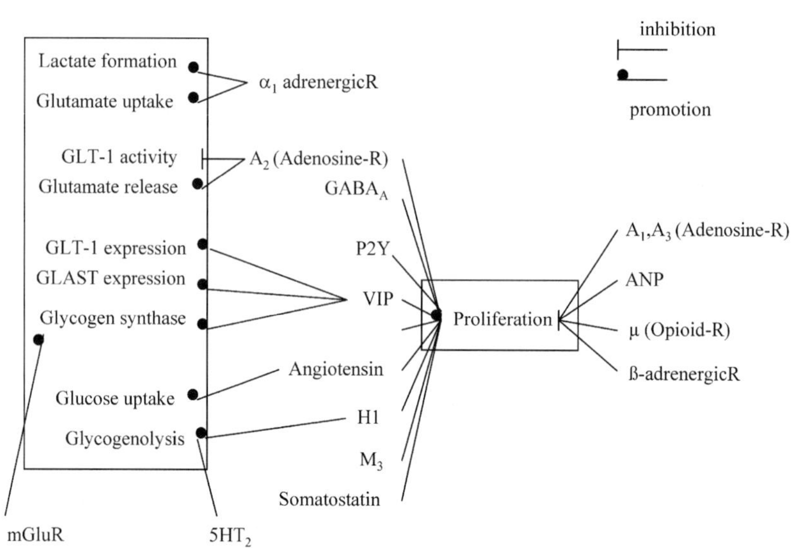

FIGURE 10.2 This figure summarizes the influence of different astrocytic receptors on glutamate and glucose metabolism and transport and combines this with its influence on proliferation. It is evident that only proliferation-promoting receptors also control glutamate or glucose metabolism and transport, in contrast to receptors that inhibit astrocyte proliferation. ANP: atrial natriuretic peptide; GLAST: glutamate-asparate transporter; $GABA_A$: γaminobutyric acid$_A$; GLT-1: glutamate transporter 1; 5-HT_2: 5-hydroxytryptamine-2; mGluR: metabotropic glutamate receptor; VIP: vasoactive intestinal polypeptide.

bellum, in freshly isolated astrocytes from cortex and hippocampus, and in Müller cells and astrocytes from the retina. P2Y receptor activation leads to a G_q-PLC-mediated increase in IP_3 and Ca^{2+} release from intracellular stores. Moreover, these receptors are coupled to pertussis toxin (PTX)-sensitive G_i/G_o proteins linked to the synthesis of phospholipase A2, arachidonic acid and protein kinase C (PKC), extracellular signal-regulated kinase (ERK), and cyclooxygenase 2 (COX 2), release of arachidonic acid and prostaglandin E2, stimulation of mitogen-activated protein kinases (MAPKs) and induction of immediate early genes. Astrocytes of the postnatal hippocampus express the $P2Y_1$ and $P2Y_2$ receptor subtypes, with $P2Y_2$ increasing during development (Zhu and Kimelberg, 2001). P2Y-induced signaling in astrocytes plays an important role in the spread of Ca^{2+} waves, first established in cultured cells (Cotrina et al., 1998) and subsequently in the freshly isolated retina (Li et al., 2001; Newman, 2001) and in slices of the corpus callosum (Schipke et al., 2001a). Accordingly, ATP is considered to be released from astrocytes and acts on P2Y receptors to propagate the wave. In addition, P2Y receptor activation was reported to enhance the proliferation rate in cultured astrocytes (Rathbone et al., 1992) (Fig. 10.2) and is involved in the induction of astrogliosis *in vivo* (Franke et al., 2001). Thus, P2Y receptors play an important role for astrocyte signaling and for the responses of these cells to injury.

Glycine Receptors

Functional glycine receptors have been detected in astrocytes from spinal cord slices. Reverse transcriptase–polymerase chain reaction (RT-PCR) revealed the expression of $\alpha 1$ and β subunits. As in neurons, glycine activated a Cl^- conductance (Kirchhoff et al., 1996). Interestingly, glycine receptor expression has not been reported for cultured astrocytes and is also not a common property of astrocytes *in situ*: Bergmann glial cells, for instance, do not express functional glycine receptors.

Acetylcholine Receptors

Recently, α-bungarotoxin-sensitive nicotinic acetylcholine receptors (nACh) containing the $\alpha 7$ subunit were described for cultured astrocytes. Receptor activation led to Ca^{2+} influx and Ca^{2+}-induced Ca^{2+} release from caffeine-sensitive stores (Sharma and Vijayaraghavan, 2001). In addition, nAch was localized on astrocytes of human cerebellum *in situ* (Graham et al., 2002). The expression of muscarinic ACh (mACh) receptors by astrocytes is well established (reviewed by Porter and McCarthy, 1997; Verkhratsky et al., 1998). There is evidence for the expression of transcripts for the mACh receptor subtypes, M_1 to M_5, in cultured astrocytes. Acetylcholine induces IP_3 formation and release of Ca^{2+} from cytoplasmic stores and inhibits adenylate cyclase. As tested in culture, acetylcholine induced an increase in astroglial proliferation due to activation of M_3 receptors (Fig. 10.2) and phosphorylation of MAPK. Neuronal activity can activate astrocytic mACh receptors: Stimulating cholinergic fibers triggered Ca^{2+} responses in hippocampal astrocytes via mACh receptors (Araque et al., 2002). Excessive neuronal activity leads to upregulation of mACh receptors *in vivo*, as has been shown in amygdala kindling (Beldhuis et al., 1992), indicating that neuronal activity can regulate astrocyte receptor expression. During development, mACh receptor responses and receptor protein expression are upregulated.

Oxytocin and Vasopressin Receptors

Both vasopressin and oxytocin can trigger Ca^{2+} responses in astrocytes. Neuronal production and release of TGF-β led to an increase in astroglial oxytocin receptor mRNA in astrocytes, indicating that neurons were able to upregulate the astrocyte receptor (Mittaud et al., 2002). V_{1A} vasopressin receptors were identified by binding and biochemical studies. There is evidence that vasopressin is important for Cl^- homeostasis and volume regulation of astrocytes. Increased Cl^- uptake was observed upon vasopressin application, presumably mediated by V_{1A} receptors. Observation in acute slices demonstrated that astrocytes express high levels of a water channel, aquaporin-4. Indirect evidence suggested that the activity of aquaporin-4 is regulated by vasopressin. This interaction between vasopressin receptors and water channels is considered to be an important control element for volume regulation in the brain (Niermann et al., 2001).

Vasoactive Intestinal Polypeptide Receptors

Vasoactive intestinal polypeptide (VIP) receptors are expressed by astrocytes, and the activation leads to Ca^{2+} signaling (see reviews by Magistretti et al., 1998; Verkhratsky et al., 1998). All three subtypes of VIP receptors have been identified in cultured astrocytes. Activation of VIP receptors induces release of IL-6 and neurotrophic factors and stimulates proliferation (Fig. 10.2). There is a link between receptor activation and glutamate uptake: Stimulation of VIP receptors leads to the promotion of GLT-1 and GLAST expression (Figiel and Engele, 2000). This finding is in line with another study showing that VIP enhances glutamate uptake in astrocytes (Fig. 10.2). Together, these data indicate that VIP can increase the strength of glutamate-mediated neurotransmission. In addition, VIP receptors may play an important role in regulating energy metabolism. Vasoactive intestinal polypeptide depletes astrocyte glycogen initially, followed by delayed reaccumulation to a level beyond baseline (Fig. 10.2). These effects are mediated by regulating a number of related genes such as glycogen synthase via the transcription factor family CCAAT/enhancer-binding protein (C/EBP). However, at present there is no convincing evidence of the presence of VIP receptors in astrocytes *in situ*.

Adrenergic Receptors

Both α- and β-adrenergic receptors have been described in astrocytes in culture and *in situ* (reviewed by Porter and McCarthy, 1997; Verkhratsky et al., 1998). The α_1 receptors trigger the release of Ca^{2+} from internal stores. They affect astrocyte function by inhibiting gap junction coupling via PLC. This is in line with the finding that mechanically induced Ca^{2+} waves in hippocampal astroglial cells are inhibited after stimulation of α_1 receptors (Muyderman et al., 1998). Moreover, α_{1b} receptor activation stimulated glutamate uptake in cultured astrocytes. There is also an indication of the control of metabolic activity by α_1 receptors because receptor activation induced lactate formation (Fig. 10.2). The α_1 receptors regulate expression of α_2 receptors and thus form a complex feedback circuit. Both α_1 and α_2 receptors have been identified *in situ*. In the hippocampus, α_2 receptors are located on astroglial processes near terminals, forming asymmetric excitatory synapses (Milner et al., 1998). Neuronal stimulation in acute cerebellar slices leads to the release of noradrenaline from afferent fibers and activation of α_1 receptors in Bergmann glial cells (Kulik et al., 1999).

Both subtypes of β receptors, β_1 and β_2, are expressed by astrocytes *in situ*, with β_2 being most prominently expressed under pathological conditions. In astrocytes of rat visual cortex, β receptors appear after the second postnatal week. In the injured brain, adrenergic receptors are differentially regulated. While α_1 receptor density decreases in areas of neuronal degeneration and gliosis, β receptors are upregulated. The change in β receptor density and astrogliosis seems to be functionally linked. Blockade of β receptors suppressed glial scar formation, indicating that adrenergic receptors are part of the cascade leading to astrocyte activation (Griffith and Sutin, 1996). This suggestion is substantiated by the finding that β_2 receptors are activated or upregulated in the transected optic nerve *in vivo*, confirming that β-adrenergic signaling is an important feature of the astrocyte response to injury. Further support comes from the observation that stimulation of β receptors leads to astrogliosis and cell proliferation in the optic nerve *in vivo*. This effect might be mediated via the control of growth factor expression [e.g. fibroblast growth factor 1, 2 (FGF1, FGF2), brain-derived neurotrophic factor (BDNF), ciliary neuronotrophic factor (CNTT)]. In contrast, inhibition of proliferation upon β-adrenergic stimulation was observed in cultured astrocytes (Fig. 10.2), which, however, does not contradict gliosis. The involvement of β receptors in pathological processes is further substantiated by the finding that their stimulation leads to production of APP, changes in morphology, and increase in glial fibrillary acidic protein (GFAP) (Lee et al., 1997). Stimulation of β_1 receptors is also accompanied by enhanced glycogen levels that could be part of the gliotic response. The observation that β-adrenergic receptor stimulation leads to a cAMP-mediated inhibition of astroglial inwardly rectifying K^+ channels points to a role in the regulation of extracellular K^+ homeostasis (Roy and Sontheimer, 1995).

Angiotensin Receptors

Expression of angiotensin receptors in astrocytes *in situ* seems to be restricted to white matter (see reviews by Sumners et al., 1994; Verkhratsky et al., 1998). Antibody staining identified AT_1 and AT_2 receptors in astrocytes of white matter tracts in cerebellum and subcortical regions, in the optic nerve, and in the corpus callosum; no immunoreactivity was found in gray matter. The diversity in expression is also reflected when astrocytes are harvested from different brain areas: AT_1 receptors were found in astrocytes from medulla oblongata and cerebellum, whereas astrocyte cultures from hypothalamus and cortex did not express functional receptors. Activation of astroglial angiotensin receptors stimulates phosphoinositide (PI) hydrolysis and PKC and triggers Ca^{2+} release from internal stores. Receptor activation stimulates proliferation, increases glucose uptake, and induces prostaglandin release in cultured astrocytes (Fig. 10.2).

Somatostatin Receptors

Prominent expression of somatostatin receptors in astrocytes of hippocampus, amygdala, and hypothalamus *in situ* has been identified in binding studies on brain slices (reviewed by Porter and McCarthy, 1997). In culture it is evident that astrocytes express the sst_{2A} splice variant. Receptor activation is linked to inhibition of cAMP accumulation and leads to enhanced proliferation rates (Fig. 10.2). Moreover, it leads to a reduction in forskolin-induced IL-6 release.

Serotonin Receptors

Reverse transcriptase–polymerase chain reaction in human and rat brain cultures revealed that astrocytes can express various serotonin receptors (see reviews by Verkhratsky et al., 1998; Azmitia, 2001). In cell culture, stimulation of 5-hydroxytryptamine-2 (5-HT_2) led to PI hydrolysis, cAMP accumulation, and upregulation of glycogenolysis (Fig. 10.2). A distinct expression of 5-HT subtypes also occurs *in situ* since the subtypes

5-HT_{1A}, 5-HT_{2A}, and 5-HT_{5A} have been identified in different brain areas. 5-Hydroxytryptamine receptors have been speculated to be involved in pathogenesis. The 5-HT_{5A} subtype is upregulated in gliosis and the 5-HT_{2A} subtype is enhanced in schizophrenia. Stimulation of 5-HT receptors leads to the release of S100β from astrocytes, and this release was hypothesized to have an impact on the ongoing pathological event. Transcripts of 5-HT_{5A} are developmentally regulated: Receptor mRNA is detected prior to birth, and expression peaks at postnatal day 20 in the rat.

Atrial Natriuretic Peptide Receptors

All three types of atrial natriuretic peptide (ANP) receptors have been identified in cultured astrocytes: ANP_A and ANP_B (biological receptor) as well as ANP_C (clearance receptor) (reviewed by Sumners et al., 1994). So far, only the ANP_A receptor has been unequivocally identified *in situ* (in the brain stem). Atrial natriuretic peptide receptors, without subtype specification, have been found in several other brain structures including olfactory bulb, hippocampus, and amygdala. Culture studies suggest that the clearance receptor is important for astrocyte function: ANP inhibits MAPKs via ANP_C (Prins et al., 1996). MAPK is stimulated by growth factors such as endothelin-3 (ET-3) or platelet-derived growth factor (PDGF) and thus ANP_C counteracts their activation. This antimitogenic action of ANP in astrocytes is mediated via inhibition of ET-3-induced G-protein activation. In consequence, since these growth factors stimulate proliferation, ANP acts as an antiproliferative substance on astrocytes (Fig. 10.2). Accordingly, if astrocytes are stimulated with a proliferative agent such as angiotensin-2 or other growth factors, ANP acts as an antagonist to restrict cell number. Atrial natriuretic peptide has been shown to stimulate cyclic guanosine monophosphate (cGMP) production and activate guanylate cyclase in astrocytes.

Tachykinin Receptors

Cultured astrocytes express all subtypes of tachykinin receptors, from NK_1 to NK_3. Activation of NK_1 receptors leads to membrane depolarization due to blockade of a constitutive K^+ conductance and opening of Cl^- channels (Backus et al., 1991). Receptor localization on the light and electron microscopic levels in different species, including humans, has identified NK_2 and NK_3 receptors in astrocytes of various areas of the CNS, such as spinal cord, cortex, and hippocampus. NK_2 receptors have been found to cluster close to axon terminals in spinal cord. The ligand substance P enhances secretion of IL-6 and prostaglandin E2 (PGE2) upon IL-1β stimulation in cultured spinal cord astrocytes (Palma et al., 1997). Moreover, lipopolysaccharide (LPS)-induced secretion of tumor necrosis factor-α (TNFα) and IL-1 from astrocytes was augmented by substance P (Luber-Narod et al., 1994). A proinflammatory function of tachykinin receptors in reactive astrocytes has been suggested, since upregulation of the receptors was observed in astrocytes of transected optic nerve *in vivo*. Tachykinin receptors are expressed not only in mature astrocytes but as early as embryonic day 13 in rat.

Bradykinin Receptors

So far, functional bradykinin receptors (B_1 and B_2) have been identified only in cultured astrocytes. Receptor activation leads to a release of Ca^{2+} from intracellular stores and to a blockade of a constitutive K^+ conductance via B_2 receptors (Gimpl et al., 1992). B_2 receptors trigger the release of glutamate and aspartate from astrocytes (Parpura et al., 1994).

Thyrotropin-Releasing Hormone Receptors

Astrocytes express the thyrotropin-releasing hormone$_1$ (TRH_1) subtype in culture and *in situ*. Expression *in situ* is stronger in white compared to gray matter in the adult rat spinal cord. The receptors are present in TRH-synthesizing astrocytes, indicating that this hormone acts in an autocrine and paracrine fashion.

Opioid Receptors

Early work indicated the presence of opioid receptors on tanycytes and pituicytes. There is evidence for the expression of all three subtypes of the opioid receptors, μ, δ, and κ, both in cell culture and *in situ* (reviewed by Verkhratsky et al., 1998). Activation of μ and κ receptors inhibited DNA synthesis, proliferation, and astroglial growth (Fig. 10.2). Interestingly, the inhibitory action of opioids on astrocyte proliferation was restricted to GFAP-positive astrocytes, while S100β-positive cells were not affected. κ and δ receptors are linked to Ca^{2+} signaling, and their stimulation inhibited forskolin-induced cAMP stimulation. Circumstantial evidence indicates that the effect of opioids on astroglial proliferation is Ca^{2+}-dependent. μ and δ receptors were shown to be preferentially expressed on astrocytic processes *in situ*. While μ receptors are more frequently present on immature astrocytes, the expression of δ and κ receptors is increased in adult tissue.

Histamine Receptors

In cultured astrocytes, binding sites for H_1 and H_2 subtypes of histamine receptors have been identified (reviewed by Inagaki and Wada, 1994) that couple to G_q and G_s types of G-proteins, respectively. Accordingly,

H_1 receptors couple to PLC, leading to IP_3 production and Ca^{2+} release, while H_2 receptor activation in astrocytes is linked to adenylate cyclase and intracellular cAMP accumulation. H_1 receptors were found mainly on the processes of astrocytes, and stimulation led to locally restricted Ca^{2+} responses. Histamine acts as a mitogen in cortical astrocytes. Activation of H_1 receptors has been shown to stimulate glycogen breakdown (Fig. 10.2). Although *in situ* hybridization did not unequivocally associate histamine receptors with astrocytes, pharmacological studies indicate their expression in cerebellum and hippocampus. Histamine triggered an increase in $[Ca^{2+}]_i$ due to release from thapsigargin-sensitive intracellular pools; the response was inhibited by H_1 receptor–specific antagonists (Jung et al., 2000). In acute rat hippocampal slices, functional H_1 receptors linked to Ca^{2+} signaling are upregulated after postnatal day 8 (Shelton and McCarthy, 2000). Ultrastructural studies demonstrate astrocytic apposition to histaminergic neurons in hippocampus.

Dopamine Receptors

Cultured astrocytes express D_1 and D_2 subtypes of dopamine receptors, as evidenced by autoradiography, pharmacological experiments (see Hösli and Hösli, 1993), and transcript analysis. D_1 receptor activation leads to PTX-sensitive cAMP formation via protein kinase A (PKA) stimulation. Prolonged receptor activation led to a reduction of astroglial dopamine sensitivity (Reuss and Unsicker, 2001). D_2 receptors in astrocytes are linked to the actin cytoskeleton via interaction with filamin A. A recent study provided the first evidence for the presence of dopamine receptors on astrocytes *in vivo*. Ligand binding and ultrastructural analysis found strong expression of D_2 receptors linked to Ca^{2+} signaling in GFAP-positive cortical astrocyte processes surrounding interneurons. These receptors were indeed functional since their activation induced intracellular Ca^{2+} elevations in the astrocytes (Khan et al., 2001).

OLIGODENDROCYTES

Glutamate Receptors

Glutamate responses were first noted in oligodendrocytes cultured from spinal cord when the membrane potential was recorded with sharp microelectrodes: Application of glutamate depolarized the cells (Kettenmann et al., 1984). Today we know that oligodendrocytes express glutamate receptors of the AMPA and kainate subtypes, and physiological responses have been observed under different culture conditions as well as in cells from acute slices of corpus callosum or spinal cord (Berger et al., 1992; Ziak et al., 1998). In cell culture, RT-PCR indicated the expression of the AMPA receptor subunits GluR2–GluR4 and the kainate receptor subunits GluR6, GluR7, KA1, and KA2 in oligodendrocytes. AMPA receptors are also expressed by oligodendrocyte progenitor cells from both early postnatal and adult nervous system (reviewed by Verkhratsky and Steinhäuser, 2000). AMPA receptor activation leads to secondary effects, namely, a blockade of voltage-gated potassium channels and an increase in cytosolic Ca^{2+}. The increase in Ca^{2+} is triggered by the depolarization of the membrane and subsequent activation of voltage-gated Ca^{2+} channels. Secondly, receptor activation triggers a transient blockade of transient and delayed rectifying potassium conductances that are constitutively expressed by oligodendrocytes (Borges et al., 1994). The blockade of the K^+ channels is due to entry of Na^+ through the AMPA receptor pore, and the resulting high intracellular Na^+ concentration blocks the K^+ channels from inside (Fig. 10.3). The Na^+ dependence of the K^+ channels was supported by the observation that elevation of intracellular Na^+ alone led to a blockade of the outward K^+ currents. K^+ channel blockade was not mediated by the increase in intracellular Ca^{2+}. In conclusion, AMPA and/or kainate receptor activation leads to an influx of Na^+ via the ionotropic receptor, and the intracellular Na^+ increase blocks voltage-gated K^+ channels in a G-protein–independent fashion (Borges and Kettenmann, 1995). This interesting interaction has important implications for oligodendrocyte development. As shown in cerebellar cultures, glutamate receptor activation inhibited cell proliferation in oligodendrocyte progenitor cells and prevented lineage progression, an effect mimicked by K^+ channel blockers. This indicates that K^+ channel activity controls oligodendrocyte development (Yuan et al., 1998).

Studies *in vitro* and *in vivo* have demonstrated that chronic activation of AMPA receptors results in oligodendrocyte death; as a consequence, excessive activation of iGluRs will decrease the oligodendrocyte population (Matute et al., 1997). A recent study indicates that this vulnerability occurs at a defined developmental stage (Itoh et al., 2002). Early oligodendrocyte precursor cells lack the GluR2 subunit and thus express AMPA receptors with high Ca^{2+} permeability. In more mature oligodendroglial cells, GluR2 is expressed and confers low Ca^{2+} permeability to the receptor complex. Thus, oligodendrocytes tune their vulnerability to glutamate by regulating the AMPA receptor subunit composition. Interestingly, mGluRs are also expressed and limit AMPA receptor-mediated oligodendrocyte progenitor cell death, as indicated by pharmacological studies.

In most preparations, cells of the oligodendrocyte lineage failed to respond to NMDA, indicating a lack of functional NMDA receptors. In an *in vitro* assay using neurohypophyseal explants, NMDA receptor blockers

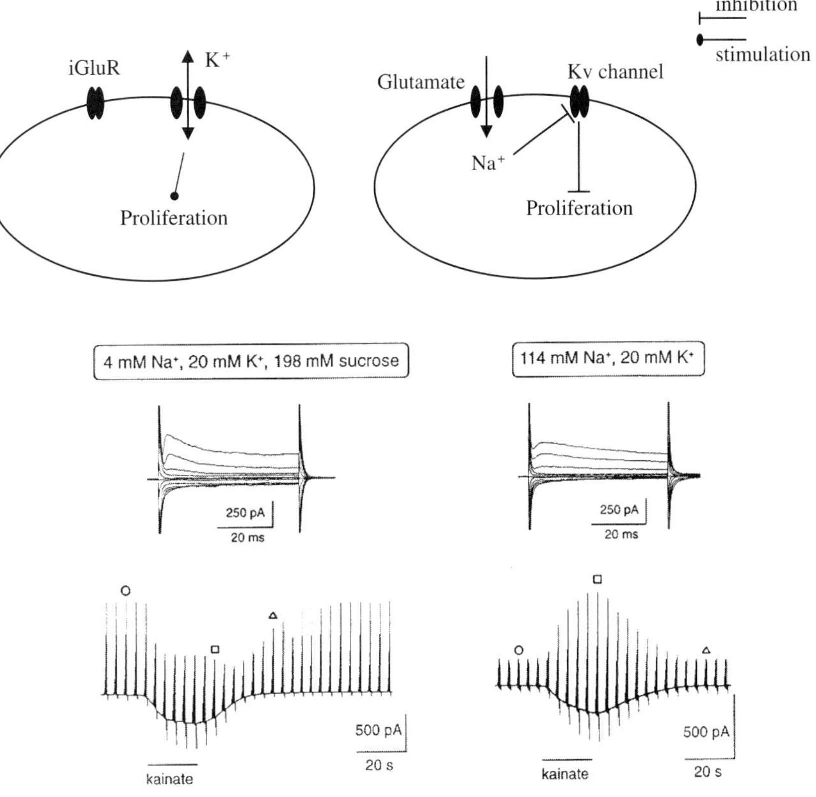

FIGURE 10.3 The upper scheme illustrates the link between glutamate receptors and proliferation in oligodendrocytes. Glutatmate receptor activation leads to an increase in intracellular sodium, which results in a block of potassium channels. The activity of the K^+ channels is linked to proliferation control. The lower set of experiments illustrates the dependence of an increasing K^+ current on levels of intracellular sodium on potassium currents. On the left, kainate triggers a prominent blockade of the resting potassium conductance when the intracellular sodium level is low. In contrast, on the right, with an experimentally increased intracellular sodium level, the resting conductance is lower and kainate induces only a catonic conductance increase without affecting the resting potassium conductance. For details see Borges et al. (1994). ; GluR: ionotropic glutamate receptor.

led to diminished migration of oligodendrocyte precursor cells. The presence of NMDA receptors in this preparation is further supported by a report on NMDA-induced $[Ca^{2+}]_i$ increase. In slices of spinal cord, high concentrations of NMDA (2 mM) triggered membrane currents in oligodendrocytes and precursor cells. In contrast to the response described in neurons, the glial NMDA response was not sensitive to Mg^{2+}. There were also changes during development: NMDA responses of oligodendrocytes were more prominent than those of precursors (Ziak et al., 1998).

Ionotropic Gamma-Aminobutyric Acid Receptors

γ-Aminobutyric acid–mediated responses were first detected in cultured oligodendrocytes from spinal cord using sharp microelectrodes, where GABA triggered a membrane depolarization (Gilbert et al., 1984). The GABA response shows the typical pharmacological profile of $GABA_A$ receptors: Responses are mimicked by muscimol and blocked by bicuculline and picrotoxin. The response can be enhanced by pentobarbital and by benzodiazepines. The inverse benzodiazepine agonist, DMCM, attenuates GABA responses, as described for neuronal $GABA_A$ receptors. There is an inverse relationship between $GABA_A$ receptor density and cell maturation. In glial precursor cells GABA triggered large membrane currents, while in more mature oligodendrocytes responses were rather small. Estimates indicate that the receptor density decreases by a factor of 100 during oligodendrocyte development. A similar decrease in GABA responsiveness has also been observed in cells from corpus callosum slices (Berger et al., 1992). Furthermore, GABA responses were detected in spinal cord slices, indicating that oligodendrocytes and precursors express $GABA_A$ receptors *in situ*.

In contrast to mature neurons, GABA depolarizes astrocytes and oligodendrocytes. Thus Cl^- flows out of the cells, leading to a decrease in intracellular Cl^- activity. The prerequisite for that efflux is an accumulation of Cl^- beyond the passive distribution, and there is active Cl^- transport into oligodendrocytes (Hoppe and Kettenmann, 1989). Moreover, activation of $GABA_A$ receptors in glial progenitor cells, as studied in cell culture, led to an increase in intracellular Ca^{2+} due to activation of voltage-gated Ca^{2+} channels after GABA-induced membrane depolarization. In addition, $GABA_A$ receptors are present in oligodendrocyte progenitor cells isolated from adult rat.

Purinergic Receptors

Cultured cells of the oligodendrocyte lineage, as well as oligodendrocytes from mouse corpus callosum slices, respond to ATP with an increase in intracellular $[Ca^{2+}]$ mediated by metabotropic purinergic (P2Y) receptors. The purinergic response shows an interesting developmental regulation: ATP induces a transient increase of

Ca^{2+} in late precursors and oligodendrocytes but not in early glial precursor cells, as studied in retinal or cortical cultures and in acute corpus callosum slices. The Ca^{2+} increase was due to Ca^{2+} release from intracellular stores. Interestingly, Ca^{2+} transients were significantly larger in processes than in the soma, indicative of a subcellular compartmentalization within the oligodendrocyte (Kirischuk et al., 1995; Pastor et al., 1995).

Glycine Receptors

In slices of rat spinal cord, glial precursor cells and a subpopulation of oligodendrocytes responded to glycine. The involvement of glycine receptors is inferred from the observation that the response was blocked by the specific glycine receptor antagonist strychnine and that the induced current reversed close to the Cl^- equilibrium potential, as expected for a Cl^- channel. Glycine responses were also found in oligodendrocyte progenitors cultured from newborn rats. These glycine receptors differ from the neuronal receptors: ^{3H}strychnine binding data and the strychnine dose-inhibition curve of glycine-induced currents suggest the existence of two strychnine binding sites on the oligodendrocyte glycine receptor (Belachew et al., 1998) compared to only a single site on neurons. As with activation of GABA receptors, glycine activates voltage-gated Ca^{2+} channels, indicating that glycine also depolarizes cells.

Acetylcholine Receptors

Oligodendrocyte progenitor cells express both types of acetylcholine receptors: mACh and nACh receptors (Cohen and Almazan, 1994; Rogers et al., 2001). Reverse transcriptase–polymerase chain reaction studies revealed the expression of the nACh receptor subunits $\alpha3$, $\alpha4$, $\alpha5$, $\alpha7$, $\beta2$, and $\beta4$ in oligodendrocyte progenitors purified from rat corpus callosum. Nicotine application triggered an increase in intracellular Ca^{2+} that was sensitive to antagonists of voltage-gated Ca^{2+} channels. This implies that nACh receptor activation depolarizes the membrane beyond the threshold potential of voltage-gated Ca^{2+} channels.

Muscarinic responses were identified in rat oligodendrocyte primary cultures and could be mimicked by the specific mACh receptor agonist, carbachol. It triggered an increase in cytosolic Ca^{2+}, which depended both on the mobilization from intracellular stores and on influx of extracellular Ca^2. The mACh receptor antagonist, atropine, blocked the carbachol-triggered response. Reverse transcriptase–polymerase chain reaction implies the expression of M_1 and M_2 subtypes of mACh receptors. Activation of mACh receptors attenuates β-adrenergic stimulation of cAMP formation, indicating mutual interactions between these two receptor systems. Activation of mACh receptors leads to a PTX-sensitive inhibition of inwardly rectifying K^+ channels within less than 1 second. This mechanism could play a role in the regulation of K^+ homeostasis. Serotonin and somatostatin trigger similar responses.

Adrenergic Receptors

Pharmacological evidence indicates that oligodendrocyte progenitors express α_1 adrenoceptors, which are linked to the formation of the intracellular messenger IP3 but lack β adrenoceptors (Cohen and Almazan, 1993).

Bradykinin Receptors

Rat cortical oligodendroytes in culture respond to bradykinin with an increase in intracellular [Ca^{2+}] and a decrease in the resting K^+ conductance. Moreover, bradykinin triggers the turnover of PI, indicating that Ca^{2+} signaling is linked to Ca^{2+} release from intracellular stores (Stephens et al., 1993).

Opioid Receptors

There is evidence for mRNA expression of μ receptors by cultured cells of the oligodendrocyte lineage. Transcripts were found in oligodendrocyte progenitor cells and in immature oligodendrocytes but not in mature oligodendrocytes, indicating that receptor expression is downregulated during development (Troyen-Toth et al., 2000).

Dopamine Receptors

Cells of the oligodendrocyte lineage can express dopamine receptors of the D_3 subtype both in culture and in the corpus callosum *in vivo*. D_3 receptor expression was found in precursors and in immature oligodendrocytes but not in mature oligodendrocytes. The receptor was associated with cell bodies but not with processes. Interestingly, D_3 receptor expression correlates with the peak of myelination *in situ*. This suggests that dopamine or some other D_3 receptor ligands may play a role in oligodendrocyte differentiation and/or formation of myelin (Bongarzone et al., 1998).

MICROGLIA

Microglial cells are the immune-competent elements of the brain and express a large variety of receptors for cytokines, chemokines, and growth factors. These are described in Chapter 11. Here, we will concentrate on the classical transmitter receptors of the nervous system. A small number of recent studies have indicated that these macrophage-related cells indeed express such receptors.

Glutamate Receptors

Microglial cells express AMPA (GluR1–GluR4) and kainate (primarily GluR5) subtypes of glutamate receptors (Noda et al., 2000). Ion substitution experiments show that microglia AMPA receptors have low Ca^{2+} permeability, indicating the expression of the GluR2 subunit that controls the Ca^{2+} permeability of AMPA receptors. This was verified by RT-PCR identifying the subunits GluR2 to GluR5. Activation of these receptors enhanced the production of TNFα. Based on mRNA and protein expression, rat microglia possess group III mGluRs mGluR4, mGluR6, and mGluR8 but not mGluR7. Stimulation of these receptors reduced microglial activation by LPS, chromogranin A or amyloid beta peptides 25–35 (Taylor et al., 2003).

Purinergic Receptors

Adenosine triphosphate activates complex responses in microglial cells. As first analyzed in culture, purinergic receptor activation triggers the induction of a nonselective cationic and a K^+ conductance and leads to an increase in cytosolic [Ca^{2+}] (Walz et al., 1993; Langosch et al., 1994). Pharmacological screening indicates that microglial cells express more than one subtype of both P2Y and P2X receptors. In culture, microglia express purinergic receptors in both states of activation, while there is an attenuation of purinergic responsiveness in activated microglial cells. Similar to other immune cells, activation of $P2X_7$ receptors provokes the release of IL-1β and triggers the release of plasminogen (Ferrari et al., 1997; Honda et al., 2001). P2Y receptor activity, which can be induced by ATP or adenosine diphosphate (ADP), influences microglia chemotaxis (Honda et al., 2001). Microglia *in situ* also express different purinergic receptors including $P2X_7$ receptors (Haas et al. 1996; Boucsein et al., 2003).

Other Receptors

Carbachol, an mACh agonist, produces a transient increase in [Ca^{2+}] in cultured microglial cells. The response is atropine sensitive, confirming the involvement of mACh receptors (Zhang et al., 1998).

Using the release of the cytokine IL-12 as a bioassay, adrenergic receptor–mediated responses have been characterized. The agonist salbutamol dose-dependently inhibited LPS-induced IL-12p40 release, and the involvement of β_2 adrenoceptors was inferred by the observation that a specific antagonist abolished this inhibitory effect (Prinz et al., 2001). This study indicated that β_2 adrenoceptors control microglia chemokine release via cAMP accumulation. Furthermore, microglial proliferation is modulated by β_2 adrenoceptors via elevation of intracellular cAMP. Microglia express substance P and tachykinin receptors. The substance P receptor, NK_1, was identified at the mRNA level. The four isoforms of the preprotachykinin-A gene transcript are expressed, and microglia produce much higher levels of endogenous substance P protein than blood monocyte–derived macrophages (Lai et al. 2000).

The presence of endothelin receptors is inferred by the observation that cultured mouse microglial cells respond to endothelin with an increase in intracellular [Ca^{2+}]. This response involves the release of Ca^{2+} from cytoplasmic stores. Pharmacological screening indicates that ET_B receptors mediate the response. Moreover, transcripts encoding ET_B receptors were detected in purified microglia cultures and by single cell RT-PCR (Möller et al., 1997).

SCHWANN CELLS

Purinergic Receptors

Schwann cells express several purinergic receptors, of both the ionotropic and metabotropic subtype (Lyons et al., 1994; Colomar and Amedee, 2001). Among the ionotropic ATP receptors, the large pore-forming $P2X_7$ receptor is prominently expressed and leads to an increase of three different conductances: a nonselective cationic conductance and selective K^+ and Cl^- conductances. Moreover, activation triggers an increase in intracellular [Ca^{2+}]. The metabotropic receptor, $P2Y_1$, has been identified. Purinergic receptors have been identified in freshly isolated Schwann cells, in cells from isolated rat spinal roots, and in perisynaptic glial cells of the frog neuromuscular junction. They are expressed both in myelinating and nonmyelinating Schwann cells. The response to ATP is lost when the cells are taken into culture (Lyons et al., 1995). Direct contact of Schwann cells with neurons stabilizes the expression of purinergic receptors, as revealed in coculture experiments, suggesting a role of purinergic receptors in neuron–Schwann cell signaling. Indeed, at the frog neuromuscular junction, neuronal activity triggers a Ca^{2+} response in perisynaptic Schwann cells via purinergic receptors (Robitaille, 1995). While adenosine receptors are also present in Schwann cells, they do not play an important role in neuron-glia signaling. There is also a feedback loop from the Schwann cell to the axon: Ca^{2+} release from Schwann cell intracellular stores initiates a potentiation of synaptic transmission. Moreover, purinergic receptor activation causes release of the excitatory amino acids glutamate and aspartate from Schwann cells. This release is mediated by metabotropic purinergic receptors and requires a release of Ca^{2+} from intracellular stores. The excitatory amino acid release is not due to reversed uptake, but rather to a Ca^{2+}-sensitive release mechanism.

Endothelin and Tachykinin Receptors

Endothelin and tachykinin receptors are considered to be involved in pain perception. Two types of endothelin receptors are known: ET_A receptors play a role in acute or neuropathic pain signaling, and ET_B receptors are involved in the transmission of chronic inflammatory pain. ET_A receptors are expressed on dorsal root ganglion neurons or axons, and ET_B receptors are present on dorsal root ganglion satellite cells and nonmyelinating Schwann cells. (Pomonis et al., 2001). During development, endothelins influence survival and lineage progression of Schwann cells. By acting on ET_B receptors, they promote Schwann cell precursor survival and delay the transition of the precursor cells to more mature stages of differentiation. Thus, ET_B receptors act as negative regulators in Schwann cell maturation (Brennan et al., 2000).

Tachykinin receptors have been detected on perisynaptic Schwann cells of the frog neuromuscular junction. They trigger release of Ca^{2+} from cytoplasmic stores involving the activation of G-proteins. Signaling is mediated via NK_1 receptors, and receptor activation modulates Schwann cell Ca^{2+} signaling: Responses of Schwann cells to ATP or to nerve stimulation are significantly reduced upon tachykinin receptor activation, indicating that substance P has an impact on neuron-glia communication (Bourque and Robitaille, 1998).

Other Receptors

There is only weak evidence for the presence of acetylcholine receptors in Schwann cells, namely, a study reporting faint immunolabeling for muscarinic acetylcholine receptor subtypes M_1–M_4. Myelinating rat Schwann cells express 5-HT receptors *in vivo*, as revealed with immunocytochemistry and receptor-specific antibodies (Yoder et al., 1997). There is evidence for the expression of bradykinin receptors: Similar to ATP, bradykinin can trigger the release of excitatory amino acids such as glutamate and aspartate in cultured Schwann cells (Parpura et al., 1995). Studies of Ca^{2+} responses in cultured Schwann cells of guinea pig indicated the presence of iGluRs of the NMDA, AMPA, and kainate subtypes. The same group reported on the expression of α_1, α_2, and β adrenoceptors. However, it should be taken into account that none of these receptors have been identified in Schwann cells *in situ*.

Concluding Remarks

The studies in cell culture indicate that astrocytes have the capacity to express almost all the different transmitter receptors. Analyses in brain slices, however, indicate that there is some heterogeneity with respect to brain region and subtype of astrocyte. We could even define subtypes of astrocytes by their diverse physiological response profiles. This may be an important footprint for identifying and characterizing astrocytes *in situ*. There is increasing evidence that synaptic activity stimulates receptors in astrocytes and in Schwann cells. However, many questions remain: Are astrocytic receptors important for signal processing in the brain? What controls receptor expression, and how does neuronal activity influence the receptor pattern of astrocytes? What is the impact of altered astrocytic receptor functioning on the pathogenesis in the diseased nervous system?

The functional role of oligodendrocyte receptors is well established only for glutamate receptors that play a role in cellular differentiation. In microglia, glutamate receptor and adrenergic receptors are linked to immunological functions. These transmitter receptors could be important for mediating cross-talk between the nervous system and the immune system.

REFERENCES

Reviews

Azmitia, E.C. (2001) Modern views on an ancient chemical: serotonin effects on cell proliferation, maturation, and apoptosis. *Brain Res. Bull.* 56:413–424.

Ciccarelli, R., Ballerini, P., Sabatino, G., Rathbone, M.P., D'Onofrio, M., Caciagli, F., and Di Iorio, P. (2001) Involvement of astrocytes in purine-mediated reparative processes in the brain. *Int. J. Dev. Neurosci.* 19:395–414.

Condorelli, D.F., Conti, F., Gallo, V., Kirchhoff, F., Seifert, G., Steinhäuser, C., Verkhratsky A., and Yuan, X.Q. (1999) Expression and functional analysis of glutamate receptors in glial cells. *Adv. Exp. Med. Biol.* 468:49–67.

Fraser, D.D., Mudrick-Donnon, L.A., and MacVicar, B.A. (1994) Astrocytic GABA receptors. *Glia* 11:83–93.

Hösli, E. and Hösli, L. (1993) Receptors for neurotransmitters on astrocytes in the mammalian central nervous system. *Prog. Neurobiol.* 40:477–506.

Inagaki, N. and Wada, H. (1994) Histamine and prostanoid receptors on glial cells. *Glia* 11:102–109.

James, G. and Butt, A.M. (2002) P2Y and P2X purinoceptor mediated Ca(2+) signalling in glial cell pathology in the central nervous system. *Eur. J. Pharmacol.* 447:247–260.

Magistretti, P.J., Cardinaux, J.R., and Martin, J.L. (1998) VIP and PACAP in the CNS: regulators of glial energy metabolism and modulators of glutamatergic signaling. *Ann. NY Acad. Sci.* 865: 213–225.

Porter, J.T. and McCarthy, K.D. (1997) Astrocytic neurotransmitter receptors *in situ* and *in vivo*. *Prog. Neurobiol.* 51:439–455.

Seifert, G. and Steinhäuser, C. (2001) Ionotropic glutamate receptors in astrocytes. *Prog. Brain Res.* 132:287–299.

Steinhäuser, C. and Seifert, G. (2002) Glial membrane channels and receptors in epilepsy: impact for generation and spread of seizure activity. *Eur. J. Pharmacol.* 447:227–237.

Sumners, C., Tang, W., Paulding, W., and Raizada, M.K. (1994) Peptide receptors in astroglia: focus on angiotensin II and atrial natriuretic peptide. *Glia* 11:110–116.

Taylor, D.L., Diemel, L.T., and Pocock, J.M. (2003) Activation of microglial group III metabotropic glutamate receptors protects neurons against microglial neurotoxicity. *J. Neurosc.* 23:2150–2160.

Verkhratsky, A., Orkand, R.K., and Kettenmann, H. (1998) Glial calcium: homeostasis and signaling function. *Physiol. Rev.* 78: 99–141.

Verkhratsky, A. and Steinhäuser, C. (2000) Ion channels in glial cells. *Brain Res. Rev.* 32:380–412.

Winder, D.G. and Conn, P.J. (1996) Roles of metabotropic glutamate receptors in glial function and glial-neuronal communication. *J. Neurosci. Res.* 46:131–137.

Original Articles

Abbracchio, M.P., Rainaldi, G., Giammarioli, A.M., Ceruti, S., Brambilla, R., Cattabeni, F., Barbieri, D., Franceschi, C., Jacobson, K.A., and Malorni, W. (1997) The A3 adenosine receptor mediates cell spreading, reorganization of actin cytoskeleton, and distribution of Bcl-XL: studies in human astroglioma cells. *Biochem. Biophys. Res. Commun.* 241:297–304.

Agrawal, S.K., Theriault, E., and Fehlings, M.G. (1998) Role of group I metabotropic glutamate receptors in traumatic spinal cord white matter injury. *J. Neurotrauma* 15:929–941.

Aguado, F., Espinosa-Parrilla, J.F., Carmona, M.A., and Soriano, E. (2002) Neuronal activity regulates correlated network properties of spontaneous calcium transients in astrocytes in situ. *J. Neurosci.* 22:9430–9444.

Araque, A., Martin, E.D., Perea, G., Arellano, J.I., and Buno, W. (2002) Synaptically released acetylcholine evokes Ca^{2+} elevations in astrocytes in hippocampal slices. *J. Neurosci.* 22:2443–2450.

Aronica, E., Catania, M.V., Geurts, J., Yankaya, B., and Troost, D. (2001) Immunohistochemical localization of group I and II metabotropic glutamate receptors in control and amyotrophic lateral sclerosis human spinal cord: upregulation in reactive astrocytes. *Neuroscience* 105:509–520.

Backus, K.H., Berger, T., and Kettenmann, H. (1991) Activation of neurokinin receptors modulates K^+ and Cl^- channel activity in cultured astrocytes from rat cortex. *Brain Res.* 541:103–109.

Bekar, L.K., Jabs, R., and Walz, W. (1999) $GABA_A$ receptor agonists modulate K^+ currents in adult hippocampal glial cells in situ. *Glia* 26:129–138.

Belachew, S., Rogister, B., Rigo, J.M., Malgrange, B., Mazy-Servais, C., Xhauflaire, G., Coucke, P., and Moonen, G. (1998) Cultured oligodendrocyte progenitors derived from cerebral cortex express a glycine receptor which is pharmacologically distinct from the neuronal isoform. *Eur. J. Neurosci.* 10:3556–3564.

Beldhuis, H.J., Everts, H.G., van der Zee, E.A., Luiten, P.G., and Bohus, B. (1992) Amygdala kindling–induced seizures selectively impair spatial memory. 2. Effects on hippocampal neuronal and glial muscarinic acetylcholine receptor. *Hippocampus* 2:411–419.

Berger, T. Walz, W., Schnitzer, J., and Kettenmann, H. (1992) GABA- and glutamate-activated currents in glial cells of the mouse corpus callosum slice. *J. Neurosci. Res.* 31:21–27.

Bezzi, P., Carmignoto, G., Pasti, L., Vesce, S., Rossi, D., Rizzini, B.L., Pozzan, T., and Volterra, A. (1998) Prostaglandins stimulate calcium-dependent glutamate release in astrocytes. *Nature* 391:281–285.

Bongarzone, E.R., Howard, S.G., Schonmann, V., and Campagnoni, A.T. (1998) Identification of the dopamine D_3 receptor in oligodendrocyte precursors: potential role in regulating differentiation and myelin formation. *J. Neurosci. Res.* 60:10–20.

Borges, K., and Kettenmann, H. (1995) Blockade of K^+ channels induced by AMPA/kainate receptor activation in mouse oligodendrocyte precursor cells is mediated by Na^+ entry. *J. Neurosci. Res.* 42:579–593.

Borges, K., Ohlemeyer, C., Trotter, J., and Kettenmann, H. (1994) AMPA/kainate receptor activation in murine oligodendrocyte precursor cells leads to activation of a cation conductance, calcium influx and blockade of delayed rectifying K^+ channels. *Neuroscience* 63:135–149.

Boucsein, C., Zacharias, R., Färber, K., Pavlovic, S., Hanisch, U.-K., and Kettenmann H. (2003) Purinergic receptors on microglial cells: functional expression in acute brain slices and modulation of microglial activation in vitro, *Eur. J. Neurosci.* 17:2267–2276.

Bourque, M.J. and Robitaille, R. (1998) Endogenous peptidergic modulation of perisynaptic Schwann cells at the frog neuromuscular junction. *J. Physiol.* 512:197–209.

Bowman, C.L. and Kimelberg, H.K. (1984) Excitatory amino acids directly depolarize rat brain astrocytes in primary culture. *Nature* 311:656–659.

Brennan, A., Dean, C.H., Zhang, A.L., Cass, D.T., Mirsky, R., and Jessen, K.R. (2000) Endothelins control the timing of Schwann cell generation in vitro and in vivo. *Dev. Biol.* 227:545–557.

Chen, J.G., Backus, K.H., and Deitmer, J.W. (1997) Intracellular calcium transients and potassium current oscillations evoked by glutamate in cultured rat astrocytes. *J. Neurosci.* 17:7278–7287.

Ciccarelli, R., Di Iorio, P., Bruno, V., Battaglia, G., D'Alimonte, I., D'Onofrio, M., Nicoletti, F., and Caciagli, F. (1999) Activation of A_1 adenosine or mGlu3 metabotropic glutamate receptors enhances the release of nerve growth factor and S-100β protein from cultured astrocytes. *Glia* 27:275–281.

Cohen, R.I. and Almazan, G. (1993) Norepinephrine-stimulated PI hydrolysis in oligodendrocytes is mediated by alpha 1A adrenoceptors. *NeuroReport* 4:1115–1118.

Cohen, R.I. and Almazan, G. (1994) Rat oligodendrocytes express muscarinic receptors coupled to phosphoinositide hydrolysis and adenylyl cyclase. *Eur. J. Neurosci.* 6:1213–1224.

Colomar, A. and Amedee, T. (2001) ATP stimulation of $P2X_7$ receptors activates three different ionic conductances on cultured mouse Schwann cells. *Eur. J. Neurosci.* 14:927–936.

Cormier, R.J., Mennerick, S., Melbostad, H., and Zorumski, C.F. (2001) Basal levels of adenosine modulate mGluR5 on rat hippocampal astrocytes. *Glia* 33:24–35.

Cotrina, M.L., Lin, J.H.C., and Nedergaard, M. (1998) Cytoskeletal assembly and ATP release regulate astrocytic calcium signaling. *J. Neurosci.* 18:8794–8804.

Di Iorio, P., Kleywegt, S., Ciccarelli, R., Traversa, U., Andrew, C.M., Crocker, C.E., Werstiuk, E.S., and Rathbone, M.P. (2002) Mechanisms of apoptosis induced by purine nucleosides in astrocytes. *Glia* 38:179–190.

Ferrari, D., Chiozzi, P., Falzoni, S., Hanau, S., and Di Virgilio, F. (1997) Purinergic modulation of interleukin-1 beta release from microglial cells stimulated with bacterial endotoxin. *J. Exp. Med.* 185:579–582.

Figiel, M. and Engele, J. (2000) Pituitary adenylate cyclase–activating polypeptide (PACAP), a neuron-derived peptide regulating glial glutamate transport and metabolism. *J. Neurosci.* 20:3596–3605.

Franke, H., Krugel, U., Schmidt, R., Grosche, J., Reichenbach, A., and Illes, P. (2001) P2 receptor types involved in astrogliosis in vivo. *Br. J. Pharmacol.* 134:1180–1189.

Fraser, D.D., Duffy, S., Angelides, K.J., Perez-Velazquez, J.L., Kettenmann, H., and MacVicar, B.A. (1995) $GABA_A$/benzodiazepine receptors in acutely isolated hippocampal astrocytes. *J. Neurosci.* 15:2720–2732.

García-Barcina, J.M., and Matute, C. (1996) Expression of kainate-selective glutamate receptor subunits in glial cells of the adult bovine white matter. *Eur. J. Neurosci.* 8:2379–2387.

Gilbert, P., Kettenmann, H., and Schachner, M. (1984) Gamma-aminobutyric acid directly depolarizes cultured oligodendrocytes. *J. Neurosci.* 4:561–569.

Gimpl, G., Walz, W., Ohlemeyer, C., and Kettenmann, H. (1992) Bradykinin receptors in cultured astrocytes from neonatal brain are linked to physiological responses. *Neurosci. Lett.* 144:139–142.

Graham, A., Court, J.A., Martin-Ruiz, C.M., Jaros, E., Perry, R., Volsen, S.G., Bose, S., Evans, N., Ince, P., Kuryatov, A., Lindstrom, J., Gotti, C., and Perry, E.K. (2002) Immunohistochemical localisation of nicotinic acetylcholine receptor subunits in human cerebellum. *Neuroscience* 113:493–507.

Griffith, R. and Sutin, J. (1996) Reactive astrocyte formation in vivo is regulated by noradrenergic axons. *J. Comp. Neurol.* 371:362–375.

Haas, S., Brockhaus, J., Verkhratsky, A., and Kettenmann, H. (1996)

ATP-induced membrane currents in ameboid microglia acutely isolated from mouse brain slices. *Neuroscience* 75:257–261.

Honda, S., Sasaki, Y., Ohsawa, K., Imai, Y., Nakamura, Y., Inoue, K., and Kohsaka, S. (2001) Extracellular ATP or ADP induce chemotaxis of cultured microglia through Gi/o-coupled P2Y receptors. *J. Neurosci.* 21:1975–1982.

Hoppe, D. and Kettenmann, H. (1989) GABA triggers a Cl^- efflux from cultured mouse oligodendrocytes. *Neurosci. Lett.* 97:334–339.

Iino, M., Goto, K., Kakegawa, W., Okado, H., Sudo, M., Ishiuchi, S., Miwa, A., Takayasu, Y., Saito, I., Tsuzuki, K., and Ozawa, S. (2001) Glia-synapse interaction through Ca^{2+}-permeable AMPA receptors in Bergmann glia. *Science* 292:926–929.

Itoh, T., Beesley, J., Itoh, A., Cohen, A.S., Kavanaugh, B., Coulter, D.A., Grinspan, J.B., and Pleasure, D. (2002) AMPA glutamate receptor-mediated calcium signaling is transiently enhanced during development of oligodendrocytes. *J. Neurochem.* 81:390–402.

Jung, S., Pfeiffer, F., and Deitmer, J.W. (2000) Histamine-induced calcium entry in rat cerebellar astrocytes: evidence for capacitative and non-capacitative mechanisms. *J. Physiol. (Lond.)* 527: 549–561.

Kang, J., Jiang, L., Goldman, S.A., and Nedergaard, M. (1998) Astrocyte-mediated potentiation of inhibitory synaptic transmission. *Nat. Neurosci.* 1:683–692.

Kettenmann, H., Backus, K.H., and Schachner, M. (1984) Aspartate, glutamate and γ-aminobutyric acid depolarize cultured astrocytes. *Neurosci. Lett.* 52:25–29.

Kettenmann, H. Gilbert, P., and Schachner, M. (1984) Depolarization of cultured oligodendrocytes by glutamate and GABA. *Neurosci. Lett.* 47:271–276.

Khan, Z.U., Koulen, P., Rubinstein, M., Grandy, D.K., and Goldman-Rakic, P.S. (2001) An astroglia-linked dopamine D2-receptor action in prefrontal cortex. *Proc. Natl. Acad. Sci. USA* 98:1964–1969.

Kirchhoff, F., Mülhardt, C., Pastor, A., Becker, C.M., and Kettenmann, H. (1996) Expression of glycine receptor subunits in glial cells of the rat spinal cord. *J. Neurochem.* 66:1383–1390.

Kirischuk, S., Scherer, J., Kettenmann, H., and Verkhratsky, A. (1995) Activation of P_2-purinoreceptors triggered Ca^{2+} release from InsP3-sensitive internal stores in mammalian oligodendrocytes. *J. Physiol.* 483:41–57.

Krebs, C., Fernandes, H.B., Sheldon, C., Raymond, L.A., and Baimbridge, K.G. (2003) Functional NMDA receptor subtype 2B is expressed in astrocytes after ischemia in vivo and anoxia in vitro. *J. Neurosci.* 23:3364–3372.

Kukley, M., Barden, J.A., Steinhäuser, C., and Jabs, R. (2001) Distribution of P2X receptors on astrocytes in juvenile rat hippocampus. *Glia* 36:11–21.

Kulik, A., Haentzsch, A., Lückermann, M., Reichelt, W., and Ballanyi, K. (1999) Neuron-glia signaling via α_1 adrenoceptor-mediated Ca^{2+} release in Bergmann glial cells *in situ*. *J. Neurosci.* 19:8401–8408.

Lai, J.P., Zhan, G.X., Campbell, D.E., Douglas, S.D., and Ho, W.Z. (2000) Detection of substance P and its receptor in human fetal microglia. *Neuroscience* 101:1137–1144.

Langosch, J.M., Gebicke-Haerter, P.J., Norenberg, W., and Illes, P. (1994) Characterization and transduction mechanisms of purinoceptors in activated rat microglia. *Br. J. Pharmacol.* 113: 29–34.

Lee, R.K., Araki, W., and Wurtman, R.J. (1997) Stimulation of amyloid precursor protein synthesis by adrenergic receptors couplet to cAMP formation. *Proc. Natl. Acad. Sci. USA* 94:5422–5426.

Lee, R.K., Jimenez, J., Cox, A.J., and Wurtman, R.J. (1996) Metabotropic glutamate receptors regulate APP processing in hippocampal neurons and cortical astrocytes derived from fetal rats. *Ann. NY. Acad. Sci.* 777:338–343.

Li, Y., Holtzclaw, L.A., and Russell, J.T. (2001) Müller cell Ca^{2+} waves evoked by purinergic receptor agonists in slices of rat retina. *J. Neurophysiol.* 85:986–994.

Luber-Narod, J., Kage, R., and Leeman, S.E. (1994) Substance P enhances the secretion of tumor necrosis factor-alpha from neuroglial cells stimulated with lipopolysaccharide. *J. Immunol.* 152:819–824.

Lyons, S.A., Morell, P., and McCarthy, K.D. (1994) Schwann cells exhibit P2Y purinergic receptors that regulate intracellular calcium and are up-regulated by cyclic AMP analogues. *J. Neurochem.* 63:552–560.

Lyons, S.A., Morell, P., and McCarthy, K.D. (1995) Schwann cell ATP-mediated calcium increases in vitro and in situ are dependent on contact with neurons. *Glia* 13:27–38.

Matthias, K., Kirchhoff, F., Seifert, G., Hüttmann, K., Matyash, M., Kettenmann, H., and Steinhäuser, C. (2003) Segregated expression of AMPA-type glutamate receptors and glutamate transporters defines distinct astrocyte populations in the mouse hippocampus. *J. Neurosci.* 23:1750–1758.

Matute, C., Sanchez-Gomez, M.V., Martinez-Millan, L., and Miledi, R. (1997) Glutamate receptor-mediated toxicity in optic nerve oligodendrocytes. *Proc. Natl. Acad. Sci. USA* 94:8830–8835.

Milner, T.A., Lee, A., Aicher, S.A., and Rosin, D.L. (1998) Hippocampal α_{2A}-adrenergic receptors are located predominantly presynaptically but are also found postsynaptically and in selective astrocytes. *J. Comp. Neurol.* 395:310–327.

Mittaud, P., Labourdette, G., Zingg, H., and Guenot-Di Scala, D. (2002) Neurons modulate oxytocin receptor expression in rat cultured astrocytes: involvement of TGF-beta and membrane components. *Glia* 37:169–177.

Möller, T., Kann, O., Prinz, M., Kirchhoff, F., Verkhratsky, A., and Kettenmann, H. (1997) Endothelin-induced calcium signaling in cultured mouse microglial cells is mediated through ET_B receptors. *NeuroReport.* 8:2127–2131.

Mong, J.A., Nunez, J.L., and McCarthy, M.M. (2002) GABA mediates steroid-induced astrocyte differentiation in the neonatal rat hypothalamus. *J. Neuroendocrinol.* 14:45–55.

Mudrick-Donnon, L.A., Williams, P.J., Pittman, Q.J., and MacVicar, B.A. (1993) Postsynaptic potentials mediated by GABA and dopamine evoked in stellate glial cells of the pituitary pars intermedia. *J. Neurosci.* 13:4660–4668.

Müller, T., Fritschy, J.M., Grosche, J., Pratt, G.D., Möhler, H., and Kettenmann, H. (1994) Developmental regulation of voltage-gated K^+ channel and $GABA_A$ receptor expression in Bergmann glial cells. *J. Neurosci.* 14:2503–2514.

Müller, T., Möller, T., Berger, T., Schnitzer, J., and Kettenmann, H. (1992) Calcium entry through kainate receptors and resulting potassium-channel blockade in Bergmann glial cells. *Science* 256: 1563–1566.

Muyderman, H., Nilsson, M., Blomstrand, F., Khatibi, S., Olsson, T., Hansson, E., and Rönnbäck, L. (1998) Modulation of mechanically induced calcium waves in hippocampal astroglial cells. Inhibitory effects of α_1-adrenergic stimulation. *Brain Res.* 793: 127–135.

Newman, E.A. (2001) Propagation of intercellular calcium waves in retinal astrocytes and Muller cells. *J. Neurosci.* 21:2215–2223.

Niermann, H., Amiry-Moghaddam, M., Holthoff, K., Witte, O.W., and Ottersen, O.P. (2001) A novel role of vasopressin in the brain: modulation of activity-dependent water flux in the neocortex. *J. Neurosci.* 21:3045–3051.

Nishizaki, T., Nagai, K., Nomura, T., Tada, H., Kanno, T., Tozaki, H., Li, X.X., Kondoh, T., Kodama, N., Takahashi, E., Sakai, N., Tanaka, K., and Saito, N. (2002) A new neuromodulatory pathway with a glial contribution mediated via A_{2a} adenosine receptors. *Glia* 39:133–147.

Noda, M., Nakanishi, H., Nabekura, J., and Akaike, N. (2000) AMPA-kainate subtypes of glutamate receptor in rat cerebral microglia. *J. Neurosci.* 20:251–258.

Palma, C., Minghetti, L., Astolfi, M., Ambrosini, E., Silberstein, F.C., Manzini, S., Levi, G., and Aloisi, F. (1997) Functional characterization of substance P receptors on cultured human spinal cord astrocytes: synergism of substance P with cytokines in inducing interleukin-6 and prostaglandin E2 production. *Glia* 21:183–193.

Panenka, W., Jijon, H., Herx, L.M., Armstrong, J.N., Feighan, D., Wei, T., Yong, V.W., Ransohoff, R.M., and MacVicar, B.A. (2001) $P2X_7$-like receptor activation in astrocytes increases chemokine monocyte chemoattractant protein-1 expression via mitogen-activated protein kinase. *J. Neurosci.* 21:7135–7142.

Pannicke, T., Wolfgang, F., Biedermann, B., Schädlich, H., Grosche, J., Faude, F., Wiedemann, P., Allgaier, C., Illes, P., Burnstock, G., and Reichenbach, A. (2000) $P2X_7$ receptors in Mueller glial cells from the human retina. *J. Neurosci.* 20:5965–5972.

Parpura, V., Basarsky, T.A., Liu, F., Jeftinija, K., Jeftinija, S., and Haydon, P. G. (1994) Glutamate-mediated astrocyte-neuron signalling. *Nature* 369:744–747.

Parpura, V., Liu, F., Jeftinija, K.V., Haydon, P.G., and Jeftinija, S.D. (1995) Neuroligand-evoked calcium-dependent release of excitatory amino acids from Schwann cells. *J. Neurosci.* 15:5831–5839.

Pasti, L., Volterra, A., Pozzan, T., and Carmignoto, G. (1997) Intracellular calcium oscillations in astrocytes: a highly plastic, bidirectional form of communication between neurons and astrocytes in situ. *J. Neurosci.* 17:7817–7830.

Pastor, A., Chvátal, A., Syková, E., and Kettenmann, H. (1995) Glycine- and GABA-activated currents in identified glial cells of the developing rat spinal cord slice. *Eur. J. Neurosci.* 7:1188–1198.

Patte, C., Gandolfo, P., Leprince, J., Thoumas, J.L., Fontaine, M., Vaudry, H., and Tonon, M.C. (1999) GABA inhibits endozepine release from cultured rat astrocytes. *Glia* 25:404–411.

Pilitsis, J.G., and Kimelberg, H.K. (1998) Adenosine receptor mediated stimulation of intracellular calcium in acutely isolated astrocytes. *Brain Res.* 798:294–303.

Pomonis, J.D., Rogers, S.D., Peters, C.M., Ghilardi, J.R., and Mantyh, P.W. (2001) Expression and localization of endothelin receptors: implications for the involvement of peripheral glia in nociception. *J. Neurosci.* 21:999–1006.

Porter, J.T. and McCarthy, K.D. (1995) Adenosine receptors modulate $[Ca^{2+}]_i$ in hippocampal astrocytes in situ. *J. Neurochem.* 65:1515–1523.

Prins, B.A., Weber, M.J., Hu, R.M., Pedram, A., Daniels, M., and Levin, E.R. (1996) Atrial natriuretic peptide inhibits mitogen-activated protein kinase through the clearance receptor—potential role in the inhibition of astrocyte proliferation. *J. Biol. Chem.* 271:14156–14162.

Prinz, M., Haeusler, K.G., Kettenmann, H., and Hanisch, U.K. (2001) Beta-adrenergic receptor stimulation selectively inhibits IL-12p40 release in microglia. *Brain Res.* 899:264–270.

Rathbone, M.P., Middlemiss, P.J., Kim, J.K., Gysbers, J.W., DeForge, S.P., Smith, R.W., and Hughes, D.W. (1992) Adenosine and its nucleotides stimulate proliferation of chick astrocytes and human astrocytoma cells. *Neurosci. Res.* 13:1–17.

Reuss, B. and Unsicker, K. (2001) Atypical neuroleptic drugs downregulate dopamine sensitivity in rat cortical and striatal astrocytes. *Mol. Cell Neurosci.* 18:197–209.

Robitaille, R. (1995) Purinergic receptors and their activation by endogenous purines at perisynaptic glial cells of the frog neuromuscular junction. *J. Neurosci.* 15:7121–7131.

Rogers, S.W., Gregori, N.Z., Carlson, N., Gahring, L.C., and Noble, M. (2001) Neuronal nicotinic acetylcholine receptor expression by O2A/oligodendrocyte progenitor cells. *Glia* 33:306–313.

Roy, M.L. and Sontheimer, H. (1995) α-Adrenergic modulation of glial inwardly rectifying potassium channels. *J. Neurochem.* 64:1576–1584.

Schipke, C.G., Boucsein, C., Ohlemeyer, C., Kirchhoff, F., and Kettenmann, H. (2001a) Astrocyte Ca^{2+} waves trigger responses in microglial cells in brain slices. *FASEB J.* 16:255–257.

Schipke, C.G., Ohlemeyer, C., Matyash, M., Nolte, C., Kettenmann, H., and Kirchhoff, F. (2001b) Astrocytes of the mouse neocortex express functional *N*-methyl-D-aspartate receptors. *FASEB J.* 15: 1270–1272.

Schröder, W., Seifert, G., Hüttmann, K., Hinterkeuser, S., and Steinhäuser, C. (2002) AMPA receptor-mediated modulation of inward rectifier K^+ channels in astrocytes of mouse hippocampus. *Mol. Cell Neurosci.* 19:447–458.

Seifert, G., Weber, M., Schramm, J., and Steinhäuser, C. (2003) Changes in splice variant expression and subunit assembly of AMPA receptors during maturation of hippocampal astrocytes. *Mol. Cell. Neurosci.* 22:248–258.

Seifert, G., Hüttmann, J., Schramm, J., and Steinhäuser, C. (2004) Enhanced relative expression of GluR1 flip AMPA receptor subunits in hippocampal astrocytes of epilepsy patients with Ammon's horn sclerosis. *J. Neurosci* 24:1996–2003.

Sharma, G. and Vijayaraghavan, S. (2001) Nicotinic cholinergic signaling in hippocampal astrocytes involves calcium-induced calcium release from intracellular stores. *Proc. Natl. Acad. Sci. USA* 98:4148–4153.

Shelton, M.K. and McCarthy, K.D. (2000) Hippocampal astrocytes exhibit Ca^{2+}-elevating muscarinic cholinergic and histaminergic receptors in situ. *J. Neurochem.* 74:555–563.

Stephens, G.J., Marriott, D.R., Djamgoz, M.B., and Wilkin, G.P. (1993) Electrophysiological and biochemical evidence for bradykinin receptors on cultured rat cortical oligodendrocytes. *Neurosci. Lett.* 153:223–226.

Sul, J.-Y., Orsz, G., Givens, R.S., and Haydon, P.G. (2004) Astrocytic connectivity in the hippocampus. *Neuron Glia Biology* 1:3–11.

Taylor, D.L., Diemel, L.T., and Pocock, J.M. (2003) Activation of microglial group III metabotropic glutamate receptors protects neurons against microglial neurotoxicity. *J. Neurosci.* 23:2150–2160.

Tryoen-Toth, P., Gaveriaux-Ruff, C., and Labourdette, G. (2000) Down-regulation of mu-opioid receptor expression in rat oligodendrocytes during their development in vitro. *J. Neurosci. Res.* 60:10–20.

Walz, W., Ilschner, S., Ohlemeyer, C., Banati, R. and Kettenmann, H. (1993) Extracellular ATP activates a cation conductance and a K^+ conductance in cultured microglial cells from mouse brain. *J. Neurosci.* 13:4403–4411.

Yoder, E.J., Tamir, H., and Ellisman, M.H. (1997) Serotonin receptors expressed by myelinating Schwann cells in rat sciatic nerve. *Brain Res.* 753:299–308.

Yuan, X., Eisen, A.M., McBain, C.J., and Gallo, V. (1998) A role for glutamate and its receptors in the regulation of oligodendrocyte development in cerebellar tissue slices. *Development* 125:2901–2914.

Zhang, L., McLarnon, J.G., Goghari, V., Lee, Y.B., Kim, S.U., and Krieger, C. (1998) Cholinergic agonists increase intracellular Ca^{2+} in cultured human microglia. *Neurosci. Lett.* 255:33–36.

Zhang, J.-M., Wang, H.-K., Yem C.-Q., Ge, W., Chen, A., Jiang, Z.-L., Wu, C.-P., Poo, M.-M., and Duan, S. (2003) ATP released by astrocytes mediates glutamatergic activity-dependent heterosynaptic suppression. *Neuron* 40:971–982.

Zhu, Y. and Kimelberg, H.K. (2001) Developmental expression of metabotropic $P2Y_1$ and P2Y(2) receptors in freshly isolated astrocytes from rat hippocampus. *J. Neurochem.* 77:530–541.

Ziak, D., Chvatal, A., and Sykova, E. (1998) Glutamate-, kainate- and NMDA-evoked membrane currents in identified glial cells in rat spinal cord slice. *Physiol. Res.* 47:365–375.

11 Cytokine and chemokine receptors and signaling

DUANE R. WESEMANN AND ETTY N. BENVENISTE

Cytokines, chemokines, and growth factors are secreted proteins that influence the survival, proliferation, differentiation, and functional activity of virtually all cell types. These soluble mediators communicate with cells through transmembrane-bound receptors or receptor complexes on target cells. This initiates multiple receptor-coupled intracellular signaling pathways that dictate the timing, nature, and strength of the cellular response to the external stimulus. One consequence of this recognition is a rapid reprogramming in the pattern of genes expressed in the target cell.

A large group of cytokines use type I or type II cytokine receptors: these include interferons (IFNs), many interleukins (i.e., IL-2, -4, -6, -9, -10, -12, -15, and -21); and IL-6 family members (IL-11, OSM, LIF, CNTF, NNT-1/BSF-3, CT-1) (see Table 11.1). These mediators stimulate responses by binding to and activating a family of structurally and functionally conserved receptors. Despite the number and diversity of cytokines and growth factors, the signaling pathways used are highly conserved. As is the case for many types of receptor families, downstream signaling involves tyrosine phosphorylation events. Signaling from the receptor is initiated by receptor oligomerization that is induced by cytokine binding, which brings receptor-associated Janus kinases (JAKs) into close apposition, allowing for their cross-phosphorylation and activation. The active JAKs phosphorylate tyrosine residues on the cytoplasmic portion of the receptor, which leads to the recruitment and activation of various signal transduction proteins, most notably the signal transducers and activators of transcription (STATs) family of transcription factors. The STATs are recruited through specific interactions with phosphorylated tyrosine residues on the receptor, in turn become phosphorylated by the JAKs, dimerize, and translocate to the nucleus. Once within the nucleus, they stimulate transcription of a wide array of cytokine responsive genes (Fig. 11.1).

In this chapter, we will provide details on the activation of the JAK/STAT pathway and the mechanisms that are used to control the magnitude and duration of signaling. Specifically, we will focus on the suppressor of cytokine signaling (SOCS) family of proteins that act in a negative feedback loop to extinguish signal transduction.

We will also briefly review the other major signaling pathways that are used by tumor necrosis factor (TNF) family members and members of the transforming growth factor (TGF) family. In addition, signaling by chemokines through G-protein–coupled chemokine receptors will be described. The intent of this chapter is to provide an overview of the major signaling cascades used by cytokines, chemokines, and growth factors and to describe the expression of receptors found on glial cells (astrocytes, microglia, and oligodendrocytes), thereby providing the foundation for subsequent chapters dealing with cytokine/chemokine responses in the central nervous system (CNS).

THE JAK/STAT PATHWAY

There are four mammalian members of the JAK family of receptor-associated tyrosine kinases: JAK1, JAK2, JAK3, and TYK2 (for review see Schindler, 2002). The JAKs are kinases of approximately 1000 amino acids and have clear, nonredundant functions *in vivo*, as assessed by the analysis of mice deficient in JAK1, JAK2, JAK3, and TYK2, as well as humans deficient in JAK3. Seven STATs have been identified: STAT-1, STAT-2, STAT-3, STAT-4, STAT-5A, STAT-5B, and STAT-6. The STATs are proteins of 750–850 amino acids that contain the following domains: amino terminal, coiled coil, DNA binding domain, linker, SH2 domain, and transcriptional activation domain. Cytokines and growth factors transduce their signals through specific sets of JAKs and STATs, as indicated in Table 11.1.

One of the major contributions of the studies on IFNs has been the elucidation of the JAK/STAT pathway, whose underlying principle of signal transduction and transcriptional regulation is used by more than 50 members of cytokine and growth factor families. We

See the list of abbreviations at the end of the chapter.

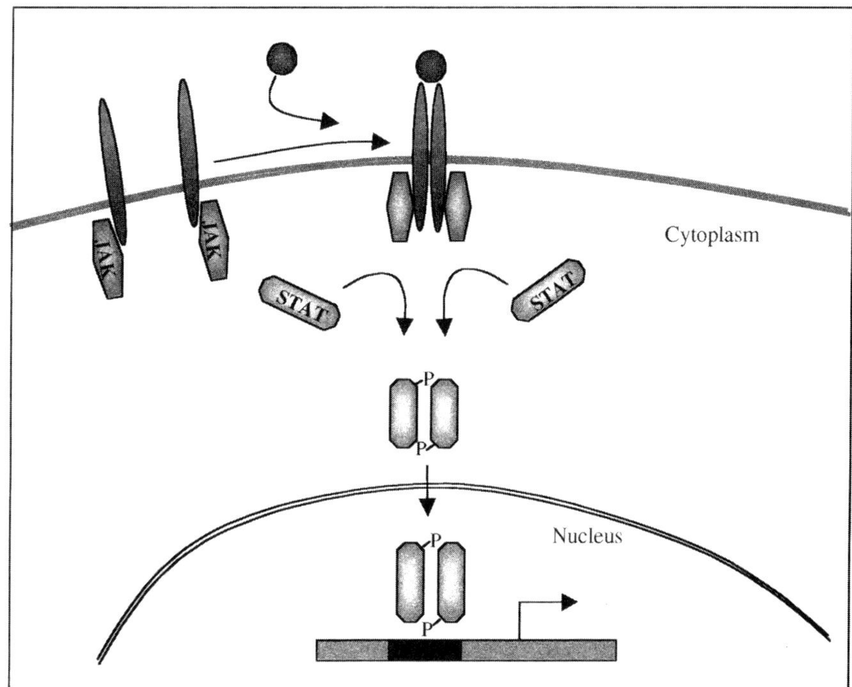

FIGURE 11.1 Generic Janus kinase/signal transducer and activator of transcription (JAK/STAT) signaling pathway. Following cytokine binding, signaling from cytokine receptors generally entails receptor oligomerization and approximation of receptor-bound JAKs, which are induced to phosphorylate receptor subunits when brought into proximity with other JAKs. Phosphorylated receptors serve as docking sites for latent STAT proteins, which in turn become targets for phosphorylation by the JAKs. Phosphorylated STATs dissociate from the receptor, dimerize, and translocate to the nucleus, where they bind to specific DNA sequences to regulate transcription of various genes.

will review the specific signaling pathways of several of these IFNs and cytokines (IFN-α/β, IFN-γ, IL-10, IL-6 family members, and IL-4). They have been chosen as examples since they have important biological effects within the CNS.

The Interferon/Interleukin-10 Receptor Family

The IFN and IL-10 receptors are related to each other and belong to the class II cytokine receptor family. The IFNs are divided into two functionally distinct groups, each of which binds to a unique receptor. Type I IFNs consist of IFN-α and IFN-β, which can be produced by most cell types. Type II IFN includes only IFN-γ, which is produced predominantly by T cells and natural killer cells. Both type I and type II IFN receptors consist of two chains that heterodimerize (IFNαRI/IFNαRII and IFNγRI/IFNγRII, respectively). The IL-10 receptor has the highest structural similarity to the IFN-γ receptor and is also composed of two subunits (IL-10RI/IL-10R2). Astrocytes, microglia, and oligodendrocytes express the receptors for type I IFNs (IFN-α and IFN-β), type II IFN (IFN-γ), and IL-10 (see Table 11.2).

Type II interferon (interferon-γ)

Interferon-γ is a pleiotropic cytokine involved in many aspects of immune responses (for review see Stark et al., 1998). As a cytokine secreted by Th1 cells, IFN-γ favors Th1 cell-mediated immune responses. Interferon-γ is a potent activator of macrophages and mi-

TABLE 11.1 *JAK/STAT Use By Selected Cytokines*

Ligands	*JAKs*	*STATs*
IFN family		
IFN-α/β	TYK2, JAK1	STAT-1, STAT-2
IFN-γ	JAK1, JAK2	STAT-1
IL-10	TYK2, JAK1	STAT-3
Gp130 family		
IL-6	JAK1, JAK2	STAT-3, (STAT-1)
IL-11	JAK1	STAT-3, (STAT-1)
OSM	JAK1, JAK2	STAT-3, (STAT-1)
LIF	JAK1, JAK2	STAT-3, (STAT-1)
CNTF	JAK1, JAK2	STAT-3, (STAT-1)
NNT-1/BSF-3	JAK1, JAK2	STAT-3, (STAT-1)
CT-1	JAK1, JAK2	STAT-3
IL-12	TYK2, JAK2	STAT-4
γC family		
IL-2	JAK1, JAK3	STAT-5, (STAT-3)
IL-4	JAK1, JAK3	STAT-6
IL-7	JAK1, JAK3	STAT-5, (STAT-3)
IL-9	JAK1, JAK3	STAT-5, (STAT-3)
IL-13	JAK1	STAT-6, (STAT-3)
IL-15	JAK1, JAK3	STAT-5, (STAT-3)
IL-21	(JAK1), JAK3	STAT-5 (STAT-1)

CNTF: ciliary neurotrophic factor; CT-1: cardiotrophin-1; IFN-α/β, γ: interferons α/β, γ; IL: interleukin; JAK: Janus kinase; LIF: leukemia inhibitory factor; NNT-1/BSF-3: novel neurotrophin-1/B-cell stimulating factor-3; OSM: oncostatin M; STAT-1 to -6: signal transducers and activators of transcription 1–6; TYK2: tyrosine kinase-2.

TABLE 11.2 *Cytokine/Chemokine Receptor Expression in Neuroglia*

Receptors	*Astrocytes*	*Microglia*	*Oligodendrocytes*
IFN family			
IFNα/β receptor	+	+	+
IFNγ receptor	+	+	+
IL-10 receptor	+	+	+
gp130 family			
gp130	+	+	+
IL-6 receptor	−	+	−
IL-11 receptor	?	+	?
OSM receptor	+	+	+
LIF receptor	+	+	+
CNTF receptor	+	+	+
γC family			
IL-4 receptor	+	+	+
TNF			
TNFR1	+	+	+
TNFRII	+	+	+
IL-1			
IL-1 receptor	+	+	+
TGF-β			
TGF-β receptor	+	+	+
Chemokines			
CCR1	+	+	?
CCR2	+	+	?
CCR3	+	+	?
CCR4	?	?	?
CCR5	+	+	?
CCR8	?	?	?
CCR9	?	?	?
CCR10	+	?	?
CCR11	+	+	?
CXCR1	?	?	+
CXCR2	+	+	+
CXCR3	+	?	?
CXCR4	+	+	?
CXCR5	?	?	?
CXC3CR1	+	+	?

CCR1–11: CC receptors 1–11; CNTF: ciliary neurotrophic factor; CXCR1–5: CXC receptors 1–5; IFNα/β, γ: interferon α/β, γ; IL: interleukin; LIF: leukemia inhibitory factor; OSM: oncostatin M; TGF: transforming growth factor; TNFR: tumor necrosis factor receptor.

croglia (the resident macrophage of the brain), leading to expression of cell surface molecules such as class II major histocompatibility complex (MHC) antigens and costimulatory molecules such as B7 and CD40, all of which are critical for immune reactivity. In addition, IFN-γ mediates the activation of macrophages by inducing respiratory burst and nitric oxide production, which greatly enhances the microbicidal activity of macrophages for many intracellular pathogens (for review see Boehm et al., 1997). Interferon-γ has also been shown to have antiviral activity as well as antiproliferative effects on tumor cells.

The IFN-γ receptor is ubiquitously but not evenly expressed (200 to 25,000 receptors per cell) on all nucleated cells, with the highest expression outside the lymphoid system (for review see Bach et al., 1997). It consists of two subunits, the 90 kDa α-chain (IFNγRI), with high ligand binding affinity, and the 65 kDa β-chain (IFNγRII), which is necessary for signaling. The IFN-γ receptor belongs to the type II cytokine receptor family and has no intrinsic kinase activity. However, it is constitutively associated with JAKs: IFNγRI with JAK1 and IFNγRII with JAK2. Binding of the IFN-γ homodimer to two IFNγRI subunits induces dimerization of IFNγRI, which then recruits two IFNγRII chains and leads to transphosphorylation and reciprocal activation of the JAKs. The activated JAKs then phosphorylate tyrosine residue 440 of IFNγRI, creating a recruitment site for latent STAT-1α. Phosphorylation of STAT-1α at position 701 by JAKs results in its dissociation from the IFN-γ receptor and the formation of STAT-1α homodimers. The STAT-1α homodimer then translocates into the nucleus, where it binds to specific gamma activation sites (GAS) in promoters of IFN-γ-inducible genes, leading to activation of transcription (see Fig. 11.2*A*). Serine phosphorylation at residue 727 has been shown to increase the transactivation potential of STAT-1α (for review see Decker and Kovarik, 2000); however, the serine kinase(s) responsible for this reaction has not been identified. STAT-1α interacts with other transcriptional regulators (transcription factors and cotransactivators) to potentiate activation of gene expression. These include NF-κB, Sp1, USF-1, PU-1, and CBP/p300. Astrocytes, microglia, and oligodendrocytes have been shown to respond to IFN-γ by various biological outcomes including induction of class II MHC, CD40, and adhesion molecule expression, STAT-1α activation, and, in the case of oligodendrocytes, by apoptosis (Benveniste et al., 1991; Lee et al., 1999; Popko and Baerwald, 1999; Nguyen and Benveniste, 2000b).

Type I interferons (interferon-α/β)

Interferon-α and IFN-β represent the prototypical type I interferons, and play a critical role in innate and early host responses to viral infection (for review see

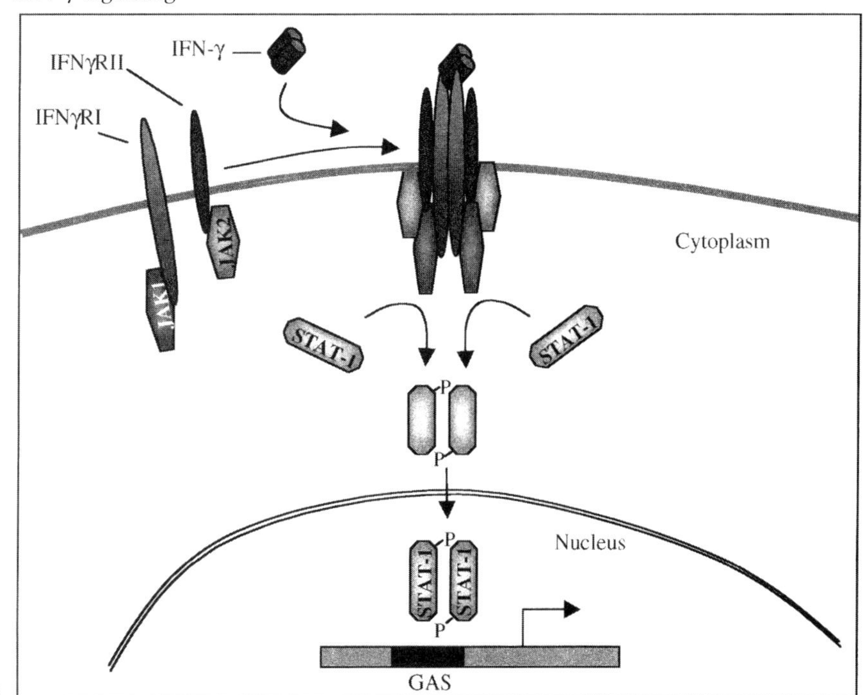

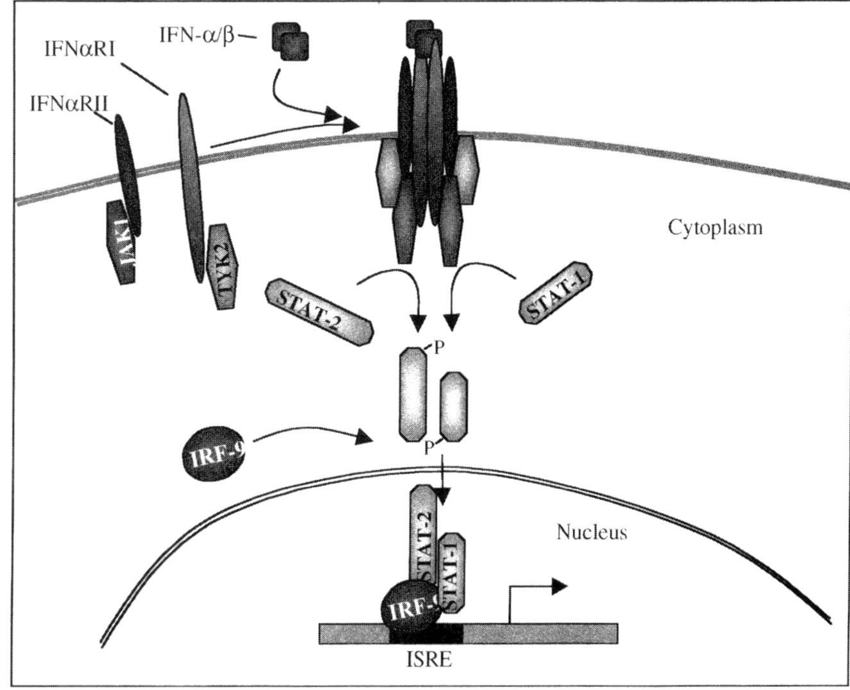

FIGURE 11.2 Interferon (IFN) signaling. *A.* Binding of the IFN-γ homodimer to two IFN-γ receptor I (IFNγRI) subunits induces dimerization of IFNγRI, which then recruits two IFNγRII chains and leads to transphosphorylation and reciprocal activation of the Janus kinases (JAKs). The activated JAKs then phosphorylate IFNγRI, creating a recruitment site for latent signal transducer and activation of transcription-1α (STAT-1α). Phosphorylation of STAT-1α by JAKs results in its dissociation from the IFN-γ receptor and the formation of STAT-1α homodimers. The STAT-1α homodimer then translocates into the nucleus, where it binds to specific gamma activation sites (GAS) in promoters of IFN-γ-inducible genes, leading to activation of transcription. *B.* Upon IFN-β or IFN-α binding, tyrosine kinase-2 (TYK2) and JAK1, which are constitutively bound to IFNαR1 and IFNαRII, respectively, are brought into proximity and transphosphorylate each other. Phosphorylated TYK2 and JAK1 are then activated to tyrosine phosphorylate IFNαR1. STAT-2 is recruited to this complex, binds to tyrosine-phosphorylated IFNαR1 via its SH2 domains, and subsequently becomes tyrosine-phosphorylated. The STAT-2 phosphotyrosine then serves as a docking site for latent STAT-1α, which then is also tyrosine-phosphorylated by the JAKs. Tyrosine-phosphorylated STAT-1α and STAT-2 form a heterodimer, dissociate from the receptor, translocate to the nucleus, and bind to IRF-9, a member of the interferon regulatory factor (IRF) family. The resulting heterotrimer, called ISGF3, binds to IFN-stimulated regulatory elements (ISRE) found in the promoters of IFN-α/β-regulated genes and activate gene expression.

Schindler, 2002). Type I IFNs also exhibit potent antiproliferative effects, particularly on tumor cells. As well, type I IFNs are used in the clinical management of malignant tumors, chronic viral hepatitis, and of multiple sclerosis (for review see Biron, 2001).

Signaling occurs through specific receptors that consist of two subunits (IFNαRI and IFNαRII) that bind either IFN-α or IFN-β. Upon ligand binding, TYK2 and JAK1, which are constitutively bound to IFNαR1 and IFNαRII, respectively, are brought into proximity and transphosphorylate each other. Phosphorylated TYK2 and JAK1 are then activated to tyrosine phosphorylate IFNαR1. STAT-2 is recruited to this complex, binds to tyrosine-phosphorylated IFNαR1 via its SH2 domains, and subsequently becomes tyrosine phosphorylated. The STAT-2 phosphotyrosine then serves as a docking site for latent STAT-1α, which then is also tyrosine-phosphorylated by the JAKs. Tyrosine-phosphorylated STAT-1α and STAT-2 form a heterodimer, dissociate from the receptor, translocate to the nucleus, and bind to IRF-9, a member of the interferon regulatory factor (IRF) family. The resulting heterotrimer, called ISGF3, binds to IFN-stimulated regulatory elements (ISRE) found in the promoters of IFN-α/β-regulated genes and activates gene expression (Fig. 11.2*B*). Within the ISGF3 complex, IRF-9 plays a critical role in recognizing ISRE sites, with STAT-1α contacting additional flanking nucleotides. STAT-2 does not interact directly with DNA. As well, STAT-1α homodimers can result from IFN-α/β stimulation, and bind to GAS elements as described above. All three glial cell types respond to IFN-α/β by activation of ISGF3, as well as by biological responses including suppression of pro-inflammatory cytokine gene expression, induction of IL-10 production, and suppression of matrix metalloproteinases (Chabot and Yong, 2000; Ma et al., 2001; Kim et al., 2002; Teige et al., 2003).

Interleukin-10

Interleukin-10 is a cytokine that has an important role in the suppression of inflammatory responses. It is produced predominantly by Th2 and Th3 cells and modulates a number of immune cell functions, especially those of macrophages and dendritic cells (for review see Strle et al., 2001). Interleukin-10 functions as a potent anti-inflammatory cytokine by inhibiting the expression of proinflammatory cytokines such as TNF-α, IL-1β, IFN-γ, IL-6, and IL-12, as well as inhibiting expression of class II MHC, CD40, and B7 molecules, thereby suppressing T-cell responsiveness. Within the CNS, both activated astrocytes and microglia are capable of producing IL-10, as well as expressing high-affinity IL-10 receptors (Ledeboer et al., 2002). Functional effects of IL-10 on astrocytes include inhibition of intercellular adhesion molecule-1 (ICAM-1) and TNF-α expression (Benveniste et al., 1995). In microglia, IL-10 is a potent inhibitor of cytokine/chemokine expression (Szczepanik et al., 2001). In oligodendrocytes, IL-10 exerts a protective effect against lipopolysaccharide/interferon-γ (LPS/IFN-γ)-induced cytotoxicity (Molina-Holgado et al., 2001).

Interleukin-10 cellular responses require the sequential assembly of two different receptor chains, IL-10R1 and IL-10R2, on the cell surface. Interleukin-10 binds to IL-10R1, and then this intermediate IL-10/IL-10R1 complex associates with IL-10R2, resulting in an active signaling complex that uses the JAK/STAT pathway. Stimulation with IL-10 results in tyrosine phosphorylation of JAK1 and TYK2, which are constitutively associated with IL-10R1 and IL-10R2, respectively. After activation, JAK1 and TYK2 phosphorylate IL-10R1 on tyrosine residues, creating docking sites for the binding of STAT proteins. STAT-3 is the protein that is predominantly activated by IL-10; however, STAT-1 and STAT-5 are activated to a lesser extent by IL-10 in certain cells. Upon tyrosine phosphorylation, STAT-3 dimerizes and translocates to the nucleus to bind to a STAT-3-specific sequence found in the promoter regions of many IL-10-responsive genes. These include cyclins, cyclin-dependent kinase inhibitors, *c-myc*, *c-pim*, *bcl-xL*, *bcl-2*, and *IL-10* itself (for review see Strle et al., 2001).

Gp130 Receptor Family

Cytokines of the gp130 family exert their diverse biological effects by forming high-affinity transmembrane receptor complexes characterized by the presence of the shared 130 kDa receptor subunit, gp130. Gp130 is ubiquitously expressed and has been detected on astrocytes, microglia, and oligodendrocytes (Table 11.2). The gp130 family of cytokines exhibit a wide range of biological functions due to the diversity of receptor complexes that can be formed. As well, they exhibit redundant functions that are dependent upon the signaling functions of the shared gp130 receptor. There are at least seven cytokine ligands that use gp130; these include IL-6, IL-11, leukemia inhibitory factor (LIF), oncostatin M (OSM), ciliary neurotrophic factor (CNTF), cardiotrophin-1 (CT-1) and novel neurotrophin-1/B-cell stimulating factor-3 (NNT-1/BSF-3). These cytokines play pivotal roles in immune, hematopoietic, nervous, cardiovascular, and endocrine systems, and also function in bone metabolism, inflammation, and acute phase responses (for review see Hirano et al., 1997).

Interleukin-6, IL-11, CNTF, and possibly CT-1 and NNT-1/BSF-3 act on target cells through interactions with a ligand-specific receptor, and induce signaling by association of this ligand/receptor complex with either a gp130/gp130 homodimer (IL-6 and IL-11) or a gp130/LIF receptor (LIFR) heterodimer (Fig. 11.3*A*). Leukemia inhibitory factor binds directly to the LIFR, with subsequent formation of the gp130/LIFR heterodimer. Oncostatin M is the only family member known to bind directly to gp130, then recruit either the oncostatin M receptor (OSMR) or LIFR to form an activated receptor complex (see Fig. 11.3*A*). Interleukin-6 will be used as an example for further explanation of the signal cascades transmitted through the gp130 receptor family.

Interleukin-6

Since its discovery, IL-6 has been shown to have diverse biological functions. Well characterized is its role

gp130 Receptor Complexes

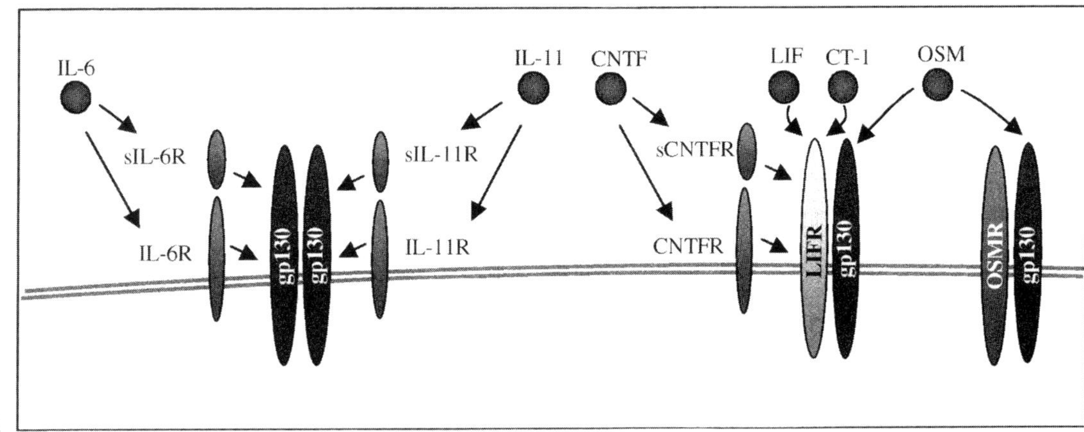

IL-6 Signaling

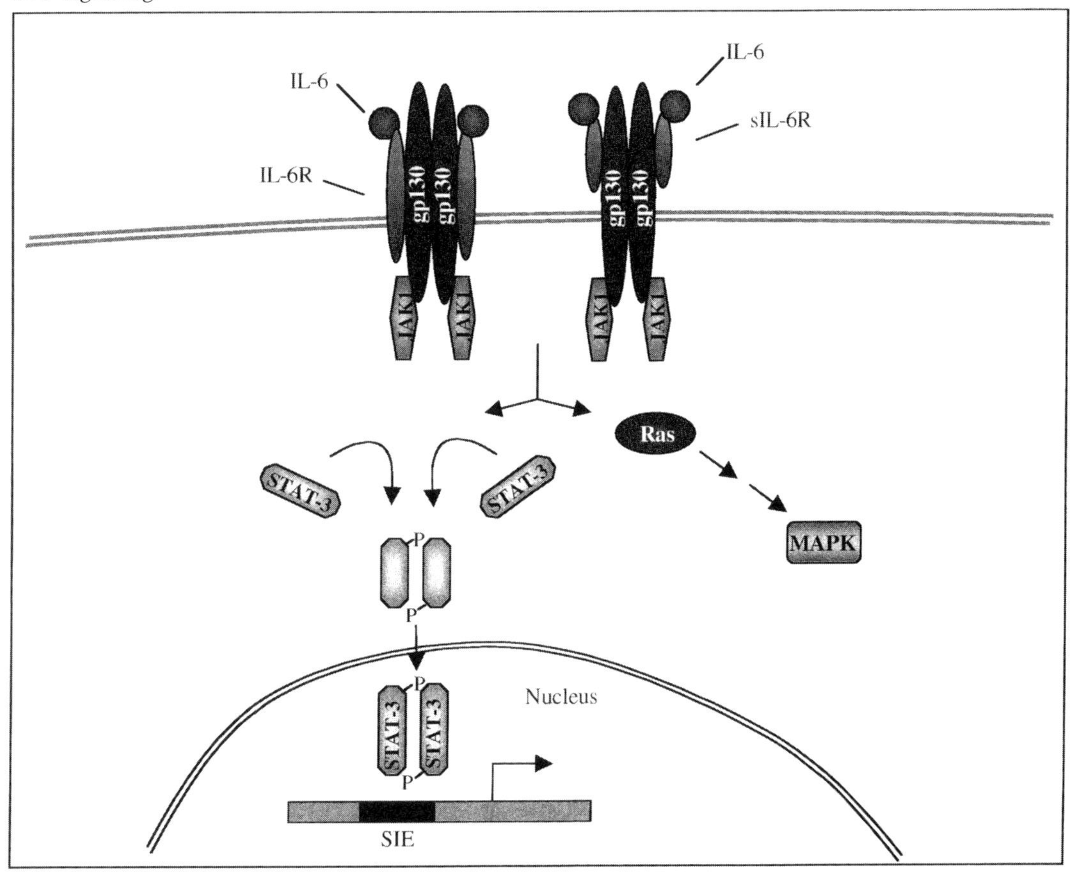

FIGURE 11.3 The gp130 receptor complexes and signaling. *A*. The interleukin-6/interleukin-6 receptor (IL-6/IL-6R) and IL-11/IL-11R induce gp130 homodimerization. Leukemia inhibitory factor (LIF), cardiotrophin-1 (CT-1), or ciliary neurotrophic factor/ciliary neurotrophic factor receptor (CNTF/CNTFR) binds to leukemia inhibitory factor receptor (LIFR), which then interacts with gp130. Oncostatin-M (OSM) binds directly to gp130, then forms a complex with either the leukemia inhibitory factor receptor (LIFR) or the oncostatin-M receptor (OSMR) in humans. Interleukin-6R, IL-11R and CNTFR are found in soluble forms. The soluble receptors can bind ligand and signal through gp130. *B*. Interleukin-6 acts on target cells through a receptor complex composed of an IL-6 binding subunit (IL-6R) or the sIL-6R and gp130. The sIL-6R, like the membrane-bound IL-6R, can complex with IL-6, bind, and signal through gp130, thus serving as an agonist of IL-6-induced responses. Initiation of IL-6 signaling occurs when IL-6 binds to the IL-6R or sIL-6R, leading to an association with gp130. Receptor activation requires formation of a hexameric complex composed of two each of IL-6, the IL-6R (or sIL-6R), and gp130. This event leads to activation of gp130-associated Janus kinases (JAKs), which phosphorylate gp130 to provide docking and activation sites for signal transducer and activator of transcription-3 (STAT-3), which then activates IL-6-responsive genes. As well, IL-6 signaling leads to activation of the mitogen-activated protein kinase (MAPK) signaling pathway.

as an immune and hematopoietic factor. In this capacity, IL-6 drives the proliferation and differentiation of B cells into plasma cells, induces the synthesis of acute phase proteins, and plays a role in T cell maturation and activation (for review see Taga and Kishimoto, 1997). Interleukin-6 requires a ligand-specific receptor, which is found in both membrane-associated and soluble forms (Fig. 11.3*B*). Interestingly, the IL-6 soluble receptor (sIL-6R) functions as an agonist of IL-6. This process, called *trans-signaling*, makes cells expressing gp130 but not the membrane-bound form of the IL-6R (which are nonresponsive to IL-6) responsive upon addition of the sIL-6R. These findings imply that sIL-6R may offer an additional level of regulation that depends on soluble receptor expression and availability. Regarding glial cells, astrocytes and oligodendrocytes do not express the membrane-bound form of the IL-6R; rather, they respond to IL-6 only in the presence of the sIL-6R (Table 11.2). Astrocytes respond to IL-6/sIL-6R by the induction of α_1-antichymotrypsin expression (Kordula et al., 1998). Microglia express the IL-6R on their cell surface and respond to IL-6 by the activation of STAT-3 (unpublished observation).

Interleukin-6 acts on target cells through a receptor complex composed of IL-6, either membrane-bound IL-6R or the sIL-6R, and gp130 (Fig. 11.3*B*). Receptor activation requires formation of a hexameric complex composed of two each of the above-mentioned proteins. This event leads to activation of gp130-associated tyrosine kinases, the JAKs. Although IL-6 has been shown to activate JAK1, JAK2, and TYK2, JAK1 is most important for signaling through gp130 (Rodig et al., 1998). The cytoplasmic domain of gp130 contains four STAT recruitment motifs that become phosphorylated by JAKs upon receptor oligomerization. STAT-1α and STAT-3 are tyrosine phosphorylated in a cell-specific manner after treatment with IL-6, with STAT-3 being dominant in this response (for review see Taga and Kishimoto, 1997). Upon phosphorylation, STAT-3 dimers translocate to the nucleus and activate transcription from target gene promoters that contain a GAS-like element known as the *sis-inducible element* (SIE). Interleukin-6 also activates STAT-1α, leading to homodimers of STAT-1α and heterodimers of STAT-1α/STAT-3. It has been demonstrated that serine phosphorylation is required for optimal transcriptional activation by STAT-3 (Wen and Darnell, 1997). Interleukin-6 signaling also leads to activation of the mitogen-activated protein kinase (MAPK) pathway (Fig. 11.3*B*).

Interleukin-2 Receptor Family

Receptors for IL-2 and other cytokines such as IL-4, IL-7, IL-9, IL-13, IL-15, and IL-21 make up the IL-2 receptor family (for review see O'Shea et al., 2002). The receptors for these cytokines are composed of at least one ligand-specific binding chain (usually termed the α chain) and a shared receptor component, the common gamma chain (γC). There are some differences in the receptor complex subunits; the receptors for IL-2 and IL-15 contain a third chain, while the IL-13 receptor consists of the IL-4 receptor α-chain and an IL-13-specific ligand binding chain. The receptors for IL-2, IL-7, IL-9, IL-15, and IL-21 transduce signals through activation of STAT-5, while the IL-4 and IL-13 receptors activate STAT-6 (Table 11.1). The IL-4 signal transduction cascade will be used as the example for signaling through the IL-2 receptor superfamily.

Interleukin-4

Interleukin-4 was originally isolated based on its ability to stimulate the proliferation and immunoglobulin G1 (IgG1) secretion of B lymphocytes, and is produced by CD4+ Th2 cells, mast cells, and basophils (for review see Nelms et al., 1999). Interleukin-4 is generally considered an anti-inflammatory cytokine due to its ability to suppress TNF-α and IL-1β production and IFN-γ-induced gene expression (class II MHC, CD40) in macrophages.

Interleukin-4 mediates its effects by binding to a heterodimeric receptor. The IL-4R is composed of a 140 kDa high-affinity α chain and a 65 kDa low-affinity receptor (the γC chain). The cytoplasmic regions of the IL-4R do not contain intrinsic kinase activity, and the tyrosine kinase activity observed when IL-4 binds to its receptor is from the constitutive association of JAK1 to IL-4Rα and JAK3 to the γC chain. JAK1 and JAK3 are activated by IL-4 cross-linking IL-4R, leading to the phosphorylation of STAT-6 (for review see Nelms et al., 1999). STAT-6 is the primary STAT activated in response to IL-4. Phosphorylated STAT-6 appears to bind preferentially to N4 STAT binding elements (SBE) (Ihle, 1996). Similar to STAT-1α, STAT-6 also interacts with a number of transcription factors/coactivators such as NF-κB, C/EBPα, and CBP (Delphin and Stavnezer, 1995; Ohmori and Hamilton, 1998; Gingras et al., 1999). The IL-4 receptor is found on astrocytes, microglia, and oligodendrocytes (Table 11.2) (Brodie et al., 1998; Wei and Jonakait, 1999; Molina-Holgado et al., 2001). Interleukin-4 exerts an immunosuppressive function on microglia by inhibiting class II MHC, CD40, and B7 expression (O'Keefe et al., 1999; Wei and Jonakait, 1999; Nguyen and Benveniste, 2000a).

NEGATIVE REGULATION OF THE JANUS KINASE/SIGNAL TRANSDUCERS AND ACTIVATORS OF TRANSCRIPTION

Signaling through the JAK/STAT pathway is critical for diverse host responses including immunological defense, cellular differentiation and proliferation, and oncogenesis. However, control of the magnitude and duration of signaling through the JAK/STAT pathway is accomplished by a variety of mechanisms. These include receptor internalization and subsequent receptor degradation; protein tyrosine phosphatases (SHP1, SHP2, CD45) that act at the level of the membrane-associated receptor-JAK complex to negatively regulate the activity of both JAKS and STATS; protein inhibitors of activated STATs (PIAS) that bind to phosphorylated STAT dimers, preventing binding to DNA; and SOCS proteins that directly antagonize STAT activation (for review see Alexander, 2002). A description of the SOCS family of proteins and their mechanism of inhibitory action follows, with an emphasis on SOCS-1.

The SOCS-1 protein is one of eight recently discovered cytokine-inducible downregulators of cytokine signaling (for review see Alexander, 2002). This protein interacts with phosphorylated JAK1 and JAK2 via its SH2 domain, thereby inhibiting their tyrosine kinase activity (Fig. 11.4). Additionally, a conserved C-terminal motif among SOCS members, known as the *SOCS box*, has been implicated in coupling proteins to proteasomal degradation (for review see Zhang et al., 1999). A multitude of studies have implicated SOCS-1 involvement in the inhibition of a number of signaling pathways (IFN-γ, IL-2, IL-4, IL-6, IFN-α) (for review see Alexander, 2002). However, it appears that the most important *in vivo* target of SOCS-1 is the IFN-γ-activated JAK/STAT pathway. This has been demonstrated by the fact that the lethal perinatal syndrome observed in SOCS-1-deficient mice, which includes fatty degeneration, necrosis of the liver, and damage to the pancreas, heart, and skin due to infiltrating T lymphocytes, macrophages, and eosinophils, is eliminated with antibodies to IFN-γ or in mice deficient in IFN-γ in addition to SOCS-1 (Alexander et al., 1999). Thus, the disease in SOCS-1-deficient mice is due to increased sensitivity to IFN-γ and elevated serum levels of this cytokine. From these studies, it has been shown that SOCS-1 is an essential physiological regulator of IFN-γ signaling that is crucial for allowing the beneficial immunological effects of IFN-γ without the damaging pathological responses (for review see Alexander, 2002). Astocytes and microglia can be activated by IFN-γ treatment to express SOCS-1. This SOCS-1 expression leads to inhibition of IFN-γ-induced class II MHC and CD40 expression in these cells (O'Keefe et al., 2001; Wesemann et al., 2002). The role of SOCS proteins in oligodendrocytes is yet to be discovered.

THE TUMOR NECROSIS FACTOR SUPERFAMILY

The TNF receptor superfamily consists of over 20 structurally related type I transmembrane proteins that are specifically activated by the corresponding superfamily of TNF-like cytokines, eliciting a wide spectrum of cellular responses including transcriptional gene activation and induction of apoptosis (for review see Chen and Goeddel, 2002). Members of this receptor superfamily are found in many cell types within the body and play key roles in many essential biological activities, including lymphoid and neuronal development, innate and adaptive immunity, development and mainte-

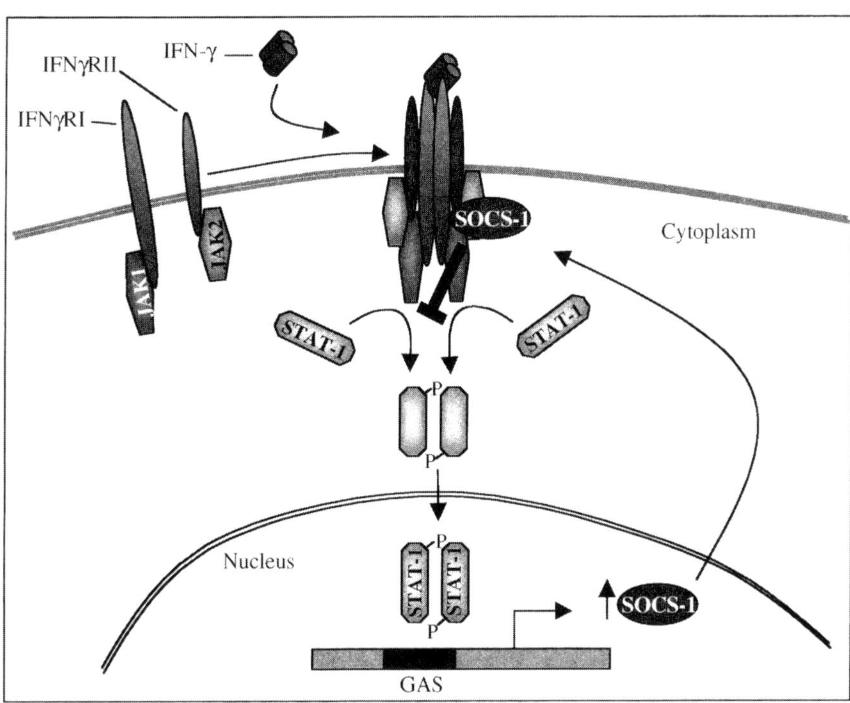

FIGURE 11.4 Mechanism of suppressor of cytokine signaling (SOCS-1) action. In a negative-feedback manner, SOCS-1 is induced by interferon-γ (IFN-γ) and binds to activated Janus kinases (JAKs) to inhibit IFN-γ-induced, JAK-mediated signal transducer and activation of transcription 1α (STAT-1α) phosphorylation. This then terminates signaling through this pathway.

nance of epithelial structures, and maintenance of homeostasis. Agents that manipulate the signaling of these receptors are being used or showing promise in the treatment and prevention of many human diseases such as rheumatoid arthritis, coronary heart disease, transplantation rejection, insulin resistance, multiple organ failure, and neoplasm (for review see Ashkenazi and Dixit, 1998).

The TNF receptor superfamily can be divided into two subgroups, depending on whether the intracellular region contains a death domain. Receptors that contain death domains are known as *death receptors* (for review see Ashkenazi and Dixit, 1998). The most well-known death receptors are the TNF receptor 1 (TNFR1) and Fas; while TNFR1 induces cell death only under certain circumstances and more often induces transcriptional gene activation, Fas is efficient in cell death induction. Many members of the TNF family of receptors do not contain death domains; these are represented by TNFR2, CD40, CD30, and many others. These receptors are involved primarily in gene transcription for cell survival, growth, and differentiation. The best-studied example of TNF signaling is TNF-α signaling through the TNFR1, which is explained in some detail below.

Tumor Necrosis Factor-α

Tumor necrosis factor-α is a pleiotropic cytokine that elicits a broad spectrum of organismal and cellular responses, including lymphocyte and leukocyte activation, fever, and an acute phase response, as well as cell proliferation, differentiation, and apoptosis (for review see Chen and Goeddel, 2002). Of the two types of TNF receptors characterized (TNFR1 and TNFR2), TNFR1 is responsible for most of the biological properties of TNF-α (for review see Chen and Goeddel, 2002). Both receptors are ubiquitously expressed on astrocytes, microglia, and oligodendrocytes (Table 11.2) (Dopp et al., 1997). The cytoplasmic domain of TNFR1, when activated by ligand binding, can recruit the adaptor protein TNFR1-associated death domain protein (TRADD). The TNFR1–TRADD complex leads to at least two opposing downstream signaling cascades. On the one hand, the TNFR1–TRADD complex can form the death-initiated signaling complex (DISC) by recruiting Fas-associated death domain protein (FADD), which leads to caspase activation and apoptosis. On the other hand, the TNFR1–TRADD complex can recruit receptor interacting protein (RIP) and/or TNFR-associated factor 2 (TRAF2), leading to JNK and NF-κB activation (Fig. 11.5). NF-κB activation is key for the expression of proinflammatory cytokines (IL-1, IL-2, IL-6, IL-12, TNF-α, LTα, LTβ, and GM-CSF), chemokines (IL-8, macrophage inflammatory protein-1α [MIP-1α], macrophage chemoattractant protein-1 [MCP-1], regulated upon activation, normal T-cell expressed and secreted [RANTES], and eotaxin), adhesion molecules (intercellular adhesion molecule-1 [ICAM], vascular cell adhesion molecule-1 [VCAM]. and E-selectin), acute phase proteins, and inducible effector molecules (inducible nitric oxide synthase [iNOS]

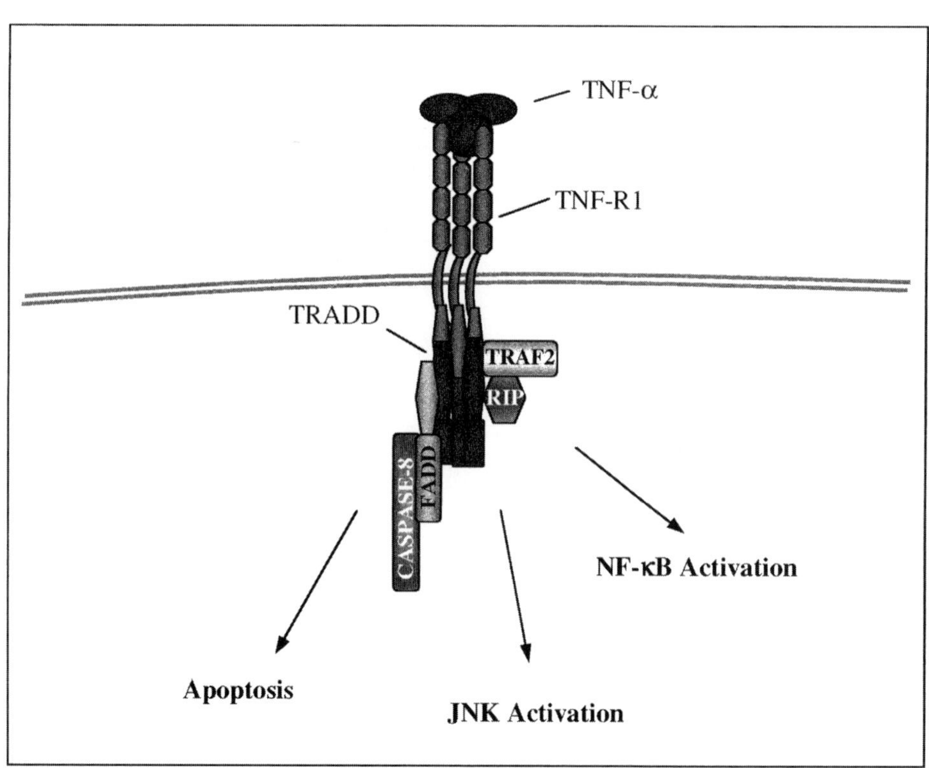

FIGURE 11.5 Tumor necrosis factor-α (TNF-α) signaling. A TNF-α homotrimer induces trimerization of tumor necrosis factor receptor 1 (TNFR1) subunits and recruits tumor necrosis factor receptor-1-associated death domain protein (TRADD) proteins to interact with the cytoplasmic portion of TNFR1. The TNFR1:TRADD complex can recruit tumor necrosis factor receptor-associated factor-2 (TRAF2) and receptor interacting protein (RIP), which are important for Janus kinase (JAK) and NF-κB activation. Alternatively, the TNFR1:TRADD complex can recruit Fas-associated death domain protein (FADD), which is an adaptor protein for caspase-8 recruitment. Subsequent caspase-8 cleavage and activation leads to the amplification of a signaling cascade that ultimately results in cellular apoptosis.

and cyclooxygenase-2 [COX-2]). Moreover, NF-κB is central to the overall immune response through its ability to activate genes coding for regulators of apoptosis and cell proliferation such as c-IAP-1, c-IAP-2, Bcl2A1, Bcl-XL, Fas ligand, c-myc, and cyclin D1. As such, modulation of NF-κB activity and action has been suggested to represent effective therapeutic strategies for combating diseases that result from hyperactivation of the immune system (for review see Ghosh and Karin, 2002).

Tumor necrosis factor-α has been shown to be directly cytotoxic to oligodendrocytes (Louis et al., 1993). For astrocytes and microglia, TNF-α is a potent inducer of cytokines, chemokines, and adhesion molecules (for review see John et al., 2003).

INTERLEUKIN-1 SIGNALING

Interleukin-1 is one of the most pleiotropic cytokines and has effects on nearly every cell in the body. Upon activation by IL-1, cells are induced to produce a large variety of mediators that regulate immune reactivity and inflammation such as cytokines, cytokine receptors, acute-phase reactants, growth factors, tissue remodeling enzymes, extracellular matrix components, and adhesion molecules (for review see O'Neill and Greene, 1998). Most of the immune and inflammatory genes induced by IL-1 are NF-κB regulated, making it a key mediator of IL-1 effects in cells. The activation of NF-κB by IL-1 involves a multiprotein complex that ultimately results in the phosphorylation of IκB followed by its ubiquitination and degradation, thereby allowing NF-κB to translocate to the nucleus and affect gene transcription.

Both IL-1α and IL-1β bind to the type I IL-1 receptor (IL-1RI), which is found on astrocytes, microglia, and oligodendrocytes (Table 11.2) (D'Souza et al., 1994; Molina-Holgado et al., 2000; Pinteaux et al., 2002). This receptor is a member of an extended family of receptors, which contains 10 members including the IL-18 receptor. The extracellular ligand-binding portion of IL-1RI contains three immunoglobulin-like domains (Ig domains), and the intracellular signal-transducing portion of the receptor contains considerable homology to the Toll family members (for review see O'Neill and Greene, 1998). A homolog of the IL-1RI, known as *IL-1R accessory protein* (AcP), forms a heterodimer with the IL-1RI to form the receptor complex necessary for signal transduction. Subsequent to IL-1 binding to IL-1RI, the IL-1RI:IL-1RAcP heterodimer is formed, which then serves as a scaffold for the recruitment of a number of proteins. Among these proteins are IL-1 receptor-associated kinases 1 and 2 (IRAK-1, IRAK-2), which bind to IL-1RAcP and IL-1RI, respectively (Fig. 11.6). Furthermore, the death

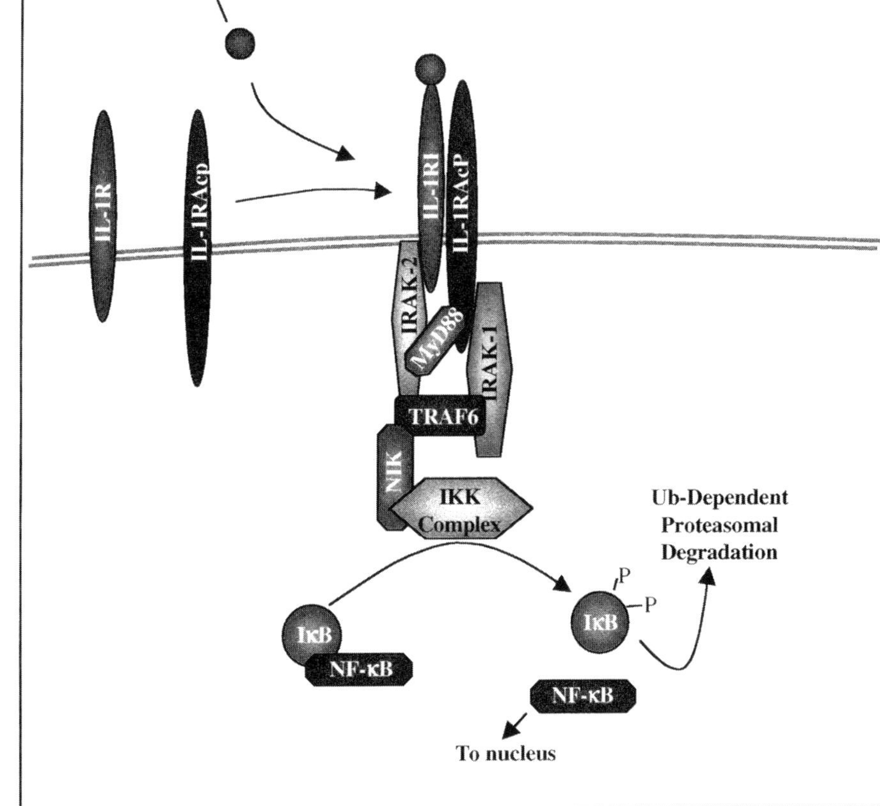

FIGURE 11.6 Interleukin-1 signaling. Subsequent to IL-1α/β binding to IL-1 receptor-I (IL-1RI), the IL-1RI:IL-1RAcP heterodimer is formed, which then serves as a scaffold for the recruitment of a number of IL-1 receptor-associated kinase (IRAK-1) and IRAK-2, which bind to IL-1RAcP and IL-1RI, respectively. Furthermore, MyD88 associates with both IL-1RAcP and IRAK-2. Tumor necrosis factor receptor-associated factor-6 (TRAF6) then binds to this complex and recruits NF-κB inducing kinase (NIK) which activates the IκB kinase complex. This leads to the subsequent phosphorylation of IκB, thereby targeting it for proteosomal degradation and allowing NF-κB to enter the nucleus and affect transcription of IL-1 target genes.

domain–containing cytosolic protein, MyD88, which is a member of the IL-1 receptor family, associates with both IL-1RAcP and IRAK-2. Tumor necrosis factor receptor–associated factor 6 (TRAF6) then binds to this complex and recruits NF-κB inducing kinase (NIK), which activates the IκB kinase complex. This leads to the subsequent phosphorylation of IκB, thereby targeting it for proteosomal degradation and allowing NF-κB to enter the nucleus, as mentioned above.

Interleukin-1β is a potent inducer of astrogliosis and also enhances expression of adhesion molecules (ICAM-1, VCAM-1) by astrocytes. Furthermore, IL-1β induces cytokine/chemokine production (TNF-α, MCP-1, IL-6, IL-8, IP-10) by astrocytes (for review see John et al., 2003).

There are two natural regulators of IL-1 activity. One is an IL-1-like ligand called the *IL-1 receptor antagonist* (IL-1Ra). The other is a membrane-bound IL-1 binding protein resembling IL-1R, called the *type II IL-1R*, that is not capable of signal transduction (for review see Mantovani et al., 2001). The IL-1 receptor antagonist resembles IL-1α and IL-1β in its amino acid sequence, three-dimensional folding pattern, and gene structure, and is located with IL-1α and IL-1β in a 430 kb gene cluster on human chromosome 2q12. The IL-1 receptor antagonist binds to IL-1RI in a slightly different manner, though with higher affinity than IL-1α and IL-1β, and fails to recruit IL-1RAcP, which is required for IL-1R signaling. Constitutive expression by microglia of the IL-1Ra is thought to contribute to immunosuppression in the normal brain. Furthermore, IL-10 enhances expression of the IL-1Ra by these cells. The type II IL-1R resembles the IL-1RI in its extracellular portion. However, it has a very short cytoplasmic tail that does not mediate any biological signals and thus functions as a decoy receptor.

TRANSFORMING GROWTH FACTORS

Transforming growth factor-β belongs to a superfamily that comprises more than 30 distinct members including various forms of TGF-β, the bone morphogenetic proteins, the nodals, and activins (for review see Attisano and Wrana, 2002). At least five genes encode distinct TGF-β proteins in vertebrates (referred to as TGF-β1-5). Mammalian cells express the TGF-β1, -β2, and -β3 isoforms, while TGF-β4 and -β5 represent a chicken and a *Xenopus laevis* isoform, respectively. Transforming growth factor-β isoforms are 25 kDa homodimers that share more than 70% sequence identity at the amino acid level and are expressed in a tissue- and development-specific manner.

Transforming growth factor-β is a pleiotropic growth factor regulating a remarkable range of biological activities. It is one of the most potent regulators of extracellular matrix (ECM) accumulation (for review see Alevizopoulos and Mermod, 1997). Transforming growth factor-β regulates cellular proliferation in a cell-specific manner. In most epithelial, endothelial, and hematopoietic cells, TGF-β is a potent inhibitor of cell proliferation by regulating the expression of cell cycle–related genes such as c-*myc*, cyclin A, and the CDK inhibitors p15 and p21 (for review see Alevizopoulos and Mermod, 1997). Mice lacking TGF-β2 have cardiac, lung, craniofacial, and urogenital defects, and mice lacking TGF-β3 have cleft palates, indicating that TGF-β plays an important role in embryonic development. Transforming growth factor-β is a potent suppressive modulator of immunological functions by inhibiting the development and differentiation of immunocompetent cells including B cells, T cells, and monocytes/macrophages, and by inhibiting production of proinflammatory cytokines such as TNF-α and IL-1 (for review see Letterio and Roberts, 1998). In addition, TGF-β represses constitutive and IFN-γ-inducible class II MHC expression in a variety of cell types (for review see Dong and Benveniste, 2001). In TGF-β1-deficient mice, levels of class II MHC mRNA are elevated and the incidence of fatal multifocal inflammatory disease is strikingly high (Shull et al., 1992), confirming the role of TGF-β as a suppressor of inflammation.

All three mammalian TGF-β isoforms signal through the same receptor, which is ubiquitously expressed on astrocytes, microglia, and oligodendrocytes (Table 11.2) (Loughlin et al., 1993; Asakura et al., 1997; De Groot et al., 1999). The TGF-βR is a serine/threonine kinase receptor composed of two type I (TGF-βRI) and two type II (TGF-βRII) receptors (for review see Attisano and Wrana, 2002). The kinase domain of the TGF-βRII is constitutively active, and phosphorylates and activates the kinase domain of the TGF-βRI when the two are brought in close proximity upon the binding of TGF-β. The activated TGF-βRI then signals to the (small) mothers against decapentaplegic (SMAD) family of intracellular mediators (for review see Attisano and Wrana, 2002); (see Fig. 11.7). The SMADs can be divided into three classes: receptor-regulated, or R-SMAD (SMAD-1, -2, -3, -5, and -8), are directly phosphorylated by TGF-βRI. The R-SMADs then form heteromeric complexes with SMAD4, which is the only member of the second class of SMADs, the co-SMADs. The activated SMAD proteins then translocate into the nucleus, where they bind to SMAD binding elements, thereby affecting transcription of TGF-β target genes. Recently, SMAD proteins have been found to interact with other known transcription factors such as AP-1 and CBP/p300 (Janknecht et al., 1998; Shen and Stavnezer, 1998; Topper et al., 1998; Zhang et al., 1998). In a sense, the SMAD signaling pathway is similar to the JAK/STAT pathway; the latent cytoplasmic

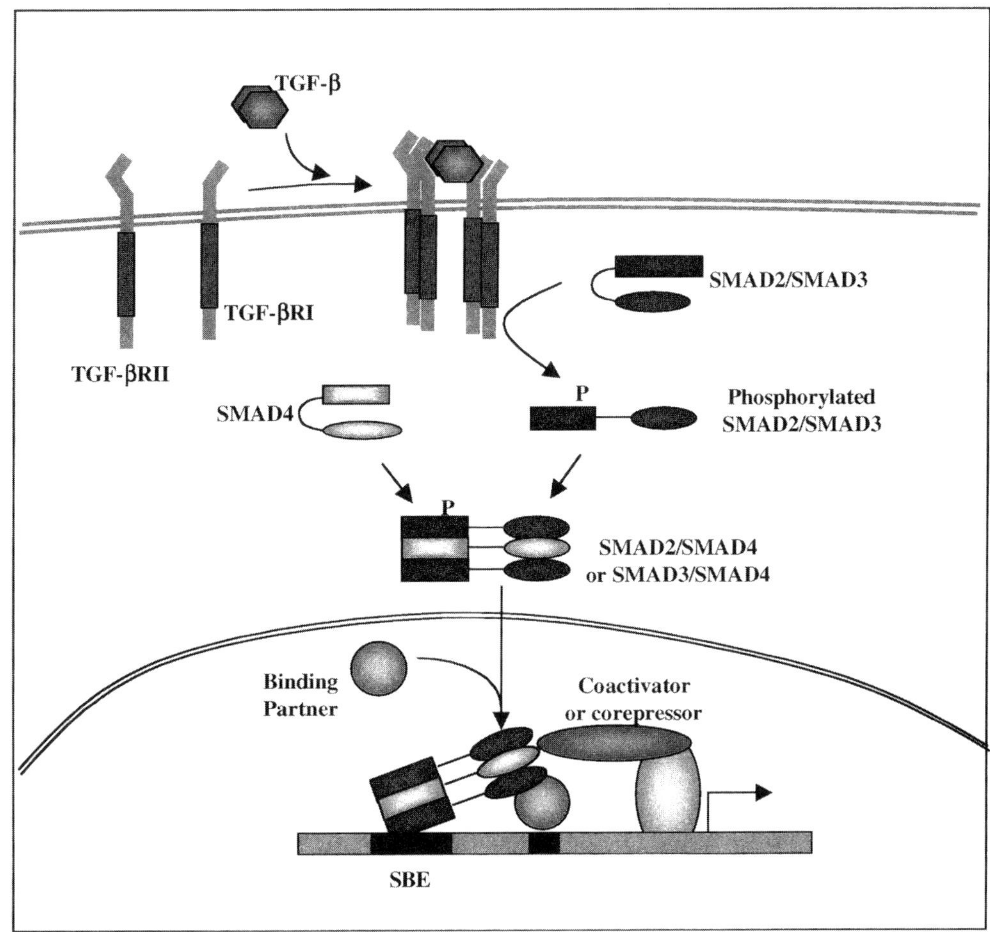

FIGURE 11.7 Transforming growth factor-β (TGF-β) signaling. Engagement of TGF-β with its receptor recruits receptor-regulated (small) Mothers against decapentaplegic (SMAD) proteins (SMAD-2/SMAD-3), which are then subsequently phosphorylated by the TGF-β receptor-I (TGF-βRI) and form heteromeric complexes with SMAD-4, translocate to the nucleus, and affect the transcription of TGF-β target genes containing SMAD binding elements (SBE). SMADs have been shown to interact with a number of transcriptional regulators and can serve to activate or repress target genes.

factors (SMADs or STATs) are activated by phosphorylation, form higher-ordered complexes, translocate into the nucleus, and then interact with other transcription factors to regulate gene expression. Indeed, SMAD-1 has been shown to interact with STAT-3 to synergistically increase gene transcription (Nakashima et al., 1999), demonstrating the existence of cross-talk between the JAK/STAT and SMAD signaling pathways.

The third class of SMADs, the inhibitory SMADs (SMAD-6 and -7), antagonize TGF-β signaling. These proteins inhibit phosphorylation of the R-SMADs or compete for their interaction with SMAD-4. Thus, the inhibitory SMADs serve an important role in silencing SMAD-mediated gene expression.

Transforming growth factor-β exerts predominantly immunosuppressive effects on astrocytes and microglia by inhibiting expression of class II MHC, B7, CD40, ICAM-1, VCAM-1, and TNF-α (for review see O'Keefe et al., 2002). The inhibitory effect of TGF-β on astrocyte class II MHC expression is mediated directly by SMAD-3 (Dong et al., 2001).

CHEMOKINES

Chemokines are a group of molecules that regulate migration of a number of cell types in a variety of physiological and pathological conditions (for review see Bajetto et al., 2002). Chemokines are small (8–14 kDa) molecules that are structurally and functionally related to form a family of proteins divided into four groups based on the relative position of their first N-terminal cysteine residues. These are the CC or β-chemokines, the CXC or α-chemokines, the CX3C or δ-chemokines, and the C or γ-chemokines. Chemokine receptors have been divided into four subfamilies: CCR, CXCR,

CX_3CR, and XCR, based on the sequence motif of the conserved cysteine residues of the chemokines that bind to them (for review see Horuk, 2001; Bajetto et al., 2002). Stimulation of cells (mainly leukocytes) with chemokines leads to a rise in intracellular free calcium concentration, the production of microbiocidal oxygen radicals and bioactive lipids, and the release of the contents of cytoplasmic storage granules, such as proteases from neutrophils and monocytes, histamine from basophils, and cytotoxic proteins from eosinophils. The induction of migration is caused by polymerization and breakdown of actin, which leads to the formation and retraction of lamellipodia, which function to move the cell through tissues toward the direction of higher chemokine concentrations. Chemokine stimulation also leads to the upregulation and activation of integrins, which cause leukocytes to adhere to endothelial cells of the vessel wall to position the cells to migrate through the vessel wall (for review see Baggiolini, 2001).

Chemokines exert their biological activity by binding to cell surface receptors that belong to the superfamily of seven-transmembrane domain receptors that signal through heterotrimeric G-proteins (for review see Baggiolini, 2001; see Fig. 11.8). Upon chemokine binding, the heterotrimeric G-protein is activated by the exchange of GDP for GTP, and dissociates into the GTP-bound α and the $\beta\gamma$ subunit. The $\beta\gamma$ subunit activates two major signal transduction enzymes: phospholipase C (PLC) and phosphatidylinositol-3-OH kinase (PI3K). Activation of PLC yields two second messengers, inositol 1,4,5-trisphosphate (IP_3) and diacylglycerol (DAG). IP_3 induces the release of Ca^{2+} from intracellular stores, leading to a transient rise of the free intracellular calcium concentration, and DAG activates several isoforms of protein kinase C (PKC). PITC rapidly generates phosphatidylinositol 3,4,5-trisphosphate (PIP_3) and initiates the activation of Akt/protein kinase B (PKB), which is an important component of the cells' prosurvival machinery. Akt leads to phosphorylation

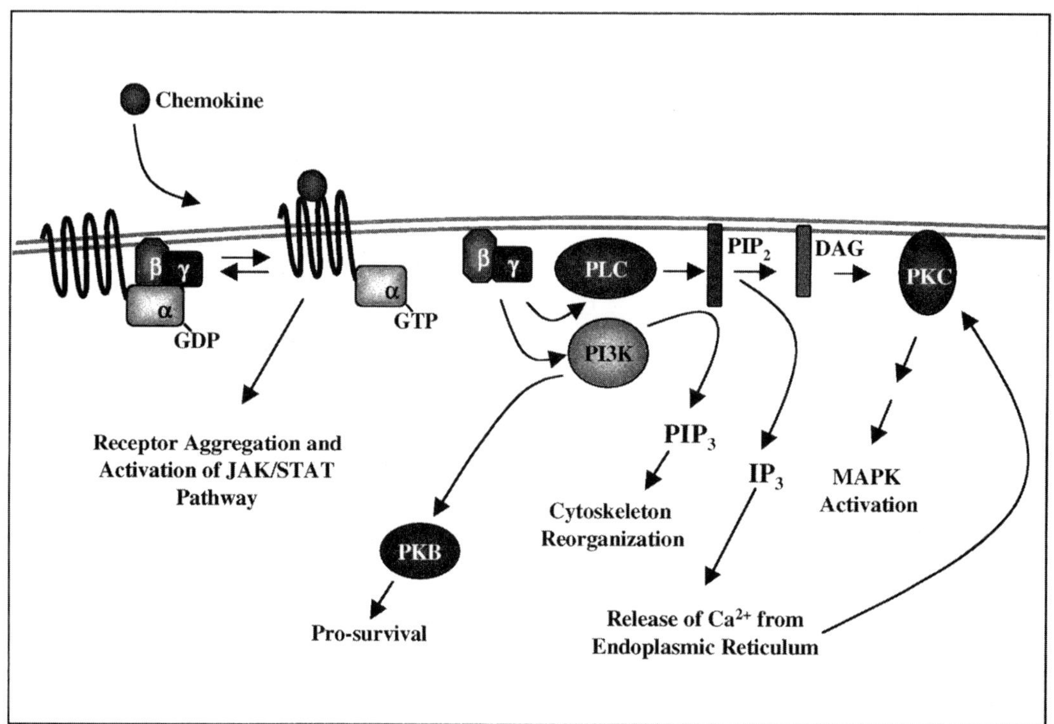

FIGURE 11.8 Chemokine signaling. Upon chemokine binding, a G-protein coupled, seven-transmembrane domain receptor is activated by the exchange of guanosine diphosphate (GDP) for guanosine triphosphate (GTP), and dissociates into the GTP-bound α and the $\beta\gamma$ subunit. The $\beta\gamma$ subunit activates phospholipase C (PLC) and phosphatidylinositol-3-OH kinase (PI3K). Activation of PLC yields two second messengers, inositol 1,4,5-trisphosphate (IP_3) and diacylglycerol (DAG). IP_3 induces the release of Ca^{2+} from intracellular stores, leading to a transient rise of the free calcium concentration, and DAG activates several isoforms of protein kinase C (PKC). Protein kinase C can lead to the subsequent activation of mitogen-activated protein kinase. Protein kinase C is also activated by the increase in Ca^{2+} concentration induced by IP_3. PI3K rapidly generates phosphatidylinositol 3,4,5-trisphosphate (PIP_3) and initiates the activation of Akt/protein kinase B (PKB). PIP_3 is thought to be important for the cytoskeleton remodeling induced by chemokines, and PKB is an important component of the cell's pro-survival machinery. In addition, select chemokines can activate the Janus kinase/signal transducer and activator of transcription (JAK/STAT) pathway.

of IκB, which allows NF-κB to translocate to the nucleus and increase the transcription of survival and proinflammatory genes. Chemokines also activate the MAPK cascade, although the precise mechanism of activation has not been elucidated. After GTP hydrolysis, the GDP-bound α subunit reassociates with the $\beta\gamma$ subunit and terminates signaling. Additionally, the Gα subunit of the heterotrimeric G-protein may regulate the activity of the $\beta\gamma$ subunits, and may also signal on its own by activating tyrosine kinases (for review see Thelen, 2001). A large number of studies have described chemokine receptor expression and function within the CNS (for review see Bajetto et al., 2002). Glial chemokine receptor expression is summarized in Table 11.2.

In addition, to the G-protein signaling involved in chemokine effector function, the JAK/STAT pathway has been demonstrated to be activated by α and β chemokines. Ligand binding causes receptor aggregation and activation of JAKs, with subsequent phosphorylation of STAT proteins. This response appears to depend on the receptor involved, as well as the cell type under study. The chemokines MCP-1, MIP-1α, RANTES, and SDF-1α have been shown to activate the JAK/STAT pathway in a variety of cell types including T cells and astrocytes (for review see Mellado et al., 2001).

Negative regulation of chemokine receptor activation is accomplished by ligand-dependent receptor phosphorylation and subsequent desensitization to further stimulation. The major mechanism for desensitization is through sequestration of the chemokine receptor via clathrin-coated pits into early endosomes. The receptor is then either recycled back to the surface or degraded and downregulated (for review see Mellado et al., 2001).

SUMMARY

This chapter provides an overview of some of the more well-studied signaling mechanisms induced by interferons, cytokines, and chemokines, and is by no means complete or comprehensive. Key to the ability of glial cells to respond to changes in the neural environment is the use of specific receptors that can sense and respond to inflammatory mediators such as interferons, cytokines, and chemokines. A common theme among signaling pathways is the activation of membrane-bound receptors upon ligand binding and subsequent engagement of an amplifying signaling cascade that usually results in the alteration of gene expression. Because such signals are critical for determining the nature and magnitude of inflammatory reactions, they are tightly regulated and are usually transient in nature. Indeed, cytokine and chemokine action in the brain can be both neuroprotective and neurodestructive, depending on the timing, magnitude, and duration of the signal. A current challenge in neuroimmunology is to understand how multiple cytokine signals are integrated within cells and the molecular mechanisms that determine cellular responses to such signals. Certainly, a deeper understanding of the cellular regulation of their responses to interferons, cytokines, and chemokines may yield insights into the pathogenesis of acute and chronic neurological diseases and uncover potential targets for therapeutic intervention.

ACKNOWLEDGMENTS

This work was supported by grants from the National Institutes of Health (NS-39954, NS-36765, MH-63650, and CA-97247). D.R.W. was previously supported by the National Institutes of Health Predoctoral Fellowship T32AI-07051 and is currently supported by a National Institutes of Health Predoctoral Fellowship NS-47051.

ABBREVIATIONS

AcP	accessory protein
Bcl	B-cell lymphoma
Bcl2A1	B-cell lymphoma protein-2-related protein A1
BSF-3	B cell-stimulating factor-3
CBP	CREB binding protein
CD	cluster of differentiation
CDK	cyclin-dependent kinase
CNS	central nervous system
CNTF	ciliary neurotrophic factor
COX-2	cyclooxygenase-2
CREB	cAMP response element binding protein
CT-1	cardiotrophin-1
DAG	diacylglycerol
DISC	death-initiated signaling complex
E-selectin	endothelial selectin
ECM	extracellular matrix
FADD	fas-associated death domain protein
GAS	interferon-γ activating site
GM-CSF	granulocyte-macrophage colony-stimulating factor
GDP	guanosine diphosphate
GTP	guanosine triphosphate
IAP	inhibitor of apoptosis protein
ICAM-1	intercellular adhesion molecule-1
IFN-γ	interferon-γ

IFN-γR	interferon-γ receptor
IgG	immunoglobulin G
IL	interleukin
iNOS	inducible nitric oxide synthase
IP_3	inositol trisphosphate
IP-10	interferon-γ inducible protein-10 kDa
IRAK	IL-1 receptor-associated kinase
IRF-1	interferon regulatory factor-1
ISRE	IFN-stimulated regulatory elements
JAK	Janus kinase
JNK	c-jun N-terminal kinase
LIF	leukemia inhibitory factor
LIFR	leukemia inhibitory factor receptor
LPS	lipopolysaccharide
LT	lymphotoxin
MAPK	mitogen-activated protein kinase
MCP-1	monocyte chemoattractant protein-1
MHC	major histocompatibility complex
MIP-1α	macrophage inflammatory protein-1α
NF	nuclear factor
NIK	NF-κB inducing kinase
NNT-1	Novel neurotrophin-1
OSM	oncostatin-M
OSMR	oncostatin-M receptor
PI3K	phosphatidylinositol-3-OH kinase
PIAS	protein inhibitor of activated STAT
PKB	Protein kinase B
PKC	Protein kinase C
PLC	phospholipase C
RANTES	regulated upon activation, normal T cell expressed and secreted
RIP	receptor interacting protein
SHP	SH2 domain-containing protein tyrosine phosphatase
sIL-6R	soluble IL-6 receptor
SOCS	suppressor of cytokine signaling
STAT	signal transducer and activator of transcription
TGF	transforming growth factor
TNF-α	tumor necrosis factor-α
TNFR	tumor necrosis factor receptor
TRADD	tumor necrosis factor receptor-1-associated death domain protein
TRAF2	tumor necrosis factor receptor-associated factor-2
TYK2	tyrosine kinase-2
USF-1	upstream stimulatory factor
VCAM-1	vascular cell adhesion molecule-1

REFERENCES

Alevizopoulos, A. and Mermod, N. (1997) Transforming growth factor-3: the breaking open of a black box. *BioEssays* 19:581–591.

Alexander, W.S. (2002) Suppressors of cytokine signalling (SOCS) in the immune system. *Nat. Rev. Immunol.* 2:410–416.

Alexander, W.S., Starr, R., Fenner, J.E., Scott, C.L., Handman, E., Sprigg, N.S., Corbin, J.E., Cornish, A.L., Darwiche, R., Owczarek, C.M., Kay, T.W.H., Nicola, N.A., Hertzog, P.J., Metcalf, D., and Hilton, D.J. (1999) SOCS1 is a critical inhibitor of interferon γ signaling and prevents the potentially fatal neonatal actions of this cytokine. *Cell* 98:597–608.

Asakura, K., Hunter, S.F., and Rodriguez, M. (1997) Effects of transforming growth factor-β and platelet-derived growth factor on oligodendrocyte precursors: insights gained from a neuronal cell line. *J. Neurochem.* 68:2281–2290.

Ashkenazi, A. and Dixit, V.M. (1998) Death receptors: signaling and modulation. *Science* 281:1305–1308.

Attisano, L. and Wrana, J.L. (2002) Signal transduction by the TGF-β superfamily. *Science* 296:1646–1647.

Bach, E.A., Aguet, M., and Schreiber, R.D. (1997) The IFNγ receptor: a paradigm for cytokine receptor signaling. *Annu. Rev. Immunol.* 15:563–591.

Baggiolini, M. (2001) Chemokines in pathology and medicine. *J. Intern. Med.* 250:91–104.

Bajetto, A., Bonavia, R., Barbero, S., and Schettini, G. (2002) Characterization of chemokines and their receptors in the central nervous system: physiopathological implications. *J. Neurochem.* 82:1311–1329.

Benveniste, E.N., Tang, L.P., and Law, R.M. (1995) Differential regulation of astrocyte TNF-α expression by the cytokines TGF-β, IL-6 and IL-10. *Int. J. Dev. Neurosci.* 13:341–349.

Benveniste, E.N., Vidovic, M., Panek, R.B., Norris, J.G., Reddy, A.T., and Benos, D.J. (1991) Interferon-γ induced astrocyte class II major histocompatibility complex gene expression is associated with both protein kinase C activation and Na^+ entry. *J. Biol. Chem.* 266:18119–18126.

Biron, C.A. (2001) Interferons α and β as immune regulators—a new look. *Immunity* 14:661–664.

Boehm, U., Klamp, T., Groot, M., and Howard, J.D. (1997) Cellular responses to interferon-γ. *Annu. Rev. Immunol.* 15:749–795.

Brodie, C., Goldreich, N., Haiman, T., and Kazimirsky, G. (1998) Functional IL-4 receptors on mouse astrocytes: IL-4 inhibits astrocyte activation and induces NGF secretion. *J. Neuroimmunol.* 81:20–30.

Chabot, S. and Yong, V.W. (2000) Interferon beta-13 increases interleukin-10 in a model of T cell-microglia interaction—revelance to MS. *Neurology* 55:1497–1505.

Chen, G. and Goeddel, D.V. (2002) TNF-R1 signaling: a beautiful pathway. *Science* 296:1634–1635.

D'Souza, S.D., Antel, J.P., and Freedman, M.S. (1994) Cytokine induction of heat shock protein expression in human oligodendrocytes: an interleukin-1-mediated mechanism. *J. Neuroimmunol.* 50:17–24.

De Groot, C.J., Montagne, L., Barten, A.D., Sminia, P., and Van Der Valk, P. (1999) Expression of transforming growth factor (TGF)-beta1, -beta2, and -beta3 isoforms and TGF-beta type I and type II receptors in multiple sclerosis lesions and human adult astrocyte cultures. *J. Neuropathol. Exp. Neurol.* 58:174–187.

Decker, T. and Kovarik, P. (2000) Serine phosphorylation of STATs. *Oncogene* 19:2628–2637.

Delphin, S. and Stavnezer, J. (1995) Characterization of an interleukin 4 (IL-4) responsive region in the immunoglobulin heavy chain germline e promoter: regulation by NF-IL-4, a C/EBP family member and NF-κB/p50. *J. Exp. Med.* 181:181–192.

Dong, Y. and Benveniste, E.N. (2001) Immune function of astrocytes. *Glia* 36:180–190.

Dong, Y., Tang, L. , Letterio, J.J., and Benveniste, E.N. (2001) The Smad3 protein is involved in TGF-β inhibition of class II transactivator and class II MHC expression. *J. Immunol.* 167:311–319.

Dopp, J.M., Mackenzie-Graham, A., Otero, G.C., and Merrill, J.E. (1997) Differential expression, cytokine modulation, and specific functions of type-1 and type-2 tumor necrosis factor receptors in rat glia. *J. Neuroimmunol.* 75:104–112.

Ghosh, S. and Karin, M. (2002) Missing pieces in the NF-κB puzzle. *Cell* 109 Suppl.:S81–S96.

Gingras, S., Simard, J., Groner, B., and Pfitzner, E. (1999) p300/CBP is required for transcriptional induction by interleukin-4 and interacts with Stat6. *Nucleic Acids Res.* 27:2722–2729.

Hirano, T., Nakajima, K., and Hibi, M. (1997) Signaling mechanisms through gp130: a model of the cytokine system. *Cytokine Growth Factor Rev.* 8:241–252.

Horuk, R. (2001) Chemokine receptors. *Cytokine Growth Factor Rev.* 12:313–335.

Ihle, J.N. (1996) STATs: signal transducers and activators of transcription. *Cell* 84:331–334.

Janknecht, R., Wells, N.J., and Hunter, T. (1998) TGF-β-stimulated cooperation of Smad proteins with the coactivators CBP/p300. *Genes Dev.* 12:2114–2119.

John, G.R., Lee, S.C., and Brosnan, C.F. (2003) Cytokines: powerful regulators of glial cell activation. *Neuroscientist* 9:10–22.

Kim, M.-O., Si, Q., Zhou, J.N., Pestell, R.G., Brosnan, C.F., Locker, J., and Lee, S.C. (2002) Interferon-β activates multiple signaling cascades in primary human microglia. *J. Neurochem.* 81:1361–1371.

Kordula, T., Rydel, R.E., Brigham, E.F., Horn, F., Heinrich, P.C., and Travis, J. (1998) Oncostatin M and the interleukin-6 and soluble interleukin-6 receptor complex regulate α_1-antichymotrypsin expression in human cortical astrocytes. *J. Biol. Chem.* 273:4112–4118.

Ledeboer, A., Brevé, J.J., Wierinckx, A., van der Jagt, S., Bristow, A.F., Leysen, J.E., Tilders, F.J.H., and Van Dam, A.-M. (2002) Expression and regulation of interleukin-10 and interleukin-10 receptor in rat astroglial and microglial cells. *Eur. J. Neurosci.* 16:1175–1185.

Lee, S.J., Park, J.Y., Hou, J., and Benveniste, E.N. (1999) Transcriptional regulation of the intercellular adhesion molecule-1 gene by proinflammatory cytokines in human astrocytes. *Glia* 25:21–32.

Letterio, J.J. and Roberts, A.B. (1998) Regulation of immune responses by TGF-β. *Annu. Rev. Immunol.* 16:137–161.

Loughlin, A.J., Woodroofe, M.N., and Cuzner, M.L. (1993) Modulation of interferon-γ-induced major histocompatibility complex class II and Fc receptor expression on isolated microglia by transforming growth factor-β1, interleukin-4, noradrenaline and glucocorticoids. *Immunology* 79:125–130.

Louis, J.-C., Magal, E., Takayama, S., and Varon, S. (1993) CNTF protection of oligodendrocytes against natural and tumor necrosis factor-induced death. *Science* 259:689–692.

Ma, Z., Qin, H., and Benveniste, E.N. (2001) Transcriptional suppression of matrix metalloproteinase-9 gene expression by IFN-γ and IFN-β: critical role of STAT-1α. *J. Immunol.* 167:5150–5159.

Mantovani, A., Locati, M., Vecchi, A., Sozzani, S., and Allavena, P. (2001) Decoy receptors: a strategy to regulate inflammatory cytokines and chemokines. *Trends Immunol.* 22:328–336.

Mellado, M., Vila-Coro, A.J., Martínez-A., C., and Rodríguez-Frade, J.M. (2001) Receptor dimerization: a key step in chemokine signaling. *Cell. Mol. Biol.* 47:575–582.

Molina-Holgado, E., Ortiz, S., Molina-Holgado, F. and Guaza, C. (2000) Induction of COX-2 and PGE(2) biosynthesis by IL-1β is mediated by PKC and mitogen-activated protein kinases in murine astrocytes. *Br. J. Pharmacol.* 131:152–159.

Molina-Holgado, E., Vela, J.M., Arevalo-Martin, A., and Guaza, C. (2001) LPS/IFN-gamma cytotoxicity in oligodendroglial cells: role of nitric oxide and protection by the anti-inflammatory cytokine IL-10. *Eur. J. Neurosci.* 13:493–502.

Nakashima, K., Yangagisawa, M., Arakawa, H., Kimura, N., Histasune, T., Kawabata, M., Miyazono, K., and Taga, T. (1999) Synergistic signaling in fetal brain by STAT3-Smad1 complex bridged by p300. *Science* 284:479–482.

Nelms, K., Keegan, A.D., Zamorano, J., Ryan, J.J., and Paul, W.E. (1999) The IL-4 receptor: signaling mechanisms and biologic functions. *Annu. Rev. Immunol.* 17:701–738.

Nguyen, V. and Benveniste, E.N. (2000a) Interleukin-4 activated STAT-6 inhibits IFN-γ induced CD40 gene expression in macrophages/microglia. *J. Immunol.* 165:6235–6243.

Nguyen, V.T. and Benveniste, E.N. (2000b) Involvement of STAT-1α and ets family members in interferon-γ induction of CD40 transcription in macrophages/microglia. *J. Biol. Chem.* 271:23674–23684.

O'Keefe, G.M., Nguyen, V.T., and Benveniste, E.N. (1999) Class II transactivator and class II MHC gene expression in microglia: modulation by the cytokines TGF-β, IL-4, IL-13, and IL-10. *Eur. J. Immunol.* 29:1275–1285.

O'Keefe, G.M., Nguyen, V.T., and Benveniste, E.N. (2002) Regulation and function of class II major histocompatibility complex, CD40, and B7 expression in macrophages and microglia: implications in neurological diseases. *J. Neurovirol.* 8:496–512.

O'Keefe, G.M., Nguyen, V.T., Tang, L.P., and Benveniste, E.N. (2001) IFN-γ regulation of class II transactivator promoter IV in macrophages and microglia: involvement of the suppressors of cytokine signaling-1 protein. *J. Immunol.* 166:2260–2269.

O'Neill, L.A.J. and Greene, C. (1998) Signal transduction pathways activated by the IL-1 receptor family: ancient signaling machinery in mammals, insects, and plants. *J. Leuk. Biol.* 63:650–657.

O'Shea, J.J., Gadina, M., and Schreiber, R.D. (2002) Cytokine signaling in 2002. New surprises in the Jak/STAT pathway. *Cell* 109 Suppl.:S121–S131.

Ohmori, Y. and Hamilton, T.A. (1998) STAT6 is required for the anti-inflammatory activity of interleukin-4 in mouse peritoneal macrophages. *J. Biol. Chem.* 273:29202–29209.

Pinteaux, E., Parker, L.C., Rothwell, N.J., and Luheshi, G.N. (2002) Expression of interleukin-1 receptors and their role in interleukin-1 actions in murine microglial cells. *J. Neurochem.* 83:754–763.

Popko, B. and Baerwald, K.D. (1999) Oligodendroglial response to the immune cytokine interferon gamma. *Neurochem. Res.* 24:331–338.

Rodig, S.J., Meraz, M.A., White, J.M., Lampe, P.A., Riley, J.K., Arthur, C.D., King, K.L., Sheehan, K.C.F., Yin, L., Pennica, D., Johnson, E.M, Jr., and Schreiber, R.D. (1998) Disruption of the *Jak1* gene demonstrates obligatory and nonredundant roles of the Jaks in cytokine-induced biologic responses. *Cell* 93:373–383.

Schindler, C.W. (2002) JAK-STAT signaling in human disease. *J. Clin. Invest.* 109:1133–1137.

Shen, C.-H. and Stavnezer, J. (1998) Interaction of Stat6 and NF-κB: direct association and synergistic activation of interleukin-4-induced transcription. *Mol. Cell. Biol.* 18:3395–3404.

Shull, M.M., Ormsby, I., Kier, A.B., Pawlowski, S., Diebold, R.J., Yin, M., Allen, R., Sidman, C., Proetzel, G., Calvin, D., Annunziata, N., and Doetschman, T. (1992) Targeted disruption of the mouse transforming growth factor-β1 gene results in multifocal inflammatory disease. *Nature* 359:693–699.

Stark, G.R., Kerr, I.M., Williams, B.R., Silverman, R.H., and Schreiber, R.D. (1998) How cells respond to interferons. *Annu. Rev. Biochem.* 67:227–264.

Strle, K., Zhou, J.-H., Shen, W.-H., Broussard, S.R., Johnson, R.W.,

Freund, G.G., Dantzer, R., and Kelley, K.W. (2001) Interleukin-10 in the brain. *Crit. Rev. Immunol.* 21:427–449.

Szczepanik, A.M., Funes, S., Petko, W., and Ringheim, G.E. (2001) IL-4, IL-10, and IL-13 modulate Aβ(1–42)-induced cytokine and chemokine production in primary murine microglia and a human monocyte cell line. *J. Neuroimmunol.* 113:49–62.

Taga, T. and Kishimoto, T. (1997) gp130 and the interleukin-6 family of cytokines. *Annu. Rev. Immunol.* 15:797–819.

Teige, I., Treschow, A., Teige, A., Mattsson, R., Navikas, V., Leanderson, T., Holmdahl, R., and Issazadeh-Navikas, S. (2003) IFN-β gene deletion leads to augmented and chronic demyelinating experimental autoimmune encephalomyelitis. *J. Immunol.* 170:4776–4784.

Thelen, M. (2001) Dancing to the tune of chemokines. *Nat. Immunol.* 2:129–134.

Topper, J.N., DiChiara, M.R., Brown, J.D., Williams, A.J., Falb, D., Collins, T., and Gimbrone, M.A., Jr. (1998) CREB binding protein is a required coactivator for Smad-dependent, transforming growth factor β transcriptional responses in endothelial cells. *Proc. Natl. Acad. Sci. USA* 95:9506–9511.

Wei, R. and Jonakait, G.M. (1999) Neurotrophins and the anti-inflammatory agents interleukin-4 (IL-4), IL-10, IL-11 and transforming growth factor-β1 (TGF-β1) downregulate T cell costimulatory molecules B7 and CD40 on cultured rat microglia. *J. Neuroimmunol.* 95:8–18.

Wen, Z. and Darnell, J.E., Jr. (1997) Mapping of Stat3 serine phosphorylation to a single residue (727) and evidence that serine phosphorylation has no influence on DNA binding of Stat1 and Stat3. *Nucleic Acids Res.* 25:2062–2067.

Wesemann, D., Dong, Y., O'Keefe, G.M., Nguyen, V.T., and Benveniste, E.N. (2002) Suppressor of cytokine signaling 1 inhibits cytokine induction of CD40 expression in macrophages. *J. Immunol.* 169:2354–2360.

Zhang, J.-G., Farley, A., Nicholson, S.E., Willson, T.A., Zugaro, L.M., Simpson, R.J., Moritz, R.L., Cary, D., Richardson, R., Hausmann, G., Kile, B.J., Kent, S.B.H., Alexander, W.S., Metcalf, D., Hilton, D.J., Nicola, N.A., and Baca, M. (1999) The conserved SOCS box motif in suppressors of cytokine signaling binds to elongins B and C and may couple bound proteins to proteasomal degradation. *Proc. Natl. Acad. Sci. USA* 96:2071–2076.

Zhang, Y., Feng, X.-H., and Derynck, R. (1998) Smad3 and Smad4 cooperate with c-Jun/c-Fos to mediate TGF-β-induced transcription. *Nature* 394:909–913.

12 Mechanisms of solute transport in glia

NEVILLE BROOKES

SPEAKING THE LANGUAGE OF TRANSPORT

The question of how neuroglia control the extracellular milieu that they share with neurons directed attention early to the transport of ions, neurotransmitters, and other vital solutes across the glial plasma membrane. The term *transporter* can be used in a broad sense to include channels, but in this chapter transporters are defined more exclusively to distinguish them from channels. Even the simplest transporter differs from a channel in that the binding site for the transported substrate is not accessible from both sides of the membrane at the same time. As a result, the maximum flux of the substrate across the biomembrane is limited by the rate at which its binding site alternates between inward and outward orientations. The simplest transporter, or *simple carrier*, facilitates the passive migration of a substrate down its electrochemical gradient, a process called *facilitated diffusion*. Adopting terminology from prokaryotic research, the simple carrier is also called a *uniporter*. When different substrates for the same uniporter are located on opposite sides of the membrane, these substrates can undergo *exchange diffusion* via the uniporter.

However, the cardinal feature of transporters, which distinguishes them from channels, is their ability to move solutes *against* an electrochemical gradient, and thereby indeed to generate electrochemical gradients. Ion-translocating adenosine triphosphatases (ATPases) harness the free energy of ATP hydrolysis to generate transmembrane electrochemical gradients, most commonly of H^+, Na^+, and K^+, in a process known as *primary active transport*. The transmembrane gradient of H^+, Na^+, or K^+ created by primary transport constitutes an ion-motive force that can be tapped by a large variety of secondary active transporters to move other ions and solutes against an electrochemical gradient. In energetic and mechanistic terms, the uphill translocation of solute is *coupled* to a driving force produced either by a metabolic reaction (primary transport) or by the downhill movement of the driving ions (secondary transport). Coupled fluxes of the driving ion and the driven species in the same direction across a membrane are termed *cotransport* or *symport*, whereas the term *countertransport* or *antiport* applies to coupled fluxes in opposing directions.

The *stoichiometry* of transport refers to the number of ions or molecules of each transported species that is translocated by one complete cycle of transport. Together with the number and sign of the charges carried by each transported ion, the stoichiometry determines whether one complete cycle of transport results in a net transfer of electric charge from one side of the membrane to the other. If so, then this transport is described as *electrogenic* because it elicits a flow of current across the membrane. Transport currents are characteristically much smaller than channel currents. Ions must negotiate the "turnstile" of the transporter cycle rather than streaming through the aqueous pore of an open channel. Electrogenic transport, unlike electroneutral transport, is coupled to the transmembrane potential difference as an additional driving force.

A transporter therefore may couple solute flux to multiple, sometimes opposing, driving forces. The net amplitude and direction of solute flux are described by established thermodynamic relationships that accurately predict how changes in the driving electrochemical gradients and transmembrane potential can modulate or reverse the driven solute flux. This aspect of transport modulation and reversal is especially relevant to transport in the central nervous system (CNS), where wide fluctuations of ion-motive forces are integral to communication between cells. However, in the rapid time frame of synaptic events, which can be brief compared to that of a single transport cycle, the steady-state energetics may be less important than *transporter kinetics*, meaning the rates of transition between intermediate transporter conformations.

The molecular identification of transporters made it possible to measure the currents associated with their individual expression in *Xenopus oocytes* or suitable mammalian cell lines. An unexpected outcome of this

See the list of abbreviations at the end of the chapter.

TABLE 12.1 *Selected Transporters of Ions and Other Solutes in Mammalian Astrocytes (A), Oligodendrocytes (O), and Microglia (M)*

Transporter Family	*Human Gene Family*[a]	*Prominent Isoforms or Subunits*	*Representative Evidence, Preparation, Glial Cell Type*[b]	*Reference*[c]
Ion-translocating ATPases				
F-ATPase	*ATP5*	Not known	Inhibitor, *culture*, A	Almeida et al. (2001)
V-ATPase	*ATP6*	c, a1, A	rtPCR, *culture*, A	Philippe et al. (2002)
		c	rtPCR, *in situ*, glioma	Philippe et al. (2002)
P-type ATPases				
Na^+,K^+-ATPase	*ATP1*	α_1, α_2, β_2	Immunostain, *in situ*, A	Knapp et al. (2000)
		α_1, α_2, β_3	Immunostain, *in situ*, O	Martin-Vasallo et al. (2000)
Ca^{2+}-ATPase (SERCA)	*ATP2A*	SERCA2	Immunostain, *culture*, A	Blaustein et al. (2002)
		Not known	Inhibitor, *in situ*, A	Nett et al. (2002)
Ca^{2+}-ATPase (PMCA)	*ATP2B*	PMCA1,2,4	Immunoblot, *culture*, A	Fresu et al. (1999)
ATP-binding cassette transporters				
Multidrug resistance (MDR)	*ABCB*	MDR1(P-gp)	Immunostain, *in situ*, A	Golden and Pardridge (1999)
MDR-associated proteins	*ABCC*	MRP1,3,4,5	rtPCR, *culture*, A, O, M	Hirrlinger et al. (2002)
Endogenous lipid transport	*ABCA*	ABCA2	Immunostain, *in situ*, O	Tanaka et al. (2003)
Secondary transport of inorganic ions				
Cation-chloride cotransporters	*SLC12*	NKCC1	Immunostain, *in situ*, O	Plotkin et al. (1997)
		NKCC1, KCC1	Hybridization, *in situ*, glia[d]	Kanaka et al. (2001)
Bicarbonate transporters	*SLC4*	NBC1	Immunostain, *in situ*, A	Schmitt et al. (2000)
		AE3	Immunostain, *retinal Müller*	Kobayashi et al. (1994)
Sodium/hydrogen exchangers	*SLC9*	NHE1,2	rtPCR, *culture*, A	Benos et al. (1994)
		NHE1	Immunoblot, *culture*, glioma	McLean et al. (2000)
Sodium/calcium exchangers	*SLC8*	NCX1,2,3	rtPCR, *culture*, A,O	Quednau et al. (1997)
Transporters of organic solutes				
Facilitative glucose transporters	*SLC2*	GLUT1	Immunostain, *in situ*, A,O	Yu and Ding (1998)
		GLUT5	Immunostain, *in situ*, M	Payne et al. (1997)
		HMIT	Immunostain, *in situ*, A	Uldry and Thorens (2004)
Monocarboxylate transporters	*SLC16*	MCT1,2	Immunostain, *in situ*, A	Hanu et al. (2000)
		MCT4	Immunostain, *in situ*, A	Bergersen et al. (2002)
Sodium- and chloride-dependent neurotransmitter transporters	*SLC6*	GAT1,2,3	Immunostain, *in situ*, A	Gadea and Lopez-Colome (2001)
		BGT1	rtPCR, *culture*, A	Bitoun and Tappaz (2000)
		TAUT2	Immunostain, *in situ*, A	Pow et al. (2002)
		SERT	Immunostain, *in situ*, A	Pickel and Chan (1999)
		GLYT1	Immunostain, *in situ*, A	Zafra et al. (1995)
Sodium-dependent glutamate transporters	*SLC1*	GLT-1, GLAST	Immunostain, *in situ*, A	Chaudhry et al. (1995)
		GLAST	Immunostain, *in situ*, O	Domercq et al. (1999)
		GLT-1	Immunostain, *in situ*, M	Lopez-Redondo et al. (2000)
		ASCT1	Immunostain, *in situ*, A	Sakai et al. (2003)
		ASCT2	rtPCR, *culture*, A	Bröer et al. (1999a)
Cationic and heterodimeric amino acid transporters	*SLC7*	CAT1	Hybridization, *in situ*, A	Braissant et al. (1999)
		CAT2(B)	Hybridization, *in situ*, O	Braissant et al. (2001)
		CAT2	RNA blot, *culture*, M	Kawahara et al. (2001)
		y^+LAT2	rtPCR, *culture*, A	Bröer et al. (2000)
		xCT	Immunostain, *in situ*, A	Pow (2001)
Sodium-coupled neutral amino acid transporters	*SLC38*	SNAT3	Immunostain, *in situ*, A	Boulland et al. (2003)
Type I phosphate/vesicular glutamate transporters	*SLC17*	VGLUT3	Immunostain, *in situ*, A	Fremeau, Jr. et al. (2002)

[a]Human gene symbols are designated by the Human Genome Organization Gene Nomenclature Committee (*SLC*, solute carrier gene families).

[b]Multiple lines of evidence make the case for functional transporter expression in astrocytes (A), oligodendrocytes (O) or microglia (M). Only a single representative example of the evidence is cited in this table. Citation of evidence in cell *culture* indicates that *in situ* studies of sufficient resolution were not found (rtPCR: reverse transcriptase polymerase chain reaction).

[c]In some cases the cited reference is not itself a primary source of the data, but provides access to primary sources.

[d]Glial cell type not identified.

approach has been the discovery that many transporters also function as ion channels, mediating substantial constitutive or solute-gated ion fluxes that are *not* coupled to transport. These channel-mediated currents can readily mask, or can be misinterpreted as, transport-generated currents. Thus do versatile proteins thwart our attempts to categorize them.

What follows is a survey of the properties of selected transporter families (Table 12.1) that have prominent roles in the functions of neuroglia detailed in other chapters of this book, especially the interactions of glia with neurons. The purpose of this chapter is to examine how transport mechanisms may subserve glial functions.

ION-TRANSLOCATING ADENOSINE TRIPHOSPHATASES

F_1F_0-Type ATPase (F-ATPase)

Mitochondrial F_1F_0-type ATPase (F-ATPase), acting in reverse mode as ATP synthase, is the main source of ATP production in most cells. Oxidative phosphorylation generates a steep gradient of H^+, and a large potential difference, across the inner membrane of mitochondria. This proton-motive force drives ATP synthesis by F-ATPase. In astrocytes, an estimated 25%–30% of ATP production is normally derived from cytosolic glycolysis (Silver and Erecińska, 1997), yet ATP levels do not fall when mitochondrial respiration is blocked. Under these conditions, the ATP supply is sustained by a compensatory stimulation of glycolysis, and F-ATPase now acts as a proton pump, consuming ATP to generate the mitochondrial proton-motive force. Neurons were found to lack the glycolytic response observed in glia, so that interruption of the respiratory chain in neurons leads to ATP depletion, depolarization of the mitochondrial inner membrane, and ultimately apoptotic cell death (Almeida et al., 2001).

Mammalian F-ATPase is a large complex assembled from 16–18 polypeptide subunits. The proton-transporting F_0 domain of the complex spans the mitochondrial inner membrane. Two stalks connect the globular, catalytic F_1 domain to F_0 on the matrix side of the membrane. Rotation of the central stalk is responsible for bidirectional energy transfer between F_0 and F_1 (Itoh et al., 2004). The second stalk serves as a stationary anchor to prevent futile rotation of F_1.

Vacuolar H^+-ATPase (V-ATPase)

The function of intracellular organelles that participate in endocytotic and secretory pathways depends critically upon an acidic luminal pH relative to cytosol. This proton electrochemical gradient is generated by vacuolar H^+-ATPase (V-ATPase), the ubiquitous proton pump of vacuolar membrane. V-ATPase is a large multimeric complex phylogenetically related to F-ATPase and similar to it structurally. A membrane-embedded V_0 component is similarly coupled to a catalytic V_1 component, but the coupling is unidirectional and V-ATPase is unable to synthesize ATP. *Slippage* of proton transport through V_0 is believed to be responsible for the lack of bidirectional coupling, and for proton electrochemical gradients smaller in amplitude than those generated by F-ATPase.

Redox conditions modulate V-ATPase activity by reversible disulfide bond formation between cysteine residues in the catalytic V_1 head. A further regulatory mechanism involves reversible dissociation of the V_0 and V_1 components, which contrasts with the stability of the F_1F_0 complex. V-ATPase and F-ATPase activities can be discriminated by their susceptibility to high-affinity block by the macrolide antibiotics bafilomycin and oligomycin, respectively. About 25% of the V-ATPase expressed in cultured C6 glioma and astrocytic cells is present and functional in the glial *plasma membrane* (Fig. 12.1), suggesting a role for this transporter in cytosolic and extracellular pH regulation as well as in organelle acidity (Philippe et al., 2002).

P-Type ATPases

The defining characteristic of the P-type ATPases is the association of conformational change with the phosphorylation of a conserved aspartate residue in the cat-

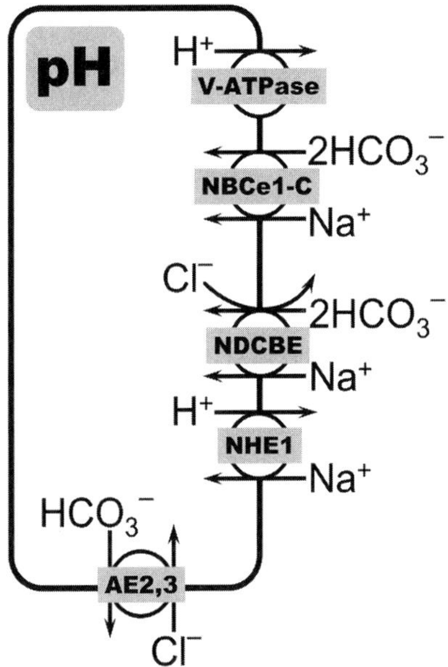

FIGURE 12.1 pH-Regulating transporters in astrocytes. Acid-extruding transport includes vacuolar H^+-ATPase (V-ATPase), sodium bicarbonate cotransport (NBCe1-C), sodium-driven chloride/bicarbonate exchange (NDCBE), and sodium/hydrogen exchange (NHE1). Acid-loading transport includes chloride/bicarbonate exchange (AE2 and AE3).

alytic domain. In marked contrast to F- and V-ATPases, the catalytic, transport, and coupling functions of P-type ATPases are all expressed in a single polypeptide. Prominent among the P-type ATPases in neuroglia are the sodium pump (Na^+,K^+-ATPase) and the calcium pumps of endoplasmic reticulum (sarcoplasmic/endoplasmic reticulum Ca^{2+}-ATPase, SERCA) and plasma membrane (plasma membrane Ca^{2+}-ATPase, PMCA). The crystal structure of SERCA has been resolved in Ca^{2+}-bound and Ca^{2+}-free conformations (Toyoshima and Nomura, 2002). There are 10 membrane-spanning helices and a large cytoplasmic region composed of three domains called *actuator* (A), *nucleotide-binding* (N), and *phosphorylation* (P). The molecular mechanism by which P-type ATPases couple ATP hydrolysis to concentrative transport is likely to emerge from such structural advances.

Both astrocytic and neuronal plasma membranes are rich in Na^+,K^+-ATPase, an essential generator of the membrane potential and cation gradients that drive intercellular communication and secondary active transport. One cycle of transport moves $3Na^+$ out of the cell and $2K^+$ inward for the hydrolysis of one ATP molecule. The net outward movement of one positive charge per cycle makes the transport electrogenic. In the absence of a stimulus to pump activity, Na^+,K^+-ATPase consumes about 20% of astrocytic ATP production (Silver and Erecińska, 1997). However, when Na^+ cotransport, for example, increases the cytosolic Na^+ concentration, astrocyte glucose consumption accelerates markedly in cell cultures to meet the increased demand for ATP (Loaiza et al., 2003). By comparison, the elevations of extracellular [K^+] associated with neuronal activity elicit only modest increases in glucose consumption in these same culture models. This insensitivity to extracellular [K^+] may not necessarily reflect function *in situ*, but rather the expression *in vitro* of Na^+,K^+-ATPase isoforms with K^+ affinity too high to respond in the physiological range of extracellular [K^+] (Peng et al., 1998).

The functional unit of Na^+,K^+-ATPase is a heterodimer composed of an α and a β subunit. Catalytic and transport activity, and the binding site for glycoside inhibitors such as ouabain, all reside in the α subunit. The β subunit, a glycoprotein with a single membrane-spanning region, serves as an essential *chaperone* for the routing and maturation of the α subunit. Four α and three β isoforms are known. The $\alpha1$ subunit is ubiquitous, whereas certain other isoforms are expressed preferentially in neuroglial subtypes (Table 12.1).

The levels of expression of the $\alpha2$ and $\beta2$ subunits in astrocytes are regulated by environmental cues that may not be present *in vitro* (Peng et al., 1998). The low K^+ affinity of the $\alpha2\beta2$ dimer makes it responsive to physiologically relevant increases in extracellular [K^+] and therefore potentially significant for the clearance of K^+ released from active neurons. There is evidence that the kinetic properties of Na^+,K^+-ATPase are also regulated by interaction with tissue factors. Such factors include members of the FXYD family of small membrane-spanning polypeptides that are named for a conserved sequence in their N termini. Notably, FXYD7 is a brain-specific isoform, expressed both in neurons and in astroglia, that lowers the K^+ affinity of $\alpha1\beta$ dimers (Beguin et al., 2002). Resolving the main features of isoform composition, distribution, and modulation of the Na^+,K^+-ATPase heterodimers in the CNS will be key to understanding their roles.

ATP-BINDING CASSETTE (ABC) TRANSPORTERS

The ATP–binding cassette (ABC) transporters are a large superfamily of ATPases that export a remarkably broad range of substrates from cells against an electrochemical gradient. This is primary transport energized by hydrolysis of ATP. Prominent among the substrates for ABC transporters are xenobiotics (including dietary toxins and drugs), conjugates of xenobiotics, and endogenous lipids. The xenobiotic-exporting ABC transporters were first identified as P-glycoproteins that confer multidrug resistance (MDR) on cancer cells. It is now thought that drug resistance reflects the wider role of MDR1 P-glycoprotein, and related isoforms, in protecting tissues including brain from toxins. MDR1 P-glycoprotein is richly expressed in the capillary endothelial cells of the blood–brain barrier, and also in the remnants of astroglial endfeet attached to isolated human brain capillaries (Golden and Pardridge, 1999). Multidrug resistance of some gliomas, and of human immunodeficiency virus-1 (HIV-1)–infected microglia, potentially relates to P-glycoprotein expression. Also, the overexpression of glial P-glycoprotein in epileptogenic brain tissue is associated with multidrug resistance in epilepsy.

Neuroglia can also detoxify xenobiotics by conjugating them with glutathione to form negatively charged conjugates that are exported most efficiently by members of another ABC transporter subfamily, typified by MRP1 (multidrug resistance-associated protein 1). Among the MRPs detected in glia are nucleotide transporters that may serve as efflux pathways for ATP, which has emerged as a significant neuromodulator released by astrocytes (Hirrlinger et al., 2002).

ABCA1, a widespread exporter of cholesterol and phospholipids from cells, is representative of lipid transporters drawn from several subfamilies of ABC transporters. Expression of these transporters is highly regulated by nuclear receptors responsive to oxysterols and fatty acid metabolites. The ABCA2 isoform is distributed primarily in brain and neural tissues. In the developing rat brain, a rapid increase in ABCA2 expression coincides spatially and temporally with the onset of myelination (Tanaka et al., 2003). Little is known about the roles of the ABC transporters in neuroglia, but appreciation of their significance is sure to grow.

SECONDARY TRANSPORT OF INORGANIC IONS

Cation-Chloride Cotransporter (CCC) Family

The cation-chloride cotransporter (CCC) gene family encodes the Na^+-K^+-$2Cl^-$ cotransporters (NKCC), the K^+-Cl^- cotransporters (KCC), and a renal Na^+-Cl^- cotransporter (NCC). They have well-documented roles in the transport of NaCl and/or KCl, accompanied by water, across epithelia, and in the regulatory responses of cells to changes in volume. The regulation of cell volume is particularly significant in glia (Fig. 12.2) because of its critical impact on intracranial pressure (Chapter 44).

Neuroglia, like most other cells, express the "housekeeping" isoform 1 of the Na^+-K^+-$2Cl^-$ cotransporter (NKCC1) and of the K^+-Cl^- cotransporter (KCC1) (Kanaka et al., 2001). These cotransporters mediate obligatorily coupled, electroneutral fluxes of cation and chloride that are inhibited by loop diuretics. Bumetanide is more potent than furosemide as an inhibitor of NKCC, whereas the relative inhibitory potency of these loop diuretics is reversed and reduced for KCC. The prevailing electrochemical gradients of Na^+ and K^+ drive an inward flux of cation chloride via NKCC1 but an outward flux via KCC1. The osmotic effect of any net flux of cation chloride across the cell membrane results in a corresponding movement of water. Accordingly, increased extracellular [K^+] causes swelling of normal astrocytes from wild-type mice, a response that is absent in astrocytes from NKCC1-null mice (Su et al., 2002).

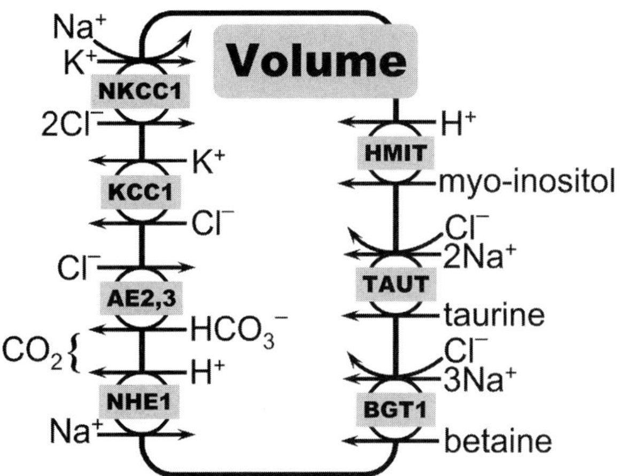

FIGURE 12.2 Volume-regulating transporters in astrocytes. Inorganic osmolyte transport includes sodium-potassium-chloride cotransport (NKCC1), potassium-chloride cotransport (KCC1), and chloride/bicarbonate exchange (AE2 and AE3) combined with sodium/hydrogen exchange (NHE1). Organic osmolyte transport includes hydrogen-coupled myo-inositol transport (HMIT), taurine transport (TAUT), and betaine transport by the betaine/GABA transporter (BGT1).

It is thought that opposing ion fluxes via NKCC1 and KCC1 are normally small under euvolemic conditions, and that they are activated selectively by cell shrinkage or swelling, respectively. For example, astrocytes from wild-type mice showed a regulatory volume increase after hypertonic shrinkage, and this response was abolished in NKCC1-null mice (Su et al., 2002). However, activation of KCC by hypotonic challenge is not obvious in cultured astrocytes (Parkerson and Sontheimer, 2003). Much interest attaches therefore to the signaling mechanisms that coordinate the activation of these transporters. Distinct pathways for regulation of NKCC activity involve phosphorylation/dephosphorylation by multiple kinases/phosphatases, protein-protein interactions, and cytosolic [Cl^-].

Bicarbonate Transporter Superfamily

The bicarbonate transporter superfamily includes the protein families that mediate chloride/bicarbonate anion exchange (AE), sodium bicarbonate cotransport (NBC), and sodium-driven chloride/bicarbonate exchange (NDCBE) (Boron, 2001). The task of regulating pH in neural tissue is shared primarily by these bicarbonate transporters acting in concert with sodium/hydrogen exchangers (NHE) and V-ATPase (Fig. 12.1). Much evidence implicates pH as a prominent intercellular signal and as a modulator of neuronal excitability and glial metabolism (Chapter 26). Anion transport is typically inhibited by disulfonic stilbene derivatives such as 4,4′-diisothiocyanatostilbene-2,2′-disulfonic acid (DIDS). However, these inhibitors are relatively nonselective and do not discriminate usefully between bicarbonate transporter subfamilies.

It is a well-established property of astrocytes that the cytosol is alkalinized by membrane depolarization, for example, in response to K^+ released by active neurons (Chesler, 2003). This linkage between neural activity and astrocytic pH is mediated by electrogenic sodium bicarbonate cotransport across the plasma membrane of astrocytes. Coupled transport of two HCO_3^- with each Na^+ results in a net flux of negative charge. Thus, any reduction of the inside-negative transmembrane potential increases the electrochemical gradient for HCO_3^- influx. The interaction of entering HCO_3^- with H^+ to form CO_2 and water raises cytosolic pH. This process is greatly facilitated by carbonic anhydrase activity that catalyzes the rapid interconversion between H_2CO_3 and CO_2. Because HCO_3^- influx obligates dissociation of extracellular H_2CO_3 with formation of H^+, the effect of this cotransport can be described as *acid extrusion* to the extracellular space. However, there is evidence that the "resting" membrane potential of astrocytes can be large enough to drive HCO_3^- *efflux* via the cotransporter, so that membrane depolarization *reverses* HCO_3^- flux from *acid loading* to *acid extruding* (Brookes and Turner, 1994).

The electrogenic Na^+-HCO_3^- cotransporter in astrocytes has been identified as a splice variant of NBC isoform 1, designated NBCe1-C (Boron, 2001). Observations in oligodendrocytes, which do not exhibit depolarization-induced alkalinization, suggest that they express a different, *electroneutral*, variant of NBC. The stoichiometry of the kidney variant NBCe1-A is normally 3 HCO_3^- : 1 Na^+, which results in HCO_3^- *efflux* at physiological membrane potentials. However, phosphorylation of the carboxy terminus of NBCe1-A changes the stoichiometry from 3:1 to 2:1 (Gross et al., 2002), which raises the possibility that the activity of glial variants might be modulated similarly. Protein-protein interactions, particularly with intracellular carbonic anhydrase II (CAII) and extracellular CAIV, also are found to regulate the activity of the bicarbonate transporters.

The recovery of glia from an intracellular *alkaline* load is facilitated by bicarbonate extrusion via AE transporters in electroneutral exchange for chloride. The widely expressed AE2 isoform, and also AE3, are the variants most likely to be found in glia, as the well-known band 3 protein AE1 is confined almost entirely to erythrocytes. Chloride/bicarbonate exchangers can participate in glial volume regulation when they act in concert with the Na^+/H^+ exchangers (Fig. 12.2). The influx of Na^+ plus Cl^- in exchange for H^+ plus HCO_3^- via these combined transporters results in the net import of inorganic osmolyte without effect on pH.

The Na^+-driven chloride/bicarbonate exchanger NDCBE couples influx of 1 Na^+ and 2 HCO_3^- to efflux of 1 Cl^- under normal physiological conditions, thus mediating electroneutral extrusion of acid. NDCBE, which is structurally closer to NBC than to AE, appears to be the primary regulator of pH in some neurons (Boron, 2001). This transport activity is detectable in astrocyte culture, although not yet shown to be a major determinant of glial pH.

Sodium/Hydrogen Exchangers (NHE)

Sodium/hydrogen exchange contributes prominently to the recovery of glial cytosol from an acid load (Chesler, 2003). The inward electrochemical gradient of Na^+ can potentially drive intracellular pH substantially above extracellular pH by 1:1 electroneutral exchange of Na^+ for H^+. Yet this thermodynamic equilibrium is not attained because NHE activity is inhibited when intracellular pH rises to a *setpoint* normally of about pH 7.2. NHE can also act in combination with AE to regulate cell volume (Fig. 12.2). The ubiquitous housekeeping isoform NHE1 is the predominant form expressed in rat astrocyte cultures (Benos et al., 1994). However, expression of this and other members of the NHE family, which comprises NHE1–5 plus mitochondrial variant NHE6, shows marked regional variation in the intact brain (Douglas et al., 2001). Isoforms NHE1-2 are inhibited by amiloride and its derivatives at lower concentrations than are NHE3–5, which consequently are called *amiloride resistant*. Sodium/hydrogen exchange in astrocytes was reported to be amiloride resistant in some studies but not others, possibly reflecting the expression of more than one isoform (Touyz et al., 1997).

As a result of its well-documented functions in the control of cytosolic pH and cell volume, and also as a membrane anchor for cytoskeletal actin, the NHE1 transporter influences cell proliferation, migration, and shape (Putney et al., 2002). In human malignant gliomas, for example, there is evidence of increased NHE1 activity associated with alkalinization of the cytosol and extracellular acidification. The N-terminal, ion-translocating domain of NHE1 contains pH sensing sites in addition to the binding site for amiloride and related inhibitors. However, pH-sensing is subject to modulation by the large cytoplasmic C-terminal region of the protein. Neurohormones, cytokines, and growth factors are able to raise the pH setpoint of NHE1, and thereby activate NHE1 transport, by the convergence of multiple signaling pathways on specialized zones of the regulatory C terminus (Putney et al., 2002). The C-terminal sequence is less conserved among NHE isoforms than is the ion-translocating domain, and the regulatory responses of different isoforms are correspondingly varied. Inactivation of the NHE1 gene in the mouse is not lethal, but results in seizures and ataxia (Counillon and Pouyssegur, 2000). Thus, despite the apparent redundancy built into the regulation of cell pH and volume, NHE1 is essential for normal CNS function.

Sodium/Calcium Exchangers (NCX)

The task of Ca^{2+} extrusion across the astrocytic plasma membrane is shared by sodium/calcium exchangers (NCX) and plasma membrane Ca^{2+}-ATPase (PMCA) (Chapter 17). NCX has a lower affinity for Ca^{2+} than does PCMA, but a faster transport cycle. In the plasma membrane of cultured mouse astrocytes, PCMA is distributed diffusely, whereas NCX is confined to small membrane patches corresponding to underlying endoplasmic reticulum, suggesting that NCX activity may be restricted to specialized compartments of the glial cytoplasm (Lencesova et al., 2004). Most studies indicate a stoichiometry of $3Na^+:1Ca^{2+}$ such that Ca^{2+} extrusion is accompanied by inward current. However,

NCX may adopt multiple transport modes (Kang and Hilgemann, 2004). High intracellular Na^+ or low intracellular Ca^{2+} inactivates NCX allosterically.

Transcripts of all three NCX genes are expressed in the mammalian brain, but regional expression levels of NCX1–3 vary greatly (Canitano et al., 2002). The NCX polypeptide sequence contains membrane-spanning domains at both termini joined by a large cytoplasmic loop involved in regulating transport activity. NCX1 undergoes alternative splicing in the cytoplasmic loop region by differing combinations of six exons labeled A through F, exons A and B being mutually exclusive. In culture, astrocytes express exon B–containing variants of NCX1, whereas neurons express exon A–containing variants (He et al., 1998). These variants differ significantly in the regulation of transport when expressed in heterologous cell systems. However, recent findings suggest that the regulatory properties of NCX1 are also dependent on coexpression of, and complex formation with, a group of cell-specific regulatory proteins (Schulze et al., 2003).

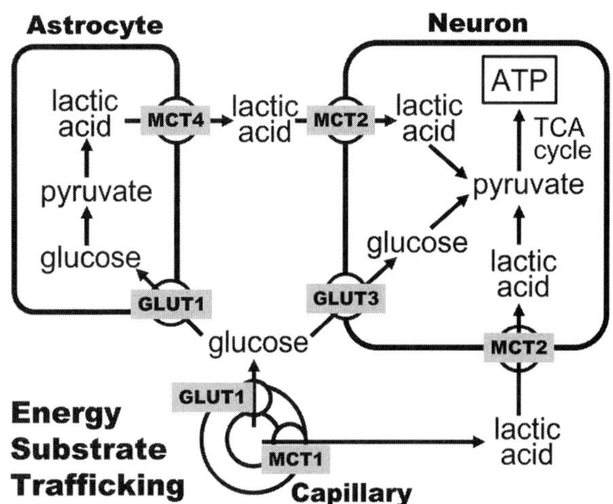

FIGURE 12.3 Transporters participating in energy substrate trafficking include facilitative glucose transporter isoforms (GLUT) and monocarboxylate transporter isoforms (MCT) adapted for their specific roles. This simplified scheme is based upon Uldry and Thorens (2004). ATP: adenosine triphosphate; TCA: tricarboxylic acid.

TRANSPORTERS OF ORGANIC SOLUTES

Facilitative Glucose Transporters (GLUT)

The entry of glucose into brain cells, as in other tissues, is mediated by sodium-independent glucose transporter (GLUT) isoforms acting as simple carriers facilitating glucose diffusion down the transmembrane concentration gradient (Fig. 12.3). The major participants are the class I isoforms GLUT1–4, which are inhibitable by cytochalasin B. High levels of GLUT1 are found in neuroglia and in the microvascular endothelium of the blood–brain barrier, whereas GLUT3, which exhibits higher substrate affinity and a faster transport cycle, predominates in neurons. The kinetics of GLUT1- and GLUT3-mediated transport are asymmetric, meaning that the alternating conformations of the unloaded transporter differ in energetic stability, resulting typically in higher K_m and V_{max} values for efflux of glucose than for influx (Uldry and Thorens, 2004). GLUT2 is a component of the *glucose-sensing* complex that regulates insulin release from pancreatic beta cells. Evidence suggests that GLUT2 may also play a glucose-sensing role in subpopulations of astrocytes (Leloup et al., 1994) and in hypothalamic ependymal-glial cells (Garcia et al., 2003). GLUT4, the isoform associated with insulin-responsive tissues, is detected in several brain regions, but the extent of glial expression is unclear. Cells that express GLUT4 contain endosomes rich in GLUT4 protein that fuse rapidly with the plasma membrane in response to stimulation by insulin, dramatically increasing the velocity of glucose uptake.

Glucose is not the preferred substrate of all GLUT transporters. GLUT5 is a fructose transporter that poorly recognizes glucose. In human brain, GLUT5 is confined exclusively to microglia, where its primary substrate and function remain unknown (Uldry and Thorens, 2004). The H^+-coupled myo-inositol transporter (HMIT) is a class III GLUT family transporter expressed predominantly in the brain and detected in both neurons and astrocytes *in situ*. Myo-inositol is a significant glial osmolyte and is the metabolic precursor of phophatidylinositol. In common with the other class III GLUT transporters, the HMIT sequence contains targeting motifs, and much HMIT protein is intracellular, suggesting that HMIT traffic to and from the plasma membrane regulates transport.

Monocarboxylate Transporters (MCT)

Because of their capacity for glycolysis, astrocytes are generators of lactate that can be used by neurons as an energy source (Chapter 29). A flux of lactate from astrocytes to neurons may be of particular importance, for example, during periods of increased neuronal activity or hypoxia. The H^+-coupled monocarboxylate transporters (MCT) expressed in the plasma membranes of glia and neurons mediate this lactate flux (Fig. 12.3). Of the 14 MCT genes identified in the human genome, the MCT1–4 products have been studied in most detail (Halestrap and Meredith, 2004), and MCT8 encodes a specific thyroid hormone transporter expressed in the brain (Friesema et al., 2003).

MCT1, which is expressed in most tissues, recognizes several monocarboxylates other than lactate with equal or greater affinity, including acetate, propionate, and pyruvate, and is characteristically inhibited by α-cyano-

4-hydroxycinnamate. Vectorial transport of monocarboxylate is coupled to the cotransport of H^+, whereas substrate exchange is mediated without the transfer of protons. Monocarboxylate export via MCT1 is accelerated when cytosolic pH falls or when extracellular pH rises. In comparison to MCT1, the MCT2 isoform has a higher affinity for lactate and pyruvate, and so is more specialized for uptake (Bröer et al., 1999b). MCT4 has greater specificity than MCT1 for lactate but lower binding affinity, and thus is better adapted for lactate export (Dimmer et al., 2000). Coexpression of a common cell surface glycoprotein, CD147, is a requirement for the anchoring of MCT1 and MCT4 in the plasma membrane. The distribution of MCT1, MCT2, and MCT4 visualized at subcellular resolution in cerebellum was found to be consistent with lactate export from astrocytes via MCT4 and uptake into neurons via MCT2, with MCT1 found predominantly in microvascular endothelium (Bergersen et al., 2002).

Sodium- and Chloride-Dependent Neurotransmitter Transporters (GAT/NET Transporters)

The neurotransmitter transporter family is also named for its prototype members, the γ-aminobutyric acid (GABA) transporter (GAT) and the norepinephrine transporter (NET). Central synapses are increasingly viewed as functionally *tripartite* structures in which glial processes in close proximity to pre- and postsynaptic neuronal elements participate actively in shaping synaptic communication (Chapter 28). There is a substantial body of evidence that neuroglia participate in the termination of synaptic transmission and/or extrasynaptic *spillover* by active uptake of released neurotransmitters (Chen et al., 2004).

GABA transporter (GAT) subfamily

Gamma-aminobutyric acid is the principal inhibitory neurotransmitter of the CNS. Three GABA transporter isoforms, GAT1–3, are distributed in both neurons and astrocytes in most regions of the brain (Gadea and Lopez-Colome, 2001). GAT1, the predominant and most extensively studied variant, mediates the cotransport of GABA, Na^+, and Cl^- with a stoichiometry of 1:2:1 and an apparent K_m for GABA in the low micromolar range. The resulting inward current associated with GABA uptake has a nonlinear relationship to membrane potential, tending to saturate with increasing hyperpolarization. In the absence of GABA, GAT1 still produces a transient capacitative current because Na^+ binding, and a consequent electrogenic conformational transition of the transporter, precede the binding of GABA (Lu and Hilgemann, 1999).

The measurement of glial transporter currents evoked by synaptically released GABA *in situ* provides valuable insights into the role of glial transport. In neocortical astrocytes these GABA transporter currents are very slow in onset and decay (seconds) compared to the time course of inhibitory postsynaptic currents (IPSC) (Kinney and Spain, 2002). Thus, in cortex it appears that most glial GABA transporters are remote from inhibitory synapses and do not shape IPSC decay, and that extrasynaptic GABA levels remain elevated for an extended time after the initiating synaptic event. Significance also attaches to the conditions under which GAT-mediated transport can be induced to reverse and release GABA to the extracellular space. Reversed transport of GABA is demonstrable in partially depolarized Bergmann glia *in situ* when they are perfused intracellularly with 10 mM each of Na^+ and GABA (Barakat and Bordey, 2002), but it is unresolved whether glial transport reverses in any physiological or pathophysiological conditions. Prolonged exposure of cells to GABA has been shown to upregulate GAT1 expression in the plasma membrane, whereas activation of protein kinase C promotes GAT1 internalization. The relative extent of tyrosine versus serine phosphorylation is a further determinant of the subcellular distribution of GAT1 (Quick et al., 2004).

The betaine/GABA transporter (BGT1) and taurine transporter (TAUT) are GAT subfamily members expressed in astrocytes. Betaine and taurine, like myoinositol, are considered major glial osmolytes. Taurine, which also has neuromodulatory and neuroprotective roles, is transported by TAUT with a stoichiometry and affinity that match GABA transport by GAT1. Taurine transport currents are similarly reversible when measured in Bergmann glia in cerebellar slices. By contrast, GABA transport via BGT1 is only partially chloride dependent and translocates 3 Na^+ with each GABA molecule, making it highly concentrative. However, there is as yet no indication of a role for BGT1 in shaping GABAergic neurotransmission. Of two TAUT variants, differing in C-terminal sequence, only the variant designated TAUT2 is associated primarily with glial cells in rat neural tissues (Pow et al., 2002). In common with other GAT/NET transporters, the traffic of BGT1 and TAUT to the cell surface is subject to multiple regulatory mechanisms (Chen et al., 2004).

Monoamine transporter subfamily

Because the monoamine neurotransmitters are implicated in many common neurobehavioral disorders, their transporters are intensively studied. However, the norepinephrine transporter (NET) and dopamine transporter (DAT) are exclusively neuronal, and of this subfamily only the serotonin transporter (SERT) is expressed in astrocytes as well as neurons (Pickel and Chan, 1999). The serotonin transporter translocates neither norepinephrine nor dopamine, yet these monoamines are nevertheless taken up by astrocytes. One identified pathway for this uptake in astrocyte cultures is the extraneuronal monoamine transporter (EMT), a Na^+-independent electrogenic transporter of organic cations (OCT family; *SLC22* genes) (Inazu et al., 2003).

The cotransport of 1 Na^+, 1 Cl^-, and 1 serotonin cation via SERT is coupled to the countertransport of 1 K^+, resulting in electroneutral transport. Heterologous SERT expression is associated, however, with a constitutive leakage current that is not coupled to transport and is observed in the absence of serotonin. Antidepressants related to fluoxetine, that are selective inhibitors of SERT-mediated transport, also block the leakage current. The expression level of SERT alters the ratio of leakage current to transport activity and alters the potency of inhibitors (Ramsey and DeFelice, 2002). A likely interpretation of this finding is that SERT function is regulated by an endogenous factor possessed by the host cell in limited supply. This would be consistent with the accumulating evidence of the regulation of GAT/NET transporter function by protein-protein interactions. Thus, although the SERT gene products in glia and neurons appear identical, cell-specific regulatory proteins could produce significant differences in function (Quick, 2003).

Glycine transporter (GLYT) subfamily

Glycine is the main inhibitory neurotransmitter in spinal cord and brain stem, and is an essential high-affinity coagonist at glutamatergic *N*-methyl-D-aspartate (NMDA) receptors throughout the brain. The imperative to regulate tightly the interstitial concentration of glycine in the neuromodulatory submicromolar range is met by the expression of glial and neuronal glycine transporter (GLYT) isoforms with distinctly different properties. Expression of *neuronal* GLYT2 is largely confined to spinal cord, brain stem, and cerebellum, and is concentrated in the presynaptic elements of putatively glycinergic synapses. By contrast, the CNS distribution of *glial* GLYT1 is much broader, including glial processes in the vicinity of nonglycinergic neurons (Zafra et al., 1995). The stoichiometry of GLYT2-mediated cotransport (1 glycine: 3 Na^+:1 Cl^-) is highly concentrative and necessitates extreme conditions for reversal of transport. GLYT1 stoichiometry (1 glycine: 2 Na^+: 1 Cl^-) yields less concentrative uptake that is more readily reversible. Multiple splice variants of GLYT1 are formed by combinations of two out of five exons encoding N- and C-terminal sequences with probable regulatory functions (Chen et al., 2004). GLYT1-null mice show severe motor and respiratory dysfunction at birth and die on the first postnatal day, underlining the vital role of this glial transporter (Gomeza et al., 2003).

Sodium-Dependent Glutamate Transporter Family

Excitatory amino acid transporters (EAAT)

Glutamate is the ubiquitous excitatory neurotransmitter of the mammalian brain and a key factor in synaptogenesis, but it is uniquely neurotoxic if allowed to persist in the extracellular compartment. Glutamate neurotoxicity has been implicated to some degree in many human neurodegenerative disorders. Accordingly, the transport mechanisms that take up glutamate from the extracellular space into brain cells have attracted intensive scrutiny (Chapter 27). Neuroglia play the dominant role in inactivating by uptake the glutamate released by neurons or by glia themselves (Fig. 12.4). Isoforms of excitatory amino acid transporters (EAAT) are encoded by five human genes, and two of these are considered primarily glial in the mature brain: EAAT2 (GLT-1 in rat) is richly expressed in cortical astrocytes, and EAAT1 (GLAST in rat) predominates in cerebellar and retinal glia (Chaudhry et al., 1995). In mouse hippocampus, only a subpopulation of astrocytes, which expresses both GLT-1 and GLAST, exhibits glutamate transport currents (Matthias et al., 2003). Further, two splice variants of GLT-1 show discrete nonuniform distributions over the surface of astrocytes in rat CNS (Sullivan et al., 2004).

Neuroglia take up glutamate against a steep concentration gradient by EAAT-mediated cotransport of 3 Na^+ and 1 H^+ per glutamate anion and countertransport of 1 K^+. Intense neuronal activity results not only in increased release of glutamate, but also increased extracellular K^+ and decreased extracellular Na^+. Thermodynamic considerations alone suggest

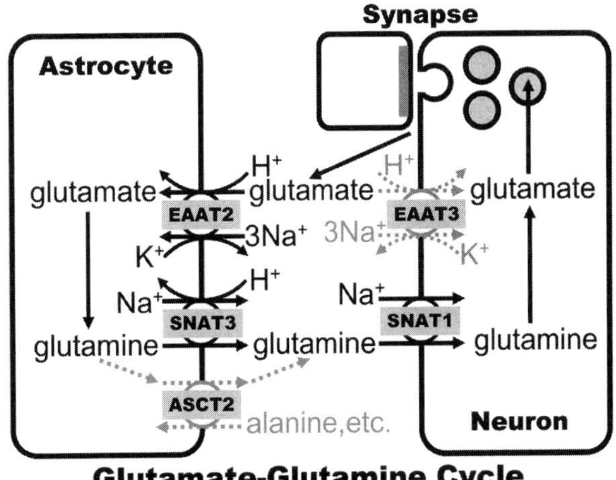

FIGURE 12.4 Transporter isoforms mediating primary (*solid arrows*) and secondary (*broken arrows*) pathways in the glutamate-glutamine cycle. Participating transport includes excitatory amino acid transport (EAAT), system N transport (SNAT3), system A transport (SNAT1), and system ASC transport (ASCT2). This is a partial, noninclusive scheme of participating transporter isoforms and their distribution.

that glutamate uptake would be impeded by these conditions. However, the coordinated activity of other ion transporters elicits compensatory adjustments, including declines in intracellular Na^+ and H^+. Extreme perturbations of extracellular Na^+ and K^+ fail to reverse glial glutamate uptake in the presence of an adequate supply of ATP. Notably, the release of glutamate observed in severely ischemic hippocampus is attributable to reversal of neuronal, but not glial, transport (Rossi et al., 2000).

In addition to the translocation of coupled charges, the binding of glutamate to EAAT activates an anion conductance pathway with the properties of a channel. The current generated by the uncoupled flux of anions is generally much larger than the coupled transport current, so it is used to monitor EAAT activity. However, the coupled and uncoupled currents are associated with different conformations of the transporter, exhibiting different activation kinetics (Bergles et al., 2002). At some synapses, glutamate transporters accelerate the decay of glutamatergic postsynaptic currents even though these currents are brief compared to the cycling time of EAAT (Mennerick et al., 1999). In this case, the transporters appear to act as buffers, reversibly binding and occluding glutamate in less time than is required for full translocation.

ASC system transporters (ASCT)

Despite substantial sequence identity with EAAT isoforms, the ASC system transporters ASCT1 and ASCT2 function as obligatory exchangers of small neutral amino acids typified by alanine, serine and cysteine. ASCT-mediated exchange is Na^+-dependent but electroneutral, since there is no net flux of Na^+. However, as in the case of EAAT, ASCT substrates activate an anion current uncoupled to transport. It should be noted that EAAT also can function in exchange mode. This is observed in the effect of EAAT inhibitors such as threo-3-hydroxyaspartate that are competitive substrates and can stimulate glutamate efflux by exchange (Mennerick et al., 1999). ASCT1 is widely expressed in brain astrocytes and neurons, and may have a specialized role in the export of serine from a subset of serine-rich astrocytes to neurons (Sakai et al., 2003). At low pH, ASCT1 recognizes and transports glutamate in the form of zwitterionic glutamic acid. It is possible that hypoxia-induced acidification recruits this mechanism in the neurotoxic release of glutamate associated with brain ischemia/hypoxia.

ASCT2, which exists as multiple variants differing in N-terminal truncation, is upregulated in immature and reactive astrocytes, but little is known of its distribution in the mature brain. Unlike ASCT1, ASCT2 recognizes glutamine as a high-affinity substrate. A flux of glutamine from astrocytes to neurons contributes to the replenishment of synaptically released glutamate and GABA. ASCT2 is likely to play a secondary role in the export of glutamine from astrocytes (Fig. 12.4) by mediating obligatory exchange of glutamine for extracellular amino acids such as alanine and serine (Bröer and Brookes, 2001).

Cationic (CAT) and Heterodimeric (HAT) Amino Acid Transporters

The dibasic amino acid arginine is the essential substrate for synthesis of nitric oxide by nitric oxide synthase (NOS). Glutamate stimulation of either neurons or glia triggers the formation of neuromodulatory nitric oxide by neuronal NOS (nNOS). In host defense reactions, astrocytes and microglia respond to cytokines and bacterial endotoxins by inducing the expression of inducible NOS (iNOS), which can generate potentially cytotoxic amounts of nitric oxide (Chapter 47). Arginine levels are much higher in glia than in neurons, and it is suspected that the neuronal pool of arginine is supplied by a flux from glia (Vega-Agapito et al., 2002). Three main transporters of arginine have been identified in astrocytes: CAT1, CAT2, and y^+LAT2. CAT1, a widely expressed dibasic amino acid transporter also known as system y^+, transports cationic arginine by Na^+-independent facilitated diffusion. This transport is concentrative in astrocytes because the normally large membrane potential acts as a driving force for the electrogenic influx of cations. It follows that membrane depolarization causes an outward redistribution of arginine to the extracellular space. The related lower-affinity CAT2 isoform, expressed as two splice variants, is coinduced in astrocytes together with iNOS (Manner et al., 2003). CAT3 expression is predominantly neuronal in mature rats.

Several heterodimeric (HAT) family transporters, including y^+LAT2, are expressed in cultured astrocytes and neurons (Bröer and Brookes, 2001). The y^+LAT2 light chain requires coexpression of, and linkage to, 4F2 heavy chain (an *SLC3* gene product) for functional expression in the plasma membrane. This transporter mediates Na^+-independent obligatory exchange of cationic amino acids but also recognizes neutral amino acids paired with Na^+. In an expression system, y^+LAT2 appears well adapted for export of arginine cation in electroneutral exchange for glutamine plus Na^+ (Bröer et al., 2000). The related transporter xCT (x_c^--system transporter), which also forms a functional heterodimer with 4F2, mediates the Cl^--dependent, electroneutral exchange of glutamate for cystine anions (Pow, 2001). This transport is a significant source of cysteine, formed by intracellular reduction of cystine, for neuroglial synthesis of glutathione.

Sodium-Coupled Neutral Amino Acid Transporters (SNAT)

Much of the neurotransmitter glutamate taken up by astrocytes is converted to glutamine by the signature glial enzyme glutamine synthase. This glutamine is thought to be exported by astrocytes and used in part for the synthesis of glutamate and GABA by neurons in a recurrent cycle named the *glutamate-glutamine cycle* (Fig. 12.4). The chief transporters positioned to mediate the traffic of glutamine from glia to neurons seem so well matched to the task that in themselves they are evidence in favor of such a cycle. These are the sodium-coupled neutral amino acid transporters, SNAT3 (previously named SN1 for system N transport), expressed selectively in astrocytes (Boulland et al., 2003), and SNAT1 (previously named SAT1, ATA1, or SA2 for system A transport), expressed selectively in neurons and ependyma (Mackenzie et al., 2003). The transporters given the consensus designation of SNAT (Mackenzie and Erickson, 2004) form a mammalian subfamily of the extensive amino acid and auxin permease (AAAP) family of eukaryotic transporters (Rubio-Aliaga et al., 2004).

Translocation of each glutamine by SNAT3 is coupled to cotransport of 1 Na^+ and countertransport of 1 H^+, yielding no net transfer of charge. Nonetheless, glutamine elicits a current in heterologous SNAT3 expression systems by activating an uncoupled flux of protons. Since the pH of glial cytosol is set by pH-regulatory transporters and is well buffered, it is unlikely to be affected by this H^+ leakage. The stoichiometry of SNAT3-mediated glutamine transport supports an approximately 20-fold steady-state concentration gradient of glutamine that matches the normal physiological distribution in astrocytes. Consequently, transport is poised for reversal and for outward redistribution of glutamine in the event that the extracellular glutamine concentration falls or increased neuronal activity causes the extrusion of H^+ from glial cytosol) (Bröer and Brookes, 2001). By contrast, the neuronal transporter SNAT1, though similarly selective for glutamine as a substrate, is an electrogenic Na^+-glutamine cotransporter not coupled to H^+, and therefore mediates a more concentrative uptake than SNAT3 that is much less readily reversed (Chaudhry et al., 2002).

Type I Phosphate/Vesicular Glutamate Transporters (VGLUT)

This family of proteins, originally identified as phosphate transporters, is now known to transport a variety of organic anions and to include the vesicular glutamate transporters (VGLUT) that mediate glutamate uptake into synaptic vesicles. Glutamate transport by VGLUT is coupled to the proton electrochemical gradient generated by V-ATPase. The observed dependence on vesicular membrane potential as well as the pH gradient indicates an electrogenic stoichiometry. Whereas isoforms VGLUT1 and VGLUT2 are largely confined to vesicular membrane in glutamatergic nerve terminals, the closely related VGLUT3 isoform localizes to subpopulations of nonglutamatergic neurons and to astrocytic processes and endfeet (Fremeau et al., 2002). This unanticipated distribution of VGLUT3 adds significantly to the accumulating evidence of exocytotic release of glutamate by astrocytes (Chapter 14).

SUMMARY AND PERSPECTIVES

It emerges convincingly, from even a partial survey, that the complement of cell surface transporters expressed in neuroglia is exquisitely adapted to glial functions and is distinctly different than that in neurons. At the same time that progress is being made in identifying a distinctive complement of transporters for each glial cell subtype, it becomes clear that the deployment of transporters in the plasma membrane is subject to a host of developmental, regional, and local cues. Individual transporters are found to possess unexpected versatility and plasticity in their properties. The properties observed upon expression of a transporter in heterologous hosts may represent only a first approximation of phenotypic transport in the glial milieu. Transporters are seen to function in the context of a cell-specific ensemble of regulatory proteins, and the regulatory repertoire is still expanding. The cogs and wheels that typified the transport models of an earlier era are now put to shame by an adaptability that challenges the ingenuity of today's modeler.

ABBREVIATIONS

AAAP	amino acid and auxin permease
ABC	ATP-binding cassette
AE	anion exchanger
ASCT	ASC-system transporter
BGT	betaine/GABA transporter
CA	carbonic anhydrase
CAT	cationic amino acid transporter
CCC	cation-chloride cotransporter
DAT	dopamine transporter
DIDS	4,4′-diisothiocyanatostilbene-2,2′-disulfonic acid
EAAT	excitatory amino acid transporter
EMT	extraneuronal monoamine transporter

F-ATPase	F_1F_0-type ATPase
GABA	γ-aminobutyric acid
GAT	γ-aminobutyric acid transporter
GLAST	glutamate/aspartate transporter isoform
GLT	glutamate transporter isoform
GLUT	sodium-independent glucose transporter
GLYT	glycine transporter
HAT	heterodimeric amino acid transporter
HMIT	H^+-coupled myo-inositol transporter
iNOS	inducible NOS
IPSC	inhibitory postsynaptic current
KCC	K^+-Cl^- cotransporter
MCT	monocarboxylate transporter
MDR	multidrug resistance
MRP	multidrug resistance-associated protein
NBC	sodium bicarbonate cotransporter
NCC	Na^+-Cl^- cotransporter
NCX	sodium/calcium exchanger
NDCBE	sodium-driven chloride/bicarbonate exchanger
NET	norepinephrine transporter
NHE	sodium/hydrogen exchanger
NKCC	Na^+-K^+-$2Cl^-$ cotransporter
NMDA	*N*-methyl-D-aspartate
nNOS	neuronal NOS
NOS	nitric oxide synthase
OCT	organic cation transporter
PMCA	plasma membrane Ca^{2+}-ATPase
SERCA	sarcoplasmic/endoplasmic-reticulum Ca^{2+}-ATPase
SERT	serotonin transporter
SLC	solute carrier
SNAT	sodium-coupled neutral amino acid transporter
TAUT	taurine transporter
V-ATPase	vacuolar H^+-ATPase
VGLUT	vesicular glutamate transporter
xCT	x_c^--system transporter
y^+LAT	y^+L-system amino acid transporter

REFERENCES

Almeida, A., Almeida, J., Bolanos, J.P., and Moncada, S. (2001) Different responses of astrocytes and neurons to nitric oxide: the role of glycolytically generated ATP in astrocyte protection. *Proc. Natl. Acad. Sci. USA* 98:15294–15299.

Barakat, L. and Bordey, A. (2002) GAT-1 and reversible GABA transport in Bergmann glia in slices. *J. Neurophysiol.* 88:1407–1419.

Beguin, P., Crambert, G., Monnet-Tschudi, F., Uldry, M., Horisberger, J.D., Garty, H., and Geering, K. (2002) FXYD7 is a brain-specific regulator of Na,K-ATPase alpha 1-beta isozymes. *EMBO J.* 21:3264–3273.

Benos, D.J., McPherson, S., Hahn, B.H., Chaikin, M.A., and Benveniste, E.N. (1994) Cytokines and HIV envelope glycoprotein gp120 stimulate Na^+/H^+ exchange in astrocytes. *J. Biol. Chem.* 269:13811–13816.

Bergersen, L., Rafiki, A., and Ottersen, O.P. (2002) Immunogold cytochemistry identifies specialized membrane domains for monocarboxylate transport in the central nervous system. *Neurochem. Res.* 27:89–96.

Bergles, D.E., Tzingounis, A.V., and Jahr, C.E. (2002) Comparison of coupled and uncoupled currents during glutamate uptake by GLT-1 transporters. *J. Neurosci.* 22:10153–10162.

Bitoun, M. and Tappaz, M. (2000) Gene expression of the transporters and biosynthetic enzymes of the osmolytes in astrocyte primary cultures exposed to hyperosmotic conditions. *Glia* 32:165–176.

Blaustein, M.P., Juhaszova, M., Golovina, V.A., Church, P.J., and Stanley, E.F. (2002) Na/Ca exchanger and PMCA localization in neurons and astrocytes: functional implications. *Ann. N.Y. Acad. Sci.* 976:356–366.

Boron, W.F. (2001) Sodium-coupled bicarbonate transporters. *J. Pancreas (Online)* 2:176–181.

Boulland, J.L., Rafiki, A., Levy, L.M., Storm-Mathisen, J., and Chaudhry, F.A. (2003) Highly differential expression of SN1, a bidirectional glutamine transporter, in astroglia and endothelium in the developing rat brain. *Glia* 41:260–275.

Braissant, O., Gotoh, T., Loup, M., Mori, M., and Bachmann, C. (1999) L-Arginine uptake, the citrulline-NO cycle and arginase II in the rat brain: an in situ hybridization study. *Brain Res. Mol. Brain Res.* 70:231–241.

Braissant, O., Gotoh, T., Loup, M., Mori, M., and Bachmann, C. (2001) Differential expression of the cationic amino acid transporter 2(B) in the adult rat brain. *Brain Res. Mol. Brain Res.* 91:189–195.

Bröer, S., Bröer, A., Schneider, H.P., Stegen, C., Halestrap, A.P., and Deitmer, J.W. (1999b) Characterization of the high-affinity monocarboxylate transporter MCT2 in *Xenopus laevis* oocytes. *Biochem. J.* 341:529–535.

Bröer, S. and Brookes, N. (2001) Transfer of glutamine between astrocytes and neurons. *J. Neurochem.* 77:705–719.

Bröer, A., Brookes, N., Ganapathy, V., Dimmer, K.S., Wagner, C.A., Lang, F., and Bröer, S. (1999a) The astroglial ASCT2 amino acid transporter as a mediator of glutamine efflux. *J. Neurochem.* 73:2184–2194.

Bröer, A., Wagner, C.A., Lang, F., and Bröer, S. (2000) The heterodimeric amino acid transporter 4F2hc/y^+LAT2 mediates arginine efflux in exchange with glutamine. *Biochem. J.* 349:787–795.

Brookes, N. and Turner, R.J. (1994) K^+-induced alkalinization in mouse cerebral astrocytes mediated by reversal of electrogenic Na^+-HCO_3^- cotransport. *Am. J. Physiol.* 267:C1633–C1640.

Canitano, A., Papa, M., Boscia, F., Castaldo, P., Sellitti, S., Taglialatela, M., and Annunziato, L. (2002) Brain distribution of the Na^+/Ca^{2+} exchanger-encoding genes NCX1, NCX2, and NCX3 and their related proteins in the central nervous system. *Ann. N.Y. Acad. Sci.* 976:394–404.

Chaudhry, F.A., Lehre, K.P., van Lookeren, C.M., Ottersen, O.P., Danbolt, N.C., and Storm-Mathisen, J. (1995) Glutamate transporters in glial plasma membranes: highly differentiated localizations revealed by quantitative ultrastructural immunocytochemistry. *Neuron* 15:711–720.

Chaudhry, F.A., Schmitz, D., Reimer, R.J., Larsson, P., Gray, A.T., Nicoll, R., Kavanaugh, M., and Edwards, R.H. (2002) Glutamine uptake by neurons: interaction of protons with system A transporters. *J. Neurosci.* 22:62–72.

Chen, N.H., Reith, M.E., and Quick, M.W. (2004) Synaptic uptake and beyond: the sodium- and chloride-dependent neurotransmitter transporter family SLC6. *Pflugers Arch.* 447:519–531.

Chesler, M. (2003) Regulation and modulation of pH in the brain. *Physiol Rev.* 83:1183–1221.

Counillon, L. and Pouyssegur, J. (2000) The expanding family of eucaryotic Na^+/H^+ exchangers. *J. Biol. Chem.* 275:1–4.

Dimmer, K.S., Friedrich, B., Lang, F., Deitmer, J.W., and Bröer, S. (2000) The low-affinity monocarboxylate transporter MCT4 is adapted to the export of lactate in highly glycolytic cells. *Biochem. J.* 350:219–227.

Domercq, M., Sanchez-Gomez, M.V., Areso, P., and Matute, C. (1999) Expression of glutamate transporters in rat optic nerve oligodendrocytes. *Eur. J. Neurosci.* 11:2226–2236.

Douglas, R.M., Schmitt, B.M., Xia, Y., Bevensee, M.O., Biemesderfer, D., Boron, W.F., and Haddad, G.G. (2001) Sodium-hydrogen exchangers and sodium-bicarbonate cotransporters: ontogeny of protein expression in the rat brain. *Neuroscience* 102:217–228.

Fremeau, R.T., Jr., Burman, J., Qureshi, T., Tran, C.H., Proctor, J., Johnson, J., Zhang, H., Sulzer, D., Copenhagen, D.R., Storm-Mathisen, J., Reimer, R.J., Chaudhry, F.A., and Edwards, R.H. (2002) The identification of vesicular glutamate transporter 3 suggests novel modes of signaling by glutamate. *Proc. Natl. Acad. Sci. USA* 99:14488–14493.

Fresu, L., Dehpour, A., Genazzani, A.A., Carafoli, E., and Guerini, D. (1999) Plasma membrane calcium ATPase isoforms in astrocytes. *Glia* 28:150–155.

Friesema, E.C., Ganguly, S., Abdalla, A., Manning Fox, J.E., Halestrap, A.P., and Visser, T.J. (2003) Identification of monocarboxylate transporter 8 as a specific thyroid hormone transporter. *J. Biol. Chem.* 278:40128–40135.

Gadea, A. and Lopez-Colome, A.M. (2001) Glial transporters for glutamate, glycine, and GABA: II. GABA transporters. *J. Neurosci. Res.* 63:461–468.

Garcia, M.A., Millan, C., Balmaceda-Aguilera, C., Castro, T., Pastor, P., Montecinos, H., Reinicke, K., Zuniga, F., Vera, J.C., Onate, S.A., and Nualart, F. (2003) Hypothalamic ependymal-glial cells express the glucose transporter GLUT2, a protein involved in glucose sensing. *J. Neurochem.* 86:709–724.

Golden, P.L. and Pardridge, W.M. (1999) P-glycoprotein on astrocyte foot processes of unfixed isolated human brain capillaries. *Brain Res.* 819:143–146.

Gomeza, J., Hulsmann, S., Ohno, K., Eulenburg, V., Szoke, K., Richter, D., and Betz, H. (2003) Inactivation of the glycine transporter 1 gene discloses vital role of glial glycine uptake in glycinergic inhibition. *Neuron* 40:785–796.

Gross, E., Pushkin, A., Abuladze, N., Fedotoff, O., and Kurtz, I. (2002) Regulation of the sodium bicarbonate cotransporter kNBC1 function: role of Asp(986), Asp(988) and kNBC1-carbonic anhydrase II binding. *J. Physiol.* 544:679–685.

Halestrap, A.P. and Meredith, D. (2004) The SLC16 gene family—from monocarboxylate transporters (MCTs) to aromatic amino acid transporters and beyond. *Pflugers Arch.* 447:619–628.

Hanu, R., McKenna, M., O'Neill, A., Resneck, W.G., and Bloch, R.J. (2000) Monocarboxylic acid transporters, MCT1 and MCT2, in cortical astrocytes *in vitro* and *in vivo*. *Am. J. Physiol. Cell Physiol.* 278:C921–C930.

He, S., Ruknudin, A., Bambrick, L.L., Lederer, W.J., and Schulze, D.H. (1998) Isoform-specific regulation of the Na^+/Ca^{2+} exchanger in rat astrocytes and neurons by PKA. *J. Neurosci.* 18:4833–4841.

Hirrlinger, J., Konig, J., and Dringen, R. (2002) Expression of mRNAs of multidrug resistance proteins (Mrps) in cultured rat astrocytes, oligodendrocytes, microglial cells and neurones. *J. Neurochem.* 82:716–719.

Inazu, M., Takeda, H., and Matsumiya, T. (2003) Expression and functional characterization of the extraneuronal monoamine transporter in normal human astrocytes. *J. Neurochem.* 84:43–52.

Itoh, H., Takahashi, A., Adachi, K., Noji, H., Yasuda, R., Yoshida, M., and Kinosita, K. (2004) Mechanically driven ATP synthesis by F1-ATPase. *Nature* 427:465–468.

Kanaka, C., Ohno, K., Okabe, A., Kuriyama, K., Itoh, T., Fukuda, A., and Sato, K. (2001) The differential expression patterns of messenger RNAs encoding K-Cl cotransporters (KCC1,2) and Na-K-2Cl cotransporter (NKCC1) in the rat nervous system. *Neuroscience* 104:933–946.

Kang, T.M. and Hilgemann, D.W. (2004) Multiple transport modes of the cardiac Na^+/Ca^{2+} exchanger. *Nature* 427:544–548.

Kawahara, K., Gotoh, T., Oyadomari, S., Kajizono, M., Kuniyasu, A., Ohsawa, K., Imai, Y., Kohsaka, S., Nakayama, H., and Mori, M. (2001) Co-induction of argininosuccinate synthetase, cationic amino acid transporter-2, and nitric oxide synthase in activated murine microglial cells. *Brain Res. Mol. Brain Res.* 90:165–173.

Kinney, G.A. and Spain, W.J. (2002) Synaptically evoked GABA transporter currents in neocortical glia. *J. Neurophysiol.* 88:2899–2908.

Knapp, P.E., Itkis, O.S., and Mata, M. (2000) Neuronal interaction determines the expression of the alpha-2 isoform of Na, K-ATPase in oligodendrocytes. *Brain Res. Dev. Brain Res.* 125:89–97.

Kobayashi, S., Morgans, C.W., Casey, J.R., and Kopito, R.R. (1994) AE3 anion exchanger isoforms in the vertebrate retina: developmental regulation and differential expression in neurons and glia. *J. Neurosci.* 14:6266–6279.

Leloup, C., Arluison, M., Lepetit, N., Cartier, N., Marfaing-Jallat, P., Ferre, P., and Penicaud, L. (1994) Glucose transporter 2 (GLUT 2): expression in specific brain nuclei. *Brain Res.* 638:221–226.

Lencesova, L., O'Neill, A., Resneck, W.G., Bloch, R.J., and Blaustein, M.P. (2004) Plasma membrane-cytoskeleton-endoplasmic reticulum complexes in neurons and astrocytes. *J. Biol. Chem.* 279:2885–2893.

Loaiza, A., Porras, O.H., and Barros, L.F. (2003) Glutamate triggers rapid glucose transport stimulation in astrocytes as evidenced by real-time confocal microscopy. *J. Neurosci.* 23:7337–7342.

Lopez-Redondo, F., Nakajima, K., Honda, S., and Kohsaka, S. (2000) Glutamate transporter GLT-1 is highly expressed in activated microglia following facial nerve axotomy. *Brain Res. Mol. Brain Res.* 76:429–435.

Lu, C.C. and Hilgemann, D.W. (1999) GAT1 ($GABA:Na^+:Cl^-$) cotransport function. Steady state studies in giant Xenopus oocyte membrane patches. *J. Gen. Physiol.* 114:429–444.

Mackenzie, B. and Erickson, J.D. (2004) Sodium-coupled neutral amino acid (System N/A) transporters of the SLC38 gene family. *Pflugers Arch.* 447:784–795.

Mackenzie, B., Schafer, M.K., Erickson, J.D., Hediger, M.A., Weihe, E., and Varoqui, H. (2003) Functional properties and cellular distribution of the system A glutamine transporter SNAT1 support specialized roles in central neurons. *J. Biol. Chem.* 278:23720–23730.

Manner, C.K., Nicholson, B., and MacLeod, C.L. (2003) CAT2 arginine transporter deficiency significantly reduces iNOS-mediated NO production in astrocytes. *J. Neurochem.* 85:476–482.

Martin-Vasallo, P., Wetzel, R.K., Garcia-Segura, L.M., Molina-Holgado, E., Arystarkhova, E., and Sweadner, K.J. (2000) Oligodendrocytes in brain and optic nerve express the beta3 subunit isoform of Na,K-ATPase. *Glia* 31:206–218.

Matthias, K., Kirchhoff, F., Seifert, G., Huttmann, K., Matyash, M., Kettenmann, H., and Steinhauser, C. (2003) Segregated expression of AMPA-type glutamate receptors and glutamate transporters defines distinct astrocyte populations in the mouse hippocampus. *J. Neurosci.* 23:1750–1758.

McLean, L.A., Roscoe, J., Jorgensen, N.K., Gorin, F.A., and Cala, P.M. (2000) Malignant gliomas display altered pH regulation by NHE1 compared with nontransformed astrocytes. *Am. J. Physiol Cell Physiol.* 278:C676–C688.

Mennerick, S., Shen, W., Xu, W., Benz, A., Tanaka, K., Shimamoto, K., Isenberg, K.E., Krause, J.E., and Zorumski, C.F. (1999) Substrate turnover by transporters curtails synaptic glutamate transients. *J. Neurosci.* 19:9242–9251.

Nett, W.J., Oloff, S.H., and McCarthy, K.D. (2002) Hippocampal astrocytes in situ exhibit calcium oscillations that occur independent of neuronal activity. *J. Neurophysiol.* 87:528–537.

Parkerson, K.A. and Sontheimer, H. (2003) Contribution of chloride channels to volume regulation of cortical astrocytes. *Am. J. Physiol. Cell Physiol.* 284:C1460–C1467.

Payne, J., Maher, F., Simpson, I., Mattice, L., and Davies, P. (1997) Glucose transporter Glut 5 expression in microglial cells. *Glia* 21:327–331.

Peng, L., Arystarkhova, E., and Sweadner, K.J. (1998) Plasticity of Na,K-ATPase isoform expression in cultures of flat astrocytes: species differences in gene expression. *Glia* 24:257–271.

Philippe, J.M., Dubois, J.M., Rouzaire-Dubois, B., Cartron, P.F., Vallette, F., and More, N. (2002) Functional expression of V-ATPases in the plasma membrane of glial cells. *Glia* 37:365–373.

Pickel, V.M. and Chan, J. (1999) Ultrastructural localization of the serotonin transporter in limbic and motor compartments of the nucleus accumbens. *J. Neurosci.* 19:7356–7366.

Plotkin, M.D., Snyder, E.Y., Hebert, S.C., and Delpire, E. (1997) Expression of the Na-K-2Cl cotransporter is developmentally regulated in postnatal rat brains: a possible mechanism underlying GABA's excitatory role in immature brain. *J. Neurobiol.* 33:781–795.

Pow, D.V. (2001) Visualising the activity of the cystine-glutamate antiporter in glial cells using antibodies to aminoadipic acid, a selectively transported substrate. *Glia* 34:27–38.

Pow, D.V., Sullivan, R., Reye, P., and Hermanussen, S. (2002) Localization of taurine transporters, taurine, and ^{3}H taurine accumulation in the rat retina, pituitary, and brain. *Glia* 37:153–168.

Putney, L.K., Denker, S.P., and Barber, D.L. (2002) The changing face of the Na^+/H^+ exchanger, NHE1: structure, regulation, and cellular actions. *Annu. Rev. Pharmacol. Toxicol.* 42:527–552.

Quednau, B.D., Nicoll, D.A., and Philipson, K.D. (1997) Tissue specificity and alternative splicing of the Na^+/Ca^{2+} exchanger isoforms NCX1, NCX2, and NCX3 in rat. *Am. J. Physiol.* 272: C1250–C1261.

Quick, M.W. (2003) Regulating the conducting states of a mammalian serotonin transporter. *Neuron* 40:537–549.

Quick, M.W., Hu, J., Wang, D., and Zhang, H.Y. (2004) Regulation of a gamma-aminobutyric acid (GABA) transporter by reciprocal tyrosine and serine phosphorylation. *J. Biol. Chem.* 279: 15961–15967

Ramsey, I.S. and DeFelice, L.J. (2002) Serotonin transporter function and pharmacology are sensitive to expression level: evidence for an endogenous regulatory factor. *J. Biol. Chem.* 277:14475–14482.

Rossi, D.J., Oshima, T., and Attwell, D. (2000) Glutamate release in severe brain ischaemia is mainly by reversed uptake. *Nature* 403:316–321.

Rubio-Aliaga, I., Boll, M., Vogt Weisenhorn, D.M., Foltz, M., Kottra, G., and Daniel, H. (2004) The proton/amino acid cotransporter PAT2 is expressed in neurons with a different subcellular localization than its paralog PAT1. *J. Biol. Chem.* 279:2754–2760.

Sakai, K., Shimizu, H., Koike, T., Furuya, S., and Watanabe, M. (2003) Neutral amino acid transporter ASCT1 is preferentially expressed in L-Ser-synthetic/storing glial cells in the mouse brain with transient expression in developing capillaries. *J. Neurosci.* 23:550–560.

Schmitt, B.M., Berger, U.V., Douglas, R.M., Bevensee, M.O., Hediger, M.A., Haddad, G.G., and Boron, W.F. (2000) Na/HCO_3 cotransporters in rat brain: expression in glia, neurons, and choroid plexus. *J. Neurosci.* 20:6839–6848.

Schulze, D.H., Mughal, M., Lederer, W.J., and Ruknudin, A.M. (2003) Sodium/calcium exchanger (NCX1) macromolecular complex. *J. Biol. Chem.* 278:28849–28855.

Silver, I.A. and Erecińska, M. (1997) Energetic demands of the Na^+/K^+ ATPase in mammalian astrocytes. *Glia* 21:35–45.

Su, G., Kintner, D.B., Flagella, M., Shull, G.E., and Sun, D. (2002) Astrocytes from Na^+-K^+-Cl^- cotransporter-null mice exhibit absence of swelling and decrease in EAA release. *Am. J. Physiol Cell Physiol.* 282:C1147–C1160.

Sullivan, R., Rauen, T., Fischer, F., Wiessner, M., Grewer, C., Bicho, A., and Pow, D.V. (2004) Cloning, transport properties, and differential localization of two splice variants of GLT-1 in the rat CNS: Implications for CNS glutamate homeostasis. *Glia* 45: 155–169.

Tanaka, Y., Yamada, K., Zhou, C.J., Ban, N., Shioda, S., and Inagaki, N. (2003) Temporal and spatial profiles of ABCA2-expressing oligodendrocytes in the developing rat brain. *J. Comp. Neurol.* 455:353–367.

Touyz, R.M., Picard, S., Schiffrin, E.L., and Deschepper, C.F. (1997) Cyclic GMP inhibits a pharmacologically distinct Na^+/H^+ exchanger variant in cultured rat astrocytes via an extracellular site of action. *J. Neurochem.* 68:1451–1461.

Toyoshima, C. and Nomura, H. (2002) Structural changes in the calcium pump accompanying the dissociation of calcium. *Nature* 418:605–611.

Uldry, M. and Thorens, B. (2004) The SLC2 family of facilitated hexose and polyol transporters. *Pflugers Arch.* 447:480–489.

Vega-Agapito, V., Almeida, A., Hatzoglou, M., and Bolanos, J.P. (2002) Peroxynitrite stimulates L-arginine transport system y^+ in glial cells. A potential mechanism for replenishing neuronal L-arginine. *J. Biol. Chem.* 277:29753–29759.

Yu, S. and Ding, W.G. (1998) The 45 kDa form of glucose transporter 1 (GLUT1) is localized in oligodendrocyte and astrocyte but not in microglia in the rat brain. *Brain Res.* 797:65–72.

Zafra, F., Aragon, C., Olivares, L., Danbolt, N.C., Gimenez, C., and Storm-Mathisen, J. (1995) Glycine transporters are differentially expressed among CNS cells. *J. Neurosci.* 15:3952–3969.

13 Gap junctions and hemichannels

BRUCE R. RANSOM AND ZU-CHENG YE

An intriguing form of intercellular communication is mediated by large channels called *gap junctions* that directly link the cytoplasmic interiors of cells. Most mammalian cells express gap junctions except mature skeletal muscle, spermatozoa, and erythrocytes. Loewenstein (1981) has summarized the history of how these channels were discovered, which began with the observation of electrical coupling between heart cells in 1952. Electrical coupling between glial cells was first noted in the leech central nervous system (CNS) (Kuffler and Potter, 1964). In the mammalian CNS, gap junctions are most abundantly expressed by glial cells, and the characteristics and possible functions of these channels in glial cells are the focus of this review. First, however, some important general principles about these channels and the proteins that make them will be discussed. A wealth of new information about gap junctions, and "half" gap junctions called *hemichannels* has accumulated since the first edition of this book and will be emphasized.

The channels comprising a gap junction are large-diameter aqueous pores that extend from one cell, across the extracellular space, into an adjacent cell. These channels allow all inorganic ions and small organic molecules to diffuse freely from the interior of one cell into the interior of another cell. The discovery of gap junctional communication challenged the fundamental concept of classical cell theory, which states that individual cells are autonomous functional units. When cells are connected with their neighboring cells by gap junctions, the functional unit is no longer the individual cell of classical cell theory but rather the large aggregate of cells that are so joined, because they share so much of their cytoplasmic contents (Loewenstein, 1981).

GENERAL FEATURES OF GAP JUNCTIONS

Gap Junction Structure

In electron micrographs, gap junctions appear as discrete areas where the cell membranes of adjacent cells closely approach one another, leaving a narrow gap of only about 2.5 nm (normal width = ~20 nm) (Fig. 13.1). These junctions have a seven-layer appearance because a small layer of extracellular space can be seen between the three-layered cell membranes under high-power magnification (Fig. 13.1*B*). Using the freeze fracture technique, gap junctions appear as clusters of intramembrane particles on the cytoplasmic fracture face of the plasma membranes (Fig. 13.2). Each particle represents a gap junction hemichannel or connexon. X-ray diffraction experiments show that each connexon is composed of six symmetrical subunits called *connexins* (Fig. 13.1*C*). It is now established that each connexin is a separate protein molecule (see below). A gap junction channel is formed when a connexon in one cell aligns with another connexon in an adjacent cell. Each macroscopic gap junction is an aggregate of many, often hundreds of, tightly packed gap junction channels (Fig. 13.2).

The three-dimensional structure of gap junction channels is elegantly revealed by electron crystallography on recombinant cardiac gap junctions [i.e., connexin-43 (Cx43)] (Unger et al., 1999) (Fig. 13.1*D*). Each connexon consists of 24 *rods* that correspond to the transmembrane spanning, alpha-helical portions of the six constituent connexins. The extracellular loops of two hemichannels mesh to form a high-density extracellular docking area consistent with a structural *tight seal* guaranteeing that the extracellular portion of the channel will not leak (Fig. 13.1*D*). The union of two hemichannels appears to be stabilized by hydrophobic interactions; covalent bonds are not involved. It has been shown that a 30 degree relative rotation between the two docking connexins is required to form a secure gap junction channel that is tight to the extracellular space (Perkins et al., 1998). The overall shape of a gap junction channel suggests an hourglass. The limiting diameter of the central pore is about 1.5 nm, with slight narrowing of the opening on the extracellular side of the membrane (Fig. 13.1*D*).

Connexins

Significant progress has been made in the isolation and characterization of the proteins, that is, connexins, that form gap junctions. More than 20 putative connexin proteins have been identified in mammalian tissues (Hua et al., 2003; Saez et al., 2003a) (Fig. 13.3*B*), with

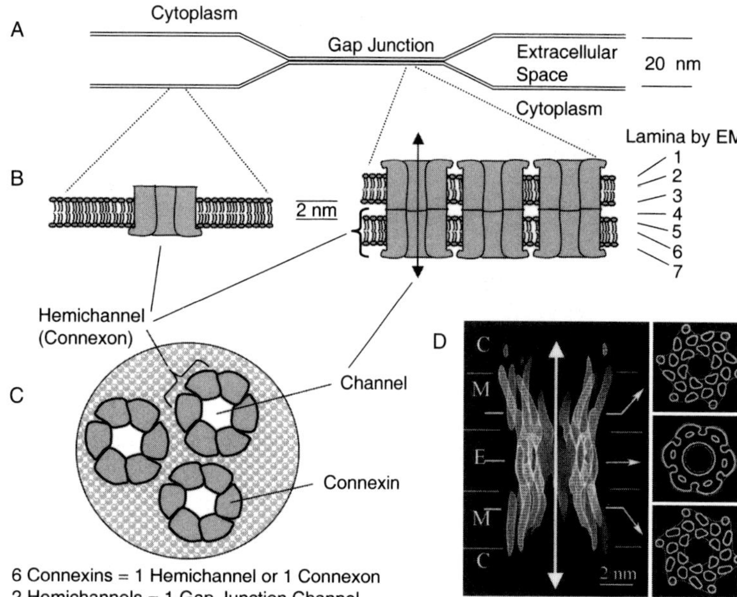

FIGURE 13.1 Gap junction and hemichannel structure. *A*. Schematic drawing of a gap junction as visualized by electron microscopy (*EM*). The junction appears to have five layers. *B*. Hemichannels are unopposed connexons. This is the only possible configuration when a connexon is inserted into the membrane outside the junction area. At higher magnification, the small slit of extracellular space remaining between cells at gap junctions causes them to have a seven-layered appearance. *C*. Gap junctions are composed of two hemichannels, or connexons, each formed from six connexin proteins. Two hemichannels dock with one another and bridge the extracellular space, forming a gap junction. *D*. Three-dimensional structure of a recombinant connexin-43 gap junction channel determined by electron crystallography. Longitudinal and cross-sectional views are shown. C: cytoplasm; E: extracellular space; M: membrane. (From Unger et al., 1999 with permission.)

the molecular mass of cloned connexins ranging from 25 to 62 kDa. The commonly used nomenclature for connexins is based on predicted molecular weight (e.g., Cx43 for a predicted mass of ~43 kDa, and so on). Connexins are derived from ancient proteins, and different connexins share significant sequence homology. Connexins are not found in invertebrates, although these animals have abundant gap junctions. Instead, invertebrates contain functionally analogous but sequence-unique proteins termed *innexins* (Phelan and Starich, 2001). Curiously, innexin-like proteins called *pannexins* have been detected in mammals and may mediate coupling between hippocampal pyramidal neurons and perhaps elsewhere (Bruzzone et al., 2003).

All cloned connexins have four transmembrane domains (M1–M4) and belong to a class of proteins that includes innexins, claudins, and occludins (Hua et al., 2003); claudins and occludins form tight junctions. The N terminal (NT) and C terminal (CT) segments of connexins are both intracellular, resulting in two extracellular loops (EL1 and EL2) and one cytoplasmic loop (CL) (Fig. 13.3*A*). The transmembrane domains are highly conserved, while the CT and CL vary in length and amino acid sequence between different connexins. The differences in connexin molecular weights are mainly reflected in the length of the CT. The functional gating of gap junctions is primarily mediated by the CL and CT, which have sites for phosphorylation and other protein-protein interactions. The extracellular loops mediate the end-to-end docking of paired connexons, and their confirmations are stabilized by conserved cysteine residues (Harris, 2001).

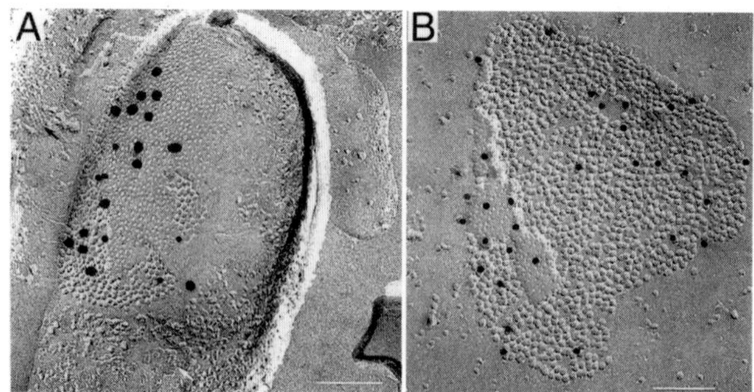

FIGURE 13.2 Freeze fracture–immunogold imaging of glial gap junctions. *A*. A freeze fracture view of a gap junction linking two astrocyte processes in the supraoptic nucleus. Gold-labeled connexin-483 (Cx43) antibodies (*large black dots*) and Cx30 antibodies (*smaller black dots*) stain the protein particles making up the junction. Note that Cx43 staining predominates. *B*. A freeze fracture view of an oligodendrocyte gap junction in the cerebellum. Gold-labeled Cx32 antibodies (*black dots*) stain the protein particles in this junction. (From Rash et al., 2001, with permission.)

All connexins are phosphoproteins, except for Cx26. Connexins are phosphorylated at a number of different sites by multiple mechanisms; this can affect connexin trafficking, assembly, membrane insertion, channel gating, and degradation (Saez et al., 2003a). While the importance of phosphorylation events for connexin function is understood, we are early in the process of understanding the biochemical and functional intricacies.

Most connexins have a half-life of several hours (Saez et al., 2003a). Creatively tagging old and newly synthesized Cx43 with different colors reveals that newly synthesized connexons are added to the periphery of established gap junctions; "old" gap junction plaques are endocytosed and destroyed (Gaietta et al., 2002). The fast turnover rate of connexins means that processes regulating their synthesis and/or degradation effectively modulate the level and function of gap junctions.

Structural studies indicate that hundreds of gap junc-

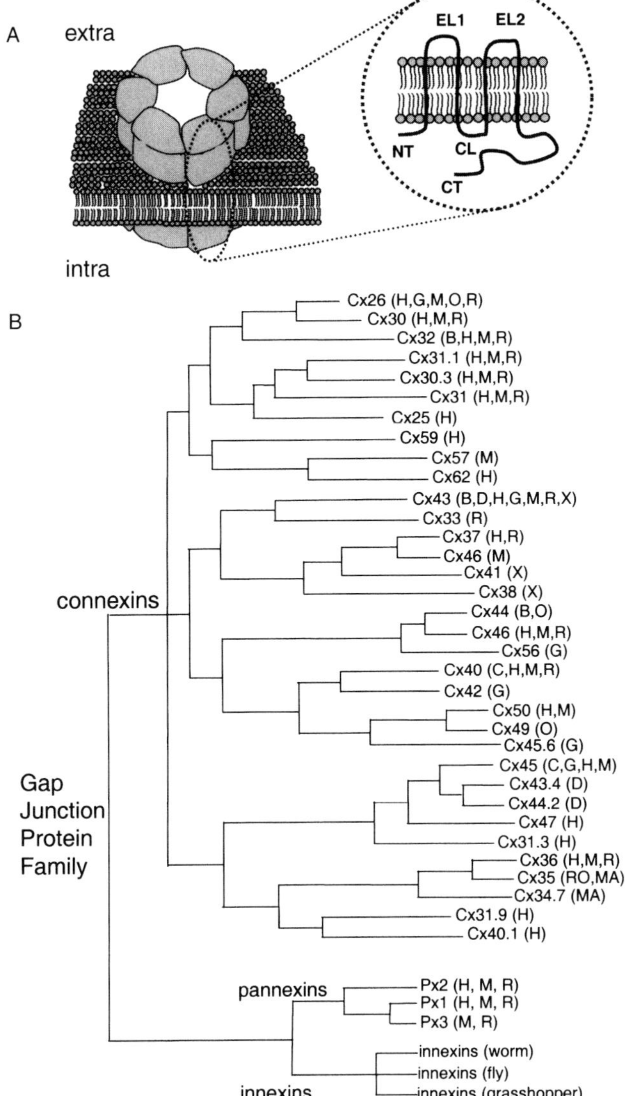

FIGURE 13.3 *A*. Schematic drawing of a hemichannel. Each component connexin has four-transmembrane-spanning domains with both the C-terminal (*CT*) and N-terminal (*NT*) ends within the cytoplasm. This creates a cytoplasmic loop (*CL*) and two extracellular loops (*EL*). *B*. Phylogenetic tree of gap junction proteins in vertebrate (connexins and pannexins) and invertebrate (innexins) animal cells (Bruzzone et al., 2003; Hua et al., 2003). B: *Bos taurus* (cow); C: *Canis familiaris* (dog); D: *Danio rerio* (zebrafish); G: *Gallus gallus* (chicken); H: *Homo sapiens* (human); MA: *Morone americana* (white perch); M: *Mus musculus* (mouse); O: *Ovis aries* (sheep); R: *Rattus norvegicus* (rat); RO: *Raja ocellata* (skate); X: *Xenopus laevis* (frog).

tion channels may aggregate at a gap junction plaque (Fig. 13.2). The size of gap junction plaques varies, but studies show that a plaque needs to reach a certain size (a minimum of a few hundred channels) to form electrically permeable channels (Bukauskas et al., 2000). It is possible that the aggregation of gap junctions generates forces that stabilize the docking of hemichannels. On the other hand, this suggests that only a small percentage of gap junctions, that is, those with hundreds of channels, are functionally open and raises the question of other roles for nonconducting gap junctions, perhaps cell adhesion or cell survival (Lin et al., 2003). Conversely, adhesion molecules like cadherins, which bring adjacent membranes into close apposition, may facilitate the formation of gap junctions (Fujimoto et al., 1997).

It is well established that nonsimilar cells, that is, from different organs or different species, may form gap junctions with one another (Harris, 2001) (see Fig. 13.4). Moreover, most cells express more than one type of connexin (Table 13.1). These observations suggest, and subsequent experiments have proven, that hemichannels of different protein composition may form functional gap junction channels with one another. The six connexins forming a hemichannel can be identical, forming a homomeric hemichannel, or can consist of more than one isoform of connexin, forming a heteromeric hemichannel (Fig. 13.4*A*). A gap junction formed from identified homomeric hemichannels is called homotypic. A gap junction formed of two different homomeric hemichemicals is called heterotypic. The best-characterized heterotypic gap junctions are

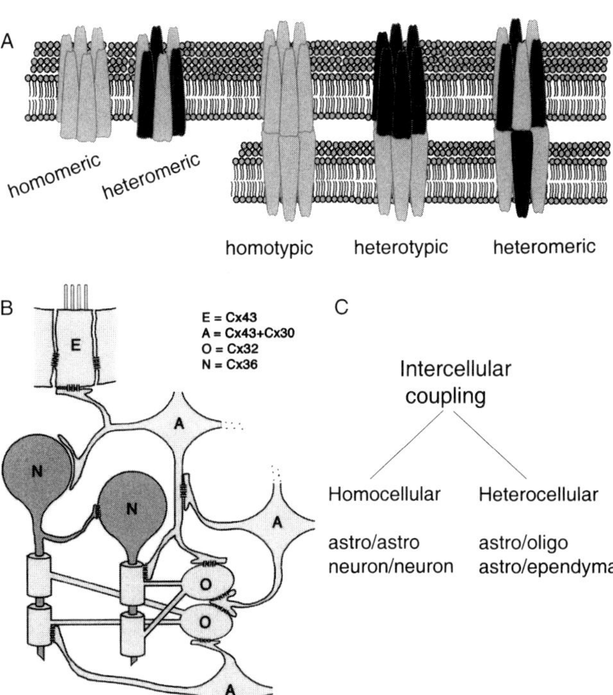

FIGURE 13.4 *A*. Cartoon illustrating the nomenclature for hemichannel and gap junction composition. Hemichannel subunits of different shading represent different connexin (Cx) proteins. (Modified from Phelan and Starich, 2001.) *B*. Summary diagram of the central nervous system cell types that form gap junctions *in vivo*. Astrocyte-astrocyte and astrocyte–oligodendrocyte gap junctions are most common. A: astrocyte; O: oligodendrocyte; N: neuron; E: ependymal cell. (From Rash et al., 2001, with permission.) *C*. Diagram showing types of intercellular coupling.

TABLE 13.1 *Gap Junction Coupling in Mammalian Glial Cells*

Glial Cell Pair	*Relative Coupling Strength*	*Connexin Pairing*
Astrocytes	++++ (Dermietzel et al., 1991; Sontheimer et al., 1991)	Cx43–Cx43, CX43–Cx30, Cx30–Cx30, Cx30–Cx26, Cx26–Cx26 (Dermietzel et al., 1991; Harris, 2001)
Astrocyte-Oligodendrocyte	+ (Ransom and Kettenmann, 1990)	Cx43–Cx47, Cx30–Cx32, CX26–Cx32 (Nagy et al., 2003)
Oligodendrocytes	++ (Von Blankenfeld et al., 1993; Kettenmann and Ransom, 1988; Butt and Ransom, 1989)	Cx32–Cx32, (Bergoffen et al., 1993), Cx29–Cx29 (Altevogt et al., 2002)
Schwann cells	++ (Konishi, 1990)	Cx32–Cx32, (Altevogt et al., 2002)
Microglia	+ (upregulated by cytokines)	Cx43–Cx43 (Eugenin et al., 2001)
Müller cells	++ (Ceelen et al., 2001)	Cx43–Cx43, Cx43–Cx45, Cx45–Cx45 (Dermietzel et al., 2000b; Zahs et al., 2003)
Müller cell–astrocyte	++ (Ceelen et al., 2001)	Cx43–Cx43, Cx43–Cx45, Cx45–Cx45 (Dermietzel et al., 2000b; Zahs et al., 2003)
Ependymal cells	+++ (Connors and Ransom, 1987)	Cx43–Cx43 (Ochalski et al., 1997)
Astrocyte-neuron	+ (Alvarez-Maubecin et al., 2000)	Cx43–Cx43 (Froes et al., 1999; but see Rash et al., 2001)

those formed between astrocytes and oligodendrocytes. Astrocytes express Cx43, Cx30, and Cx26, whereas oligodendrocytes express Cx29, Cx32, and Cx47 (Nagy et al., 2003). This lack of overlap between the types of connexins in astrocytes and oligodendrocytes determines that the junctions between them can only be heterotypic. There appears to be some selectivity in the formation of heterotypic gap junctions. For example, Cx32 hemichannels form junctions with Cx30 and Cx26 hemichannels but not with Cx43 hemichannels (Elfgang et al., 1995) (Fig. 13.4*B*). Coupling between different hemichannels is primarily determined by the compatibility of connexin extracellular loops (Harris, 2001). These preferences in hemichannel pairing can be useful in surmising the connexin composition of junctions between different cell types, for example, astrocyte-oligodendrocyte junctions. Details about the biophysical function of these heterologous channels are still forthcoming, but such channels may have unique permeability characteristics (Robinson et al., 1993; Harris, 2001)(see below).

Biophysical Properties of Gap Junctions

The minimal diameter of the gap junction channel in vertebrates is about 1.5 nm (Unger et al., 1999). These pores are permeable to molecules up to a molecular mass of about 1 kDa, largely independent of charge (Loewenstein, 1981). As a consequence, coupled cells are able to exchange a wide range of biologically important molecules including cyclic nucleotides, small molecules of intermediate metabolism, vitamins, and inorganic ions. This does not necessarily imply that coupled cells will have identical concentrations of all permeable molecules; the concentration of a given permeable molecule in each cell depends on the transmembrane fluxes, and on production and removal of the molecule in question, in addition to the gap junction permeability of that molecule. Obviously, the tendency for coupled cells to have the same concentration of a cytoplasmic constituent will increase with the strength of coupling (Rose and Ransom, 1997).

Electrophysiological analysis of single gap junction channels indicates that they abruptly open and close in a manner similar to that of other ion channels (Bennett et al., 1991; Harris, 2001). Some gap junction channels have subconductance states (Harris, 2001). As channels with a huge pore diameter and apparent lack of a selection gate, gap junctions have commonly been regarded as the least selective channel. Each of the different connexin isoforms, however, "produces channels with distinct unitary conductance, molecular permeability, and electrical and chemical gating sensitivities" (Harris, 2001). For example, the unitary conductance of connexin channels varies from 15 to over 300 pS, and charge selectivity varies from slightly anion-selective to highly cation-selective. The rank order of unitary conductance, from highest to lowest, according to connexin composition of homomeric channels, is Cx37 > Cx40 = Cx46 > Cx43 = Cx26 > Cx32 > Cx45.

Channels formed by different connexins have different limiting pore diameters, determined by fluorescent probes varying in size. They also differ in their permeability to cytoplasmic molecules, but not in a manner consistently predicted by pore size. Cx43 channels are much more permeable to adenosine triphosphate (ATP) and adenosine diphosphate (ADP), and to glutamate and glutathione than Cx32 channels, even though they are equally permeable to calcein. In addition, Cx43 channels are more permeable to ATP and ADP than to the smaller molecules glutamate and glutathione (Harris, 2001). This suggests that the pore may interact "chemically" with cytoplasmic molecules in a manner that selectively affects permeability. Even for structurally related compounds, such as adenosine, adenosine monophosphate (AMP), and ATP, channels composed of Cx32 and Cx43 show marked differences in permeability: Adenosine is 12-fold more permeable through Cx32 versus Cx43 channels. Conversely, AMP and ATP are 8-fold and 300-fold, respectively, more permeable through Cx43 versus Cx32 channels (Goldberg et al., 2002). Indeed, recent experiments indicate that astrocyte hemichannels (i.e., Cx43) may mediate ATP release (Cotrina et al., 1998; Stout et al., 2002).

The permeability of gap junction channels is influenced by physiological variables, including transjunctional voltage (V_j), and by the intracellular concentrations of H^+ and Ca^{2+}. Macroscopic junctional conductance is maximal when V_j is zero; typically, junctional conductance decreases with hyperpolarization or depolarization of either cell, but the degree of voltage sensitivity varies among different connexins (Harris, 2001).

Increases in intracellular concentrations of either H^+ or Ca^{2+} rapidly decrease junctional conductance and permeability to large molecules (Bennett et al., 1991; Harris, 2001). Coupling conductance is sensitive to changes in intracellular pH that are within the physiological range of this variable (i.e., 6.5 ± 0.5 pH). Gating by pH depends on the CT. Truncation of the CT eliminates pH sensitivity. It is believed that pH changes induce the CT to interact with a portion of the CL to close the channel in a fashion analogous to a "ball and chain." The increases in intracellular Ca^{2+} that result in decreased junctional conductance are high (e.g., ≥ 10 μM), and this variable is not likely to affect coupling under normal physiological conditions; cell injury causes large increases in intracellular [Ca^{2+}] that could lead to uncoupling. A site sensitive to near-millimolar calcium is located on the extracellular portion of the pore (Gomez-Hernandez et al., 2003). This explains how hemichannels are held in the closed position by high extracellular calcium.

Lipophilic agents such as the higher-order alcohols heptanol and octanol, and the anesthetic halothane, block gap junction channels, but the mechanism of blockade by these agents is not clearly understood (Rozental et al., 2001). The sensitivity of junctional conductance to octanol varies considerably among astrocytes from different brain regions (Lee et al., 1994), even though they would be expected to express the same connexin proteins.

Second messengers have complex effects on gap junctional conductance (Bennett et al., 1991; Harris, 2001). In some systems, cyclic monophosphates show high-affinity, selective binding to connexins resulting in channel inhibition (Harris, 2001). In other systems, an increase of cyclic AMP (cAMP) increases junctional conductance over a period of hours; this effect can be prevented by blocking mRNA or protein synthesis, suggesting that channels are being newly synthesized. These second messenger effects, which may be initiated by a wide range of agents including hormones and neurotransmitters, imply an important degree of plasticity in the control of physiological events mediated by gap junction communication. Several excellent reviews may be consulted for more detailed general information about the molecular biology and biophysics of gap junctions (Bennett et al., 1991; Goodenough et al., 1996; Harris, 2001).

Properties of Hemichannels

Hemichannels have not traditionally been thought of as stand-alone ion channels. The presumption was that these channels existed only transiently in membranes before being incorporated into gap junctions. Moreover, to the extent that unpaired hemichannels existed, they would always be in the closed state because of high extracellular [Ca^{2+}] ([$Ca^{2+}]_o$). Recently, however, the concept of hemichannels as unopposed functional channels has gained ground. Because unopposed hemichannels connect cell cytoplasm to the extracellular space, the roles of hemichannels and traditional gap junctions are fundamentally different.

Unlike gap junctions, hemichannels are directly exposed to extracellular ions and thus can be effectively gated by extracellular, as well as intracellular, ionic changes. A wide range of factors influence hemichannel gating (Contreras et al., 2002; Saez et al., 2003b; Ye et al., 2003) (Fig. 13.5*A*). For example, divalent-cation free solution opens these channels in astrocytes (Ye et al., 2003). Open hemichannels are detected by uptake of appropriate marker dyes like Lucifer Yellow CH (LY) and by the release of molecules like glutamate, and both events are blocked by gap junction blockers (Fig. 13.5*B*). Hemichannels have been primarily studied in cultured cells, but functional hemichannels can also be demonstrated *in situ*. Acutely isolated rat optic nerve exposed to divalent-cation free solution releases glutamate, probably from astrocytes, and this is blocked by the gap junction blocker carbenoxolone (Fig. 13.5*C*).

Hemichannels can open under pathological conditions and may release glutamate that could contribute to excitotoxic injury (Contreras et al., 2002). It also seems likely that a small fraction of these channels may be open under normal physiological conditions or may be gated open in a controlled manner during normal activity. If this is true, the implications for CNS physiology, ranging from synaptic transmission to development, are obvious but remain largely unexplored.

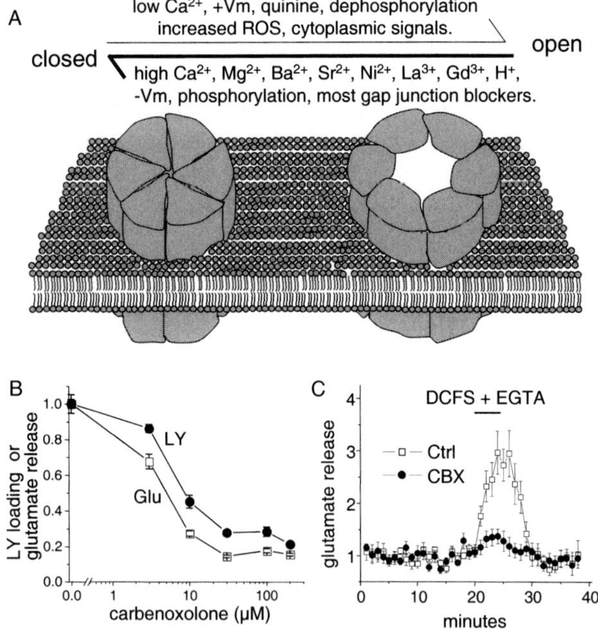

FIGURE 13.5 *A*. Cartoon showing some of the factors that influence gating of hemichannels. ROS: reactive oxygen species. (Modified from Saez et al., 2003b.) *B*. Astrocytes show LY loading and glutamate (Glu) release in divalent cation free solution (DCFS) that is blocked in a concentration-dependent manner by carbenoxolone (Ye and Ransom, unpublished data). *C*. Glutamate is released from freshly isolated adult mouse optic nerve in divalent cation free solution [*DCFS* plus ethylene glycol tetraacetic acid (*EGTA*)]. Consistent with release from hemichannels, release is blocked by carbenoxolone (*CBX*), a gap junction blocker. (Modified from Ye et al., 2003.)

GAP JUNCTIONS IN GLIAL CELLS

Connexins are variably expressed by virtually all mammalian glial cells. Microglial cells were the sole exception to this statement, but recent studies reveal that they too can express Cx43 and form gap junctions (Eugenin et al., 2001). The functions of connexins, and the channels that they form (both gap junctions and hemichannels), are still debated and undoubtedly vary by cell type.

Several methods have been used to study glial gap junctions or hemichannels: (*1*) ultrastructural visualization of gap junctions using electron microsopy (EM) or freeze fracture techniques; (*2*) injection or uptake of small fluorescent dyes, like LY (molecular weight of 443 Da), that permeate gap junctions or hemichannels but not classic ion channels; (*3*) electrophysiological techniques, including dual pipette recordings to measure gap junction currents and whole cell patch clamp recording to characterize hemichannels; (*4*) gap-FRAP (gap junction–mediated fluorescent recovery after photo-bleaching); laser light bleaches and destroys fluorescent dye molecules in an individual cell, and the strength of gap junction coupling to adjacent cells is judged by the speed with which dye diffuses back into this cell from nearby cells; (*5*) immunohistochemistry for connexins in combination with freeze fracturing (Fig. 13.2); this technique is essential for characterizing the *in vivo* connexin composition of gap junctions in specific cells; and (*6*) genetic modulations, including knockouts and knockins of specific connexin isoforms (Scemes et al., 1998).

Distribution and Anatomy

Gap junction coupling and connexin expression in mammalian glial cells is summarized in Table 13.1. The EM and freeze fracture features of glial gap junctions are similar to those described in other cells (Fig. 13.2). Astrocytes are the most robustly coupled glial cells. Astrocytes of various types (e.g., protoplasmic, fibrous, Bergmann glia) form homotypic gap junctions with other astrocytes and heterotypic (and heterocellular) junctions with oligodendrocytes and ependymal cells. Astrocytes, as well as other glial cells, express several different connexins that may be regulated during development (Kunzelmann et al., 1999) and affected by injury (Saez et al., 2003a). There are intriguing reports indicating that astrocytes form gap junctions with neurons (Froes et al., 1999; Alvarez-Maubecin et al., 2000). However, these junctions may be limited to immature cells and occur only during development (Rash et al., 2001).

Nonmammalian glial cells

Direct electrical communication between nonmammalian glial cells was first established in the leech CNS and the mud-puppy optic nerve (Kuffler and Potter, 1964). In fish, gap junctions are seen between the somata of oligodendrocytes and between the processes of astrocytes, and fish astrocytes are dye-coupled *in vitro* (for review see, Ransom, 1995).

Astrocytes

Mammalian astrocytes *in situ* typically show widespread dye coupling with each other. When LY is injected into individual cortical astrocytes, as many as 100 adjacent cells are stained (Gutnick et al., 1981). White matter astrocytes are also highly dye-coupled *in situ* (Butt and Ransom, 1989). Type 2 astrocytes from the rat optic nerve are devoid of coupling (Sontheimer et al., 1990) and do not express connexins. The existence of a unique astrocyte in the mammalian CNS similar to the type 2 astrocyte defined *in vitro,* however, remains controversial.

Astrocytes grown *in vitro* are not always dye-coupled. A maximum of ~50% of hippocampal astrocytes and ~80% of optic nerve astrocytes (Sontheimer et al., 1990) are coupled. Rat cortical astrocytes in confluent monolayer cultures are strongly coupled electrically (Kettenmann and Ransom, 1988). All astrocytes within 300 μm of one another are coupled and the average coupling ratio (i.e., voltage change in the current-injected cell divided by the voltage change in a nearby cell) of astrocytes within 100 μm of each other is 0.44.

Astrocytes express Cx43, Cx30, and Cx26; they may also express small amounts of Cx40, Cx45, and Cx46 (Dermietzel et al., 2000a). The predominant connexin is Cx43, but its expression varies by brain region. Hypothalamic astrocytes *in vitro* express four times more Cx43 than striatal astrocytes and are more highly coupled (Batter et al., 1992). Connexin-43 is least expressed in spinal white matter (Nagy et al., 1992). There are also regional differences in the way astrocyte gap junctions respond to molecular modulations (Reuss et al., 2000), including their sensitivity to gap junction blockers (Lee et al., 1994).

Connexin-43 is distributed in a plaque-like manner between astrocytes and is also located elsewhere in these cells compatible with cytoplasmic pools or hemichannels. Connexin-43 appears postnatally, while Cx30 develops several weeks after birth and remains less abundant than Cx43 (Kunzelmann et al., 1999). Patch-clamp recordings of coupled astrocyte pairs reveal a unitary conductance of single channels of 50–60 pS. In general, astrocyte gap junctions behave similarly to Cx43 gap junctions studied in other tissues (Spray et al., 1999).

Norepinephrine and arachidonic acid, apparently acting through phospholipase C (PLC), reduce gap junction communication between striatal astrocytes (Giaume et al., 1991). Gap junctions can also be regulated by other stimuli that act by modulating protein kinase C (PKC) or mitogen-activated protein kinase (MAPK) (for review see (Saez et al., 2003a). Astrocyte dye-coupling can be increased by application of glutamate or high [K^+] solutions (Enkvist and McCarthy, 1994) or hyposmotic shock (Scemes and Spray, 1998). The K^+-induced upregulation of gap junction communication may involve the calmodulin kinase pathway (De Pina-Benabou et al., 2001). Glutamate effects on gap junction may contribute to neuronal activity-dependent control of Cx43 expression in astrocytes (Rouach et al., 2000). In contrast to the effect of neuronal activity, brain macrophages can reduce Cx43 expression in astrocytes (Rouach et al., 2002; Faustmann et al., 2003). Other naturally occurring molecules, including endothelins and inflammatory cytokines (Duffy et al., 2000), have also been shown to downregulate astrocytic gap junction expression and function.

Brief applications of high [K^+] solutions did not increase coupling between oligodendrocytes and astrocytes (Ransom and Kettenmann, 1990). Glutamate or high [K^+] solution causes membrane depolarization, and this might be linked to changes in coupling via changes in intracellular pH. Depolarization produces an alkaline shift in astrocytes that could enhance coupling (Ransom, 1992). The effects of pH on coupling can be persistent; intracellular acidification mediated by lactate results in irreversible uncoupling if the acidification persists for 30 minutes (Anders, 1988).

Oligodendrocytes

Few, if any, gap junctions are found between oligodendroctes in white matter of the cat, although gap junctions are abundant between oligodendrocytes and astrocytes. Based on ultrastructural data, it is proposed that communication between oligodendrocytes is mediated by connections through the astrocytic syncytium (Rash et al., 2001) (Fig. 13.4*B*). However, gap junctions have been seen between purified rat oligodendrocytes, and physiological coupling can be demonstrated directly between oligodendrocytes *in vitro* (Ransom and Kettenmann, 1990; Von Blankenfeld et al., 1993) and *in situ* (Butt and Ransom, 1993; Robinson et al., 1993).

Myelinating oligodendrocytes *in situ* typically (i.e., 75% fills) show dye-coupling to other oligodendrocytes (Butt and Ransom, 1993). The number of dye-coupled cells is small, usually between two and four, and coupling appears to occur at contacts between adjacent cell bodies (Butt and Ransom, 1993). Oligodendrocytes in the rabbit retina also show dye-coupling (Robinson et al., 1993), but immature oligodendrocytes in mouse corpus callosum are not dye-coupled (Berger et al., 1991). About 20% of oligodendrocytes in spinal cord gray matter are coupled, but coupling between these cells is never seen in spinal cord white matter (Pastor et al., 1998). The significance of these regional differences is not known.

Mouse spinal cord oligodendrocyte studied *in vitro* show electrical coupling in about 75% of cell pairs tested (Kettenmann and Ransom, 1988). The coupling between oligodendrocytes is less intense than between astrocytes; coupled oligodendrocytes within 100 μm of each other have an average coupling ratio of 0.11. As with astrocytes, the application of either Cs^+ or Ba^{2+} enhances electrical coupling (Kettenmann and Ransom, 1988). Oligodendrocytes therefore appear to be widely coupled by junctions that allow only weak electrical interaction, in accordance with the ultrastructural observation that interoligodendrocytic gap junctions are much less frequent than gap junctions between astrocytes (Rash et al., 2001).

Gap junctions are common between astrocytes and oligodendrocytes, and coupling between astrocytes and oligodendrocytes has been demonstrated *in vitro* (Ransom and Kettenmann, 1990) and *in situ* (Robinson et al., 1993). In comparison to the strength of coupling between astrocytes and between oligodendrocytes, electrical coupling between cultured spinal cord astrocytes and oligodendrocytes is weak (Ransom and Kettenmann, 1990). The average coupling ratio for cells within 100 μm of one another is 0.04. Under optimal conditions for the detection of coupling (i.e., in the presence of Ba^{2+} or Cs^+, which increases the coupling ratio 3- to 5-fold), coupling is seen in about 80% of the contiguous cell pairs tested (Ransom and Kettenmann, 1990). In rabbit retina, dye is able to flow more freely from astrocytes into oligodendrocytes than from oligodendrocytes into astrocytes (Robinson et al., 1993; see also Zahs, 1998). This interesting observation of unidirectional coupling, or *chemical rectification*, may be the consequence of a gap junction composed of two hemichannels, each composed of a different connexin. Astrocytes express Cx26, Cx30, and Cx43, and the oligodendrocytes express Cx29, Cx32, Cx45, or Cx47 (Nagy et al., 2003) (see Table 13.1). Interestingly, the most abundant connexins in these two cell types, Cx43 and Cx32, do not readily pair with each other (Elfgang et al., 1995). The most frequent coupling between astrocytes and oligodendrocytes is likely formed by Cx43 or Cx30 in astrocytes with Cx47 in oligodendrocytes (Nagy et al., 2003). Unlike Cx43 or Cx32, Cx45 displays very strong voltage dependency, very low permeability to anions, and very small single-channel conductance (~30 pS). Because it is preferentially anion permeable, Cx45 may aid in transferring K^+ from oligodendrocytes to astrocytes (see below). It is not yet clear if unidirectional coupling is a general feature of astrocyte-oligodendrocyte junctions, but to the extent that it is, it suggests the possibility of a hierarchical arrangement for the flow of some metabolic signals (Robinson et al., 1993).

Schwann cells

Proliferating Schwann cells, during early development or after peripheral nerve crush injury, primarily express Cx46 and are coupled to one another. Cytokines may be involved in the injury-related switch from Cx32 to Cx46 (Chandross, 1998). Nonmyelinating Schwann cells *in vitro* exhibit dye-coupling that disappears when they begin to make myelin (Konishi, 1990). Myelinating Schwann cells stop expressing Cx46 but increase expression of Cx32, which is confined to paranodal regions and Schmidt-Lanterman incisures. At these sites, so-called "reflexive" gap junctions connect the paranodal folds, perhaps facilitating ion and small molecule movements to and from the tight periaxonal space (Balice-Gordon et al., 1998). The X-linked form of the hereditary neuropathy known as *Charcot-Marie-Tooth disease* is associated with mutations in the Cx32 gene (Bergoffen et al., 1993). In this condition, Cx32 is also depressed in the CNS but oligodendrocytes appear normal and have been found to express another connexin, Cx29 (Altevogt et al., 2002). These observations indicate that connexins expressed in Schwann cells play a critical role in peripheral nerve integrity and function.

Other glial cells

Ependymal cells, specialized glia that line the ventricles, have gap junctions and exhibit physiological properties similar to those of astrocytes (Connors and Ransom, 1987). Turtle ependymal cells are extensively coupled to one another and are uncoupled by exposure to elevated CO_2 (Connors and Ransom, 1987). Gap junctions in ependyma are constructed of Cx26 and Cx43. Ependymal cells also form gap junctions with astrocytes (Rash et al., 2001).

Nonmammalian Müller cells exhibit gap junction communication. Müller cells in the salamander retina show strong coupling to one another, with coupling ratios as high as 0.2 at distances of 200 μm. Theoretical calculations indicate that electrical coupling in this system may contribute significantly to lateral movement of accumulated K^+ within the retina (Mobbs et al., 1988). Mammalian Müller cells are not coupled to each other but seem to be coupled to nearby astrocytes. The coupling is unidirectional; dye passes readily from astrocytes to Müller cells but not from Müller cells to astrocytes (Zahs and Newman, 1997).

Bergmann glial cells of the cerebellum are coupled to each other *in situ*. Activation of AMPA receptors on Bergmann glia reduced coupling in a Ca^{2+}-dependent manner, suggesting that Ca^{2+} entry mediated the gap junction closure (Müller et al., 1996).

Glial cells of the intermediate lobe of the pituitary, called *stellate glia*, are strongly coupled to one another (Mudrick-Donnon et al., 1993). These unique cells receive synapse-like contacts from neurons and exhibit stimulus-evoked, synaptic-like potentials mediated by the inhibitory transmitter gamma-aminobutyric acid (GABA).

Microglia in their resting state do not express connexins. Activated microglia, however, express Cx43 and show dye-coupling *in vitro* (Eugenin et al., 2001). Interestingly, activated microglia can downregulate Cx43 expression and functional coupling in nearby astrocytes (Faustmann et al., 2003), suggesting that astrocyte communication may be reduced at sites of brain injury where microglia would assume their activated phenotype.

Functions of Gap Junctions and Hemichannels

Several functions have been proposed for gap junctions based on their physiological properties (Loewenstein, 1981; Bennett et al., 1991; Harris, 2001; Saez et al., 2003a). They may coordinate the electrical and metabolic activities of cell populations, amplify the consequences of signal transduction, control intrinsic proliferative capacity, and help to orchestrate the complex events of embryonic morphogenesis. In some tissues, like the heart, the practical significance of intercellular coupling is clear (i.e., coordination of contraction). The role of gap junctions in glial cells is not as well understood, but plausible hypotheses may be formulated that are variations on the general themes listed above. In addition, recent discoveries indicate that connexins can have functions apart from forming gap junctions; they can form functional hemichannels (Contreras et al., 2002; Saez et al., 2003b; Ye et al., 2003), and connexin expression appears to influence cell survival (Lin et al., 2003). Further insights into connexin functions should derive from analysis of diseases associated with connexin mutations (this large topic is beyond the scope of our review; e.g., see Saez et al., 2003a) and from studies on specific connexin knockouts.

The pattern and strength of coupling among different types of glial cells should be kept in mind as possible functions of these cells are discussed. Available evidence indicates that astrocytes are strongly coupled to one another, while coupling between oligodendrocytes is weak and heterologous coupling between astrocytes and oligodendrocytes is weaker still (see however Rash et al., 2001). Astrocytes, therefore, are likely to participate more vigorously than oligodendrocytes in functions related to intercellular coupling. The heterotypic coupling between astrocytes and oligodendrocytes creates, in essence, a *panglial syncytium* (Rash et al., 2001).

$[K^+]_o$ homeostasis and extracellular potential generation

The spatial buffer hypothesis states that glial cells participate in moving extracellular K^+ from areas where it accumulates secondary to neural activity to distant areas where the K^+ is not elevated (Orkand et al., 1966). Strong astrocytic coupling would extend the distance over which this K^+ distribution system could operate and, perhaps, increase its efficiency (Mobbs et al., 1988). Glial cells also minimize the extent of K^+ accumulation occurring with neural activity by uptake and sequestration of K^+ (Rose and Ransom, 1996). Glial coupling might benefit this process by creating a functionally larger intracellular volume that would tend to minimize changes in intracellular K^+ concentration that could occur with K^+ uptake.

The significance of coupling between astrocytes and oligodendrocytes remains obscure. Astrocytic processes that project to nodes of Ranvier are frequently connected by gap junctions to the terminal paranodal loops of nearby myelinating oligodendrocytes (Black and Waxman, 1988). This specialized arrangement could mediate an axon-specific type of K^+ spatial buffering.

It is well established that glial cells participate in the production of extracellular field potentials seen with neural activity (Somjen, 1970). This has been most elegantly studied in the mud puppy optic nerve, where the consequences of direct glial depolarization on surface potential can be quantitatively analyzed (Cohen, 1970). It is apparent from this work that interglial coupling is critical for determining the distribution of extracellular field potentials (Cohen, 1970).

Intracellular metabolic homeostasis

Glial gap junctions may be important for metabolic coordination within the coupled aggregate. In the case of cells that are strongly coupled, this tends to ensure uniform cellular concentrations of junction-permeant molecules. For example, coupled astrocytes tend to have similar intracellular $[Na^+]$ ($[Na^+]_i$), but $[Na^+]_i$s diverge when coupling is blocked (Rose and Ransom, 1997) (Fig. 13.6). Gap junctions, therefore, can cause a group of individual cells to function almost as one in terms of metabolism and membrane potential (Fig. 13.7*A*).

The capacity for small molecules to diffuse freely between coupled cells offers a theoretical advantage for the operation of the high-affinity glutamate uptake system in glia. The rate of glutamate uptake will be affected by the transmembrane gradients of glutamate and the ions that are cotransported or countertransported. Strong glial coupling, by providing a larger effective intracellular volume, would minimize changes in the intracellular concentrations of the transmitter

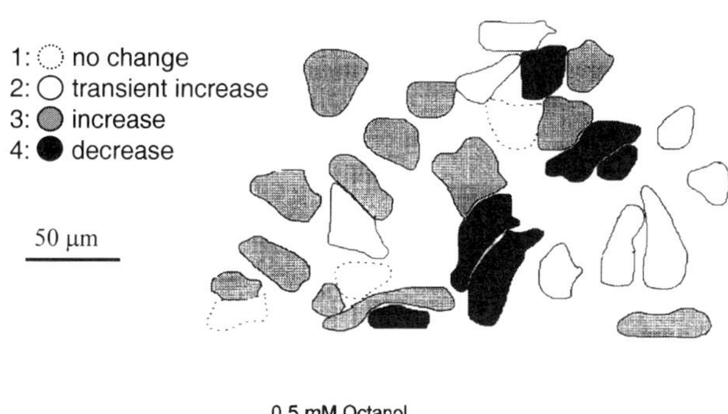

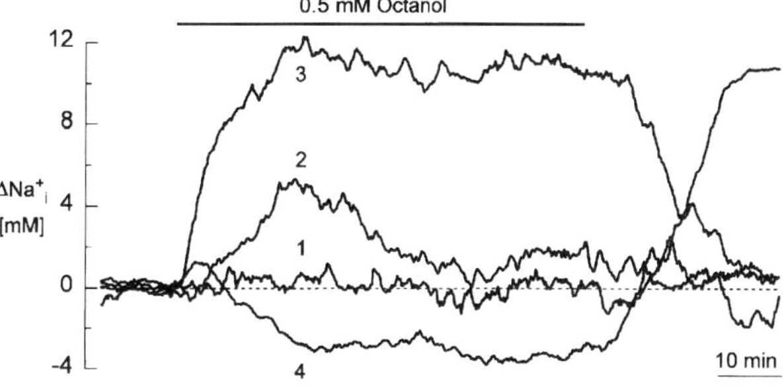

FIGURE 13.6 Gap junctions equalize intracellular ion concentrations in coupled astrocytes. The $[Na^+]_i$ is similar and stable in coupled astrocytes, but $[Na^+]_i$s diverge when gap junctions are blocked with octanol (*lower panel*). The changes in $[Na^+]_i$ that occur in a group of cultured astrocytes during application of octanol are shown in the top panel. (From Rose and Ransom, 1997, with permission.)

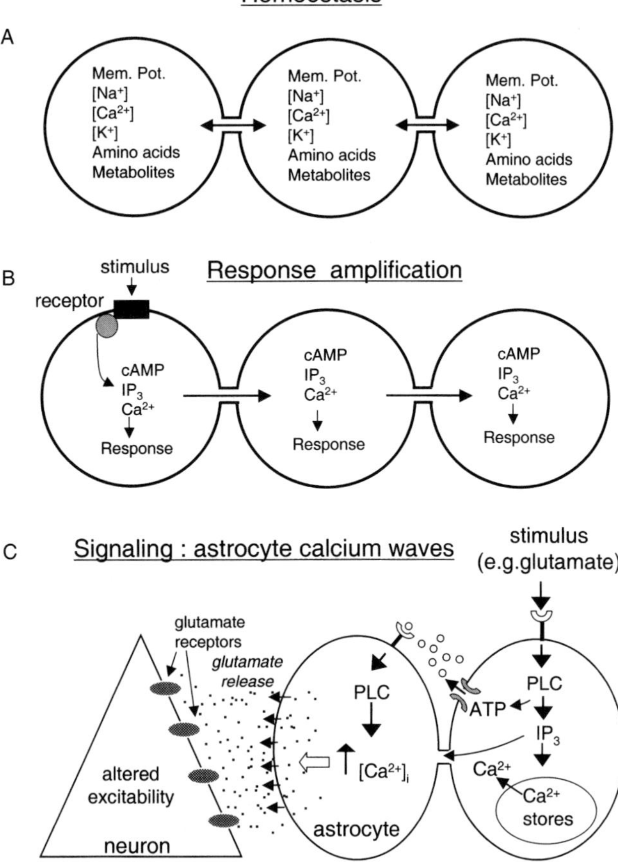

FIGURE 13.7 Schematic illustration of possible functions of gap junctions and hemichannels. *A*. In strongly coupled cell aggregates, the intracellular concentrations of ions and molecules less than ~1 kDa in size (including amino acids, sugars, and second messenger molecules) tend to be similar due to free exchange across gap junctions. *B*. Coupling can amplify the physiological consequences of a chemical stimulus (i.e., hormone, neurotransmitter) acting upon a single cell. Such stimuli often cause the production of second messenger molecules [i.e., Ca^{2+}, inositol 1,4,5-triphosphate (*IP3*), cyclic adenosine monophosphate (cAMP)] that can move easily into adjacent cells via gap junctions; the coupled cells are then recruited to respond. *C*. Gap junctions and hemichannels participate in astrocyte Ca^{2+} waves. Astrocytes can be provoked to exhibit Ca^{2+} waves in many ways, such as the application of glutamate. Effective stimuli activate phospholipase C (*PLC*) and IP3-dependent pathways that cause Ca^{2+} release from Ca^{2+} stores. Ca^{2+} and IP3 can diffuse to adjacent cells through gap junctions. Astrocytes also release adenosine triphosphate (*ATP*) upon activation, probably through hemichannels. In turn, ATP activates purinergic receptors on nearby astrocytes, and this is the predominant mode by which Ca^{2+} waves spread (but see Hofer et al., 2002). Increase in astrocyte $[Ca^{2+}]_i$ causes glutamate release, which modulates the excitability of neighboring neurons.

and associated ions from occurring with uptake, maximizing the efficiency of this process.

Signal transfer

Another functional consequence of intercellular coupling is divergence of signal transmission (Fig. 13.7*B*). Consider the case of a cell stimulated to produce an intracellular second messenger molecule [e.g., cAMP, inositol 1,4,5-triphosphate (IP_3), Ca^{2+}] by binding a specific ligand. If the cell is not connected to its neighbors by gap junctions, it will act in isolation. But if the cell is widely coupled to other cells, the diffusible, junction-permeable second messenger has the potential to affect many cells (Loewenstein, 1981).

Traveling waves of increased cytoplasmic $[Ca^{2+}]$ are elicited in astrocytes by a variety of stimuli including glutamate application (Finkbeiner, 1992; Cotrina et al., 1998). As the wave passes through astrocytes, it can elicit glutamate release and alter the behavior of adjacent neurons; in essence, this event is a slow form of signaling (Haydon, 2001). Ca^{2+} wave propagation is dependent on both gap junctions and extracellular signaling pathways, including hemichannel-mediated ATP release (Cotrina et al., 1998; Giaume and Venance, 1998; Guthrie et al., 1999); the relative contribution of these two mechanisms may vary in different brain regions (Hofer et al., 2002) (Fig. 13.7C). Gap junction blockers also block spreading depression, suggesting the involvement of gap junctions (Martins-Ferreira et al., 2000). An important caveat should be mentioned, however. Because astrocytes express functional hemichannels that can mediate glutamate release (see below), this raises the possibility that gap junction blockers might be acting on hemichannels, not gap junctions, changing the interpretation of these results.

Proliferative activity and development

The role of gap junctional communication during development has been discussed at length (Levin, 2002). Embryos exhibit widespread gap junctional communication, which may be important in establishing developmental fields critical for morphogenesis. For example, developing cortical neurons are transiently coupled together in columnar groups, and this may influence organization of the cortex (Lo Turco and Kriegstein, 1991). Coupling in glia, however, develops as these cells mature, precluding a role during development. One can speculate that glial coupling might help determine, and perhaps maintain, the final cellular phenotype.

Considerable evidence indicates that gap junctions can restrict cell proliferation. Neoplastic transformation is accompanied by loss of gap junctions, and most malignant cells are not coupled (Trosko et al., 1990). Most primary brain tumors derive from glial cells, and the possibility that loss of gap junctions contributes to their neoplastic transformation is intriguing. The absence of gap junctions in C6 glioma cells and highly malignant human gliomas (Tani et al., 1973) would support this concept. Moreover, proliferation is reduced in glioma cells induced to express Cx43

(Sanchez-Alvarez et al., 2001). How gap junctions suppress mitotic activity is not clear.

Possible functions of hemichannels

Recent studies suggest that hemichannels can act as unopposed membrane channels (e.g., Contreras et al., 2002; Ye et al., 2003). Most factors that regulate gap junctions, but probably not all, have similar effects on hemichannels. The ELs of an unopposed hemichannel, for example, are far more exposed than the same loops of two aligned hemichannels forming a gap junction, making these ELs a prime candidate site for differential modulation. For now, however, caution is needed when interpreting results obtained with agents that block gap junctions, because these would probably also block hemichannels. Hemichannels may also be confused with a few other membrane ion channels that have very large pores such as the $P2X_7$ purinergic receptor channel (Surprenant et al., 1996).

We are early in our understanding of the neurobiological roles of glial hemichannels. Proposed roles for hemichannels include (*1*) release of signaling molecules such as ATP (Cotrina et al., 1998; Stout et al., 2002) or glutamate (Ye et al., 2003), (*2*) modulation of membrane potential or ion gradients in a manner similar to that of conventional ion channels, (*3*) transmembrane movement of small molecules not permeable to conventional ion channels, and (*4*) mediation of cell injury under pathological conditions like ischemia (Contreras et al., 2002).

CONCLUSIONS

Connexins and the special forms of transmembrane communication that they mediate have been extensively investigated in the past four decades since their discovery. Our knowledge about gap junctions and hemichannels is impressive but incomplete. This is especially so in the brain, where these channels are widely expressed in glial cells but where we lack conclusive insight about how they participate in brain function. The situation, however, should be viewed optimistically because glial cell gap junctions and hemichannels are sufficiently well characterized that reasonable hypotheses about their function can now be formulated and tested. Research prospects in this area are also brighter due to the availability of important new information about the biophysics, genetics, and disease associations of connexins. These developments place in our hands powerful new tools and strategies for further experimental analysis.

ACKNOWLEDGMENTS

This work was supported by grants from NIH and Eastern Paralyzed Veterans of America.

REFERENCES

Altevogt, B.M., Kleopa, K.A., Postma, F.R., Scherer, S.S., and Paul, D.L. (2002) Connexin29 is uniquely distributed within myelinating glial cells of the central and peripheral nervous systems. *J. Neurosci.* 22:6458–6470.

Alvarez-Maubecin, V., Garcia-Hernandez, F., Williams, J.T., and Van Bockstaele, E.J. (2000) Functional coupling between neurons and glia. *J. Neurosci.* 20:4091–4098.

Anders, J.J. (1988) Lactic acid inhibition of gap junctional intercellular communication in in vitro astrocytes as measured by fluorescence recovery after laser photobleaching. *Glia* 1:371–379.

Balice-Gordon, R.J., Bone, L.J., and Scherer, S.S. (1998) Functional gap junctions in the Schwann cell myelin sheath. *J. Cell Biol.* 142:1095–1104.

Batter, D.K., Corpina, R.A., Roy, C., Spray, D.C., Hertzberg, E.L., and Kessler, J.A. (1992) Heterogeneity in gap junction expression in astrocytes cultured from different brain regions. *Glia* 6:213–221.

Bennett, M.V., Barrio, L.C., Bargiello, T.A., Spray, D.C., Hertzberg, E., and Saez, J.C. (1991) Gap junctions: new tools, new answers, new questions. *Neuron* 6:305–320.

Berger, T., Schnitzer, J., and Kettenmann, H. (1991) Developmental changes in the membrane current pattern, K^+ buffer capacity, and morphology of glial cells in the corpus callosum slice. *J. Neurosci.* 11:3008–3024.

Bergoffen, J., Scherer, S.S., Wang, S., Scott, M.O., Bone, L.J., Paul, D.L., Chen, K., Lensch, M.W., Chance, P.F., and Fischbeck, K.H. (1993) Connexin mutations in X-linked Charcot-Marie-Tooth disease. *Science* 262:2039–2042.

Black, J.A. and Waxman, S.G. (1988) The perinodal astrocyte. *Glia* 1:169–183.

Bruzzone, R., Hormuzdi, S.G., Barbe, M.T., Herb, A., and Monyer, H. (2003a) Pannexins, a family of gap junction proteins expressed in brain. *Proc. Natl. Acad. Sci. USA* 100:13644–13649.

Bukauskas, F.F., Jordan, K., Bukauskiene, A., Bennett, M.V., Lampe, P.D., Laird, D.W., and Verselis, V.K. (2000) Clustering of connexin 43–enhanced green fluorescent protein gap junction channels and functional coupling in living cells. *Proc. Natl. Acad. Sci. USA* 97:2556–2561.

Butt, A.M. and Ransom, B.R. (1989) Visualization of oligodendrocytes and astrocytes in the intact rat optic nerve by intracellular injection of lucifer yellow and horseradish peroxidase. *Glia* 2:470–475.

Butt, A.M. and Ransom, B.R. (1993) Morphology of astrocytes and oligodendrocytes during development in the intact rat optic nerve. *J. Comp. Neurol.* 338:141–158.

Ceelen, P.W., Lockridge, A., and Newman, E.A. (2001) Electrical coupling between glial cells in the rat retina. *Glia* 35:1–13.

Chandross, K.J. (1998) Nerve injury and inflammatory cytokines modulate gap junctions in the peripheral nervous system. *Glia* 24:21–31.

Cohen, M.W. (1970) The contribution by glial cells to surface recordings from the optic nerve of an amphibian. *J. Physiol.* 210:565–580.

Connors, B.W. and Ransom, B.R. (1987) Electrophysiological properties of ependymal cells (radial glia) in dorsal cortex of the turtle, *Pseudemys scripta*. *J. Physiol.* 385:287–306.

Contreras, J.E., Sanchez, H.A., Eugenin, E.A., Speidel, D., Theis, M., Willecke, K., Bukauskas, F.F., Bennett, M.V., and Saez, J.C. (2002) Metabolic inhibition induces opening of unapposed connexin 43 gap junction hemichannels and reduces gap junctional communication in cortical astrocytes in culture. *Proc. Natl. Acad. Sci. USA* 99:495–500.

Cotrina, M.L., Lin, J.H., Alves-Rodrigues, A., Liu, S., Li, J., Azmi-Ghadimi, H., Kang, J., Naus, C.C., and Nedergaard, M. (1998) Connexins regulate calcium signaling by controlling ATP release. *Proc. Natl. Acad. Sci. USA* 95:15735–15740.

De Pina-Benabou, M.H., Srinivas, M., Spray, D.C., and Scemes, E. (2001) Calmodulin kinase pathway mediates the K^+-induced increase in gap junctional communication between mouse spinal cord astrocytes. *J. Neurosci.* 21:6635–6643.

Dermietzel, R., Gao, Y., Scemes, E., Vieira, D., Urban, M., Kremer, M., Bennett, M.V., and Spray, D.C. (2000a) Connexin43 null mice reveal that astrocytes express multiple connexins. *Brain Res. Brain Res. Rev.* 32:45–56.

Dermietzel, R., Hertberg, E.L., Kessler, J.A., and Spray, D.C. (1991) Gap junctions between cultured astrocytes: immunocytochemical, molecular, and electrophysiological analysis. *J. Neurosci.* 11:1421–1432.

Dermietzel, R., Kremer, M., Paputsoglu, G., Stang, A., Skerrett, I.M., Gomes, D., Srinivas, M., Janssen-Bienhold, U., Weiler, R., Nicholson, B.J., Bruzzone, R., and Spray, D.C. (2000b) Molecular and functional diversity of neural connexins in the retina. *J. Neurosci.* 20:8331–8343.

Duffy, H.S., John, G.R., Lee, S.C., Brosnan, C.F., and Spray, D.C. (2000) Reciprocal regulation of the junctional proteins claudin-1 and connexin43 by interleukin-1beta in primary human fetal astrocytes. *J. Neurosci.* 20:RC114.

Elfgang, C., Eckert, R., Lichtenberg-Frate, H., Butterweck, A., Traub, O., Klein, R.A., Hulser, D.F., and Willecke, K. (1995) Specific permeability and selective formation of gap junction channels in connexin-transfected HeLa cells. *J. Cell Biol.* 129:805–817.

Enkvist, M.O. and McCarthy, K.D. (1994) Astroglial gap junction communication is increased by treatment with either glutamate or high K^+ concentration. *J. Neurochem.* 62:489–495.

Eugenin, E.A., Eckardt, D., Theis, M., Willecke, K., Bennett, M.V., and Saez, J.C. (2001) Microglia at brain stab wounds express connexin 43 and in vitro form functional gap junctions after treatment with interferon-gamma and tumor necrosis factor-alpha. *Proc. Natl. Acad. Sci. USA* 98:4190–4195.

Faustmann, P.M., Haase, C.G., Romberg, S., Hinkerohe, D., Szlachta, D., Smikalla, D., Krause, D., and Dermietzel, R. (2003) Microglia activation influences dye coupling and Cx43 expression of the astrocytic network. *Glia* 42:101–108.

Finkbeiner, S. (1992) Calcium waves in astrocytes-filling in the gaps. *Neuron* 8:1101–1108.

Froes, M.M., Correia, A.H., Garcia-Abreu, J., Spray, D.C., Campos de Carvalho, A.C., and Neto, M.V. (1999) Gap-junctional coupling between neurons and astrocytes in primary central nervous system cultures. *Proc. Natl. Acad. Sci. USA* 96:7541–7546.

Fujimoto, K., Nagafuchi, A., Tsukita, S., Kuraoka, A., Ohokuma, A., and Shibata, Y. (1997) Dynamics of connexins, E-cadherin and alpha-catenin on cell membranes during gap junction formation. *J. Cell Sci.* 110(Pt 3):311–322.

Gaietta, G., Deerinck, T.J., Adams, S.R., Bouwer, J., Tour, O., Laird, D.W., Sosinsky, G.E., Tsien, R.Y., and Ellisman, M.H. (2002) Multicolor and electron microscopic imaging of connexin trafficking. *Science* 296:503–507.

Giaume, C., Marin, P., Cordier, J., Glowinski, J., and Premont, J. (1991) Adrenergic regulation of intercellular communications between cultured striatal astrocytes from the mouse. *Proc. Natl. Acad. Sci. USA* 88:5577–5581.

Giaume, C. and Venance, L. (1998) Intercellular calcium signaling and gap junctional communication in astrocytes. *Glia* 24:50–64.

Goldberg, G.S., Moreno, A.P., and Lampe, P.D. (2002) Gap junctions between cells expressing connexin 43 or 32 show inverse permselectivity to adenosine and ATP. *J. Biol. Chem.* 277: 36725–36730.

Gomez-Hernandez, J.M., de Miguel, M., Larrosa, B., Gonzalez, D., and Barrio, L.C. (2003) Molecular basis of calcium regulation in connexin-32 hemichannels. *Proc. Natl. Acad. Sci. USA* 100: 16030–16035.

Goodenough, D.A., Goliger, J.A., and Paul, D.L. (1996) Connexins, connexons, and intercellular communication. *Annu. Rev. Biochem.* 65:475–502.

Guthrie, P.B., Knappenberger, J., Segal, M., Bennett, M.V., Charles, A.C., and Kater, S.B. (1999) ATP released from astrocytes mediates glial calcium waves. *J. Neurosci.* 19:520–528.

Gutnick, M.J., Connors, B.W., and Ransom, B.R. (1981) Dye-coupling between glial cells in the guinea pig neocortical slice. *Brain Res.* 213:486–492.

Harris, A.L. (2001) Emerging issues of connexin channels: biophysics fills the gap. *Q. Rev. Biophys.* 34:325–472.

Haydon, P.G. (2001) GLIA: listening and talking to the synapse. *Nat. Rev. Neurosci.* 2:185–193.

Hofer, T., Venance, L., and Giaume, C. (2002) Control and plasticity of intercellular calcium waves in astrocytes: a modeling approach. *J. Neurosci.* 22:4850–4859.

Hua, V.B., Chang, A.B., Tchieu, J.H., Kumar, N.M., Nielsen, P.A., and Saier, M.H., Jr. (2003) Sequence and phylogenetic analyses of 4 TMS junctional proteins of animals: connexins, innexins, claudins and occludins. *J. Membr. Biol.* 194:59–76.

Kettenmann, H. and Ransom, B.R. (1988) Electrical coupling between astrocytes and between oligodendrocytes studied in mammalian cell cultures. *Glia* 1:64–73.

Konishi, T. (1990) Dye coupling between mouse Schwann cells. *Brain Res.* 508:85–92.

Kuffler, S.W. and Potter, D.D. (1964) *Glia* in the leech central nervous system: physiological properties and neuron-glia relationship. *J. Neurophysiol.* 27:290–320.

Kunzelmann, P., Schroder, W., Traub, O., Steinhauser, C., Dermietzel, R., and Willecke, K. (1999) Late onset and increasing expression of the gap junction protein connexin30 in adult murine brain and long-term cultured astrocytes. *Glia* 25:111–119.

Lee, S.H., Kim, W.T., Cornell-Bell, A.H., and Sontheimer, H. (1994) Astrocytes exhibit regional specificity in gap-junction coupling. *Glia* 11:315–325.

Levin, M. (2002) Isolation and community: a review of the role of gap-junctional communication in embryonic patterning. *J. Membr. Biol.* 185:177–192.

Lin, J.H., Yang, J., Liu, S., Takano, T., Wang, X., Gao, Q., Willecke, K., and Nedergaard, M. (2003) Connexin mediates gap junction-independent resistance to cellular injury. *J. Neurosci.* 23:430–441.

Lo Turco, J.J. and Kriegstein, A.R. (1991) Clusters of coupled neuroblasts in embryonic neocortex. *Science* 252:563–566.

Loewenstein, W.R. (1981) Junctional intercellular communication: the cell-to-cell membrane channel. *Physiol. Rev.* 61:829–913.

Martins-Ferreira, H., Nedergaard, M., and Nicholson, C. (2000) Perspectives on spreading depression. *Brain Res. Brain Res.* Rev 32:215–234.

Mobbs, P., Brew, H., and Attwell, D. (1988) A quantitative analysis of glial cell coupling in the retina of the axolotl (*Ambystoma mexicanum*). *Brain Res.* 460:235–245.

Mudrick-Donnon, L.A., Williams, P.J., Pittman, Q.J., and MacVicar, B.A. (1993) Postsynaptic potentials mediated by GABA and dopamine evoked in stellate glial cells of the pituitary pars intermedia. *J. Neurosci.* 13:4660–4668.

Müller, T., Moller, T., Neuhaus, J., and Kettenmann, H. (1996) Electrical coupling among Bergmann glial cells and its modulation by glutamate receptor activation. *Glia* 17:274–284.

Nagy, J.I., Ionescu, A.V., Lynn, B.D., and Rash, J.E. (2003) Coupling of astrocyte connexins Cx26, Cx30, Cx43 to oligodendrocyte Cx29, Cx32, Cx47: implications from normal and connexin32 knockout mice. *Glia* 44:205–218.

Nagy, J.I., Yamamoto, T., Sawchuk, M.A., Nance, D.M., and Hertzberg, E.L. (1992) Quantitative immunohistochemical and biochemical correlates of connexin43 localization in rat brain. *Glia* 5:1–9.

Ochalski, P.A., Frankenstein, U.N., Hertzberg, E.L., and Nagy, J.I. (1997) Connexin-43 in rat spinal cord: localization in astrocytes and identification of heterotypic astro-oligodendrocytic gap junctions. *Neuroscience* 76:931–945.

Orkand, R.K., Nicholls, J.G., and Kuffler, S.W. (1966) Effect of nerve impulses on the membrane potential of glial cells in the central nervous system of amphibia. *J. Neurophysiol.* 29:788–806.

Pastor, A., Kremer, M., Moller, T., Kettenmann, H., and Dermietzel, R. (1998) Dye coupling between spinal cord oligodendrocytes: differences in coupling efficiency between gray and white matter. *Glia* 24:108–120.

Perkins, G.A., Goodenough, D.A., and Sosinsky, G.E. (1998) Formation of the gap junction intercellular channel requires a 30 degree rotation for interdigitating two apposing connexons. *J. Mol. Biol.* 277:171–177.

Phelan, P. and Starich, T.A. (2001) Innexins get into the gap. *Bioessays* 23:388–396.

Ransom, B.R. (1992) Glial modulation of neural excitability mediated by extracellular pH: a hypothesis. *Prog. Brain Res.* 94:37–46.

Ransom, B.R. (1995) Gap junctions. In: Kettenmann, H. and Ransom, B.R., eds. *Neuroglia*. New York: Oxford University Press, pp. 299–318.

Ransom, B.R. and Kettenmann, H. (1990) Electrical coupling, without dye coupling, between mammalian astrocytes and oligodendrocytes in cell culture. *Glia* 3:258–266.

Rash, J.E., Yasumura, T., Dudek, F.E., and Nagy, J.I. (2001) Cell-specific expression of connexins and evidence of restricted gap junctional coupling between glial cells and between neurons. *J. Neurosci.* 21:1983–2000.

Reuss, B., Hertel, M., Werner, S., and Unsicker, K. (2000) Fibroblast growth factors-5 and -9 distinctly regulate expression and function of the gap junction protein connexin43 in cultured astroglial cells from different brain regions. *Glia* 30:231–241.

Robinson, S.R., Hampson, E.C., Munro, M.N., and Vaney, D.I. (1993) Unidirectional coupling of gap junctions between neuroglia. *Science* 262:1072–1074.

Rose, C.R. and Ransom, B.R. (1996) Intracellular sodium homeostasis in rat hippocampal astrocytes. *J. Physiol.* 491(Pt 2):291–305.

Rose, C.R. and Ransom, B.R. (1997) Gap junctions equalize intracellular Na^+ concentration in astrocytes. *Glia* 20:299–307.

Rouach, N., Calvo, C.F., Glowinski, J., and Giaume, C. (2002) Brain macrophages inhibit gap junctional communication and downregulate connexin 43 expression in cultured astrocytes. Eur *J. Neurosci.* 15:403–407.

Rouach, N., Glowinski, J., and Giaume, C. (2000) Activity-dependent neuronal control of gap-junctional communication in astrocytes. *J. Cell Biol.* 149:1513–1526.

Rozental, R., Srinivas, M., and Spray, D.C. (2001) How to close a gap junction channel. Efficacies and potencies of uncoupling agents. *Meth. Mol. Biol.* 154:447–476.

Saez, J.C., Berthoud, V.M., Branes, M.C., Martinez, A.D., and Beyer, E.C. (2003a) Plasma membrane channels formed by connexins: their regulation and functions. *Physiol. Rev.* 83:1359–1400.

Saez, J.C., Contreras, J.E., Bukauskas, F.F., Retamal, M.A., and Bennett, M.V. (2003b) Gap junction hemichannels in astrocytes of the CNS. *Acta Physiol. Scand.* 179:9–22.

Sanchez-Alvarez, R., Tabernero, A., Sanchez-Abarca, L.I., Orfao, A., Giaume, C., and Medina, J.M. (2001) Proliferation of C6 glioma cells is blunted by the increase in gap junction communication caused by tolbutamide. *FEBS Lett* 509:202–206.

Scemes, E., Dermietzel, R., and Spray, D.C. (1998) Calcium waves between astrocytes from Cx43 knockout mice. *Glia* 24:65–73.

Scemes, E. and Spray, D.C. (1998) Increased intercellular communication in mouse astrocytes exposed to hyposmotic shocks. *Glia* 24:74–84.

Somjen, G.G. (1970) Evoked sustained focal potentials and membrane potential of neurons and of unresponsive cells of the spinal cord. *J. Neurophysiol.* 33:562–582.

Sontheimer, H., Minturn, J.E., Black, J.A., Waxman, S.G., and Ransom, B.R. (1990) Specificity of cell-cell coupling in rat optic nerve astrocytes in vitro. *Proc. Natl. Acad. Sci. USA* 87:9833–9837.

Sontheimer, H., Minturn, J.E., Ransom, B.R., Black, J.A., Cornell-Bell, A.H., and Waxman, S.G. (1991) Cell coupling is restricted to subpopulations of astrocytes cultured from rat hippocampus and optic nerve. *Ann. NY Acad. Sci.* 633:592–596.

Spray, D.C., Duffy, H.S., and Scemes, E. (1999) GAP junctions in glia. Type, roles and plasticity. *Adv. Exp. Med. Biol.* 468:339–359.

Stout, C.E., Costantin, J.L., Naus, C.C., and Charles, A.C. (2002) Intercellular calcium signaling in astrocytes via ATP release through connexin hemichannels. *J. Biol. Chem.* 277:10482–10488.

Surprenant, A., Rassendren, F., Kawashima, E., North, R.A., and Buell, G. (1996) The cytolytic P2Z receptor for extracellular ATP identified as a P2X receptor (P2X7). *Science* 272:735–738.

Tani, E., Nishiura, M., and Higashi, N. (1973) Freeze-fracture studies of gap junctions of normal and neoplastic astrocytes. *Acta Neuropathol. (Berl.)* 26:127–138.

Trosko, J.E., Chang, C.C., Madhukar, B.V., and Klaunig, J.E. (1990) Chemical, oncogene and growth factor inhibition gap junctional intercellular communication: an integrative hypothesis of carcinogenesis. *Pathobiology* 58:265–278.

Unger, V.M., Kumar, N.M., Gilula, N.B., and Yeager, M. (1999) Three-dimensional structure of a recombinant gap junction membrane channel. *Science* 283:1176–1180.

Von Blankenfeld, G., Ransom, B.R., and Kettenmann, H. (1993) Development of cell-cell coupling among cells of the oligodendrocyte lineage. *Glia* 7:322–328.

Ye, Z.C., Wyeth, M.S., Baltan-Tekkok, S., and Ransom, B.R. (2003) Functional hemichannels in astrocytes: a novel mechanism of glutamate release. *J. Neurosci.* 23:3588–3596.

Zahs, K.R. (1998) Heterotypic coupling between glial cells of the mammalian central nervous system. *Glia* 24:85–96.

Zahs, K.R., Kofuji, P., Meier, C., and Dermietzel, R. (2003) Connexin immunoreactivity in glial cells of the rat retina. *J. Comp. Neurol.* 455:531–546.

Zahs, K.R. and Newman, E.A. (1997) Asymmetric gap junctional coupling between glial cells in the rat retina. *Glia* 20:10–22.

14 Quantal release of transmitter: not only from neurons but from astrocytes as well?

ANDREA VOLTERRA AND JACOPO MELDOLESI

ASTROCYTES RELEASE GLUTAMATE

The status of astrocytes has changed profoundly during the past 15 years, going from a cell scaffold and metabolic-trophic reservoir offering neurons a necessary, yet only passive, support to a full actor, working in collaboration with other glial cells and with the surrounding neurons by the continuous exchange of chemical messengers including glutamate, a classical neurotransmitter (Volterra et al., 2002). The existence of communication systems between astrocytes and other brain cells was first hypothesized at the end of the 1980s, based on the observation that glial cells synthesize and release a variety of compounds. At the time, however, critical issues, such as the timing and mechanisms of release, were not investigated. Release of glutamate from glial cells, taking place, however, by molecular, nonquantal mechanisms and independent of the cytosolic concentration of Ca^{2+}, $[Ca^{2+}]_i$, (see Nedergaard et al., 2002), was first shown by two groups in 1990. Attwell and associates, working by whole-cell patch-clamping on cultured Müller glial cells from the salamander retina, demonstrated that the inwardly directed glutamate current turns outward as external K^+ rises, provided that enough Na^+ and glutamate are present intracellularly (Szatkowski et al., 1990). Concomitantly, the Kimelberg group, investigating the effects of swelling on astrocytes, demonstrated release of glutamate and other negatively charged amino acids occurring via the opening of volume-activated anion channels (hypo-osmotic release, HOR) (Kimelberg et al., 1990). The significance of these findings is still discussed. A physiological, regulatory role of HOR has been recently proposed (Hussy et al., 2000). In addition, both HOR and reverse transport release may participate in multiple pathological conditions, contributing to the buildup of toxic extracellular concentrations of excitatory amino acids (Kimelberg and Mongin, 1998; Rossi et al., 2000).

Recently, two additional molecular pathways of glutamate release have emerged. The Ransom group demonstrated that hemichannels of gap junctions can act as functional, glutamate-permeable channels. Release of the amino acid through these channels, however, was blocked by divalent cations present in physiological fluids (Ye et al., 2002). Glutamate release was also shown to take place via $P2X_7$, a purinergic receptor expressed by astrocytes (Duan et al., 2003). This pathway is interesting because the putative ligand of the receptor, adenosine triphosphate (ATP), is known to be released by astrocytes. Moreover, the HOR and ATP-dependent mechanisms seem to function synergistically (Mongin and Kimelberg, 2002). Also at $P2X_7$ channels divalent cations seem to play a modulatory role (Duan et al., 2003).

Glutamate release from astrocytes does not seem to take place by molecular mechanisms only, however. Evidence for the existence of regulated exocytosis activated in response to binding of endogenous ligands to cell surface receptors began to emerge in the early 1990s (Parpura et al., 1994; Jeftinija et al., 1996). Exocytosis differs from molecular release in a variety of properties, notably in its dependence on $[Ca^{2+}]_i$ (demonstrated by the inhibitory effect of intracellular Ca^{2+} chelators such as 1,2-bis(2-aminophenoxy)-ethane-N,N,N′,N′-tetraacetic acid [BAPTA]). The vesicular nature of the process was first hypothesized based on the effects of specific blockers in cultures (Jeftinija et al., 1997; Bezzi et al., 1998). A Ca^{2+}-dependent release process distinct from exocytosis in neuronal terminals was observed in hippocampal slices (Bezzi et al., 1998, 2001), suggesting that this pathway is also operative in the intact brain.

CONSTITUTIVE AND REGULATED FORMS OF EXOCYTOSIS

Exocytosis, that is, membrane fusion of intracellular membranes with the plasmalemma, is a general property of eukaryotic cells. Traditionally, nonsecretory cells are believed to express only constitutive secretion, where fusions take place continuously, independent of regulatory signals. By constitutive secretion, cells discharge to the extracellular space a variety of products to be integrated in the extracellular matrix, such as various filamentous proteins and proteoglycans. The latter products, first accumulated in the Golgi complex/trans-Golgi network (TGN), are quickly picked up by organelles (vesicles and tubules, still poorly known in molecular terms) destined to reach the plasma membrane, discharge their content with no delay, and finally recycle their membrane to the Golgi area (Keller and Simons, 1997). Similar to classical constitutive secretion is recycling to the plasmalemma of membranes that, after internalization by various forms of endocytosis, had undergone complex molecular and structural rearrangements along well-defined intracellular pathways.

Secretion that for decades has attracted the highest interest is, however, regulated secretion, the form taking place in response to specific stimuli acting most often through the generation of $[Ca^{2+}]_i$ signals. Until recently, competence in this function was believed to be restricted to specialized cells: exocrine cells, endocrine cells, and neurons. Results obtained during the past decade have revealed, however, that some forms of regulated exocytosis also exist in nonsecretory cells. Thus, electrophysiological studies carried out initially in fibroblasts and in a defective clone of pheochromocytoma PC12 cells (Coorsens et al., 1996; Ninomyia et al., 1996; Kasai et al., 1999), and later extended to other cell types, have identified new vesicles, the enlargeosomes, competent for rapid (hundreds of milliseconds), $[Ca^{2+}]_i$-dependent exocytosis, whose discharge induces significant (up to 10%–20%) increases of the cell surface area. This exocytic system, which is insensitive to tetanus toxin (see the sections "Expression of Neurosecretion-Specific Proteins" and "Clostridial Neurotoxins"), seems to be involved not in secretion but in the control of membrane enlargement, as it occurs during cell differentiation (Borgonovo et al., 2002).

A form of exocytosis even closer to classical neurosecretion has been described in various types of cells (*Xenopus* myocytes, cultured fibroblasts) after loading with acetylcholine (Dan and Poo, 1992; Morimoto et al., 1995). Small but appreciable transmitter quanta were discharged by these cells both spontaneously and in response to depolarization and $[Ca^{2+}]_i$ rise. Compared to synaptic release, the depolarization-evoked responses of these cells developed after some delay (20–30 msec), and their rate of failures was very high.

The most interesting processes of regulated secretion are still those taking place in *bona fide* secretory cells. In the resting state, the main property of these cells is the accumulation within the cytoplasm of specific organelles destined to be promptly exocytized upon stimulation. This property is particularly impressive at neuronal synapses, where a pool of neurotransmitter-filled clear vesicles (CV), the so-called readily releasable pool, can be discharged very quickly (within a few hundred microseconds) after $[Ca^{2+}]_i$ rise. In neurosecretory cells, discharge of clear vesicles, the synaptic-like microvesicles (SLMV), is not as rapid; however, it remains considerable. In contrast, exocytoses of the second type of synaptic and neurosecretory vesicles, the dense-core granules (DCG), are slower. In spite of these kinetic differences, the molecular machinery of membrane fusion and recycling of both CVs/SLMVs and DCGs is similar, at least in large part. In the following sections the process, defined as *neurosecretion*, will be considered as a whole and employed as reference to discuss quantal transmitter release as it appears to occur from astrocytes.

ASTROCYTES AS NEUROSECRETORY CELLS

The observations of Parpura et al. (1994) and subsequent reports by others strongly suggest that the Ca^{2+}-dependent astrocyte release of glutamate, and possibly also of other products, takes place by quantal exocytic process(es) resembling neurosecretion. In this section, starting with the profound knowledge existing on nerve cells, we will deal with the proteins, organelles, mechanisms, and regulation processes existing in astrocytes as they have emerged from the studies of the past decade.

Expression of Neurosecretion-Specific Proteins

In eukaryotic cells, all processes of membrane fusion require the activation of molecular machineries assembled around a core complex composed of specific proteins, the "soluble N-ethylmaleimide-sensitive factor (NSF)-associated protein receptors, (SNAREs). At synapses and neurosecretory cells the core complex includes three SNAREs that in the course of the fusion process become bound to each other by the strict interconnection of four hydrophilic α helices. One of these SNAREs, vesicle-associated membrane protein 2 (VAMP2) (also called *synaptobrevin II*), is exposed at the vesicle surface and is therefore defined as a vSNARE; the other two, SNAP25 (synaptosome-associated protein of 25 KDa) and syntaxin, protrude from the plasmalemma into the cytoplasm and are defined as target SNAREs (tSNAREs). Fusion is believed to be triggered by the activation of another vesicle protein, synaptotagmin I, working as a Ca^{2+} sensor, while among regulatory proteins, located primarily in the cytosol, are Munc18a, needed for syntaxin1 integration into the core; the G protein rab3a; complexins; and many others (Madison et al., 1996). In nonneurosecretory cells, exocytosis depends not on the above SNAREs and regulatory proteins, but on analogs playing similar roles, although with different functional properties (Jahn et al., 2003).

For many years VAMP2, syntaxin1, and SNAP25 were believed to be specific of neurons and neurosecretory cells. The results of Parpura et al. (1995a), showing expression in long-term astrocyte cultures [analyzed by Western blot, reverse transcriptase–polymerase chain reaction (RT-PCR) and immunocytochemistry] of VAMP2 together with the homolog cellubrevin (VAMP3), were therefore a surprise. Of the other SNAREs, Parpura et al. identified syntaxin1; SNAP25 could not be detected. Hepp et al. (1999) confirmed the expression of cellubrevin and syntaxin1 as well as the absence of SNAP25, replaced by a homolog, SNAP23a, present also in oligodendrocytes, microglia, and the precursor cells positive for the A2B5 marker. The assembly of SNAP23 into a SNARE complex with cellubrevin and syntaxin1 was suggested by coimmunoprecipitation results obtained with specific antibodies.

Expression of SNAREs in cultured astrocytes was found to change over time, however. Maienschein et al. (1999) reported that after 2 days *in vitro*, most cells expressing the classical astrocyte marker, glial fibrillary acidic protein (GFAP), were also positive for neurosecretory proteins: not only VAMP2 and syntaxin but also SNAP25, the vesicle proteins synaptotagmin I and synaptophysin, as well as rab3a and the scaffold protein of the vesicle storage compartment, synapsin I. Later (after 20 days), expression of many of these proteins had declined or become inappreciable. Proteins expressed by astrocyte cultures are not only those of SLMV. A secretory protein of the granin family, typical of DCG and abundant in neurons and neuroendocrine cells, secretogranin II, was also found to be present (Fischer-Colbrie et al., 1993; Calegari et al., 1999).

Summing up, the state of astrocytes in terms of neurosecretion-specific proteins appears not yet fully clarified. Many of these proteins were found to be expressed (see Table 14.1), however, not by all astrocytes and not at all stages of their life. Moreover, proteins that in neurosecretory cells are directly involved in exocytic membrane fusion could be replaced by analogs also expressed by nonneurosecretory cells. We conclude that, in spite of their widely purported nonneurosecretory nature, astrocytes appear to share at least part of the secretion machinery typical of neurons and endocrine cells.

Neurosecretory Organelles

The information about neurosecretory protein composition can be extended to the intracellular organelle level. By immunofluorescence, numerous puncta positive for VAMP2 and cellubrevin were observed particularly at the Golgi/TGN complex (Parpura et al., 1995a; Maienschein et al., 1999), with some concentration over large (protoplasmic cells) and fine (fibrous cells) processes. Double immunofluorescence results at cell boundaries and filopodia showed VAMP and rab3a partially overlapping glutamate-specific puncta (Anlauf and Derouiche, 2002).

At the level of conventional electron microscopy, the properties of astrocyte SLMVs known so far appear short for direct identification. In particular, clustering at discrete sites, as observed in presynaptic terminals, was never reported. This property, however, is not unique to astrocytes but resembles that described both in immature neurons, where transmitters are released by exocytosis not at the terminals but from the surface of axons

TABLE 14.1 *Proteins of the Exocytic Apparatus Expressed in Astrocytes*

Type of Protein	*Role in Exocytosis*	*References*
Synaptobrevin II (VAMP2)	v-SNARE[a]	Parpura et al. (1995[a]), Jeftinija et al. (1997), Maienschein et al. (1999), Araque et al. (2000), Pasti et al. (2001), Anlauf and Derouiche (2002)
Cellubrevin (VAMP3)	v-SNARE	Parpura et al. (1995a), Jeftinija et al. (1997), Hepp et al. (1999), Maienschein et al. (1999)
TI-VAMP[b] (VAMP8)	v-SNARE	Calegari et al. (1999)
Syntaxin 1	t-SNARE[c]	Parpura et al. (1995a), Jeftinija et al. (1997), Calegari et al. (1999), Hepp et al. (1999), Maienschein et al. (1999)
SNAP23	t-SNARE	Calegari et al. (1999), Hepp et al. (1999)
SNAP25	t-SNARE	Maienschein et al. (1999)
Synaptotagmin I	Ca^{2+} sensor	Maienschein et al. (1999)
Synapsin I	Cytoskeleton-vesicle interaction	Maienschein et al. (1999)
Rab3 (a and b)[d]	Vesicle trafficking	Madison et al. (1996), Maienschein et al. (1999), Anlauf and Derouiche (2002)
Secretogranin II	Stored within dense-core granules	Fischer-Colbrie et al. (1993), Calegari et al. (1999)

[a]v-SNARE: protein of synaptic vesicles involved in formation of the soluble N-ethylmalimide-sensitive factor (NSF)-associated protein receptors (SNARE) complex.

[b]TI-VAMP: tetanus neurotoxin-insensitive vesicle-associated membrane protein (VAMP).

[c]t-SNARE: protein of the plasma membrane (of synaptic terminals in neurons) involved in the formation of the SNARE complex.

[d]rab3: small guanosine triphosphate-binding protein.

(Zakharenko et al., 1999), and in neurosecretory cells, where exocytic release of SLMVs is still defined according to biochemical/physiological rather than morphological evidence. Identification of astrocyte SLMVs therefore requires immunogold labeling of specific markers (see the section "Present Conclusions and Ongoing Developments"). Maienschein et al. (1999) used gold particles addressed to VAMP2 and synaptophysin in 4-day-old astrocytic cultures, labeling mostly clear organelles between 100 and 700 nm in diameter. Other organelles, capped or with an electron-dense core, were labeled occasionally. Heterogeneity was confirmed by density gradient centrifugation since markers distributed over a broad range of sucrose concentrations.

As far as DCGs are concerned, 3week-old astrocyte cultures from the hippocampus (but not from the cerebral cortex and the cerebellum), investigated by immunocytochemistry at the fluorescence and electron microscopic levels, were found to possess structures positive for a secretory granin, secretogranin II, localized partly in the Golgi/TGN complex and partly in vesicles (with an average diameter of 110 nm), similar to DCGs of PC12 cells, a widely used neurosecretory cell model (Calegari et al., 1999). Consistently, when homogenates of these cultured astrocytes were analyzed by sucrose gradients, about 50% of the secretogranin II was recovered in fractions coinciding with the DCG fractions of PC12, while the rest was distributed into lighter fractions also labeled by Golgi markers. When investigated by classical pulse-chase experiments with radioactive amino acids, only a small fraction of the newly synthesized granin was found to be discharged to the medium from resting cells (constitutive secretion), while a much larger fraction was discharged during stimulation in the presence (but not in the absence) of Ca^{2+} into the medium (regulated secretion). In particular, the combination of bradykinin, dibutyryl cyclic adenosine monophosphate (cAMP), and the activator of protein kinase C, phorbol myristate acetate, yielded synergistic responses (Calegari et al., 1999).

Recently, the evidence in astrocytes for a *bona fide* DCG-like secretory pathway has been strengthened. Sucrose density analysis has revealed that the secretogranin II-containing granules also store ATP, suggesting that, as in neurons and neurosecretory cells, the nucleotide and the protein are coreleased by exocytosis (Coco et al., 2003). Moreover, atrial natriuretic peptide release from astrocytes transfected with the precursor occurred not by constitutive secretion, as it does from nonsecretory cells, but by a regulated pathway resembling that of neuronal DCGs (Krzan et al., 2003). Evidence along the same line was obtained in the glial cells of a mollusk, *Lymnea stagnalis*. A 24 kDa protein, acetylcholine-binding protein, was shown to segregate into a population of dense-core vesicles distributed both in the Golgi area and in long processes intermingled with neuronal axon terminals (Smit et al., 2001). Finally, a proteomic analysis of the medium bathing cultured astrocytes revealed release of numerous proteins, that was partially blocked by brefeldin A, a drug that inhibits the assembly of DCG (Lafon-Cazal et al., 2003). Taken together, these results support the existence and functioning of a true DCG system in astrocytes from at least some areas of the brain, in culture and possibly also in the intact tissue. Moreover, they suggest that astrocytes, like neurons and neurosecretory cells, express more than one type of secretory organelle.

Glutamate Release from Astrocytes Is Stimulated/Blocked by Agents Specifically Active on Neurons and Neurosecretory Cells

The most direct evidence of the neurosecretory properties of astrocytes comes from the effects of agents, mostly natural toxins, universally known as highly specific for neurons and endocrine cells.

α-Latrotoxin

Alpha-latrotoxin, the main toxin of the black widow spider venom, is known to induce massive release of neurotransmitter from synapses of both the central and peripheral nervous systems and from neurosecretory cells such as PC12. Other endocrine cells and all exocrine cells are insensitive to the toxin (Rosenthal and Meldolesi, 1989; Sudhof, 2001). The specificity of the toxin's action is due to its binding to at least two types of receptors expressed by target cells: one, neurexin, Ca^{2+}-dependent; the other, latrophilin, Ca^{2+}-independent. Expression of a member of the neurexin family has been described in glial cells of *Drosophila* (Yuan and Ganetzky, 1999).

The mechanism of action of α-latrotoxin is complex. On the one hand, the toxin triggers Ca^{2+} influx via activation of Ca^{2+}-permeable channel(s) in the plasmalemma; on the other hand, it stimulates intracellular Ca^{2+} release and possibly activates directly the exocytic system, inducing responses that do persist in Ca^{2+}-free media (Sudhof, 2001). Parpura et al. (1995b) tested the effects of α-latrotoxin on cultured astrocytes and observed a considerable stimulation of glutamate release, which faded slowly in Ca^{2+}-free medium.

Clostridial neurotoxins

These toxins, produced by bacteria of the genus *Clostridium*, have been known for centuries because of their effects in humans and animals: spastic (tetanus) and flaccid (botulism) paralyses, due to the blockade of transmitter release at different nerve terminals. The molecular mechanism of these effects is now known. Tetanus neurotoxin (TeNT) and the seven serotypes of botulinum neurotoxins (BoNT A–G), are proteins consisting of two chains, a light one (about 50 kDa) and a heavy one (about 100 kDa), linked by a disulfide bond. After binding to specific membrane acceptors at the surface of target presynaptic terminals, BoNTs and TeNT are internalized via endocytosis. Within endosomes the toxins are rearranged, with insertion of the heavy chains into the membrane lipid bilayer. Oligomerization of the transmembrane heavy chains leads to the assembly of channels through which light chains, which are Zn^{2+}-dependent endopeptidases, are translocated to the cytosol, gaining access to their targets; one of the three SNAREs of the exocytic machinery of neurons. In particular, TeNT and BoNT-B cleave VAMP2 and cellubrevin, BoNT-A cleaves SNAP25, and BoNT-C cleaves syntaxin 1. The exquisite selectivity of the toxins is due to highly conserved motives in the amino acid sequence of their targets.

Within synapses, clostridial neurotoxins have free access to their substrates only for a short time, when SNARE proteins are no longer protected by association with chaperones and not yet assembled into the fusogenic core complex. Once assembled in the latter complex, SNAREs become protected from the proteolytic attack of the toxins. This is why, shortly after intoxication, transmitter release can proceed for some time, apparently unaffected. When, in contrast, SNAREs are cleaved, transmitter release is blocked. In neurosecretory cells the intracellular events induced by clostridial toxins are the same as in neurons; however, high-affinity toxin binding sites are not expressed at the surface. Uptake is therefore much less effective, and longer treatments with high toxin concentrations are needed to induce a block of regulated exocytosis (see Humeau et al., 2000, and Schiavo et al., 2000, for reviews).

The effect of clostridial toxins on Ca^{2+}-dependent glutamate release was investigated in cultured astrocytes, and the results resembled those in neurosecretory cells. Jeftinija et al. (1997) observed that long incubations (16 hours) with either BoNT-A, -B, -C or TeNT are needed to inhibit glutamate release in response to bradykinin. Moreover, in the cells poisoned with BoNT-B or TeNT the VAMP2 immunostaining appeared reduced. Bezzi et al. (1998) found that the concomitant activation of astrocyte group I metabotropic (mGlu) and (S)-12-amino-3-hydroxy-5-methyl-4-isoxazolepropionic acid (AMPA) receptors induces Ca^{2+}-dependent release of glutamate. Preincubation of the cells with TeNT resulted in an inhibition of this release, appreciable after 8 hours and complete after 20–24 hours. While slow, the toxin's effect is specific because two forms of nonexocytic glutamate release, by reversed transport and HOR, are unaffected (Jeftinija et al., 1997; Bezzi et al., 1998, 2001). Interestingly, Verderio et al. (1999), working with cultured astrocytes pulse-labeled with the BoNT-B holotoxin conjugated with Texas Red, observed toxin internalized into endosomes first scattered throughout the cytoplasm and later concentrated in the perinuclear area. Transfer to the cytosol seems therefore to take place not at an early but at a late stage of the endosome cycle, a fact that could explain the delayed efficacy of the toxins. Indeed, Araque et al. (2000) showed that BoNT-B can act quickly in astrocytes, provided that the dissociated light chain is microinjected intracellularly. The observed time differences between neurons and astrocytes therefore are due not to the action, but to the distinct uptake and intracellular processing systems for the toxins.

Bafilomycin A1

Bafilomycins, a family of natural macrolide antibiotics, are inhibitors of ion adenosine triphosphatases (ATPases). Bafilomycin A1 is highly selective for a class of these pumps, the vacuolar ATPases (vATPases), which serve for the acidification of intracellular membrane-bound compartments. At synapses, the proton gradient generated by the vATPase provides the driving force for the uptake and accumulation of transmitters into synaptic vesicles. The vesicular uptake of glutamate (Takamori et al., 2000; Herzog et al., 2001), and thus synaptic transmission at hippocampal synapses (Nett et al., 2002), are inhibited by bafilomycin A1. In addition, bafilomycin A1 blocks glutamate release from astrocytes (Araque et al., 2000). Therefore, although involving a profoundly different mechanism, the inhibitory effect of the antibiotic ultimately resembles that of clostridial toxins (Bezzi et al., 2001; Pasti et al., 2001).

Quantal Properties of Astrocyte Glutamate Release

The comprehensive evidence reported so far strongly suggests the existence in astrocytes of a vesicular glutamate release process operating by a molecular and structural machinery similar to that of neurons and neurosecretory cells. A question that remained open, however, was whether this process does induce in target cells the rapid and discrete electrical events definable as quanta according to the classical nomenclature of synaptic transmission. To answer this question Pasti et al. (2001) used a coculture approach. Astrocytes were stimulated by L-quisqualate, and their glutamate release was revealed by cocultured *sniffer cells*, that is, cells of the HEK 293 line stably transfected with the 1–2A subunits of the glutamatergic *N*-methyl-D aspartate (NMDA) receptor, which is not expressed by cultured astrocytes. Patch-clamping of sniffer cells revealed the appearance of discrete, pulsatile inward current events, similar in terms of kinetics (rise and decay constants) and blockade (by amino phosphonovaleric acid) to the excitatory current pulses recorded at NMDA receptor-expressing synapses, which are universally attributed to the exocytic fusion of individual synaptic vesicles. Glutamate release by astrocytes therefore appears fully competent to trigger in target cells the generation of signals considered until now specific for synapses.

STIMULUS-SECRETION COUPLING IN ASTROCYTES

As already discussed in the sections "Astrocytes Release Glutamate" and "Astrocytes as Neurosecretory Cells," quantal release of glutamate from astrocytes may occur by exocytosis of specific vesicles, regulated by appropriate changes of $[Ca^{2+}]_i$. Compared to neurons and neurosecretory cells, however, an important difference exists since only a fraction of astrocytes displays voltage-dependent Ca^{2+} currents (Akopian et al., 1996), the others being unable to respond to stimulation with rapid voltage-dependent $[Ca^{2+}]_i$ rises (Carmignoto et al., 1998). The main process of stimulus-secretion coupling known to take place in excitable cells, and especially at synapses, that is, depolarization-induced Ca^{2+} influx, does not occur in most astrocytes. In the latter, therefore, coupling depends primarily on intracellular Ca^{2+} release triggered by the second messenger, inositol 1,4,5-trisphosphate (IP_3), generated by receptor activation.

Astrocyte Stimulation

Table 14.2 lists the agonists and corresponding astrocyte receptors known to elicit glutamate release responses sensitive to blockers of exocytosis. The considerable number of these agents documents the high degree of responsiveness of astrocytes and suggests that their glutamate release process plays a key role in the network of brain intercellular communication pathways.

An unexpected property of astrocyte signal transduction is complexity. Activation of a single receptor appears to increase $[Ca^{2+}]_i$ and stimulate glutamate release not only per se but also via the release of multiple autocrine/paracrine mediators, acting apparently as spatiotemporal amplifiers of the responses. In particular, release of prostaglandin E_2 (PGE_2) was observed following coactivation of group I mGlu and AMPA receptors (Bezzi et al., 1998; Sanzgiri et al., 1999) and release of tumor necrosis factor-α (TNFα), leading to release of PGE_2, following activation of the chemokine receptor, CXCR4 (Bezzi et al., 2001). In either case, selective blockade of the mediators dramatically reduced glutamate release (Bezzi et al., 1998, 2001; Pasti et al., 2001).

Ca^{2+} Dependence

At presynaptic terminals, release of neurotransmitters is known to be triggered at very high (50–100 μM) $[Ca^{2+}]_i$ microdomains induced around docked synaptic vesicles by the opening of strategically located voltage-gated Ca^{2+} channels. The molecular machinery of the fusion has been largely clarified (see the section "Expression of Neurosecretion-Specific Proteins"). In contrast, information

TABLE 14.2 *Agents Stimulating Regulated Release of Glutamate from Astrocytes*

		GLUTAMATE RELEASE SENSITIVE TO:			
Mediator	*Receptor*	*Ca^{2+} Chelators*[a]	*Clostr. NTxs*[b]	*Baf A1*[c]	*References*
Bradykinin	B2	EGTA BAPTA/AM	BoNT-A/B/C TeNT	N.T.[d]	Jeftinija et al. (1996, 1997)
Glutamate	Group I mGluR + AMPA receptors	EGTA BAPTA/AM	TeNT	Yes	Bezzi et al. (1998), Pasti et al. (2001)
PGE_2[e]	EP?	BAPTA/AM	TeNT	Yes	Bezzi et al. (1998, 2001), Sanzgiri et al. (1999)
ATP	P2Y?	BAPTA/AM	N.T.	N.T.	Bezzi et al. (1999), Jeremic et al. (2001)
SDF-1α[f]	CXCR4	BAPTA/AM	TeNT	Yes	Bezzi et al. (2001)
TNFα[g]	p55-TNF receptor	BAPTA/AM	TeNT	Yes	Bezzi et al. (2001)
BDNF[h]	Trk B	EGTA, BAPTA/AM	TeNT	N.T.	Pascual et al. (2001)
NO[i]		EGTA, BAPTA/AM	BoNT-C	N.T.	Bal-Price et al. (2002)

[a]Ca^{2+} chelators: chelators of intracellular free calcium [1,2-bis(2-aminophenoxy)-ethane-N,N,N′,N′-tetraacetic acid/tetrakis (acetoxymethyl) ester (BAPTA/AM)] or extracellular free calcium [ethylene glycol tetraacetic acid (EGTA), often added in nominal 0 Ca^{2+} media].

[b]Clostr. NTxs: clostridial neurotoxins: botulinum neurotoxin, BoNT; tetanus neurotoxin, TeNT.

[c]Baf A1: bafilomycin A1.

[d]N.T.: not tested.

[e]PGE_2: prostaglandin E_2, a cyclooxygenase metabolite of arachidonic acid.

[f]SDF-1α: stromal cell-derived factor 1α, a chemokine.

[g]TNFα: tumor necrosis factor-α.

[h]BDNF: brain-derived neurotrophic factor.

[i]NO: nitric oxide.

about Ca^{2+} signals regulating glutamate release from astrocytes is still scarce. Since in most astrocytes these signals originate not from the plasma membrane but from intracellular stores, $[Ca^{2+}]_i$ levels at release sites are expected to be lower, and therefore a higher Ca^{2+} sensitivity of the exocytic process is expected. Actual values, however, are still debated. Studies carried out in cultured astrocytes by photolysis of a caged Ca^{2+} compound, NP-EGTA, suggested that $[Ca^{2+}]_i$ elevations were very modest (in the range of 80–140 nM; Parpura and Haydon, 2000). Part of the stimulated cells, after the first response, failed to release glutamate following further elevations of $[Ca^{2+}]_i$. Others, however, responded to step-like increases of $[Ca^{2+}]_i$ (up to 300 nM) accompanied by graded glutamate release. It should be emphasized, however, that Ca^{2+} photolysis is an approach mimicking neither the spatiotemporal nor the mechanistic properties of $[Ca^{2+}]_i$ elevations elicited via endogenous mechanisms. Results obtained by this approach, therefore, should be considered with caution.

In an alternative approach (Pasti et al., 2001), application of a glutamate analog was shown to induce $[Ca^{2+}]_i$ elevations, either oscillations or single spikes followed by plateaus, in astrocytes cocultured with snifer cells (see the section "Quantal Properties of Astrocyte Glutamate Release"). Oscillations exceeding 500 nM (measured as $[Ca^{2+}]_i$ peak at the soma) almost always were accompanied by episodes of glutamate release, whereas oscillations of lower amplitude often failed to induce any release. With the peak-plateau signal, release was observed. However, it was associated only with the initial peak, with no response during the plateau. When studied as cell-averaged $[Ca^{2+}]_i$ elevation, the threshold for glutamate release in response to physiological stimuli therefore seems higher than that reported by Parpura and Haydon (2000). Moreover, the stimulus-secretion coupling of astrocytes appears to operate not according to a stereotyped mode, but rather depending on the amplitude and spatiotemporal properties of $[Ca^{2+}]_i$ transients, which in turn depend on the kinetics of the underlying signaling mechanisms.

ROLE IN PHYSIOLOGY AND PATHOLOGY

The role that regulated secretion from astrocytes plays in brain physiology is still little understood. An interesting exception concerns the control of cholinergic transmission in the mollusk *Lymnea stagnalis* (Smit et al., 2001). Glial cells respond to presynaptic release of acetylcholine by releasing their acetylcholine-binding protein into the synaptic cleft (see the section "Neurosecretory Organelles"). The protein acts as a scavenger of the neuronally released transmitter, thus inducing a progressive depression of synaptic transmission. In the case of glutamate, both the homeostasis of the transmitter and the cellular effects are more complex. At astrocytes, the released glutamate pool, regardless of its astrocytic or neuronal origin, acts by activation of specific glutamatergic receptors (group I mGlu receptors, leading to generation of IP_3 and $[Ca^{2+}]_i$ rise; ionotropic AMPA receptors). By acting on neighboring astrocytes, these events could induce regenerative waves of glutamate release and sustain long-range communication events in the glial network (Innocenti et al., 2000). As far as neurons are concerned, glutamate released from astrocytes may have various effects. Studies in cell cultures demonstrate the potential of the astrocyte pool to affect both neuronal excitability and synaptic transmission. Thus, the astrocyte-released glutamate evokes slow inward currents and stimulates spontaneous synaptic transmission by enhancing the frequency of miniature postsynaptic currents (mPSCs) in cocultured hippocampal neurons. When, in contrast, release from astrocytes was induced while synaptic activity was evoked, the postsynaptic current (PSC) responses were reduced, independently of whether synapses were excitatory or inhibitory. These two distinct modulatory effects have been explained by the interaction of astrocyte-released glutamate with neuronal receptors of distinct type and localization: presynaptic mGlu receptors for the reduction of evoked PSCs; NMDA receptors, probably located extrasynaptically in the presynaptic neuron, for the enhancement of mPSC frequency (Araque et al., 1998a, 1998b). Studies in hippocampal and thalamic slices confirm that astrocyte-released glutamate can activate neuronal ionotropic receptors, particularly the NMDA receptors, generating inward currents and $[Ca^{2+}]_i$ increases (Pasti et al., 1997; Bezzi et al., 1998; Parri et al., 2001). During brain development, astrocyte-derived inputs could play a role in neuronal maturation, in the strengthening of synaptic connections, and in the establishment of neuronal pathways. Studies performed with acutely isolated retinas demonstrate that Ca^{2+} waves, mechanically evoked in glial cells, modulate photoreceptor-induced ganglion cell activity (Newman and Zahs, 1998). Even if the mechanisms involved in these effects are probably multiple, sensitivity to AMPA and NMDA receptor antagonists suggests that glial glutamatergic transmission is implicated in the modulation of retinal integration. Moreover, release of glutamate from astrocytes was proposed to participate in a form of synaptic plasticity of the CA1 hippocamapal pyramidal cells (Kang et al., 1998). In this system, stimulation of GABAergic interneurons elevates astrocytic Ca^{2+} and leads to a long-term facilitation of the interneuron-pyramidal cell synapse (documented by the enhancement of miniature inhibitory post-synaptic current (mIPSC) frequency), an effect blocked by ionotropic glutamate receptor antagonists. Taken together, the present results suggest that glutamate release from astrocytes, in coordination with neuronal glutamate release, may take part in a variety of fundamental processes of brain physiology.

Glutamate has a role not only in physiology but also in pathology. Excess extracellular neurotransmitter is known in fact to participate in the development of neurotoxicity, a basic process of brain lesions. Studies by Bezzi et al. (2001) have demonstrated that neurotoxicity in neuronal dysfunction can be accompanied by alterations of astrocyte stimulus-secretion coupling. The severity of these alterations depends on the synergistic interactions between astrocytes and microglia, the macrophagic brain cells established at reactive foci of brain infection or injury. The mechanisms of this synergism rely on the complex regulation of glutamate release from astrocytes, stimulated by $[Ca^{2+}]_i$ rises and greatly potentiated by the cytokine TNFα, released autocrinally by the cell (see the section "Astrocyte Stimulation"). Following activation of $[Ca^{2+}]_i$-raising receptors such as the chemokine CXCR4, which are expressed by both astrocytes and microglial cells, TNFα is released from both cell types and reaches high levels, strongly potentiating the release of astrocytic glutamate, which can become excitotoxic for the surrounding neurons. Whether the concentration of chemokines or other receptor agents in the brain rises high enough to trigger the above sequence of events is unknown. Unfortunately, however, CXCR4 is activated not only by its physiological agonist but also by human immunodeficiency virus-1 (HIV-1) coat protein, gp120, and by the HIV-1 progeny virions released in the brain of acquired immune deficiency syndrome (AIDS) patients by infected microglial cells (Zheng et al., 1999; reviewed by Kaul et al., 2001). Therefore, although neurons are not directly infected by the virus, they appear to undergo excitotoxicity sustained by HIV-dependent activation of CXCR4 and ensuing release of glutamate by astrocytes. This might be one of the mechanisms by which AIDS dementia is established in a considerable fraction of HIV patients (Bezzi et al., 2001).

PRESENT CONCLUSIONS AND ONGOING DEVELOPMENTS

A large body of converging evidence strongly suggests the existence in astrocytes of the quantal transmitter release process. Ongoing developments are providing further support for this conclusion and may ultimately clarify aspects of the issue that now remain unclear.

The first and most worrying such aspect is that so far, almost all studies have been performed with astrocyte cultures, where properties of the cells are known to be influenced by the *in vitro* conditions and may change with time (Maienschein et al., 1999). At the moment, only indirect evidence exists of glutamate exocytosis from astrocytes *in situ* (Bezzi et al., 1998, 2001). In addition, astrocytes have often been considered as a homogeneous population in terms of transmitter release, in spite of their clear heterogeneity observed, for example, in cultures from the hippocampus with respect to those from the cerebral and cerebellar cortices (e.g., see Calegari et al., 1999). Therefore, studies on cultures need to be extended to tissues from various areas of the brain and to specific neuron-glia circuits. Characterization of the elusive glutamate-containing vesicles in tissue astrocytes is underway by post-embedding immunogold electron microscopy addressed to specific markers, in particular the expanding family of vesicular glutamate transporters (VGLUTs), today comprising three molecular isoforms. Indeed at least one of these isoforms, VGLUT3, is known to be expressed not only by neurons but also by subsets of tissue astrocytes (Fremeau et al., 2002). The other two, VGLUT1 and VGLUT2, have been recently detected in

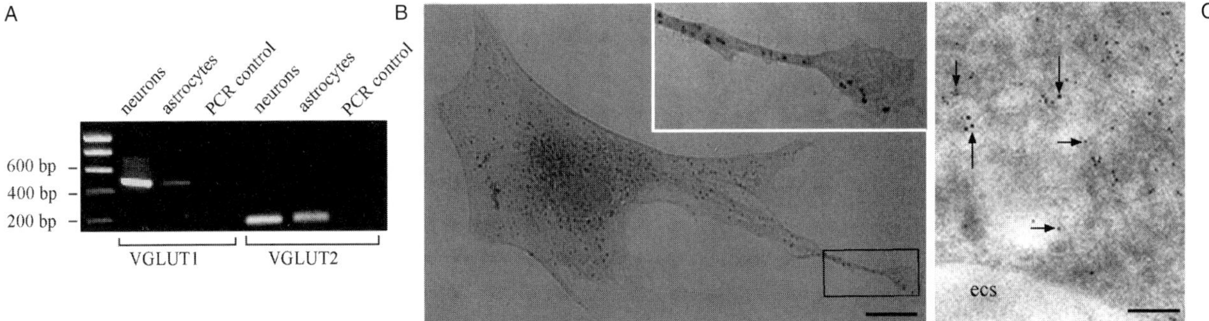

FIGURE 14.1 Vesicular glutamate transporters (VGLUT) are expressed in cultured astrocytes: cellular and ultrastructural localization. *A*. Vesicular glutamate transporter-1 (VGLUT1) and VGLUT2 mRNAs are present in cultured neurons and astrocytes from the rat cerebral cortex. PCR: polymerase chain reaction. *B*. Immunoperoxidase staining of VGLUT2 reveals a punctate pattern in the cell body, along the cell boundaries, and in the processes (*inset*). Bar: 20 μm. C. Ultrastructural localization of VGLUT1 (small gold particles, some indicated by *short arrows*) and VGLUT2 (large gold particles, *long arrows*) in a cell process. Particles label to groups of faintly appearing, small, clear vesicular organelles near the plasma membrane. Ecs: extracellular space. Bar: 100 nm. (Parts *A*, *B*, and *C* are courtesy of Drs. J.L. Galbete, E. Pilati, and V. Gundersen, respectively.)

cultured astrocytes (Fig. 14.1). According to ultrastructural immunogold labeling, they appear to be located in clear synaptic-like vesicular organelles (about 30 nanometers). Importantly, VGLUT1 and VGLUT2 labeling associated with similar vesicle-like structures is found also in thin astrocytic processes ensheathing excitatory synapses in the intact hippocampus (Bezzi et al., 2004).

Other aspects of astrocyte secretion remain undefined even in cell cultures. One is the cell biological and dynamic properties of astrocytic transmitter release vesicles. Very little is known about their biogenesis, intracellular transport, and precise intracellular distribution; about the possible existence of multiple pools (as in neurons); or about release sites, rates of exocytosis and endocytosis, and so on. This is true both for SLMVs that release glutamate (Bezzi et al., 2004) and for DCGs containing secretogranin II (Calegari et al., 1999), ATP (Coco et al., 2003), and probably several other proteins (Lafon-Cazal et al., 2003).

Another issue is the molecular identity and functional properties of the components in the exocytic machinery, also in relation to the specificity of the astrocyte process with respect to its neuronal counterpart. A well-known property of various SNARE isoforms is their ability to replace each other. It is therefore possible that two homologous SNARE proteins, for example SNAP25 and SNAP23, both play a role in astrocyte exocytosis, depending on their level of expression. Also, VAMP2 and cellubrevin are both expressed in cultured astrocytes, and future studies will clarify whether they play distinct or interchangeable roles.

Even more complex is the situation of synaptotagmins, a family of proteins believed to work as Ca^{2+} sensors that includes multiple isoforms of different Ca^{2+} affinity, located both in the membrane of vesicles and in the presynaptic membrane (Sugita et al., 2002). In astrocyte cultures, immunocytochemistry has revealed the expression of synaptotagmin I (Maienschein et al., 1999), the same isoform localized in neuronal synaptic vesicles and DCG. In the latter organelles, however, Ca^{2+} binding by synaptotagmin is known to be of low affinity, taking place at the very high $[Ca^{2+}]_i$ domains generated by activation of voltage-gated Ca^{2+} channels strategically located close to vesicle fusion sites (Sugita et al., 2002). In astrocytes, where vesicle exocytosis is mostly activated by Ca^{2+} release from the internal stores, the sensor is likely to be of higher affinity. Whether this role is played by another synaptotagmin isoform, by synaptotagmin I associated with a regulatory protein, or by another type of Ca^{2+}-sensing mechanism remains to be determined.

Dynamic imaging approaches appear particularly promising for answering the above questions. By allowing visualization of single vesicles, they will help to directly demonstrate transmitter exocytosis, generating information about the kinetics of SLMV and DCG fusions. Toward these goals, Krzan et al. (2003) have recently used confocal microscopy and atrial natriuretic peptide fused to emerald green fluorescent protein

A

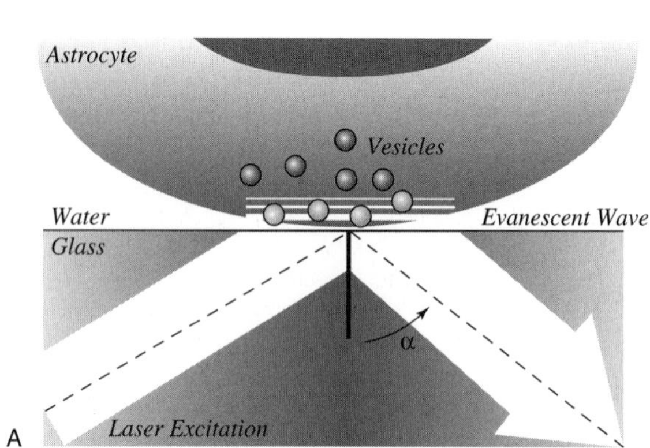

B

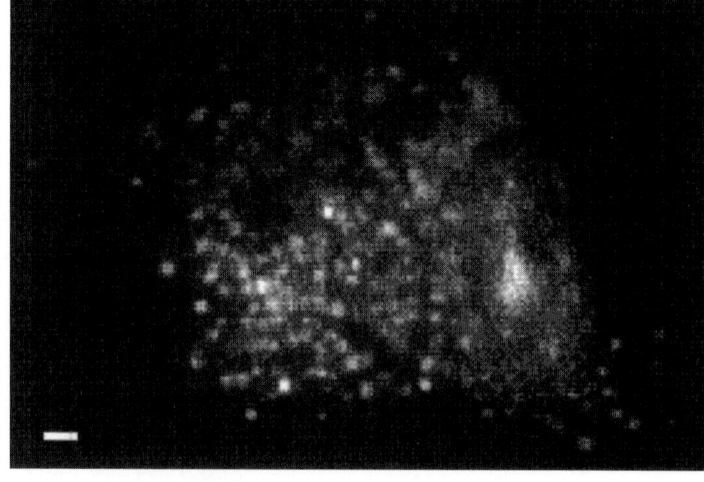

FIGURE 14.2 Studying glutamate vesicle dynamics in astrocytes by total internal reflection fluorescence (TIRF) microscopy. *A*. The principle of TIRF microscopy: a laser beam (white) undergoes total internal reflection at the interface between two media with different refractive indexes (glass and water/cell environment) when the angle of incidence, α, exceeds a critical value. As a consequence, a thin zone of electromagnetic energy, called an *evanescent wave*, (white lines), is generated in the medium with a lower refractive index (water/cell environment). Such a wave, typically on the order of tens to hundreds of nanometers, can selectively excite fluorophores present very close to the glass surface. In this case, an astrocyte has been transfected with a vesicular glutamate transporter (VGLUT)-enhanced green fluorescent protein (EGFP) chimeric protein, which highlights vesicles (bright dots) when excited at 488 nm (see *B*). *B*. The TIRF image reveals a homogeneous population of VGLUT-expressing vesicles (bright dots) present just beneath the plasma membrane of a cultured astrocyte. Bar: 1 μm. (Courtesy of Dr. P. Bezzi.)

(EGFP) to approach the study of peptide-containing organelles, most likely DCGs, while Volterra's group has fused with EGFP a VGLUT expressed by cultured astrocytes. As shown in Figure 14.2, VGLUT-EGFP labels in astrocytes a population of vesicular organelles, most likely SLMVs, whose dynamics is being studied in real time by total internal reflection fluorescence (TIRF) microscopy (Bezzi et al., 2004). This is a recent advance in fluorescence imaging technology that allows focusing on cellular events occurring within tens to hundreds of nanometers from the plasma membrane (see Fig. 14.2). This approach is therefore ideal for studying the dynamics of the various steps of exocytosis (transport, docking, fusion) at the level of individual vesicles. In addition, TIRF has important advantages over classical confocal microscopy, including higher temporal resolution and longer-lasting monitoring of events (Steyer and Almers, 2001). An additional approach, fluorescence resonance energy transfert (FRET) imaging, is being used to investigate dynamic and molecular aspects of the SNARE core complex assembly (Parpura and Hwang, 2002). Cyan and yellow GFPs fused to the N termini of SNAP-23 and VAMP2, respectively, have been coexpressed in astrocytes. When secretion is stimulated with a calcium ionophore, an increase in the FRET signal indicates a molecular interaction between the two SNAREs, with assembly of the complex. This approach appears appropriate to answer questions related to the specificity of SNAREs and the precise role in the exocytic fusion of the various members of the SNARE core complex and of their modulatory proteins.

In conclusion, until a few years ago, definition of astrocytes according to our present knowledge would have been considered a paradox: a "nonexcitable" cell that, however, is competent for neurotransmitter release, a function usually envisaged as strictly dependent on excitability. Indeed, astrocytes may well be considered excitable cells, except that their excitability exhibits properties distinct from those of neurons, neurosecretory cells, and muscle cells, being based on chemical rather than electrical signals. As a whole, astrocyte signaling appears more complex and elaborate than that operating in typical nonexcitable cells (e.g. fibroblasts, epithelial cells) since, in addition to active stimulus-secretion coupling via receptors, intracellular Ca^{2+} stores, messengers, and kinases, it relies on numerous extracellular messengers and on synergistic interactions with microglia and neurons. The peculiar aspects of astrocyte signaling have not been investigated in detail in other types of cells. Comparative studies of astrocyte/nonastrocyte cells may therefore increase understanding of new, important aspects of cell function and intercellular communication that at the moment remain obscure or incompletely known, both in the normal and in the diseased brain.

ACKNOWLEDGMENTS

The original work presented in this chapter was supported by grants from the European Community (QLK6-CT1999-02203 and QLRT-200-02233), OFES (00.0553), FNRS (3100A0-100850/1), MIUR-Italy (Cofin 2000-01 and 053389_003, and FIRB), and ISS-Italy (National Programs on Alzheimer's Disease and AIDS).

REFERENCES

Akopian, G., Kressin, K., Derouiche, A., and Steinhauser, C. (1996) Identified glial cells in the early postnatal mouse hippocampus display different types of Ca^{2+} currents. *Glia* 17:181–194.

Anlauf, E. and Derouiche, A. (2002) Exocytosis markers label glutamate-containing vesicles in cultured astrocytes. *Glia* Suppl. 1:S33.

Araque, A., Li, N., Doyle, R.T., and Haydon, P.G. (2000) SNARE protein-dependent glutamate release from astrocytes. *J. Neurosci.* 20:666–673.

Araque, A., Parpura, V., Sanzgiri, R.P., and Haydon, P.G. (1998a) Glutamate-dependent astrocyte modulation of synaptic transmission between cultured hippocampal neurons. *Eur. J. Neurosci.* 10:2129–2142.

Araque, A., Sanzgiri, R.P., Parpura, V., and Haydon, P.G. (1998b) Calcium elevation in astrocytes causes an NMDA receptor-dependent increase in the frequency of miniature synaptic currents in cultured hippocampal neurons. *J. Neurosci.* 18:6822–6829.

Bal-Price, A., Moneer, Z., and Brown, G.C. (2002) Nitric oxide induces rapid, calcium-dependent release of vesicular glutamate and ATP from cultured rat astrocytes. *Glia* 40:312–323.

Bezzi, P., Carmignoto, G., Pasti, L., Vesce, S., Rossi, D., Lodi Rizzini, B., Pozzan, T., and Volterra, A. (1998) Prostaglandins stimulate calcium-dependent glutamate release in astrocytes. *Nature* 391: 281–285.

Bezzi, P., Domercq, M., Brambilla, L., Galli, R., Schols, D., De Clercq, E., Vescovi, A., Bagetta, G., Kollias, G., Meldolesi, J., and Volterra, A. (2001) CXCR4-activated astrocyte glutamate release via TNFα: amplification by microglia triggers neurotoxicity. *Nat. Neurosci.* 4:702–710.

Bezzi, P., Gravaghi, C., Grohovaz, F., and Volterra, A. (1999) Cyclooxygenase activity is critical for $[Ca^{2+}]_i$ elevation leading to glutamate release in astrocytes in response to neuroligands. *SFN Annual Meeting Abs.* Program n. 600.5, pp. 1506.

Bezzi, P., Gundersen, V., Galbete, J.L., Seifert G., Steinhäuser C., Pilati, E., and Volterra, A. (2004) Astrocytes contain a vesicular compartment competent for regulated exocytosis of glutamate. *Nat. Neurosci.*, in press.

Borgonovo, B., Cocucci, E., Racchetti, G., Podini, P., Bachi, A., and Meldolesi, J. (2002) Regulated exocytosis: a novel, widely expressed system. *Nat. Cell Biol.* 4:955–962.

Calegari, F., Coco, S., Taverna, E., Bassetti, M., Verderio, C., Corradi, N., Matteoli, M., and Rosa, P. (1999) A regulated secretory pathway in cultured hippocampal astrocytes. *J. Biol. Chem.* 274: 22539–22547.

Carmignoto, G., Pasti, L., and Pozzan, T. (1998) On the role of voltage-dependent calcium channels in calcium signaling of astrocytes in situ. *J. Neurosci.* 18:4637–4645.

Coco, S., Calegari, F., Pravettoni, E., Pozzi, D., Taverna, E., Rosa, P., Matteoli, M., and Verderio, C. (2003) Storage and release of ATP from astrocytes in culture. *J. Biol. Chem.* 278:1354–1362.

Coorssen, J.R., Schmitt, H., and Almers, W. (1996) Ca^{2+} triggers massive exocytosis in Chinese hamster ovary cells. *EMBO J.* 15:3787–3791.

Dan, Y. and Poo, M-M. (1992) Quantal transmitter secretion from myocytes loaded with acetylcholine. *Nature* 359:733–736.

Duan, S., Anderson, C.M., Keung, E.C., Chen, Y., Chen, Y., and

Swanson, R.A. (2003) $P2X_7$ receptor-mediated release of excitatory amino acids from astrocytes. *J. Neurosci.* 23:1320–1328.

Fischer-Colbrie, R., Kirchmair, R., Schobert, A., Olenik, C., Meyer, D.K., and Winkler, H. (1993) Secretogranin II is synthesized and secreted in astrocyte cultures. *J. Neurochem.* 60:2312–2314.

Fremeau, R.T., Jr., Burman, J., Qureshi, T., Tran, C.H., Proctor, J., Johnson, J., Zhang, H., Sulzer, D., Copenhagen, D.R., Storm-Mathisen, J., Reimer, R.J., Chaudhry, F.A., and Edwards, R.H. (2002) The identification of vesicular glutamate transporter 3 suggests novel modes of signaling by glutamate. *Proc. Natl. Acad. Sci. USA* 99:14488–14493.

Hepp, R., Perraut, M., Chasserot-Golaz, S., Galli, T., Aunis, D., Langley, K., and Grant, N.J. (1999) Cultured glial cells express the SNAP-25 analogue SNAP-23. *Glia* 27:181–187.

Herzog, E., Bellenchi, G.C., Gras, C., Bernard, V., Ravassard, P., Bedet, C., Gasnier, B., Giros, B., and El Mestikawy, S. (2001) The existence of a second vesicular glutamate transporter specifies subpopulations of glutamatergic neurons. *J. Neurosci.* 21:RC181.

Humeau, Y., Doussau, F., Grant, N.J., and Poulain, B. (2000) How botulinum and tetanus neurotoxins block neurotransmitter release. *Biochimie* 82:427–446.

Hussy, N., Deleuze, C., Desarménien, M.G., and Moos, F.C. (2000) Osmotic regulation of neuronal activity: a new role for taurine and glial cells in a hypothalamic neuroendocrine structure. *Prog. Neurobiol.* 62:113–134.

Innocenti, B., Parpura, V., and Haydon, P.G. (2000) Imaging extracellular waves of glutamate during calcium signaling in cultured astrocytes. *J. Neurosci.* 20:1800–1806.

Jahn, R., Lang, T., and Sudhof, T.C. (2003) Membrane fusion. *Cell* 112:519–533.

Jeftinija, S.D., Jeftinija, K.V., and Stefanovic, G. (1997) Cultured astrocytes express proteins involved in vesicular glutamate release. *Brain Res.* 750:41–47.

Jeftinija, S.D., Jeftinija, K.V., Stefanovic, G., and Liu, F. (1996) Neuroligand-evoked calcium-dependent release of excitatory amino acids from cultured astrocytes. *J. Neurochem.* 66:676–684.

Jeremic, A., Jeftinija, K., Stevanovic, J., Glavaski, A., and Jeftinija, S. (2001) ATP stimulates calcium-dependent glutamate release from cultured astrocytes. *J. Neurochem.* 77:664–675

Kang, J., Jiang, L., Goldman, S.A., and Nedergaard, M. (1998) Astrocyte-mediated potentiation of inhibitory synaptic transmission. *Nat. Neurosci.* 1:683–692.

Kasai, H., Kishimoto, T., Liu, T.T., Miyashita, Y., Podini, P., Grohovaz, F., and Meldolesi, J. (1999) Multiple and diverse forms of regulated exocytosis in wild-type and defective PC12 cells. *Proc. Natl. Acad. Sci. USA* 96:945–949.

Kaul, M., Garden, G.A., and Lipton, S.A. (2001) Pathways to neuronal injury and apoptosis in HIV-associated dementia. *Nature* 410:988–994.

Keller, P. and Simons, K. (1997) Post-Golgi biosynthetic trafficking. *J. Cell Sci.* 110:3001–3009.

Kimelberg, H.K., Goderie, S.K., Higman, S., Pang, S., and Waniewski, R.A. (1990) Swelling-induced release of glutamate, aspartate, and taurine from astrocyte cultures. *J. Neurosci.* 10:1583–1591.

Kimelberg, H.K. and Mongin, A.A. (1998) Swelling-activated release of excitatory amino acids in the brain: relevance for pathophysiology. *Contrib. Nephrol.* 123:240–257.

Krzan, M., Stenovec, M., Kreft, M., Pangrsic, T., Grilc, S., Haydon, P.G., and Zorec, R. (2003) Calcium-dependent exocytosis of atrial natriuretic peptide from astrocytes. *J. Neurosci.* 23:1580–1583.

Lafon-Cazal, M., Adjali, O., Galeotti, N., Poncet, J., Jouin, P., Homburger, V., Bockaert, J., and Marin, P. (2003) Proteomic analysis of astrocytic secretion in the mouse. Comparison with the cerebrospinal fluid proteome. *J. Biol. Chem.* 278:24438–24448.

Madison, D.L., Kruger, W.H., Kim, T., and Pfeiffer, S.E. (1996) Differential expression of rab3 isoforms in oligodendrocytes and astrocytes. *J. Neurosci. Rev.* 45:258–268.

Maienschein, V., Marxen, M., Volknandt, W., and Zimmermann, H. (1999) A plethora of presynaptic proteins associated with ATP-storing organelles in cultured astrocytes. *Glia* 26:233–244.

Mongin, A.A. and Kimelberg, H.K. (2002) ATP potently modulates anion channel-mediated excitatory amino acid release from cultured astrocytes. *Am. J. Physiol. Cell Physiol.* 283:C569–C578.

Morimoto, T., Popov, S., Buckley, K.M., and Poo, M.-M. (1995) Calcium-dependent transmitter secretion from fibroblasts: modulation by synaptotagmin I. *Neuron* 15:689–696.

Nedergaard, M., Takano, T., and Hansen, A.J. (2002) Beyond the role of glutamate as a neurotransmitter. *Nat. Rev. Neurosci.* 3:748–754.

Nett, W.J., Oloff, S.H., and McCarthy, K.D. (2002) Hippocampal astrocytes in situ exhibit calcium oscillations that occur independent of neuronal activity. *J. Neurophysiol.* 87:528–537.

Newman, E.A. and Zahs, K.R. (1998) Modulation of neuronal activity by glial cells in the retina. *J. Neurosci.* 18:4022–4028.

Ninomiya, Y., Kishimoto, T., Miyashita, Y., and Kasai, H. (1996) Ca^{2+}-dependent exocytotic pathways in Chinese Hamster Ovary fibroblasts revealed by a caged-Ca^{2+} compound. *J. Biol. Chem.* 271:17751–17754.

Parpura, V., Basarsky, T.A., Liu, F., Jeftinija, K., Jeftinija, S., and Haydon, P.G. (1994) Glutamate-mediated astrocyte-neuron signalling. *Nature* 369:744–747.

Parpura, V., Fang, Y., Basarsky, T., Jahn, R., and Haydon, P.G. (1995a) Expression of synaptobrevin II, cellubrevin and syntaxin but not SNAP-25 in cultured astrocytes. *FEBS Lett.* 377:489–492.

Parpura, V. and Haydon, P.G. (2000) Physiological astrocytic calcium levels stimulate glutamate release to modulate adjacent neurons. *Proc. Natl. Acad. Sci. USA* 97:8629–8634.

Parpura, V. and Hwang, H.J. (2002) Imaging of SNARE complexes in cultured astrocytes. *Biophys. J. Ann. Meeting Abstr.* 82:11a.

Parpura, V., Liu, F., Brethorst, S., Jeftinija, K., Jeftinija, S., and Haydon, P.G. (1995b) α-Latrotoxin stimulates glutamate release from cortical astrocytes in cell culture. *FEBS Lett.* 360:266–270.

Parri, H.R., Gould, T.M., and Crunelli, V. (2001) Spontaneous astrocytic Ca^{2+} oscillations in situ drive NMDA receptor-mediated neuronal excitation. *Nat. Neurosci.* 4:803–812.

Pascual, M., Climent, E., and Guerri, C. (2001) BDNF induces glutamate release in cerebrocortical terminals and in cortical astrocytes. *NeuroReport* 12:2673–2677.

Pasti, L., Volterra, A., Pozzan, T., and Carmignoto, G. (1997) Intracellular calcium oscillations in astrocytes: a highly plastic, bidirectional form of communication between neurons and astrocytes *in situ*. *J. Neurosci.* 17:7817–7830.

Pasti, L., Zonta, M., Pozzan, T., Vicini, S., and Carmignoto, G. (2001) Cytosolic calcium oscillations in astrocytes may regulate exocytotic release of glutamate. *J. Neurosci.* 21:477–484.

Rosenthal, L. and Meldolesi, J. (1989) Alpha-latrotoxin and related toxins. *Pharmacol. Ther.* 42:115–134.

Rossi, D.J., Oshima, T., and Attwell, D. (2000) Glutamate release in severe brain ischemia is mainly by reversed uptake. *Nature* 403:316–321.

Sanzgiri, R.P., Araque, A., and Haydon, P.G. (1999) Prostaglandin E_2 stimulates glutamate receptor-dependent astrocyte neuromodulation in cultured hippocampal cells. *J. Neurobiol.* 41:221–229.

Schiavo, G., Matteoli, M., and Montecucco, C. (2000) Neurotoxins affecting neuroexocytosis. *Physiol. Rev.* 80:717–766.

Smit, A.B., Syed, N.I., Schaap, D., van Minnen, J., Klumperman, J., Kits, K.S., Lodder, H., van der Schors, R.C., van Elk, R., Sorgedrager, B., Brejc, K., Sixma, T.K., and Geraerts, W.P.M. (2001) A glia-derived acethylcholine-binding protein that modulates synaptic transmission. *Nature* 411:261–268.

Steyer, J.A. and Almers, W. (2001) A real-time view of life within

100 nm of the plasma membrane. *Nat. Rev. Mol. Cell Biol.* 2:268–275.

Sudhof, T.C. (2001) Alpha-latrotoxin and its receptors: neurexins and CIRL/latrophilins. *Annu. Rev. Neurosci.* 24:933–962.

Sugita, S., Shin, O.H., Han, W., Lao, Y., and Sudhof, T.C. (2002) Synaptotagmins form a hierarchy of exocytotic Ca^{2+} sensors with distinct Ca^{2+} affinities. *EMBO J.* 21:270–280.

Szatkovski, M., Barbour, B., and Attwell, D. (1990) Non-vesicular release of glutamate from glial cells by reversed electrogenic glutamate uptake. *Nature* 348:443–446.

Takamori, S., Rhee, J.S., Rosenmund, C., and Jahn, R. (2000) Identification of a vesicular glutamate transporter that defines a glutamatergic phenotype in neurons. *Nature* 407:189–194.

Verderio, C., Coco, S., Rossetto, O., Montecucco, C., and Matteoli, M. (1999) Internalization and proteolytic action of botulinum toxins in CNS neurons and astrocytes. *J. Neurochem.* 73:372–379.

Volterra, A., Magistretti, P.J., and Haydon, P.G. (eds.). (2002) *The Tripartite Synapse: Glia in Synaptic Transmission.* Oxford: Oxford University Press. pp. 282.

Ye, Z.C., Wyeth, M.S., Baltan-Tekkok, S., and Ransom, B.R. (2002) Functional hemichannels in astrocytes: a novel mechanism of glutamate release. *J. Neurosci.* 23:3588–3596.

Yuan, L-L. and Ganetzky, B. (1999) A glial-neuronal signaling pathway revealed by mutations in a neurexin-related protein. *Science* 283:1343–1345.

Zakharenko, S., Chang, S., O'Donoghue, M., and Popov, S.V. (1999) Neurotransmitter secretion along growing nerve processes: comparison with synaptic vesicle exocytosis. *J. Cell Biol.* 144:507–518.

Zheng, J., Ghorpade, A., Niemann, D., Cotter, R.L., Thylin, M.R., Epstein, L., Swartz, J.M., Shepard, R.B., Liu, X., Nukuna, A., and Gendelman, H.E. (1999) Lymphotropic virions affect chemokine receptor-mediated neural signaling and apoptosis: implications for human immunodeficiency virus type 1-associated dementia. *J. Virol.* 73:8256–8267.

15 Enzymes of carbohydrate and energy metabolism

BERND HAMPRECHT, STEPHAN VERLEYSDONK, AND HEINRICH WIESINGER

The present update on enzymes of carbohydrate and energy metabolism in glial cells has its foundation in two chapters of the first edition of this handbook (Hamprecht and Dringen, 1995; Wiesinger, 1995). The enzymes covered are (*1*) those involved in the metabolism of the carbohydrates glucose and glycogen, (*2*) the carboanhydrase isoforms dealing with the CO_2 generated in oxidative metabolism of these carbohydrates, and (*3*) those of cellular energization. The last comprise creatine kinase, carnitine palmitoyltransferase, and ion-transporting adenosine triphosphatases (ATPases), especially Na^+, K^+-ATPase. Table 15.1 provides an overview of the enzymes covered in this chapter, and of the metabolic engagement of these enzymes. Naturally, such an overview cannot be complete. Many enzymes were left out since they occur more or less ubiquitously or their assignment to brain cell types is not sufficiently developed.

Since the first edition of this handbook, experimental approaches to the allocation of enzymes to cell types have been refined, in particular using techniques of image analysis such as high-resolution laser-scanning microscopy. On the other hand, underlying principles such as immunohistochemistry, immunocytochemistry, and *in situ* hybridization in cell culture or tissue have not been abandoned. However, the gain in sensitivity rewards those who have to cope with the difficult task of proving the absence of enzyme expression from a specific cell type. One particular technique, the generation of transgenic animals and the possibility of cell type–specific deletion of a protein, is enhancing our knowledge about the functional implications of enzyme expression in a certain cell type and not in others. It is important to point out the increasing evidence for the necessity to interprete mRNA abundance data with great caution since translational control mechanisms may prevent the synthesis of protein despite the existence of ample mRNA. Thus, the appearance of a certain mRNA is not a sufficient criterion for expression of the corresponding gene and therefore cannot be equated with gene expression.

ENZYMES OF CARBOHYDRATE METABOLISM

Enzymes of Glucose Metabolism

Focus will be on enzymes of the three main pathways of glucose metabolism: glycolysis, the pentose phosphate pathway, and gluconeogenesis. Of these, glycolysis is the paradigm household pathway and, therefore, is expected to be present in practically all mammalian cells. Thus, if brain cells were to differ qualitatively in the expression of individual glycolytic enzymes, they could differ from each other only by using different isoforms of a given enzyme (isozyme).

Glycolytic enzymes

In mammals the introductory enzyme of the glycolytic pathway, hexokinase, exists in four isoforms, types I–IV (Wilson, 1995, 2003). Using immunocytochemical techniques, two of the isoforms, types I and III, have been definitely shown to occur in brain (Preller and Wilson, 1992). Type I can exist as cytosolic enzyme and can be bound to porin of the outer mitochondrial membrane (Wilson, 1983, 1997) and to tubulin (Wagner et al., 2001). There it has direct access to mitochondrially generated adenosine triphosphate (ATP) and cannot use cytosolic ATP (de Cerqueira Cesar and Wilson, 1998). It has been clearly detected in neurons and astrocytes of various brain regions (Wilkin and Wilson, 1977), in ventricular ependymal cells and in choroid plexus cells (Wilkin and Wilson, 1977), but hardly in oligodendrocytes (Kao-Jen and Wilson, 1980). In this context, it is amazing that the corresponding mRNA could not be detected in ependymal cells by *in situ* hybridization (Jacobsson and Meister, 1994). Also, the muscle isozyme of hexokinase, isoform type II, might be associated with the nervous system. At least in cultured astroglial cells it is induced by deprivation of glucose (Niitsu et al., 1999). The assignment of type III to certain cell types of the brain parenchyma has turned out to be difficult, with the exception of

TABLE 15.1 *Alphabetical List of the Enzymes Covered and Their Occurrence in Neural Cell Types*

ENZYME			*Occurrence in Neural Cell Type*	*Reference(s) Providing Access to Literature*
Name	*Isoform*	*Action In*		
Aldolase	C	Carbohydrate metabolism (glycolysis)	A, N	Kumanishi et al. (1985)
Branching enzyme	—	Glycogen metabolism (synthesis)	(A)	Schröder et al. (1993)
Ca^{2+}-ATPase (plasma membrane-bound)	PMCA1	Cation transport	A	Fresu et al. (1999)
	PMCA2		A, N	Fresu et al. (1999)
	PMCA3		N	Fresu et al. (1999)
	PMCA4		A	Fresu et al. (1999)
Carbonic anhydrase	CA-I	Carbon dioxide metabolism	—	—
	CA-II (=CA-C)		A, CPC, (M), (N), O, P	Roussell et al. (1979) Cammer and Tansey (1987/1988); Ghandour et al. (1989), Agnati et al. (1995)
	CA-III		CPC, M	—
	CA-IV		—	—
	CA-VA		—	—
	CA-VB		A, N	Ghandour et al. (2000)
	CA-VI		—	—
	CA-VII		CPC, N	Lokkis et al. (1997)
	CA-IX		—	—
	CA-XII		—	—
	CA-XIV		N	Parkkila et al. (2001)
Carnitine palmitoyltransferase CPT1	—	Fatty acid metabolism	A	Blazquez et al. (1999)
Creatine kinase	CK-BB	Cellular energization	A	Hemmer et al. (1994)
	CK-MM		N	Hemmer et al. (1994)
	sMt-CK		N	Kaldis et al. (1996)
Enolase	γ	Carbohydrate metabolism (glycolysis)	A, N, O, S	Sensenbrenner et al. (1997)
Fructokinase	—	Carbohydrate metabolism (fructose metabolism)	—	Bergbauer et al. (1996)
Fructose-1,6-bisphosphatase	Liver type	Carbohydrate metabolism (gluconeogenesis)	A	Schmoll et al. (1995a)
Glucose-6-phosphatase	—	Carbohydrate metabolism (gluconeogenesis)	A	Bell et al. (1993)
Glucose-6-phosphate dehydrogenase	—	Carbohydrate metabolism (pentose phosphate pathway)	A, CPC, O, N, P, S	Philbert et al. (1991) Rust et al. (1991)
Glycogen phosphorylase	BB	Glycogen metabolism (degradation)	A, E, N	Pfeiffer-Guglielmi et al. (2003)
	MM		A	Pfeiffer-Guglielmi et al. (2003)
Glycogen synthase	B	Glycogen metabolism (synthesis)	A (mRNA), N (mRNA)	Pellegri et al. (1996)
Hexokinase	I	Carbohydrate metabolism (glycolysis)	A, CPC, E, N	Wilson (1995)
	II		A	Niitsu et al. (1999)
	III		CPC, E	Preller and Wilson (1992)
Lactate dehydrogenase	LDH1	Carbohydrate metabolism (glycolysis)	A, N	Poitry-Yamate et al. (1995)
	LDH5		A	Poitry-Yamate et al. (1995)
Na^+, K^+-ATPase	α_1	Cation transport	A, N	McGrail et al. (1991)
	α_2		A	McGrail et al. (1991), Peng et al. (1998)
	α_3		N	Wetzel et al. (1999)
	α_4		—	—
	β_1		A, N	Fink et al. (1996)
	β_2		A, N	Wetzel et al. (1999)
	β_3		O, N	Martin-Vasallo et al. (2000)
Phosphoprotein phosphatase/PTG	—	Glycogen metabolism (degradation, synthesis)	A	Allaman et al. (2000), Newgard et al. (2000)

TABLE 15.1 *Continued*

ENZYME			*Occurrence in Neural Cell Type*	*Reference(s) Providing Access to Literature*
Name	*Isoform*	*Action In*		
Phosphorylase kinase	Muscle	Glycogen metabolism (degradation)	A, E, N	Psarra et al. (1998)
Pyruvate carboxylase	—	Carbohydrate metabolism (gluconeogenesis)	A, P	Cesar and Hamprecht (1995), Miller et al. (2002)

Note. The arrangement of enzymes listed generally follows the sequence of their appearance in the text. In the column "Occurrence in Neural Cell Type" a letter in parentheses indicates that the expression of the enzyme in this cell type occurs in very few cells of this type or that the evidence for its presence is indirect, or that the enzyme is expressed in this cell type only transiently. A dash in this column stands for absence of the isoform from the CNS. A dash in the column "Isoform" indicates that there are no isoforms or that no information on isoforms was found. A dash in the "References" column means that provision of a reference is considered unimportant. When an older reference is presented in this column, it is recommended that the Science Citation Index be used to find the more recent literature that addresses various details. The references do not always refer to a particular isoform, but may refer to the enzyme without emphasizing an isoform.

A: astrocyte; CPC: choroid plexus cell; E: ependymal cell; M: microglial cell; N: neuron; O: oligodendrocyte; P: PNS satellite cell; PTG: protein targeting to glycogen; S: Schwann cell.

ventricular ependymal cells and choroid plexus cells, where the enzyme was clearly localized in the nuclear periphery (Preller and Wilson, 1992). More information is needed before this isoform can be considered as a marker for ependymal cells.

Aldolase C, an isoform of the fourth enzyme acting in the course of glycolysis, can be considered an isozyme restricted to the brain. There it is located in astrocytes and Purkinje cells, as shown immunocytochemically (Thompson et al., 1982; Kumanishi et al., 1985). The presence of the isozyme in astrocytes is supported by results of an *in situ* hybridization study focusing on aldolase C mRNA (Walther et al., 1998). It is important to note that subventricular zone cells of apparent astrocyte lineage already strongly express aldolase C at a stage when they do not yet contain glial fibrillary acidic protein (GFAP) or vimentin (Staugaitis et al., 2001). Consequently, the enzyme could be a valuable marker for such astrocyte precursor cells. On the other hand, such cellular markers must be used with caution, since it has been shown that the classical neuronal markers neuron-specific enolase (NSE; γ-enolase) and growth-associated protein 43 (GAP-43) are also transiently expressed, during development in culture and *in situ*, in oligodendroglial cells, astroglial cells, and Schwann cell precursors (Sensenbrenner et al., 1997).

Brain can also use mannose or fructose instead of glucose. While the former would be introduced into metabolism by hexokinase, the latter could choose principally between hexokinase and fructokinase. Since no brain cell contains fructokinase (Bergbauer et al., 1996), it is hexokinase that channels fructose into brain metabolism.

In skeletal muscle the glycolytic breakdown of glucose ends in the formation of lactate from the pyruvate and reduced nicotinamide adenine dinucleotide (NADH) that are generated in the course of the pathway. The enzyme catalyzing this reaction is one from the classical set of isozymes, that is lactate dehydrogenase (LDH). Isozyme LDH5 is typically expressed in tissues that very actively produce lactic acid from glucose. Therefore, it is also called the *muscle-type* isozyme. In contrast, isoform LDH1 is called the *heart-type* isozyme, since it is characteristic of tissues that consume lactic acid, such as the heart and the liver. By immunocytochemistry, neurons were found to contain only LDH1, while astrocytes contained both isoforms (Bittar et al., 1996). The authors interpreted this finding as support for the idea of lactate flux (Hamprecht and Dringen, 1995; Poitry-Yamate et al., 1995) from astrocytes to neurons (Dringen et al., 1993a; Tsacopoulos and Magistretti, 1996). The presence in astrocytes of LDH1 supports the notion that astrocytes, as well as glucose, also consume lactate, especially in glyconeogenesis (Hamprecht and Dringen, 1995).

Enzymes of the pentose phosphate pathway

As an alternative to entering glycolysis, glucose-6-phosphate can also serve as a substrate of the first enzyme of the oxidative part of the pentose phosphate pathway, glucose-6-phosphate dehydrogenase. Apparently this reduced nicotinamide adenine dinucleotide phosphate (NADPH)–generating enzyme that has no isoform is present in practically all cell types of the body, including all neural cells (Philbert et al., 1991; Rust et al., 1991). This is not surprising since NADPH-dependent reduction reactions are ubiquitous cellular requirements. Representative of these are the reduction of oxidized glutathione in the defense against reactive oxygen species, the biosynthesis of long-chain fatty acids and cholesterol for building up membranes, and the generation of deoxyribonucleotides as building blocks for DNA synthesis. Nevertheless, there are considerable quantitative differences in the level of expression of the enzyme, with oligodendrocytes especially abounding in this enzyme activity (Kugler, 1994).

Enzymes of gluconeogenesis

Glyconeogenesis is the *de novo* synthesis from gluconeogenic precursors of the glucosyl residues of glycogen. This pathway is identical to the sum of two pathways, gluconeogenesis to glucose-6-phosphate and the glycogen synthetic pathway starting with glucose-6-phosphate. The glyconeogenic pathway is used by astroglial cells in culture (Dringen et al., 1993b; Schmoll et al., 1995b; Bernard-Helary et al., 2002). In agreement therewith, two of the key gluconeogenic enzymes, pyruvate carboxylase (Cesar and Hamprecht, 1995) and fructose-1,6-bisphosphatase (Schmoll et al., 1995a), have been detected immunocytochemically in astrocytes but not in neurons, using antibodies against the enzymes isolated from liver. The presence, besides that of glutamine synthetase and glutamate dehydrogenase, of pyruvate carboxylase in peripheral nervous system (PNS) satellite cells of dorsal root ganglia (Miller et al., 2002) stresses the relatedness between these cells and central nervous system (CNS) astrocytes. Fructose-1,6-bisphosphatase exists in two isoforms, the muscle and the liver isotype. The mRNA of the muscle isotype, but not of the liver isotype, has been found in brain astrocytes by an *in situ* hybridization technique (Löffler et al., 2001). Lack of isozyme specificity of the antiserum raised against the liver enzyme was used as a convincing argument against a contradiction between the results from the *in situ* hybridization (Löffler et al., 2001) and the immunocytochemistry experiments (Schmoll et al., 1995a) as far as astrocytes are concerned. The former authors found the message for the liver isoform in neurons only. The corresponding protein was not found in brain neurons (Schmoll et al., 1995a). Also, this is no contradiction, since Löffler et al. (2001) did not try to demonstrate that the mRNA for the liver isoform was indeed translated in the neurons. Alternatively, the enzyme protein may be expressed so weakly in neurons that it could not be detected by the monoclonal antibody used (Schmoll et al., 1995a). The physiological function of astrocytic glyconeogenesis is seen in the removal of lactic acid released into the extracellular space by neurons that perform rapid anaerobic glycolysis as a consequence of high electrical activity. This disposition would prevent a local acidosis by transforming the carboxyl protons of lactic acid molecules into secondary alcohol protons of the glucosyl residues of glycogen (Hamprecht and Dringen, 1995; Schmoll et al., 1995b).

As the liver paradigm has shown, gluconeogenic activity could result principally in two products, free glucose or the glucosyl residues of glycogen. The idea has generally been found highly attractive that astrocytes provide gluconeogenically produced glucose to neighboring cells by engaging in a local Cori cycle with them. However, in spite of many efforts to prove it, the generation of free glucose by astrocytes has not been unequivocally demonstrated. The formation of free glucose hinges on the activity of the glucose-6-phosphatase system. In fact, the presence of glucose-6-phosphatase in brain and cultured astrocytes has been demonstrated by immunological techniques, and the corresponding enzyme activity was reported to be present in cultured astrocytes (Bell et al., 1993; Forsyth et al., 1993). More recently, however, a study carried out under somewhat different conditions virtually ruled out the presence of glucose-6-phosphatase in cultured astrocytes (Gotoh et al., 2000). Thus, the function of the glucose-6-phosphatase protein contained in astrocytes remains unclear. This is the more so, since a new isoform of the enzyme has been cloned from human brain mRNA (Guionie et al., 2003).

Enzymes of Glycogen Metabolism

Glycogen is a polycondensate of glucose and serves as glucose store with essentially no osmotic activity. Liver stores glycogen in an altruistic way mainly for the benefit of other tissues, since it contains glucose-6-phosphatase, which hydrolytically breaks down to glucose and phosphate, the glucose-6-phosphate emerging from glycogenolysis. The ensuing glucose is released into the bloodstream and transported to cells and tissues in need of glucose. Due to the lack of glucose-6-phosphatase, muscle uses in an egotistic way the glucose-6-phosphate resulting from degradation of glycogen for local generation of energy. Astrocytes appear to behave like muscle. They process glucose-6-phosphate in the glycolytic pathway to lactate with a net gain of 3 ATP per mol of glycogen-glucosyl residue. The resulting lactate they forward to other brain cells as valuable fuel material for the oxidative production of energy (Dringen et al., 1993a). It has turned out that there is also another purpose glycogen can serve in astrocytes. The glucose-6-phosphate derived from it enters the oxidative part of the pentose phosphate pathway to produce NADPH if NADP is available. This is the case under oxidative stress exerted by peroxides, since NADPH is consumed in regenerating reduced glutathione from oxidized glutathione (Rahman et al., 2000).

Enzymes of glycogen breakdown

The glycogen-degrading enzyme glycogen phosphorylase (GP) exists in three homodimeric isoforms: liver (LL), muscle (MM), and brain (BB) isozymes. They are closely related in their primary structures, the L chain having 80% sequence identity with the M and B chains and the B chain having 83% sequence identity with the M chain (Newgard et al., 1988). In the nervous system, immunoreactivity has been detected in Müller cells of the retina (Pfeiffer et al., 1994), in brain astrocytes, and in ependymal cells (for review see Hamprecht and Dringen, 1995; Wiesinger, 1995). It was also found in sensory neurons, but not in oligodendrocytes, microglial cells, or capillary endothelial cells (Pfeiffer et al., 1995; Richter et al., 1996). It has been known for more than a quarter century that brain contains two GP isoforms, the brain (fetal) type and the muscle type (Sato et al., 1976; Richter et al., 1983; Crerar et al., 1988), whereas the occurrence of the liver isoform has been reported by one laboratory (Crerar et al., 1988) but not by other laboratories (Sato et al., 1976; Richter et al., 1983). A more detailed analysis, including reverse transcriptase–polymerase chain reaction, confirmed the coexistence in brain of the brain and muscle isozymes (Pfeiffer-Guglielmi et al., 2000). The distribution of these isoforms in the glycogen-containing (Oksche 1958, 1961; Cavalcante et al., 1996) and GP-expressing brain cells, that is, astrocytes, ependymal cells, and sensory neurons, was clarified after non-cross-reacting antibodies against isoform-specific peptides were developed.

Throughout the brain, astrocytes contain the brain and muscle isoforms (Pfeiffer-Guglielmi et al., 2003), but it is not known whether the protomers of the isoforms exist as a combination of the two homodimers or as heterodimers, or as a mixture of both. Consistent with the occurrence of the muscle isoform in astrocytes is the observation that deficiency in this isozyme in a patient suffering from McArdle's disease is accompanied by an increased level of cerebral glycogen (Salvan et al., 1997). In contrast to astrocytes, ependymal cells and sensory neurons in brain express the BB isozyme only, and so do astroglial cells in culture (Pfeiffer-Guglielmi et al., 2003). In this context, it is important to note that the MM isoform is more prominently activated by neurohormone-induced phosphorylation, whereas the BB isoform is preferentially activated by adenosine monophosphate (AMP) (Newgard et al., 1989). Thus, in astrocytes, glycogen breakdown catalyzed by isoform MM could be evoked in an anticipatory mechanism by neurotransmitters released from processes of far-projecting neurons such as the noradrenergic neurons of the locus coeruleus. Activation of GP *in situ* by neuronal input has indeed been reported (Folbergrova, 1995; Harley et al., 1995). In cases of rapid depletion of ATP during phases of high energy demand, the ensuing AMP would activate isoform BB in astrocytes, ependymal cells, and sensory neurons. Thereby the cells could meet the energy requirements in the fastest possible way biochemically, by mobilizing the glucosyl residues of their glycogen stores for glycolytic breakdown. Initiation of energy generation this way would be more rapid and efficient than uptake of glucose followed by hexokinase-catalyzed phosphorylation to glucose-6-phosphate.

Besides glycogen phosphorylase, glycogen breakdown requires the action of glycogen debranching enzyme. This enzyme is present in brain, albeit in an isoform that differs from that in liver and muscle (Narahara et al., 2001). Especially noteworthy is that, besides glycogen phosphorylase, this isoform is likely to include another regulatory site for glycogen breakdown, since it is inhibited by ATP (Narahara et al., 2001). It is important to find out if the peripheral isoform is also expressed in brain and if debranching enzyme is indeed contained in the cell types in which it is expected to be required, that is, those cells containing glycogen phosphorylase.

All GP isozymes can be activated by phosphorylase kinase–catalyzed phosphorylation, although the maximal extent of activation differs, dependent on the presence of AMP (Newgard et al., 1989). Therefore, it is reassuring rather than surprising that phosphorylase kinase could be immunocytochemically detected only in GP-containing cells in neural cell cultures as well as in brain (Psarra et al., 1998). This may also be considered evidence against extrapolating from *in vitro* findings that phosphorylase kinase could have substrates other than GP (Paudel et al., 1993) *in vivo*.

Enzymes of glycogen synthesis

As in glycogen degradation, several enzymes and proteins are involved in the synthesis of glycogen, and they also occur in isoforms. The cDNA of the brain isoform of glycogen synthase has been cloned from mouse brain. It has 96% amino acid identity with the muscle isozyme and a somewhat lower level of identity with the liver isozyme. Surprisingly, by *in situ* hybridization, the corresponding mRNA has been found not only in astrocytes but also in neurons (Pellegri et al., 1996) throughout the brain that do not contain GP. It is important to see if these findings can be corroborated by immunocytochemistry with antibodies against brain glycogen synthase. In retina, apparently two isoforms exist (Curtino and Lacoste, 2000), with their molecular characterization and their cellular allocation awaiting elucidation.

Glycogen synthase can start building up the polysaccharide part of the glycogen particles (which in fact is a glycoprotein) only, if the apoprotein glycogenin has made use of its Mn^{2+}-dependent glucosyltransferase activity and has autoglucosylated itself on a particular tyrosyl residue up to an octasaccharide chain (Alonso et al., 1995; Roach and Skurat, 1997). Thus far, the presence of glycogenin in astrocytes has been inferred only from results of studies on cultured astrocytes (Lomako et al., 1993). The identification of glycogenin expected to be present in glycogen-containing brain cells has still to be carried out. This task will have to include the determination of the isotype present. Thus far two isoforms have become known, the muscle (Rodriguez and

Whelan, 1985; Pitcher et al., 1988) and liver (Mu et al., 1997) isoforms, the structure of the former has been solved at 0.19 nm resolution (Gibbons et al., 2002).

For the generation of the 1,6-glycosidically linked branches in glycogen, branching enzyme is needed. The enzyme was partially purified from rat brain (Tolmasky et al., 1998). The deposition of polyglucosan bodies in astrocytes of patients with a complete deficiency of branching enzyme (Schröder et al., 1993) is the only—albeit indirect—evidence for the presence of this enzyme in glial cells.

It is textbook knowledge that cellular glycogen levels are hormonally regulated by processes involving protein kinases and phosphoprotein phosphatases. Thus, phosphorylation of glycogen phosphorylase results in activation of glycogen synthase and in inactivation of the respective enzyme. These phosphorylations can be reversed by phosphoprotein phosphatase 1 (PP1), resulting in increased levels of glycogen by opening the synthetic pathway and closing the degradative pathway. Four isoforms of a protein are known that bind to PP1 and target it to glycogen: glycogen synthase, glycogen phosphorylase, and phosphorylase kinase (Printen et al., 1997; Newgard et al., 2000). The mRNA of one of these isoforms, protein targeting to glycogen (PTG), has been found to be present in cultured astrocytes and to be induced by noradrenaline and vasoactive intestinal peptide (Allaman et al., 2000), neurohormones known to raise cyclic AMP levels in these cells (for review see Hamprecht and Dringen, 1995). Indeed, cyclic AMP–mimetic agents could simulate the effect of the hormones (Allaman et al., 2000). In this context it is noteworthy that also the β_1-isoform of the energy deficiency sensing $\alpha\beta\gamma$-trimeric AMP kinase targets this enzyme to glycogen (Polekhina et al., 2003).

CARBONIC ANHYDRASES

Carbonic anhydrase (CA) catalyzes the reversible addition of water to carbon dioxide. Besides being required for respiration, this reaction is important for homeostatic regulation of tissue pH, for proton symport processes, for the secretion of HCl in the stomach and of cerebrospinal fluid by the ventricular choroid plexus, and for the provision of bicarbonate that is to serve as substrate for enzymatically catalyzed reactions (Henry, 1996; Breton, 2001). Since the previous survey on glial enzymes (Wiesinger, 1995), the number of known CA isoforms has doubled. In humans there are 11 enzymatically active carbonic anhydrase isozymes (CA I–IV, VA, VB, VI, VII, IX, XII, and XIV; Hewett-Emmett, 2000) and 3 carboanhydrase-related proteins (CA VIII, X, XI; Taniuchi et al., 2002a), which are inactive due to an incomplete Zn^{2+} binding site. Isozyme CA XIV is a recently discovered isozyme (Fujikawa-Adachi et al., 1999a; Mori et al., 1999) that joins the group of carboanhydrase ectoenzymes thus far represented by the membrane-spanning isozymes CA IX and CA XII, and by lipid-anchored CA IV. Also, CA VI is active extracellularly since it is the only secreted form, appearing in body fluids such as saliva and tears (Sly and Hu, 1995; Henry, 1996; Kivela et al., 1999). Isozymes CA VA (Nagao et al., 1994) and CA VB (Fujikawa-Adachi, 1999b) are isoforms located in the inner mitochondrial membrane, with their active centers facing the matrix.

In brain, where CAI and VI are missing and CA III occurs only in choroid plexus (Nogradi et al., 1993) and microglial cells (Nogradi, 1993), the most abundant carboanhydrase isoform is CA II (Parkkila A. et al., 1995; Parkkila S., 2000), also called *carbonic anhydrase C*. The fact that mental retardation is among the symptoms accompanying CA II deficiency stresses the importance of this enzyme (Ocal et al., 2001). In rat brain CA II has been immunocytochemically (Roussel et al., 1979; Agnati et al., 1995; Tong et al., 2000) detected in oligodendrocytes and astrocytes and in the choroid plexus, but definitely not in neurons. In the oligodendrocytes, staining was found restricted to the cytoplasm of the soma and did not appear in the compact myelin.

The presence of CA II in oligodendrocytes and choroid plexus and the absence from neurons also occurs in mouse (Kumpulainen and Korhonen, 1982) and human (Kumpulainen and Nystrom, 1981) brain. Conflicting reports exist in regard to the expression of CA II in brain astrocytes. While some researchers have found the isozyme by immunocytochemical techniques in mouse (Tong et al., 2000) and rat (Roussel et al., 1979; Agnati et al, 1995) brain astrocytes, others have not (Ghandour et al., 1980; Kumpulainen and Korhonen, 1982; Ridderstrale and Wistrand, 2000), nor not in human brain (Kumpulainen and Nystrom, 1981). In fact, since CA II could not be detected in any other cell of brain parenchyma but oligodendrocytes, it was proposed as a marker for these myelin-forming cells (Ghandour et al., 1980; Langley et al., 1980). The controversy also pertained to rat glial cell cultures. Although there was agreement on the presence of the CA II in oligodendroglial cells, the isozyme was found to be absent (Delaunoy et al., 1980) or present (Kimelberg et al., 1982; Hazen et al., 1997; Cammer, 1998) in GFAP-positive astroglial cells. Differences in culture conditions and antisera are likely to account for the difference in results. In an early effort to resolve the controversy (Delaunoy et al., 1980, vs. Kimelberg et al., 1982) on the presence of CA II in astrocytes at least for brain, double labeling studies were carried out on rat brain using antibodies against the astrocyte markers glutamine synthetase and GFAP. They led to the conclusion that CA II is present in some astrocytes in the mammalian CNS, but not all (Cammer and Tansey, 1988). The same pattern is found in chicken cerebral cortex, where CA II immunoreactivity is encountered not only in oligodendrocytes but also in glutamine synthetase–positive astrocytes. In addition, CA II is strongly present in some neurons (Linser, 1985). In summary, CA II cannot be safely used as a marker for astrocytes in brain.

The doubt that the CA immunoreactivity could be due to CA isoforms other than CA II has been eliminated by immunocytochemical analysis of CA II knockout mice. In comparison to wild-type brains, the brains of CA II–deficient mice do not stain positively for CA II in oligodendrocytes, myelin, and astrocytes (Ghandour et al., 1989; Cammer and Zhang, 1991). Also, the staining around neuronal cell bodies disappears, obviously due to CA II in fine astrocytic lamellae. On the other hand, it became clear that histochemical staining in neuronal processes, not perikarya, must be due to a membrane-bound CA isoform rather than CA II (Ridderstrale and Wistrand, 2000). In addition, this report confirms an earlier communication (Hazen et al., 1997) that CA III is not present in brain parenchyma. In accord with this notion is the observation that in microglia CA II is expressed only transiently during early postnatal development of rats (Cammer and Zhang, 1996).

In retina of chicken, CA II appears transiently in neurons (Linser and Moscona, 1981) and continues to be expressed in the Müller glia cells *in situ* (Linser and Moscona, 1981; Kumpulainen and Korhonen, 1982), as well as in culture (Linser and Moscona, 1983).

In contrast to brain, there are some neurons in the PNS of rodents that do contain CA II. However, the isozyme is immunocytochemically detected not only in a subpopulation of sensory neurons (Kazimierczak et al., 1986; Cammer and Tansey, 1987; Carr et al., 1989; Robertson and Grant, 1989; Persson et al., 1995), but also in satellite cells and their processes (Cammer and Tansey, 1987).

Of the mitochondrially located isoforms, CA VA is expressed only in liver, heart, kidney, and skeletal muscle (Vaananen et al., 1991), whereas isoform CA VB mRNA occurs in other tissues (Shah et al., 2000), including spinal cord (Fujikawa-Adachi et al., 1999b) and brain (Ghandour et al., 2000). In brain CA VB was shown by immunocytochemistry to be present in astrocytes and neurons but absent in oligodendrocytes (Ghandour et al., 2000). The location in astrocytes stresses the provision of bicarbonate for the action of the anaplerotic and gluconeogenic enzyme pyruvate carboxylase and for carbamoyl phosphate synthetase in pyrimidine synthesis (for review see Wiesinger, 1995). In this context it must be mentioned, however, that such an ancillary function in pyruvate carboxylation has also been assigned to CA II on the basis (*1*) that in cultured astrocytes CA II, but not CA III–V, could be detected (Hazen et al., 1997), and (*2*) that in exocrine pancreas CA II but not CA V is colocalized with the two enzymes (Sato et al., 2002).

By *in situ* hybridization the mRNA of CA VII, one of the soluble intracellular CA isoforms, was detected not only in pia mater and choroid plexus but also in neurons of various brain regions. It was not found in glial cells (Lakkis et al., 1997).

The provision of H^+ also appears to be a function of plasma membrane-bound CA isozymes. Lactate can serve as a fuel for neurons (for review see Hamprecht and Dringen, 1995). Since it is cotransported with a proton, uptake of lactate into neurons requires the immediate availability of H^+. Obviously this is achieved by extracellularly located CA since a non-membrane-permeant CA inhibitor was able to block lactate uptake into cultured astrocytes and pyramidal neurons freshly isolated from hippocampus (Svichar and Chesler, 2003). Apparently C IV is physically and functionally closely associated with the electrogenic Na^+/HCO_3^- cotransporter (Alvarez et al., 2003). Of the four plasma membrane–associated CA isozymes, only CA IV and CA XIV have been detected in brain. CA IV is a marker of brain capillary endothelial cells (Ghandour et al., 1992) and appears as a compensatory isoform in oligodendrocytes of CA II–deficient mice (Brion et al., 1994). The newly discovered isozyme CA XIV (Mori et al., 1999) is located on the plasma membrane of neuronal cell bodies and axons in a wide variety of regions in mouse and human brain (Parkkila S. et al., 2001). Therefore, it is this isoform that most likely furnishes the protons for cotransport with lactate.

The enzymatically inactive isoforms CA VIII, X, and XI are also more correctly referred to as *CA-related proteins* (CA-RP VIII, X, XI). All three of them are found in brain in the somata and neurites of neurons throughout the human (Taniuchi et al., 2002a) and murine (Taniuchi et al., 2002b) brain. Carbonic anhydrase–related protein X is a constituent of the myelin sheath and CA-RP XI of astrocytes in restricted brain areas (Taniuchi et al., 2002a). Carbonic anhydrase–related proteins VIII and XI appear also in choroid plexus epithelium and in neuroprogenitors of the subventricular zone (Taniuchi et al., 2002a). In accord with the immunocytochemical observations in mouse brain, CA-RP VIII mRNA was detected by *in situ* hybridization in neurons of various brain regions, and in pia mater and choroid plexus (Lakkis et al., 1997).

ENZYMES OF CELLULAR ENERGIZATION

Creatine Kinase

Creatine phosphate is no longer considered primarily as an energy reserve to be used for the regeneration of

ATP from the adenosine diphosphate (ADP) that is produced at an elevated rate during high cellular demand of energy. Rather, due to its lower molecular mass and therefore 50% higher diffusion coefficient (Hubley et al., 1995) in comparison to that of ATP, creatine phosphate is considered as a shuttle for fast transfer of energy-rich phosphate from the mitochondria to the locations of energy consumption (Bessman and Carpenter, 1985; Kraft et al., 2000). Creatine kinase (CK), the enzyme that catalyzes the reversible transfer of a phosphoryl residue between creatine phosphate and ADP, exists as four different protomers. Two of these form the cytosolic isozymes characteristic for brain (CK-BB, homodimer), muscle (CK-MM, homodimer), and heart (CK-MB, heterodimer). The other two constitute the mitochondrial homoactameric isozymes that can attach to the outer mitochondrial membrane and are called *sarcomeric mitochondrial* (sMt-CK) and *ubiquitous mitochondrial* (uMt-CK) CK (for review, see Wallimann et al., 1998). Of all tissues, CK is by far most abundant in brain. As revealed immunocytochemically by applying isozyme-specific antibodies to cerebellar sections, CK-BB was found in radial Bergmann glial cells and in stellate astrocytes, whereas CK-MM was located exclusively in Purkinje neurons (Hemmer et al., 1994). In rat brain, all three cytosolic CK isoforms (MM, MB, BB) have been described, their distribution depending on the developmental state and the sex of the animal (Ramirez and Jimenez, 2002). The mitochondrial isoform Mt-CK has been detected in the glomerular structures of the granule cell layer, in Purkinje cells, layer Va pyramidal cells, thalamic nuclei and hippocampal interneurons, also dependent on the ontogenic state of the brain (Hemmer et al., 1994; Boero et al., 2003). Compatible with the presence of the muscle type of cytosolic CK, Purkinje cells also contain the corresponding mitochondrial isoform, sMt-CK (Kaldis et al., 1996). Consistent with the finding obtained in brain is the occurrence of high levels of CK-BB mRNA in cultured astrocytes and levels more than one order of magnitude lower in cultured neurons, whereas cultured oligodendrocytes contain levels as high as those of cultured astrocytes (Molloy et al., 1992). On the other hand, the same group has reported high concentrations of CK-BB and its mRNA in cultured cerebellar granule cells (Shen et al., 2002). This finding is corroborated by results from *in situ* hybridization experiments, in which CK-BB mRNA was detected in neurons, but not in clearly identified glial cells, and only occasionally in ependymal cells (Bergen et al., 1993). In retina CK-BB was detected in the outer segments of photoreceptor cells and, as would be expected from the regional restriction of the mitochondrial clusters in these cells, mitochondrial isozyme immunoreactivity could be localized in the inner segments (Hemmer et al., 1993).

Apparently the findings concerning the cellular expression of CK-BB presented above (Hemmer et al., 1994; Kaldis et al., 1996) are not unequivocal, since another group reported the opposite: the presence of CK-BB in neurons but not in glial cells, and in the inner rather than the outer segments of photoreceptor cells (Sistermans et al., 1995). It is noteworthy that, in development of rat brain, CK-BB first appears postnatally and increases in concentration strongly during gliogenesis and myelination. Expression of CK-BB is especially high in dividing astrocytes, where intense nuclear staining for the isozyme is likely to reflect an important function of CK in the energization of nucleic acid synthesis (Manos and Bryan, 1993). The reason for the number of discrepancies between the various reports may lie in different specificities of the antibodies used or in the different brain regions investigated. Alternatively, it may reside in species differences, since the brains of chicken, mice, rats, rabbits, and humans were analyzed. Elucidation of the divergent results by revisiting the problem of cellular allocation is highly desirable. This would be the prerequisite for assessing the role of CK in various disease processes of the brain (e.g., Alzheimer's disease), where CK-BB has been identified as one of the proteins subject to targeted protein oxidation (Castegna et al., 2002).

Carnitine Palmitoyltransferase

Two carnitine palmitoyltransferase (CPT) isozymes are involved in the translocation of long-chain fatty acyl residues from the cytosol into the mitochondrial matrix. This delivery is required for β-oxidation, which, in turn, is the prerequisite for the generation of energy and of ketone bodies from such fatty acids. The cytosolically located isoform CPT1 was shown to be active in cultured astrocytes and to be subject to regulation by the metabolic feedback inhibitor malonyl-coenzyme A and by cyclic AMP (Blazquez et al., 1998, 1999). Except for the demonstration of CPT activity in cultured neurons (Arduini et al., 1994), comparable studies on other types of brain cells appear to be missing. Also, it remains to be determined which of the cytosolic isotypes of CPT1, the liver or the muscle isotype, is involved in the regulatory events described by Blazquez et al. (1999). The cellular location of a recently described (Price et al., 2002) novel brain- and testis-specific CPT1-related protein has not yet been determined. The possibility that these isozymes and isotypes could be used as cellular markers is a subject for future research.

Na^+,K^+-Adenosine Triphosphatase

The transmembrane enzyme Na^+,K^+-adenosine triphosphatase (Na^+,K^+-ATPase), which actively transports Na^+ and K^+ in opposite directions through the plasma membrane, is an $\alpha\beta$ heterodimer. In addition, a family of FXYD proteins, among them the renal γ subunit, regulate transport activity in a tissue-specific manner (Geering et al., 2003). All the functional properties associated with the name of the enzyme and the heart glycoside binding site reside in the α subunit. The α-subunit is also the site of intermolecular interaction between Na^+, K^+-ATPase and glycogen phosphorylase, which also regulates the activity of the pump (Takeyasu et al., 2003). The β subunit is important for rendering the α subunit active. Furthermore, besides performing other functions (Kaplan, 2002), it participates in the occlusion of K^+ and regulates the alkali ion affinity of the α subunit. In mammalian cells there exist the four α-isoforms (α-protomers) α_1, α_2, α_3, and α_4, in addition to the three β-isoforms (β-protomers) β_1, β_2, and β_3 (Blanco and Mercer, 1998; Woo et al., 2000; Kaplan, 2002). Whereas the $\alpha_1\beta_1$ isozyme is ubiquitous in mammalian tissues, other isozymes, which can arise from the free combination of the various α- and β-protomers, display more specific cellular affiliations (Mobasheri et al., 2000), especially in the nervous system (Sweadner, 1992). The only one of the seven α- and β-protomers that has not been detected in mammalian CNS is α_4, which thus far appears to be sperm cell and testis specific (Blanco et al., 2000).

In the CNS the cellular allocation of the protomer isoforms of Na^+,K^+-ATPase has been carried out on brain and retina, whereas information on spinal cord and the PNS is still missing. The major methods used were immunocytochemistry and *in situ* hybridization. At the level of individual neural cell types the studies have apparently been concentrating on neurons, astrocytes, and oligodendrocytes. There is some information on Schwann cells but probably no explicit report on ependymal, microglial, and olfactory ensheathing cells. Studies on the appearance of the protomeric isoforms during development have started (Wetzel et al., 1999).

In accordance with the α_1-protomer's reputation of being part of a ubiquitous household isozyme, α_1 is found in many neurons and astroglial cell types. In the retina it was detected in horizontal cells and Müller cells (Wetzel et al., 1999). In cultures of rat brain cells the α_1-protomer has been found in various kinds of neurons (Brines and Robbins, 1993a; Cameron et al., 1994). By *in situ* hybridization carried out on brain slices, the corresponding mRNA has been detected in neurons (Hieber et al., 1991; Chauhan and Siegel, 1996). The α_1 subunit is the only α-protomer found this way in granule cells of the cerebellar cortex (Hieber et al., 1991). As for brain glial cells, the presence of the ATPase protomer has been analyzed in cultured cells and *in situ*. As one would expect, the α_1-protomer was found in astrocytes in brain (McGrail et al., 1991) and in culture (Brines and Robbins, 1993a; Cameron et al., 1994; Fink et al., 1996). The brain-specific γ subunit homologue, FXYD7, has been immunohistochemically shown to be expressed in neurons and astrocytes, where it regulates the activity of the α_1-containing isoforms of the Na^+,K^+-ATPase (Beguin et al., 2002). Oligodendrocytes appear to lack α_1 (Knapp et al., 2000), as do Schwann cells (Kawai et al., 1997).

Equivocal information exists on the necessity of the presence of neurons for cultured astrocytes to contain α_2 (Corthesy-Theulaz et al., 1990; Brines and Robbins, 1993a; Fink et al., 1996). But there is no doubt that brain astrocytes do contain α_2 (McGrail et al., 1991; Hartford et al., 2004). Other reports confirm the importance of the copresence of neurons and point out a strong species difference, with mouse astrocytes in culture expressing α_2 at a much higher level than their rat counterparts (Peng et al., 1997). In addition, there are considerable regional differences, such that astrocytes cultured from cortex express α_2 more frequently than those from cerebellum (Peng et al., 1998). Obviously, regulatory influences from neighboring neurons are important in α_2 expression. In this context, it may also be of interest that glutamate upregulates the levels of both α_1 and α_2 in astrocytes only, if neurons are also present (Brines and Robbins, 1993b). While neuronal α_2 expression appears to be scarce in the adult, it occurs widely during gestation and has been shown to be critical for survival (Moseley et al., 2003). The intricacy of Na^+, K^+-ATPase regulation in the brain is emphasized by the region-specific expression of another FXYD family member, phospholemman. Immunoreactivity has been detected in ependymal cells of the choroid plexus, in tanycytes and most abundantly in cerebellar neurons. The interaction between the regulator and the transporter does apparently not depend on the type of α-subunit expressed (Feschenko et al., 2003).

Since α_3 appears to be exclusively a neuronal isoform both in retina (Wetzel et al., 1999) and in brain (Hieber et al., 1991; McGrail et al., 1991; Brines and Robbins, 1993a; Cameron et al., 1994; Chauhan and Siegel, 1996), it will not be discussed here.

Besides occurring in granule cells both in culture and *in situ* (Peng et al., 1997), and in retinal (Wetzel et al., 1999) and other neurons (Lecuona et al., 1996), the protomer β_1 is contained in astrocytes at a level considerably lower than that of α_2 (Cameron et al., 1994; Fink et al., 1996; Peng et al., 1997).

A similar distribution is encountered for β_2, which is not only present in neurons such as bipolar and photoreceptor cells in the retina (Wetzel et al., 1999) and cerebellar granule cells (Peng et al., 1997). It is also expressed in glial cells, that is, Müller cells of the retina (Wetzel et al., 1999), astrocytes in brain (Lecuona et al., 1996) and in culture (Cameron et al., 1994; Fink et al., 1996; Peng et al., 1998), and Schwann cells (Kawai et al., 1997). Developmental aspects of the expression of the β_2-protomer, which has been found to be identical to adhesion molecule on glia (AMOG; Gloor et al., 1990), have been studied intensively. Also, the β_3-protomer is not a peculiarity of neurons or glial cells; it is found both in the inner segment of photoreceptor cells (Wetzel et al., 1999) and in oligodendrocytes (Martin-Vasallo et al., 2000).

Other Adenosine Triphosphatases

There are at least four isoforms of the Ca^{2+}-extruding plasma membrane Ca^{2+}-ATPase (PMCA) that are encoded by four different genes. The isoforms PMCA1 and PMCA4 occur almost ubiquitously in mammalian cells (Krizaj et al., 2002), whereas expression of PMCA2 and PMCA3 appear to be a domain of neurons (Stauffer et al., 1997; Krizaj et al., 2002). More recently, the presence of all PMCA isoforms except PMCA3 has been described in cultured astrocytes (Fresu et al., 1999).

The vacuolar H^+-transporting ATPases (V-ATPases) are high molecular weight complexes made up of 13 protomers, at least some of which can exist in several isoforms. They create proton gradients across the membranes of cell organelles and are essential for a multitude of cellular processes such as protein processing and degradation, receptor-mediated endocytosis, and intracellular membrane shuffling. There are promising indications that immunological techniques and techniques of qualitative and quantitative assessment of protomer mRNAs may be useful in identifying cell types and diagnosing glial brain tumors (Philippe et al., 2002).

REFERENCES

Agnati, L.F., Tinner, B., Staines, W.A., Vaananen, K., and Fuxe, K. (1995) On the cellular localization and distribution of carbonic anhydrase II immunoreactivity in the rat brain. *Brain Res.* 676:10–24.

Allaman, I., Pellerin, L., and Magistretti, P.J. (2000) Protein targeting to glycogen mRNA expression is stimulated by noradrenaline in mouse cortical astrocytes. *Glia* 30:382–391.

Alonso, M.D., Lomako, J., Lomako, W.M., and Whelan, W.J. (1995) Catalytic activities of glycogenin additional to autocatalytic self-glucosylation. *J. Biol. Chem.* 270:15315–15319.

Alvarez, B.V., Loiselle, F.B., Supuran, C.T., Schwartz, G.J., and Casey, J.R. (2003) Direct extracellular interaction between carbonic anhydrase IV and the human NBC1 sodium/bicarbonate co-transporter. *Biochemistry* 42:12321–12329.

Arduini, A., Denisova, N., Virmani, A., Avrova, N., Federici, G., and Arrigoni-Martelli, E. (1994) Evidence for the involvement of carnitine-dependent long-chain acyltransferases in neuronal triglyceride and phospholipid fatty acid turnover. *J. Neurochem.* 62: 1530–1538.

Beguin, P., Crambert, G., Monnet-Tschudi, F., Uldry, M., Horisberger, J.D., Garty, H., and Geering, K. (2002). FXYC7 is a brain-specific regulator of Na, K-ATPase alpha 1-beta isozymes. *EMBO J.* 21:3264–3273.

Bell, J.E., Hume, R., Busuttil, A., and Burchell, A. (1993) Immunocytochemical detection of the microsomal glucose-6-phosphatase in human brain astrocytes. *Neuropathol. Appl. Neurobiol.* 19: 429–435.

Bergbauer, K., Dringen, R., Verleysdonk, S., Gebhardt, R., Hamprecht, B., and Wiesinger, H. (1996) Studies on fructose metabolism in cultured astroglial cells and control hepatocytes: lack of fructokinase activity and immunoreactivity in astrocytes. *Dev. Neurosci.* 18:371–379.

Bergen, H.T., Pentecost, B.T., Dickerman, H.W., and Pfaff, D.W. (1993) In situ hybridization for creatine kinase-B messenger RNA in rat uterus and brain. *Mol. Cell Endocrinol.* 92:111–119.

Bernard-Helary, K., Ardourel, M., Magistretti, P., Hevor, T., and Cloix, J.F. (2002) Stable transfection of cDNAs targeting specific steps of glycogen metabolism supports the existence of active gluconeogenesis in mouse cultured astrocytes. *Glia* 37:379–382.

Bessman, S.P. and Carpenter, C.L. (1985) The creatine-creatine phosphate energy shuttle. *Annu. Rev. Biochem.* 54:831–862.

Bittar, P.G., Charnay, Y., Pellerin, L., Bouras, C., and Magistretti, P.J. (1996) Selective distribution of lactate dehydrogenase isoenzymes in neurons and astrocytes of human brain. *J. Cereb. Blood Flow Metab.* 16:1079–1089.

Blanco, G. and Mercer, R.W. (1998) Isozymes of the Na-K-ATPase: heterogeneity in structure, diversity in function. *Am. J. Physiol.* 275:F633–F650.

Blanco, G., Sanchez, G., Melton, R.J., Tourtellotte, W.G., and Mercer, R.W. (2000) The alpha4 isoform of the Na,K-ATPase is expressed in the germ cells of the testes. *J. Histochem. Cytochem.* 48:1023–1032.

Blazquez, C., Sanchez, C., Velasco, G., and Guzman, M. (1998) Role of carnitine palmitoyltransferase I in the control of ketogenesis in primary cultures of rat astrocytes. *J. Neurochem.* 71:1597–1606.

Blazquez, C., Woods, A., De Ceballos, M.L., Carling, D., and Guzman, M. (1999) The AMP-activated protein kinase is involved in the regulation of ketone body production by astrocytes. *J. Neurochem.* 73:1674–1682.

Boero, J., Qin, W., Cheng, J., Woolsey, T.A., Strauss, A.W., and Khuchua, Z. (2003) Restricted neuronal expression of ubiquitous mitochondrial creatine kinase: changing patterns in development and with increased activity. *Mol. Cell. Biochem.* 244:69–76.

Breton, S. (2001) The cellular physiology of carbonic anhydrases. *J. Pancreas* 2(Suppl. 4):159–164.

Brines, M.L., and Robbins, R.J. (1993a) Cell-type specific expression of Na^+,K^+-ATPase catalytic subunits in cultured neurons and glia: evidence for polarized distribution in neurons. *Brain Res.* 631:1–11.

Brines, M.L. and Robbins, R.J. (1993b) Glutamate up-regulates alpha 1 and alpha 2 subunits of the sodium pump in astrocytes of mixed telencephalic cultures but not in pure astrocyte cultures. *Brain Res.* 631:12–21.

Brion, L.P., Suarez, C., Zhang, H., and Cammer, W. (1994) Up-regulation of carbonic anhydrase isozyme IV in CNS myelin of mice genetically deficient in carbonic anhydrase II. *J. Neurochem.* 63:360–366.

Cameron, R., Klein, L., Shyjan, A.W., Rakic, P., and Levenson, R. (1994) Neurons and astroglia express distinct subsets of Na,K-ATPase alpha and beta subunits. *Brain Res. Mol. Brain Res.* 21:333–343.

Cammer, W. (1998) Glial-cell cultures from brains of carbonic anhydrase II–deficient mutant mice: delay in oligodendrocyte maturation. *Neurochem. Res.* 23:407–412.

Cammer, W. and Tansey, F.A. (1987) Immunocytochemical localization of carbonic anhydrase in myelinated fibers in peripheral nerves of rat and mouse. *J. Histochem. Cytochem.* 35:865–870.

Cammer, W. and Tansey, F.A. (1988) Carbonic anhydrase immunostaining in astrocytes in the rat cerebral cortex. *J. Neurochem.* 50:319–322.

Cammer, W. and Zhang, H. (1991) Comparison of immunocytochemical staining of astrocytes, oligodendrocytes, and myelinated fibers in the brains of carbonic anhydrase II-deficient mice and normal littermates. *J. Neuroimmunol.* 34:81–86.

Cammer, W. and Zhang, H. (1996) Carbonic anhydrase II in microglia in forebrains of neonatal rats. *J. Neuroimmunol.* 67:131–136.

Carr, P.A., Yamamoto, T., Karmy, G., Baimbridge, K.G., and Nagy, J.I. (1989). Analysis of parvalbumin and calbindin D28k-immunoreactive neurons in dorsal root ganglia of rat in relation to their cytochrome oxidase and carbonic anhydrase content. *Neuroscience* 33:363–371.

Castegna, A., Aksenov, M., Aksenova, M., Thongboonkerd, V., Klein, J.B., Pierce, W.M., Booze, R., Markesbery, W.R., and Butterfield, D.A. (2002) Proteomic identification of oxidatively modified proteins in Alzheimer's disease brain. Part I: creatine kinase BB, glutamine synthase, and ubiquitin carboxy-terminal hydrolase L-1. *Free Radic. Biol. Med.* 33:562–571.

Cavalcante, L.A., Barradas, P.C., and Vieira, A.M. (1996) The regional distribution of neuronal glycogen in the opossum brain, with special reference to hypothalamic systems. *J. Neurocytol.* 25:455–463.

Cesar, M. and Hamprecht, B. (1995) Immunocytochemical examination of neural rat and mouse primary cultures using monoclonal antibodies raised against pyruvate carboxylase. *J. Neurochem.* 64:2312–2318.

Chauhan, N.B. and Siegel, G.J. (1996) In situ analsyis of Na, K-ATPase alpha1- and alpha3-isoform mRNAs in aging rat hippocampus. *J. Neurochem.* 66:1742–1751.

Corthesy-Theulaz, I., Merillat, A.M., Honegger, P., and Rossier, B.C. (1990) Na(+)-K(+)-ATPase gene expression during in vitro development of rat fetal forebrain. *Am. J. Physiol.* 258:C1062–C1069.

Crerar, M.M., Hudson, J.W., Matthews, K.E., David, E.S., and Golding, G.B. (1988) Studies on the expression and evolution of the glycogen phosphorylase gene family in the rat. *Genome* 30:582–590.

Curtino, J.A. and Lacoste, E.R. (2000) Two glycogen synthase activities associated with proteoglycogen in retina. *Neurochem. Res.* 25:129–132.

De Cerqueira Cesar, M. and Wilson, J.E. (1998) Further studies on the coupling of mitochondrially bound hexokinase to intramitochondrially compartmented ATP, generated by oxidative phosphorylation. *Arch. Biochem. Biophys.* 350:109–117.

Delaunoy, J.P., Hog, F., Devilliers, G., Bansart, M., Mandel, P., and Sensenbrenner, M. (1980) Developmental changes and localization of carbonic anhydrase in cerebral hemispheres of the rat and in rat glial cell cultures. *Cell Mol. Biol.* 26:235–240.

Dringen, R., Gebhardt, R., and Hamprecht, B. (1993a) Glycogen in astrocytes: possible function as lactate supply for neighboring cells. *Brain Res.* 623:208–214.

Dringen, R., Schmoll, D., Cesar, M., and Hamprecht, B. (1993b) Incorporation of radioactivity from [14C]lactate into the glycogen of cultured mouse astroglial cells. Evidence for gluconeogenesis in brain cells. *Biol. Chem. Hoppe-Seyler* 374:343–347.

Feschenko, M.S., Donnet, C., Wetzel, R.K., Asinovski, N.K., Jones, L.R., and Sweadner, K.J. (2003) Phospholemman, a single-span membrane protein, is an accessory protein of Na,K-ATPase in cerebellum and choroid plexus. *J. Neurosci.* 23:2161–2169.

Fink, D., Knapp, P.E., and Mata, M. (1996) Differential expression of Na,K-ATPase isoforms in oligodendrocytes and astrocytes. *Dev. Neurosci.* 18:319–326.

Folbergrova, J. (1995) Glycogen phosphorylase activity in the cerebral cortex of rats during development: effect of homocysteine-induced seizures. *Brain. Res.* 694:128–132.

Forsyth, R.J., Bartlett, K., Burchell, A., Scott, H.M., and Eyre, J.A. (1993) Astrocytic glucose-6-phosphatase and the permeability of brain microsomes to glucose 6-phosphate. *Biochem. J.* 294:145–151.

Fresu, L., Dehpour, A., Genazzani, A.A., Carafoli, E., and Guerini, D. (1999) Plasma membrane calcium ATPase isoforms in astrocytes. *Glia* 28:150–155.

Fujikawa-Adachi, K., Nishimori, I., Taguchi, T., and Onishi, S. (1999a) Human carbonic anhydrase XIV (CA 14): cDNA cloning, mRNA expression, and mapping to chromosome 1. *Genomics* 61:74–81.

Fujikawa-Adachi, K., Nishimori, I., Taguchi, T., and Onishi, S. (1999b) Human mitochondrial carbonic anhydrase VB. cDNA cloning, mRNA expression, subcellular localization, and mapping to chromosome X. *J. Biol. Chem.* 274:21228–21233.

Geering, K., Beguin, P., Garty, H., Karlish, S., Fuzesi, M., Horisberger, J.D., and Crambert, G. (2003) FXYD proteins: new tissue- and isoform-specific regulators of Na, K-ATPase. *Ann. N.Y. Acad. Sci.* 986:388–394.

Ghandour, M.S., Langley, O.K., Vincendon, G., Gombos, G., Filippi, D., Limozin, N., Dalmasso, D., and Laurent, G. (1980) Immunochemical and immunohistochemical study of carbonic anhydrase II in adult rat cerebellum: a marker for oligodendrocytes. *Neuroscience* 5:559–571.

Ghandour, M.S., Langley, O.K., Zhu, X.L., Waheed, A., and Sly, W.S. (1992) Carbonic anhydrase IV on brain capillary endothelial cells: a marker associated with the blood–brain barrier. *Proc. Natl. Acad. Sci. USA* 89:6823–6827.

Ghandour, M.S., Parkkila, A.K., Parkkila, S., Waheed, A., and Sly, W.S. (2000) Mitochondrial carbonic anhydrase in the nervous system: expression in neuronal and glial cells. *J. Neurochem.* 75:2212–2220.

Ghandour, M.S., Skoff, R.P., Venta, P.J., and Tashian, R.E. (1989) Oligodendrocytes express a normal phenotype in carbonic anhydrase II-deficient mice. *J. Neurosci. Res.* 23:189–190.

Gibbons, B.J., Roach, P.J., and Harley, T.D. (2002) Crystal structure of the autocatalytic initiator of glycogen biosynthesis, glycogenin. *J. Mol. Biol.* 319:463–467.

Gloor, S., Antonicek, H., Sweadner, K.J., Pagliusi, S., Frank, R., Moos, M., and Schachner, M. (1990) The adhesion molecule on glia (AMOG) is a homologue of the beta subunit of the Na,K-ATPase. *J. Cell Biol.* 110:165–174.

Gotoh, J., Itoh, Y., Kuang, T.Y., Cook, M., Law, M., and Sokoloff, L. (2000) Negligible glucose-6-phosphatase activity in cultured astroglia. *J. Neurochem.* 74:1400–1408.

Guionie, O., Clottes, E., Stafford, K., and Burchell, A. (2003) Identification and characterization of a new human glucose-6-phosphatase isoform. *FEBS Lett.* 551:159–164.

Hamprecht, B. and Dringen, R. (1995) Energy metabolism. In: Ransom, B. and Kettenmann, H., eds. *Neuroglia.* New York and Oxford: Oxford University Press, pp. 488–499.

Harley, C.W., Milway J.S., and Fara-On, M. (1995) Medial forebrain bundle stimulation in rats activates glycogen phosphorylase in layers 4, 5b and 6 of ipsilateral granular neocortex. *Brain Res.* 685:217–223.

Hartford, A.K., Messer, M.L., Moseley, A.E., Lingrel, J.B., and Delamere, N.A. (2004) Na, K-ATPase alpha2 inhibition alters calcium responses in optic nerve astrocytes. *Glia* 43:229–237.

Hazen, S.A., Waheed, A., Sly, W.S., Lanoue, K.F., and Lynch, C.J. (1997) Effect of carbonic anhydrase inhibition and acetoacetate on anaplerotic pyruvate carboxylase activity in cultured rat astrocytes. *Dev. Neurosci.* 19:162–171.

Hemmer, W., Riesinger, I., Wallimann, T., Eppenberger, H.M., and Quest, A.F. (1993) Brain-type creatine kinase in photoreceptor cell outer segments: role of a phosphocreatine circuit in outer segment energy metabolism and phototransduction. *J. Cell Sci.* 106:671–683.

Hemmer, W., Zanolla, E., Furter-Graves, E.M., Eppenberger, H.M., and Wallimann, T. (1994) Creatine kinase isoenzymes in chicken cerebellum: specific localization of brain-type creatine kinase in Bergmann glial cells and muscle-type creatine kinase in Purkinje neurons. *Eur. J. Neurosci.* 6:538–549.

Henry, R.P. (1996) Multiple roles of carbonic anhydrase in cellular transport and metabolism. *Annu. Rev. Physiol.* 58:523–538.

Hewett-Emmett, D. (2000) Evolution and distribution of the carbonic anhydrase gene families. In: Chegwidden, W.R., Carter, N.D., and Edwards, Y.H., eds. *The Carbonic Anhydrases: New Horizons*. Basel: Birkhäuser, pp. 29–76.

Hieber, V., Siegel, G.J., Fink, D.J., Beaty, M.W., and Mata, M. (1991) Differential distribution of (Na, K)-ATPase alpha isoforms in the central nervous system. *Cell Mol. Neurobiol.* 11:253–262.

Hubley, M.J., Rosanske, R.C., and Moerland, T.S. (1995) Diffusion coefficients of ATP and creatine phosphate in isolated muscle: pulsed gradient 31P NMR of small biological samples. *NMR-Biomed.* 8:72–78.

Jacobsson, G. and Meister, B. (1994) Hexokinase I messenger RNA in the rat central nervous system. *Mol. Cell. Neurosci.* 5:658–677.

Kaldis, P., Hemmer, W., Zanolla, E., Holtzman, D., and Wallimann, T. (1996) "Hot spots" of creatine kinase localization in brain: cerebellum, hippocampus and choroid plexus. *Dev. Neurosci.* 18:542–554.

Kao-Jen, J. and Wilson, J.E. (1980) Localization of hexokinase in neural tissue: electron microscopic studies of rat cerebellar cortex. *J. Neurochem.* 35:667–678.

Kaplan, J.H. (2002) Biochemistry of Na,K-ATPase. *Annu. Rev. Biochem.* 71:511–535.

Kawai, H., Yasuda, H., Terada, M., Omatsu-Kanbe, M., and Kikkawa, R. (1997) Axonal contact regulates expression of alpha2 and beta2 isoforms of Na^+, K^+-ATPase in Schwann cells: adhesion molecules and nerve regeneration. *J. Neurochem.* 69: 330–339.

Kazimierczak, J., Sommer, E.W., Philippe, E., and Droz, B. (1986) Carbonic anhydrase activity in primary sensory neurons. I. Requirements for the cytochemical localization in the dorsal root ganglion of chicken and mouse by light and electron microscopy. *Cell Tissue Res.* 245:487–495.

Kimelberg, H.K., Stieg, P.E., and Mazurkiewicz, J.E. (1982) Immunocytochemical and biochemical analysis of carbonic anhydrase in primary astrocyte cultures from rat brain. *J. Neurochem.* 39:734–742.

Kivela, J., Parkkila, S., Parkkila, A.K., Leinonen, J., and Rajaniemi, H. (1999) Salivary carbonic anhydrase isoenzyme VI. *J. Physiol.* 520:315–320.

Knapp, P.E., Itkis, O.S., and Mata, M. (2000) Neuronal interaction determines the expression of the alpha-2 isoform of Na, K-ATPase in oligodendrocytes. *Brain Res. Dev. Brain Res.* 125:89–97.

Kraft, T., Hornemann, T., Stolz, M., Nier, V., and Wallimann, T. (2000) Coupling of creatine kinase to glycolytic enzymes at the sarcomeric I-band of skeletal muscle: a biochemical study in situ. *J. Muscle Res. Cell Motil.* 21:691–703.

Krizaj, D., Demarco, S.J., Johnson, J., Strehler, E.E., and Copenhagen, D.R. (2002) Cell-specific expression of plasma-membrane calcium ATPase isoforms in retinal neurons. *J. Comp. Neurol.* 451:1–21.

Kugler, P. (1994) Glucose-6-phosphate dehydrogenase is enriched in oligodendrocytes of the rat spinal cord. Enzyme histochemical and immunocytochemical studies. *Histochemistry* 101:143–153.

Kumanishi, T., Watabe, K., and Washiyama, K. (1985) An immunohistochemical study of aldolase C in normal and neoplastic nervous tissues. *Acta Neuropathol. (Berl.)* 67:309–314.

Kumpulainen, T. and Korhonen, L.K. (1982) Immunohistochemical localization of carbonic anhydrase isoenzyme C in the central and peripheral nervous system of the mouse. *J. Histochem. Cytochem.* 30:283–292.

Kumpulainen, T. and Nystrom, S.H. (1981) Immunohistochemical localization of carbonic anhydrase isoenzyme C in human brain. *Brain Res.* 220:220–225.

Lakkis, M.M., O'Shea, K.S., and Tashian, R.E. (1997) Differential expression of the carbonic anhydrase genes for CA VII (Car7) and CA-RP VIII (Car8) in mouse brain. *J. Histochem. Cytochem.* 45:657–662.

Langley, O.K., Ghandour, M.S., Vincendon, G., and Gombos, G. (1980) Carbonic anhydrase: an ultrastructural study in rat cerebellum. *Histochem. J.* 12:473–483.

Lecuona, E., Luquin, S., Avila, J., Garcia-Segura, L.M., and Martin-Vasallo, P. (1996) Expression of the beta 1 and beta 2 (AMOG) subunits of the Na,K-ATPase in neural tissues: cellular and developmental distribution patterns. *Brain Res. Bull.* 40:167–174.

Linser, P.J. (1985) Multiple marker analysis in the avian optic tectum reveals three classes of neuroglia and carbonic anhydrase-containing neurons. *J. Neurosci.* 5:2388–2396.

Linser, P. and Moscona, A.A. (1981) Carbonic anhydrase C in the neural retina: transition from generalized to glia-specific cell localization during embryonic development. *Proc. Natl. Acad. Sci. USA* 78:7190–7194.

Linser, P. and Moscona, A.A. (1983) Hormonal induction of glutamine synthetase in cultures of embryonic retina cells: requirement for neuron-glia contact interactions. *Dev. Biol.* 96:529–534.

Löffler T., Al-Robaiy, S., Bigl, M., Eschrich, K., and Schliebs, R. (2001) Expression of fructose-1,6-bisphosphatase mRNA isoforms in normal and basal forebrain cholinergic lesioned rat brain. *Int. J. Dev. Neurosci.* 19:279–285.

Lomako, J., Lomako W.M., Whelan, W.J., Dombro, R.S., Neary, J.T., and Norenberg, M.D. (1993) Glycogen synthesis in the astrocyte: from glycogenin to proglycogen to glycogen. *FASEB J.* 7:1386–1393.

Manos, P. and Bryan, G.K. (1993) Cellular and subcellular compartmentation of creatine kinase in brain. *Dev. Neurosci.* 15: 271–279.

Martin-Vasallo, P., Wetzel, R.K., Garcia-Segura, L.M., Molina-Holgado, E., Arystarkhova, E., and Sweadner, K.J. (2000) Oligodendrocytes in brain and optic nerve express the beta3 subunit isoform of Na,K-ATPase. *Glia* 31:206–218.

McGrail, K.M., Phillips, J.M., and Sweadner, K.J. (1991) Immunofluorescent localization of three Na,K-ATPase isozymes in the rat central nervous cystem: both neurons and glia can express more than one Na,K-ATPase. *J. Neurosci.* 11:381–391.

Miller, K.E., Richards, B.A., and Kriebel, R.M. (2002) Glutamine-, glutamine synthetase-, glutamate dehydrogenase- and pyruvate carboxylase-immunoreactivities in the rat dorsal root ganglion and peripheral nerve. *Brain Res.* 945:202–211.

Mobasheri, A., Avila, J., Cozar-Castellano, I., Brownleader, M.D., Trevan, M., Francis, M.J., Lamb, J.F., and Martin-Vasallo, P. (2000) Na+, K+-ATPase isozyme diversity; comparative biochemistry and physiological implications of novel functional interactions. *Biosci. Rep.* 20:51–91.

Molloy, G.R., Wilson, C.D., Benfield, P., De Vellis, J., and Kumar, S. (1992) Rat brain creatine kinase messenger RNA levels are high in primary cultures of brain astrocytes and oligodendrocytes and low in neurons. *J. Neurochem.* 59:1925–1932.

Mori, K., Ogawa, Y., Ebihara, K., Tamura, N., Tashiro, K., Kuwahara, T., Mukoyama, M., Sugawara, A., Ozaki, S., Tanaka, I., and Nakao, K. (1999) Isolation and characterization of CA XIV, a novel membrane-bound carbonic anhydrase from mouse kidney. *J. Biol. Chem.* 274:15701–15705.

Moseley, A.E., Lieske, S.P., Wetzel, R.K., James, P.F., He, S., Shelly, D.A., Paul, R.J., Boivin, G.P., Witte, D.P., Ramirez, J.M., Sweadner, K.J., and Lingrel, J.B. (2003) The Na, K-ATPase alpha 2 isoform is expressed in neurons, and its absence disrupts neuronal activity in newborn mice. *J. Biol. Chem.* 278:5317–5324.

Mu, J., Skurat, A.V., and Roach, P.J. (1997) Glycogenin-2, a novel self-glucosylating protein involved in liver glycogen biosynthesis. *J. Biol. Chem.* 272:27589–27597.

Nagao, Y., Srinivasan, M., Platero, J.S., Svendrowski, M., Waheed, A., and Sly, W.S. (1994) Mitochondrial carbonic anhydrase (isozyme V) in mouse and rat: cDNA cloning, expression, subcellular localization, processing, and tissue distribution. *Proc. Natl. Acad. Sci. USA* 91:10330–10334.

Narahara, E., Makino, Y., and Omichi, K. (2001) Glycogen debranching enzyme in bovine brain. *J. Biochem. (Tokyo)* 130:465–470.

Newgard, C.B., Brady, M.J., Odoherty, R.M., and Saltiel, A.R. (2000) Organizing glucose disposal—Emerging roles of the glycogen targeting subunits of protein phosphatase-1. *Diabetes* 49: 1967–1977.

Newgard, C.B., Hwang, P.K., and Fletterick, R.J. (1989) The family of glycogen phosphorylases: structure and function. *Crit. Rev. Biochem. Mol. Biol.* 24:69–99.

Newgard, C.B., Littman, D.R., Van Genderen, C., Smith, M., and Fletterick, R.J. (1988) Human brain glycogen phosphorylase: cloning, sequence analysis, chromosomal mapping, tissue expression, and comparison with the human liver and muscle isozymes. *J. Biol. Chem.* 263:3850–3857.

Nogradi, A. (1993) Differential expression of carbonic anhydrase isoenzymes in microglial cell types. *Glia* 8:133–142.

Nogradi, A., Kelly, C., and Carter, N.D. (1993) Localization of acetazolamide-resistant carbonic anhydrase III in human and rat choroid plexus by immunocytochemistry and in situ hybridization. *Neurosci. Lett.* 151:162–165.

Ocal, G., Berberoglu, M., Adiyaman, P., Cetinkaya, E., Ekim, M., Aycan, Z., and Evliyaoglu, O. (2001) Osteoporosis, renal tubular acidosis without urinary concentration abnormality, cerebral calcification and severe mental retardation in three Turkish brothers. *J. Pediatr. Endocrinol. Metab.* 14:1671–1677.

Niitsu, Y., Hori, O., Yamaguchi, A., Bando, Y., Ozawa, K., Tamatani, M., Ogawa, S., and Tohyama, M. (1999) Exposure of cultured primary rat astrocytes to hypoxia results in intracellular glucose depletion and induction of glycolytic enzymes. *Brain Res. Mol. Brain Res.* 74:26–34.

Oksche, A. (1958) Histologische Untersuchungen über die Bedeutung des Ependyms, der Glia und der plexus choroidei für den Kohlenhydratstoffwechsel des ZNS. *Z. Zellforschung* 48:74–129.

Oksche, A. (1961) Der histochemisch nachweisbare Glycogenaufbau und abbau in den Astrocyten und Ependymzellen als Beispiel einer funktionsabhängigen Stoffwechselaktivität der Neuroglia. *Z. Zellforschung* 54:307–361.

Parkkila, A.K., Herva, R., Parkkila, S., and Rajaniemi, H. (1995) Immunohistochemical demonstration of human carbonic anhydrase isoenzyme II in brain tumours. *Histochem. J.* 27:974–982.

Parkkila, S. (2000) Carbonic anhydrase isoforms and their expression in mammals. In: Chegwidden, W.R., Carter, N.D., and Edwards, Y.H., eds. *The Carbonic Anhydrases, New Horizons.* Basel: Birkhäuser, pp. 79–93.

Parkkila, S., Parkkila, A.K., Rajaniemi, H., Shah, G.N., Grubb, J.H., Waheed, A., and Sly, W.S. (2001) Expression of membrane-associated carbonic anhydrase XIV on neurons and axons in mouse and human brain. *Proc. Natl. Acad. Sci. USA* 98:1918–1923.

Paudel, H.K., Zwiers, H., and Wang, J.H. (1993) Phosphorylase kinase phosphorylates the calmodulin-binding regulatory regions of neuronal tissue-specific proteins B-50 (GAP-43) and neurogranin. *J. Biol. Chem.* 268:6207–6213.

Pellegri, G., Rossier, C., Magistretti, P.J., and Martin, J.L. (1996) Cloning, localization and induction of mouse brain glycogen synthase. *Brain. Res. Mol. Brain. Res.* 38:191–199.

Peng, L., Arystarkhova, E., and Sweadner, K.J. (1998) Plasticity of Na,K-ATPase isoform expression in cultures of flat astrocytes: species differences in gene expression. *Glia* 24:257–271.

Peng, L., Martin-Vasallo, P., and Sweadner, K.J. (1997) Isoforms of Na, K-ATPase alpha and beta subunits in the rat cerebellum and in granule cell cultures. *J. Neurosci.* 17:3488–3502.

Persson, J.K., Lindh, B., Elde, R., Robertson, B., Rivero-Melian, C., Eriksson, N.P., Hokfelt, T., and Aldskogius, H. (1995) The expression of different cytochemical markers in normal and axotomised dorsal root ganglion cells projecting to the nucleus gracilis in the adult rat. *Exp. Brain Res.* 105:331–344.

Pfeiffer, B., Buse, E., Meyermann, R., and Hamprecht, B. (1995) Immunocytochemical localization of glycogen phosphorylase in primary sensory ganglia of the peripheral nervous system of the rat. *Histochem. Cell Biol.* 103:69–74.

Pfeiffer, B., Grosche, J., Reichenbach, A., and Hamprecht, B. (1994) Immunocytochemical demonstration of glycogen phosphorylase in Muller (glial) cells of the mammalian retina. *Glia* 12:62–67.

Pfeiffer-Guglielmi, B., Broer, S., Broer, A., and Hamprecht, B. (2000) Isozyme pattern of glycogen phosphorylase in the rat nervous system and rat astroglia-rich primary cultures: electrophoretic and polymerase chain reaction studies. *Neurochem. Res.* 25:1485–1491.

Pfeiffer-Guglielmi, B., Fleckenstein, B., Jung, G., and Hamprecht, B. (2003) Immunocytochemical localization of glycogen phosphorylase isozymes in rat nervous tissues by using isozyme-specific antibodies. *J. Neurochem.* 85:73–81.

Philbert, M.A., Beiswanger, C.M., Roscoe, T.L., Waters, D.K., and Lowndes, H.E. (1991) Enhanced resolution of histochemical distribution of glucose-6-phosphate dehydrogenase activity in rat neural tissue by use of a semipermeable membrane. *J. Histochem. Cytochem.* 39:937–943.

Philippe, J.M., Dubois, J.M., Rouzaire-Dubois, B., Cartron, P.F., Vallette, F., and Morel, N. (2002) Functional expression of V-ATPases in the plasma membrane of glial cells. *Glia* 37:365–373.

Pitcher, J., Smythe, C., and Cohen, P. (1988) Glycogenin is the priming glucosyltransferase required for the initiation of glycogen biogenesis in rabbit skeletal muscle. *Eur. J. Biochem.* 176:391–395.

Poitry-Yamate, L.L., Poitry, S., and Tsacopoulos, M. (1995) Lactate released by Muller glial cells is metabolized by photoreceptors from mammalian retina. *J. Neurosci.* 15:5179–5191.

Polekhina, G., Gupta, A., Michell, B.J., van Denderen, B., Murthy, S., Feil, S.C., Jennings, I.G., Campbell, D.J., Witters, L.A., Parker, M.W., Kemp, B.E., and Stapleton, D. (2003) AMPK beta subunit targets metabolic stress sensing to glycogen. *Curr. Biol.* 13:867–871.

Preller, A. and Wilson, J.E. (1992) Localization of the type III isozyme of hexokinase at the nuclear periphery. *Arch. Biochem. Biophys.* 294:482–492.

Price, N., van der Leij, F., Jackson, V., Corstorphine, C., Thomson, R., Sorensen, A., and Zammit, V. (2002) A novel brain-expressed protein related to carnitine palmitoyltransferase I. *Genomics* 80:433–442.

Printen, J.A., Brady, M.J., and Saltiel, A.R. (1997) PTG, a protein phosphatase 1-binding protein with a role in glycogen metabolism. *Science* 275:1475–1478.

Psarra, A.M., Pfeiffer, B., Giannakopoulou, M., Sotiroudis, T.G., Stylianopoulou, F., and Hamprecht, B. (1998) Immunocytochemical localization of glycogen phosphorylase kinase in rat brain sections and in glial and neuronal primary cultures. *J. Neurocytol.* 27:779–790.

Rahman, B., Kussmaul, L., Hamprecht, B., and Dringen, R. (2000) Glycogen is mobilized during the disposal of peroxides by cultured astroglial cells from rat brain. *Neurosci. Lett.* 290:169–172.

Ramirez, O. and Jimenez, E. (2002) Sexual dimorphism in rat cerebrum and cerebellum: different patterns of catalytically active creatine kinase isoenzymes during postnatal development and aging. *Int. J. Dev. Neurosci.* 20:627–639.

Richter, F., Böhme, H.J., and Hofmann, E. (1983) Developmental changes of glycogen phosphorylase b isozymes in rat tissues. *Biomed. Biochim. Acta* 42:1229–1235.

Richter, K., Hamprecht, B., and Scheich, H. (1996) Ultrastructural localization of glycogen phosphorylase predominantly in astrocytes of the gerbil brain. *Glia* 17:263–273.

Ridderstrale, Y. and Wistrand, P.J. (2000) Membrane-associated carbonic anhydrase activity in the brain of CA II-deficient mice. *J. Neurocytol.* 29:263–269.

Roach, P.J. and Skurat, A.V. (1997) Self-glucosylating initiator proteins and their role in glycogen biosynthesis. *Prog. Nucleic Acid Res. Mol. Biol.* 57:289–316.

Robertson, B. and Grant, G. (1989) Immunocytochemical evidence for the localization of the GM1 ganglioside in carbonic anhydrase-containing and RT 97-immunoreactive rat primary sensory neurons. *J. Neurocytol.* 18:77–86.

Rodriguez, I.R. and Whelan, W.J. (1985) A novel glycosyl-amino acid linkage: rabbit-muscle glycogen is covalently linked to a protein via tyrosine. *Biochem. Biophys. Res. Commun.* 132:829–836.

Roussel, G., Delaunoy, J.P., Nussbaum, J.L., and Mandel, P. (1979) Demonstration of a specific localization of carbonic anhydrase C in the glial cells of rat CNS by an immunohistochemical method. *Brain Res.* 160:47–55.

Rust, R.S., Jr., Carter, J.G., Martin, D., Nerbonne, J.M., Lampe, P.A., Pusateri, M.E., and Lowry, O.H. (1991) Enzyme levels in cultured astrocytes, oligodendrocytes and Schwann cells, and neurons from the cerebral cortex and superior cervical ganglia of the rat. *Neurochem. Res.* 16:991–999.

Salvan, A.M., Vion-Dury, J., Confort-Gouny, S., Dano, P., and Cozzone, P.J. (1997) Increased cerebral glycogen detected by localized ^{1}H-magnetic resonance spectroscopy in a patient with suspected McArdle's disease. *Eur. Neurol.* 37:251–253.

Sato, K., Satoh, K., Sato, T., Imai, F., and Morris, H.P. (1976) Isozyme patterns of glycogen phosphorylase in rat tissues and transplantable hepatomas. *Cancer Res.* 36:487–495.

Sato, T., Kashima, K., Gamachi, A., Daa, T., Nakayama, I., and Yokoyama, S. (2002) Immunohistochemical localization of pyruvate carboxylase and carbamyl-phosphate synthetase I in normal and neoplastic human pancreatic tissues. *Pancreas* 25:130–135.

Schmoll, D., Cesar, M., Fuhrmann, E., and Hamprecht, B. (1995a) Colocalization of fructose-1,6-bisphosphatase and glial fibrillary acidic protein in rat brain. *Brain Res.* 677:341–344.

Schmoll, D., Fuhrmann, E., Gebhardt, R., and Hamprecht, B. (1995b) Significant amounts of glycogen are synthesized from 3-carbon compounds in astroglial primary cultures from mice with participation of the mitochondrial phosphoenolpyruvate carboxykinase isoenzyme. *Eur. J. Biochem.* 227:308–315.

Schröder, J.M., May, R., Shin, Y.S., Sigmund, M., and Nase-Huppmeier, S. (1993) Juvenile hereditary polyglucosan body disease with complete branching enzyme deficiency (type IV glycogenosis). *Acta Neuropathol. (Berl)* 85:419–430.

Sensenbrenner, M., Lucas, M., and Deloulme, J.C. (1997) Expression of two neuronal markers, growth-associated protein 43 and neuron-specific enolase in rat glial cells. *J. Mol. Med.* 75:653–663.

Shah, G.N., Hewett-Emmett, D., Grubb, J.H., Migas, M.C., Fleming, R.E., Waheed, A., and Sly, W.S. (2000) Mitochondrial carbonic anhydrase CA VB: differences in tissue distribution and pattern of evolution from those of CA VA suggest distinct physiological roles. *Proc. Natl. Acad. Sci. USA* 97:1677–1682.

Shearer, J. and Graham, T.E. (2002) New perspectives on the storage and organization of muscle glycogen. *Can. J. Appl. Physiol.* 27:179–203.

Shen, W., Willis, D., Zhang, Y., Schlattner, U., Wallimann, T., and Molloy, G.R. (2002) Expression of creatine kinase isoenzyme genes during postnatal development of rat brain cerebellum: evidence for transcriptional regulation. *Biochem. J.* 367:369–380.

Sistermans, E.A., De Kok, Y.J., Peters, W., Ginsel, L.A., Jap, P.H., and Wieringa, B. (1995) Tissue- and cell-specific distribution of creatine kinase B: a new and highly specific monoclonal antibody for use in immunohistochemistry. *Cell Tissue Res.* 280:435–446.

Sly, W.S. and Hu, P.Y. (1995) Human carbonic anhydrases and carbonic anhydrase deficiencies. *Annu. Rev. Biochem.* 64:375–401.

Stauffer, T.P., Guerini, D., Celio, M.R., and Carafoli, E. (1997) Immunolocalization of the plasma membrane Ca^{2+} pump isoforms in the rat brain. *Brain Res.* 748:21–29.

Staugaitis, S.M., Zerlin, M., Hawkes, R., Levine, J.M., and Goldman, J.E. (2001) Aldolase C/zebrin II expression in the neonatal rat forebrain reveals cellular heterogeneity within the subventricular zone and early astrocyte differentiation. *J. Neurosci.* 21:6195–6205.

Svichar, N. and Chesler, M. (2003) Surface carbonic anhydrase activity on astrocytes and neurons facilitates lactate transport. *Glia* 41:415–419.

Sweadner, K.J. (1992) Overlapping and diverse distribution of Na-K ATPase isozymes in neurons and glia. *Can. J. Physiol. Pharmacol.* 70 Suppl.: S255–S259.

Takeyasu, K., Kawase, T., and Yoshimura, S.H. (2003) Intermolecular interaction between Na+/K+-ATPase alpha subunit and glycogen phosphorylase. *Ann. N.Y. Acad. Sci.* 986:522–524.

Taniuchi, K., Nishimori, I., Takeuchi, T., Fujikawa-Adachi, K., Ohtsuki, Y., and Onishi, S. (2002a) Developmental expression of carbonic anhydrase-related proteins VIII, X and XI in the human brain. *Neuroscience* 112:93–99.

Taniuchi, K., Nishimori, I., Takeuchi, T., Ohtsuki, Y., and Onishi, S. (2002b) cDNA cloning and developmental expression of murine carbonic anhydrase-related proteins VIII, X and XI. *Brain Res. Mol. Brain Res.* 109:207–215.

Thompson, R.J., Kynoch, P.A., and Willson, V.J. (1982) Cellular localization of aldolase C subunits in human brain. *Brain Res.* 232:489–493.

Tolmasky, D.S., Labriola, C., and Krisman, C.R. (1998) Glycogen brain branching enzyme. *Cell. Mol. Biol.* 44:455–460.

Tong, C.K., Cammer, W., and Chesler, M. (2000) Activity-dependent pH shifts in hippocampal slices from normal and carbonic anhydrase II-deficient mice. *Glia* 31:125–130.

Tsacopoulos, M. and Magistretti, P.J. (1996) Metabolic coupling between glia and neurons. *J. Neurosci.* 16:877–885.

Vaananen, H.K., Carter, N.D., and Dodgson, S.J. (1991) Immunocytochemical localization of mitochondrial carbonic anhydrase in rat tissues. *J. Histochem. Cytochem.* 39:451–459.

Wagner, G., Kovacs, J., Low, P., Orosz, F., and Ovadi, J. (2001) Tubulin and microtubule are potential targets for brain hexokinase binding. FEBS Lett. 509:81–84.

Wallimann, T., Dolder, M., Schlattner, U., Eder, M., Hornemann, T., O'Gorman, E., Ruck, A., and Brdiczka, D. (1998) Some new aspects of creatine kinase (CK): compartmentation, structure, function and regulation for cellular and mitochondrial bioenergetics and physiology. *Biofactors* 8:229–234.

Walther, E.U., Dichgans, M., Maricich, S.M., Romito, R.R., Yang, F., Dziennis, S., Zackson, S., Hawkes, R., and Herrup, K. (1998) Genomic sequences of aldolase C (Zebrin II) direct lacZ expression exclusively in non-neuronal cells of transgenic mice. *Proc. Natl. Acad. Sci. USA* 95:2615–2620.

Wetzel, R.K., Arystarkhova, E., and Sweadner, K.J. (1999) Cellular and subcellular specification of Na,K-ATPase alpha and beta isoforms in the postnatal development of mouse retina. *J. Neurosci.* 19:9878–9889.

Wiesinger, H. (1995) Glia-specific enzyme systems. In: Ransom, B. and Kettenmann, H., eds. *Neuroglia*. New York and Oxford: Oxford University Press, pp. 488–499.

Wilkin, G.P. and Wilson, J.E. (1977) Localization of hexokinase in neural tissue: light microscopic studies with immunofluorescence and histochemical procedures. *J. Neurochem.* 29:1039–1051.

Wilson, J.E. (1983) Hexokinase. In: Lajtha, A., ed. *Handbook of Neurochemistry*, vol. 4, 2nd ed. New York: Klemm, pp. 151–172.

Wilson, J.E. (1995) Hexokinases. *Rev. Physiol. Biochem. Pharmacol.* 126:65–198.

Wilson, J.E. (1997) Homologous and heterologous interactions between hexokinase and mitochondrial porin: evolutionary implications. *J. Bioenerg. Biomembr.* 29:97–102.

Wilson, J.E. (2003) Isozymes of mammalian hexokinase: structure, subcellular localization and metabolic function. *J. Exp. Biol.* 206: 2049–2057.

Woo, A.L., James, P.F., and Lingrel, J.B. (2000) Sperm motility is dependent on a unique isoform of the Na,K-ATPase. *J. Biol. Chem.* 275:20693–20699.

16 Second messenger systems

SEAN MURPHY AND BRIAN R. PEARCE

Our understanding of signaling between astrocytes, and between glia and neurons, has increased considerably over the past decade. Such communication can be mediated by conventional ligand-receptor coupling, with the subsequent initiation of second messenger cascades, and/or ion channel opening, or via gap junctions. This area of research has been the subject of a number of recent reviews (Carmignoto, 2000; Araque et al., 2001; Bezzi and Volterra, 2001; Fields and Stevens-Graham, 2002; Gallo and Ghiani, 2000; Hansson and Ronnback, 2003). Particular aspects of signaling will be addressed in detail in the chapters concerning specific glial subtypes. Here we confine ourselves to recent developments in (predominantly astro-) glial second messenger pathways, particularly those involved in intracellular Ca^{2+} signaling. Wherever possible, we indicate how these may influence the expression and/or function of downstream targets.

Rather than be redundant or attempt the impossible (a synthesis), we have chosen to illustrate signaling cascades in glia by reference to the regulation of expression and activity of the nitric oxide synthases (NOS). The product of NOS activity, nitric oxide (NO), then interacts with numerous other molecules, including cyclooxygenase (COX)-2. Finally, we draw attention to the evidence for *assemblies* of signaling molecules. Compared with highly polarized endothelial cells and neurons, little attention has yet been paid to such *compartmentation* within glia.

SECOND MESSENGER PATHWAYS AND INTRACELLULAR Ca^{2+} RELEASE CHANNELS

Astrocytes possess an array of receptors linked to the mobilization of intracellular Ca^{2+} stores (Deitmer et al., 1998). The release of Ca^{2+} from these stores is mediated, as in other cell types, by the opening of second messenger–activated intracellular Ca^{2+} release channels that belong to either the inositol 1,4,5-trisphosphate (IP_3R) or ryanodine (RyR) receptor families, three isoforms of each being known to exist.

See the list of abbreviations at the end of the chapter.

The first step in the sequence of events leading to IP_3R activation is receptor-G-protein-coupled generation of the second messenger 1,4,5-IP_3 by phospholipase C–mediated cleavage of phosphatidylinositol 4,5-bisphosphate (PIP2). It was generally believed that 1,4,5-IP_3 was then subjected to dephosphorylation by a 5-phosphatase, thus terminating its effect. However, it is also a substrate for the enzyme 1,4,5-IP_3-3-kinase, a reaction that yields inositol 1,3,4,5-tetrakisphosphate (1,3,4,5-IP_4). Two isoforms of the 3-kinase are known to exist (A and B), the B isoform being present in astrocytes, where its activity was found to be regulated by protein kinase C and Ca^{2+}-calmodulin-dependent kinase II (Communi et al., 1999). Previous studies on other cell types have shown this isoform to be located at the endoplasmic reticulum (Soriano et al., 1997), but Communi et al. (1999) reported translocation to the particulate fraction upon receptor stimulation in astrocytes. The function(s) of 1,3,4,5-IP_4 remain to be fully elucidated in these cells, as in many others. Nonetheless, some intriguing possibilities have been suggested (Irvine, 2001): protection of 1,4,5-IP_3 from 5-phosphatase hydrolysis and enhancement of Ca^{2+} mobilization; regulation of Ca^{2+} influx in response to store depletion; inhibition of the IP_3Rs contribution to the generation of Ca^{2+} oscillations; a precursor for more highly phosphorylated "messenger" IPs.

There is some controversy over the subtype of IP_3R expressed by astrocytes. Immunohistochemical studies in intact tissue have either shown the presence of IP_3R3 but not types 1 or 2 (Yamamoto-Hino et al., 1995) or predominantly IP_3R2 (Sharp et al., 1999). The latter group also reported the expression of IP_3R2 in cultured astrocytes (Sheppard et al., 1997), yet using reverse transcriptase–polymerase chain reaction (RT-PCR) analysis, one of us (B.P.) found mRNA for only IP_3R1 in similar cultures (K. Brickley, F.A. Lai, and B. Pearce, unpublished observations).

The first observation of RyR-mediated Ca^{2+} mobilization in cultured cortical astrocytes was made by Langley and Pearce (1994), who showed that RyRs were not expressed by all cells in these cultures and that responses were not mimicked by caffeine. This suggested that astrocytes might possess the RyR3 isoform, a proposal that was subsequently confirmed by RT-PCR analysis of mRNA isolated from both cultured cells and astrocytes acutely dissociated from adult brain (Brickley et al., 1998; Matyash et al., 2002). However, Russell and coworkers have rarely observed RyR-mediated Ca^{2+} transients in type 1 astrocytes but have found them in populations of type 2 astrocytes (Simpson et al., 1995, 1998a). They argue that this may be due to the poor colocalization of RyRs and calreticulin, a Ca^{2+} binding protein known to be involved in Ca^{2+} storage and release from the endoplasmic reticulum (Simpson et al., 1998b). Indeed, more recent studies have shown that cultured astrocytes possess structurally distinct components of the endoplasmic reticulum that might be accessed independently by either RyR or IP_3R activation (Golovina and Blaustein, 2000). There may, however, be a more simple explanation for this apparent discrepancy. The Russell group routinely uses astrocyte cultures that have been maintained *in vitro* for approximately 7–10 days. The RT-PCR results from one of our laboratories (B.P.) indicated that cortical astrocytes only possess mRNA for RyR3 after some 21 days *in vitro* (K. Brickley, F.A. Lai, and B. Pearce, unpublished observations).

Using a wound-healing model in cultures prepared from RyR3 knockout mice, Matyash et al. (2002) found astrocyte migration into the damaged area to be impaired. This suggested a role for RyR3 in astrocyte motility; however, it was found not to be involved in chemokine-mediated chemotaxis (Matyash et al., 2002). Whether RyR3 is involved in other aspects of astrocyte biology remains to be established, as does the intracellular signaling molecule responsible for its activation. One candidate for this role is cyclic ADP-ribose (cADPr), which is synthesized from nicotinamide adenine dinucleotide by adenosine diphosphate (ADP) ribosyl cyclase and is known to activate RyRs in various cell types (Higashida et al., 2001). Early reports showed this enzyme to be present in astrocytes, but on the extracellular face of the plasma membrane (Pawlikowska et al., 1996). More recently, Hotta et al. (2000) have confirmed this, but have also demonstrated that these cells are capable of generating intracellular cADPr and that enzyme activity can be increased by β-adrenoceptor stimulation. It is interesting to note that there is little evidence for cADPr-mediated activation of RyR3 (Fulceri et al., 2001). With nicotinamide adenine dinucleotide phosphate as a substrate, ADP ribosyl cyclase also generates nicotinic acid adenine dinucleotide phosphate (NAADP), another Ca^{2+}-mobilizing signal molecule that has been shown to act at sites distinct from both RyRs and IP_3Rs. The release of Ca^{2+} from NAADP-sensitive stores may prime further Ca^{2+} release from IP_3- and/or cADPr-sensitive stores (Genazzi and Galione, 1997; Churchill and Galione, 2001; Genazzi and Billington, 2002). To our knowledge, there is no evidence for NAADP-mediated Ca^{2+} signaling in astrocytes.

NITRIC OXIDE SYNTHASES

Changes in intracellular Ca^{2+} have important consequences for cell signaling, including the generation of NO. The NOS enzymes catalyze an oxidation reaction whereby NO is generated from L-arginine, with L-citrulline as the coproduct. The three isoforms of NOS, while products of distinct genes, share 50%–60% homology at the nucleotide and amino acid levels. Two of these gene products, NOS-1 and NOS-3, are constitutively expressed enzymes that are Ca^{2+}-calmodulin dependent and produce small amounts of NO in response to transient elevations in intracellular Ca^{2+}. However, NOS-2 is transcriptionally induced and functions independently of a rise in intracellular Ca^{2+} (Murphy, 2000). In contrast to the constitutive isoforms, NOS-2 has calmodulin bound at all times, maintaining the enzyme in a tonically active state and therefore capable of producing a continuous flux of NO in the presence of adequate substrate (L-arginine) and cofactors.

All central nervous system (CNS) parenchymal cells, together with the smooth muscle and endothelium of the cerebral vessel wall, can express NOS activity. *In vitro* and *in vivo* evidence suggests that all three NOS isoforms can be expressed in astrocytes. The evidence for NOS-2 expression in microglia is well established, and expression of NOS-2 in oligodendrocytes has been reported. To date, there is no firm evidence for any constitutive expression of NOS in oligodendrocytes or microglia (Murphy, 2000).

Activation of Constitutive Nitric Oxide Synthase Isoforms

Simply put, the activities of NOS-1 and NOS-3 are regulated by changes in intracellular Ca^{2+}. In addition, both isoforms display signature motifs in the N-terminal regions to permit interactions with proteins in lipid domains.

Nitric oxide synthase-3

This protein is targeted to plasmalemmal caveolae (Shaul, 2002) through dual acylation by myristate (irreversible) and palmitate (reversible). First described more than 40 years ago, caveolae have distinct physical features, such as the caveolin proteins 1–3 and cholesterol (see Table 16.1). Lipid rafts have lipid compositions similar to those of caveolae but do not contain caveolin. Flotillin in caveolar membranes can replace caveolin in lipid domains. We shall not discuss whether caveolae are biochemically distinct from lipid rafts, though there is evidence to support this conclusion (Sowa et al., 2001).

Much attention and debate has centered on lipid domains in highly polar cells such as endothelium and

TABLE 16.1 *Typical Components of Lipid Rafts*

Cholesterol
Sphingomyelin
Glyco-sphingolipids (GM1)
Phosphoinositides (PIP2)
Caveolins-1, -2, and -3
Flotillins-1 and -2
Glycosyl-phospharidylinositol (GPI)-linked proteins (e.g., Thy-1)
Src-family tyrosine kinases
G-proteins
Nitric oxide synthase-3
H-Ras
RAGE receptor
Receptor tyrosine kinases (e.g., insulin-receptor, epidermal growth factor receptor, platelet-derived growth factor receptor)
Hepta-helical receptors (e.g., endothelin receptor)

neurons (Tsui-Pierchala et al., 2002). The apparent lack of caveolae and the caveolin proteins in the nervous system has delayed their appreciation (Masserini et al., 1999), coupled with the lack of any distinct CNS phenotype in caveolin-1 and -3 knockout mice (Razani and Lisanti, 2001). However, the transient expression or downregulation of caveolin may explain why these proteins are not readily reported in the CNS.

Concerning glia, the first report of caveolae in astrocytes was by Lawrence and Raisman (1987), subsequently supported by evidence obtained using electron microscopy (Cameron et al., 1997). Plasma membrane invaginations with the morphological appearance of caveolae are also present in cells forming the perineurial sheath of the peripheral nervous system (PNS). Mikol et al. (1999) reported caveolin-1 immunoreactivity in rat sciatic nerve, and also in Schwann cells and derived cell lines, with a possible role in integrin signaling. They went on to show that caveolin expression is tightly linked to the myelinating phenotype, and speculated that loss of caveolin by Schwann cells after axotomy enables the switch from dedifferentiated to a proliferative cell type (Mikol et al., 2002). As the targeted downregulation of caveolin-1 apparently promotes cell transformation and tumorigenicity, Cameron et al. (2002) looked at levels in transformed glia and a series of human glioma–derived cell lines. However, the process of transformation did not reduce caveolin expression, nor did its expression prevent transformation.

Caveolins function as scaffolding proteins to organize signaling molecules, concentrating components related to each other, allowing interaction, and modulating function (often negatively) (Smart et al., 1999). Caveolin-binding sequence motifs are found in the enzymatically active catalytic domain of a given signaling molecule. Caveolin inhibits NOS-3 activity, and this is reversed by increases in cell Ca^{2+}. Depalmitoylation causes translocation of NOS-3 to the cytoplasm, where phosphorylation may terminate enzyme activity. Interestingly, in caveolin-1 knockout mice, there is decreased vascular tone. This presumably results from constitutive NOS-3 activity in the absence of the negative regulator, caveolin-1. It is not yet known whether this extends to the cerebral vasculature or to changes in NOS-3 function in astrocytes.

Tyrosine kinase receptors, mono- and heterotrimeric G proteins, src-like tyrosine kinases, protein kinase C (PKC) and cyclic AMP–dependent protein kinase (PKA), adenylyl cyclase, phospholipase D-1, mitogen-activated protein kinase kinase (MEK), the integrins, interleukin-6 (IL-6) receptor gp130, interferon-γ receptor (IFNγR) alpha chain, and signal transducers and activators of transcription (STATS) 1 and 3 are all associated with caveolae. In the vasculature, NOS-3 activity can also be increased independent of cell calcium, for example in response to vascular endothelial growth factor (VEGF), insulin, and shear stress, presumably through the near-neighbor receptors (Shaul, 2002). These signal through the phosphatidylinositol 3-kinase (PI 3-K) pathway and its downstream effector Akt (protein kinase B), which phosphorylates NOS-3 on a serine residue at position 1179. While NOS-1 is not normally a substrate for Akt, it becomes both membrane-associated and a substrate for Akt if engineered to contain the N-myristoylation site. Whether NOS-3 in astrocytes colocalizes with similar signaling molecules is unknown.

Nitric oxide synthase-1

The structure of the NOS-1 gene is very diverse. The identification of multiple NOS-1 promoter sites, RNA splice variants, and alternate translation products suggest that NOS-1 expression is highly regulated. The major NOS-1 transcript, nNOSα, is a product of the splicing of variant exons 1 to a common exon 2. The genetic analysis of NOS-1 knockouts, generated by the deletion of exon 2, has revealed the expression of two additional transcripts (nNOSβ, nNOSγ), each with a unique exon 1 and spliced into exon 3. Later studies demonstrated that truncated proteins are translated and enzymatically functional in wild-type mice. The NOS-1α protein (but not β or γ) displays a single interactive PDZ domain (see the section "Assemblies of Signaling Molecules") in the N-terminal region, which permits direct targeting to membrane receptors, such as serotonin 2B and the melatonin receptor, and in neurons is a component of the synaptic assembly (Sheng and Sala, 2001).

Activation of astrocyte NOS-1 is via α1-adrenergic and glutamate receptors (coupled to PIP_2 hydrolysis and intracellular calcium elevation), and also calcium-permeable AMPA receptors. However, the NOS-1 described in cultured astrocytes does not appear to be membrane-associated (Arbones et al., 1996) and therefore might be a variant, such as β or γ. Indeed, Catania et al. (2001) have described up-regulation of β and γ in reactive astrocyes.

Transcriptional activation of nitric oxide synthase-2

The expression of NOS-2 in all glia can be promoted by extracellular signals, such as cytokines [IL-1β, tumor necrosis factor-α (TNF-α), IFN-γ] and bacterial lipopolysaccharide (LPS), via activation of transcription factors such as NFκB (Murphy, 2000). Evidence is now accumulating that this process can be regulated by a complex interplay between intracellular signaling pathways involving both protein kinases and phosphatases. Reversible protein phosphorylation regulates a wide array of cellular functions. The identification and possible roles of protein kinases in glial biology have expanded dramatically over the past decade, yet little attention has been paid to their counterparts the protein phosphatases.

Mammalian mitogen-activated protein kinase (MAPK) pathways involve either extracellular regulated protein kinases (ERKs), p38 MAPK, or Jun-NH_2-terminal kinase (JNK). Each kinase is activated by an upstream MAPK kinase (MEK), and all have been described in glial cells *in situ*. Several studies reveal that some of these kinases regulate NOS-2 expression. For example, Bhat et al. (1998, 2002) demonstrated the involvement of both p38 MAPK and ERK in rat astrocytes and microglia, while Hua et al. (2002) showed that inhibition of p38 MAPK and JNK, but not ERK, prevented IL-1β-mediated NOS-2 induction in human astrocytes. It is clear, however, that other signaling pathways impinge upon the MAPK cascade to regulate NOS-2 expression in these cells. Pahan et al. (1999, 2000) showed that blockade of PI 3-kinase potentiated LPS- and IL-1β-stimulated NOS-2 induction in rat and human primary astrocytes; in C6 glioma, neither stimulus is able to promote induction when used alone. Interestingly, despite their inability to induce NOS-2 expression, these agents were found to stimulate MAPK and NFκB activity in the glioma cell line (Pahan et al., 1999). These findings point to a PI 3-kinase-mediated negative regulation of NOS-2 expression at some point(s) in the cascade of events leading to this response. The precise mechanism has yet to be established; however, a downstream target of PI 3-kinase (via Akt) is NOS-3, which is activated by this kinase (see the section "Nitric Oxide Synthase-3"), suggesting that a reduction in tonic NO production within the cell contributes in some way to the expression of NOS-2.

Negative regulation can also be achieved by the activation of PKA. Agents that increase intracellular cyclic adenosine monophosphate (cAMP) concentrations have been shown to decrease both NOS-2 expression and NFκB activation in astrocytes (Pahan et al., 1997), supporting much earlier work showing that the same effect can be achieved by activating β-adrenoceptors (Feinstein et al., 1993). Pahan et al. (1999) suggest that PKA may exert its effect upstream of MAPK by phosphorylating Raf and thus preventing the interaction with Ras. However, these findings might also be explained by the recent observation that β-adrenoceptor activation increases the expression of IκBα (the inhibitory regulator of NFκB) in primary astrocytes, C6 glioma, and the intact brain (Gavrilyuk et al., 2002). Like Akt, PKA also activates NOS-3 (Michell et al., 2001) but inactivates NOS-1 (Butt et al., 2000). Interestingly, NOS-3 activation involves phosphorylation and dephosphorylation of particular serine and threonine residues, respectively, suggesting the additional involvement of a phosphatase, probably protein phosphatase 1 (PP1) (Michell et al., 2001).

With regard to NOS-2 induction in glia, Pahan et al. (1998b) have shown that okadaic acid, an inhibitor of PP1 and PP2A, promotes NFκB activity and NOS-2 expression in LPS- and cytokine-treated astrocytes. It could be that the removal of PP1-mediated dephosphorylation of constitutive NOS prevents its activation and allows for NOS-2 induction. Alternatively, the blockade of PP2A-mediated phosphatase activity with okadaic acid might result in increased MEK and/or IκB kinase activity, as both are tonically inhibited by the enzymatic action of PP2A (Millward et al., 1999). It is known that MEK is important in NOS-2 induction, and stimulation of IκB kinase would result in the phosphorylation and degradation of IκB, thus allowing the activation of NFκB, which is required for NOS-2 transcription in glia.

The induction of NOS-2 in these cells is further complicated by the involvement of another signaling cascade that appears to impinge upon the components of the pathways described previously. Simmons and Murphy (1994) showed that phorbol ester-stimulated PKC activation–induced NOS-2 expression in astrocytes; however, neither PKC inhibition nor its downregulation prevented LPS- or cytokine-stimulated induction. Later work by Chen et al. (1998) indicated that LPS-induced NOS-2 expression was indeed due to PKC activation but that the isoform-involved (PKCη) is not subject to downregulation by prolonged phorbol ester treatment. Various extracellular signal molecules, including IL-1β and TNFα, initiate sphingomyelin breakdown via the activation of sphingomyelinase. The product, ceramide, in turn activates targets such as ceramide-activated protein kinase, PKC ζ, ceramide-activated protein phosphatase (a member of the PP2A family), and the stress-activated protein kinase (SAPK)/JNK cascade (Mathias et al., 1998). Astrocytes are known to be capable of synthesizing endogenous ceramide (Riboni et al., 1994) and respond to the application of exogenous ceramide and/or sphingomyelinase in a number of ways. Among these is the finding that, despite having no effect alone, these treatments potentiate the effects of LPS and cytokines on NFκB activity and NOS-2 expression in astrocytes and C_6 glioma (Pahan et al., 1998a). Once again, these authors present evidence to suggest that targets upstream of MAPK, possibly Ras and/or MEK, mediate the effects of ceramide, but there is no clear indication of which elements of the ceramide pathway are involved.

PROTEIN KINASES

It is evident from the above that NOS-2 induction can be regulated by several pathways, some of which merge at common points (Fig. 16.1). A major goal for the future is to establish which pathways are activated and under what conditions in the intact brain.

Glia display a wide variety of protein kinase cascades. Protein kinase C is one of the better-known kinases in terms of its role(s) in glial cells. A study by Slepko et al. (1999) attempted to characterize the PKC isoforms expressed in astrocyte and microglial cultures by Western blot analysis. Although there were differences in the abundance of particular PKC isoforms, both cell types were found to express examples of the classical, novel, and atypical isoforms. However, PKC isoforms α and ε were not detected in microglia, and PKC γ was absent from both microglia and astrocytes. A less well known protein kinase, particularly with regard to the CNS, is AMP-activated protein kinase (AMPK). It is activated under conditions of metabolic stress by an increase in the intracellular concentration of AMP and phosphorylation by an upstream kinase kinase. It is a heterotrimer ($\alpha\beta\gamma$; the catalytic subunit is α) with two isoforms of each subunit (Kemp et al., 1999). *In situ* immunocytochemical analysis showed that some astrocytes were labeled with antibodies against $\alpha 1$, $\beta 1$, and $\beta 2$ subunits ($\alpha 2$ being the most intense) in some brain regions (hippocampus, cerebellum, and spinal cord) but not others (cerebral cortex). Although Bergmann glia contained the $\gamma 2$ subunit, no $\alpha 1$, $\gamma 1$ and $\gamma 2$ immunoreactive astrocytes were found in any region (Turnley et al., 1999). Interestingly, these authors also reported an increase in $\alpha 2$ and $\beta 2$ subunit expression in activated astrocytes in the hippocampus and corpus callosum of transgenic mice exhibiting gliosis in white matter tracts. Activity of AMPK has also been demonstrated in cultured astrocytes (Cox et al., 1997) and has been found to be much greater than that in cultured neurons (Blásquez et al., 1999). Whether this relates to the upregulation of the $\alpha 2$ subunit in activated astrocytes *in situ* (see above) remains to be established. Blásquez et al. (1999) also showed that AMPK activation caused increased ketone body formation in cultured astrocytes and in the intact brain. They concluded that ketone bodies may serve as a substrate for neuronal oxidative metabolism during hypoxia. In a later study, this group reported that AMPK activation prevented ceramide synthesis and apoptosis in cultured astrocytes (Blásquez et al., 2001). Given the high metabolic demands of the CNS and its susceptibility to hypoxia, the role(s) played by AMPK and the mechanisms by which its activity is regulated are key areas for future investigation.

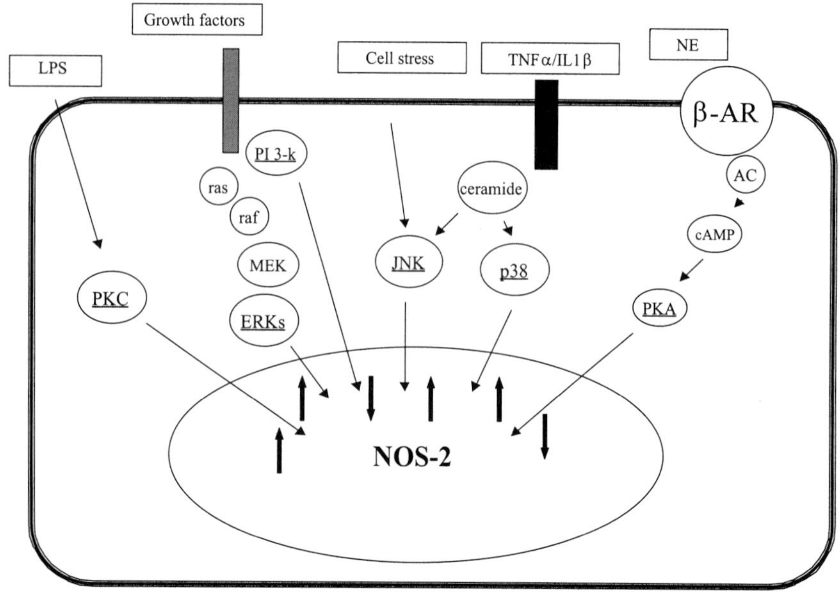

FIGURE 16.1 The role of kinases in transcriptional activation of the astrocyte nitric oxide synthase-2 (NOS-2) gene by a variety of stimuli. AC: adenylate cyclase; β-AR: β-adrenergic receptor; cAMP: cyclic adenosine monophosphate; ERK: extracellular regulated protein kinase; JNK: jun kinase; LPS: lipopolysaccharide; MET: mitogen-activated protein kinase kinase; NE: norepinephrine; PI 3-K: phosphatidylinositol 3-kinase; PKA, PKC: protein kinase A, C; TNFα/IL1β: tumor necrosis factor-α/interleukin-1β.

PROTEIN PHOSPHATASES

As indicated earlier, little attention has been paid to glial functions regulated by protein phosphatases. Apart from the involvement of these enzymes in NOS-2 induction, they also appear to play roles in other events, some of which will be reviewed here.

The two main families of protein phosphatases are directed toward either serine/threonine or tyrosine residues in target proteins. The serine/threonine phosphatases can be divided into two classes according to their amino acid sequences. The best characterized of these are phosphatases PP1, PP2A, and PP2B (calcineurin), which belong to the PPP class, and the structurally unrelated phosphatase PP2C, which belongs to the PPM family (Millward et al., 1999). There are four families of tyrosine phosphatases, with the cytoplasmic PTP class probably being the most relevant in the context of this review. The PTP class contains phosphatases, such as SHP-1 and SHP-2, which are bound to cellular partners via SH-2 domains, and PTP1B and PTPH1 that are targeted to the endoplasmic reticulum and actin cytoskeleton, respectively.

Mice that are genetically lacking SHP-1 (moth-eaten) show glial deficits, such as reduced numbers of astrocytes and microglia (Wishcamper et al., 2001) and aberrant myelination (Massa et al., 2000), suggesting that SHP-1 is involved in regulating the normal differentiation and distribution of glia in the CNS. These findings are somewhat surprising, given that SHP-1 is known to regulate mitosis negatively in other cell types. On this basis, one might expect the deletion of SHP-1 to promote glial proliferation. However, the way in which SHP-1 is involved in cell division may depend upon the stimulus for that event and the intracellular signaling pathways activated. Astrocyte proliferation is a common response to injury in the CNS; however, Lurie et al. (2000) have shown the existence of a small population of astrocytes that do not proliferate following deafferentation of the chicken auditory brain stem. Interestingly, these cells were found to be labeled positively with an antibody against SHP-1. Studies on cultured astrocytes have revealed that SHP-1 is associated with phospholipase C (PLC) $\gamma 1$, an important target for many growth factors, and that its role may be to prevent these cells from responding to certain mitogens (Machide et al., 2000). SHP-1 also appears to be an important component of cytokine signaling through the Janus kinase (JAK)/STAT pathway. Astrocytes from SHP-1-deficient mice show increased NFκB expression and associated gene products, including NOS-2, following exposure to certain cytokines (Massa and Wu, 1998). Thus, SHP-1 may serve more than one function in glia. It may play a role in normal glial development, but also acts to prevent glia, or certain populations of glia, from responding to mitogenic and/or inflammatory signals in the damaged brain.

The identification of functional roles for the serine/threonine protein phosphatases has been aided by availability of membrane-permeant inhibitors such as the marine toxin okadaic acid. Okadaic acid inhibits both PP1 and PP2A, with IC_{50} values of approximately 0.1 nM and 10 nM, respectively. Micromolar concentrations of the toxin are required to inhibit PP2B, while PP2C is unaffected (Cohen et al., 1990). The differential sensitivities of the enzymes to okadaic acid have been used to designate cellular responses to particular phosphatase species. However, as Cohen et al. (1990) point out, caution should always be exercised when attempting to do this in intact cells.

It is well known that glial fibrillary acidic protein (GFAP) can be phosphorylated by a variety of serine/threonine protein kinases and that this results in depolymerization, an event associated with mitosis. Vinadé and Rodnight (1996) have reported that the dephosphorylation of GFAP is mediated primarily by PP1. They also propose a role for PP2B in this process but suggest that its effect may be indirect, perhaps via the dephosphorylation of inhibitor-1 (an endogenous inhibitor of PP1), which is active in its phosphorylated state. The upregulation of GFAP expression is considered to be a hallmark characteristic of reactive astrocytes. Pei et al. (1997) have shown increases in both GFAP levels and numbers of astrocytes immunoreactive for phosphatases PP2A and PP2B in the brains of Alzheimer's disease patients. Relatedly, cultured astrocytes can be induced to adopt a stellate morphology when exposed to β-amyloid (a major component of senile plaques in Alzheimer's disease) and that this change in shape can be blocked by PP2A inhibition but enhanced by inhibition of PP2B (Salinero et al., 1997). These findings may suggest a role for protein phosphatases in the induction of the reactive phenotype often found associated with senile plaques in Alzheimer's disease. Studies employing okadaic acid have also implicated PP1 and/or PP2A in the regulation of nerve growth factor expression and secretion (Pshenichkin and Wise, 1995) and glutamate transport (Daniels and Vickroy, 1999) in astrocytes.

INTERACTIONS BETWEEN NITRIC OXIDE AND CYCLOOXYGENASE

Cyclooxygenase catalyzes the conversion of arachidonic acid to prostaglandin G_2 and then to prostaglandin H_2, which, in turn, is converted to the biologically active prostanoids [prostaglandins (PGs) and thromboxane A_2] by the appropriate isomerases. Like NOS, COX exists in both constitutive (COX-1) and inducible (COX-2) isoforms, and their products play roles in both physiological and pathological conditions (O'Banion, 1999). The stimuli, and intracellular signaling pathways responsible for promoting COX-2 expression in cultured glia (LPS, cytokines, and phorbol esters), and glia *in situ* (ischemic and chemical insults), are remarkably similar to those known to upregulate NOS-2 expression (Bauer et al., 1997; Hirst et al., 1999; Levi et al., 1998; Luo et al., 1998; Minghetti and Levi, 1998; Pistritto et al., 1999; Molina-Holgado et al., 2000; Strauss et al., 2000).

The coinduction of NOS-2 and COX-2 has been demonstrated in a number of peripheral cell types and in animal models of inflammation (Salvemini, 1997). These studies have pointed to a functional relationship between these enzymes in the initiation, progression, and resolution of the inflammatory response and have prompted investigators to determine whether NO and the prostanoids are involved in the reciprocal regulation of enzyme expression and/or activity. To date, the weight of evidence favors the idea that NO produced by NOS-2 activates COX-2 and thus amplifies the inflammatory response (Salvemini, 1997). Regulation of NOS by the prostanoids, on the other hand, is more controversial, with evidence that they can either inhibit or stimulate the release of NO. If we focus on the activation of COX-2 by NO, two questions need to be addressed in the context of this chapter: What is the molecular mechanism underlying this interaction, and does it hold true for cells, and glia in particular, in the CNS?

The precise mechanism by which NO potentiates COX-2 activity remains to be elucidated. Nonetheless, a survey of the potential points of interaction between these molecules suggests that NO itself is incapable of increasing the catalytic capacity of COX-2, and that certain interactions should result in enzyme inhibition rather than activation (Goodwin et al., 1999). The most convincing evidence for COX-2 activation by NO involves the generation of $ONOO^-$ (peroxynitrite). Goodwin et al. (1999) suggest that the increased O_2^- (superoxide) levels are provided by enhanced NADPH oxidase activity in inflammatory cells and that $ONOO^-$ then acts as a peroxidase substrate to oxidize the iron haem moiety in COX-2, thus releasing the tyrosyl radical required for the oxygenation of arachidonic acid.

Nogawa et al. (1998) have shown that COX-2 and NOS-2 expression is upregulated in neurons and neutrophils, respectively, at the periphery of infarcts elicited in a rodent model of focal cerebral ischemia. In addition, the associated increase in extracellular PG levels was attenuated by the administration of an NOS-2 inhibitor and was not evident in animals with a deletion of the NOS-2 gene. This finding tends to support the view that NO activates COX-2 in the CNS as well as in peripheral cells, but it suggests no involvement of glia. This is somewhat surprising given the numerous reports of upregulated COX-2 and NOS-2 expression in glia (both microglia and astrocytes) in the vicinity of ischemic infarcts and other CNS injuries in both animals and humans (Maslinska et al., 1999; O'Banion, 1999; Stoll and Jander, 1999; Tomimoto et al., 2000). Work in this area has, however, been carried out on cultured cells.

Using microglia obtained from neonatal rat brains, Minghetti et al. (1996) showed that LPS-induced COX-2 expression and activity in these cells is subject to downregulation by endogenous NO synthesis and by NO donors. In a comparative study, Guastadisegni et al. (1997) demonstrated that the opposite was true in a macrophage cell line, suggesting clear differences in the regulation of COX-2 in central microglia compared to cells that resemble their peripheral counterparts. Inhibition of NOS was also found to attenuate PG release from human microglia stimulated with a combination of IL-1β and IFN-γ (Janabi et al., 1996). Interestingly, these authors reported no upregulated NOS-2 activity in these cells following cytokine treatment, suggesting the involvement of NO generated from a constitutive NOS isoform in this response. Whether this points to a species difference in the pathway(s) controlling COX-2 expression remains to be established. In this regard, it is worth noting that Minghetti et al. (1996) showed that IFN-γ attenuated LPS-stimulated PG production in rat microglia via an NO-independent mechanism, whereas the cytokine promoted PG production in human microglia when used in conjunction with IL-1β (Janabi et al., 1996). Interferon-γ was also found to inhibit COX-2 expression and activity in LPS-treated mouse astrocytes, again via an NO-independent mechanism (Hewett, 1999), but in combination with IL-β it promoted both PG and NO synthesis in human astrocytes (Janabi et al., 1996). A role for NO in the activation of COX-2 activity has, however, been reported both in LPS-treated mouse astrocytes (Molina-Holgado et al., 1995) and in an astrocyte cell line of human origin treated with a combination of IL-1β and TNF-α (Mollace et al., 1998). As far as rodent glia are concerned, it would appear that NO inhibits COX-2 activity in microglia but enhances it in astrocytes. Exactly how this occurs has not been established, but there is no evidence for the involvement of cyclic guanosine monophosphate (GMP). The inhibition of COX-2 seems the most likely response given the accumulating evidence that NO suppresses NFκB activation in glia and that COX-2 is a target for this transcription factor (Colasanti and Persichini, 2000). So what is the explanation for this difference between microglia and astrocytes? One possibility centers on the tools used to investigate the interaction between NO and COX. Vidwans et al. (2001) have shown that NO donors that release either $NO^{\cdot}$ or NO^- enhanced COX-2 activity in LPS-treated astrocytes, while those releasing $ONOO^-$ caused an inhibition. The characteristics of the compounds used and the prevailing redox environment of the cells are, therefore, potentially important determinants of the effect NO may have on COX activity. Another consideration is the isoform of COX affected. Recent work on resting and LPS-treated macrophages and on fibroblast cell lines deficient in either COX-1 or COX-2 has demonstrated that NO activates COX-1 but inhibits COX-2 (Clancy et al., 2000). Given that cultured astrocytes express COX-1 constitutively (Luo et al., 1998) and that COX-1-containing microglia accumulate at sites of CNS injury (Schwab et al., 2000a, 2000b), more attention should be paid to the isoform of COX expressed by particular glial cell types as well as their state of activation. It may be that relatively subtle changes in any of the parameters discussed above may alter the way in which NO and COX interact so that inflammatory responses in the brain are either exacerbated or attenuated as required.

ASSEMBLIES OF SIGNALING MOLECULES—EVIDENCE FOR PROTEIN-PROTEIN ASSOCIATIONS IN GLIA

The complexity of the molecular interactions described thus far suggests that mechanisms must exist to exert fine control over intracellular events. No longer are cells considered to possess an internal environment unregulated or noncompartmentalized beyond that of intracellular organelles. Protein-protein interactions, and the specific targeting of components of signaling cascades, allow the control of intracellular events to be confined, as appropriate, to particular domains.

An important consideration in our understanding of the roles played by protein phosphorylation in the biology of glia, and other cell types, is the targeting of kinases and phosphatases to specific locations and to other proteins within the cell. It is becoming increasingly clear that this is necessary to achieve coordinated control over cellular functions so that the appropriate response is initiated when the cell is exposed to particular extracellular cues.

One of the best-described interactions is that of one protein acting as a ligand for the PSD-95/discs large/zona occludens-1 (PDZ) domain of another (Sheng and Sala, 2001). The PDZ is a domain of ~90 amino acids found in proteins derived from a variety of species. This suggestion, that PDZ domains are modules through which proteins interact, arose in the mid-1990s from studies of the PSD-95 protein associating with Shaker-type K^+ channels and *N*-methyl-D-aspartate (NMDA) receptor NR2 subunits, and the tyrosine phosphatase PTP1E associating with the receptor Fas. Consensus sequences of four amino acid residues in the C termini of these receptors/channels bind to their respective PDZ domains, and phosphorylation of component residues can regulate this binding. Some proteins express 1 PDZ domain (NOS-1), while others display multiple (13 domains in MUPP1). There are examples of proteins (such as NOS-1) in which a conformationally constrained internal sequence binds to a PDZ domain of another protein (PSD-95), and also of PDZ domains on different proteins interacting with each other.

A number of signaling molecules and receptor types known to be present in glia interact with partner proteins (Table 16.2). Whether the PDZ partner proteins PICK1, NHERF, Shank, and GRIP are expressed in glial cells is not known. Furthermore, glial cells express other receptors, monovalent cation channels, the serine esterase neuroligin, the neurexin Caspr3, and the proteoglycans syndecan-2, all of which have associated partners, but not yet proven in glia (Table 16.2). The C terminus of the GLAST glutamate transporter has a sequence similar to that of ion channels that associate with PDZ partners, and perturbation of this sequence affects transporter current (Marie and Attwell, 1999). Once again, the protein partner is unknown.

At least we can document that glial cells do express proteins with PDZ domains. In two cases, identity of

TABLE 16.2 *Association of Ligand Proteins and Proteins with PDZ Domains, Drawn from Studies of a Variety of Cell Types*

Ligand Protein	*Associated PDZ Protein*
PKCα (this Ch.)	PICK1
β2-Adrenergic receptor (Ch. 10)	NHERF
Glutamate receptor, subunit mGluR5	Shank (ProSAP)
AMPA receptor, subunit GluR2	PICK1, GRIP
NMDAR, subunits NR2A/B	PSD-95
Fas receptor (Ch. 11)	FAP-1 (PTP1E)
ErbB4 (Ma et al., 1999)	PSD-95
ErbB2 (Morris et al., 1999)	Erbin
Neuroligin (Gilbert et al., 2001)	PSD-95
Syndecan-2 (Bansal et al., 1996)	CASK
Caspr3 (Spiegel et al., 2002)	Mint1
Voltage-gated Na^+ channel (Ch. 9)	Syntrophin
Kir4.1 K+ channel	CIPP1
Shaker K+ channel	PSD-95
Kir2.2 (**Leonoudakis et al., 2001**)	SAP97
?	Mint3 (Okamato et al., 2001)
?	L/S periaxins (Gillespie et al., 1994)
GLAST glutamate transporter (Marie and Attwell, 1999)	?

See Sheng and Sala, 2001.

Note. Reference to glial expression of a specific protein is given (chapter/primary citation).

The citation in boldface indicates that this association has been demonstrated in glia. PDZ: PSD-95/discs large/zona occludens-1.

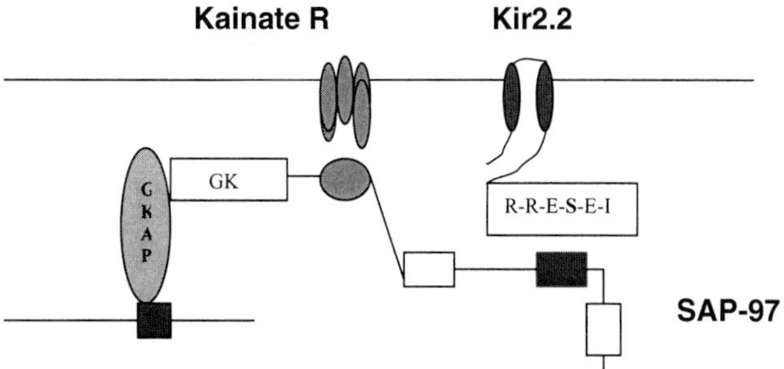

FIGURE 16.2 The association of inwardly rectifying K channel 2.2 (Kir 2.2) with synapse-associated protein-97 (SAP-97) in glial cells. The PSD-95/discs large/zona occludens-1 (PDZ) domains are indicated as small boxes and the SH3 domain of SAP-97 as an ellipse. Association of the kainate receptor and guanylate kinase associated protein (GKAP) with SAP-97 have been reported in neurons but not yet in glia. In addition, GKAP is shown as potentially interacting with the PDZ domain of another protein.

the ligand protein is not yet clear. The mint proteins contain two PDZ domains. Mint1 and mint2 are neuronal isoforms, whereas mint3 is also expressed in glial and ependymal cells, where it is believed to regulate the transport, endocytosis, and metabolism of amyloid precursor protein (Okamoto et al., 2001). Interestingly, the neurexin Caspr3, which is expressed in axons and oligodendrocytes, associates with mint1 in neurons. The periaxins (long and short forms) have a PDZ domain at the N terminus, which is believed to recruit proteins at the Schwann cell surface (Gillespie et al., 1994).

In a third case, we do know both the PDZ protein and its ligand (Table 16.2). In some partner proteins, the PDZ domains are found together with other interaction domains such as SH3, guanylate kinase, WW, LIM, Ca^{2+}/calmodulin-dependent protein kinase-like domains, ankyrin, and leucine-rich repeats. For example, SAP97 is a ubiquitously expressed protein related to the more spatially restricted PSD-95, and both are members of the MAGUK (membrane-associated guanylate kinase) family. In addition to PDZ domains, these proteins express an SH3 domain and a catalytically inactive guanylate kinase-like domain. Leonoudakis et al. (2001) found that the K^+ channel Kir2.2 and SAP97 coimmunoprecipitate, and colocalize in cerebellar Bergmann glia and in astrocytes of the granule cell layer. It appears to be the middle PDZ domain of SAP97 that associates with Kir2.2, leaving the adjacent PDZ domains free to bind to other components (Fig. 16.2). By analogy with PSD-95, the SH3 domain of SAP97 could interact with a membrane receptor, and the GUK domain may provide additional links to a cytoskeletal matrix by binding proteins such as GKAP, which could then interact with other PDZ domains.

SUMMARY AND PERSPECTIVES

In the same way as any other cell type, glia display complex signaling cascades that regulate and control the expression and activity of specific proteins. Though little is yet known in glia, the molecular components of these cascades appear to associate via specific recognition domains into discrete cellular compartments. With reference to similar arrangements in neurons and extraneural cell types, we can then begin to search for partner proteins in glia.

These molecular assemblies are dynamic structures, and their localization changes depending on the activity state of the cell. Developments in imaging, such as fluorescence correlation spectroscopy, now make it possible to track molecular interactions in single identified cells over time and space. Similarly, advances in gene modification allow components of assemblies to be either temporarily overexpressed, excised, or rendered incapable of interacting with their partners. In this way, we can start to understand the significance of discrete *associations* to specific cellular functions, certainly *in vitro* and possibly *in vivo*.

Over the past decade, our appreciation of glial-neuronal interactions has blossomed, and has provided insight into the myriad ways that glia contribute to neuronal differentiation and function, both in health and in disease. In some ways, glial cells are more dynamic than neurons, able to undergo hypertrophy and hyperplasia in response to extracellular signals. How this metamorphosis is brought about, what this means for glial signaling, and where glia contribute to or ameliorate the damage resulting from specific pathologies are important questions that now have a reasonable chance of being answered.

ACKNOWLEDGMENTS

Past and present support of the authors' laboratories by the USPHS-National Institutes of Health, American Heart Association, Biotechnology and Biological Sciences Research Council (UK), and the Wellcome Trust is gratefully acknowledged.

This chapter is dedicated to Gary R. Dutton, mentor and friend, on his retiring from neuroscience for the tranquility (and riches!) of the desert.

ABBREVIATIONS

AC	adenylyl cyclase
Akt	protein kinase B
AMPK	adenosine monophosphate–activated protein kinase
AR	adrenergic receptor
CAMKII	calcium calmodulin-activated protein kinase II

cADPr	cyclic ADP-ribose
CASK	calcium-calmodulin dependent serine kinase
COX	cyclooxygenase
ERK	extracellular regulated protein kinase
GFAP	glial fibrillary acidic protein
GK	guanylate kinase
GKAP	guanylate kinase associated protein
GLAST	glutamate transporter
GPI	glycosylphosphatidylinositol
IFN	interferon
IκB	inhibitory factor κB
IL	interleukin
IP_3	inositol trisphosphate
IP_3R	inositol trisphosphate receptor
JAK	Janus kinase
JNK	jun kinase
Kir	inwardly rectifying K channel
LPS	lipopolysaccharide
MAGUK	membrane-associated guanylate kinase
MAPK	mitogen-activated protein kinase
MEK	mitogen-activated protein kinase kinase
NAADP	nicotinic acid adenine dinucleotide phosphate
NE	norepinephrine
NFκB	nuclear factor kappa B
NO	nitric oxide
NOS	nitric oxide synthase
$ONOO^-$	peroxynitrite
O_2^-	superoxide
PDZ	PSD-95/discs large/zona occludens-1
PG	prostaglandin
PICK1	protein interacting with C kinase
PI 3-K	phosphatidylinositol 3-kinase
PIP2	phosphatidylinositol 4,5-bisphosphate
PK	protein kinase
PLC	phospholipase C
PP	protein phosphatase
PSD-95	postsynaptic density protein
RT-PCR	reverse transcriptase–polymerase chain reaction
RyR	ryanodine receptor
SAP	synapse-associated protein
SAPK	stress-activated protein kinase
SH3	src homology 3
STAT	signal transducer and activator of transcription
TNF	tumor necrosis factor
VEGF	vascular endothelial growth factor

REFERENCES

Araque, A., Carmignoto, G., and Haydon, P.G. (2001) Dynamic signalling between astrocytes and neurons. *Annu. Rev. Physiol.* 63:795–813.

Arbones, M.L., Ribeira, J., Agullo, L., Baltrons, M.A., Casanovas, A., Riveros-Moreno, V., and Garcia, A. (1996) Characteristics of nitric oxide synthase type-1 of rat cerebellar astrocytes. *Glia* 18:224–232.

Bansal, R., Kumar, M., Murray, K., and Pfeiffer, S.E. (1996) Developmental and FGF-2 mediated regulation of sydecans (1–4) and glypican in oligodendrocytes. *Mol. Cell. Neurosci.* 7:276–288.

Bauer, M.K., Lieb, K., Schulze-Osthoff, K., Berger, M., Gebicke-Haerter, P.J., Bauer, J., and Fiebich, B.L. (1997) Expression and regulation of cyclooxygenase-2 in rat microglia. *Eur. J. Biochem.* 243:726–731.

Bezzi, P. and Volterra, A. (2001) A neuron-glia signalling network in the active brain. *Curr. Opin. Neurobiol.* 11:387–394.

Bhat, N.R., Zhang, P., Lee, J.C., and Hogan, E.L. (1998) Extracellular signal-regulated kinase and p38 subgroups of mitogen-activated protein kinases regulate inducible nitric oxide synthase and tumour necrosis factor-α gene expression in endotoxin-stimulated glial cultures. *J. Neurosci.* 18:1633–1641.

Bhat, R.B., Feinstein, D.L., Shen, Q., and Bhat, A.N. (2002) p38 MAPK-mediated transcriptional activation of iNOS in glial cells. *J. Biol. Chem.* 277:29584–29592.

Blásquez, C., Geelen, M.J.H., Velasco, G., and Guzmán, M. (2001) The AMP-activated protein kinase prevents ceramide synthesis de novo and apoptosis in astrocytes. *FEBS Lett.* 489:149–153.

Blásquez, C., Woods, A., de Caballos, M.L., Carling, D., and Guzmán, M. (1999) The AMP-activated protein kinase is involved in the regulation of ketone body production by astrocytes. *J. Neurochem.* 73:1674–1682.

Brickley, K., Pearce, B., and Lai, F.A. (1998) Ryanodine receptor (RyR) expression in cultured rat cortical glia. In: Petersen, O.H. and Verkhratsky, A., eds. *Calcium Signalling in the Nervous System—Proceedings of the Symposium.* Proc. Sarr. Meet. 3rd Europ. Forum Neurosci, Bogesee, Germany, p. 29.

Butt, E., Bernhard, M., Smolenski, A., Kotsonis, P., Frölich, L.G., Sickman, A., Meyer, H.E., Lohmann, S.M., and Schmidt, H.H.H.W. (2000) Endothelial nitric oxide synthase (type III) is activated and becomes calcium independent upon phosphorylation by cyclic nucleotide-dependent protein kinases. *J. Biol. Chem.* 275:5179–5187.

Cameron, P.L., Liu, C., Smart, D.K., Hantus, S.T., Fick, J.R., and Cameron, R.S. (2002) Caveolin-1 expression is maintained in rat and human astroglioma cell lines. *Glia* 37:275–290.

Cameron, P.L., Ruffin, J.W., Bollag, R., Rasmussen, H., and Cameron, R.S. (1997) Identification of caveolin and caveolin-related proteins in the brain. *J. Neurosci.* 14:3139–3155.

Carmignoto, G. (2000) Reciprocal communication between astrocytes and neurones. *Prog. Neurobiol.* 62:561–581.

Catania, M.V., Aronica, E., Yankaya, B., and Troost, D. (2001) Increased expression of nNOS spliced variants in reactive astrocytes of amyotrophic lateral sclerosis human spinal cord. *J. Neurosci.* 21:RC148.

Chen, C.-C., Wang, J.-K., Chen, W.-C., and Lin, S.-B. (1998) Protein kinase C mediates lipopolysaccharide-induced nitric oxide synthase expression in primary astrocytes. *J. Biol. Chem.* 273: 19424–19430.

Churchill, G.C. and Galione, A. (2001) NAADP induces Ca^{2+} oscillations via a two-pool mechanism by priming IP_3- and cADPr-sensitive Ca^{2+} stores. *EMBO J.* 20:2666–2671.

Clancy, R., Varenika, B., Huang, W., Ballou, L., Attur, M., Amin, A.R., and Abramson, S.B. (2000) Nitric oxide synthase/COX cross-talk: nitric oxide activates COX-1 but inhibits COX-2-derived prostaglandin production. *J. Immunol.* 165:1582–1587.

Cohen, P., Holmes, C.F.B., and Tsukitani, Y. (1990) Okadaic acid: a new probe for the study of cellular regulation. *Trends Biochem. Sci.* 15:98–102.

Colasanti, M. and Persichini, T. (2000) Nitric oxide: an inhibitor of NF-κB/Rel system in glial cells. *Brain Res. Bull.* 52:155–161.

Communi, D., Dewaste, V., and Erneux, C. (1999) Calcium-calmodulin-dependent protein kinase II and protein kinase C-mediated phosphorylation and activation of D-myo-inositol 1,4,5-trisphosphate 3-kinase B in astrocytes. *J. Biol. Chem.* 274:14734–14742.

Cox, S.E., Pearce, B., and Munday, M.R. (1997) AMP-activated protein kinase in astrocytes. *Biochem. Soc. Trans.* 25:S583.

Daniels, K.K. and Vickroy, T.W. (1999) Reversible activation of glutamate transport in rat brain glia by protein kinase C and an okadaic acid-sensitive phosphoprotein phosphatase. *Neurochem. Res.* 24:1017–1025.

Deitmer, J.W., Verkhratsky, A.J., and Lohr, C. (1998) Calcium signalling in glial cells. *Cell Calcium* 24:405–416.

Fields, R.D. and Stevens-Graham, B. (2002) New insights into neuron-glia communication. *Science* 298:556–562.

Feinstein, D.L., Galea, E., and Reis, D.J. (1993) Norepinephrine suppresses inducible nitric oxide synthase activity in rat astroglial cultures. *J. Neurochem.* 60:1945–1948.

Fulceri, R., Rossi, R., Bottinelli, R., Conti, A., Intravaia, E., Galione, A., Benedetti, A., Sorrentino, V., and Reggiani, C. (2001) Ca^{2+} release induced by cyclic ADP ribose in mice lacking type 3 ryanodine receptor. *Biochem. Biophys. Res. Commun.* 288:697–702.

Gallo, V. and Ghiani, C.A. (2000) Glutamate receptors in glia. *Trends Pharmacol. Sci.* 21:252–258.

Gavrilyuk, V., Dello Russo, C., Heneka, M.T., Pelligrino, D., Weinberg, G., and Feinstein, D.L. (2002) Norepinephrine increases IκBα expression in astrocytes. *J. Biol. Chem.* 277:29662–29668.

Genazzi, A.A. and Billington, R.A. (2002) NAADP: an atypical Ca^{2+} release messenger? *Trends Pharmacol. Sci.* 23:165–167.

Genazzi, A.A. and Galione, A. (1997) A Ca^{2+} release mechanism gated by the novel pyridine nucleotide, NAADP. *Trends Pharmacol. Sci.* 18:108–110.

Gilbert, M., Smith, J., Roskams, A.-J., and Auld, V.J. (2001) Neuroligin 3 is a vertebrate gliotactin expressed in the olfactory ensheathing glia, a growth-promoting class of macroglia. *Glia* 34: 151–164.

Gillespie, C.S., Sherman, D.L., Blair, G.E., and Brophy, P.J. (1994) Periaxin, a novel protein of myelinating Schwann cells with a possible role in axonal ensheathment. *Neuron* 12:497–508.

Golovina, V.A. and Blaustein, M.P. (2000) Unloading and refilling of two classes of spatially resolved endoplasmic reticulum Ca^{2+} stores in astrocytes. *Glia* 31:15–28.

Goodwin, D.C., Landino, L.M., and Marnett, L.J. (1999) Effects of nitric oxide and nitric oxide-derived species on prostaglandin endoperoxide synthase and prostaglandin biosynthesis. *FASEB J.* 13:1121–1136.

Guastadisegni, C., Minghetti, L., Nicolini, A., Polazzi, E., Ade, P., Balduzzi, M., and Levi, G. (1997) Prostaglandin E_2 synthesis is differentially affected by reactive nitrogen intermediates in cultured rat microglia and RAW 264.7 cells. *FEBS Lett.* 413:314–318.

Hansson, E. and Ronnback, L. (2003) Glial neuronal signaling in the CNS. *FASEB J.* 17:341–348.

Hewett, S.J. (1999) Interferon-γ reduces cyclooxygenase-2-mediated prostaglandin E_2 production from primary mouse astrocytes independent of nitric oxide formation. *J. Neuroimmunol.* 94:134–143.

Higashida, H., Hashii, M., Yokoyama, S., Hoshi, N., Asai, K., and Kato, T. (2001) Cyclic ADP-ribose as a potential second messenger for neuronal Ca^{2+} signaling. *J. Neurochem.* 76:321–331.

Hirst, W.D., Young, K.A., Newton, R., Allport, V.C., Marriott, D.R., and Wilkin, G.P. (1999) Expression of COX-2 by normal and reactive astrocytes in the adult rat central nervous system. *Mol. Cell. Neurosci.* 13:57–68.

Hotta, T., Asai, K., Fujita, K., Kato, T., and Higashida, H. (2000) Membrane-bound form of ADP-ribosyl cyclase in rat cortical astrocytes in culture. *J. Neurochem.* 74:669–675.

Hua, L.L., Zhao, M.-L., Cosenza, M., Kim, M.-O., Huang, H., Tanowitz, H.B., Brosnan, C.F., and Lee, S.C. (2002) Role of mitogen-activated protein kinases in inducible nitric oxide synthase and TNFα expression in human foetal astrocytes. *J. Neuroimmunol.* 126:180–189.

Irvine, R.F. (2001) Inositol phosphates: does IP_4 run a protection racket? *Curr. Biol.* 11:172–174.

Janabi, N., Chabrier, S., and Tardieu, M. (1996) Endogenous nitric oxide activates prostaglandin $F_{2\alpha}$ production in human microglial cells but not in astrocytes. *J. Immunol.* 157:2129–2135.

Kemp, B.E., Mitchelhill, K.I., Stapleton, D., Michell, B.J., Chen, Z.-P., and Witters, L.A. (1999) Dealing with energy demand: the AMP-activated protein kinase. *Trends Biochem. Sci.* 24:22–25.

Langley, D. and Pearce, B. (1994) Ryanodine-induced intracellular Ca^{2+} mobilisation in cultured astrocytes. *Glia* 12:128–134.

Lawrence, J.M. and Raisman, G. (1987) Membrane specializations and extracellular material associated with host astrocytes in peripheral neural transplants. *Neuroscience* 20:1031–1041.

Leonoudakis, D., Mailliard, W.S., Wingerd, K.L., Clegg, D.O., and Vandenberg, C.A. (2001) Inward rectifier potassium channel Kir2.2 is associated with SAP-97. *J. Cell Sci.* 114:987–998.

Levi, G., Minghetti, L., and Aloisi, F. (1998) Regulation of prostanoid synthesis in microglial cells and effects of prostaglandin E_2 on microglial functions. *Biochimie* 80:899–904.

Luo, J., Lang, J.A., and Miller, M.W. (1998) Transforming growth factor β1 regulates the expression of cyclooxygenase in cultured cortical astrocytes and neurons. *J. Neurochem.* 71:526–534.

Lurie, D.I., Solca, F., Fischer, E.F., and Rubel, E.W. (2000) Tyrosine phosphatase SHP-1 immunoreactivity increases in a subset of astrocytes following deafferentation of the chicken auditory brainstem. *J. Comp. Neurol.* 421:199–214.

Ma, Y.J., Hill, D.K., Creswick, K.E., Costa, M.E., Cornea, A., Lioubin, M.N., Plowman, G.D., and Ojeda, S.R. (1999) Neuregulins signaling via a glial ErbB2–ErbB4 receptor complex contribute to the neuroendocrine control of mammalian sexual development. *J. Neurosci.* 19:9913–9927.

Machide, M., Kamitori, K., and Kohsaka, S. (2000) Hepatocyte growth factor-induced differential activation of phospholipase C and phosphatidylinositol 3-kinase is regulated by tyrosine phosphatase SHP-1 in astrocytes. *J. Biol. Chem.* 275:31392–31398.

Marie, H., and Attwell, D. (1999) C-terminal interactions modulate the affinity of GLAST glutamate transporters in salamander retinal glial cells. *J Physiol. (Lond.)* 520:393–397.

Maslinska, D., Wozniak, R., Kaliszek, A., and Modelska, I. (1999) Expression of cyclooxygenase-2 in astrocytes of human brain after global ischaemia. *Folia Neuropathol.* 37:75–79.

Massa, P.T., Saha, S., Wu, C., and Jarosinski, K.W. (2000) Expression and function of the protein tyrosine phosphatase SHP-1 in oligodendrocytes. *Glia* 29:376–385.

Massa, P.T. and Wu, C. (1998) Increased inducible activation of NFκB and responsive genes in astrocytes deficient in the protein tyrosine phosphatase SHP-1. *J. Interferon Cytokine Res.* 18:499–507.

Masserini, M., Palestini, P., and Pitto, M. (1999) Glycolipid-enriched caveolae and caveolae-like domains in the nervous system. *J. Neurochem.* 73:1–11.

Mathias, S., Pea, L.A., and Kolesnick, R.N. (1998) Signal transduction of stress via ceramide. *Biochem. J.* 335:465–480.

Matyash, M., Matyash, V., Nolte, C., Sorrentino, V., and Kettenmann, H. (2002) Requirement of functional ryanodine receptor type 3 for astrocyte migration. *FASEB J.* 16:84–86.

Michell, B.J., Chen, Z., Tiganis, T., Stapleton, D., Katsis, F., Power, D.A., Sim, A.T., and Kemp, B.E. (2001) Coordinated control of endothelial nitric oxide synthase phosphorylation by protein kinase C and the cAMP-dependent protein kinase. *J. Biol. Chem.* 276:17625–17628.

Mikol, D.D., Hong, H.L., Cheng, H.-L., and Feldman, E.L. (1999) Caveolin-1 expression in Schwann cells. *Glia* 27:39–52.

Mikol, D.D., Scherer, S.S., Duckett, S.J., Hing, H.L., and Feldman, E.L. (2002) Schwann cell caveolin-1 expression increases during myelination and decreases after axotomy. *Glia* 38:191–199.

Millward, T.A., Zolnierowicz, S., and Hemmings, B.A. (1999) Regulation of protein kinase cascades by protein phosphatase 2A. *Trends Biochem. Sci.* 24:186–191.

Minghetti, L. and Levi, G. (1998) Microglia as effector cells in brain damage and repair: focus on prostanoids and nitric oxide. *Prog. Neurobiol.* 54:99–125.

Minghetti, L., Polazzi, E., Nicolini, A., Créminon, C., and Levi, G. (1996) Interferon-γ and nitric oxide down-regulate lipopolysaccharide-induced prostanoid production in cultured rat microglial cells by inhibiting cyclooxygenase-2 expression. *J. Neurochem.* 66:1963–1970.

Molina-Holgado, F., Lledó, A., and Guaza, C. (1995) Evidence for cyclooxygenase activation by nitric oxide in astrocytes. *Glia* 15: 167–172.

Molina-Holgado, E., Ortiz, S., Molina-Holgado, F., and Guaza, C. (2000) Induction of COX-2 and PGE_2 biosynthesis by IL-1β is mediated by PKC and mitogen-activated protein kinases in murine astrocytes. *Br. J. Pharmacol.* 131:152–159.

Mollace, V., Colasanti, M., Muscoli, C., Lauro, G.M., Iannone, M., Rotiroti, D., and Nistico, G. (1998) The effect of nitric oxide on cytokine-induced release of PGE_2 by human cultured astroglial cells. *Br. J. Pharmacol.* 124:742–746.

Morris, J.K., Lin, W., Hauser, C., Marchuk, Y., Getman, D., and Lee, K-F. (1999) Rescue of the cardiac defect in ErbB2 mutant mice reveals essential roles of ErbB2 in peripheral nervous system development. *Neuron* 23:273–283.

Murphy, S. (2000) Production of nitric oxide by glial cells: regulation and potential roles in the CNS. *Glia* 29:1–14.

Nogawa, S., Forster, C., Zhang, F., Nagayama, M., Ross, M.E., and Iadecola, C. (1998) Interaction between inducible nitric oxide synthase and cyclooxygenase-2 after cerebral ischaemia. *Proc. Natl. Acad. Sci. USA* 95:10966–10971.

O'Banion, M.K. (1999) Cyclooxygenase-2: molecular biology, pharmacology and neurobiology. *Crit. Rev. Neurobiol.* 13:45–82.

Okamoto, M., Nakajima, Y., Matsuyama, T., and Sugita, M. (2001) Amyloid precursor protein associates independently and collaboratively with PTB and PDZ domains of MINT on vesicles and at cell membrane. *Neuroscience* 104:653–665.

Pahan, K., Liu, X., Wood, C., and Raymond, J.R. (2000) Expression of a constitutively active form of phosphatidylinositol 3-kinase inhibits the induction of nitric oxide synthase in human astrocytes. *FEBS Lett.* 472:203–207.

Pahan, K., Namboordiri, A.M.S., Sheikh, F.G., Smith, B.T., and Singh, I. (1997) Increasing cAMP attenuates induction of inducible nitric oxide synthase in rat primary astrocytes. *J. Biol. Chem.* 272:7786–7791.

Pahan, K., Sheikh, F.G., Khan, M., Namboordiri, A.M.S., and Singh, I. (1998a) Sphingomyelinase and ceramide stimulate the expression of inducible nitric oxide synthase in rat primary astrocytes. *J. Biol. Chem.* 273:2591–2600.

Pahan, K., Sheikh, F.G., Namboordiri, A.M.S., and Singh, I. (1998b) Inhibitors of protein phosphatase 1 and 2A differentially regulate the expression of inducible nitric oxide synthase in rat astrocytes and macrophages. *J. Biol. Chem.* 273:12219–12226.

Pahan, K., Raymond, J.R., and Singh, I. (1999) Inhibition of phosphatidylinositol 3-kinase induces nitric oxide synthase in lipopolysaccharide- or cytokine-stimulated C_6 glial cells. *J. Biol. Chem.* 274:7528–7536.

Pawlikowska, L., Cotterell, S.E., Harms, M.B., Li, Y., and Rosenberg, P.A. (1996) Extracellular synthesis of cADP-ribose from nicotinamide-adenine dinucleotide by rat cortical astrocytes in culture. *J. Neurosci.* 16:5372–5381.

Pei, J.-J., Grundke-Iqbal, I., Iqbal, K., Bogdanovic, N., Winblad, B., and Cowburn, R.F. (1997) Elevated protein levels of protein phosphatases PP2A and PP2B in astrocytes of Alzheimer's disease temporal cortex. *J. Neural Transm.* 104:1329–1338.

Pistritto, G., Franzese, O., Pozzoli, G., Mancuso, C., Tringali, G., Preziosi, P., and Navarra, P. (1999) Bacterial lipopolysaccharide increases prostaglandin production by rat astrocytes via inducible cyclooxygenase: evidence for the involvement of nuclear factor κB. *Biochem. Biophys. Res. Commun.* 263:570–574.

Pshenichkin, S.P. and Wise, B.C (1995) Okadaic acid increases nerve growth factor secretion, mRNA stability, and gene transcription in primary cultures of cortical astrocytes. *J. Biol. Chem.* 270: 5994–5999.

Razani, B. and Lisanti, M.P. (2001) Caveolin-deficient mice. *J. Clin. Invest.* 108:1553–1561.

Riboni, L., Prinetti, A., Bassi, R., and Tettamanti, G. (1994) Formation of bioactive sphingoid molecules from exogenous sphingomyelin in primary cultures of neurons and astrocytes. *FEBS Lett.* 352:323–326.

Salinero, O., Moreno-Flores, M.T., and Wandosell, F. (1997) Okadaic acid modulates the cytoskeletal changes induced by amyloid peptide (25-35) in cultured astrocytes. *NeuroReport* 8:3333–3338.

Salvemini, D. (1997) Regulation of cyclooxygenase enzymes by nitric oxide. *Cell. Mol. Life Sci.* 53:576–582.

Schwab, J.M., Brechtel, K., Nguyen, T.D., and Schluesener, H.J. (2000a) Persistent accumulation of cyclooxygenase-1 (COX-1) expressing microglia/macrophages and upregulation by endothelium following spinal cord injury. *J. Neuroimmunol.* 111:122–130.

Schwab, J.M., Nguyen, T.D., Postler, E., Meyermann, R., and Schluesener, H.J. (2000b) Selective accumulation of cyclooxygenase-1-expressing microglial cells/macrophages in lesion of human focal cerebral ischaemia. *Acta Neuropathol.* 99:609–614.

Sharp, A.H., Nucifora, F.C., Blondel, O., Sheppard, C.A., Zhang, C., Snyder, S.H., Russell, J.T., Ryugo, D.K., and Ross, C.A. (1999) Differential cellular expression of isoforms of inositol 1,4,5-trisphosphate receptors in neurons and glia in brain. *J. Comp. Neurol.* 406:207–220.

Shaul, P.W. (2002) Regulation of eNOS. *Annu. Rev. Physiol.* 64: 749–774.

Sheng, M. and Sala, C. (2001) PDZ domains and the organization of supramolecular complexes. *Annu. Rev. Neurosci.* 24:1–29.

Sheppard, C.A., Simpson, P.B., Sharp, A.H., Nucifora, F.C., Ross, C.A., Lange, G.D., and Russell, J.T. (1997) Comparison of type 2 inositol 1,4,5-trisphosphate receptor distribution and subcellular Ca^{2+} release sites that support Ca^{2+} waves in cultured astrocytes. *J. Neurochem.* 68:2317–2327.

Simmons, M.L. and Murphy, S. (1994) Roles for protein kinases in the induction of nitric oxide synthase in astrocytes. *Glia* 11:227–234.

Simpson, P.B., Holtzclaw, L.A., Langley, D.B., and Russell, J.T. (1998a) Characterization of ryanodine receptors in oligodendrocytes, type 2 astrocytes, and O-2A progenitors. *J. Neurosci. Res.* 52:468–482.

Simpson, P.B., Mehotra, S., Langley, D.B., Sheppard, C.A., and Russell, J.T. (1998b) Specialized distributions of mitochondria and endoplasmic reticulum proteins define Ca^{2+} wave amplification sites in cultured astrocytes. *J. Neurosci. Res.* 52:672–683.

Simpson, P.B., Sheppard, C.A., and Russell, J.T. (1995) Properties of Ca^{2+} stores in type 1 and type 2 astrocytes. *Soc. Neurosci. Abstr.* 21:1129.

Slepko, N., Patrizio, M., and Levi, G. (1999) Expression and translocation of protein kinase C isoforms in rat microglial and astroglial cultures. *J. Neurosci. Res.* 57:33–38.

Smart, E.J., Graf, G.A., McNiven, M.A., Sessa, W.C., Engelman, J.A., Scherer, P.E., Okamoto, T., and Lisanti, M.P. (1999) Caveolins, liquid-ordered domains, and signal transduction. *Mol. Cell Biol.* 19:7289–7304.

Soriano, S., Thomas, S., High, S., Griffiths, G., D'Santos, C., Cullen, P., and Banting, G. (1997) Membrane association, localization and topology of rat inositol 1,4,5-trisphosphate 3-kinase B: implications for membrane traffic and Ca^{2+} homeostasis. *Biochem. J.* 324:579–589.

Sowa, G., Pypaert, M., and Sessa, W.C. (2001) Distinction between signaling mechanisms in lipid rafts vs. caveolae. *Proc. Natl. Acad. Sci. USA* 98:14072–14077.

Spiegel, I., Salomon, D., Erne, B., Schaeren-Wiemers, N., and Peles, E. (2002) Caspr3 and Caspr4, two novel members of the Caspr family are expressed in the *nervous system and interact with PDZ domains. Mol. Cell. Neurosci.* 20:283–297.

Stoll, G. and Jander, S. (1999) The role of microglia and macrophages in the pathophysiology of the CNS. *Prog. Neurobiol.* 58:233–247.

Strauss, K.I., Barbe, M.F., Marshall, R.M., Raghupathi, R., Mehta, S., and Narayan, R.K. (2000) Prolonged cyclooxygenase-2 induction in neurons and glia following traumatic brain injury in the rat. *J. Neurotrauma* 17:695–711.

Tomimoto, H., Akiguchi, I., Wakita, H., Lin, J.-X., and Budka, H. (2000) Cyclooxygenase-2 is induced in microglia during chronic cerebral ischaemia in humans. *Acta Neuropathol.* 99:26–30.

Tsui-Pierchala, B.A., Encinas, M., Milbrandt, J., and Johnson, E.M., Jr. (2002) Lipid rafts in neuronal signaling and function. *Trends Neurosci.* 25:412–417.

Turnley, A.M., Stapleton, D., Mann, R.J., Witters, L.E., Kemp, B.E., and Bartlett, P.F. (1999) Cellular distribution and developmental expression of AMP-activated protein kinase isoforms in mouse central nervous system. *J. Neurochem.* 72:1707–1716.

Vidwans, A.S., Uliasz, T.F., Hewett, J.A., and Hewett, S.J. (2001) Differential modulation of prostaglandin H synthase-2 by nitric oxide-related species in intact cells. *Biochemistry* 40:11533–11542.

Vinadé, L. and Rodnight, R. (1996) The dephosphorylation of glial fibrillary acidic protein (GFAP) in the immature rat hippocampus is catalysed primarily by a type 1 protein phosphatase. *Brain Res.* 732:195–200.

Wishcamper, C.A., Coffin, J.D., and Lurie, D.I. (2001) Lack of protein tyrosine phosphatase SHP-1 results in decreased numbers of glia within the motheaten (me/me) mouse brain. *J. Comp. Neurol.* 441:118–133.

Yamamoto-Hino, M., Miyawaki, A., Kawano, H., Sugiyama, T., Furuichi, T., Hasegawa, M., and Mikoshiba, K. (1995) Immunohistochemical study of inositol 1,4,5-trisphosphate receptor type 3 in rat central nervous system. *NeuroReport* 6:273–276.

17 Intracellular calcium control mechanisms in glia

MARIA LUISA COTRINA AND MAIKEN NEDERGAARD

Glial cells, like all eukaryotic cells, relay on calcium ions to display a large variety of signaling capabilities inside the cell and among neighboring cells. These calcium activities are key to regulate not only the growth and survival of glial cells but also the communication with neurons. As glial cells are not electrically excitable, calcium signaling, specially in astrocytes, is particularly important to understand how glia regulate synaptic activity and brain function. In this chapter, we will discuss the evidence for the existence of calcium signaling in glia, the different mechanisms of glial calcium signaling, its spatial and temporal resolution, and how glial cells make use of this diverse array of activities to modulate neuronal function.

CALCIUM HOMEOSTASIS IN ASTROCYTES

Calcium signaling is largely based on the existence of a strong calcium gradient between the extracellular and intracellular environments. The tight regulation of this gradient is key to ensure the efficacy and reliability of calcium signaling. The way astrocytes achieve this cellular control is common to many other cell types and denotes a high degree of conservancy among nonexcitable cell types.

Influx Pathways versus Intracellular Stores

The free calcium concentration inside astrocytic cells is approximately 50–200 nM compared with 1 mM in the extracellular space. Several stimuli can promote a rapid, transient increase in cytosolic calcium, which can reach levels as high as 1 μM or more. In principle, any channel that allows the passage of calcium ions through the plasma membrane will promote this intracellular calcium rise. As such, voltage-gated and ligand-gated ion channels or nonspecific cation channels can contribute to the entrance of calcium from the extracellular milieu. Although the presence of voltage-gated channels of the L and T types has been documented in cultured astrocytes, especially under pathophysiological conditions (Westenbroek et al., 1998), astrocytes *in situ* do not seem to use this mechanism as the main pathway for extracellular calcium entry (Fig. 17.1). Likewise, ligand-gated ion channels, like glutamate and acetylcholine receptors, which may contribute to calcium influx in cultured astrocytes, seem to have a minor role in astrocytes *in situ* (Shelton and McCarthy, 1999). Indeed, glutamate-evoked currents recorded in outside-out patches from physiologically identified astrocytes are unaffected by glutamate receptor antagonists (Bergles and Jahr, 1998) but attenuated by glutamate transport inhibitors, suggesting that uptake rather than channel activation mediates some astrocytic responses. In contrast, glutamate evoked-currents in Bergmann glia exhibit an alpha-amino-3-hydroxy-5-methyl-4-isoxazolepropionate (AMPA) (NBQX-sensitive) component (Bergles and Jahr, 1997), supporting the idea of heterogeneity of receptor expression among astrocytes.

The primary mechanism of increases in astrocytic cytosolic calcium is release from intracellular stores, specifically from the endoplasmic reticulum (ER). Calcium concentrations in the ER are kept in the high micromolar range. Many different transmitters and hormones coupled to a membrane-associated G-protein stimulate the release of calcium from the ER via the activation of phospholipase C (PLC). This enzyme cleaves phosphatidylinositol 4,5-bisphosphate (PIP_2) to generate diacylglycerol (DAG) and inositol 1,4,5-trisphosphate (IP_3). Binding of IP_3 to the IP_3 receptors (IP_3Rs) of the ER will open these channels and allow the efflux of calcium into the cytosol. Ryanodine receptors (RyRs), mostly sensitive to ryanodine and caffeine, are another type of calcium channel that also serves as conduit of calcium release from the ER. In astrocytes, the association of RyRs with calcium activity has often been debated, as calcium release sensitive to caffeine has been difficult to show. However, RyR type 3, a RyR insensitive to caffeine, has been identified in these cells (Matyash et al., 2001), and calcium mobilization in response to ryanodine has been found in cultured astrocytes (Langley and Pearce 1994). It has been recently

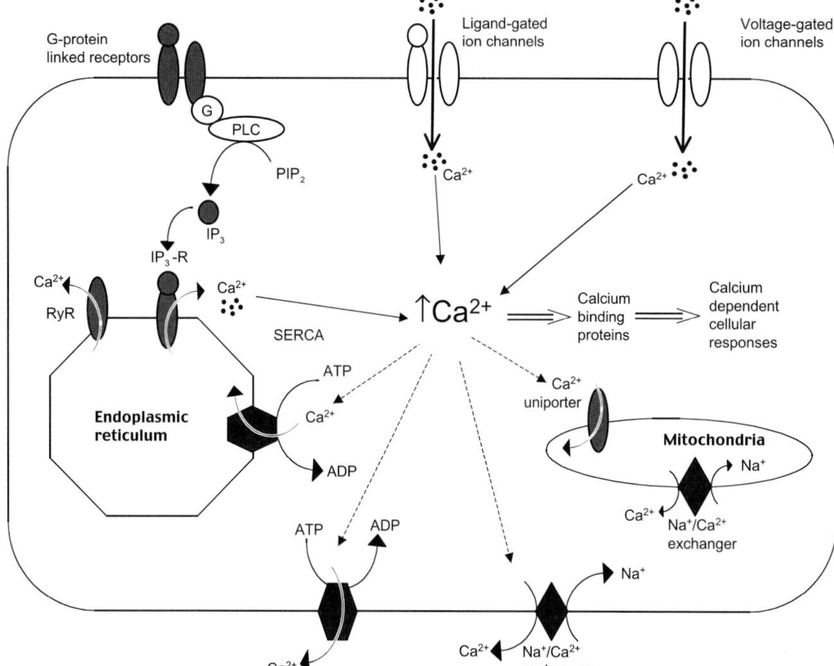

FIGURE 17.1 Diagram of major pathways involved in control of cytosolic Ca^{2+} in astrocytes. ADP: adenosine diphosphate; ATP: adenosine triphosphate; IP_3: inositol 1,4,5-trisphosphate; IP_3R: IP_3 receptor; PIP_2: phosphatidylinositol 4,5-bisphosphate; PLC: phospholipase C; RyR: ryanodine receptor; SERCA: sarco-endoplasmic reticulum Ca^{2+}-ATP.

demonstrated that cyclic adenosine diphosphate–ribose (cADP-r), another modulator of RyRs, can also promote calcium increases in astrocytes (Verderio et al., 2001), evidencing the potential for RyRs in astrocytic signaling. However, the activity of the RyRs is relatively low compared to the activity of the IP_3Rs in astrocytes.

Amplification of the Initial Calcium Signal

Both RyRs and IP_3Rs have a crucial role in the type of calcium response cells will exhibit upon stimulation. This response will be determined by their particular abundance and subcellular localization, and by their association to other mechanisms that allow either amplification or decay of the signal. On the one hand, initial calcium increases from the ER can be followed by further calcium release, mainly mediated by the RyRs (Berridge et al., 2000). This mechanism of calcium-induced calcium release (CICR) has been recently shown in cultured hippocampal astrocytes but, as mentioned before, the extent of this calcium activity in astrocytes needs to be investigated further. On the other hand, ER calcium release can be followed by calcium entry across the plasma membrane through store-operated calcium channels (SOCs), the identity of which is not clear yet. These channels are activated when the ER calcium stores are depleted. The calcium influx through these calcium-release-activated channels (CRACs), also known as *capacitative calcium entry* (CCE), provides a means for a more sustained calcium increase into the cytosol as long as the ER calcium stores remain empty. Cortical and cerebellar astrocytes exhibit CCE upon depletion of ER stores with thapsigargin and cyclopiazonic acid, two inhibitors of the sarcoendoplasmic reticulum calcium adenosine triphosphatases (ATPases) (Wu et al., 1999), although non-CCE has also been described for the latter. However, it is important to keep in mind that complete depletion of the intracellular calcium stores under normal conditions is rare and that the exact role of this calcium current needs to be considered with smaller reductions in ER calcium. It has been recently found that, in the presence of energized mitochondria capable of maintaining active calcium uptake, CRACs can be activated under more physiological conditions (Gilabert and Parekh, 2000), although this has not been shown for astrocytes.

Calcium Buffering and Calcium Extrusion

Once intracellular calcium levels have increased, extrusion channels, buffering proteins, and intracellular organelles are critical to cancel these initial calcium bursts, which, if sustained for too long, might trigger nonspecific, potentially harmful events. First, high-affinity calcium-binding proteins, generally members of the EF-hand family such as troponin C, parvalbumin, calcineurin, and calmodulin in the cytosol, or non-EF-hand proteins, like calreticulin and calsequestrin in the ER, rapidly chelate calcium ions (Kawasaki et al., 1998). However, all of these proteins are present in limited amounts and function more as effectors to trigger calcium-dependent cellular responses. This implies that cytosolic calcium clearance is more efficiently achieved by other means. For example, activation of sarco-endoplasmic reticulum Ca^{2+}-ATPases (SERCAs) pump calcium back into the ER, whereas plasma membrane Ca^{2+}-ATPases (PMCAs) and Na^{+}/Ca^{2+} exchangers extrude calcium to the extracellular space. Astrocytes contain all three types of protein, and the relative contribution of each one to calcium clearance depends on the relative calcium concentrations of the cytosolic/intracellular pools. Mitochondria are also activated by ER calcium release. Calcium uptake in this organelle relies on the activity of a low-affinity uniporter. Hence it is important that mitochondria be located close to the ER, where the local concentration of released calcium is higher.

Mitochondria as Sources of Calcium Signals

It is been recently recognized that mitochondria can not only buffer calcium levels, but also promote calcium signals on their own. Mitochondrial calcium release is slowly achieved through Na^{+}-dependent and -independent exchangers but also through a permeability transition pore (PTP). We must appreciate that mitochondrial activity makes a slightly different contribution than that of the ER to the dynamics of calcium signals. Whereas mitochondria buffering initially reduces the size of calcium peaks of the signals generated by the ER, it has the ability to sustain these signals by its slow release through the calcium exchangers (Hoth et al., 2000). By rapidly taking up calcium, mitochondria can also activate CRACs, preventing the quick refill of ER stores.

CALCIUM SIGNALING PATHWAYS

Many cells can display calcium activity in various modes, depending not only on the stimuli that initiates the signal, but also on the type of intracellular receptor involved (either IP_3 or RyR), its abundance, its location, and its proximity to amplification or attenuation mechanisms. These parameters will determine both the spatial and temporal properties of the calcium signal, which in turn, will decide the physiological outcome of the initial stimuli.

Spatial Properties of Calcium Signaling: Intracellular versus Intercellular Calcium Signaling

When cells exhibit a single, brief calcium spike in response to extracellular stimuli, the response is known as *monophasic*. These responses usually occur in most cell types mediated by entry through extracellular pathways, whereas activation of intracellular release gives rise to more complex patterns of calcium activity. If small groups of IP_3Rs or RyRs are opened, the calcium signals are known as *puffs* or *sparks*, respectively (reviewed in Berridge et al., 2000) (Box 17.1). Depending on the number of channels involved, the amplitudes of the signals will vary and will give rise to more global responses that spread throughout the cell from the initial stimulation point in the form of intracellular calcium waves. These waves require the activation of neighboring channels by a CICR mechanism.

Rather than limiting its range to individual cells, calcium signals can spread over long distances and affect groups of cells, evoking intercellular calcium waves. The mechanisms involved in this type of calcium signaling are widely debated but are very relevant for the implications of astrocytic signaling. They will be discussed in detail later.

Temporal Aspects of Calcium Signaling: Calcium Oscillations

Calcium spikes can give rise to a variety of responses on their own. However, in some circumstances, longer

Box 17.1 Calcium Signaling in Neurons

Calcium signaling in neurons contrasts to that in astrocytes because of differences in the use of their calcium machinery and because neurons are electrically excitable. Neurons make strong use of the voltage-operated calcium channels (L, P/Q, and N type, mainly) to increase their intracellular calcium levels, especially during synaptic activity. *N*-methyl-D-aspartate and AMPA receptors also contribute largely to the entry of extracellular calcium upon activation with the neurotransmitter glutamate. In addition, internal calcium stores are mobilized by activation of the IP_3R (types 1 and 3 but not type 2, as in astrocytes) but also by opening RyRs in the ER. All these differences are translated into alternative temporal and spatial calcium activities compared to those of astrocytes. For example, some forms of synaptic plasticity depend on very localized calcium activities in dendritic microdomains (Yuste et al., 2000). Neurotransmitter release also depends on a particular disposition of the calcium machinery, the presynaptic vesicle-release complex (t-SNARE proteins) and proteins on the vesicle membrane (v-SNARE proteins) (SNARE: soluble NSF-associated protein receptor) (Sheng et al., 1998). Calcium waves in neurons are significantly faster than those of astrocytes (100–200 vs. 10–20 μm/s) and depend on the presence of extracellular calcium (Charles et al., 1996). At the nuclear level, the efficient decodification of the various calcium signals via different calcium targets (adenylyl cyclase, mitogen-activated protein kinase, calcium/calmodulin-dependent protein kinase) promotes changes in gene transcription that contribute to alterations in synaptic plasticity (reviewed in West et al., 2002). Most of the intracellular pathways that have been discovered in neuronal calcium signaling remain to be explored in astrocytic calcium signaling.

periods of signaling are required and calcium spikes are repeated over time, giving rise to the so-called calcium oscillations. A peculiarity of this mode of signaling is that information can be coded by the specific frequency at which oscillations are generated. This has been shown in detail in cells of the immune system, in which particular frequencies of calcium activity promoted both qualitative and quantitative differences in the pattern of gene expression compared with what is obtained with stimuli that produce a steady level of calcium (Li et al., 1998). An important aspect of frequency-coded information is the requirement for specific cellular *decoders* that are capable of translating the calcium information into a cellular response. The two most widely studied calcium-sensitive proteins that are involved in decoding calcium signals are Ca^{2+} calmodulin-dependent (CaM) kinase and protein kinase C (PKC), although only the latter has been evaluated in astrocytes. Thus, it seems that glutamate-induced astrocytic calcium oscillations depend on the periodic translocation and activation of PKC, which, in turn, responds to the oscillating DAG and Ca^{2+} concentrations (Codazzi et al., 2001).

ASTROCYTIC CALCIUM OSCILLATIONS

Astrocytes can respond to a large range of neuroligands with a calcium increase. The type of agonist determines whether the calcium response will be sustained or oscillating. The concentration of the agonist can also determine the outcome of the calcium signal. For example, cultured hippocampal astrocytes can respond to a particular concentration of glutamate with sustained oscillations, lasting for more than 5 minutes; to a higher concentration with damped oscillations, which decay within 6 minutes of initiation; or to a higher one by exhibiting a single response of elevated calcium (Cornell-Bell et al., 1990).

Occurrence and Significance

The calcium response of astrocytes to glutamate has been one of the most widely studied behaviors of calcium signaling in glia since glutamate is the major excitatory neurotransmitter in the brain. A critical question is therefore whether astrocytes exhibit similar calcium activities in response to glutamate released by neurons. Dani and coworkers (1992) explored this possibility by monitoring calcium activities in intact hippocampal astrocytic networks of organotypic brain slices. They found that, upon neuronal stimulation, astrocytes exhibited irregular cytoplasmic calcium oscillations, with periods ranging between 16 and 30 seconds, which recovered to a resting level as soon as neuronal stimulation was terminated. These observations have been corroborated in astrocytic cultures (Murphy et al., 1993), and it has been further shown that the frequency of the calcium oscillations can be modulated by the frequency of glutamate stimulation (Pasti et al., 1995). The use of acute brain slices has revealed additional information about the signaling capabilities of astrocytes *in situ*. Astrocytes in hippocampal and cortical brain slices are capable of responding to neuronal activity with calcium oscillations, and these astrocytes exhibit calcium oscillations that are modulated by the frequency of the neuronal stimulation and that can persist over a period of time after the neuronal stimuli. These oscillations involve synaptically released glutamate and the activation of the metabotropic glutamate receptor (mGluR) in astrocytes (Pasti et al., 1997). More important, calcium oscillations are accompanied by similar oscillations in adjacent neurons; these neuronal oscillations depend on the activation of ionotropic glutamate. So, astrocytes and neurons can establish a bidirectional form of communication based on their specific patterns of calcium oscillations.

What are the implications of astrocytic calcium oscillations? Since astrocytic calcium increases can trigger glutamate signaling in adjacent neurons (Araque et al., 1998), an appealing hypothesis is that a repetitive pattern of calcium increases contributes to transient episodes of glutamate release. Astrocytic glutamate release may, by activation of presynaptic mGluR, inhibit neuronal glutamate release and thereby function as a negative feedback mechanism that dampens local excitation. Astrocytic calcium oscillations may also participate in activity-dependent increases in cerebral blood flow by release of a diffusible agent, possibly prostaglandins (Zonta et al., 2003), again supporting the idea of astrocytic calcium oscillations as a major mechanism to control the release of neuromodulatory transmitters.

But astrocytes not only produce calcium oscillations in response to neuronal activity. Two studies have uncovered spontaneous calcium oscillations in thalamic (Parri et al., 2001) and hippocampal (Nett et al., 2002) astrocytes *in situ*. These oscillations follow the same pattern as the neuron-induced oscillations that are observed in culture and in slices, are developmentally regulated, require release from IP_3-sensitive intracellular stores, and depend on store refilling via the plasma membrane calcium channel. The challenge now is to decipher the functional significance of these spontaneous, neuron-independent astrocytic activities. Calcium oscillations in early-developing neurons have been associated with neurotransmitter differentiation, axonal growth, and establishment of neuronal networks (Yuste et al., 1992; Gu and Spitzer, 1995). It is therefore possible that glial cells require this mode of activity for proper maturation and formation of the glial syncitium. But what makes these observations more striking is the possibility that they may contribute directly to the proper establishment of neuronal networking during early development, when synaptic connectivity is not yet in place.

ASTROCYTIC CALCIUM WAVES

In addition to calcium oscillations, astrocytes display propagating calcium waves. Cornell-Bell and coworkers (1990) were the first to note that astrocytes generated propagating calcium waves when exposed to glutamate. The discovery that astrocytes possess a mechanism for long-distance communication had a profound impact on the field and brought into question the view that astrocytes are passive support cells. Later studies showed that astrocytic Ca^{2+} waves evoked large spike-like increases in neuronal cytosolic Ca^{2+}, suggesting that astrocytes may participate directly in neurotransmission (Fig. 17.2) (Nedergaard, 1994; Parpura et al., 1994). It was subsequently confirmed that astrocytic calcium signaling modulates the strength of synaptic transmission: stimulation of astrocytes led to a decrease in synaptic failure rate between pairs of synaptically coupled interneurons and CA1 pyramidal cells (Kang et al., 1998). Astrocytic calcium waves modulate the firing frequency of ganglion cells in dissected eyecup retinas and in hippocampal cultures (Newman and Zahs, 1998). Similarly, Schwann cells regulate neuromuscular transmission in a pathway that requires intracellular calcium signaling (Robitaille, 1998). Together these observations identified a new signaling loop between neurons and astrocytes: astrocytes can modulate the Ca^{2+} level, and thereby the firing pattern, of neurons in their surroundings. In turn, neurons can trigger astrocytic Ca^{2+} signaling by releasing glutamate.

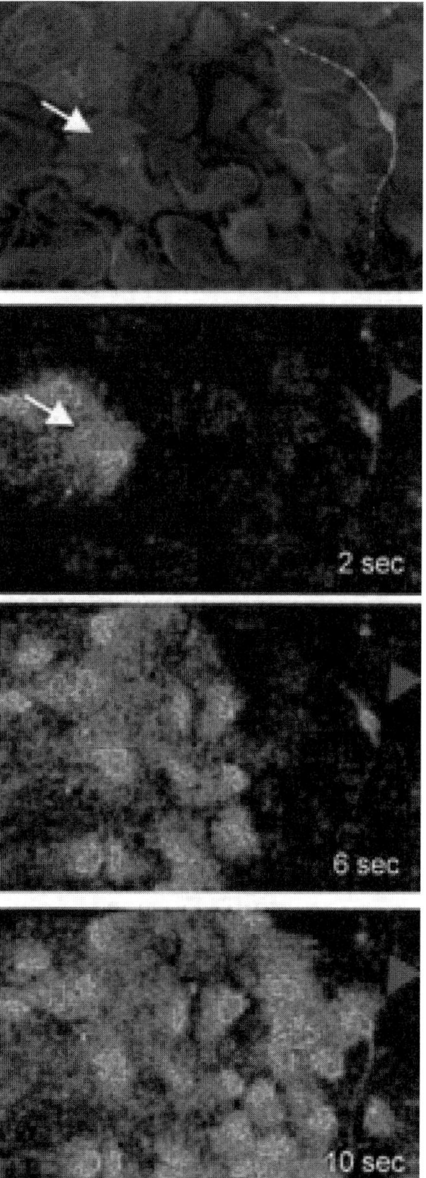

FIGURE 17.2 An astrocytic Ca^{2+} wave triggers an increase in neuronal cytosolic Ca^{2+}. Upper panels show a mixed culture stained against glial fibrillary acidic protein (GFAP) (gray) and microtubulin-associated protein-2 (MAP2) (white). The three lower panels show the same field of cells loaded with the Ca^{2+} indicator, fluo-3. A Ca^{2+} wave (electrical field stimulation, *white arrow*) propagates slowly across the field and triggers an increase in neuronal cytosolic Ca^{2+} (*gray arrowheads*).

Mechanism of Astrocytic Ca^{2+} Waves

Astrocytic Ca^{2+} waves have been intensively studied over the past decade, and the view on the mechanism underlying their intercellular expansion has undergone several important revisions. Ca^{2+} waves can, in cultured astrocytes, be evoked by receptor activation (glutamate, ATP, or endothelin-1), by lowering of extracellular calcium, or by intense neuronal firing in cultured organotypic slices (Zanotti and Charles, 1997; Arcuino et al., 2002). Most studies have, however, focused on the properties of waves evoked by mechanical and electrical stimulation of cultured astrocytes due to the precision with which the waves can be initiated (Venance and Giaume, 1997). A general feature of Ca^{2+} waves is that they propagate with a velocity of ~20 μm/s and expand over a maximal radius of ~300 to 400 μm, thereby engaging 30–60 cells in a single wave (Cornell-Bell et al., 1990). Despite controversies with regard to the mechanism of propagation, it is clear that Ca^{2+} waves require activation of phospholipase C (PLC), which produces IP_3. In turn, IP_3, mobilizes Ca^{2+}

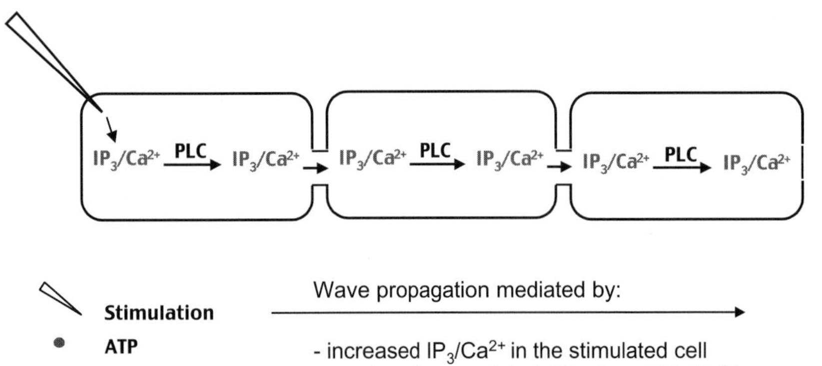

FIGURE 17.3 Gap junction mediated propagation of astrocytic Ca^{2+} waves. Phospholipase C (PLC) activation triggers an increase in inositol 1,4,5-trisphosphate (IP_3), which causes a release of Ca^{2+} from intracellular stores. Diffusion of IP_3 and/or Ca^{2+} across gap junctions trigger activation of PLC and a regenerative increase of IP_3 and Ca^{2+} in the neighboring cells, leading to propagation of a Ca^{2+} wave. ATP: adenosine triphosphate.

from intracellular stores, resulting in further activation of PLC (Boitano et al., 1992).

Model 1: gap junction–mediated Ca^{2+} signaling

The first model of astrocytic calcium signaling proposed that IP_3 and/or Ca^{2+} diffuses through the gap junction channels and initiates a cascade that requires PLC activation and results in Ca^{2+} increases in neighboring cells (Sanderson et al., 1990) (Fig. 17.3). A critical argument for the model was that C6 glioma cells, which are gap junction–deficient cells, could not propagate calcium waves. However, transfection and overexpression of the gap junction protein connexin 43 (Cx43) enabled the cells to transmit long-distance Ca^{2+} waves (>200 μm) (Zanotti and Charles, 1997). Later studies confirmed this observation by showing that overexpression of Cx32 in C6 glioma cells or in HeLa cells greatly enhanced the distance of Ca^{2+} wave propagation (Co-trina et al., 1998a).

Model 2: adenosine triphosphate–mediated regenerative Ca^{2+} waves

The role of gap junctions in Ca^{2+} wave propagation was first questioned by a study reporting that astrocytes with no physical contact with other astrocytes can engage in Ca^{2+} waves (Hassinger et al., 1996), indicating that an extracellular component mediates intercellular Ca^{2+} signaling. Using several pharmacological approaches, ATP was subsequently identified as the diffusible messenger (Cotrina et al., 1998a; Guthrie et al., 1999) (Fig. 17.4). Parallel studies in other systems established that ATP also mediates calcium waves in osteoblasts, liver, epithelial cells, and heart. Because astrocytes express P2Y1, P2Y2, P2Y4, and P2X7 receptors (John et al., 1999), it is likely that several members of the purinergic rceptors contribute to wave propagation in astrocytes. The revised model for calcium waves (Model 2) stated that ATP release was regenerative and calcium dependent.

Model 3: point source adenosine triphosphate release

Although observations by several groups confirmed that long-distance Ca^{2+} waves are mediated by purinergic signaling, it remained to be established how ATP was released and to which extent ATP release was regenerative. The fact that Cx expression greatly enlarged calcium waves led to the speculation that Cx hemichannels mediate ATP release. This suggestion was supported experimentally by the observation that several

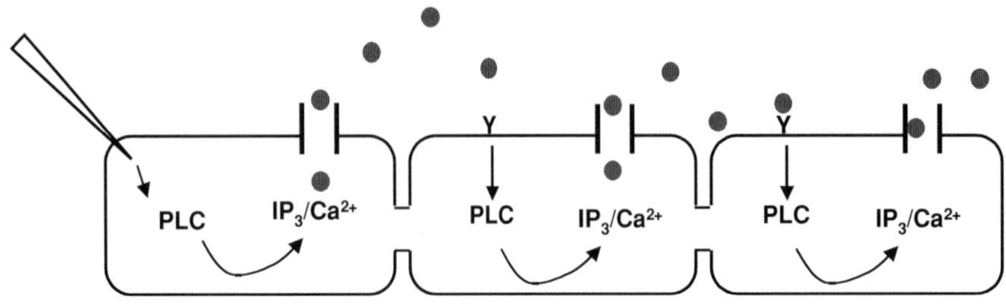

FIGURE 17.4 Regenerative purinergic receptor-mediated Ca^{2+} wave. Stimulation results in activation of phospholipase C (PLC) and an increase in cytosolic inositol 1,4,5-trisphosphate (IP_3) and Ca^{2+}, which trigger release of adenosine triphosphate (ATP). Activation of P_2Y receptors on neighboring cells mediates an increase in calcium and additional ATP release. The wave is propagated in a regenerative fashion by calcium-dependent ATP release.

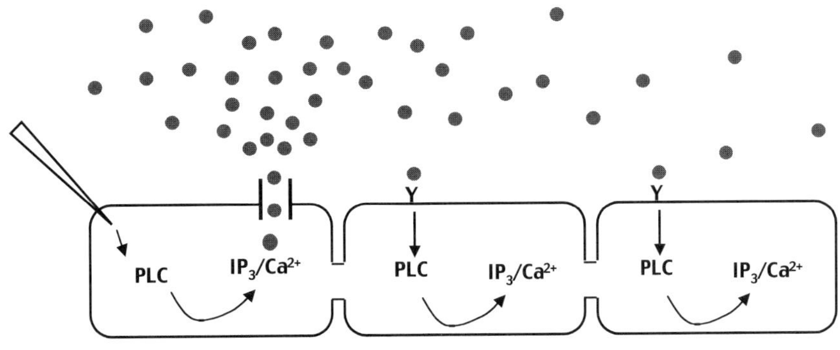

FIGURE 17.5 Nonregenerative calcium signaling as a mediator of calcium waves. Adenosine triphosphate (ATP) release from a single cell results in diffusion of ATP from a point source. P_2Y receptors on neighboring cells are activated by ATP, resulting in an increase in cytosolic Ca^{2+} concentration. The wave is not actively propagated by neighboring cells because no additional ATP is released. IP_3: inositol 1,4,5-trisphosphate; PLC: phospholipase C.

cell lines expressing Cx43, Cx32, or Cx26 released 5- to 20-fold more ATP than mock-transfected, Cx-deficient control cells (Cotrina et al., 1998a). In other words, Cx expression enlarged calcium waves by potentiating adenine triphosphate (ATP) release rather than by increasing intercellular coupling. Gap junction channels, which are composed of two hemichannels from adjacent cells, have an inner pore diameter of 10–12 Å and are freely permeable to large anions, including adenine diphosphate (ADP) and ATP. Open hemichannels may therefore direct the efflux of cytosolic ATP. Later studies documented that ATP release occurs concomitant with an increase in whole-cell current (Arcuino et al., 2002), supporting the concept of channel-mediated ATP release. Other lines of evidence have suggested, on the basis of cellular fractionation, that ATP is released by calcium-dependent exocytosis of ATP-containing vesicles (Queiroz et al., 1999). It is possible that astrocytes can release ATP by several mechanisms, but addi-

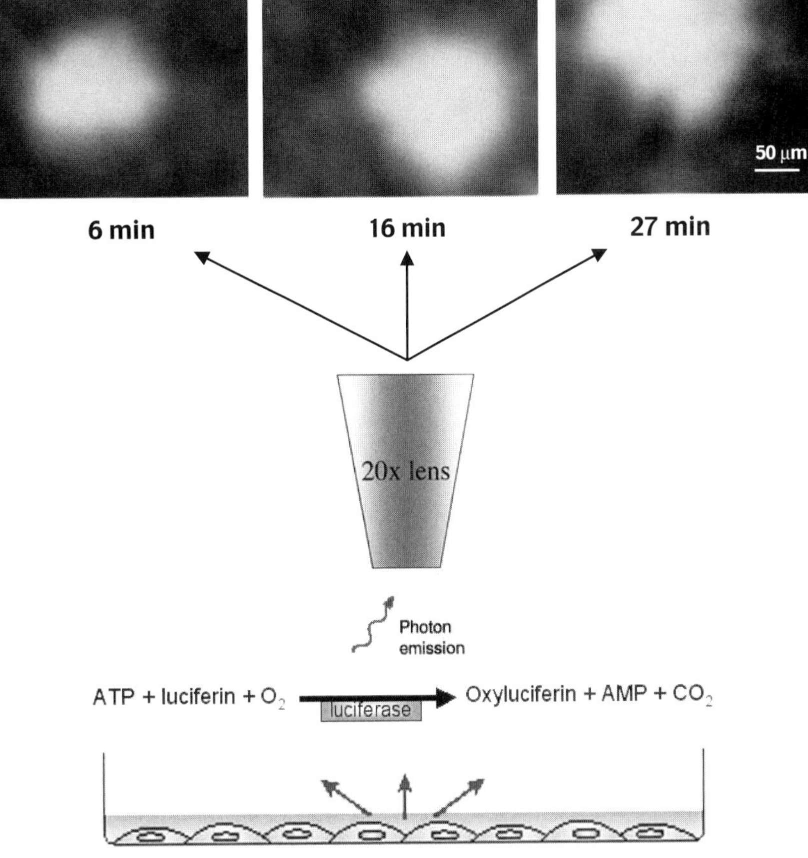

FIGURE 17.6 Bioluminescence imaging of adenosine triphosphate (ATP) from cultured astrocytes. A mixture of luciferin/luciferase is added to the recording solution. By this method, ATP release can be monitored by light emissions resulting from the ATP-triggered luciferase breakdown of luciferin, both at the single-cell level and in real time, using a liquid nitrogen–cooled CCD camera. At baseline, the majority of the astrocytes grown in a confluent monolayer exhibited no photodetectable ATP release. Stimulation of calcium signaling resulted in frequent point-source bursts of light emission. These ATP bursts were highly variable in their duration and extent of spatial expansion, but were abrupt in onset and spherical in spread, likely reflecting ATP diffusion from a point source. Three examples of ATP burst activity from a single field are shown. The ATP burst releases occurred spontaneously at 6, 16, and 27 minutes. AMP: adenosine monophosphate.

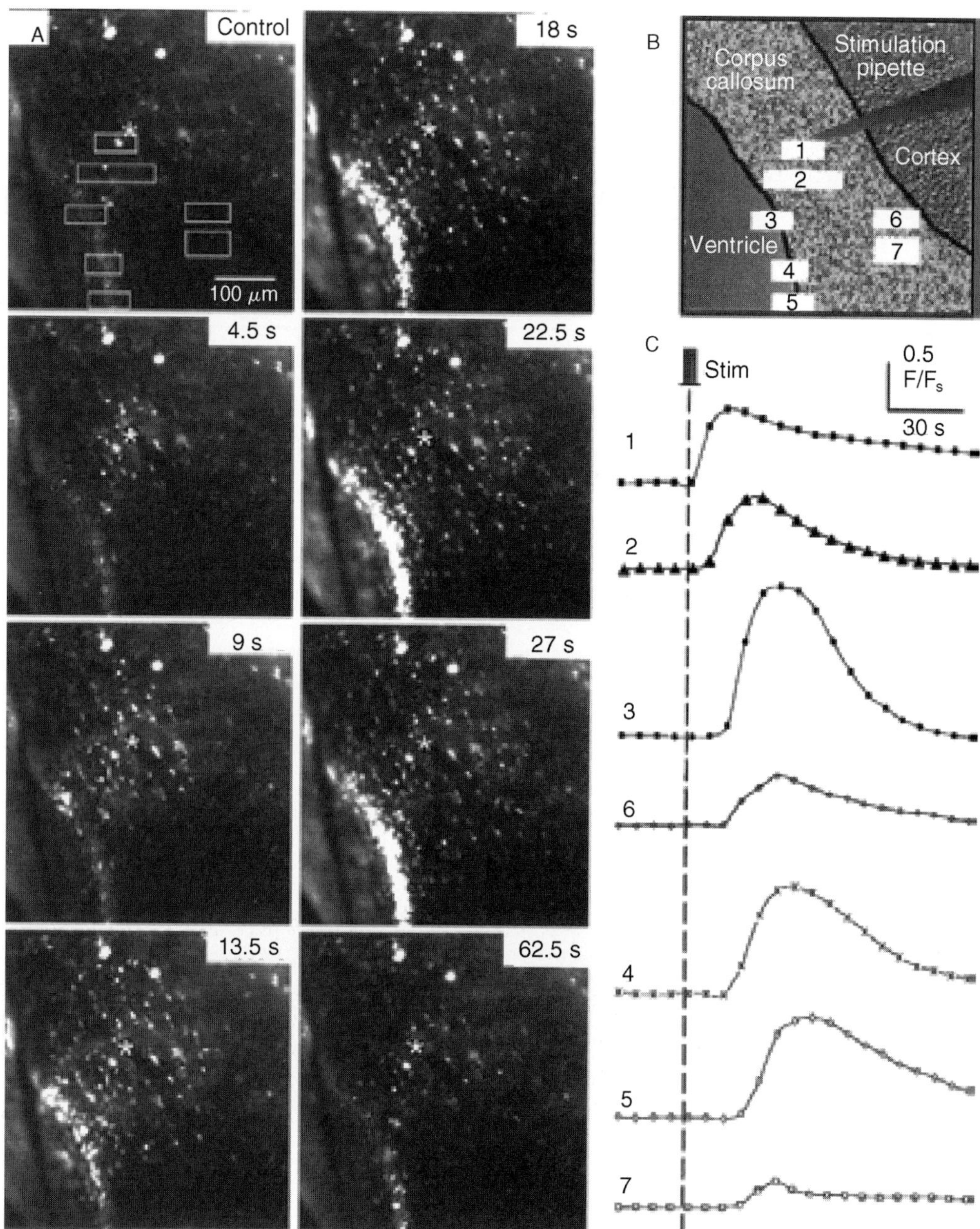

FIGURE 17.7 Propagation of Ca^{2+} waves in an acute brain slice. A series of fluorescence images just before (control) and at defined times (as indicated) after electrical stimulation illustrate the spread of the Ca^{2+} signal within a slice (*A*). The position of the stimulation electrode is marked by the asterisk. *B*. Outline of the anatomical structures of the fluorescence images. Transient changes in Ca^{2+} are displayed in panel *C*. In area 1, close to the stimulation pipette, the increase in fluorescence (F/Fo) occurred right after stimulation (indicated by the *vertical line*). At more distant areas the delay amounted to several seconds.

tional studies are needed to establish the coexistence of these mechanisms which are not necessarily mutually exclusive.

A strong argument against regenerative ATP release proposed in Model 2 (Fig. 17.4) was that calcium waves never expand more than 300 to 400 μm beyond their point of origin and therefore are not truly regenerative. In fact, real-time bioluminescence imaging of extracellular ATP failed to support the concept of regenerative ATP release during calcium wave propagation. Adenosine triphosphate was consistently released by a single cell or from a point source only (Arcuino et al., 2002) (Fig. 17.5). So, the propagating wave front reflects diffusion of ATP rather than sequential ATP release, as proposed in Model 3. Neighboring cells increase intracellular Ca^{2+} in response to P2Y receptor activation but do not actively participate in wave propagation with release of additional ATP (Fig. 17.6).

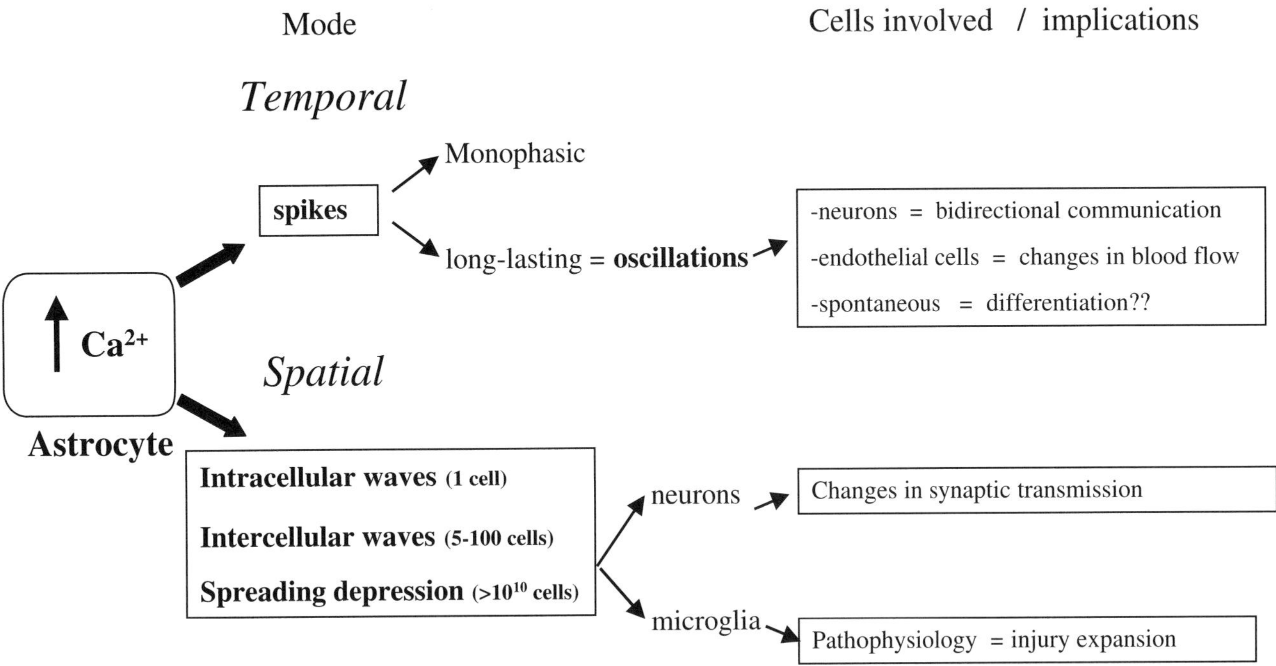

FIGURE 17.8 Schematic representation of the major Ca^{2+} signaling pathways in astrocytes.

Astrocytes in Intact Tissue Support Propagation of Calcium Waves and Possibly of Spreading Depression

The studies discussed so far on calcium wave propagation were based on observations in cultured astrocytes or organotypic slices. Calcium waves have also been observed in the retina following mechanical stimulation (Newman, 2001), and a recent report documented that intact brain tissue supported the propagation of calcium waves (Schipke et al., 2002) (Fig. 17.7 and Box 17.2). Electrical field stimulation (4 seconds at 10 Hz) triggered calcium waves, which migrated with a velocity of 14 μm/s and expanded more than 500 μm in coronal slices from 5- to 8-day-old mice. The characteristics of these calcium waves in brain slices were strikingly similar to those of astrocytic calcium waves *in vitro*. For example, depletion of internal calcium stores with thapsigargin attenuated the waves, while removal of extracellular Ca^{2+} potentiated wave propagation. Most important, purinergic receptor blockers strongly inhibited the expansion of long-distance calcium waves in the slice preparation (Schipke et al., 2002).

So, astrocytes in brain slices support the idea that calcium wave propagation depends on purinergic receptors. However, it remains an open question whether calcium waves are initiated by physiological stimuli in brain slices. In fact, several lines of evidence may point to the opposite conclusion because intense neuronal or local application of neurotransmitters triggers astrocytic calcium oscillations but not propagating calcium waves (Porter and McCarthy, 1996; Pasti et al., 1997; Kang et al., 1998). Because induction of astrocytic calcium waves requires powerful stimulation, this type of signaling might relate to pathophysiological events rather than normal brain physiology. In fact, astrocytic calcium waves share several features with spreading depression, a slowly moving wave of tissue depolarization that is evoked in ischemia and brain trauma (Nedergaard and Hansen, 1993) (Fig. 17.8). Spreading depression propagates with a velocity of 15–35 μm/s, and is associated with a transient cessation of electri-

Box 17.2 Calcium Signaling in Schwann Cells, Oligodendrocytes, and Microglia

Although calcium signaling in glial cells has been explored mostly in astrocytes, many studies suggest that other glial cell types are also capable of calcium responses similar to those of astrocytes. Ligand- and voltage-gated ion channels, CRAC channels, RyR, and IP_3R of type 2 have all been described in oligodendrocytes and microglial cells. Similarly, calcium dynamics in these glial cells have profound physiological implications for neural function. For example, calcium changes in oligodendrocytes and oligodendrocyte precursors might regulate myelin formation (Agrawal et al., 2000), microglial calcium increases in response to astrocytic signaling seem to be a generalized way to communicate injury (Verderio and Matteoli, 2001; Schipke et al., 2002), calcium waves in Müller cells of the retina can alter ganglion cells excitability (Newman and Zahs, 1997), and calcium increases within Schwann cells modulate transmitter release of motor neuron axons (Robitaille, 1998).

cal activity and depolarization of both neurons and astrocytes. The depolarization wave of spreading depression is preceded by a wave of astrocytic calcium increases. The increase in astrocytic calcium concentration spreads with the same velocity as spreading depression, but is ahead of neuronal depolarization by 6–16 seconds. It is therefore possible that astrocytic calcium signaling mediates the propagating wave front of spreading depression, but more studies are needed to define the role of astrocytes in the process. In particular, the contribution of gap junctions versus purinergic signaling in spreading depression is not fully understood. A systematic dissection of the mechanism underlying astrocytic calcium oscillations and calcium waves, as well as a clear definition of their role in normal and pathological events, is warranted. We anticipate that these insights may lead to development of drugs targeted for a broad range of neurological diseases, including migraine, stroke, and head trauma, which involve abnormal manifestations of astrocytic calcium signaling.

REFERENCES

Agrawal, S.K., Nashmi, R., and Fehlings, M.G. (2000) Role of L- and N-type calcium channels in the pathophysiology of traumatic spinal cord white matter injury. *Neuroscience* 99:179–188.

Araque, A., Parpura, V., Sanzgiri, R.P., and Haydon, P.G. (1998) Glutamate-dependent astrocyte modulation of synaptic transmission between cultured hippocampal neurons. *Eur. J. Neurosci.* 10:2129–2142.

Arcuino, G., Lin, J.H., Takano, T., Liu, C., Jiang, L., Gao, Q, Kang, J., and Nedergaard, M. (2002) Intercellular calcium signaling mediated by point-source burst release of ATP. *Proc. Natl. Acad. Sci. USA* 99:9840–9845.

Bergles, D.E. and Jahr, C.E. (1997) Synaptic activation of glutamate transporters in hippocampal astrocytes. *Neuron* 19:1297–1308.

Bergles, D.E. and Jahr, C.E. (1998) Glial contribution to glutamate uptake at Schaffer collateral-commissural synapses in the hippocampus. *J. Neurosci.* 88:7709–7716.

Berridge, M.J., Lipp, P., and Bootman, M.D. (2000) The versatility and universality of calcium signaling. *Nat. Rev. Mol. Cell Biol.* 1:11–22.

Boitano, S., Dirksen, E.R., and Sanderson, M.J. (1992) Intercellular propagation of calcium waves mediated by inositol trisphosphate. *Science* 258:292–295.

Charles, A.C., Kodali, S.K., and Tyndale, R.F. (1996) Intercellular calcium waves in neurons. *Mol. Cell. Neurosci.* 7:337–353.

Codazzi, F., Teruel, M.N., and Meyer, T. (2001) Control of astrocyte Ca^{2+} oscillations and waves by oscillating translocation and activation of protein kinase C. *Curr. Biol.* 11:1089–1097.

Cornell-Bell, A.H., Finkbeiner, S.M., Cooper, M.S., and Smith, S.J. (1990) Glutamate induces calcium waves in cultured astrocytes: long-range glial signaling. *Science* 247:470–473.

Cotrina, M.L., Lin, J.H., Alves-Rodrigues, A., Liu, S., Li, J., Azmi-Ghadimi, H., Kang, J., Naus, C.C., and Nedergaard, M. (1998a) Connexins regulate calcium signaling by controlling ATP release. *Proc. Natl. Acad. Sci. USA* 95:15735–15740.

Cotrina, M.L., Lin, J.H., and Nedergaard, M. (1998b) Cytoskeletal assembly and ATP release regulate astrocytic calcium signaling. *J. Neurosci.* 18:8794–8804.

Dani, J.W., Chernjavsky, A., and Smith, S.J. (1992) Neuronal activity triggers calcium waves in hippocampal astrocyte networks. *Neuron* 8:429–440.

Gilabert, J.A. and Parekh, A.B. (2000) Respiring mitochondria determine the pattern of activation and inactivation of the store-operated Ca^{2+} current I_{CRAC}. *EMBO J.* 19:6401–6407.

Gu, X. and Spitzer, N.C. (1995) Distinct aspects of neuronal differentiation encoded by frequency of spontaneous Ca^{2+} transients. *Nature* 375:784–787.

Guthrie, P.B., Knapperberger, J., Segal., M., Bennett, M.V., Charles, A.C., and Kater, S.B. (1999) ATP released from astrocytes mediates glial calcium waves. *J. Neurosci.* 19:520–528.

Hassinger, T.D., Guthrie, P.B., Atkinson, P.B., Bennett, M.V., and Kater, S.B. (1996) An extracellular signaling component in propagation of astrocytic calcium waves. *Proc. Natl. Acad. Sci. USA* 93:13268–13273.

Hoth, M., Button, D.C., Lewis, R.S. (2000) Mitochondrial control of calcium-channel gating: a mechanism for sustained signaling and transcriptional activation in T lymphocytes. *Proc. Natl. Acad. Sci. USA* 97:10607–10612.

John, G.R., Scemes, E., Suadicani, S.O., Liu, J.S., Charles, P.C., Lee, S.C., Spray, D.C., and Brosnan, C.F. (1999) IL-1 beta differentially regulates calcium wave propagation between primary human fetal astrocytes via pathways involving P2 receptors and gap junction channels. *Proc. Natl. Acad. Sci. USA* 96:11613–11618.

Kang, J., Jiang, L., Goldman, S.A., and Nedergaard, M. (1998) Astrocyte-mediated potentiation of inhibitory synaptic transmission. *Nat. Neurosci.* 1:683–692.

Kawasaki, H., Nakayama, S., and Kretsinger, R.H. (1998) Classification and evolution of EF-hand proteins. *Biometals* 11:277–295.

Langley, D. and Pearce, B. (1994) Ryanodine-induced intracellular calcium mobilization in cultured astrocytes. *Glia* 12:128–134.

Li, W., Llopis, J., Whitney, M., Zlokarnik, G., and Tsien, R.Y. (1998) Cell-permeant caged $InsP_3$ ester shows that Ca^{2+} spike frequency can optimize gene expression. *Nature* 392:936–941.

Matyash, M., Matyash, V., Nolte, C., Sorrentino, V., and Kettenmann, H. (2001) Requirement of functional ryanodine receptor type 3 for astrocyte migration. *FASEB J.* 16:84–86.

Murphy, T.H., Blatter, L.A., Wier, W.G., and Baraban, J.M. (1993) Rapid communication between neurons and astrocytes in primary cortical cultures. *J. Neurosci.* 13:2672–2679.

Nedergaard, M. (1994) Direct signaling from astrocytes to neurons in cultures of mammalian brain cells. *Science* 263:1768–1771.

Nedergaard, M. and Hansen, A.J. (1993) Characterization of cortical depolarization evoked in focal cerebral ischemia. *J. Cereb. Blood Flow Metab.* 13:568–574.

Nett, W.J., Oloff, S.H., and McCarthy, K.D. (2002) Hippocampal astrocytes in situ exhibit calcium oscillations that occur independent of neuronal activity. *J. Neurophysiol.* 87:528–537.

Newman, E.A. (2001) Propagation of intercellular calcium waves in retinal astrocytes and Muller cells. *J. Neurosci.* 21:2215–2223.

Newman, E.A. and Zahs, K.R. (1997) Calcium waves in retinal glial cells. *Science* 275:844–847.

Newman, E.A. and Zahs, K.R. (1998) Modulation of neuronal activity by glial cells in the retina. *J. Neurosci.* 18:4022–4028.

Parpura, V., Basarsky, T.A., Liu, F., Jeftinija, K., Jeftinija, S., and Haydon, P.G. (1994) Glutamate-mediated astrocyte-neuron signaling. *Nature* 369:744–747.

Parri, H.R., Gould, T.M., and Crunelli, V. (2001) Spontaneous astrocytic calcium oscillations in situ drive NMDAR-mediated neuronal excitation. *Nat. Neurosci.* 4:803–812.

Pasti, L., Pozzan, T., and Carmignoto, G. (1995) Long-lasting changes of calcium oscillations in astrocytes. *J. Biol. Chem.* 270: 15203–15210.

Pasti, L., Volterra, A., Pozzan, T., and Carmignoto, G. (1997) Intracellular calcium oscillations in astrocytes: a highly plastic, bidirectional form of communication between neurons and astrocytes *in situ*. *J. Neurosci.* 17:7817–7830.

Porter, J.T. and McCarthy, K.D. (1996) Hippocampal astrocytes in situ respond to glutamate released from synaptic terminals. *J. Neurosci.* 16:5073–5081.

Queiroz, G., Meyer, D.K., Meyer, A., Starke, K., and von Kugelgen, I. (1999) A study of the mechanism of the release of ATP from rat cortical astroglial cells evoked by activation of glutamate receptors. *Neuroscience* 91:1171–1181.

Robitaille, R. (1998) Modulation of synaptic efficacy and synaptic depression by glial cells at the frog neuromuscular junction. *Neuron* 21:847–855.

Sanderson, M.J., Charles, A.C., and Dirksen, E.R. (1990) Mechanical stimulation and intercellular communication increases intracellular Ca^{2+} in epithelial cells. *Cell Regul.* 1:585–596.

Schipke, C.G., Boucsein, C., Ohlemeyer, C., Kirchhoff, F., and Kettenmann, H. (2002) Astrocyte calcium waves trigger responses in microglial cells in brain slices. *FASEB J.* 16:255–257.

Shelton, M.K. and McCarthy, K.D. (1999) Mature hippocampal astrocytes exhibit functional metabotropic and ionotropic glutamate receptors in situ. *Glia* 26:1–11.

Sheng, Z.H. et al. (1998) Physical link and functional coupling of presynaptic calcium channels and synaptic vesicle docking/fusion machinery. *J. Bioenerg. Biomembr.* 30:335–345.

Venance, L., Stella, N., Glowinski, J., and Giaume, C. (1997) Mechanism involved in initiation and propagation of receptor-induced intercellular calcium signaling in cultured rat astrocytes. *J. Neurosci.* 17:1981–1992.

Verderio, C. and Matteoli, M. (2001) ATP mediates calcium signaling between astrocytes and microglial cells: modulation by IFN-γ. *J. Immunol.* 166:6383–6391.

Verderio, C., Bruzzone, S., Zocchi, E., Fedele, E., Schenk, U., De Flora, A., and Matteoli, M. (2001) Evidence of a role for cyclic ADP-ribose in calcium signaling and neurotransmitter release in cultured astrocytes. *J. Neurochem.* 78:646–657.

West, A.E., Griffith, E.C., and Greenberg, M.E. (2002) Regulation of transcription factors by neuronal activity. *Nat. Rev. Neurosci.* 3:921–931.

Westenbroek, R.E., Bausch, S.B., Lin, R.C.S., Franck, J.E., Noebels, J.L., and Catterall, W.A. (1998) Upregulation of L-type Ca^{2+} channels in reactive astrocytes after brain injury, hypomyelination, and ischemia. *J. Neurosci.* 18:2321–2334.

Wu, M.L., Chen, W.H., Liu, I.H., Tseng, C.D., and Wang, S.M. (1999) A novel effect of cyclic AMP on capacitative Ca^{2+} entry in cultured rat cerebellar astrocytes. *J. Neurochem.* 73:1318–1328.

Yuste, R., Majewska, A., and Holthoff, K. (2000) From form to function: calcium compartmentalization in dendritic spines. *Nat. Neurosci.* 3:653–659.

Yuste, R., Peinado, A., and Katz, L.C. (1992) Neuronal domains in developing neocortex. *Science* 257:665–669.

Zanotti, S. and Charles, A. (1997) Extracellular calcium sensing by glial cells: low extracellular calcium induces intracellular calcium release and intercellular signaling. *J. Neurochem.* 69:594–602.

Zonta, M., Angulo, M.C., Gobbo, S., Rosengarten, B., Hossmann, K., Pozzan, T., and Carmignoto, G. (2003) Neuron-to-astrocyte signaling is central to the dynamic control of brain microcirculation. *Nat. Neurosci.* 6:43–50.

18 Cytoskeletal proteins in astroglia

LAWRENCE F. ENG AND YUEN LING LEE

The cytoskeleton is essential for many cellular processes, including mechanical strength, movement, adhesion, polarity, and intracellular trafficking. The cytoplasm of animal cells is structured by scaffolding composed of actin filaments (microfilaments), microtubules, and intermediate filaments (IFs) all joined by cross-linking proteins such as plakins (Yang et al., 1999). The chemistry, biology, and structure of the cytoskeleton have been extensively reviewed (Goldman and Steinert, 1990). In contrast to microfilaments and microtubules, whose components are highly conserved evolutionarily and similar within cells of a particular species, IFs display considerable diversity in their number, sequences, and abundance; are ubiquitous constituents of virtually all eukaryotic cells; and are present in both the nucleus (as the nuclear lamina) and the cytoplasm.

INTERMEDIATE FILAMENTS

In humans, IFs are composed of a large family of more than 50 gene products that polymerize into approximate 10 nm diameter filaments. Some form a single type of protein chain (homopolymers), while others form only as a combination with more than one type of protein (heteropolymers). Usually IFs are concentrated in the perinuclear region and radiate throughout the cytoplasm, where they are associated with the cell membrane. Intermediate filaments constitute approximately 1% of the total protein in most cells; however, in some cells, such as epidermal keratinocytes and neurons, they can account for up to 85% of the total protein in fully differentiated cells. The extent of sequence homology, the pattern of cell type–specific expression, and the similarity of intron positions of their genes are properties that have been used to classify IF proteins into six different types (Fuchs and Weber, 1994).

The neuroglia type III IF proteins are vimentin and glial fibrillary acidic protein (GFAP). These proteins are capable of polymerizing into hompolymer IFs. Vimentin is unique in that it can form a scaffold IF network before the expression and assembly of differentiation-specific GFAP. The type VI IF protein nestin is an early developmental protein of neuroepithelial cells (Lendahl et al., 1990) that cannot form IF on its own but is capable of copolymerizing with type III vimentin and type IV α-internexin chains to form filaments. Nestin can be reexpressed in reactive astrocytes of the adult central nervous system (CNS) in response to cellular stress at the site of injury, including blunt focal skull trauma, nerve graft, CNS ischemia, kainic acid lesions, and neoplastic transformation (Almqvist et al., 2002).

INTERMEDIATE FILAMENTS IN ASTROGLIA

Vimentin

Vimentin was first demonstrated in chicken fibroblasts as the major subunit of filaments and is expressed mainly in cells of mesenchymal origin. Immunohistology showed that vimentin was present in a variety of cultured cells and permanent cell lines from other tissues. Cells of different embryological origin produce vimentin when grown *in vitro*. Vimentin is also expressed during the differentiation of various cell lineages. Most cells *in situ* express only one type of IF. Exceptions include some glial cells, aortic smooth muscle cells, and neurons. For example, vimentin coexists with GFAP in immature astrocyte, in Bergmann glia, in tanycyte processes, and in Müller fibers of degenerating retinae. It is thought that expression of vimentin is correlated with a less differentiated state. By immunofluorescence and electron microscopy, vimentin IFs have been found to occur as single filaments or gently curving, loose bundles. The genomes of various vertebrate cell types are known to have a single copy of a gene for vimentin but this gene appears to make at least two mRNA species (Zehner and Paterson, 1983).

Vimentin in development and astrogliosis

Developmental expression of cytoskeletal IFs has been studied in a number of experimental models. In the developing chick embryo, vimentin is present in virtually all of the replicating neuroepithelial cells in the early neural tube. As the cells mature, neurofilaments replace vimentin in the postmitotic neuron and GFAP replaces vimentin in the mature astrocyte. Vimentin decreases and GFAP increases in differentiating rodent glial cells. Vimentin and GFAP have been reported to coexist in varying proportions in cultured astrocytes, in Bergmann radial glial fibers of the adult cerebellum, and in the corpus callosum. Intermediate filament heteropolymers consisting of alternating GFAP and vimentin monomers have been demonstrated by immunoelectron microscopy in human glial tumors and cultured mouse astrocytes.

Schiffer et al. (1986) studied astrocytic reactions to injury under two experimental conditions in the rat CNS: brains injured by laser irradiation and brain tumors induced with the chemical carcinogen, ethylnitrosourea. After immunostaining with antibodies to GFAP and vimentin, GFAP antibodies labeled all of the reactive astrocytes, whereas vimentin antibody staining was found in astrocytes at the periphery of the lesion. The authors suggested that vimentin was expressed only in the astrocytes undergoing proliferation. Subsequently, the reexpression of nestin and vimentin was demonstrated in reactive astrocytes in many types of injury, stress and disease.

Glial Fibrillary Acidic Protein

The term *glial fibrillary acidic protein* (GFAP) evolved from *plaque protein* to *glial fibrillary protein*, to *GFAP* or *GFA protein* and was originally based on its high acidic amino acid content and its morphological fibrous appearance. Other protein preparations containing GFAP or its proteolytic degradation products are astroprotein and α-albumin. Studies of the GFAP protein stemmed from our lipid studies in brains of multiple sclerosis (MS) patients. Multiple sclerosis is a demyelinating disease of the CNS characterized by demyelination, intense reactive gliosis, and formation of a scar composed of bare axons surrounded by astrocytes filled with glial filaments. The amino acid composition of purified GFAP was first determined in the Neurochemistry Laboratory of Dr. Eric Shooter at the Stanford Medical Center and was presented at a round table on "Brain-Specific Proteins" organized by Dr. Elizabeth Roboz-Einstein at the second international meeting of the International Society for Neurochemistry held in Milan on September 3, 1969 (Eng et al., 1971; Eng and Lee, 1995; Eng et al., 2000) (Figure 18.1).

Identification and biochemical properties of GFAP that have impeded its characterization are its insolubility in aqueous solvents, tendency to aggregate or polymerize, susceptibility to neutral proteases, highly specific and antigenic epitopes, and wide distribution of GFAP-containing astrocytes. Only a very small pool of aqueous soluble GFAP could be detected at any age in development of the rat brain, in cultured astrocytes, and in rat spinal cord. Early reports of a soluble GFAP fraction used human postmortem tissue and animal tissue where the time between death and homogenization

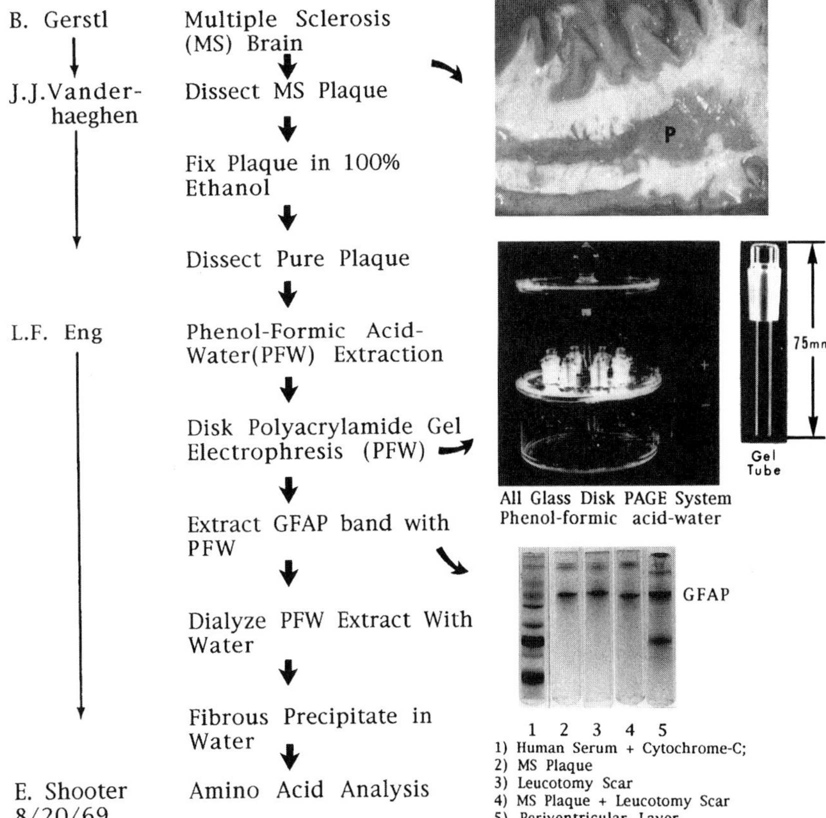

FIGURE 18.1 Diagram illustrates the isolation of glial fibrillary acidic protein (GFAP) from a multiple sclerosis (MS) plaque for amino acid. [This figure was previously published as Fig. 4.1 on page 72 of an article entitled "Glial Responses to Injury, Disease, and Aging" in the book edited by H.M. Schipper entitled *Brain Aging and Neurodegeneration* (1998) with permission from R.G. Landes Company.]

of the tissue was not controlled. The low molecular weight soluble forms in these cases are probably due to a calcium-activated neutral proteinase, which has high substrate specificity for vimentin and desmin.

Glial fibrillary acidic protein shows species-specific amino acid sequence heterogeneity, and its molecular weight ranges from 48,000 for mouse, to 49,000 for human, to 50,000 for bovine and to 51,000 for rat. *In vitro* translation of mRNA from normal and mutant rodent CNS and from a human glioma–derived cell line in culture or as a solid tumor yielded single molecular weight polypeptides that showed ionic charge differences among two or three spots with an isoelectric pH range of 5.7–5.9. Except for small interspecies polypeptide sequences variations, GFAP appears to been unaffected by CNS mutations (Jimpy mouse) or oncological events (human glioma). The relatively slow metabolic turnover rate for GFAP is consistent with a structural role for glial filaments in the cytoplasm.

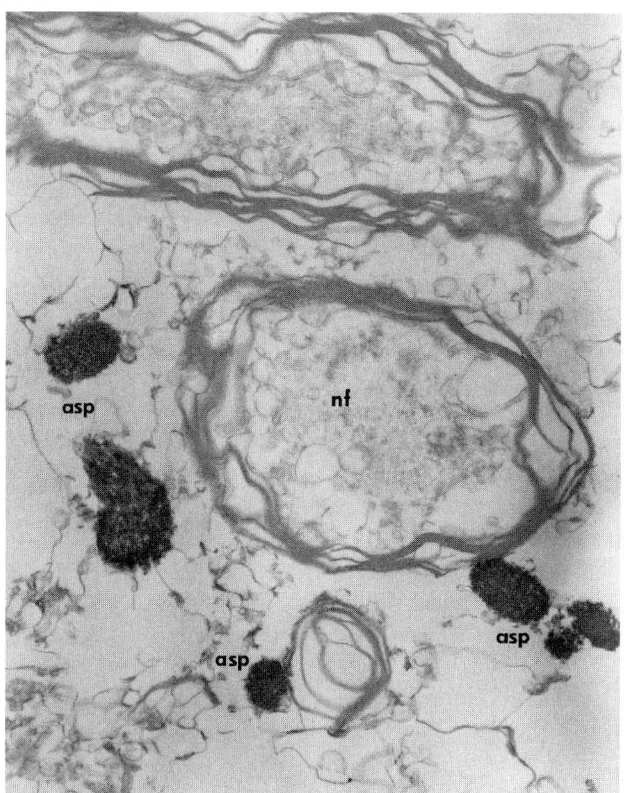

FIGURE 18.2 Bovine myelinated axon preparation immunochemically stained for glial fibrillary acidic protein (GFAP) showing strong positive staining of the astrocytic process (*asp*) adjacent to axons. Note the lack of staining at any intra-axonal structures including neurofilaments (*nf*). ×30,000.

Controversy regarding glial fibrillary acidic protein

In the past, considerable confusion existed regarding the chemical and immunological relationships between the glial filament, neurofilament, and neurotubule proteins. Since astrocytes are intimately associated with all of the cells and structures in the CNS, isolated subcellular fractions, organelles, or cells are associated with varying amounts of GFAP filaments from the disrupted astrocytes. This has led to confusion about the relationship between neurotubules, neurofilaments, and GFAP. Neurotubules had been reported to have chemical properties similar to those of glial filaments and GFAP. Neurotubules had also been reported to share common properties with neurofilaments. Still other studies had suggested that neurofilament proteins had chemical and immunological properties similar to those of GFAP and glial filaments. Our early reports, which indicated that GFAP from astrocytes were not related to neurofilaments, were controversial but subsequently were confirmed by numerous studies (Eng et al., 2000). An ultrastructural image of a GFAP-immunostained section of a myelinated axon preparation shows that GFAP astrocyte processes are heavily stained, but not the neurofilaments within the myelinated axon (Fig. 18.2).

Assembly/disassembly of glial fibrillary acidic protein

Glial fibrillary acidic protein is composed of three distinct regions: an amino-terminal head region, a central rod region, and a carboxy-terminal tail region. The rod regions are highly conserved among IF proteins, while the size and amino acid sequences of the head and tail regions vary. The head region of porcine GFAP is composed of 35 amino acid residues and has a β-turn structure. It contains eight arginine residues that characterize this highly basic region. Phosphorylation and dephosphorylation of specific amino acid residues on the head region are involved in the regulation of GFAP assembly. The rod region of GFAP is composed of 345 amino acid residues containing long tandem repeats of seven amino acid sequences called *heptad repeats*. This region is essential for the packing of the α-helical coil, which is important for the formation of 10 nm filaments. The tail region, consisting of about 50 amino acid residues, has a globular structure and may be involved in the interactions between IF and other proteins.

Under physiological conditions, the majority of GFAP proteins assemble to form 10 nm filaments *in vitro*. *In vitro* reconstitution studies show that assembly and morphology of GFAP filaments are affected by various physical factors, such as GFAP concentration, pH, divalent cations, ionic strength, amino acids, and temperature. The suitable pH range for *in vitro* assembly is around pH 7.

Phosphorylation/dephosphorylation of glial fibrillary acidic protein

Posttranslational modification to the N- and C-terminal domains of IFs are common, while those within the central α-helical domain are rare. The posttranslational modification of greatest functional and structural significance arises from the action of various kinases on serine and threonine embedded within specific recognition sequences. The phosphorylation events that have a regulatory role in the assembly and turnover of most IFs *in vivo* are confined to the N- and C-terminal domains of the chains (Parry and Steinert, 1999). Phosphatases, which dephosphorylate the chains, have an equally important role in governing assembly and function. In cytokeratins, vimentin, and lamins, the effect of phosphorylation is to disassemble the IFs, whereas dephosphorylation allows spontaneous self-assembly to proceed. These changes typically occur during cell division.

Phosphorylation and dephosphorylation of the IF head regions have a critical role for the maintenance and reconstruction of IFs. Glial fibrillary acidic protein filaments disassemble into a soluble form when the amino acids in the head are phosphorylated. The head region of GFAP is positively charged due to the many arginine residues. The mechanism of GFAP assembly regulation may be related to regulation of the electric charge in the head domain by phosphorylation. The sites of second messenger–dependent protein kinases have been identified in the head region of GFAP. Four serines (Ser-8, Ser-13, Ser-14, Ser-34) and one threonine (Thr-7) are known to be phosphorylated by different protein kinases; cyclic adenosine monophosphate (AMP)–dependent protein kinase (A kinase), Ca^{2+} calmodulin–dependent kinase II (CaM kinase II), C kinase, and Rho-kinase. A kinase phosphorylates Thr-7, Ser-8, Ser-13, and Ser-34 residues of the HEAD region. Ca^{2+} calmodulin-dependent kinase II phosphorylates Ser-8, Ser-17, Ser-34, and Ser-389. cdc2 Kinase phosphorylation of GFAP did not cause disassembly, while CaM kinase II phosphorylation did induce disassembly of the filament (Inagaki et al., 1994). The phosphorylation of vimentin and GFAP by Rho-kinase inhibits filament formation *in vitro*. The phosphorylation sites of GFAP are Thr-7, Ser-13, and Ser-34, cleavage furrow the same sites that (CF) kinase phosphorylates at the cleavage furrow during cytokinesis. Rho-kinase is a likely candidates for CF kinase phosphorylation of IFs at the cleavage furrow during cytokinesis (Matsuzawa et al., 1998).

A GFAP human wild-type knockin mouse was generated in which the coding region of the HEAD domain of GFAP was replaced with the corresponding human sequences. Employing a series of monoclonal antibodies (mAbs) reactive to human phospho-GFAP, phosphorylated at Thr-7, Ser-8, and/or Ser-13, the distribution of phospho-GFAP was determined by immunocytochemistry *in vivo* in mice and was shown to increase postnatally in the CNS. Limited populations of GFAP-positive astrocytes were labeled with anti-phospho-GFAP mAbs in most brain areas, while almost all the astrocytes in the optic nerve and spinal cord were labeled. Astrocytes in the ventricular zone and the rostral migratory stream preferentially contained phospho-GFAP. In a cold injury model of the cerebral cortex, phospho-GFAP was detected in reactive astrocytes 2–3 weeks following injury. The authors of this study suggest that the phosphorylation of GFAP plays a role in nondividing astrocytes *in vivo* (Takemura et al., 2002).

Glial fibrillary acidic protein antisense studies

Antisense oligonucleotides to GFAP have been widely used to study neuron-glial interactions. The human astrocytoma cell line, U251, was used to demonstrated a requirement for the GFAP in the formation of stable astrocytic processes in response to neurons. Cells expressing the antisense oligonucleotides could no longer extend stable processes in the presence of granule cell neurons. Subsequent studies reintroducing a fully encoding rat brain GFAP cDNA into these cells resulted in the appearance of rat GFAP as a filamentous network and the ability of these astrocytoma cells to form stable processes when cocultured with neurons. *In vitro* studies with neuron-astrocyte cocultures have shown that inhibition in GFAP synthesis leads to a reduction of astroglial hypertrophy and relieves the blockade of neuritic outgrowth that normally is observed after a lesion develops. These studies also showed that the mechanisms might involve changes in the secretion of extracellular matrix molecules by astrocytes.

Since GFAP accumulation is a prominent feature of astrocytic gliosis, our group focused on inhibiting GFAP synthesis using antisense oligonucleotides in the belief that this might delay scar formation resulting from a CNS injury. The delay in the formation of a physical barrier might allow the neurons and oligodendrocytes to reestablish a functional environment. We delivered antisense GFAP RNA complexed with lipofectin (LF), a cationic liposome, into cerebral astrocytes in culture and tested the feasibility of inhibiting GFAP synthesis. Our results demonstrated that LF facilitated antisense RNA uptake into astrocytes, and cultures treated with antisense GFAP showed a decrease in GFAP content after treatment (Yu et al., 1991). We also demonstrated that the increase in GFAP content in scratch wound injured astrocytes (which are hyperplastic, hypertrophic, and show increased GFAP content) can be inhibited by incubating the scratched culture with liposome complexed with 3′ or 5′ antisense oligonucleotides (20 nt) in the coding region of mouse GFAP (Yu et al., 1993). We have also used a recombinant retrovirus expressing antisense GFAP RNA in controlling the response of mechanically injured astrocytes. A 650 bp fragment from the coding region of mouse GFAP cDNA was cloned in the antisense orientation under the control of the long-terminal repeat (LTR) promoter of Moloney murine leukemia virus. Increase in GFAP, as detected by immunocytochemical staining in injured astrocytes, was inhibited by treatment with retrovirus expressing antisense GFAP RNA. Also, astrocytes at the site of injury in these scratched cultures did not show cell body hypertrophy compared to astrocytes in control cultures. These observations demonstrate that the increase in GFAP at the site of injury can be inhibited using retroviral treatment and indicate the potential of retrovirus-mediated gene transfer in modulating scar formation in the CNS *in vivo*. These studies also shed light on the role of GFAP in maintaining the morphology of astrocytes (Ghirnikar et al., 1994).

Glial fibrillary acidic protein antisense oligonucleotides have also been used to study the growth, invasion, and adhesion of human astrocytoma cells. The antisense GFAP–transfected cells demonstrated marked morphological alterations in the form of flat epithelioid cells devoid of long astrocytic glial processes. The antisense GFAP–transfected clones demonstrated a greater degree of cell crowding and piling at confluence; enhanced proliferative potential; formed larger and more numerous colonies when tested for anchorage-independent growth in soft agar; were less adherent to their substratum; and more readily penetrated Matrigel-coated filters. Antisense GFAP–transfected astrocytoma clones also showed a marked increase in vimentin, actin microfilaments, CD44 levels (Rutka et al., 1998), and nestin (Rutka et al., 1999).

Molecular biology of glial fibrillary acidic protein

Glial fibrillary acidic protein gene and promoter. The molecular cloning of the mouse gene by the Cowan laboratory (Lewis et al., 1984) opened a new and productive area for GFAP studies. The potential for these studies has been highlighted in past reviews (Brenner, 1994; Brenner and Messing, 1996). Genomic clones have been obtained from human, mouse, and rat GFAP genes. Each gene is composed of nine exons distributed over about 10 kb of DNA and yields a mature mRNA of about 3 kb. The coding sequences for the three genes are highly homologous. Strong homology also extends upstream of the RNA start site for about 200 bp, recurs between about −1300 and 1700 (RNA startpoint = +1), and is present in some intronic regions. The primary sites for the initiation of RNA and protein synthesis are essentially identical for the three genes, and each site contains a TAT-like sequence (CATAAA or AATAA) in the expected 5′-flanking position. In addition to GFAP-α, two additional mRNAs that start at different sites have been identified, GFAP-β and GFAP-γ. The different tissue distributions of GFAP-α, -β, and -γ mRNAs suggest that the synthesis of each is subject to unique control. All transcriptional studies to date either have explicitly measured GFAP-α or have not distinguished among the possible mRNA isotypes. In the peripheral nervous system, GFAP-β mRNA is thought to be the predominant form of GFAP, whereas GFAP-α is the predominant form in the CNS. The GFAP-γ mRNA has been found in both CNS and non-CNS tissues including mouse bone marrow and spleen. A recent report suggests the possible existence in rat brain of a novel GFAP mRNA isoform, GFAP-δ, that differs in the carboxy-terminal tail domain. Transgenes of GFAP have been used extensively to study signaling pathways that operate during development, disease, and injury—all states that increase GFAP gene activity (Brenner, 1994; Brenner and Messing, 1996).

Uses of the glial fibrillary acidic protein promoter. A major contribution of GFAP transcription studies has been the identification of DNA sequences that can target transgene expression to astrocytes in mice. Brenner and Messing (1996) have shown that their gfa2 promoter has this ability, and Mucke's laboratory has done the same for a similar fragment of the mouse GFAP gene, as well as for an entire genomic clone (Mucke and Rockenstein, 1993). Brenner has provided his GFAP promoter to over 170 investigators for various studies. This ability has initated a range of studies, including *in vivo* tests of various gene products on astrocyte function, use of astrocytes as factories for bioactive molecules, and creation of disease models. For example, the gfa2 promoter was used to express the receptor for avian leukosis virus (ALV) in transgenic mice, permitting recombinant ALV to be targeted to astrocytes and the use of this system to demonstrate that fibroblast growth factor-2 (FGF-2) induces proliferation and migration of glial cells *in vivo* without the induction of gliomas. The gfa2 promoter was used to express human nerve growth factor in mice. This study showed that epidermal growth factor (EGF)–responsive stem cells that secrete human nerve growth factor (hNGF) exhibited in vitro and *in vivo* properties similar to those seen following other methods of NGF delivery. The study also showed that these hNGF-secreting stem cells could prevent the degeneration of striatal neurons in a rodent model of Huntington's disease. Studies with GFAP-NGF mice have also been used to demonstrate a connection between the endogenous ectopic overexpression of NGF and neuropathic pain behavior and sympathetic sprouting in the dorsal root ganglia. A gfa2–lacZ transgene delivered by a modified herpes simplex virus was shown to be expressed primarily in astrocytes, suggesting that this promoter is a potential candidate for directing toxic genes to gliomas. A plasmid containing the herpes simplex virus thymidine kinase gene (HSV-TK) gene, driven by the gfa2 promotor, was lipofected into glioma cell lines and into an ovarian cancer cell line. Treatment with ganciclovir showed efficient killing of glioma cells but no effect on ovarian cells. The gfa2 promoter expressing HSV-TK was used to examine the role of astrocytes in development. Other experiments with mice expressing HSV-TK from the GFAP promoter have shown that genetic targeting can be used to ablate scar-forming astrocytes. These studies demonstrate roles for astrocytes in regulating leukocyte trafficking, repairing the blood–brain barrier (BBB), protecting neurons, and restricting nerve fiber growth after injury in the adult CNS. Transgene studies with beta-gal linked to the GFAP promoter have also been used to study neuron-glia interactions and to demonstrate that neuron-glia interaction may induce the astrocytic differentiation program. Two groups used the gfa2 promoter to drive expression of apolipoprotein E alleles E3 and E4 in mice to study their involvement in Alzheimer's disease. AP-lacZ transgenic mice have also been used to study astrocyte fate in embryonic neural grafts. Astrocyte-specific expression of hamster prion protein has shown that prion protein knockout mice are susceptible to hamster scrapie, suggesting that astrocytes could play an important role in scrapie pathogenesis. A mouse model for hydrocephalus was developed by expressing transforming growth factor-β (TGFβ) from the GFAP promoter, and others have obtained behavioral relief in a rat model of Parkinson's disease by lipofection of a gfa2-tyrosine hydroxylase transgene. Studies using the GFAP promoter metallothionein-1 (MT-1) transgene have been used to demonstrate MT protection against acute methylmercury cytotoxicity. Integrative studies using GFAP-cytokine transgenic mice such as interferon-α (IFNα), interleukin 1 (IL-1), and IL-1 receptor antagonist have provided a more thorough understanding of the actions of cytokines in the CNS.

ALEXANDER'S DISEASE

Alexander's disease (AxD) is a rare disease of unknown origin that has been the only candidate for a primary disease of astrocytes. It is a fatal disease of infants, juveniles, and adults. The pathological hallmark of AxD is the presence of Rosenthal fibers, cytoplasmic inclusions in astrocytes that contain increased amounts of GFAP in association with stress proteins (Iwaki et al., 1993). Six lines of transgenic mice have been generated that carry added copies of the human GFAP (hGFAP) gene to determine the properties of astrocytes containing increased GFAP without external stimulation and activation (Messing et al., 1998). Mice in lines that expressed high levels of the hGFAP gene died of the transgene, whereas mice in lines that expressed lower levels of the transgene survived and attained adulthood. The high over expressors showed increased amounts of stress proteins and Rosenthal fibers similar to those found in AxD astrocytes. We prepared primary astrocyte cultures from the cortex of newborn mice of the low-expressing line. Our studies with these cultures demonstrated that the cytoplasmic inclusion bodies in the cultured astrocytes exhibit the biochemical and morphological properties of the Rosenthal fibers found in AxD (Figs. 18.3, 18.4) (Eng et al., 1998). These results suggested that misexpression of the GFAP gene may be responsible for AxD and prompted Brenner and

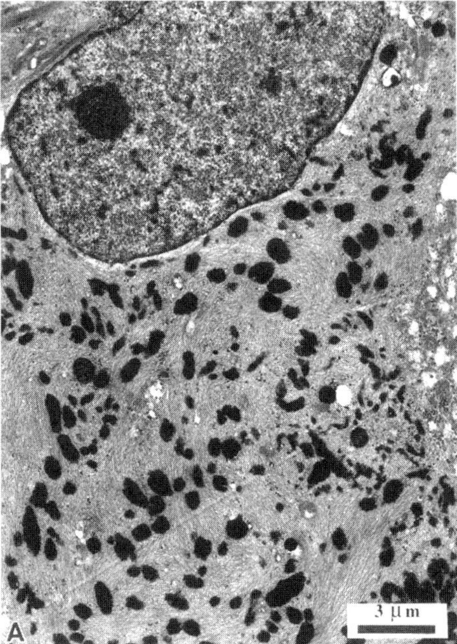

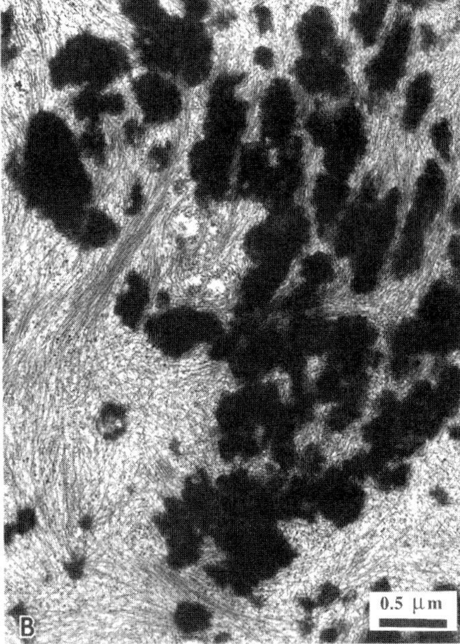

FIGURE 18.3 Astrocytes in culture for 20 days from a Tg73.2 mouse were analyzed at the ultrastructural level. Note the dense Rosenthal fibers among the glial filaments. (This was previously published as Figure 4 from Eng et al., 1998, with permission from Wiley-Liss, Inc.)

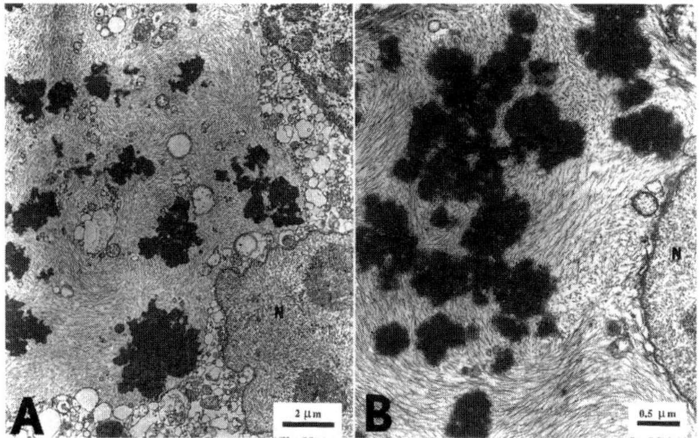

FIGURE 18.4 Astrocytes from the brain of a 17-month-old infant with Alexander's disease were examined at the ultrastructural level. Note the densed deposits in the astrocyte cell body, which are identical to those seen in the Tg73.2 astrocyte cultures in Figure 18.3. (This was previously published as Figure 5 from Eng et al., 1998, with permission from Wiley-Liss, Inc.)

associates to sequence the GFAP gene of AxD patients. DNA from 10 of 11 unrelated AxD patients contained heterozygous mutations predicting nonconservative animo acid changes in the GFAP protein. Seven different mutations were observed, with the most common occurring in four patients. None of the mutations were found in 100 control chromosomes tested. The heterezygosity of the mutations suggests that they are dominant. These results indicate that the mutations in the GFAP gene are responsible for the majority of AxD cases; that the infantile, juvenile, and adult forms may share a common basis; and that AxD is the only known primary disease of astrocytes (Brenner et al., 2001; Eng and Lee, 2004; Messing et al., 2001).

INTERMEDIATE FILAMENT KNOCKOUT MICE

Glial Fibrillary Acidic Protein Knockout Mice

Recently, the technique of gene knockout (KO) has been used to examine IFs in mice and has provided the first evidence that IFs are directly involved in cell resilience and the maintenance of tissue integrity. To investigate the structural role of GFAP *in vivo*, mice carrying a null mutation in GFAP have been generated (Gomi et al., 1995; Pekny et al., 1995; Liedtke et al., 1996; McCall et al., 1996).

In vitro studies with GFAP−/− astrocytes have shown that they are capable of stellation when cocultured with neurons and exhibit increased cell saturation density. At the ultrastructural level the amount of IFs, as revealed by transmission electron microscopy, was reduced in GFAP−/− astrocytes compared to that in GFAP+/+ astrocytes. GFAP−/− astrocytes retained the ability to form processes in response to neurons in mixed astrocyte/neuron cultures from the cerebellum. Glial fibrillary acidic protein−/− astrocyte–enriched primary cultures exhibited an increased final cell saturation density. These observations have led to the speculation that the loss of GFAP expression observed focally in a proportion of human malignant gliomas may reflect tumor progression toward a more rapidly growing and malignant phenotype (Pekny et al., 1998a). In addition, GFAP−/− astrocytes fail to induce a significant restriction to the passage of potassium and hydrophilic drugs (sucrose, 8-SPT) and fail to induce transendothelial resistance values comparable to those of control cocultures. These cells are, however, capable of inducing exclusion of Evans blue by endothelial cells, suggesting that GFAP may play a role in the induction of BBB properties in non-BBB endothelial cells (Pekny et al., 1998b). Glial fibrillary acidic protein−/− mice did not exhibit altered incubation times from untargeted control mice following inoculation with prion protein, suggesting that GFAP did not participate in the pathogenesis of the disease or in the production of prion scrapie protein (Tatzelt et al., 1996).

Homozygous mice created by disrupting the GFAP gene by gene targeting in embryonic stem cells were completely devoid of GFAP but exhibited normal development and showed no obvious anatomical abnormalities in the CNS (Gomi et al., 1995). When these animals were inoculated with scrapie prions, they exhibited neuropathological changes typical of the disease. The degree of accumulation of the prion protein in the various brain regions was similar between the mutant and control mice. These studies suggest that GFAP is not essential for the morphogenesis of the CNS and does not play a role in the pathogenesis of prion disease. Studies examining anatomy and synaptic function of the cerebellum in GFAP-deficient mice have shown that long-term depression (LTD) is clearly deficient in the GFAP mutant cerebellum without any detectable anatomical abnormalities. Furthermore, GFAP mutant mice exhibited a significant impairment of eyeblink conditioning without any detectable deficits in motor coordination tasks. These results suggest that GFAP is required for communications between Bergmann glia and Purkinje cells during LTD induction and maintenance (Shibuki et al., 1996).

In 7/14 mutant animals older than 18 months of age produced by Liedtke et al. (1996), hydrocephalus associated with white matter loss was detected. Mutant mice displayed abnormal myelination including the presence of actively myelinating oligodendrocytes in adults, nonmyelinated axons in optic nerve, and reduced myelin thickness in spinal cord. White matter was poorly vascularized, and the BBB was structurally and functionally impaired. Astrocytic structure and function were abnormal, consisting of shortened astrocytic cell processes, decreased septation of white matter, and increased CNS extracellular space. These studies suggested that GFAP expression is essential for normal white matter architecture and BBB integrity, and its absence leads to late-onset CNS dysmyelination. Studies examining the astroglial response in GFAP−/− mice with autoimmune encephalomyelitis (EAE), a model for MS, showed that clinically, the monophasic disease was more severe in GFAP−/− mice than in wild-type littermates despite increased remyelination in the former (Liedtke et al., 1998). The investigators observed an infiltrative EAE lesion in GFAP−/− mice. Glial fibrillary acidic protein−/− astrocytes had reduced cytoarchitectural stability, as evidenced by less abundant and irregularly spaced hemidesmosomes. The blunt GFAP−/− astrocyte processes possessed IFs consisting mainly of vimentin, though to a lesser degree than in the wild type. In contrast, in wild type littermates, GFAP was most abundant and nestin occurred at lower levels. These studies suggest that GFAP plays an important role in the control of clinical disease associated with formation of a clearly defined edge to the EAE lesion and that GFAP is operative in the regulation of the IF components in reactive fibrillary astrogliosis.

Glial fibrillary acidic protein null mice generated by McCall et al. (1996) using homologous recombination in embryonic stem cells showed subtle changes in astrocyte morphology and in addition showed enhanced long term potentiation (LTP) in hippocampal neurons. These data suggest that GFAP is important for astrocyte-neuron interactions and that astrocyte processes play a vital role in modulating synaptic efficacy in the CNS. Studies on percussive head injury in these GFAP-null mice with a weight drop device showed that when mice were positioned on a foam bed that allowed head movement on impact, all 14 wild-type mice tested survived but 12 of 15 GFAP-null mice died within a few minutes. When the foam bed was replaced by a firm support, both the GFAP-null and wild-type mice survived. These results indicate that mice lacking GFAP are hypersensitive to cervical spinal cord injury caused by sudden acceleration of the head and demonstrate the importance of GFAP for maintaining cell structure (Nawashiro et al., 1998). Studies on axonal and non-neuronal cell responses to spinal cord injury in these mice have shown that the absence of GFAP in reactive astrocytes does not alter axonal sprouting or regeneration. In addition, in these animals, chondroitin sulfate proteoglycan labeling was generally less intense in the gray matter, but the expression of various ECM molecules appeared unaltered in the GFAP−/− mice (Wang et al., 1997).

Vimentin Knockout Mice

Animals homozygous for the vimentin knockout (vim−/−) mouse develop and reproduce without an obvious phenotype (Colucci-Guyon et al., 1994) but show a cerebellar defect and impaired motor coordination (Colucci-Guyon et al., 1999). Fibroblasts derived from these mice are also mechanically weak and severely disabled in their capacity to migrate and to contact a three-dimensional collagen network. Wounds in the vim− adult animal showed delayed migration of fibroblasts into the wound site (Eckes et al., 2000). The GFAP network in the vim− mice disrupted GFAP and failed to assemble into a filamentous network in astrocytes that normally coexpress GFAP and vimentin, that is, corpus callosum and Bergmann glia (Galou et al., 1996).

Glial Acidic Fibrillary Protein and Vimentin Double Knockout Mice

In studies on the reaction to injury in the CNS in GFAP−/−, vimentin−/−, or GFAP−/−vim−/− mice, glial scar formation appeared normal after spinal cord or brain lesioning in GFAP−/− or vimentin−/− mice but was impaired in GFAP−/−vim−/− mice that developed less dense scars, frequently accompanied by bleeding (Pekny et al., 1999b). These studies suggest that GFAP and vimentin are required for proper glial scar formation in the injured CNS and that some degree of functional overlap exists between these IF proteins. Reactive astrocytes devoid of IFs exhibit clear morphological changes and profound defects in cell motility (Lepekhin et al. 2001). Culture studies have shown that astrocytes in mice deficient in both GFAP and vimentin (GFAP−/−vim−/−) cannot form IFs even when nestin is expressed and are thus devoid of IFs in their reactive state (Eliasson et al., 1999). Additional studies with the double mutant have suggested a role for the cytoskeleton in astrocyte volume regulation and the involvement of IFs in the process (Ding et al., 1998). The rate of glucose uptake through facilitative hexose transporters was not affected by the depletion of GFAP or vimentin, nor was ascorbate uptake and efflux. However, glutamine levels appeared to correlate inversely with GFAP and the effect of GFAP was dose-dependent, since the glutamine concentration in GFAP+/− astrocytes falls between those in wild-type and GFAP−/− astrocytes (Pekny et al., 1999a).

GENERATION OF GLIAL FIBRILLARY ACIDIC PROTEIN ANTISERUM

Glial fibrillary acidic protein and the other IFs share some chemical properties and common intramolecular polypeptide domains; however, GFAP also has some unique, highly immunogenic epitopes. It has proven to be a reliable marker for normal and neoplastic cells of glial lineage. Rabbit antiserum to human GFAP was first prepared by Uyeda et al. (1972). High-affinity polyclonal antisera and monoclonal antibodies prepared from human and bovine GFAP detect these GFAP-specific epitopes. Glial fibrillary acidic protein immunoreactivity in the mature CNS is restricted to glial filaments within protoplasmic astrocytes in gray matter, fibrous astrocytes in white matter, radial glia in the cerebellum (Bergmann glia), and subependymal astrocytes adjacent to the cerebral ventricles. At the surface of the brain, GFAP immunoreactivity is especially concentrated in astrocytes, which form the outer limiting membrane, the glia limitans. Mild tissue processing methods (i.e., unfixed, frozen, or freeze-substituted sections) and more sensitive detection procedures (immunogold labeling) have demonstrated GFAP-like immunoreactivity in regenerating Telecast spinal cord, in a subset of Schwann cells, glia-like cells in the myenteric plexus, Kupffer cells of the liver, salivary tumors, a pineal astrocytoma, and cells in the pineal gland. Glial fibrillary acidic protein immunoreactivity has also been demonstrated in epiglottic cartilage, pituicytes and pituitary adenomas, immature oligodendrocytes, papillary meningiomas, and metastasizing renal carcinomas. Mouse lens epithelium reacts with both polyclonal and monoclonal anti-GFAP antibodies. Polyclonal and monoclonal antibodies to GFAP have been used extensively for immunochemical and immunocytochemical studies (Eng and Lee, 1995; Eng et al., 2000).

GLIAL FIBRILLARY ACIDIC PROTEIN IN REACTIVE GLIOSIS

Astroglia in the CNS and peripheral nervous system (PNS) react to injury by hypertrophy and, some cases, by proliferation. The functions of reactive astroglia are still not well understood. A common feature of these cells is expression of GFAP (Eng and Ghirnikar, 1994; Kalman, 2004). In the CNS of higher vertebrates, following injury as a result of either trauma, disease, genetic disorders, or chemical insult, astrocytes become reactive and respond in a typical manner, termed *astrogliosis*. Reactive astrogliosis is a prominent feature of astrocytes adjacent to injury. Astrogliosis is also characterized by rapid synthesis of GFAP IFs. Numerous *in vitro* and *in vivo* studies on the molecular profiles of substances, that are upregulated during astrocyte activation document the complex and varied responses of astrocytes to injury (Eddleston and Mucke, 1993). Increased protein content or immunostaining of GFAP has been found in experimental models involving gliosis. These include the cryogenic lesion in the brain, stab wounds, EAE, hyperthermia, electrically induced seizures, and toxic lesions [ibotenic acid, trimethyl tin, 1,1,1-trichloroethane, xylene, dichloromethane, triethyl tin methyl mercury, colchicine, and kainate, 6-hydroxydopamine, 1-methyl-4-phenyl-1,2,3,6-tetrahydropyridine (MPTP)], ethanol, and 3,3′ iminodipropionitrile. O'Callaghan (1991) has proposed that GFAP is a sensitive and early biomarker of neurotoxicity. Increase of GFAP mRNA has been associated with scrapie, Alzheimer's disease, and Creutzfeldt-Jakob disease. It was also observed in a 6-hydroxydopamine lesion of the substantia nigra in rat, in a mechanical lesion to rat cerebral cortex, in entorhinal cortex lesions, in corticospinal axotomy, in EAE, in the lesioned dentate gyrus, and in cerebral freeze-injury.

Increase of GFAP in astrocytes occurs gradually throughout the adult life of mice, rat, and humans. Since GFAP normally increases with age and since there is wide variation in the collection and processing of human brain tissue, it is difficult to demonstrate mild gliosis by immunocytochemistry. In such cases, all aldehyde-fixed tissue samples require protease treatment in the staining protocol, and results need to be compared with those in age-matched normal controls. Three diseases that show intense gliosis are MS, an inflammatory demyelinating disease characterized by demyelinating plaques composed of bare axons and extensive reactive astrogliosis; adrenoleukodystrophy, a hereditary disorder of lipid metabolism; and AxD, which is characterized by extensive gliosis and Rosenthal fiber deposits. Reactive gliosis occurs with any type of insult to the CNS. The anatomical region, severity of gliosis, and developmental time sequence vary in amyotrophic lateral sclerosis (ALS), in Gerstmann-Straussler syndrome and Down's syndrome, and in Huntington's, Wilson's, Pick's, Parkinson's, and Alzheimer's diseases. Astrocytic gliosis is a prominent neuropathological change in Alzheimer's disease. Numerous reports have shown reactive astrocytes in Alzheimer's disease brains, most frequently in association with neuritic plaques.

SUMMARY

Glial fibrillary acidic protein is the IF protein found in differentiated astrocytes in the CNS. The rapid advances in molecular biology and newer techniques such as knockout mice, the use of the gfa-2 promoter to prepare transgenes, antisense RNA methodology, and DNA sequencing have greatly increased our knowledge of GFAP function in CNS development, injury, and disease. Mutations in the rod or TAIL domain of GFAP have been shown to cause the first known genetic defect in human astrocytes, AxD. The potential functions and GFAP response in astrocytes to stress and injury have been under continuous investigation since GFAP was first identified in 1969. The astrocyte reacts to any type of insult, whether physical, biochemical, chemical, or disease, by enhanced expression of GFAP, a process called *astrogliosis*. This astrocytic response serves as a microsensor of the injured microenvironment at any location in the CNS. The precise mechanism of this response is still unknown. Growth factors, hormones, cytokines, and chemokines have been implicated, but no one common factor has been identified. Immunostaining for GFAP is a sensitive method for identifying reactive astrocytes, whether they are due to filament disassembly as a result of kinase activation or to an increase in GFAP synthesis. Polyclonal and monoclonal antibodies have been used extensively to study astrocytes in CNS development, disease, glial tumors, and experimental injury models (Eng et al., 2000). Based on GFAP, vimentin, and double knockout mice studies, Pekny (2001) has provided a concise review on the possible functions of glial filaments. Besides providing structural support, reactive astrogliosis, and scar formation, there is now evidence that GFAP is involved with LTD, LTP, the circadian rhythm, cell volume, cell motility, and the promotion of normal BBB formation.

ACKNOWLEDGMENTS

This work was supported by the Department of Veterans Affairs Medical Research Service.

REFERENCES

Almqvist, P.M., Mah, R., Lendahl, U., Jacobsson, B., and Hendson, G. (2002) Immunohistochemical detection of nestin in pediatric brain tumors. *J. Histochem. Cytochem.* 50:147–158.

Brenner, M. (1994) Structure and transcription of the GFAP gene. *Brain Pathol.* 4:245–257.

Brenner, M., Johnson, A.B., Boespflug-Tanguy, O., Rodriguez, D., Goldman, J.E., and Messing, A. (2001) Mutation in GFAP encoding glial fibrillary acidic protein are associated with Alexander's disease. *Nat. Genet.* 27:117–120.

Brenner, M. and Messing, A. (1996) GFAP transgenic mice. *Methods* (companion to *Meth. Enzymol*). 10:351–364.

Colucci-Guyon, E., Gimenez y Ribotta, M., Maurice, T., Babinet, C., and Privat, A. (1999) Cerebellar defect and impaired motor coordination in mice lacking vimentin. *Glia* 25:33–43.

Colucci-Guyon, E., Portier, M-M., Dunia, I., Paulin, D., Pournin, S., and Babinet, C. (1994) Mice lacking vimentin develop and reproduce without obvious phenotype. *Cell* 79:679–694.

Ding, M., Eliasson, C., Betsholtz, C., Hamberger, A., and Pekny, M. (1998) Altered taurine release following hypotonic stress in astrocytes from mice deficient for GFAP and vimentin. *Brain Res. Mol. Brain Res.* 62:77–81.

Eckes, B., Colucci-Guyon, E. Smola, H., Nodder, S., Babinet, C., Krieg, T., and Martin, P. (2000) Impaired wound healing in embryonic and adult mice lacking vimentin. *J. Cell. Sci.* 113:2455–2462.

Eddleston, M. and Mucke, L. (1993) Molecular profile of reactive astrocytes: implications for their role in neurologic diseases. *Neuroscience* 54:15–36.

Eliasson, C., Sahlgren, C., Berthold, C.-H., Stakeberg, J., Celis, J.E., Betholtz, C., Eriksson, J.E., and Pekny, M. (1999) Intermediate filament protein partnership in astrocytes. *J. Biol. Chem.* 274: 23996–24006.

Eng, L.F. and Ghirnikar, R.S. (1994) GFAP and astrogliosis. *Brain Pathol.* 4:229–237.

Eng, L.F. and Lee, Y.L. (2004) Alexander disease: a primary disease of astrocytes. In: Hertz, L., ed. *Advances in Molecular Biology, 3-III, Non-neuronal Cells of the Nervous system: Function and Dysfunction, Part III, Pathological Conditions*. Amsterdam: Elsevier B.V., pp. 773–785.

Eng, L.F., Ghirnikar, R.S., and Lee, Y.L. (2000) Glial fibrillary aidic protein:GFAP-thirty-one years (1969–2000). *Neurochem. Res.* 25:1439–1451.

Eng, L.F. and Lee, Y.L. (1995) Intermediate filaments in astrocytes. In: Ransom, B.R. and Kettenmann, H., eds. *Neuroglial Cells*. New York: Oxford University Press, pp. 650–667.

Eng, L.F., Lee, Y.L., Kwan, H., Brenner, M., and Messing, A. (1998) Astrocytes cultured from transgenic mice carrying the added human glial fibrillary acidic protein gene contains Rosenthal fibers. *J. Neurosci. Res.* 53:353–360.

Eng, L.F., Vanderhaeghen, J.J., Bignami, A., and Gerstl, B. (1971) An acidic protein isolated from fibrous astrocytes. *Brain Res.* 28:351–354.

Fuchs, E. and Weber, K. (1994) Intermediate filaments: structure, dynamics, function, and disease. *Annu. Rev. Biochem.* 63:345–382.

Galou, M., Colucci-Guyon, E., Ensergueix, D., Ridet, J.L., Gimenez y Ribotta, M., Privat, A., Babinet, C., and Dupouey, P. (1996) Disrupted glial fibrillary acidic protein network in astrocytes from vimentin knockout mice. *J. Cell Biol.* 133:853–863.

Ghirnikar, R.S., Yu, A.C., and Eng, L.F. (1994) Astrogliosis in culture: III. Effect of recombinant retrovirus expressing antisense glial fibrillary acidic protein RNA. *J. Neurosci. Res.* 38:376–85.

Goldman, R.D. and Steinert, P.M. (eds.) (1990) *Cellular and Molecular Biology of Intermediate Filaments*. New York: Plenum Press.

Gomi, H.,Yokoyama, T., Fujimoto, K., Ikeda, T., Katoh, A., Itoh, T., and Itohara, S. (1995) Mice devoid of the glial fibrillary acidic protein develop normally and are susceptible to scrapie prions. *Neuron* 14:29–41.

Inagaki, M., Nakamura, Y., Takeda, M., Nishimura, T., and Inagaki, N. (1994) Glial fibrillary protein: dynamics property and regulation by phosphorylation. *Brain Pathol.* 4:139–243.

Iwaki, T., Kume-Iwaki, A., Liem, R.K.H., and Goldman, J.E. (1993) Alpha-beta crystallin and 27-kd heat shock protein are regulated by stress conditions in the central nervous system and accumulate in Rosenthal fibers. *Am. J. Pathol.* 143:487–495.

Kalman, M. (2004) Glial reactions and reactive glia. In: Hertz, L., ed. *Advances in Molecular Biology, 3-III, Non-neuronal Cells of the Nervous System: Function and Dysfunction, Part III, Pathological Conditions*. Amsterdam: Elsevier B.V., pp. 787–835.

Lendahl, U., Zimmerman, L.B., and McKay, R.D.G. (1990) CNS stem cells express a new class of intermediate filament protein. *Cell* 60:585–595.

Lepekhin, E.A., Eliasson, C., Berthold-Clae, H., Berezin, V., Bock, E., and Pekny, M. (2001) Intermediate filaments regulate astrocyte motility. *J. Neurochem.* 79:617–625.

Lewis, S.A., Balcarek, J.M., Krek, V., Shelanski, M., and Cowan, N.J. (1984) Sequence of a cDNA clone encoding mouse glial fibrillary acidic protein: structural conservation of intermediate filaments. *Proc. Natl. Acad. Sci. USA* 81:2743–2746.

Liedtke, W., Edelmann, W., Bieri, P., Chiu, F-C., Cowan, N.J., Kucheriapati, R., and Raine, C.S. (1996) GFAP is necessary for the integrity of CNS white matter architecture and long-term maintenance of myelination. *Neuron* 17:607–615.

Liedtke, W., Edelmann, W., Chiu, F.-C., Kucheriapati, R., and Raine, C.S. (1998) Experimental autoimmune encephalomyelitis in mice lacking glial fibrillary acidic protein is characterized by a more severe clinical course and an infiltrative central nervous system lesion. *Am. J. Pathol.* 152:251–259.

Matsuzawa, K., Kosako, H., Azuma, I., Inagaki, N., and Inagaka, M. (1998) Possible regulation of intermediate proteins by Rho-binding kinases. In: Herrmann, H. and Harris, R., eds. *Subcellular Biochemistry*, Vol. 31: *Intermediate Filaments*. New York: Plenum Press, pp. 423–435.

McCall, M.A., Gregg, R.G., Behringer, R.R., Brenner, M., Delaney,

C.J., Galbreath, E.J., Zhang, C.L., Pearce, R.A., Chiu, S.Y., and Messing, A. (1996) Targeted deletion in astrocyte intermediate filament (GFAP) alters neuronal physiology. *Proc. Natl. Acad. Sci. USA* 93:6361–6366.

Messing, A., Goldman, J.E., Johnson, A.B., and Brenner, M. (2001) Alexander's disease: new insights from genetics. *J. Neuropathol. Expt. Neurol.* 60:563–573.

Messing, A., Head, M.W., Galles, K., Galbreath, E.J., Goldman, J.E., and Brenner, M. (1998) Fatal encephalopathy with astrocyte inclusions in GFAP transgenic mice. *Am. J. Pathol.* 152:391–398.

Mucke, L. and Rockenstein, E.M. (1993) Prolonged delivery of transgene products to specific brain regions by migratory astrocyte grafts. *Transgene* 1:3–9.

Nawashiro, H., Messing, A., Azzam, N., and Brenner, M. (1998) Mice lacking glial fibrillary acidic protein are hypersensitive to traumatic cerebrospinal injury. *NeuroReport* 9:1691–1696,

O'Callaghan, J.P. (1991) Assessment of neurotoxicity: use of glial fibrillary acidic protein as a biomarker. *Biomed. Environ. Sci.* 4:197–206.

Parry, D.A.D. and Steinert, P.M. (1999) Intermediate filaments: molecular architecture, assembly, dynamics, and polymorphism. *Q. Rev. Biophys.* 32:97–187.

Pekny, M. (2001) Astrocytic intermediate filaments: lessons from GFAP and vimentin knock-out mice. *Prog. Brain Res.* 132:23–30.

Pekny, M., Eliasson, C., Chien, C.-L., Kindblom, L.G., Liem, R., Hamberger, A., and Betsholtz, C. (1998a) GFAP-deficient astrocytes are capable of stellation in vitro when cocultured with neurons and exhibit a reduced amount of intermediate filaments and an increased cell saturation density. *Exp. Cell Res.* 239:332–343.

Pekny, M., Eliasson, C., Siushansian, R., Ding, M., Dixon, S.J., Pekna, M., Wilson, J.X., and Hamberger, A. (1999a) The impact of genetic removal of GFAP and/or vimentin on glutamine levels and transport of glucose and ascorbate in astrocytes. *Neurochem. Res.* 24:1357–1362.

Pekny, M., Johannsson, C.B., Eliasson, C., Stakeberg, J., Wallen, A., Perlmannn, T., Lendahl, U., Betsholtz, C., Berthold, C.-H., and Frisen, J. (1999b) Abnormal reaction to central nervous system injury in mice lacking glial fibrillary acidic protein and vimentin. *J. Cell Biol.* 145:503–514.

Pekny, M., Leveen, P., Pekna, M., Eliasson, C., Berthold, C-H., Westermark, B., and Betsholtz, C. (1995) Mice lacking glial fibrillary acidic protein display astrocytes devoid of intermediate filaments but develop and reproduce normally. *EMBO J.* 14:1590–1598.

Pekny, M., Stanness, K., Eliasson, C., Betsholtz, C., and Janigro, D. (1998b) Impaired induction of blood–brain barrier properties in aortic endothelial cells by astrocytes from GFAP-deficient mice. *Glia* 22:390–400.

Rutka, J.T., Ackerley, C., Hubbard, S.L., Tilup, A., Dirks, P.B., Jung, S., Ivanchuk, S., Kurimoto, M., Tsugu, A., and Becker, L.E. (1998) Characterization of glial filament-cytoskeletal interactions in human astrocytomas: an immuno-ultrastructural analysis. *Eur. J. Cell Biol.* 76(4):279–287.

Rutka, J.T., Ivanchuk, S., Mondal, S., Taylor, M., Sakai, K., Dirks, P., Jun, P., Jung, S., Becker, L.E., and Ackerley, C. (1999) Co-expression of nestin and vimentin intermediate filaments in invasive human astrocytoma cells. *Int. J. Dev. Neurosci.* 17:503–515.

Schiffer, D., Giordana, M.T., Migheli, A., Giaccone, G., Pezzotta, S., and Mauro, A. (1986) Glial fibrillary acidic protein and vimentin in the experimental glial reaction of the rat brain. *Brain Res.* 374:110–118.

Shibuki, K., Gomi, H., Chen, L., Wakatsuki, F., Fujimoto, K., Katoh, A., Ikeda, T., Chen, C., Thompson, R.F., and Itohara, S. (1996) Deficient cerebellar long-term depression, impaired eyeblink conditioning, and normal motor coordination in GFAP mutant mice. *Neuron* 16:587–599.

Takemura, M., Nishiyama, H., and Itohara, S. (2002) Distribution of phosphorylated glial fibrillary acidic protein in the mouse central nervous system. *Genes Cells* 7:295–307.

Tatzelt, J., Maeda, N., Pekny, M., Yang, S.L., Betsholtz, C., Eliasson, C., Cayetano, J., Camerino, A.P., DeArmond, S.J., and Prusiner, S.B. (1996) Scrapie in mice deficient in apolipoprotein E or glial fibrillary acidic protein. *Neurology* 47:449–453.

Uyeda, C.T., Eng, L.F., and Bignami, A. (1972) Immunological study of the glial fibrillary acidic protein. *Brain Res.* 37:81–89.

Wang, X., Messing, A., and David, S. (1997) Axonal and nonneuronal cell responses to spinal cord injury in mice lacking glial fibrillary acidic protein. *Exp. Neurol.* 148:568–576.

Yang, Y., Bauer, C., Strasser, G., Wollman, R., Julien, J.-P., and Fuchs, E. (1999) Integrators of the cytoskeleton that stabilizes microtubules. *Cell* 98:229–238.

Yu, A.C., Lee, Y.L., and Eng, L.F. (1991) Inhibition of GFAP synthesis by antisense RNA in astrocytes. *J. Neurosci Res.* 30:72–79.

Yu, A.C., Lee Y.L., and Eng, L.F. (1993) Astrogliosis in culture: I. The model and the effect of antisense oligonucleotides on glial fibrillary acidic protein synthesis. *J. Neurosci. Res.* 34:295–303.

Zehner, Z.E. and Paterson, B.M. (1983) Characterization of the chicken vimentin gene: single copy gene producing multiple mRNAs. *Proc. Natl. Acad. Sci. USA* 80:911–915.

II | FUNCTIONS OF NEUROGLIAL CELLS

19 Molecular biology of myelination

ANTHONY T. CAMPAGNONI

Myelination is a developmentally regulated event that begins postnatally in the rat and mouse brain and within the third fetal trimester in the human spinal cord. The expression and assembly of myelin proteins into the membrane is a complex event involving many steps. Regulation of the expression of these genes occurs at a number of different levels, including (*1*) promoter choice, (*2*) transcription, (*3*) splicing, (*4*) mRNA stability, (*5*) translation, and (*6*) posttranslational processing. In this chapter I present a brief overview of the molecular biology of the myelin protein genes and their expression into mRNA and protein. Length constraints prevent a comprehensive review of the topic. The reader is referred to a number of recent reviews for further information (Ikenaka and Kagawa, 1995; Griffiths, 1996; Johns and Bernard, 1999; Jetten and Suter, 2000; Wegner, 2000; Campagnoni and Skoff, 2001; Mirsky et al., 2001; Yoshikawa, 2001).

Historically, the myelin basic protein (MBP) and proteolipid protein (PLP) were among the first nervous system proteins to be isolated in pure form, biochemically characterized, and sequenced because of their high abundance in nervous tissue. It is not surprising, then, that they also were among the first cDNAs to be cloned. Since then, the gene for virtually every myelin protein, major or minor, has been cloned, mapped, and in many cases found to be responsible for a genetic disorder of the nervous system.

CLASSIC MYELIN BASIC PROTEINS AND *GOLLI* PROTEINS

Structure of the Myelin Basic Protein Gene

A partial structure of the *MBP* gene was first elucidated by Takahashi et al. (1985), who identified the most distal seven exons of the gene distributed over a 32 kb stretch of chromosome 18 in mouse. This partial structure accounted for the four known forms of the "classic" MBPs. Additional exons and products of the *MBP* gene were subsequently identified in both mouse and human, and the gene was determined to be substantially larger than was originally thought—105 kb in mice and 180 kb in humans (for review, see Campagnoni and Skoff, 2001). The complete structure of the mouse gene is shown in Figure 19.1, along with the numbering to include all of the known exons. Many authors who study only the classic MBPs still number the gene according to the old numbering system, which is formally incorrect.

The gene encodes two families of proteins, produced from three transcription start sites, whose activities are regulated by three separate promoters. The two downstream transcription start sites (tss2 and tss3) produce the classic, myelin-associated MBPs, which arise from the alternative splicing of exons 6, 9, and 10. These alternatively spliced MBP mRNAs encode classic MBP isoforms that range in molecular size between 14 kDa and 21 kDa. The splicing of these transcripts is developmentally regulated in oligodendrocytes in the central nervous system (CNS), and both promoters appear to confer the same developmental regulation.

The second family of proteins encoded by the *MBP* gene is the *golli-MBP* proteins, which are generated from the first transcription start site and are under entirely different cell, tissue, and developmental regulation. The golli products are generated by alternative splicing encompassing the entire transcription unit of 105 kb in the mouse and ~180 kb in the human. Transcription start site 1 expresses several *golli* mRNA splice products that contain exons 1, 2, and 3 of the gene spliced into MBP-encoding exons (Fig. 19.1). The two major *golli* mRNA splice products (BG21 and J37) splice in frame so that the products contain a 133 amino acid golli domain spliced into a classic MBP domain of varying length. This makes the two families of proteins antigenically and immunologically related, which has become of great relevance in establishing mechanisms of tolerance development in experimental allergic encephalomyelitis (EAE) (Huseby and Goverman, 2000).

The promoters governing the activity of the *MBP* gene transcription start sites appear to operate independently. The first and third promoters have been

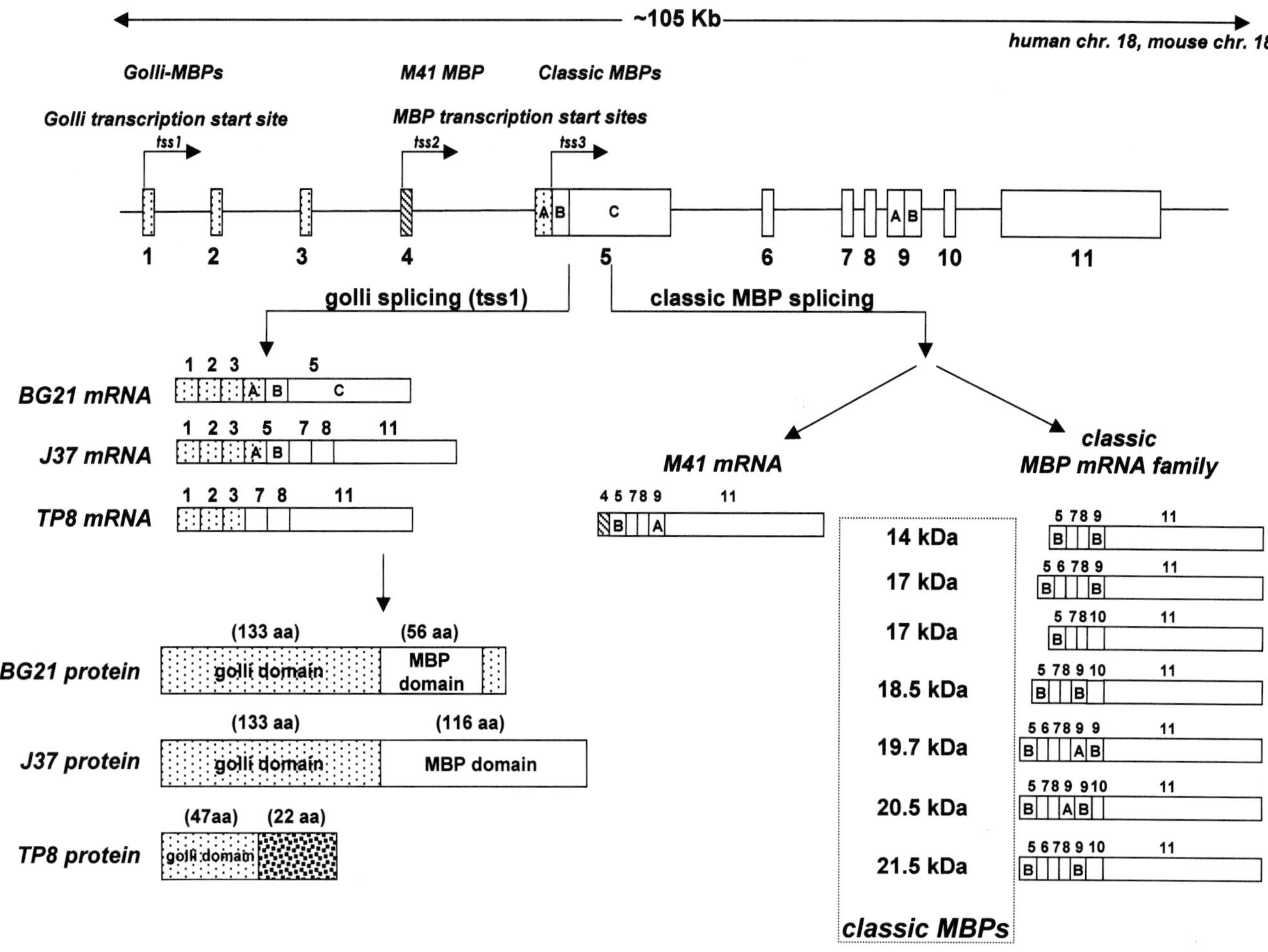

FIGURE 19.1 Structure of the myelin basic protein (*MBP*) gene illustrating the multiple promoters and splicing patterns giving rise to the two families of MBP gene products—the golli proteins and the classic MBPs.

studied most extensively. The third promoter, which includes exon 5A and governs expression of the classic MBPs, can target expression of reporter genes to oligodendrocytes in transgenic mice with remarkable cellular and developmental specificity. Sequences within intron 4 have been reported to modulate expression of the classic MBPs in Schwann cells *in vivo*. Downstream regions of intron 4 + exon 5A have been used to drive expression of classic MBP in *shiverer* mice (which have a deletion of exons 7–11), with a subsequent reduction in the clinical signs of the neurological disorder caused by the mutation.

Less is known about the regulation of the first (*golli*, tss1) or second (tss2) promoters of the *MBP* gene. Based upon the steady-state levels of the M41-MBP mRNA, which encodes the classic 14 kDa MBP, it would appear that the classic MBP promoter at tss2 is substantially less active than the major classic MBP promoter at tss3 in the nervous system. With regard to tss1, a fragment consisting of sequences 1.1 kb upstream and 0.2 kb downstream of tss1 has been used to drive transgenes in transgenic mice. While not as specific as the classic MBP promoter, this fragment appears to target expression to a limited number of neuronal populations, including cortical preplate neurons, cortical subplate neurons, olfactory neurons, and neurons within the dorsal root ganglia. It does not target expression to the immune system or to glia, such as oligodendrocytes, where expression of the *golli* proteins has been observed. The elements that regulate expression in these cells and tissues have not yet been identified.

Transcriptional Regulation

Identification of the cis genetic elements and the trans-acting factors regulating the tissue, cell, and developmental specificity of the *MBP* gene has drawn the attention of several laboratories in recent years. It has generally been felt that the regulation of the gene is complex, involving multiple sites within the region upstream of tss3, which encompasses exon 5A of the gene, where trans-acting factors that bind to different parts of the promoter interact to regulate the activity of the MBP transcription unit (see Wegner, 2000, for a general review). Accordingly, this region has been isolated, analyzed, and used to define putative regulatory elements. The MBP promoter does not contain conventional TATA or CAAT boxes, that is, regulatory sequences common to all promoters and believed to be involved in the binding of general transcription factors. A number of sequences have been reported to confer either tissue or cellular specificity to the expression of the gene.

Several factors have been identified that regulate the transcription of the classic MBP mRNAs. *Pur alpha*, *MyEF-2*, and *MyEF-3*, bind to a GC-rich region between −14 and −50 nt downstream of tss3. *Myelinating glial enriched binding activity* (MEBA) consists of at least two proteins that bind to a region just upstream of, and overlap, the NF1 site at −149 to −102 upstream of tss3. Myelinating glial enriched binding activity can activate the MBP promoter in oligodendrocytes but not Cos cells. The NF1 site has been reported to be essential for cyclic adenosine monophosphate (cAMP) induction of the classic MBP promoter.

A thyroid response element has been identified between −163 and −183, as has a NFκB site between −570 and −562 that may be responsible for the stimulation of the MBP promoter by tumor necrosis factor-α (TNFα). A protein kinase C (PKC)–responsive element has been identified at the distal end of a 1.3 Kb MBP (tss3) promoter fragment, which was responsible for the inhibition of cAMP activation of the promoter. Mutation of an AP-1-like site between −1240 and −1230 results in an increase in reporter activity in CG4 cells in differentiation media.

While the 1.3 kb upstream region of the classic MBP transcription site (tss3) is able to confer the correct developmental expression of the *MBP* gene in oligodendrocytes, there is some evidence that it does not completely restrict its expression to neural tissue and expresses at minor levels in other tissues, such as the kidney and testes. A reporter construct containing 1.9 kb downstream of tss3 has been reported to target expression solely to oligodendrocytes in transgenic mice. Schwann cell expression could be conferred by a 0.6 kb fragment that is 9 kb upstream from the third transcription initiation site.

Posttranscriptional Regulation

There is evidence that expression of the classic MBPs may be regulated at the posttranscriptional level. Several groups have reported posttranscriptional regulation by steroids or thyroid hormone by mechanisms including MBP mRNA stabilization or direct effects on translation rates. Products of the *QKI* gene, principally QKI-6 and QKI-7, can interact with classic MBP mRNAs in myelinating oligodendrocytes. The QKI proteins are RNA binding proteins that bind to the classic MBP mRNAs in an isoform-dependent fashion. They are absent in oligodendrocytes in *quaking* mice, and their loss has been postulated to be responsible for destabilization of the classic MBP mRNAs as well as defective translocation in this mutant.

One of the most interesting posttranscriptional events associated with *MBP* gene expression is the well-documented phenomenon of MBP mRNA translocation (for review, see Barbarese et al., 1999). The MBPs are highly cationic polypeptides that can interact with virtually any negatively charged molecule. Therefore, a mechanism is required for targeting MBPs to the oligodendrocyte processes without inappropriate interactions of MBP polypeptides with other cellular components. This is accomplished through the translocation of MBP mRNAs from oligodendrocyte cell somas to their processes and channels that infiltrate the myelin sheath. *In situ* hybridization data clearly show localization of MBP mRNAs within oligodendrocyte cell bodies, processes, and myelin sheaths.

Trafficking of the MBP mRNAs appears to occur through trafficking sequences in the 3′ untranslated region (3′-UTR) that serve to direct the binding of cellular proteins involved in message transport from nucleus to perikaryon. One of these is hn-RNP A2. In the perikaron, other proteins associate with the complex to form granules, which are transported along microtubules to the distal processes of the oligodendrocytes and to the myelin sheath. Several other proteins that bind to MBP mRNA have been identified, and these may play a role in the stabilization and transport of the MBP messages in the oligodendrocyte. The importance of the microtubules in this process is underscored by an analysis of the *taiep* rat, which accumulates excessive microtubules, and in which MBP mRNA transport appears to be disrupted.

MYELIN PROTEOLIPID PROTEINS

Structure and Localization

The myelin proteolipid proteins, PLP and DM-20, are quantitatively the major proteins in the myelin sheath in the CNS, constituting about 50% of the total protein content. The amino acid sequences of the PLPs, deduced from their corresponding cDNAs in many species, indicate a strong conservation of protein sequence among species.

The *PLP/DM20* gene, located on the X chromosome in mouse, rat, and human, is ~17 kb in length (Fig. 19.2). In addition to the myelin PLP, the gene also encodes the DM20 protein, originally identified and named in the early 1970s. Molecular biological stud-

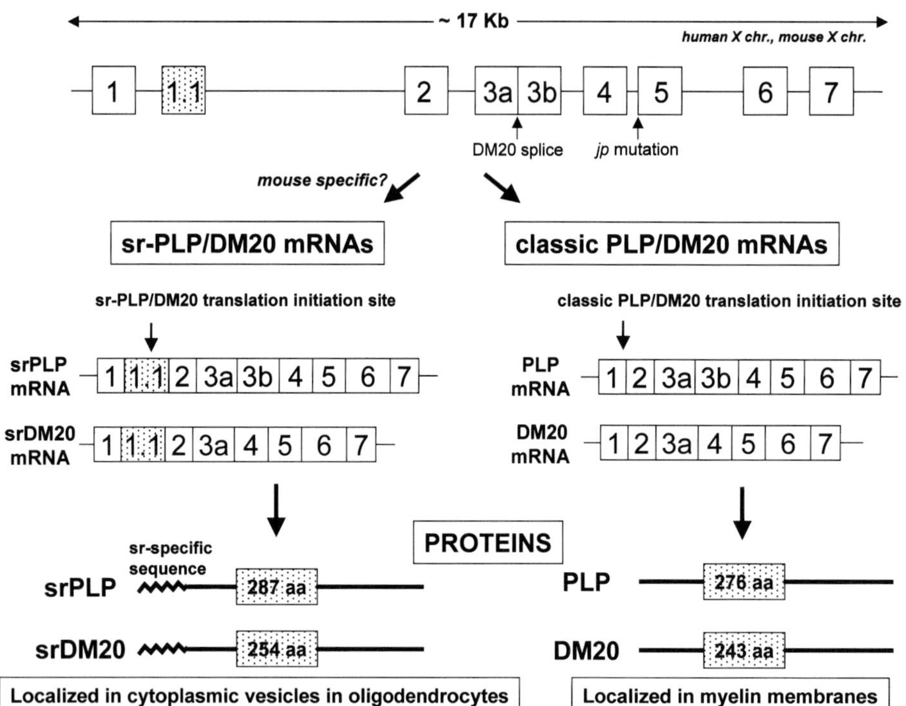

FIGURE 19.2 Structure of the mouse *PLP/DM20* gene illustrating splicing patterns giving rise to the four splice products of the gene, including the classic PLP/DM20 and the more recently described srPLP/DM20. PLP: proteolipid protein.

ies subsequently established the location of a 35 amino acid deletion in the protein. This region is encoded by exon 3B of the gene.

The *PLP/DM20* gene is alternatively spliced to produce two major mRNA products that encode the PLP and DM20 polypeptides. The gene also possesses three polyadenylation signals within the last exon encoding the 3′-UTR of the mRNA. The use of any or all of these sites generates a family of PLP/DM20 mRNAs of ~1.6 kb, ~2.4 kb, and ~3.2 kb. The proportions of these size classes of mRNAs varies among species. All three size classes appear to contain mRNAs encoding both PLP and DM20 polypeptides.

The structure of a relatively stable PLP pre-mRNA of ~4.6 kb, containing an intact intron 3, which is localized in the nucleus, has been noted by two groups.

Recently, an additional exon, lying between exons 1 and 2 of the gene (i.e., exon 1.1), has been identified in the mouse that is found within two additional mRNAs of ~3.4 kb, which encode proteolipids that contain an additional 12 amino acids at the N terminus of PLP and DM20 (Bongarzone et al., 1999). These products are derived from alternative splicing of the gene (Fig. 19.2). These proteolipids (called sr-PLP and sr-DM20) contain exon 1.1 of the gene, which is absent in the classic PLP and DM20 mRNAs. The inclusion of exon 1.1 in the mRNA alters the translation start site, such that the resulting protein products are identical to those of the classic PLP and DM20 except that they contain a unique 12 amino acid sequence at their N termini. Because immunohistochemical results showed that antibodies against the sr-proteolipids stained cell soma and not myelin sheaths, they were named sr-PLP/DM20 for "somal-restricted."

Transcriptional Regulation

Five regions in the human PLP promoter that bind nuclear proteins have been identified, and a few have been characterized. Site 4 (from −246 to −277) contains overlapping regions for the transcription factors, Myt 1 and Myt 2, which are localized in oligodendrocyte progenitors and may represent regulators of the *PLP* gene at early stages in oligodendrocyte maturation. Myt 1 is a Cys2HisCys zinc finger protein. Myt 2, a DNA binding protein that can be secreted, is highly homologous to the cerebrospinal fluid (CSF) protein cerebrin-50. Its mRNA has an unusual 1.2 kb 5′-UTR that contains an Internal Ribosome Entry Site (IRES) allowing internal initiation of translation.

Mutation of site 3 (from −104 to −127) greatly reduced promoter activity in glial cells, and was found to contain the binding site for a ubiquitous Kruppel family, zinc finger transcription factor, Yin Yang 1.

In addition, there is a thyroid response element between +18 and +31 that requires both a peroxisome proliferator-activated receptor (PPAR) and thyroid hormone receptor beta for activation. The PPARs are a family within the nuclear hormone receptor superfamily that has been shown to regulate oligodendrocyte (OL) differentiation.

Multiple binding sites have been found on both the MBP and PLP promoters for Gtx, an oligodendrocyte-specific homeodomain protein. Cotransfection experiments with an optimal Gtx-binding reporter suggest that Gtx acts as a repressor of transcription, although it had no activity on either PLP or MBP promoter-driven reporters in a cotransfection system.

Elements in the 8140 bp intron region between exons 1 and 2 have been examined extensively *in vitro*. Negative regulatory regions have been identified at bp 324–809 and at bp 7299–7615 and an oligodendrocyte-specific region at bp 7826–8068. In addition a cis-acting anti-silencing region between bp 1083 and bp 1203 has been found that stimulates the transcription of a PLP-lac z reporter when inserted in either the forward or reverse direction behind a 2.4 kb promoter-exon 1 region. These *in vitro* results have been confirmed in two transgenic mouse lines. In one line, lac z has been driven by 2.4 kb of the PLP upstream promoter + exon 1 + the first 37 bp of exon 2. In the second line, lac z was driven by the same 2.4 kb promoter + exon 1 + *intron 1* + the first 37 bp of exon 2. Ribonuclease protection experiments indicated that expression of both transgenes was restricted to the same tissues, suggesting that the mouse 2.4 kb promoter was sufficient to direct correct tissue expression of PLP. However, the level of lac z message in the transgenic mice generated with the construct missing intron 1 was low and changed relatively little over postnatal development. In contrast, the level of lac z message in the transgenic mice with the construct containing intron 1 increased significantly from 2 days to 20 days, and exhibited a developmental profile very similar to that of native PLP mRNA expression. These results suggest that intron 1 of the *PLP* gene is essential for correct temporal expression of the gene in the nervous system.

Expression

The *PLP/DM20* gene expresses two alternatively spliced mRNAs that encode a 30 kDa (PLP) and a 25 kDa (DM20) protein. In the brain, the splicing of the *PLP/DM20* gene primary transcript appears to be developmentally regulated. The developmental appearance of the DM20 protein precedes that of the myelin PLP in several species. During the early stages of myelination the expression of the DM20 splice product predominates, gradually declining with development. At later stages, the PLP splice product becomes the major form that is expressed. Interestingly, the same pattern of expression of spliced products also is found in the developmental expression of the srDM20 and srPLP isoforms.

The biological role of the DM20 protein has been unclear since its discovery almost 20 years ago, and several possible roles for the gene have been suggested. Evidence that products of the *PLP/DM20* gene may be involved in processes other than myelination first came from cell biological studies on *jimpy*, a mutation in a splice site of exon 5 of the *PLP/DM20* gene. This *PLP/DM20* gene mutation results in a number of developmental abnormalities including, for example, premature cell death of oligodendrocytes, which may be brought about through an activation of the caspase cascade.

Several studies have now identified expression of the *DM20/PLP* gene in nonmyelinating cells in the peripheral nervous system (PNS), embryonic CNS, heart, and immune system. In most cases the DM20 isoform is expressed in nonmyelinating cells, but the expression of PLP and DM20 has been observed in the mouse and human immune systems, and srDM20 cDNA was first isolated from the thymus. Furthermore, the sr-PLP/DM20 proteins appear to be expressed in a greater array of cells within the postnatal brain than the classic PLPs, including many types of neurons.

The expression of products of the *PLP/DM20* gene in so many nonmyelinating cells and the more recent discovery of the srPLP/DM20 isoforms clearly indicate functions for the *PLP/DM20* gene in addition to encoding a myelin structural protein. Indeed, there is evidence that the sr-proteolipids are associated with endosomes and recycling vesicles within oligodendrocytes, and that classic PLP interacts with integrins in oligodendrocytes and may be involved in signaling.

In situ hybridization with PLP probes or PLP promoter elements driving reporter genes have been used to study the location and earliest expression in the CNS. The expression of PLP/DM20 transcripts in midembryonic development suggests that products of the *PLP/DM20* gene may have a role in migration of OL progenitors from proliferative zones into future white and gray matter zones of brain and spinal cord. OL progenitors migrate long distances from their origins in the ventricular zone to their terminal field of differentiation during late embryonic and early postnatal development, and all subfamilies of PLP/DM20 and MBP mRNAs are abundantly expressed in the perikaryon and processes of these cells. All these studies underscore the more varied role the *DM20/PLP* gene may play in the cells in which it is expressed.

2′,3′-CYCLIC NUCLEOTIDE-3′-PHOSPHODIESTERASE

Structure and Localization of the Gene

2′,3′-Cyclic nucleotide-3′-phosphodiesterase (CNP) activity is found in many tissues, but it is particularly active in the CNS. The enzyme is localized within oligodendrocytes in the CNS and within Schwann cells in the PNS. It is one of the earliest markers of cells in the oligodendrocyte lineage, and it is widely used in cell biological studies as a marker for this purpose. Two CNP mRNAs have been identified in rat brain, and a CNP mRNA of a different size has been identified in rat thymus. Two CNP genetic loci, which hybridize to the rat CNP cDNA probes, have been reported on mouse chromosomes 3 and 11. The CNP locus on chromosome 11 appears to contain all the DNA sequences necessary to encode alternatively spliced CNP mRNAs. However, it is not clear if both genetic loci give rise to CNP mRNAs (perhaps in different tissues) or if the chromosome 3 locus is a pseudogene. The human gene maps to chromosome 17.

Promoters, Splicing, and Developmental Expression

Complementary DNAs from several different species have been isolated, and the structures of the mouse and human CNP genes have been determined. They are ~6 kb and ~9 kb in length, respectively, and each consists of four exons (Fig. 19.3). Both transcripts arise from a single gene. The mouse gene contains two transcription start sites at the beginning of the first (i.e., exon 0) and second exons (i.e., exon 1) that appear to be responsible for giving rise to two CNP mRNAs. The mRNA produced from the upstream transcription start site (at exon 0) is smaller than the one produced from the downstream start site (at exon 1), and each encodes a separate isoform of the enzyme. Exon 0 splices into the interior of exon 1 to produce the smaller CNP mRNA (Fig. 19.3). These mRNAs give rise to two isoforms of CNP. The longer 2.6 kb mRNA encodes CNP-1, a 46 kDa isoform; and the shorter 2.4 kb mRNA encodes the larger CNP-2 isoform of 48 kDa, as well as the CNP-1 isoform. The larger CNP-2 is identical to CNP-1 except for an additional 20 amino acids at its N terminus.

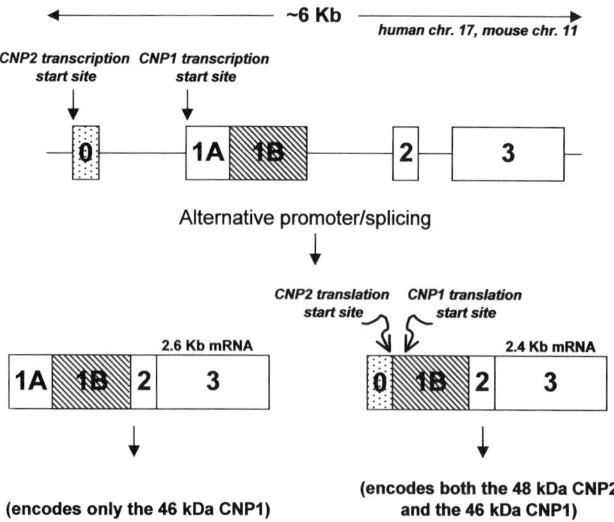

FIGURE 19.3 The *CNP* gene indicating the two transcription start sites (at exons 0 and 1A) and the two translation start sites (within exon 1B) that give rise to the CNP 1 and CNP 2 mRNAs. CNP: 2′,3′-cyclic nucleotide-3′-phosphodiesterase.

The two transcripts appear to be under the control of different promoters that are regulated in a temporally independent fashion during oligodendrocyte development. The 2.4 kb CNP-2 mRNA is the only form that appears to be expressed by oligodendrocyte precursors, but both CNP-1 and CNP-2 mRNAs are expressed at the time of oligodendrocyte differentiation. During oligodendrocyte maturation both promoters are active.

Transcriptional Regulation

Approximately a 4 kb of sequence upstream of exon 1 can drive *lac z* transgenes with correct spatial and temporal expression in transgenic mice. The element drives expression at high levels in the CNS but also in lower amounts in testis and thymus, where the gene is known to be expressed. This promoter can be a very useful element for driving oligodendrocyte-specific expression throughout the course of oligodendrocyte development.

Relatively little is known about the transcriptional regulation of the two promoter elements, but increased cAMP appears to have a relatively more pronounced influence upon the expression of the CNP1 mRNA compared to the CNP2 mRNA. They have also identified a region between exons 0 and 1 was essential for this induction of CNP-1 mRNA.

MYELIN-ASSOCIATED/OLIGODENDROCYTE BASIC PROTEIN

The myelin-associated/oligodendrocyte basic protein (MOBP) is a relatively newly described family of small proteins ranging in length from 69 to 170 amino acids. These CNS-specific myelin proteins are fairly abundant, second only to MBPs and the PLPs. cDNAs for MOBP-170 and MOBP-70 were first isolated from rat and human cDNA libraries, and several other isoforms were subsequently identified. By convention, the isoforms are named MOBP followed by a number indicating the number of amino acids in the polypeptide, followed by a letter in cases where there are distinct isoforms with the same number of amino acids. All isoforms share the first 68 amino acids at their N termini followed by variations in sequence.

The *MOBP* gene consists of eight exons spanning 15 kb in the mouse, and the various isoforms are derived by alternative splicing of the gene (Fig. 19.4). To date, eight isoforms have been identified: MOBP-69, -71, -81A, -81B, -99, -155, -169 and -170.

The MOBPs share some physicochemical and biological properties with the MBPs. They are small, basic soluble proteins, and the most abundant MOBP isoforms contain a clustering of cationic amino acids within their primary structure. The MOBPs are ex-

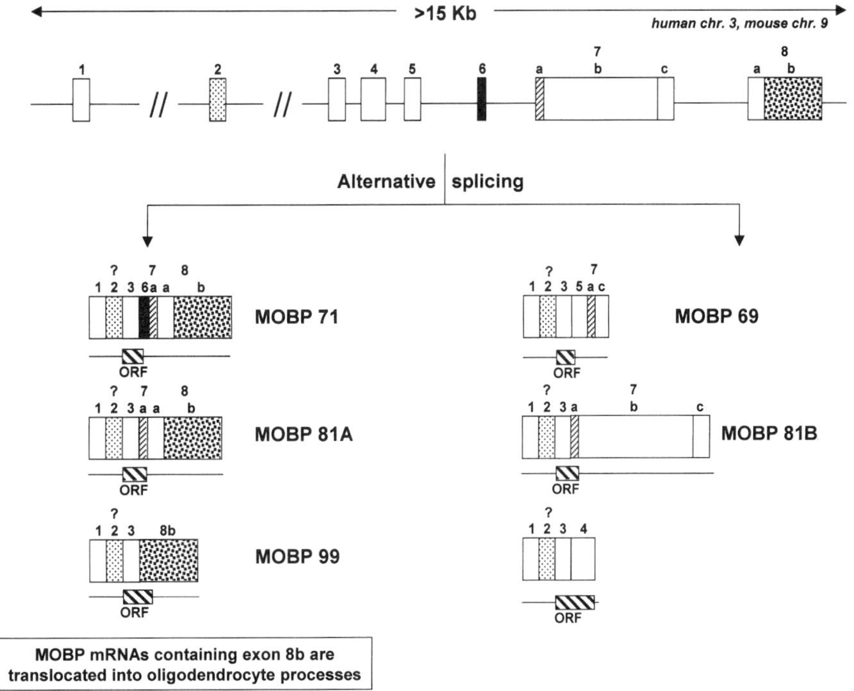

FIGURE 19.4 The *MOBP* gene and the splicing patterns that give rise to six of the myelin-associated/oligodendrocyte basic protein (MOBP) mRNAs. Those mRNAs containing exon 8b are translocated into oligodendrocyte processes because of a transport signal located in the 3-untranslated region of the mRNA encoded by exon 8b. ORF, open reading frame (i.e., coding region).

pressed exclusively in oligodendrocytes in the CNS, and they have been localized to the major dense line of myelin, like the classic MBPs. Some of the MOBP mRNAs are translocated to the processes and myelin assembly sites within the oligodendrocytes in a fashion similar to that of the classic MBP mRNA mRNAs. Interestingly, those MOBP mRNAs containing exon 8b (i.e., MOBP-71, -81A, -99, and -169) are enriched in myelin, and exon 8b contains an RNA transport signal similar to that found in the 3′-UTR of the classic MBPs. The localization of this signal in exon 8b presumably is responsible for the translocation of those MOBP mRNA isoforms.

The MOBPs and the MBPs are developmentally regulated. Expression of the MOBPs occurs in the late stages of myelination, significantly after expression of the classic MBPs. This late expression, the similarity of MOBPs to the classic MBPs, and the localization of

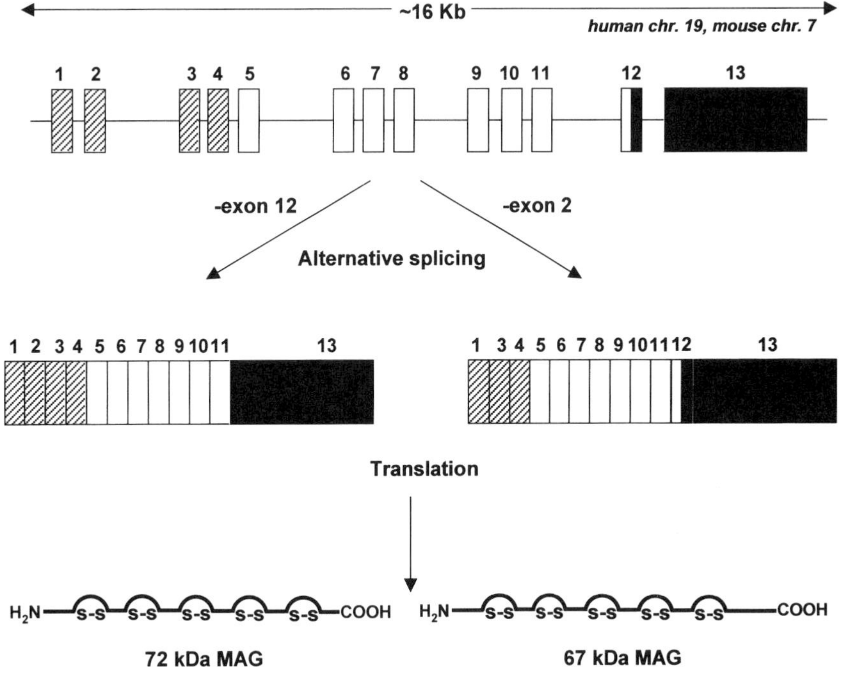

FIGURE 19.5 The *MAG* gene showing alternative splicing to produce two mRNAs and two myelin-associated glycoprotein (MAG) protein isoforms. The protein diagrams emphasize the immunoglobulin domains within their structure.

MOBPs within the major dense line of myelin have led several groups to speculate that the function of MOBPs is to aid in the compaction of myelin. In the *shiverer* mouse, which cannot express classic MBPs, one of the major isoforms of MOBP is poorly incorporated into myelin, leading to the notion that MBP expression is important for assembly of MOBP into myelin. In this regard, classic MBP and MOBP-81A have been reported to interact with the cytoskeleton, suggesting that this might mediate anchoring of these mRNAs after translocation to the subcellular site of translation.

Different MOBP isoforms have been found to localize to different subcellular locations. In transient transfection studies, MOBP-81 has been observed, by immunostaining, to localize to the perinuclear region of Cos7 cells and to the microtubular cytoskeletal network. Also, MOBP partitions with cytoskeletal fractions isolated from myelin. In contrast, transiently transfected MOBP-170 was not found to colocalize with the cytoskeleton. The results suggest more than one function for the MOBP isoforms.

Two groups have generated MOBP knockout mice with slightly differing phenotypes. The knockout mice produced by Yoshikawa and colleagues have been reported to have an increase in axonal diameter and numbers of myelin lamellae in the MOBP-null mice as well as alterations in the radial component of myelin (Yoshikawa, 2001). The phenotype of the MOBP knockout produced by Yool et al. (2002) with a different null construct was reported to be the same as that of wild-type mice, including axonal diameter. Neither group observed a difference between control and null animals in the appearance of compact myelin.

The MOBPs also share immunological properties with the MBPs in the sense that both families of proteins are encephalitogenic in mice. Encephalitogenic peptides from both mouse and human MOBP have been used to induce EAE in mice. It also appears that lymphocytes from patients with multiple sclerosis exhibit autoreactivity to MOBP.

MYELIN-ASSOCIATED GLYCOPROTEIN

The myelin-associated glycoprotein (MAG) has been the subject of intense investigation over the past decade (for reviews, see Schachner and Bartsch, 2000; McKerracher and Winton, 2002; Quarles, 2002). Although it is only a minor protein component of myelin, it is the principal glycoprotein of CNS myelin and consists of two isoforms with apparent molecular masses of 67 kDa (also called S-MAG) and 72 kDa (also called L-MAG). Theoretical analysis of the amino acid sequence data generated from cDNA clones indicate that MAG is a member of the immunoglobulin (Ig) gene superfamily. It has also been designated siglec-4a, as a member of a subgroup of sialic acid-binding proteins of the Ig superfamily with a characteristic extracellular domain. This group also includes CD22 (siglec-2), CD33 (siglec-3), and others, all of which appear to play important roles in the immune and nervous systems (see Kelm and Schauer, 1997; Schachner and Barsch, 2000).

As shown in Figure 19.5, the *MAG* gene consists of 13 exons distributed over ~16 kb in the rat and has a similar structure in the mouse. Exons 2 and 12 are alternatively spliced to produce the two MAG mRNAs in the rat. Exons 1–4 of the gene encode the 5′-UTR, and exons 5–9 each encode one Ig domain, a feature common with genes of the Ig superfamily. The mRNA encoding the 72 kDa MAG polypeptide is composed of all the exons of the gene except exon 12, and the mRNA encoding the 67 kDa MAG is composed of all the exons of the gene except exon 2 (Fig. 19.4). Exon 12 contains a termination signal that creates a shorter coding region in the mRNA than would be present in its absence, thereby encoding the smaller, 67 kDa MAG polypeptide. The absence of exon 2 (encoding the 5′-UTR) has no effect on the size of the protein.

The proportions of the two MAG isoforms appear to be developmentally regulated in the CNS and PNS. Studies have shown that L-MAG expression peaks early in both the CNS and PNS and declines thereafter, such that in the adult, S-MAG is the predominant isoform.

Myelin-associated glycoprotein appears to have a number of interesting functions with respect to myelin formation, maintenance, and repair. Immunohistochemical localization and analysis of the MAG null mice suggest that MAG plays an important role during the initial phases of myelination, perhaps through stabilization of glial axonal interactions. There also is evidence from the MAG null mice that MAG may play a role in the long-term maintenance of myelin. There has been a great deal of interest in the role of MAG as an inhibitor of remyelination and of neurite outgrowth (see McKerracher, 2002, for a short review). It seems paradoxical that MAG is important in the initial phases of myelination, yet also serves as an inhibitor of remyelination. This appears to result from a developmental switch in neuronal responses to MAG such that embryonic neurons are not inhibited by MAG but neurite outgrowth in adult neurons is inhibited. It has recently been found that three inhibitors of neuronal outgrowth, MAG, Nogo (see Brittis and Flanagan, 2001, for review) and oligodendrocyte-myelin glycoprotein (Omgp), bind to the same receptor (Wang et al., 2002).

MYELIN/OLIGODENDROCYTE GLYCOPROTEIN

The myelin/oligodendrocyte glycoprotein (MOG) is a quantitatively minor membrane protein found on the surface of oligodendrocytes and the external lamellae of the myelin sheath. It was first observed with an anonymous monoclonal antibody raised against rat cerebellar glycoproteins. Subsequently, the monoclonal was used to clone a cDNA encoding the MOG protein with a predicted size of 25 kDa. On sodium dodecyl sulfate–polyacrylamide gel electrophoresis (SDS-PAGE) immunoblots MOG runs as a 26–28 kDa doublet that upon deglycosylation runs as a single 25 kDa polypeptide, leading to the conclusion that MOG polypeptides undergo at least two different types of glycosylation to give rise to two posttranslationally modified forms of the protein. Although expression of MOG is developmentally regulated and it appears generally with the onset of myelination, it is one of the last myelin protein genes to be expressed, making it a marker of mature oligodendrocytes.

Myelin/oligodendrocyte glycoprotein has been cloned from a number of species including mouse, rat, bovine, and human. The gene in mouse and human is approximately ~12.5 kb and ~17 kb, respectively. The human gene is slightly more complex than the mouse gene and appears to generate a number of splice variants, whereas the mouse gene does not appear to undergo alternative splicing. From an analysis of the structure through translation of the cDNA, MOG has been characterized as a unique member of the immunoglobulin superfamily, and the mouse and human peptide sequences are highly conserved. Both the mouse and human MOG genes map to major histocompatibility complex (MHC) regions on chromosome 6 of the human and chromosome 17 of the mouse.

The function of MOG is not yet known. Nonetheless, it has received considerable attention because of its potential role in autoimmune-mediated demyelinating events (see Johns and Bernard, 1999). Because the protein is localized at the external surfaces of the myelin sheath and oligodendrocytes, anti-MOG antibodies can cause demyelination *in vivo* and *in vitro*. Myelin/oligodendrocyte glycoprotein has been used to generate a useful model of EAE in rodents (see Stefferl et al., 2000).

OLIGODENDROCYTE-MYELIN GLYCOPROTEIN

Oligodendrocyte-myelin glycoprotein (OMgp) is a membrane glycoprotein that appears in the CNS at the time of myelination, and it has been immunolocalized in both oligodendrocytes and neurons. The function of the protein is not known, but it has been found to have growth inhibitor activity when overexpressed in fibroblasts by altering platelet-derived growth factor (PDGF) signaling in these cells. In the nervous system OMgp has been found to be another myelin component, like MAG, that inhibits neurite outgrowth and exerts its action through binding to the Nogo receptor.

The OMgp was initially discovered and isolated from the human CNS as a 120 kDa glycoprotein that bound to peanut agglutinin. It is one of the "minor" protein components of myelin that appears in the CNS during myelination. It is highly glycosylated, and it appears to be specific to oligodendrocyte and myelin membranes in the CNS since it has not been found in Schwann cells or PNS myelin. The protein is anchored to the membrane through a glycosylphosphatidylinositol intermediate. A subpopulation of OMgp molecules from human brain appears to contain the HNK-1 carbohydrate, which has been implicated in mediating cell-cell interactions in the nervous system. A human cDNA corresponding to the OMgp mRNA predicts a polypeptide sequence of 433 amino acids, including a 17 amino acid leader sequence. The size of the nascent polypeptide backbone with the leader removed is predicted to be 46 kDa. Analysis of the predicted protein structure suggests the presence of four domains that includes a series of tandem leucine repeats that have been implicated in adhesive processes in other proteins. The presence of the HNK-1 carbohydrate in a subpopulation of OMgp molecules, the presence of a tandem leucine repeat domain in the predicted polypeptide sequence, and the apparent presence of OMgp at the paranodal regions of the myelin sheath have led to the notion that it functions as an adhesion molecule.

The human and mouse *OMgp* genes are small (~3 kb), consisting of two exons. In human the gene maps to human chromosome 17 q11–12. The mouse gene is similar in size and structure, and there is a high degree of homology of the gene in the two species. An unusual feature of the *OMgp* gene is that it is included, along with two other unrelated genes of similar simple structure, within intron 27b of the neurofibromatosis type 1 gene (Viskochil et al., 1991). Interestingly, all three of these genes have a transcriptional orientation opposite to that of the neurofibromatosis gene (i.e., they are transcribed off the opposite strand).

PERIPHERAL MYELIN PROTEIN ZERO

Peripheral myelin protein zero (P0) is the major protein of the PNS. It accounts for over 50% of the protein in peripheral nerve myelin (see Quarles, 2002, for a review). The sequence has been deduced by conventional protein sequencing techniques for the bovine protein and from the cDNAs isolated from many species including the human, rat, chicken, and shark. The protein is synthesized with a signal sequence and undergoes posttranslational glycosylation. It is a 30 kDa transmembrane glycoprotein with a glycosylated extracellular domain, a single membrane-spanning region, and a highly basic intracellular domain. The P0 extracellular domain has received considerable attention and analysis. It is generally thought to play an important role in the compaction of myelin through the homotypic interaction of molecules on adjacent myelin lamellae and stabilization of the intraperiod line of myelin (Lemke, 1988). This notion is supported by transfection studies of P0 cDNA constructs into cells in culture and several other studies (Quarles, 2002). For example, expression of anti-sense P0 mRNA impairs the ability of Schwann cells to myelinate dorsal root ganglion cells in cocultures, and P0 knockout mice exhibit severe hypomyelination. As with PLP, gene dosage effects suggest that appropriate levels of the protein are necessary for proper myelination, since overexpression of P0 causes a variable dysmyelinating phenotype ranging from transient hypomyelination to an arrest of myelination.

The *P0* gene consists of six exons distributed over 7 kb in rats and mice, and the gene maps to mouse chromosome 1 and to human chromosome 1. Expression of the *P0* gene is highly restricted to Schwann cells, unlike expression of many of the other myelin protein genes (e.g., *MBP*, *PLP*, *MAG*) that are expressed in both oligodendrocytes and Schwann cells as well as other cell types. The elements regulating this expression appear to reside within a 1.1 kb 5′ flanking region of the gene based upon transgenic experiments.

In recent years, there has been intense interest in the gene among geneticists since mutations in the gene appear to be responsible for Charcot-Marie-Tooth neuropathy type 1B. Charcot-Marie-Tooth neuropathies are associated with mutations and duplications of three genes—*P0*, *PMP22*, and *connexin 32*. There is a large literature on this subject, and the reader is referred to recent reviews for more information (for example, Chance, 2001). Mutations in *P0* also appear to be responsible for Dejerine-Sottas neuropathy. Isolation of the peripheral myelin proteins genes, such as *P0* and *PMP22* as well as *connexin 32*, has led to the development of a number of animal models of peripheral neuropathies (Martini, 1997; Previtali et al., 2000).

PERIPHERAL NERVE P2 PROTEIN

The peripheral nerve P2 protein (P2 protein) was first isolated from bovine nerve roots and was sequenced from many species. The P2 protein has been of immunological interest because it induces experimental allergic neuritis, a demyelinating disease of the PNS in animals, and has been used as an animal model of Guillain-Barré syndrome. The P2 protein bears sequence homology to cellular retinol and retinoic acid-binding proteins, and it has been shown to have a high affinity for oleic acid, retinoic acid, and retinol. It is considered to be a member of the fatty acid-binding protein (FABP) family, in which it is designated MFABP. These proteins are believed to be involved in intracellular fatty acid transport. cDNAs encoding the P2 protein have been isolated and characterized from rabbit sciatic nerve and human fetal spinal cord. The P2 mRNA has been detected in rabbit sciatic nerve, in spinal cord, and to a lesser extent in brain. The mRNA levels of P2 parallel myelination during development as well as the levels of microsomal enzymes involved in fatty acid elongation. These results have prompted the suggestion that the P2 protein may be involved in fatty acid elongation or in the transport of very long chain fatty acids to myelin.

The structure of the mouse *P2* gene appears to be similar to that of other members of the FABP family of genes. The *P2* gene is rather small (~4.5 kb) and consists of four exons. Phylogenetic studies suggest that the *P2* gene belongs to an ancient family of FABPs that diverged into two major subfamilies: one comprising the genes for mammalian liver FABP and gastrotropin, and a second comprising the genes for the retinol-binding proteins, cellular retinoic acid-binding protein, the adipocyte and heart FABPs, and the P2 protein. The *P2* gene is similar to the *PLP/DM20* gene in that they are both members of an ancient family of proteins that have been highly conserved through evolution.

PERIPHERAL NERVOUS SYSTEM MYELIN PROTEIN

Early studies indicated the existence of several glycoproteins in myelin isolated from mammalian peripheral nerve. Some of these were identified as MAG and the P0 protein. In addition to these, low molecular weight proteins in the 19–23 kDa range were identified. Initially, these glycoproteins were thought to be breakdown products of the P0 protein until it was shown that a 19 kDa band was not related to the P0 glycoprotein and probably corresponded to the (PAS II) protein described by Kitamura et al. (1976).

Predicted protein sequences derived from analysis of the first peripheral nervous system myelin protein (PMP-22) cDNAs showed high homology to the growth arrest–specific mRNA, gas 3, and the PAS II glycoprotein. The polypeptide encoded by these cDNAs was named PMP-22 and corresponded to PAS II. A human PMP-22 cDNA has also been isolated. As with the other peripheral myelin protein genes, the expression of PMP-22 mRNA is downregulated after the nerve is crushed or transected. The rat PMP-22 mRNA is ~1.8 kb in length, and its analysis indicates that it encodes a polypeptide of 160 amino acid residues with a predicted molecular mass of ~18 kDa. The polypeptide also contains a predicted leader sequence of 26 residues at its N terminus. It has four hydrophobic regions that represent membrane-spanning domains in the molecule, and it contains a single site for N-linked glycosylation.

The *PMP-22* gene maps to mouse chromosome 11, and a point mutation in this gene is responsible for the autosomal dominant mutation *Trembler* (*Tr*). In humans the gene maps to chromosome 17, and duplication, point mutations, and deletions of the gene appear to be responsible for several forms of peripheral neuropathies including Charcot-Marie Tooth type 1A and Dejerine-Sottas syndrome.

The rat *PMP-22* gene is developmentally regulated in the Schwann cell, its expression coinciding with myelination. Its expression appears to be largely confined to the PNS, although low levels of expression (0.1–0.01) can be detected in the lung, brain, and colon.

In conclusion, there has been substantial progress in our understanding of the molecular biology and genetics of myelin protein genes in recent years. The work has shown that some of the genes, such as the *MBP* and *OMgp* genes, are part of large, complex genetic loci. In many cases, the myelin protein genes are expressed in tissues outside the nervous system, including the immune system, where they may be involved in neuroimmunological diseases. The studies have suggested additional functions of the myelin protein genes beyond that of encoding structural proteins of myelin, and some of these functions are beginning to be defined. Identification of mutations in the myelin protein genes have been shown to be responsible for a number of neurological diseases of both the CNS and PNS. In spite of these advances, relatively little is known about the functions of these many proteins both within the oligodendrocyte and myelin and in other cells in tissues. It is likely that in the future, much more will be learned about the cellular function of these proteins beyond the myelin sheath.

ACKNOWLEDGMENTS

I wish to thank Celia Campagnoni, for assistance and critical comments on this manuscript, and Michael Marshall for help in its preparation. This work was supported, in part, by research grants from the National Institutes of Health and a grant from the National Multiple Sclerosis Society.

REFERENCES

Barbarese, E., Brumwell, C., Kwon, S., Cui, H., and Carson, J.H. (1999) RNA on the road to myelin. *J. Neurocytol.* 28:263–270.

Bongarzone, E.R., Campagnoni, C.W., Kampf, K., Jacobs, E., Handley, V.W., Schonmann, V., and Campagnoni, A.T. (1999) Identification of a new exon in the myelin proteolipid protein gene encoding novel protein isoforms that are restricted to the somata of oligodendrocytes and neurons. *J. Neurosci.* 19:8349–8357.

Brittis, P.A. and Flanagan, J.G. (2001) Nogo domains and a Nogo receptor: implications for axon regeneration. *Neuron* 30:11–14.

Campagnoni, A.T. and Skoff, R.P. (2001) The pathobiology of myelin mutants reveal novel biological functions of the *MBP* and *PLP* genes. *Brain. Pathol.* 11:74–91.

Chance, P.F. (2001) Molecular basis of hereditary neuropathies. *Phys. Med. Rehibil. Clin. North Am.* 12:277–291.

Griffiths, I.R. (1996) Myelin mutants: model for the study of normal and abnormal myelination. *Bioessays* 18:789–797.

Huseby, E.S. and Goverman, J. (2000) Tolerating the nervous system: a delicate balance. *J. Exp. Med.* 191:757–760.

Ikenaka, K. and Kagawa T. (1995) Transgenic systems in studying myelin gene expression. *Dev. Neurosci.* 17:127–136.

Jetten, A.M. and Suter, U. (2000) The peripheral myelin protein 22 and epithelial membrane protein family. *Prog. Nucleic Acid Res.* 64:97–129.

Johns, T.G. and Bernard, C.C.A. (1999) The structure and function of myelin oligodendrocyte glycoprotein. *J. Neurochem.* 72:1–9.

Kelm, S. and Schauer, R. (1997) Sialic acids in molecular and cellular interactions. *Int. Rev. Cytol.* 175:137–240.

Kitamura, K., Suzuki, M., and Uyemura, K. (1976) Purification and partial characterization of two glycoproteins in bovine peripheral nerve myelin membrane. *Biochim. Biophys. Acta* 455:806–816.

Lemke, G. (1988) Unwrapping the genes of myelin. *Neuron* 1:535–543.

Martini, R. (1997) Animal models for inherited peripheral neuropathies. *J. Anat.* 191:321–336.

McKerracher, L. and Winton, M.J. (2002) Nogo on the go. *Neuron* 36:345–348.

Mirsky, R., Parkinson, D.B., Dong, Z., Meier, C., Calle, E., Brennan, A., Topilko, P., Harris, B.S., Stewart, H.J., and Jessen, K.R. (2001) Regulation of genes involved in Schwann cell development and differentiation. *Prog. Brain Res.* 132:3–11.

Previtali, S.C., Quattrini, A., Fasolini, M., Panzeri, M.C., Villa, A., Filbin, M.T., Li, W., Chiu, S.-Y., Messing, A., Wrabetz, L., and Feltri, M.L. (2000) Epitope-tagged P_0 glycoprotein causes Charcot-Marie-Tooth-like neuropathy in transgenic mice. *J. Cell Biol.* 151:1035–1045.

Quarles, R.H. (2002) Myelin sheaths: glycoproteins involved in their formation, maintenance and degeneration. *Cell. Mol. Life Sci.* 59:1851–1871.

Schachner, M. and Bartsch, U. (2000) Multiple functions of the myelin-associated glycoprotein MAG siglec-4a) in formation and maintenance of myelin. *Glia* 29:154–165.

Stefferl, A., Brehm, U., and Linington, C. (2000) The myelin oligodendrocyte glycoprotein (MOG): a model for antibody-mediated demyelination in experimental autoimmune encephalomyelitis and multiple sclerosis. *J. Neural. Transm. Suppl.* 58:123–133.

Takahashi, N., Roach, A., Teplow, D.B., Prusiner, S.B., and Hood, L. (1985) Cloning and characterization of the myelin basic protein gene from mouse: one gene can encode both 14 kd and 18.5 kd MBPs by alternate use of exons. *Cell* 42:139–148.

Viskochil, D., Cawthon, R., O'Connell, P., Xu, G., Stevens, J., Culver, M., Carey, J., and White, R. (1991) The gene encoding the oligodendrocyte-myelin glycoprotein is embedded within the neurofibromatosis type 1 gene. *Mol. Cell. Biol.* 11:906–912.

Wang, K.C., Koprivica, V., Kim, J.A., Sivasankaran, R., Guo, Y., Neve, R.L., and He, Z. (2002) Oligodendrocyte-myelin glycoprotein is a Nogo receptor ligand that inhibits neurite outgrowth. *Nature* 417:941–944.

Wegner, M. (2000) Transcriptional control in myelinating glia: flavors and spices. *Glia* 31:1–14.

Yool, D., Montague, P., McLaughlin, M., McCulloch, M.C., Edgar, J.M., Nave, K.A., Davies, R.W., Griffiths, I.R., and McCallion, A.S. (2002) Phenotypic analysis of mice deficient in the major myelin protein MOBP, and evidence for a novel Mobp isoform. *Glia* 39:256–267.

Yoshikawa, H. (2001) Myelin-associated oligodendrocytic basic protein modulates the arrangement of radial growth of the axon and the radial. *Med. Electron Microsc.* 34:160–164.

20 Factors controlling myelin formation

LYNN D. HUDSON

Myelin formation is the culmination of a parade of events with a constellation of characters, beginning with the commitment of cells to a Schwann cell or oligodendrocyte lineage, followed by the selection of target axons by developing glial cells, and crowned by the industrial-scale synthesis and assembly of myelin constituents. The resultant engineering feat, the myelin sheath, is an achievement on several fronts, including the integration of a bevy of occasionally conflicting signals. Factors regulating myelin formation operate at each step in the transcription, translation, and transport of myelin constituents. The identity of some of these factors, as well as the manner in which they influence myelination, have yielded to scrutiny. Rather than surveying the rapidly expanding list of participants, this chapter will focus on emerging checkpoints in myelin formation.

TRANSCRIPTIONAL CONTROLS EXERTED ON THE SPECIFICATION AND DIFFERENTIATION OF MYELIN-FORMING CELLS

In response to extracellular cues, neural stem cells activate a subset of genes that commit their progeny to the execution of the myelin program. To examine transcriptional controls on myelination, one must start early in the lineage, long before the formation of the myelin sheath. This early focus is mandated not only because commitment to the Schwann cell or oligodendrocyte lineage is a prerequisite for myelin formation, but also since a subset of myelin genes are transcriptionally activated in precursor cells. Committed Schwann cell precursors express the *P0* myelin gene (reviewed in Chapter 7), while oligodendrocyte precursors activate the 2′,3′-cyclic nucleotide-3′-phosphodiesterase (*CNP*) (Chandross et al., 1999; Genoud et al., 2002) and proteolipid protein (*PLP*) genes (Thomas et al., 2000; Mallon et al., 2002). This curious early transcriptional activation of a few myelin genes is probably not related to any function(s) of these myelin proteins, as the absence of detectable P0, CNP, or PLP protein in precursors indicates that the transcripts are not translated. Nor do the levels of transcripts approach those maintained by actively myelinating glial cells. Perhaps the awakening of a handful of myelin loci in committed Schwann cell and oligodendrocyte precursors serves to mobilize the transcriptional machinery for the ensuing large-scale synthesis of myelin transcripts. This would be consistent with the recruitment of splicing domains to the *PLP* locus as development proceeds (Nielsen et al., 2002). The *PLP* gene appears geographically fixed at the periphery of the nuclear membrane at all stages of the oligodendrocyte lineage, a property that calls for redistribution of the necessary transcription and splicing factors to these defined domains within the nucleus. Transcriptional controls differ between Schwann cells and oligodendrocytes, which is illustrated by the contrasting expression of myelin promoter driven reporters in the peripheral nervous system (PNS) and central nervous system (CNS) of transgenic mice. Myelin basic protein (MBP) is synthesized by both oligodendrocytes and Schwann cells, but portions of the *MBP* promoter that drive appropriate expression levels at the correct time and place in the CNS are insufficient in the PNS (Gow et al., 1992; Forghani et al., 2001). These differences are attributable in part to a distinct but overlapping array of transcription factors in Schwann cells and oligodendrocytes. For a review of the transcription factors active in Schwann cells, see Chapter 7.

Transcription Factors Directing the Genetic Program of Myelination in Oligodendrocytes

What transcription factors direct the commitment of neural stem cells to the oligodendrocyte lineage? Two classes of transcription factors, the basic helix-loop-helix (bHLH) proteins and the homeodomain proteins, act in concert to control the neuron versus glial fate and neuronal subtype decisions in the embryonic spinal cord. Essential for oligodendrocyte specification are the bHLH proteins Olig1 and Olig2 (Lu et al., 2000, 2002; Zhou et al., 2001; Zhou and Anderson, 2002; Takebayashi et al., 2002). Mice deficient in both *Olig1* and *Olig2* are devoid of oligodendrocyte progenitors. The two genes share a degree of functional redundancy, as *Olig2* nulls lack progenitors in the spinal cord, while

See the list of abbreviations at the end of the chapter.

Olig1 nulls are delayed in oligodendrocyte maturation. Despite the name, the *Olig* genes are not functionally limited to the oligodendrocyte lineage. Oligodendrocyte precursors emerge from a zone in the ventral spinal cord that is demarcated by expression of *Olig1* and *Olig2* as well as homeodomain proteins and other bHLH proteins. Prior to oligodendrogliogenesis, motoneurons are generated from cells within this domain expressing *Olig2* and another bHLH protein, Neurogenin2. In the absence of *Olig2*, no motoneurons appear. Downregulation of Neurogenin2 expression coupled with the appearance of the homeodomain protein Nkx2.2, whose expression was previously restricted to the adjacent domain (Zhou et al., 2001), accompanies the onset of oligodendrogliogenesis marked by the appearance of platelet-derived growth factor receptor alpha (PDGFRα)-positive progenitors. Nkx2.2 regulates the differentiation of oligodendrocytes but is not essential for oligodendrocyte specification (Qi et al., 2001). Nkx2.2-deficient animals display an expansion of the *Olig1/Olig2* expression domain and a concomitant increase in Olig1/Olig2/PDGFRα-positive progenitors but a subsequent loss of mature oligodendrocytes. The ability of overexpressed Nkx2.2 to induce expression from the *PLP* promoter in a heterologous transfection system (Qi et al., 2001) implicates Nkx2.2 as one of the transcription factors involved in the early activation of the *PLP* gene in oligodendrocyte progenitors. Another transcription factor whose expression closely follows *Olig1/Olig2* and precedes PDGFRα expression is the high mobility group (HMG) domain protein Sox10 (Stolt et al., 2002). Transgenic mice lacking Sox10 generate normal numbers of PDGFRα+ progenitors but suffer a subsequent derailment of oligodendrocyte development. Sox10 stimulates *MBP* and *PLP* gene expression in a transfected neural cell line, and mutations in the Sox10 binding site of the *MBP* promoter display diminished binding (Stolt et al., 2002). Sox 10 represents one of the transcription factors crucial for both the Schwann cell and oligodendrocyte lineages, albeit with differing mechanisms of action in each lineage: (*1*) Schwann cell progenitors are absent in the PNS of Sox10-deficient mice, while oligodendrocyte progenitors are relatively unaffected; (*2*) Sox10 function in the PNS is mediated by neuregulin signaling, but not in the CNS.

Together with Nkx2.2 and Sox 10, a panoply of transcription factors comes to the fore in differentiating and mature oligodendrocytes. These encompass the gamut of transcription factors classes: the POU homeodomain protein SCIP/Tst-1/Oct6, the NK homeodomain protein Nkx6.2/Gtx, the helix-loop-helix (HLH) Id (inhibitor of DNA binding) proteins, and the zinc finger proteins rKr1, rKr2, and Myt1 (reviewed in Wegner, 2000). Although a loss-of-function transgenic model of SCIP/Tst-1/Oct6 has no impact on CNS myelination or oligodendrocyte differentiation, probably because of functional redundancy with other POU homeodomain proteins (e.g., Brn-1, Brn-2) (Bermingham et al., 1996; Jaegle et al., 1996), overexpression leads to abnormal, precocious myelination (Jensen et al., 1998). While overexpression paradigms present complicated interpretations, together these experiments suggest that SCIP/Tst-1/Oct6 may function at an early stage of development in oligodendrocytes, as it does in promyelinating Schwann cells (Bermingham et al., 1996; Jaegle et al., 1996).

Overexpression has also been employed to investigate the role of the HLH Id proteins in the timing of oligodendrocyte differentiation (Kondo and Raff, 2000; Wang et al., 2001). Cells of the oligodendrocyte lineage express all four of the Id proteins. Excess Id2 or Id4 blocks oligodendrocyte differentiation, and the absence of Id2 induces premature differentiation of oligodendrocyte precursors *in vitro* (Kondo and Raff, 2000; Wang et al., 2001). Lacking the basic DNA-binding domain, the HLH Id proteins behave as dominant negative blockers of bHLH proteins through their ability to dimerize with the E protein class of bHLH proteins. The bHLH E proteins are also widely distributed, and oligodendrocytes have at least two members of this class: HEB and the E2A alternatively spliced isoform E47 (Wang et al., 2001; Sussman et al., 2002). The bHLH E proteins normally heterodimerize with a tissue-restricted class of bHLH proteins, including many of the proneural genes of the *Atonal, Nato, Olig, NeuroD, Neurogenin, Achaete-Scute*, and *Nscl* families (reviewed in Bertrand et al., 2002). These tissue-restricted bHLH are unable to bind to their targets prior to heterodimerization with E proteins. Consequently, sequestration of E proteins by Id proteins is pivotal in regulating the action of these tissue-restricted bHLH proteins. Still to be identified are the bHLH proteins active in oligodendrocytes that participate in the Id2- or Id4-mediated timing of oligodendrocyte differentiation. The Olig1 and Olig2 proteins, which are expressed throughout the oligodendrocyte lineage, are potential participants in the timing mechanism.

Transcription Factors Respond to Extracellular Cues Exerted on Precursors and Developing Oligodendrocytes

Signaling commitment to the oligodendrocyte lineage: sonic hedgehog

What controls the temporal switch in the sequential production of first motoneurons and then oligodendrocyte precursors in the developing spinal cord? Sonic hedgehog (Shh) secreted from the notochord and floor plate is critical to glial fate determination in the CNS, as shown by grafting and explant studies together with the use of Shh-deficient mice (Poncet et al., 1996;

Pringle et al., 1996; Orentas et al., 1999; Lu et al., 2000; Soula et al., 2001). The emergence of oligodendrocytes in the brain is similarly tied to expression of Shh (Alberta et al., 2001; Davies and Miller, 2001; Nery et al., 2001). Oligodendrocytes fail to develop from *Shh−/−* embryos, and the addition of Shh to CNS cultures promotes the genesis of oligodendrocyte precursors. What are the downstream targets of Shh action relevant to oligodendrocyte specification? *Olig1* appears to be one target, as Shh treament of cultured neuroepithelial cultures rapidly induces *Olig1* expression (Lu et al., 2000). Moreover, ectopic expression of *Olig1* can circumvent a need for Shh in the formation of oligodendrocyte progenitors in the forebrain and spinal cord (Alberta et al., 2001). *Olig1* and *Olig2* are classified with the set of transcription factors whose expression is induced by the graded levels of Shh present in the ventral spinal cord and discrete sites within the brain. Additional targets of Shh signaling relevant to oligodendrocytes include the differentiation-promoting transcription factor Nkx2.2 (Ericson et al., 1997) and the other homeodomain proteins Nkx6.1 and Nkx6.2/Gtx, which may act directly on or in concert with the *Olig* genes (Vallstedt et al., 2001).

A checkpoint in oligodendrocyte development: Notch signaling

Olig2 initially collaborates with the neurogenic bHLH protein Neurogenin2 during the phase of motoneuron generation. Only when the pan-neurogenic program is halted within the progenitor motor neuron domain can oligodendrogliogenesis begin. One signaling pathway that may contribute to the repression of Neurogenin1 and Neurogenin2 and the coincident coexpression of Nkx2.2 is the Notch1 pathway. Notch proteins are conserved transmembrane receptors integral to many decisions of cell fate and differentiation. When activated by ligands (Jagged1/2, Delta 1, Delta-like 1/3/4), the intracellular domain of Notch is proteolytically cleaved and translocated to the nucleus, where it activates the CSL family of transcription factors, targets of which include the bHLH *HES* gene family (reviewed by Lai, 2002). In the oligodendrocyte lineage, Notch1 participates in the correct spatial and temporal regulation of oligodendrocyte differentiation. Activation of the Notch1 signaling pathway by Jagged1 suppresses oligodendrocyte differentiation in cultured precursors (Wang et al., 1998). When Notch1 expression is selectively ablated in oligodendrocyte precursors, precocious differentiation ensues (Genoud et al., 2002). The ectopic production of immature oligodendrocytes in the gray matter of the spinal cord and the anterior forebrain of the conditional Notch1 knockout mice creates a population of oligodendrocytes more susceptible to apoptosis. Of note is the constant number of oligodendrocyte precursors and the normalcy of early oligodendrocyte development in this transgenic model, suggesting that the influence of Notch signaling is felt at the timing of oligodendrocyte differentiation (Genoud et al., 2002). In mice heterozygous for a Notch1-null mutation, additional defects in myelination were noted (Givogri et al., 2002). Most intriguing was the myelination of fibers in the molecular layer of the cerebellum, a region that is typically unmyelinated. Could Notch signaling be part of the intrinsic program that dictates which axons become myelinated? Such a role would be directly relevant to diseases of myelin insufficiency such as multiple sclerosis (MS). The discovery of astrocytes strongly expressing Jagged1 in active MS plaques lacking remyelination, while remyelinated plaques displayed negligible amounts of Jagged1, points to the possibility that activation of the Notch1 signaling pathway serves to keep the Notch1-positive oligodendrocyte precursors in an immature state in a subset of MS plaques (John et al., 2002). The Notch pathway presents a new molecular handle for therapeutic efforts aimed at stimulating oligodendrocyte precursors to myelinate in demyelinating disorders.

Signaling in migrating oligodendrocyte precursors: role of the CXCR2 and platelet-derived growth factor alpha receptors

Newly specified oligodendrocyte precursors and their progeny are highly migratory cells that travel great distances from their points of origin in the CNS. This wide dispersal is in response to the migration-stimulating effects of the platelet-derived growth factor (PDGF) ligand acting on the receptor (PDGFαR) (Armstrong et al., 1991; Frost et al., 1996). Multiple PDGFαR-initiated signals operate in oligodendrocyte development, as site-directed receptor mutations that eliminate the capacity of PDGFαR to activate either the PI3 or the Src kinase signaling pathway lead to hypomyelination in transgenic mice (Klinghoffer et al., 2002). Not all oligodendrocyte precursors are responsive to PDGF, as originally indicated by a population of precursors that lack the PDGFαR and confirmed by normal myelination in the hindbrain of mice defective in PDGFAA/PDGFαR signaling (Spassky et al., 1998; Klinghoffer et al., 2002). The stimulatory nature of PDGF on responsive oligodendrocyte precursors is countered by the action of a chemokine, CXCL1 (Tsai et al., 2002). Acting through the CXCR2 receptor on oligodendrocyte precursors, CXCL1 inhibits PDGF-stimulated chemotaxis in cultures and precursor migration in slices. Mice deficient in CXCR2 have an abnormal concentration of oligodendrocytes at the periphery of the spinal cord as well as an overall reduction in oligodendrocyte number. Miller and coworkers propose that CXCL1/CXCR2 signaling may control the patterning of oligodendrocytes in the spinal cord by arresting the PDGF-induced migration of oligodendrocyte precursors (Tsai et al., 2002). Clearly, the temporal and spatial expression of the chemokine (CXCL1) is key to this pattern generation and will be the subject of future investigation. The interplay between CXCR2 and PDGFαR is evidently only part of the migration saga, as other growth factors [possibly neurotrophin 3 (NT3), basic fibroblast growth factor (bFGF), or insulin-like growth factor I (IGF-I)] may partially compensate for the lack of CXCR2-mediated proliferation in mutant mice, and several other guidance systems (e.g., ephrins, semaphorins, netrins) probably participate in directing oligodendrocyte precursors to their destinations.

POSTTRANSCRIPTIONAL CONTROL OF MYELIN SYNTHESIS

Messenger stability figures prominently in the regulation of gene expression for at least one myelin gene, namely, *PLP*. The alternative splicing of the *PLP* gene to produce the PLP- and DM20-encoding transcripts represents one checkpoint in the nucleus, where the intron 3–containing precursor mRNA accumulates prior to the alternative splicing of exon 3 (Vouyiouklis et al., 2000). Proteolipid protein (PLP) mRNA is subjected to further controls prior to translation in Schwann cells during development and following injury. By comparing transcription rates with steady-state levels of PLP/DM20 transcripts in developing sciatic nerve, Macklin and coworkers found enhanced stability of PLP mRNA, which was conferred by the 105 nucleotide region of exon 3 that distinguishes PLP from DM20 transcripts (Jiang et al., 2000). Proteolipid protein transcript stability is regulated at least in part by axonal contact, as sciatic nerve transection or the withdrawal of forskolin in cultured Schwann cells results in a selective loss of PLP transcripts. Loss of axonal contact in the CNS is similarly accompanied by a loss of PLP transcripts in affected oligodendrocytes (Scherer et al., 1992) and may likewise involve messenger stability. Mechanisms operative in stabilizing PLP mRNAs probably apply to additional myelin genes.

TRANSLATIONAL AND POSTTRANSLATIONAL CONTROLS OF MYELIN ASSEMBLY AND MAINTENANCE

Myelination requires a constant flow of lipids and proteins to multiple peripheral domains. A prominent feature of this process is the convergence of widely scattered myelin constituents upon assembly sites in the plasma membrane. Some lipids and proteins jump-start the assembly process in the Golgi network, where patches of myelin lipids and proteins self-associate, while other constituents such as MBP procrastinate, with MBP mRNA requiring transport to assembly sites before translation and incorporation of MBP can occur. Myelin-forming cells employ a number of general trafficking pathways to haul their cargo (reviewed in Kramer et al., 2001).

The cytoskeletal network figures prominently in the delivery of some myelin components and selected mRNAs to sites of assembly. Lacking intermediate filaments, oligodendrocytes rely on an integrated system of microtubules and microfilaments. Dense bundles of microtubules in a plus-end-distal orientation extend into processes, following tracks laid down by microfilaments, which constitute the major cytoskeletal element at the leading edge of the process (Song et al., 2001a). The critical nature of the microtubule component of this cytoarchitectural meshwork is illustrated by the *taiep* mutant rat. Microtubules accumulate in the perinuclear cytoplasm of *taiep* oligodendrocytes concomitant with a failure of PLP and L-myelin-associated glycoprotein (L-MAG) transport, a phenotype magnified by the distance between the cell body and the myelin sheath (Song et al., 2001b). Myelin basic protein mRNA also accumulates in the cell body of *taiep* oligodendrocytes, indicative of a transport defect (O'Connor et al., 2000). Given the basic microtubule/microfilament framework, do myelin-forming cells employ additional, cell-restricted proteins that interact with the cytoskeleton and facilitate transport of myelin constituents? One recently recognized candidate is CNP, an established myelin protein long in search of a function. CNP has several properties that recommend it for integrating the microtubule and microfilament systems in oligodendrocytes. First, CNP acts as a microtubule-associated protein: the carboxy terminus of CNP can promote microtubule assembly *in vitro*, and deletions of the carboxy terminus lead to an abnormal microtubule distribution *in vivo* (Bifulco et al., 2002). Second, CNP is membrane-associated by virtue of two posttranslational modifications, prenylation and palmitoylation (Braun et al., 1991), and may therefore serve as a membrane anchor for microtubules. CNP associates with tubulin at the plasma membrane and perinuclear region, not in between. Within the myelin membrane, a portion (40%) of CNP is associated with detergent-insoluble, glycosphingolipid/cholesterol-enriched microdomains in myelin (Kim and Pfeiffer, 1999). Third, CNP has also been shown to associate with microfilaments (Wilson and Brophy, 1989). If CNP is one of the molecules that integrate the microtubule and microfilament systems in oligodendrocytes, how are these interactions regulated? CNP is phosphorylated *in vivo* by protein kinase C (PKC) (Agrawal et al., 1994). Phosphorylation by PKC *in vitro* reduces its ability to bind to tubulin and promote polymerization. Thus, reorganization of the cytoskeleton during process elongation, branching, and ensheathment could be modulated by agents that alter PKC.

Another mode of membrane trafficking that oligodendrocytes and Schwann cells exploit is the formation of rafts, which are glycosphingolipid-cholesterol-rich membrane domains that behave as platforms for the recruitment of a specific set of proteins. During transit through the Golgi complex, PLP selectively joins cholesterol and galactosylceramide-rich membrane domains in these small, dynamic raft structures (Simons et al., 2000). This initial stage of myelin assembly can be blocked by either cholesterol depletion or, in the case of the ceramide galactosyl transferase (CGT) knockout mice, the absence of galactosylceramide and sulfatide. Proteolipid protein still manages to reach the plasma membrane in these situations, as it does when transfected into nonglial cells that lack myelin lipids (Gow et al., 1994; Gow and Lazzarini et al., 1996; Thomson et al., 1997). Proteolipid protein may take an alternative trafficking route to the plasma membrane, namely, transcytosis, as detailed by Kramer and coworkers (2001). In this model, all membrane components proceed by "bulk flow" to the plasma membrane, where subsequent endocytic uptake, sorting, and recycling distribute myelin components to the expanding myelin sheath. Consistent with a transcytosis flow of myelin proteins, PLP appears to be routed primarily to the endosomal compartment in cultured oligodendrocytes (Kramer et al., 2001), and the predominant Rab–guanosine triphosphatases (Rab-GTPases) expressed by oligodendrocytes are of the endosomal variety (Bouverat et al., 2000). When overexpressed, PLP fails to associate with myelin rafts in the Golgi complex (Simons et al., 2002). Instead, PLP accumulates in late endosomes/lysosomes, where the overexpressed protein traps cholesterol and possibly other myelin lipids and thereby perturbs myelin assembly. Together, these studies suggest that myelin assembly begins shortly after PLP synthesis, and while assembly into raft structures is not essential for transport, the integrity of compact myelin may be adversely affected by improper ratios of myelin constituents in the Golgi complex. Rafts have also been identified in other cellular compartments of myelin-forming cells, the plasma membrane, and the myelin sheath (Kramer et al., 1997, 1999; Kim and Pfeiffer, 1999; Hasse et al., 2002; Taylor et al., 2002). Rafts offer tremendous advantages for myelin generation due to their inherent self-driven assembly. As domains enriched in axon-glial recognition proteins (e.g., contactin, NCAM120) and signaling molecules (e.g., the *src* family kinase Fyn), rafts both receive and transmit signals for the myelinating glial cell. Further segregation of myelin constituents occurs within the myelin membrane. Some of these interactions marry myelin proteins with signaling complexes, as discovered by Macklin and coworkers for a tripartite complex composed of PLP, the multifunctional Ca^{+} binding protein calreticulin, and the α_V-integrin receptor (Gudz et al., 2002).

A landmark discovery by Carson and Barbarese and their coworkers was the packaging of certain mRNAs into *granules* containing various trafficking factors and components of the translational machinery, and the subsequent transport of these trafficking intermediates to the plus ends of microtubules in the myelin compartment (reviewed in Carson et al., 2001). Those mRNAs that contain an appropriate cis-acting element are eligible for incorporation into these granules. For MBP mRNA, an 11-nucleotide cis element (GCCAAGGAGCC) is recognized by the trans-acting factor hnRNP A2 (Hoek et al., 1998), which remains associated with MBP mRNA during transport and behaves as a translational enhancer upon arrival at the distal processes (Kwon et al., 1999). Another myelin protein whose mRNA contains the heteronuclear ribonuclear protein A2 (hnRNP A2) response element is myelin-associated oligodendrocyte basic protein (MOBP) (Holz et al., 1996; Gould et al., 1999). The *MOBP* gene is alternatively spliced, and only transcripts that include exon 8b with its hnRNP A2 cis element are enriched in myelin. The *MBP* gene is also alternatively spliced, but the hnRNP A2 cis element is part of exon 7, which is present in all of the classical forms of MBP. Nonetheless, not all MBP transcripts appear to be incorporated into granules for transport to processes. Immature oligodendrocytes, in which alternative splicing favors the production of exon 2–containing MBP transcripts, retain substantial amounts of MBP transcripts in the cell soma, and the MBP protein present in the soma at these early development stages probably reflects on-site translation. Moreover, the Golli MBP protein isoforms that function in the soma and nucleus (Landry et al., 1996) are most likely translated in the soma at all developmental stages. Thus, the packaging of MBP mRNA into granules for transport along the microtubule highway represents a major regulatory checkpoint. What features control this packaging? Are additional cis elements in the form of *retention* sequences present on some MBP transcripts that override the hnRNP A2 recognition signal? Do immature cells have all of the transport machinery in hand? Perhaps the transport system is overloaded in actively myelinating oligodendrocytes, so that a portion of the transcripts will be left out, and these spillover transcripts are subsequently translated in the cell soma. A number of other mRNA species have been localized in myelin, including peptidyl arginine deiminase, ferritin heavy chain, the endocytosis protein SH3p13, the kinesin heavy chain KIF1A, a dynein light intermediate chain, and a handful of uncharacterized mRNAs (Gould et al., 2000), carbonic anhydrase II (Ghandour and Skoff, 1991), and tau (LoPresti et al., 1995). The appearance of these proteins, several of which play defined roles in myelination (e.g., peptidyl arginine deiminase acts on MBP to deiminate arginine residues during development), suggests that mRNA trafficking in oligodendrocytes may be more extensive than was originally thought. If some of these mRNAs, such as MBP, MOBP, and peptidyl arginine deiminase, are found to coassemble into the same granule, a mechanism for coordinating myelin protein synthesis within a subcellular compartment would be recognized.

Posttranslational controls on myelin formation are exerted either directly through modification of myelin constituents or indirectly through signaling pathways involved in myelination. Acylation is a prominent posttranslational modification of CNP and PLP. The attachment of fatty acids via thioester linkages to specific intracellular cysteine residues of PLP is not coupled with protein synthesis, and occurs autocatalytically with acyl-coenzyme A (acyl-CoA) esters as donor molecules (Bizzozero et al., 1987; Ross and Braun, 1988). Deacylation, however, is an active enzymatic process catalyzed by a specific myelin-associated fatty acylesterase (Bizzozero et al., 1992). The acyl moieties affect the adhesive properties of PLP/DM20, as chemical deacylation leads to decompaction of the myelin sheath (Bizzozero et al., 2001). Acylation may be key to the structural role of PLP in myelin compaction. Based on structural studies and the analysis of various transgenic PLP mutants, an intriguing model proposed by Stoffel posits that the intracytoplasmic loop of PLP associates with the adjacent myelin bilayer via the three fatty acyl chains covalently linked to the loop domain (Sporkel et al., 2002). Proteolipid protein would stably link adjacent myelin bilayers, a linkage subject to the dynamic processing of fatty acyl groups by myelin-associated fatty acylesterases. This mechanism for PLP-mediated adhesion through reversible acylation would enable the focal condensation of myelin bilayers into a compact myelin structure. Such a localized regulation of myelin compaction merits further investigations of the acylesterase pathways in oligodendrocytes.

A number of growth factors that profoundly affect oligodendrocyte development (e.g., PDGF, IGF-I, bFGF, neuregulins) act through tyrosine kinase receptors (reviewed in Chapter 6) to initiate signal transduction cascades that involve reversible cycles of phosphorylation and dephosphorylation by kinases and phosphatases, among other posttranslational modifications. One of the signaling cascades in oligodendrocytes that has recently yielded to molecular definition centers on a member of the Src family of protein tyrosine kinases, Fyn. Fyn is crucial for CNS myelination (Umemori et al., 1994; Sperber and McMorris, 2001; Sperber et al., 2001). Both growth factors and cell contact have been implicated in triggering the Fyn signaling pathway in oligodendrocytes. Fyn is required for the maturation of oligodendrocytes treated with IGF-I (Sperber and McMorris, 2001), consistent with reports that Fyn forms a functional complex with insulin receptor substrate proteins (IRS-1 and IRS-2) that transduce signals from IGF-1 and other growth factor receptors (Sun et al., 1996). Apart from participating in pathways receiving soluble extracellular cues, Fyn engages in contact-mediated signaling, as predicted by its compartmentalization with cell adhesion molecules. Fyn associates with the glycosylphosphatidylinositol (GPI)-anchored proteins NCAM120 and F3/Contactin in glycosphingolipid/cholesterol-rich microdomains, and antibody-mediated cross-linking of F3 leads to activation of Fyn within these raft structures (Kramer et al., 1999). Similarly, Fyn associates with one of the isoforms of myelin-associated glycoprotein (L-MAG) and can become activated following antibody-mediated cross-linking of MAG. The downstream targets recognized by activated Fyn include cytoskeletal proteins and their regulators. One of the substrates that Fyn phosphorylates is p190 RhoGAP, an enzyme that accelerates the intrinsic GTPase activity of Rho GTPases, a family that controls actin stress fiber assembly (Wolf et al., 2001). Fyn also interacts with the microtubule-associated protein Tau and α-Tubulin (Klein et al., 2002). Following axonal contact, activated Fyn may direct process outgrowth by the local recruitment of cytoskeletal proteins to sites of axonal contact as well as by modulation of the actin network. This sketch of Fyn-mediated interactions highlights the local nature of this regulatory network, where rapid responses do not require immediate nuclear involvement.

EMERGING CONCEPTS GOVERNING MYELIN FORMATION

The myelin sheath is an undisputedly unique structure in the vertebrate world. This peerless quality notwithstanding, the manner by which glia cells go about fashioning a sheath coopts time-honored cellular strategies. The *modus operandi* of myelination incorporates global signaling pathways (e.g., Shh, Notch, PDGF, Fyn), calls on members of transcription factor superfamilies esteemed in other cellular lineages (e.g., bHLH, homeodomain, POU-homeodomain), recruits myelin constituents into recognizable subcellular domains and structures (e.g., membrane rafts, mRNA-containing trafficking granules), and oversees operations with the usual posttranslational modifications (e.g., phosphorylation/dephosphorylation, acylation). This universality, coupled with the spillover of knowledge acquired from other cell lineages, has greatly accelerated the progress in defining some of the regulatory checkpoints leading to and guiding myelination. Myelin biologists are in a golden age where not only the cast of characters is assembling onstage, but technological advances are illuminating the script. The spotlight first recognized the local nature of controls that operate on the synthesis and assembly of myelin constituents in oligodendrocytes, a feature that accommodates the varying internodal demands of different axonal targets. Will Schwann cells play to the same crowd of translational and post-translational controls that reduce the directorial preeminence of the nucleus? Given an audience of one axon, probably not. Schwann cells and oligodendrocytes appear to be working on very different productions that each close with a myelin sheath finale.

Insights gained from transgenic mice and mutant animal models establish the existence of multiple overlapping paths at each stage of myelin formation. Each step features a cluster of ubiquitous and cell-specific constituents in different subcellular compartments, and the interworkings of these clusters are ultimately woven into the sheath. The *in vivo* results prod investigators to face the complexity preeminent in myelin formation and the emptiness of claiming one's favorite gene as "necessary and sufficient" for myelin formation. Complexity emanates from each stage of myelin formation and should govern future efforts to examine the forces operative in myelinating cells. Continuing efforts will focus on cataloging the genes expressed by myelin-forming cells and describing interactions between their products. These developments will direct a more integrated phase of research on myelin formation, one where myelination as a whole can be understood in terms of the cellular components and their interactions involved at each step of myelin synthesis, together with the signaling networks that link the individual steps.

ABBREVIATIONS

bFGF	basic fibroblast growth factor
bHLH	basic helix-loop-helix
CGT	ceramide galactosyl transferase
CNP	2′,3′-cyclic nucleotide-3′-phosphodiesterase
GPI	glycosylphosphatidylinositol
HD	homeodomain
HMG	high mobility group
Id	inhibitor of DNA binding
IGF-I	insulin-like growth factor I
hnRNP A2	heteronuclear ribonuclear protein A2
MAG	myelin-associated glycoprotein
MBP	myelin basic protein
MOBP	myelin-associated oligodendrocyte basic protein
NT3	neurotrophin 3
PDGFRα	platelet-derived growth factor receptor alpha
PKC	protein kinase C
PLP	proteolipid protein

REFERENCES

Agrawal, H.C., Sprinkle, T.J. and Agrawal, D. (1994) In vivo phosphorylation of 2′,3′-cyclic nucleotide 3′-phosphohydrolase (CNP): CNP in brain myelin is phosphorylated by forskolin- and phorbol ester-sensitive protein kinases. *Neurochem. Res.* 19: 721–728.

Ainger, K., Avossa, D., Diana, A.S., Barry, C., Barbarese, E., and Carson, J.H. (1997) Transport and localization elements in myelin basic protein mRNA. *J. Cell Biol.* 138:1077–1087.

Alberta, J.A., Park, S.K., Mora, J., Yuk, D., Pawlitzky, I., Iannarelli, P., Vartanian, T., Stiles, C.D., and Rowitch, D.H. (2001) Sonic hedgehog is required during an early phase of oligodendrocyte development in mammalian brain. *Mol. Cell. Neurosci.* 18:434–441.

Armstrong, R., Harvath, L., and Dubois-Dalcq, M. (1991) Astrocytes and O-2A progenitors migrate toward distinct molecules in a microchemotaxis chamber. *Ann. NY Acad. Sci.* 633:520–522.

Bermingham, J.R., Scherer, S.S., O'Connell, S., Arroyo, E., Kalla, K.A., Powell, F.L., and Rosenfeld, MG. (1996) Tst-1/Oct-6/SCIP regulates a unique step in peripheral myelination and is required for normal respiration. *Genes Dev.* 10:1751–1762.

Bertrand, N., Castro, D.S., and Guillemot, F. (2002) Proneural genes and the specification of neural cell types. *Nat. Rev. Neurosci.* 3:517–530.

Bifulco, M., Laezza, C., Stingo, S., and Wolff, J. (2002) 2′,3′-Cyclic nucleotide 3′-phosphodiesterase: a membrane-bound, microtubule-associated protein and membrane anchor for tubulin. *Proc. Natl. Acad. Sci. USA* 99:1807–1812.

Bizzozero, O.A., Bixler, H.A., Davis, J.D., Espinosa, A., and Messier, A.M. (2001) Chemical deacylation reduces the adhesive properties of proteolipid protein and leads to decompaction of the myelin sheath. *J. Neurochem.* 76:1129–1141.

Bizzozero, O.A., Leyba, J., and Nunez, D.J. (1992) Characterization of proteolipid protein fatty acylesterase from rat brain myelin. *J. Biol. Chem.* 267:7886–7894.

Bizzozero, O.A., McGarry, J.F., and Lees, M.B. (1987) Autoacylation of myelin proteolipid protein with acyl coenzyme A. *Biol. Chem.* 262:13550–13557.

Bouverat, B.P., Krueger, W.H., Coetzee, T., Bansal, R., and Pfeiffer, S.E. (2000) Expression of rab GTP-binding proteins during oligodendrocyte differentiation in culture. *Neurosci. Res.* 59:446–453.

Braun, P.E., De Angelis, D., Shtybel, W.W., and Bernier, L. (1991) Isoprenoid modification permits 2′,3′-cyclic nucleotide 3′-phosphodiesterase to bind to membranes. *J. Neurosci. Res.* 30:540–544.

Carson, J.H., Cui, H., and Barbarese, E. (2001) The balance of power in RNA trafficking. *Curr. Opin. Neurobiol.* 11:558–563.

Chandross, K.J., Cohen, R.I., Paras, P., Gravel, M., Braun, P., and Hudson, L.D. (1999) Identification and characterization of early glial progenitors using a transgenic selection strategy. *J. Neurosci.* 19:759–774.

Davies, J.E. and Miller, R.H. (2001) Local sonic hedgehog signaling regulates oligodendrocyte precursor appearance in multiple ventricular zone domains in the chick metencephalon. *Dev. Biol.* 233: 513–525.

Ericson, J., Rashbass, P., Schedl, A., Brenner-Morton, S., Kawakami, A., van Heyningen, V., Jessell, T.M., and Briscoe, J. (1997) Pax6 controls progenitor cell identity and neuronal fate in response to graded Shh signaling. *Cell* 90:169–180.

Forghani, R., Garofalo, L., Foran, D.R., Farhadi, H.F., Lepage, P., Hudson, T.J., Tretjakoff, I., Valera, P., and Peterson, A. (2001) A distal upstream enhancer from the myelin basic protein gene regulates expression in myelin-forming Schwann cells. *J. Neurosci.* 21:3780–3787.

Frost, E., Kiernan, B.W., Faissner, A., and ffrench-Constant, C. (1996) Regulation of oligodendrocyte precursor migration by extracellular matrix: evidence for substrate-specific inhibition of migration by tenascin-C. *Dev. Neurosci.* 18:266–273.

Genoud, S., Lappe-Siefke, C., Goebbels, S., Radtke, F., Aguet, M., Scherer, S.S., Suter, U., Nave, K.A., and Mantei, N. (2002) Notch1 control of oligodendrocyte differentiation in the spinal cord. *J. Cell Biol.* 158:709–718.

Ghandour, M.S. and Skoff, R.P. (1991) Double-labeling in situ hybridization analysis of mRNAs for carbonic anhydrase II and myelin basic protein: expression in developing cultured glial cells. *Glia* 4:1–10.

Givogri, M.I., Costa, R.M., Schonmann, V., Silva, A.J., Campagnoni, A.T., and Bongarzone, E.R. (2002) Central nervous system myelination in mice with deficient expression of Notch1 receptor. *J. Neurosci. Res.* 67:309–320.

Gould, R.M., Freund, C.M., and Barbarese, E. (1999) Myelin-associated oligodendrocytic basic protein mRNAs reside at different subcellular locations. *J. Neurochem.* 73:1913–1924.

Gould, R.M., Freund, C.M., Palmer, F., and Feinstein, D.L. (2000) Messenger RNAs located in myelin sheath assembly sites. *J. Neurochem.* 75:1834–1844.

Gow, A., Friedrich, V.L., Jr., and Lazzarini, R.A. (1992) Myelin basic protein gene contains separate enhancers for oligodendrocyte and Schwann cell expression. *J. Cell Biol.* 119:605–616.

Gow, A., Friedrich, V.L., Jr., and Lazzarini, R.A. (1994) Intracellular transport and sorting of the oligodendrocyte transmembrane proteolipid protein. *J. Neurosci. Res.* 37:563–573.

Gow, A. and Lazzarini, R.A. (1996) A cellular mechanism governing the severity of Pelizaeus-Merzbacher disease. *Nat. Genet.* 13:422—428.

Gudz, T.I., Schneider, T.E., Haas, T.A., and Macklin, W.B. (2002) Myelin proteolipid protein forms a complex with integrins and may participate in integrin receptor signaling in oligodendrocytes. *J. Neurosci.* 22:7398–7407.

Hasse, B., Bosse, F., and Muller, H.W. (2002) Proteins of peripheral myelin are associated with glycosphingolipid/cholesterol-enriched membranes. *J. Neurosci. Res.* 69:227–232.

Hoek, K.S., Kidd, G.J., Carson, J.H., and Smith, R. (1998) hnRNP A2 selectively binds the cytoplasmic transport sequence of myelin basic protein mRNA. *Biochemistry* 37:7021–7029.

Holz, A., Schaeren-Wiemers, N., Schaefer, C., Pott, U., Colello, R.J., and Schwab, M.E. (1996) Molecular and developmental characterization of novel cDNAs of the myelin-associated/oligodendrocytic basic protein. *J. Neurosci.* 16:467–477.

Jaegle, M., Mandemakers, W., Broos, L., Zwart, R., Karis, A., Visser, P., Grosveld, F., and Meijer, D. (1996) The POU factor Oct-6 and Schwann cell differentiation. *Science* 273:507–510.

Jensen, N.A., Pedersen, K.M., Celis, J.E., and West, M.J. (1998) Neurological disturbances, premature lethality, and central myelination deficiency in transgenic mice overexpressing the homeo domain transcription factor Oct-6. *J. Clin. Invest.* 101:1292–1299.

Jiang, H., Duchala, C.S., Awatramani, R., Shumas, S., Carlock, L., Kamholz, J., Garbern, J., Scherer, S.S., Shy, M.E., and Macklin, W.B. (2000) Proteolipid protein mRNA stability is regulated by axonal contact in the rodent peripheral nervous system. *J. Neurobiol.* 44:7–19.

John, G.R., Shankar, S.L., Shafit-Zagardo, B., Massimi, A., Lee, S.C., Raine, C.S., and Brosnan, C.F. (2002) Multiple sclerosis: re-expression of a developmental pathway that restricts oligodendrocyte maturation. *Nat. Med.* 8:1115–1121.

Kim, T. and Pfeiffer, S.E. (1999) Myelin glycosphingolipid/cholesterol-enriched microdomains selectively sequester the non-compact myelin proteins CNP and MOG. *J. Neurocytol.* 28:281–293.

Klein, C., Kramer, E.M., Cardine, A.M., Schraven, B., Brandt, R., and Trotter, J. (2002) Process outgrowth of oligodendrocytes is promoted by interaction of fyn kinase with the cytoskeletal protein tau. *J. Neurosci.* 22:698–707.

Klinghoffer, R.A., Hamilton, T.G., Hoch, R., and Soriano, P. (2002) An allelic series at the PDGFαR locus indicates unequal contributions of distinct signaling pathways during development. *Dev. Cell* 2:103–113.

Kondo, T. and Raff, M. (2000) The Id4 HLH protein and the timing of oligodendrocyte differentiation. *EMBO J.* 19:1998–2007.

Kramer, E.M., Klein, C., Koch, T., Boytinck, M., and Trotter, J. (1999) Compartmentation of Fyn kinase with glycosylphosphatidylinositol-anchored molecules in oligodendrocytes facilitates kinase activation during myelination. *J. Biol. Chem.* 274:29042–29049.

Kramer, E.M., Koch, T., Niehaus, A., and Trotter, J. (1997) Oligodendrocytes direct glycosyl phosphatidylinositol-anchored proteins to the myelin sheath in glycosphingolipid-rich complexes. *J. Biol. Chem.* 272:8937–8945.

Kramer, E.M., Schardt, A., and Nave, K.A. (2001) Membrane traffic in myelinating oligodendrocytes. *Microsc. Res. Tech.* 52:656–671.

Kwon, S., Barbarese, E., and Carson, J.H. (1999) The cis-acting RNA trafficking signal from myelin basic protein mRNA and its cognate trans-acting ligand hnRNP A2 enhance cap-dependent translation. *J. Cell Biol.* 147:247–256.

Lai, E.C. (2002) Keeping a good pathway down: transcriptional repression of Notch pathway target genes by CSL proteins. *EMBO J.* 3:840–845.

Landry, C.F., Ellison, J.A., Pribyl, T.M., Campagnoni, C., Kampf, K., and Campagnoni, A.T. (1996) Myelin basic protein gene expression in neurons: developmental and regional changes in protein targeting within neuronal nuclei, cell bodies, and processes. *J. Neurosci.* 16:2452–2462.

LoPresti, P., Szuchet, S., Papasozomenos, S.C., Zinkowski, R.P., and Binder, L.I. (1995) Functional implications for the microtubule-associated protein tau: localization in oligodendrocytes. *Proc. Natl. Acad. Sci. USA* 92:10369–10373.

Lu, Q.R., Sun, T., Zhu, Z., Ma, N., Garcia, M., Stiles, C.D., and Rowitch, D.H. (2002) Common developmental requirement for Olig function indicates a motor neuron/oligodendrocyte connection. *Cell* 5:75–86.

Lu, Q.R., Yuk, D., Alberta, J.A., Zhu, Z., Pawlitzky, I., Chan, J., McMahon, A.P., Stiles, C.D., and Rowitch, D.H. (2000) Sonic hedgehog-regulated oligodendrocyte lineage genes encoding bHLH proteins in the mammalian central nervous system. *Neuron* 25:317–329.

Mallon, B.S., Shick, H.E., Kidd, G.J., and Macklin, W.B. (2002) Proteolipid promoter activity distinguishes two populations of NG2-positive cells throughout neonatal cortical development. *J. Neurosci.* 22(3):876–885.

Nery, S., Wichterle, H., and Fishell, G. (2001) Sonic hedgehog contributes to oligodendrocyte specification in the mammalian forebrain. *Development* 128:527–540.

Nielsen, J.A., Hudson, L.D., and Armstrong, R.C. (2002) Nuclear organization in differentiating oligodendrocytes. *J. Cell Sci.* 115:4071–4079.

O'Connor, L.T., Goetz, B.D, Couve, E., Song, J., and Duncan, I.D. (2000) Intracellular distribution of myelin protein gene products is altered in oligodendrocytes of the taiep rat. *Mol. Cell. Neurosci.* 16:396–407.

Orentas, D.M., Hayes, J.E., Dyer, K.L., and Miller, R.H. (1999) Sonic hedgehog signaling is required during the appearance of spinal cord oligodendrocyte precursors. *Development* 126:2419–2429.

Poncet, C., Soula, C., Trousse, F., Kan, P., Hirsinger, E., Pourquie, O., Duprat, A.M., and Cochard, P. (1996) Induction of oligodendrocyte progenitors in the trunk neural tube by ventralizing signals: effects of notochord and floor plate grafts, and of sonic hedgehog. *Mech. Dev.* 60:13–32.

Pringle, N.P., Yu, W.P., Guthrie, S., Roelink, H., Lumsden, A., Peterson, A.C., and Richardson, W.D. (1996) Determination of neuroepithelial cell fate: induction of the oligodendrocyte lineage by ventral midline cells and sonic hedgehog. *Dev. Biol.* 177:30–42.

Qi, Y., Cai, J., Wu, Y., Wu, R., Lee, J., Fu, H., Rao, M., Sussel, L., Rubenstein, J., and Qiu, M. (2001) Control of oligodendrocyte differentiation by the Nkx2.2 homeodomain transcription factor. *Development* 128:2723–2733.

Ross, N.W. and Braun, P.E. (1988) Acylation in vitro of the myelin proteolipid protein and comparison with acylation in vivo: acylation of a cysteine occurs nonenzymatically. *Neurosci. Res.* 21:35–44.

Scherer, S.S., Vogelbacker, H.H., and Kamholz, J. (1992) Axons modulate the expression of proteolipid protein in the CNS. *J. Neurosci. Res.* 32(2):138–148.

Simons, M., Kramer, E.M., Macchi, P., Rathke-Hartlieb, S., Trotter, J., Nave, K.-A., and Schulz, J.B. (2002) Overexpression of the myelin proteolipid protein leads to accumulation of cholesterol and proteolipid protein in endosomes/lysosomes: implications for Pelizaeus-Merzbacher disease. *J. Cell Biol.* 157:327–336.

Simons, M., Kramer, E.M., Thiele, C., Stoffel, W., and Trotter, J. (2000) Assembly of myelin by association of proteolipid protein with cholesterol- and galactosylceramide-rich membrane domains. *J. Cell Biol.* 151:143–154.

Song, J., Goetz, B.D., Baas, P.W., and Duncan, I.D. (2001a) Cytoskeletal reorganization during the formation of oligodendrocyte processes and branches. *Mol. Cell. Neurosci.* 17:624–636.

Song, J., Goetz, B.D., Kirvell, S.L., Butt, A.M., and Duncan, I.D. (2001b) Selective myelin defects in the anterior medullary velum of the taiep mutant rat. *Glia* 33:1–11.

Soula, C., Danesin, C., Kan, P., Grob, M., Poncet, C., and Cochard, P. (2001) Distinct sites of origin of oligodendrocytes and somatic motoneurons in the chick spinal cord: oligodendrocytes arise from Nkx2.2-expressing progenitors by a Shh-dependent mechanism. *Development* 128:1369–1379.

Spassky, N., Goujet-Zalc, C., Parmantier, E., Olivier, C., Martinez, S., Ivanova, A., Ikenaka, K., Macklin, W., Cerruti, I., Zalc, B., and Thomas, J.L. (1998) Multiple restricted origin of oligodendrocytes. *J. Neurosci.* 18:8331–8343.

Sperber, B.R., Boyle-Walsh, E.A., Engleka, M.J., Gadue, P., Peterson, A.C., Stein, P.L., Scherer, S.S., and McMorris, F.A. (2001) A unique role for Fyn in CNS myelination. *J. Neurosci.* 21:2039–2047.

Sperber, B.R. and McMorris, F.A. (2001) Fyn tyrosine kinase regulates oligodendroglial cell development but is not required for morphological differentiation of oligodendrocytes. *J. Neurosci. Res.* 63:303–312.

Sporkel, O., Uschkureit, T., Bussow, H., and Stoffel, W. (2002) Oligodendrocytes expressing exclusively the DM20 isoform of the proteolipid protein gene: myelination and development. *Glia* 37:19–30.

Stolt, C.C., Rehberg, S., Ader, M., Lommes, P., Riethmacher, D., Schachner, M., Bartsch, U., and Wegner, M. (2002) Terminal differentiation of myelin-forming oligodendrocytes depends on the transcription factor Sox10. *Genes Dev.* 16:165–170.

Sun, X.J., Pons, S., Asano, T., Myers, M.G., Jr., Glasheen, E., and White, M.F. (1996) The Fyn tyrosine kinase binds Irs-1 and forms a distinct signaling complex during insulin stimulation. *J. Biol. Chem.* 271:10583–10587.

Sussman, C.R., Davies, J.E., and Miller, R.H. (2002) Extracellular and intracellular regulation of oligodendrocyte development: roles of Sonic hedgehog and expression of E proteins. *Glia* 40: 55–64.

Takebayashi, H., Nabeshima, Y., Yoshida, S., Chisaka, O., Ikenaka, K., and Nabeshima, Y. (2002) The basic helix-loop-helix factor olig2 is essential for the development of motoneuron and oligodendrocyte lineages. *Curr. Biol.* 12:1157–1163.

Taylor, C.M., Coetzee, T., and Pfeiffer, S.E. (2002) Detergent-insoluble glycosphingolipid/cholesterol microdomains of the myelin membrane. *J. Neurochem.* 81:993–1004.

Thomas, J.L., Spassky, N., Perez Villegas, E.M., Olivier, C., Cobos, I., Goujet-Zalc, C., Martinez, S., and Zalc, B. (2000) Spatiotemporal development of oligodendrocytes in the embryonic brain. *J. Neurosci. Res.* 59:471–476.

Thomson, C.E, Montague, P., Jung, M., Nave, K.A., and Griffiths, I.R. (1997) Phenotypic severity of murine Plp mutants reflects in vivo and in vitro variations in transport of PLP isoproteins. *Glia* 20:322–332.

Tsai, H.H., Frost, E., To, V., Robinson, S., Ffrench-Constant, C., Geertman, R., Ransohoff, R.M., and Miller, R.H. (2002) The chemokine receptor CXCR2 controls positioning of oligodendrocyte precursors in developing spinal cord by arresting their migration. *Cell* 110:373–383.

Umemori, H., Sato, S., Yagi, T., Aizawa, S., and Yamamoto, T. (1994) Initial events of myelination involve Fyn tyrosine kinase signalling. *Nature* 367:572–576.

Vallstedt, A., Muhr, J., Pattyn, A., Pierani, A., Mendelsohn, M., Sander, M., Jessell, T.M., and Ericson, J. (2001) Different levels of repressor activity assign redundant and specific roles to Nkx6 genes in motor neuron and interneuron specification. *Neuron* 31:743–755.

Vouyiouklis, D.A., Barrie, J.A., Griffiths, I.R., and Thomson, C.E. (2003) A proteolipid protein-specific pre-mRNA (Ppm-1) contains intron 3 and is up-regulated during myelination in the CNS. *J. Neurochem.* 74(3):940–948.

Wang, S., Sdrulla, A.D., diSibio, G., Bush, G., Nofziger, D., Hicks, C., Weinmaster, G., and Barres, B.A. (1998) Notch receptor activation inhibits oligodendrocyte differentiation. *Neuron* 21:63–75.

Wang, S., Sdrulla, A., Johnson, J.E., Yokota, Y., and Barres, B.A. (2001) A role for the helix-loop-helix protein Id2 in the control of oligodendrocyte development. *Neuron* 29:603–614.

Wegner, M. (2000) Transcriptional control in myelinating glia: the basic recipe. *Glia* 29:118–123.

Wilson, R. and Brophy, P.J. (1989) Role for the oligodendrocyte cytoskeleton in myelination. *J. Neurosci. Res.* 22:439–448.

Wolf, R.M., Wilkes, J.J., Chao, M.V., and Resh, M.D. (2001) Tyrosine phosphorylation of p190 RhoGAP by Fyn regulates oligodendrocyte differentiation. *J. Neurobiol.* 49:62–78.

Zhou, Q. and Anderson, D.J. (2002) The bHLH transcription factors OLIG2 and OLIG1 couple neuronal and glial subtype specification. *Cell* 109:61–73.

Zhou, Q., Choi, G., and Anderson, D.J. (2001) The bHLH transcription factor Olig2 promotes oligodendrocyte differentiation in collaboration with Nkx2.2. *Neuron* 31:791–807.

21 Myelin function and saltatory conduction

STEPHEN G. WAXMAN AND LAKSHMI BANGALORE

The need for rapid conduction of the nerve impulse serves as a driving force that can determine and increase animal size. For an axon without myelin, the speed of impulse conduction is proportional to the diameter$^{1/2}$. Therefore, in order to achieve a faster rate of conduction, species that lack myelin have to substantially enlarge their axons. In cephalopods such as squids, which lack myelin, single axons evolved to be as large as 400–900 μm in diameter; this fortuitous specialization enabled early electrophysiologists to study the nerve impulse through recordings on single nerve fibers. The price of this adaptation was an increase in size. Higher species, on the other hand, achieve high conduction velocities by ensheathment with myelin and by strategically positioning ion channels along the length of myelinated axons. This chapter will discuss the role of myelin in the conduction of nerve impulses within the vertebrate nervous system, pathophysiological consequences of demyelination, and the molecular reorganization within the axonal membrane following demyelination.

MORPHOLOGY OF MYELINATED FIBERS

The myelinated fiber consists of an axon and its myelin sheaths. Schwann cells in the peripheral nervous system (PNS) and oligodendrocytes in the central nervous system (CNS) produce myelin. A single Schwann cell myelinates only one axon, in contrast to oligodendrocytes, which myelinate a family of axons, with estimates ranging from 1–2 to nearly 100 axons per family (Bjartmar et al., 1994). The oligodendrocyte perikaryon in most cases does not circumferentially hug its myelin sheaths, as a Schwann cell does, but, on the contrary, maintains contact with its myelin sheaths by thin cytoplasmic bridges (Bunge et al., 1961; Hirano, 1968). This apparently tenuous connection between the genomic and biosynthetic machinery within the oligodendrocyte cell body and the myelin has been suggested to underlie the paucity of remyelination within the CNS. It appears, however, that there is local synthesis of myelin membrane in distal parts of the oligodendroglial processes close to the myelin sheaths (Waxman and Sims, 1984; Waxman et al., 1988) where polyribosomes are present (Waxman and Sims, 1984).

The high electrical resistance and low capacitance of myelin prevent current loss during action potential conduction. The myelin is punctuated by nodes of Ranvier. The internode distances ranging from less than 100 μm (small-diameter fibers) to slightly over 1 mm (larger-diameter fibers) optimize conduction velocity. Because of their specialization, both structural and molecular (myelin sheaths combined with nodes of Ranvier), myelinated fibers can conduct action potentials rapidly in a discontinuous, or saltatory manner, unlike nonmyelinated fibers, which usually conduct impulses in a slower, continuous manner (Huxley and Stämpfli, 1949; Tasaki, 1959). Conduction velocity in nonmyelinated fibers is proportional to the axon diameter$^{1/2}$, whereas in myelinated fibers, conduction velocity is approximately proportional to fiber diameter (Waxman and Bennett, 1972). Above a critical diameter where the conduction velocity–diameter relationships intersect, myelinated fibers conduct impulses more rapidly than nonmyelinated fibers of the same diameter; this critical diameter is approximately 0.2 μm and, within the CNS, it is the diameter at which myelination is first seen (Waxman and Bennett, 1972) (Fig. 21.1).

MOLECULAR ORGANIZATION OF THE MYELINATED AXON

Nonmyelinated axons generally display a uniform membrane structure that does not vary from one region to another (Black et al., 1981). In contrast, the myelinated axon membrane is highly specialized, with several types of voltage-sensitive ion channels and other proteins dis-

See the list of abbreviations at the end of the chapter.

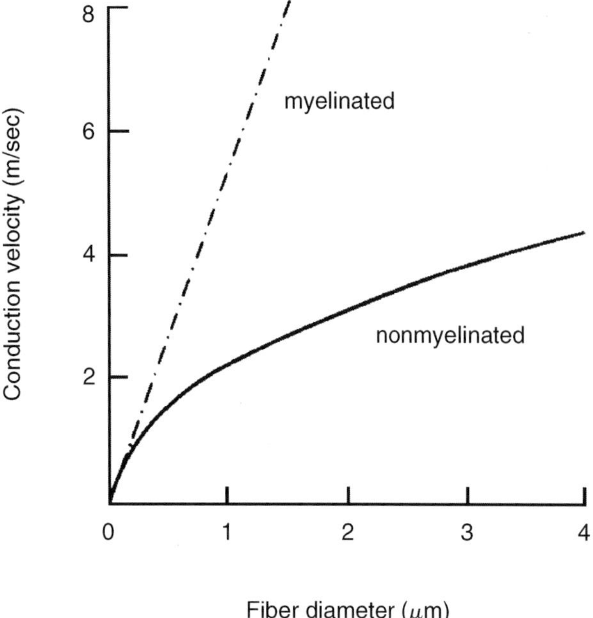

FIGURE 21.1 The relationships between conduction velocity and diameter for myelinated (*dashed line*) and nonmyelinated (*solid line*) axons are superimposed. Above a diameter of 0.2 μm, at which the two relationships cross, myelinated axons conduct more rapidly than nonmyelinated axons of the same size. In fact, 0.2 μm is the diameter of the smallest myelinated axon within the central nervous system (Modified from Waxman and Bennett, 1972.)

tributed in a spatially heterogeneous manner (Fig. 21.2). At the node of Ranvier, Na^+ channels cluster in high density (approximately $1000/\mu m^2$) in the axon membrane (Ritchie and Rogart, 1977; Waxman, 1977). In the internodal axon membrane beneath the myelin sheath, the density of Na^+ channels is much lower ($<25/\mu m^2$) (Ritchie and Rogart, 1977; Waxman, 1977), too low to support conduction under most circumstances. Nine different sodium channel subtypes have been identified so far, each with distinct molecular structures superimposed on an invariant overall motif (four similar domains, each containing six membrane-spanning segments). The identities of the sodium channel iso-

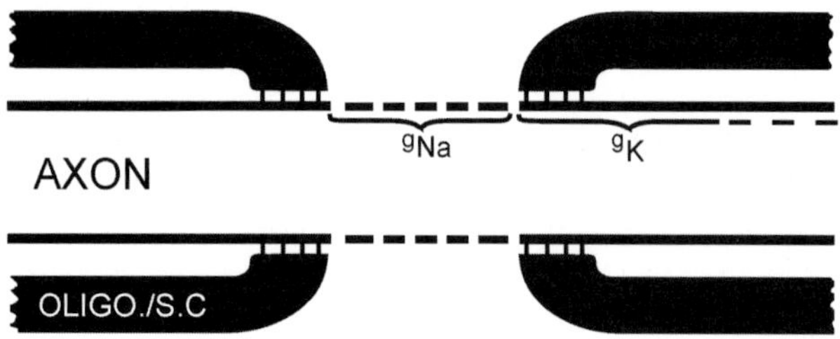

FIGURE 21.2 Schematic model of ion channel organization of the myelinated fiber g_{Na} sodium channels and g_K fast potassium channels. Sodium channels g_{Na} are clustered at the node of Ranvier. In contrast, g_K fast potassium channels, responsible for repolarization of the action potential, are present in the internodal axon membrane. Oligo/S.C.: Oligodendrocyte/Schwann cell.

forms within myelinated axons are currently under study. $Na_v1.6$ is known to be a major nodal sodium channel (Caldwell et al., 2000), but other sodium channel subtypes (e.g., $Na_v1.2$, $Na_v1.8$) are also present at some nodes (Craner et al., 2003), and $Na_v1.6$ is also present along nonmyelinated axons (Black et al., 2002a).

The sodium channel blocker, tetrodotoxin (TTX), acts specifically on sodium channels; conversely, most sodium channel isoforms are sensitive to nanomolar concentrations of TTX. Interestingly, however, two TTX-resistant (TTX-R) sodium channels, termed $Na_v1.8$/SNS (Akopian et al., 1996) and $Na_v1.9$/NaN (Dib-Hajj et al., 1998), have been cloned and characterized. $Na_v1.8$/SNS contributes to the upstroke of the action potential in cells in which it is present (Renganathan et al., 2001), while $Na_v1.9$/NaN, which is noninactivating, with substantial overlap between activation and steady-state inactivation, contributes a depolarizing influence at the resting potential and boosts subthreshold inputs (Cummins et al., 1999; Herzog et al., 2001; Baker et al., 2003). Both of these TTX-R channel isoforms are expressed preferentially in small dorsal root ganglia (DRG) neurons, and in nonmyelinated and small, myelinated axons (Fjell et al., 1997; Liu et al., 2001). Both $Na_v1.8$/SNS and $Na_v1.9$/NaN are present at nociceptive nerve terminals, suggesting that they may participate in nociceptive sensory transduction as well as impulse transmission (Black and Waxman, 2002b). $Na_v1.9$/NaN is expressed exclusively in nociceptive cells (Fang et al., 2002), making it an attractive target for drugs that might alleviate pain.

Intra-axonal recordings provide evidence for at least three types of voltage-gated potassium K^+ channels in myelinated fibers: a "fast" K^+ channel, a "slow" K^+ channel, and an inward rectifier that is permeable to both K^+ and Na^+ (Waxman and Ritchie, 1993). Fast K^+ channels can be blocked with external 4-aminopyridine (4-AP), are distributed in a pattern complementary to that of the clustered nodal Na^+ channels (i.e., in relatively low densities in the nodal axon membrane), and are present in highest density in the axon membrane beneath the myelin (Chiu and Ritchie, 1980, 1981; Ritchie et al., 1981; Foster et al., 1982; Kocsis et al., 1982; Eng et al., 1988). Voltage-clamp experiments have been interpreted as suggesting that the density of fast K^+ channels is highest in the paranode, decreasing to one-sixth of paranodal density in the node and internode (Röper and Schwarz, 1989), but this may not have accurately differentiated between the para-nodal and juxtaparanodal regions. Molecular analysis demonstrates that the Kv1.1 and Kv1.2 potassium channel subunits are localized to the juxtaparanode (Wang et al., 1993; Rasband et al., 1998; Vabnick and Shrager, 1998).

The high density of nodal Na^+ channels and the paucity of these channels in the axon membrane under the myelin, combined with the presence of fast K^+

channels in the axon membrane under the paranodal myelin, have important implications for axonal pathophysiology. Action potential electrogenesis following acute damage to the myelin is disrupted due to a low density of Na^+ channels within the exposed axon membrane and the resulting low density of inward Na^+ current (Waxman, 1982). Loss of myelin also unmasks fast K^+ channels that clamp the demyelinated axon membrane close to the K^+ equilibrium potential Ek, opposing depolarization and further impeding action potential conduction (Chiu and Ritchie, 1981).

Plasticity of the axon membrane, described below, participates in the recovery of conduction following demyelination. Recent studies have demonstrated the acquisition of a higher than normal density of Na^+ channels in some demyelinated (former internodal) axon regions, which develop the capability to support action potential conduction in the absence of myelin. The nonuniform membrane structure of the myelinated fiber also suggests the possibility of pharmacologically blocking the fast K^+ channels that are unmasked by demyelination, thereby increasing the safety factor for conduction in demyelinated axons (Bowe et al., 1987; Kocsis et al., 1987).

CONDUCTION IN MYELINATED AND DEMYELINATED AXONS

In contrast to nonmyelinated axons, in which action potentials are conducted in a continuous manner, myelinated fibers exhibit saltatory conduction in which action potentials jump from node to node in a discontinuous manner. In mammalian myelinated axons at 37°C, the time between excitation of one node and the next (internodal conduction time) is approximately 20 μs (Rasminsky and Sears, 1972). Action potential conduction is unidirectional in nature because sodium channels close soon after activation and remain refractory (due to inactivation) for a short time.

Because myelin functions as an insulator, the action current from each active node of Ranvier is shunted to subsequent nodes via the relatively low-resistance axoplasm (Fig. 21.3*A*). The safety factor (the ratio between current available to stimulate a node of Ranvier and current required to stimulate the node) is 5.0–7.7 in normal myelinated fibers, so that there is a high degree of reliability for impulse conduction (Tasaki, 1959).

When the myelin is damaged, the density of action current falls due to capacitative and resistive shunting (Fig. 21.3*B*). If the safety factor is reduced but is still greater than 1.0, the charging time for the nodal membrane will be increased so that it will take longer than normal for the axon to reach threshold, and conduction will continue but conduction velocity will be reduced. In demyelinated spinal root fibers, internodal conduction

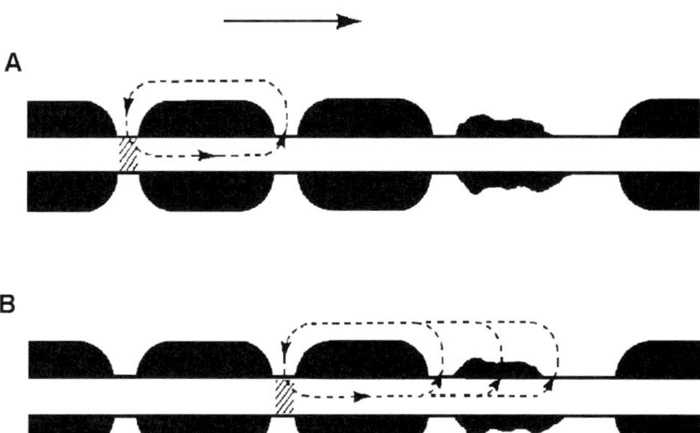

FIGURE 21.3 Diagrammatic representation of current flow associated with conduction through (*A*) normally myelinated and (*B*) demyelinated regions of an axon. The action potential is conducted from left to right (*arrow*). This idealized diagram represents the myelin as a perfect insulation. Dashed arrows illustrate current flow resulting from an action potential that is located at the crosshatched node. Current is lost in demyelinated regions as a result of capacitative and resistive shunting.

time can be increased to nearly 500 μs (Rasminsky and Sears, 1972). Thus conduction velocity is reduced. In more severely demyelinated axons, the safety factor can fall to <1.0, so that threshold will not be reached; hence conduction will fail (Waxman, 1982).

From a phenomenological point of view, demyelinated axons can display a spectrum of conduction abnormalities underlying signs and symptoms. Figure 21.4*B–E* shows conduction abnormalities that are negative in the jacksonian sense, including slowed, desynchronized, or blocked conduction. These conduction abnormalities are confined to the zone of demyelination, with normal conduction proximal and distal to the area of demyelination (Fig. 21.5). Slowed conduction appears to be less important than conduction block in producing clinical deficits (McDonald, 1963; McDonald and Sears, 1970). Temporal dispersion (loss of synchrony in tracts in which different fibers exhibit unequal degrees of conduction slowing) is a corollary of decreased conduction velocity and reflects the variability in internodal conduction times in demyelinated axons (Fig. 21.4*C*). Temporal dispersion can produce clinical abnormalities by interfering with functions such as the stretch reflex that require synchronous discharge.

Both passive and active characteristics of demyelinated fibers contribute to conduction block. In addition to capacitative current loss through injured myelin sheaths, conduction in focally demyelinated axons can fail due to impedance mismatch (Sears et al., 1978; Waxman and Brill, 1978). The low density of Na^+ channels in the demyelinated axon membrane also contributes to conduction block. Moreover, fast K^+ channels (normally covered by the myelin) are unmasked after demyelination, and because they tend to clamp the demyelinated membrane close to the potassium equlibrium potential Ek,

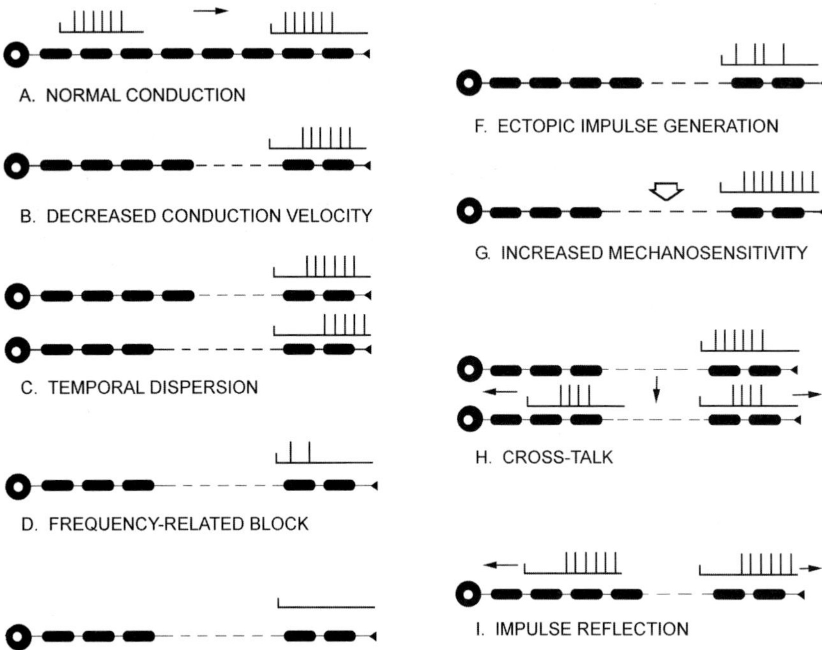

FIGURE 21.4 Conduction abnormalities in demyelinated axons. Demyelinated regions of the axon are shown diagrammatically as dashed lines. Cell bodies are located to the left and axon terminals to the right. The direction of normal conduction is indicated by the *arrow*; see text for further explanation.

they impede action potential electrogenesis (Bostock et al., 1981; Ritchie and Chiu, 1981).

Conduction failure can be frequency-related, with high-frequency impulse trains failing to propagate while low-frequency trains conduct reliably (Fig. 21.4*D*); in more severely affected fibers, conduction failure can be complete, with single action potentials failing to propagate beyond the zone of demyelination (Fig. 21.4*E*). Hyperpolarization of the axon membrane, due to electrogenic pump (Na^+, K^+-ATPase) activity, may contribute to conduction block of high-frequency impulse trains (Bostock and Grafe, 1985). Elevated intracellular Na^+ at the *driving node* (Rasminsky and Sears, 1972) and depolarization of demyelinated axons due to increases in extracellular K^+ concentration (Brismar, 1981) may also contribute to high-frequency block. Conduction abnormalities that are positive in a jacksonian sense are illustrated in Figure 21.4*F–I*. Ectopic impulse generation (Fig. 21.4*F*) has been observed, for example, in demyelinated dorsal column axons (Smith and McDonald, 1980). Abnormal cross-talk may occur between abnormally myelinated axons (Fig. 21.4*H*). Increased mechanosensitivity (Fig. 21.4*G*) probably accounts for clinical phenomena such as Tinel's and Lhermitte's signs (Smith and McDonald, 1980; Vollmer et al., 1991). Impulse reflection may occur in some focally demyelinated fibers (Burchiel, 1980) and may result in extraneous activity (e.g., paresthesia, pain, or tonic spasms). Because reflected (antidromic) impulses can collide with and abolish orthodromic impulses, impulse reflection may also interfere with normal impulse traffic.

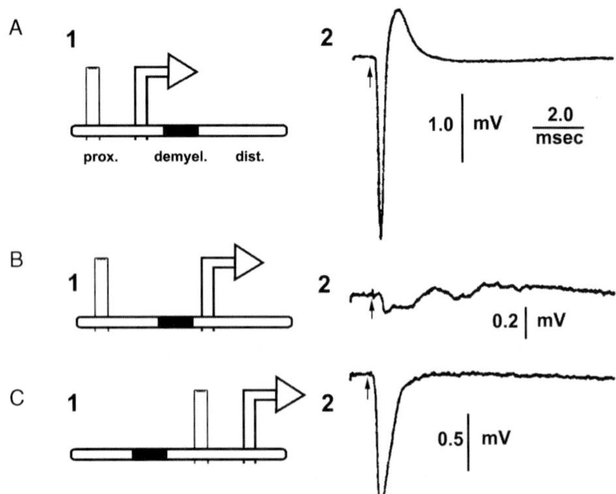

FIGURE 21.5 Recording obtained proximal to (*A*), across (*B*), and distal to (*C*) a focally demyelinated region (injected with lysophosphatidylcholine) from rat sciatic nerve. Conduction is relatively normal in proximal and distal nerve segments where myelin is intact (*A2, C2*). However, conduction slowing, block, and temporal dispersion (*B2*) are present when action potentials are conducted through the lesion site. (Modified from Kocsis and Waxman, 1985.)

A number of reports have suggested that *neuroelectric blocking factors* or *sodium channel–blocking factors* may contribute to the pathophysiology of neuroinflammatory disorders but, in general, these reports have not been confirmed by subsequent studies. It has recently been proposed that paralysis in Guillain-Barré syndrome may be due to an Na^+ channel-blocking factor in the cerebrospinal fluid (Brinkmeier et al., 1992), and that the cerebrospinal fluid of multiple sclerosis

(MS) patients contains the same factor (Brinkmeier et al., 1993). A recent study has purported to identify this blocking factor as a pentapeptide with the sequence Gln-Tyr-Asn-Ala-Asp (QYNAD) (Brinkmeier et al., 2000). QYNAD was reported to block sodium channels at concentrations as low as 10 μM by shifting steady-state inactivation to more negative potentials (Weber et al., 1999; Brinkmeier et al., 2000). Cummins et al. (2003) have, however, demonstrated that QYNAD has no sodium channel–blocking effects even at concentrations as high as 500 μM. At this time, there has been no definitive demonstration of an Na^+ channel–blocking factor that contributes to the pathophysiology of Guillain-Barré syndrome or MS.

Continuous Conduction Following Demyelination

While impulses are conducted in normal myelinated fibers by saltatory conduction with excitability apparently confined to the nodes of Ranvier (Rasminsky and Sears, 1972), continuous action potential conduction has been observed in some demyelinated axons (Bostock and Sears, 1976). Some axons can conduct with a velocity that can fall to as low as 5% of the normal saltatory conduction velocity over continuous lengths of demyelination exceeding 2 mm (several internodes) (Felts et al., 1977).

Since sodium channels are sequestered at nodes along myelinated axons, how can continuous conduction occur along previously internodal parts of the axon following demyelination? Computer simulations indicate that, in some small-caliber demyelinated axons, the density of preexisting Na^+ channels in the demyelinated region may approach the density required to support conduction (Waxman and Brill, 1978; Hines and Shrager, 1991). In very small premyelinated axons (diameter <0.25 μm) the conduction of single action potentials can be supported by Na^+ channel densities of $<10/\mu m^2$ (Waxman et al., 1989). The diameter of some demyelinated axons is reduced (Prineas and Connell, 1978; Smith et al., 1983), possibly as a result of decreased neurofilament phosphorylation and increased neurofilament packing density (De Waegh et al., 1992). Nevertheless, these results may not apply to larger axons due to their lower input impedance. For this reason, the acquisition of a higher than normal Na^+ channel density appears to be required for restoration of conduction. There is experimental evidence indicating that this does in fact occur in some demyelinated axons.

Early ultrastructural studies on experimentally demyelinated axons demonstrated the development of regions of axon membrane with cytochemical (Foster et al., 1980) and freeze-fracture (Black et al., 1987) characteristics similar to those of nodal membrane, suggesting the acquisition of a higher than normal Na^+ channel density. Additional evidence for the acquisition of increased Na^+ channel densities in the demyelinated parts of the axon membrane was provided by immunocytochemical studies. Studies on fish lateral line nerves revealed the development of relatively high densities of Na^+ channels in previously internodal regions (England et al., 1990). Similarly, immunocytochemical observations 2–3 weeks following injection of the demyelinating toxin doxorubicin suggest the expression of sodium channels at newly formed nodes along mammalian remyelinated axons (Dugandzija-Novakovic et al., 1995). These early investigations, however, relied on generic sodium channel antibodies that did not differentiate between channel subtypes.

Early studies suggested that the acquisition of higher than normal densities of Na^+ channels in demyelinated axon regions is due to a dedifferentiation of the axon membrane (see below). While the mature internodal membrane is incapable of secure conduction (Ritchie and Rogart, 1977; Waxman, 1977), the premyelinated axon membrane (including regions destined to develop into internodal membrane) is electrically excitable (Foster et al., 1982; Waxman et al., 1989). Studies on the developing internodal axon during normal ontogenesis indicate that suppression of Na^+ channel expression reduces axonal excitability and suggest that this occurs *after axons are covered by myelin*, ensuring that conduction is not compromised due to a premature loss of Na^+ channels during development (Black et al., 1986).

Recent studies at the molecular level have provided evidence that there is, in fact, a dedifferentiation of the axon membrane in some demyelinated axons. Craner et al. (2003) used subtype-specific antibodies for immunocytochemical analysis of demyelinated CNS axons in experimental allergic encephalomyelitis and observed a switch from $Na_v1.6$ to $Na_v1.2$ expression at nodes. Some demyelinated axons exhibited continuous immunostaining for $Na_v1.2$ and, less frequently, for $Na_v1.6$ channels, which extended for tens of micrometers along the fiber trajectory (i.e., as far as the axons could be followed within sections). A similar pattern of continuous $Na_v1.2$ immunostaining is seen in premyelinated axons (Boiko et al., 2001) and may provide a substrate for continuous conduction of impulses. The functional implications of a reversion to $Na_v1.2$ expression (rather than $Na_v1.6$) are not fully understood. Some evidence from patch-clamp studies (Zhou and Goldin, 2002) suggests that different functional properties may permit $Na_v1.6$ channels to support higher firing rates. Substitution of $Na_v1.2$ for $Na_v1.6$ may permit conduction to continue in demyelinated axons, but with lower reliability in terms of sustained high-frequency firing.

Nonuniform Conduction Following Demyelination

Nonuniform impulse propagation may also contribute to recovery of conduction in some demyelinated axons.

In this type of conduction, the action potential propagates nonuniformly between isolated foci of inward current generation (*phi-nodes*), which appear to be scattered aggregations of Na^+ channels that are established before remyelination (Smith et al., 1982). Phi-nodes develop several days before remyelination, consistent with the suggestion (Smith et al., 1982) that they are the precursors of nodes. Phi-nodes extend longitudinally for only several micrometers along each axon, similar to the node of Ranvier. Freeze-fracture demonstrates patches of E-face intramembranous particles with a particle size similar to those in the nodal axon at phi-nodes, consistent with the idea that these membrane foci are clusters of Na^+ channels (Rosenbluth and Blakemore, 1984). Moreover, the number of intramembranous particles in each patch is approximately the same as those of a mature node (Black et al., 1986).

MOLECULAR PLASTICITY OF THE DEMYELINATED AXON

In some demyelinated axons the sodium channel density increases so that it can support impulse invasion into the demyelinated region and continuous conduction through it (Bostock and Sears, 1978; Foster et al., 1980). While this could, in theory, reflect the redistribution of preexisting Na^+ channels from nearby nodes into the demyelinated (previously internodal) membrane, there is evidence (Hines and Shrager, 1991) that channel diffusion is not sufficient to support action potential conduction through demyelinated regions. Former nodes of Ranvier in demyelinated axons, when studied by patch-clamp, display sharp gradients in channel density, which have been interpreted as suggesting that Na^+ channels do not diffuse away from the node in large numbers following demyelination (Shrager, 1989). Radioimmunoassay studies demonstrate a significant increase in Na^+ channel concentration per weight of tissue (approximately 3-fold at 21–28 days after peripheral nerve demyelination), supporting the idea that new Na^+ channels are inserted into the demyelinated axon membrane (England et al., 1991). Quantitative autoradiography reveals a 4-fold increase in STX-binding sites in demyelinated white matter in MS patients compared with normal white matter (Moll et al., 1991). The switch from expression of $Na_v1.2$ to $Na_v1.6$ channels in demyelinated axons (Craner et al., 2003) also indicates that new channels are deployed.

The site of production of the Na^+ channels in demyelinated axons has not yet been definitively identified. Synthesis of channels in the neuronal cell body, with translocation by the axonal transport, is a clear possibility. Electrophysiological experiments have demonstrated the production of new, functional Na^+ channels by neurons after axonal transection (Kuno and Llinas, 1970), and there is evidence for axonal transport of Na^+ channels in peripheral nerves (Lombet et al., 1985). Craner et al. (2003) noted upregulated transcription of $Na_v1.2$ mRNA in neuronal cell bodies giving rise to demyelinated axons, implying that new channels are produced by the neuron.

Increased synthesis of sodium channels in demyelinated neurons does not necessarily imply that the appropriate types of sodium channels are added to the axon membrane. Following axonal transection, as shown in Figure 21.6, there are changes in the pattern of sodium channel gene activation in the affected neurons, which express abnormal combinations of sodium channel mRNA (Waxman et al., 1994; Dib-Hajj et al., 1996, 1998) and protein (Sleeper et al., 2000). For ex-

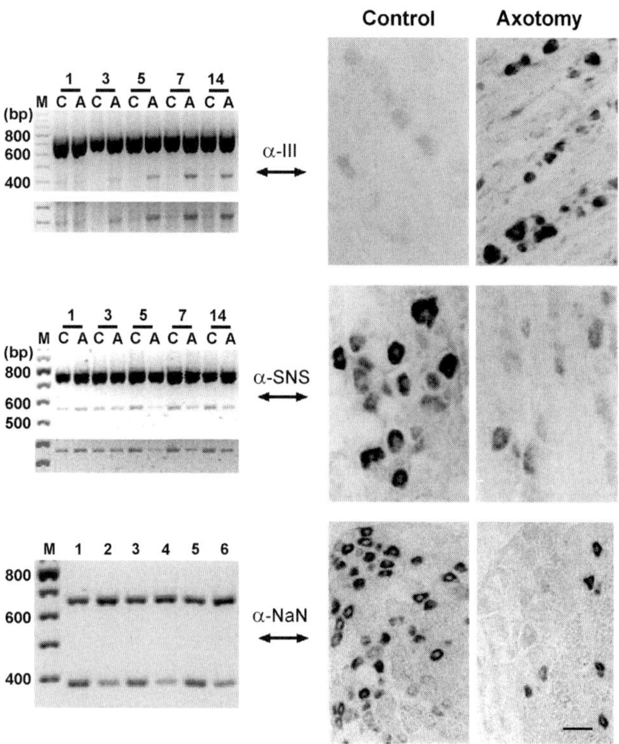

FIGURE 21.6 Na^+ channel expression can change strikingly in neurons following injury. mRNA for Na^+ channel $Na_v1.3$ (*α-III*) (*top*) is upregulated, and mRNA for $Na_v1.8$/SNS (*middle*) and $Na_v1.9$/NaN (*bottom*) are downregulated, in dorsal root ganglia (DRG) neurons following transection of their axons within the sciatic nerve. The *in situ* hybridizations (*right side*) show α-III, $Na_v1.8$ (SNS), and $Na_v1.9$ (NaN) mRNA in control DRG and at 5–7 days post-axotomy. Reverse transcriptase–polymerase chain reaction (*left side*) shows products of coamplification of α-III and SNS together with b-actin transcripts in control (C) and axotomized (*A*) DRG (days postaxotomy indicated above gels), with computer-enhanced images of amplification products shown below gels. Coamplification of NaN (392 bp) and reduced glyceraldehyde-phosphate dehydrogenase (GAPDH) (6076 bp) shows decreased expression of NaN mRNA at 7 days postaxotomy (lanes 2, 4, 6) compared to controls (lanes 1, 3, 5). (Top and middle panels modified from Dib-Hajj et al., 1996; bottom modified from Dib-Hajj et al., 1998.)

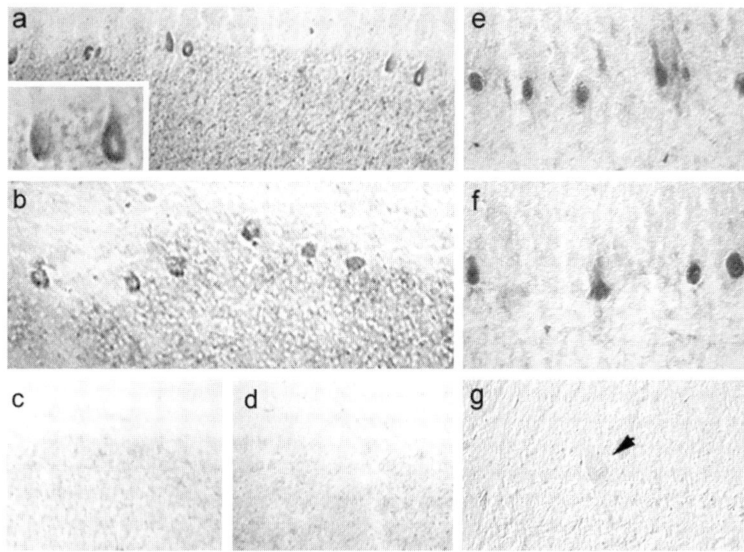

FIGURE 21.7 Expression of sodium channel $Na_v1.8$/SNS is upregulated within cerebellar Purkinje cells within brains obtained at postmortem from multiple sclerosis (MS) patients. The panels at the left show *in situ* hybridization with $Na_v1.8$-specific antisense riboprobes, and demonstrate the absence of $Na_v1.8$ (SNS) mRNA in control cerebellum (*c*) and its presence in Purkinje cells in postmortem tissue from two patients with MS (*a,b*). No signal is present following hybridization with sense riboprobe (*d*). The panels on the right show immunostaining with antibody directed against $Na_v1.8$, and illustrate the absence of $Na_v1.8$ protein in control cerebellum (*g*; *arrow* indicates Purkinje cell) and its presence in MS (*e,f*). (Modified from Black et al., 2000.)

ample, axonal transection of spinal sensory neurons results in downregulation of the expression of the TTX-R sodium channels $Na_v1.8$ and $Na_v1.9$ and an attenuation of their currents (Dib-Hajj et al., 1999; Sleeper et al., 2000). Concomitantly there is upregulated expression of $Na_v1.3$ (Waxman et al., 1994; Black et al., 1999a) that produces a rapidly repriming TTX-sensitive sodium current (Cummins and Waxman, 1997; Cummins et al., 2001).

Abnormal patterns of sodium channel expression within one particular type of neuron, the cerebellar Purkinje cell, have also been observed in several models of demyelination and in tissue from MS patients (Fig. 21.7). Sodium channel $Na_v1.8$, also termed SNS, is normally expressed only in spinal sensory and trigeminal neurons, but it is upregulated in Purkinje cells derived from patients with MS who exhibited cerebellar deficits on neurological examination (Black et al., 2000). Similar upregulation of $Na_v1.8$ was observed in the Purkinje cells of mice with chronic relapsing experimental allergic encephalomyelitis (CR-EAE), an inflammatory model of MS (Black et al., 2000). $Na_v1.8$ contributes a substantial fraction of the inward transmembrane current underlying action potential electrogenesis in cells in which it is normally present (Renganathan et al., 2001). Whether the expression of $Na_v1.8$ is adaptive (contributing to restoration of conduction along demyelinated Purkinje cell axons) or maladaptive (perturbing the pattern of impulse activity in Purkinje cells) is not clear. Evidence supporting the latter hypothesis comes from the observation that transfection with $Na_v1.8$ can substantially distort the pattern of impulse activity in cultured Purkinje neurons (Renganathan et al., 2003).

Another potential source of sodium channels that has been proposed is synthesis in glial cells, with subsequent transfer to the axon (Bevan et al., 1985; Gray and Ritchie, 1985). Perinodal astrocyte processes and Schwann cell microvilli contact the axon membrane at the node in a highly specific manner (Hildebrand, 1971; Waxman and Black, 1984). Similar glial processes are apposed to demyelinated axons at sites of Na^+ channel clustering (Black et al., 1984; Rosenbluth and Blakemore, 1984; Rosenbluth, 1985). The two specializations (glial contact and Na^+ channel clustering) usually are juxtaposed, suggesting that glial cell contact may be involved in the development of Na^+ channel clusters in the axon membrane. Patch-clamp has demonstrated that voltage-sensitive Na^+ currents in astrocytes (Bevan et al., 1985; Barres et al., 1989; Sontheimer et al., 1992) and the mRNAs for neuronal-type Na^+ channel α- and β-subunits are present (Black et al., 1994a, 1994b; Oh and Waxman, 1994). However, transfer of channels from glial cells to axons has not been demonstrated. Evidence against the *glial cell transfer* hypothesis is provided by observations of increased numbers of Na^+ channels along demyelinated axons in fish lateral line nerves after injection of doxorubicin; because Schwann cells are killed by this drug, it has been argued that glial synthesis of Na^+ channels is unlikely (England et al., 1991). Alternative functions have been proposed for astrocyte Na^+ channels [e.g., providing a return pathway for Na^+ ions that maintains astrocyte Na^+ and K^+-ATPase activity (Sontheimer et al., 1994)]. Astrocytes may also secrete extracellular molecules that target or anchor Na^+ channels at sites of aggregation (Waxman, 1992).

IMPEDANCE MISMATCH IN DEMYELINATED AXONS

A high Na^+ channel density in demyelinated axon regions does not, in itself, ensure secure conduction. Impedance mismatch due to electrical loading (largely as a result of increased membrane capacitance) can cause conduction block at sites of axonal inhomogeneity, such as the junction between myelinated and demyelinated regions (Waxman, 1978). Figure 21.8*A* shows computer-simulated action potentials (Waxman and Brill, 1978) in a fiber in which a single internode (between nodes D_1 and D_4) was focally demyelinated, in which the demyelinated axon membrane has developed a high Na^+ channel density (similar to that at nodes). Conduction block occurs at the junction between normal and demyelinated axon regions (D_1), despite the high Na^+ channel density in the demyelinated area, because impedance mismatch prevents threshold from being reached.

For action potentials to successfully invade the demyelinated zone, impedance mismatch must be overcome; that is, there must be impedance matching. Impedance matching can be achieved, as shown in Figure 21.8*B*, by the development of relatively short myelinated segments proximal to the demyelinated area (Waxman and Brill, 1978), a decrease in the axon diameter of the demyelinated region relative to the upstream myelinated segment (Sears and Bostock, 1981), the development of an increased Na^+ channel density at the node proximal to the demyelinated area, or the development of a specialized transition zone (with relatively high Na^+ channel densities or relatively low K^+ channel densities) at the border of the region of demyelination (Waxman and Wood, 1984). The short length of remyelinated myelin segments may thus serve an adaptive function by facilitating impedance matching.

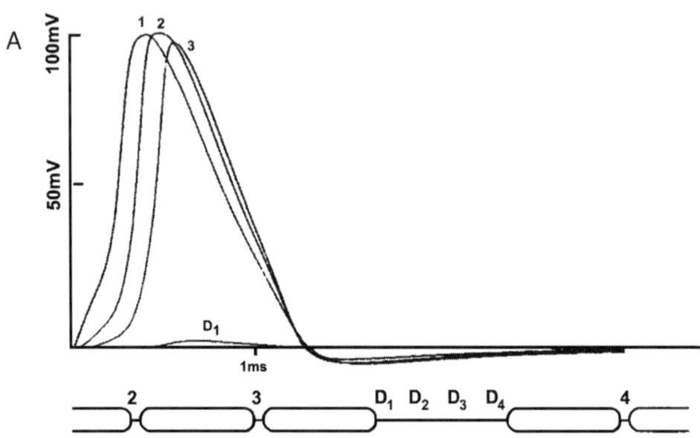

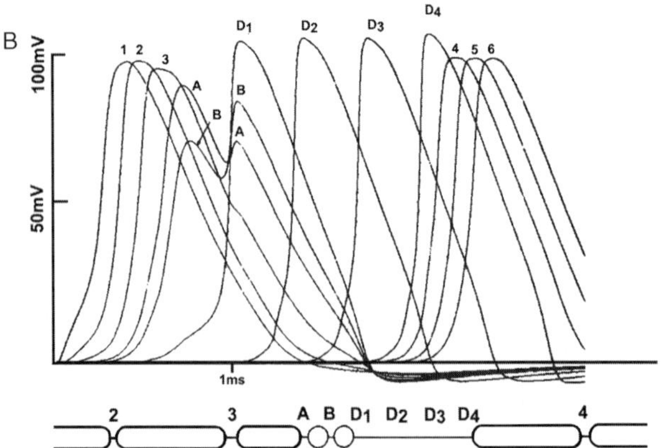

FIGURE 21.8 *A*. Computer simulations showing conduction through a focally demyelinated axon. Even in the presence of an adequate density of sodium channels in the demyelinated zone (D_1–D_4), conduction fails as a result of impedance mismatch. *B*. Interposition of two short internodes, just proximal to the demyelinated zone, provides impedance matching that facilitates conduction into, and then through, the demyelinated zone (From Waxman and Brill, 1978.)

REMYELINATION

Computer simulations suggest that remyelination with even thin or short myelin sheaths should provide a capacitative shield that promotes conduction through previously demyelinated fibers, as long as the remyelinated nodes of Ranvier develop sodium channel densities similar to those in normal fiber (Koles and Rasminsky, 1972; Waxman and Brill, 1978) and impedance mismatch is corrected. Cytochemical studies suggest that newly formed nodes acquire a high density of sodium channels (Weiner et al., 1980). Additional evidence is provided by observations on experimentally demyelinated-remyelinated axons that display an increase in STX binding that is proportional to the increase in nodal membrane area imposed by the shorter internodal spacing (Ritchie, 1982) and by immunocytochemical studies that show foci of sodium channel immunoreactivity at the newly formed nodes (Shrager, 1989).

In demyelinated peripheral nerves, conduction velocity approaches normal, and the refractory period is reduced and the ability to conduct high-frequency impulse trains is improved as remyelination occurs (Smith and Hall, 1980; Smith et al., 1981; Smith et al., 1983). Clinical recovery in rats with EAE is correlated with remyelination and the resultant restoration of conduction (Stanley and Pender, 1991). The reduced internode distances in remyelinated fibers result in conduction velocities that, while higher than those in demyelinated axons, are lower than those in normally myelinated axons (Brill et al., 1977). However, decreased conduction velocity does not necessarily, of itself, produce clinical deficits; hence, restoration of conduction as a result of remyelination would still be expected to lead to clinical improvement.

Both oligodendrocyte- and Schwann cell–mediated remyelination of CNS axons can enhance conduction. Remyelination of dorsal column axons by Schwann cells, for example, restores secure action potential conduction, characterized by a normal refractory period of transmission (but with decreased conduction velocity), and also restores the ability to conduct high-frequency impulse trains in these fibers (Blight and Young, 1989; Felts, 1991). This provides a rationale for transplantation of myelin-forming cells to the demyelinated CNS.

Transplantation of Myelin-Forming Cells

Morphological studies have shown that transplanted Schwann cells and oligodendrocytes can form myelin with a relatively normal compact structure around demyelinated axons within the CNS (Duncan et al., 1988; Gout, 1988; Rosenbluth et al., 1989). Transplanted 02-A glial progenitor cells can also differentiate and form myelin in the CNS (Groves et al., 1993). Until recently, however, the primary assay for the outcome of transplantation was structural (i.e., a determination of whether or not morphologically normal myelin was formed). As discussed above, the formation of compact myelin by transplanted cells does not, in itself, ensure improved conduction, since impedance mismatch or failure to form nodes with adequate Na^+ channel densities can lower the safety factor.

In the first physiological study of conduction properties in axons myelinated by transplanted cells, Utzschneider et al. (1994) examined myelin-deficient axons in the *md* rat spinal cord after transplantation of oligodendrocytes and demonstrated a 4-fold increase in conduction velocity, which approached myelinated control values after formation of myelin by transplanted glial cells. Ability to follow high-frequency stimulation was restored almost to normal. Moreover, action potentials could be initiated outside the transplant region, could invade and propagate into the region of demyelination, and could then propagate beyond the demyelinated region. Similar improvements in action potential conduction have been observed following transplantation of Schwann cells (Honmou et al., 1996), olfactory ensheathing cells (Imaizumi et al., 1998), *humanized* olfactory ensheathing cells from the pig (Imaizumi et al., 2000), and bone marrow stromal cells (Akiyama et al., 2002) to demyelinated lesions within the spinal cord of adult rats. Thus, there is abundant evidence that action potential conduction in demyelinated and dysmyelinated axons can be enhanced in animal models following myelination by exogenous transplanted cells. Studies currently underway are examining the effects of glial cell transplantation in other models, and the first human studies are beginning.

OVERVIEW

As summarized above, myelin plays a crucial role in action potential conduction, but the myelinated axon is more than a bare axon with myelin wrapped around it. The membrane of the myelinated axon contains aggregations of sodium channels that support saltatory conduction from node to node. The complexity of the myelinated fiber is matched by the complexity of demyelination. Passive and active properties of the axon interact to shape the conduction properties of demyelinated axon, and a variety of cellular and molecular mechanisms contribute to these properties. The multifactorial determinants of altered axonal conduction after demyelination have made it more difficult to study, but also have provided multiple therapeutic strategies that may enhance the function of demyelinated axons. These include pharmacological manipulation of K^+ channels, promotion of Na^+ channel expression in demyelinated axons, manipulation of cellular characteristics to correct impedance mismatch at the edge of the plaque, and transplantation of myelin-forming cells so that they can restore conduction in demyelinated axons.

ACKNOWLEDGMENTS

The authors' research has been supported in part by grants from the National Multiple Sclerosis Society and the Rehabilitation Research Service and Medical Research Service, Department of Veterans Affairs, as well as by gifts from the Eastern Paralyzed Veterans Association, the Paralyzed Veterans of America, and the Nancy Davis Foundation.

ABBREVIATIONS

CNS	central nervous system
DRG	dorsal root ganglia
Na_v	voltage-gated sodium channel
PNS	peripheral nervous system
MS	multiple sclerosis
TTX	tetrodotoxin

REFERENCES

Akiyama, Y., Radtke, C., and Kocsis, J.D. (2002) Remyelination of the rat spinal cord by transplantation of identified bone marrow stromal cells. *J. Neurosci.* 22:6623–6630.

Akopian, A.N., Sivilotti, L., and Wood, J.N. (1996) A tetrodotoxin-resistant voltage-gated sodium channel expressed by sensory neurons. *Nature* 379:257–262.

Baker, M., Chandra, S., Ding, Y., Waxman, S., and Wood, J. (2003) GTP-induced TTX-resistant Na^+ current regulates excitability in mouse and rat small diameter sensory neurons. *J. Physiol. (Lond.)*, 548(2):373–382.

Barres, B.A., Chun, L.L.Y., and Corey, D.P. (1989) Glial and neuronal forms of the voltage–dependent sodium channels: Characteristics and cell-type distribution. *Neuron* 2:1375–1388.

Bevan, S., Chiu, S.Y., Gray, P.T.A., and Ritchie, J.M. (1985) The presence of voltage-gated sodium, potassium and chloride channels in rat cultured astrocytes. *Proc. R. Soc. Lond.* B225:229–313.

Bjartmar, C., Hildebrand, C., and Loinder, K. (1994) Morphological heterogeneity of rat oligodendrocytes: electron microscopic studies on serial sections. *Glia* 11:235–244.

Black, J.A., Cummins, T.R., Plumpton, C., Chen, Y.H., Hormuzdiar, W., Clare, J.J., and Waxman, S.G. (1999a) Upregulation of a silent sodium channel after peripheral, but not central, nerve injury in DRG neurons. *J. Neurophysiol.* 82:2776–2785.

Black, J.A., Dib-Hajj, S., Baker, D., Newcombe, J., Cuzner, M.L., and Waxman, S.G. (2000) Sensory neuron-specific sodium channel SNS is abnormally expressed in the brains of mice with experimental allergic encephalomyelitis and humans with multiple sclerosis. *Proc. Natl. Acad. Sci. USA* 97:11598–11602.

Black, J.A., Dib-Hajj, S., McNabola, K., Jeste, S., Rizzo, M.A., Kocsis, J.D., and Waxman, S.G. (1996) Spinal sensory neurons express multiple sodium channel alpha-subunit mRNAs. *Mol. Brain Res.* 43:117–131.

Black, J.A., Fjell, J., Dib-Hajj, S., Duncan, I.D., O'Connor, L.T., Fried, K., Gladwell, Z., Tate, S., and Waxman, S.G. (1999b) Abnormal expression of SNS/PN3 sodium channel in cerebellar Purkinje cells following loss of myelin in the taiep rat. *NeuroReport* 10:913–918.

Black, J.A., Foster, R.E., and Waxman, S.G. (1981) Freeze-fracture ultrastructure of rat CNS and PNS nonmyelinated axolemma. *J. Neurocytol.* 10:981–993.

Black, J.A., Renganathan, M., and Waxman, S.G. (2002a) Sodium channel $Na_v1.6$ is expressed along nonmyelinated axons and it contributes to conduction. *Mol. Brain Res.* 105:19–28.

Black, J.A. and Waxman, S.G. (2002b) Molecular identities of two tetrodotoxin-resistant sodium channels in corneal axons. *Exp. Eye Res.* 75:193–199.

Black, J.A., Waxman, S.G., and Hildebrand, C. (1984) Membrane specialization and axo-glial association in the rat retinal nerve fiber layer: freeze-fracture observations. *J. Neurocytol.* 13:417–430.

Black, J.A., Waxman, S.G., Sims, T.J., and Gilmore, S.A. (1986) Effects of delayed myelination by oligodendrocytes and Schwann cells on the macromolecular structure of axonal membrane in rat spinal cord. *J. Neurocytol.* 15:745–762.

Black, J.A., Waxman, S.G., and Smith, M.E. (1987) Macromolecular structure of axonal membrane during acute experimental allergic encephalomyelitis in rat and guinea pig spinal cord. *J. Neuropathol. Exp. Neurol.* 46:167–184.

Black, J.A., Westenbroek, R., Ransom, B.R., Catterall, W.A., and Waxman, S.G. (1994a) Type II sodium channels in spinal cord astrocytes in situ: immunocytochemical observations. *Glia* 12: 219–227.

Black, J.A., Yokoyama, S., Waxman, S.G., Oh, Y., Zur, K.B., Sontheimer, H., Higashida, H., and Ransom, B.R. (1994b) Sodium channel mRNAs in cultured spinal cord astrocytes: in situ hybridization in identified cell types. *Mol. Brain Res.* 23:235–245.

Blight, A.R. and Young, W. (1989) Central axons in injured cat spinal cord recover electrophysiological function following remyelination by Schwann cells. *J. Neurol. Sci.* 91:15–34.

Boiko, T., Rasband, M.N., Levinson, S.R., Caldwell, J.H., Mandel, G., Trimmer, J.S., and Mattews, G. (2001) Compact myelin dictates the differential targeting of two sodium channel isoforms in the same axon. *Neuron* 30:91–104.

Bostock, H. and Grafe, P. (1985) Activity-dependent excitability changes in normal and demyelinated rat spinal root axons. *J. Physiol.* (*Lond.*) 365:239–257.

Bostock, H., and Sears, T.A. (1976) Continuous conduction in demyelinated mammalian nerve fibers. *Nature* 263:786–787.

Bostock, H., and Sears, T.A. (1978) The internodal axon membrane: electrical excitability and continuous conduction in segmental demyelination. *J. Physiol.* (*Lond.*) 280:273–301.

Bostock, H., Sears, T.A., and Sherratt, R.M. (1981) The effects of 4-aminopyridine and tetraethylammonium ions on normal and demyelinated mammalian nerve fibers. *J. Physiol.* (*Lond.*) 313: 301–315.

Bowe, C.M., Targ, E.F., Kocsis, J.D., and Waxman, S.G. (1987) Differences in the effects of 4-AP on demyelinated motor and sensory fiber. *Ann. Neurol.* 22:264–268.

Brill, M.H., Waxman, S.G., Moore, J.W., and Joyner, R.W. (1977) Conduction velocity and spike configuration in myelinated fibers: computed dependence on internode distance. *J. Neurol. Neurosurg. Psychiatry* 40:769–774.

Brinkmeier, H., Aulkemeyer, P., Wollinsky, K.H., and Rudel, R. (2000) An endogenous pentapeptide acting as a sodium channel blocker in inflammatory autoimmune disorders of the CNS. *Nat. Med.* 6:808–811.

Brinkmeier, H., Wollinsky, K.H., Hulser, P.-J., Seewald, M.J., Mehrkens H.H., and Kornhuber, H.H. (1992) The acute paralysis in Guillain-Barré syndrome is related to Na^+ channel blocking factor in the cerebrospinal. *Eur. J. Physiol.* 421:552–557.

Brinkmeier, H., Wollinsky, K.H., Seewald, M.J., Hulser, P.J., Mehrkens, H.H., Kornhuber, H.H., and Rudel, R. (1993) Factors in the cerebrospinal fluid of MS patients interfering with voltage-dependent sodium channels. *Neurosci. Lett.* 156:172–175.

Brismar, T. (1981) Specific permeability properties of demyelinated rat nerve fibers. *Acta Physiol. Scand.* 113:167–176.

Bunge, M.B., Bunge, R.P., and Pappas, G.D. (1961) Electron microscope demonstration of connections between glia and myelin sheaths in the developing mammalian central nervous system. *J. Cell Biol.* 12:448–453.

Burchiel, K. (1980) Abnormal impulse generation in focally demyelinated trigeminal roots. *J. Neurosurg.* 53:674–683.

Caldwell, J.H., Schaller, K.L., Lasher, R.S., Peles, E., and Levinson, S.R. (2000) Sodium channel Na(v)1.6 is localized at nodes of ranvier, dendrites, and synapses. *Proc. Natl. Acad. Sci. USA* 97: 5616–5620.

Chiu, S.Y. and Ritchie, J.M. (1980) Potassium channels in nodal and internodal axonal membrane in mammalian myelinated fibers. *Nature* 284:170–171.

Chiu, S.Y. and Ritchie, J.M. (1981) Evidence for the presence of potassium channels in the paranodal region of acutely demyelinated nerve fibers. *J. Physiol.* (*Lond.*) 313:415–437.

Craner, M.J., Lo, A.C., Black, J.A., and Waxman, S.G. (2003) Abnormal sodium channel distribution in optic nerve axons in a model of inflammatory demyelination. *Brain* 126:1552–1561.

Cummins, T.R., Aglieco, F., Renganathan, M., Herzog, R.I., Dib-Hajj, S.D., and Waxman, S.G. (2001) $Na_v1.3$ sodium channels: rapid repriming and slow closed-state inactivation display quantitative differences after expression in a mammalian cell line and in spinal sensory neurons. *J. Neurosci.* 21:5952–5961.

Cummins, T.R., Dib-Hajj, S.D., Black, J.A., Akopian, A.N., Wood, J.N., and Waxman, S.G. (1999) A novel persistent tetrodotoxin-resistant sodium current In SNS-null and wild type small primary sensory neurons. *J. Neurosci.* 19(24):RC43.

Cummins, T.R., Renganathan, M., Stys, P.K., Herzog, M.D., Scarfo, B.S., Horn, R., Dib-Hajj, S.D., and Waxman, S.G. (2003) The pentapeptide QYNAD does not block voltage-gated sodium channels. *Neurology* 60:224–229.

Cummins, T.R. and Waxman, S.G. (1997) Downregulation of tetrodotoxin-resistant sodium currents and upregulation of rapidly repriming tetrodotoxin-sensitive sodium current in small spinal sensory neurons after nerve injury. *J. Neurosci.* 17:3503–3514.

De Waegh, S.M., Lee, V.M., and Brady, S.T. (1992) Local modulation of neurofilament phosphorylation, axonal caliber, and slow axonal transport by myelinating Schwann cells. *Cell* 68:451–463.

Dib-Hajj, S., Black, J.A., Felts, P., and Waxman, S.G. (1996) Down-regulation of transcripts for Na channel alpha-SNS in spinal sensory neurons following axotomy. *Proc. Natl. Acad. Sci. USA* 93:14950–14954.

Dib-Hajj, S.D., Fjell, J., Cummins, T.R., Zheng, Z., Fried, K., LaMotte, R., Black, J.A., and Waxman, S.G. (1999) Plasticity of sodium channel expression in DRG neurons in the chronic constriction injury model of neuropathic pain. *Pain* 83:591–600.

Dib-Hajj, S.D., Tyrrell, L., Black, J.A., and Waxman, S.G. (1998) NaN, a novel voltage-gated Na channel, is expressed preferentially in peripheral sensory neurons and down-regulated after axotomy. *Proc. Natl. Acad. Sci. USA* 95:8963–8968.

Dugandzija-Novakovic, S., Koszowski, A.G., Levinson, S.R., and Shrager, P. (1995) Clustering of Na^+ channels and node of Ranvier formation in remyelinating axons. *J. Neurosci.* 15:492–503.

Duncan, I.D., Hammang, J.P., Jackson, K.F., Wood, P.M., Bunge, R.P., and Langford, L. (1988) Transplantation of oligodendrocytes and Schwann cells into the spinal cord of the myelin-deficient rat. *J. Neurocytol.* 17:351–360.

Eng, D.L., Gordon, T.R., Kocsis, J.D., and Waxman, S.G. (1988) Development of 4-AP and TEA sensitivities in mammalian myelinated nerve fibers. *J. Neurophysiol.* 60:2168–2179.

England, J.D., Gamboni, F., and Levinson, S.R. (1991) Increased numbers of sodium channels form along demyelinated axons. *Brain Res.* 548:334–337.

England, J.D., Gamboni, F., Levinson, S.R., and Finger, T.E. (1990) Changed distribution of sodium channels along demyelinated axons. *Proc. Natl. Acad. Sci. USA* 87(17):6777–6780.

Fang, X., Djouhri, L., Black, J.A., Dib-Hajj, S.D., Waxman, S.G., Lawson, S.N. (2002) The presence and role of the TTX resistant sodium channel $Na_v1.9$ (NaN) in nociceptive primary afferent neurons. *J. Neurosci.* 22(17):7425–7433.

Felts, P., Baker, T.A., and Smith, K.J. (1977) Conduction in segmentally demyelinated mammalian central axons. *J. Neurosci.* 17: 7267–7277.

Felts, P., and Smith, K.J. (1991) Conduction properties of central nerve fibers remyelinated by Schwann cells. *Brain Res.* 574:178–192.

Fjell, J., Dibhajj, S., Fried, K., Black, J.A., and Waxman, S.G. (1997) Differential expression of sodium channel genes in retinal ganglion cells. *Mol. Brain Res.* 50:197–204.

Foster, R.E., Connors, B.W., and Waxman, S.G. (1982) Rat optic nerve: electrophysiological, pharmacological, and anatomical studies during development. *Dev. Brain Res.* 3:361–376.

Foster, R.E., Whalen, C.C., and Waxman, S.G. (1980) Reorganization of the axonal membrane of demyelinated nerve fibers: morphological evidence. *Science* 210:661–663.

Gout, O., Gansmuller, A., Baumann, N., and Gumpel, M. (1988) Remyelination by transplanted oligodendrocytes of a demyelinated lesion in the spinal cord of the adult shiverer mouse. *Neurosci. Lett.* 87:195–199.

Gray, P.T. and Ritchie, J.M. (1985) Ion channels in Schwann and glial cells. *Trends Neurosci.* 8:411–415.

Groves, A.K., Barnett, S.C., Franklin, R.J.M., et al. (1993) Repair of demyelinated lesions by transplantation of purified 0–2A progenitor cells. *Nature* 363:453–456.

Herzog, R.I., Cummins, T.R., and Waxman, S.G. (2001) Persistent TTX-resistant Na(+) current affects resting potential and response to depolarization in simulated spinal sensory neurons. *J. Neurophysiol.* 86:1351–1364.

Hildebrand, C. (1971) Ultrastructural and light-microscopic studies of the developing feline spinal cord white matter. I. The nodes of Ranvier. *Acta Physiol. Scand. Suppl.* 364:81–101.

Hines, M. and Shrager, P. (1991) A computational test of the requirements for conduction in demyelinated axons. *Restor. Neurol. Neurosci.* 3:81–93.

Hirano, A. (1968) A confirmation of the oligodendroglial origin of myelin in the adult rat. *J. Cell Biol.* 38:637–340.

Honmou, O., Felts, P.A., Waxman, S.G., and Kocsis, J.D. (1996) Restoration of normal conduction properties in demyelinated spinal cord axons in the adult rat by transplantation of exogenous Schwann cells. *J. Neurosci.* 16:3199–3208.

Huxley, A.F. and Stämpfli, R. (1949) Evidence for saltatory conduction in peripheral myelinated nerve fibers. *J. Physiol.* (*Lond.*) 108:315–339.

Imaizumi, T., Lankford, K.L., Burton, W.V., Foder, W.L., and Kocsis, J.D. (2000) Xenotransplantation of transgenic pig olfactory ensheathing cells promotes axonal regeneration in rat spinal cord. *Nat. Biotech.* 18:949–953.

Imaizumi, T., Lankford, K.L., Waxman, S.G., Green, C.A., and Kocsis, J.D. (1998) Transplantated olfactory ensheathing cells remyelinate and enhance axonal conduction in the demyelinated dorsal columns of the rat spinal cord. *J. Neurosci.* 18:6176–6185.

Kocsis, J.D., Eng, D.L., Gordon, T.R., and Waxman, S.G. (1987) Functional differences between 4-aminopyridine and tetraethylammonium-sensitive potassium channels in myelinated axons. *Neurosci. Lett.* 75:193–198.

Kocsis, J.D., and Waxman, S.G. (1985) Demyelination: causes and mechanisms of clinical abnormality and functional recovery. In: Koetsier, J.C., ed. *Handbook of Clinical Neurology*, Vol. 3, *The Demyelinating Diseases*. Amsterdam: Elsevier, pp. 29–47.

Kocsis, J.D., Waxman, S.G., Hildebrand, C., and Ruiz, J.A. (1982) Regenerating mammalian nerve fibers: changes in action potential waveform and firing characteristics following blockage of potassium conductance. *Proc. R. Soc. Lond.* B217:277–287.

Koles, Z.J. and Rasminsky, M. (1972) A computer simulation of conduction in demyelinated nerve fibers. *J. Physiol.* (*Lond.*) 227:351–364.

Kuno, M. and Llinas, R. (1970) Enhancement of synaptic transmission by dendritic potentials in chromatolysed motoneurones of the cat. *J. Physiol.* (*Lond.*) 210:807–821.

Liu CJ, C., Dib-Hajj, S.D., Black, J.A., Greenwood, J., Lian, Z., and Waxman, S.G. (2001) Direct interaction with contactin targets voltage-gated sodium channel $Na_v1.9$/NaN to the cell membrane. *J. Biol. Chem.* 276:46553–46561.

Lombet, A., Laduron, P., Mourre, C., Jacomet, Y., and Lazdunski, M. (1985) Axonal transport of the voltage-dependent Na channel protein identified by its tetrodotoxin–binding site in rat sciatic nerves. *Brain Res.* 345:153–158.

McDonald, W.I. (1963) The effects of experimental demyelination on conduction in peripheral nerve: a histological and electrophysiological study. Electrophysiological observations. *Brain* 86:501–524.

McDonald, W.I. and Sears, T.A. (1970) The effects of experimental demyelination on conduction in the central nervous system. *Brain* 93:583–598.

Moll, C., Mourre, C., Lazdunski, M., and Ulrich, J. (1991) Increase of sodium channels in demyelinated lesions of multiple sclerosis. *Brain Res.* 556:311–316.

Oh, Y. and Waxman, S.G. (1994) The beta 1 subunit mRNA of the rat brain Na^+ channel is expressed in glial cells. *PNAS* 91:9985–9989.

Prineas, J. and Connell, F. (1978) Fine structure of chronically active multiple sclerosis plaques. *Neurology* 28:68–75.

Rasband, M., Trimmer, J.S., Schwarz, T.L., Levinson, S.R., Ellisman, M.H., Schachner, M., and Shrager, P. (1998) Potassium channel distribution, clustering, and function in remyelinating rat axons. *J. Neurosci.* 18:36–47.

Rasminsky, M. and Sears, T.A. (1972) Internodal conduction in undissected demyelinated nerve fibers. *J. Physiol.* (*Lond.*) 227:323–350.

Renganathan, M., Cummins, T.R., and Waxman, S.G. (2001) Contribution of $Na_v1.8$ sodium channels to action potential electrogenesis in DRG neurons. *J. Neurophysiol.* 86:629–640.

Renganathan, M., Gelderblom, M., Black, J.A., and Waxman, S.G. (2003) Expression of $Na_v1.8$ sodium channels perturbs the firing patterns of cerebellar Purkinje cells. *Brain Res.* 959:235–242.

Ritchie, J.M. (1982) Sodium and potassium channels in regenerating and developing mammalian myelinated nerves. *Proc. R. Soc.* B215:273–287.

Ritchie, J.M. and Chiu, S.Y. (1981) Distribution of sodium and potassium channnels in mammalian myelinated nerve. In: Waxman, S.G. and Ritchie, J.H., eds. *Demyelinating Diseases: Basic and Clinical Electrophysiology*. New York: Raven Press, pp. 329–342.

Ritchie, J.M., Rang, H.P., and Pellegrino, R. (1981) Sodium and potassium channels in demyelinated and remyelinated mammalian nerve. *Nature* 294:257–259.

Ritchie, J.M. and Rogart, R.B. (1977) The density of sodium channels in mammalian myelinated nerve fibers and the nature of the axonal membrane under the myelin sheath. *Proc. Natl. Acad. Sci. USA* 74:211–215.

Röper, J. and Schwarz, J.R. (1989) Heterogeneous distribution of fast and slow potassium channels in myelinated rat nerve fibers. *J. Physiol. (Lond.)* 416:93–110.

Rosenbluth, J. (1985) Intramembranous particle patches in myelin-deficient rat mutant. *Neurosci. Lett.* 62:19–24.

Rosenbluth, J. and Blakemore, W.F. (1984) Structural specializations in cat of chronically demyelinated spinal cord axons as seen in freeze-fracture replicas. *Neurosci. Lett.* 48:171–177.

Rosenbluth, J., Hasegawa, M., and Schiff, R. (1989) Myelin formation in myelin-deficient rat spinal cord following transplantation of normal fetal spinal cord. *Neurosci. Lett.* 97:35–40.

Sears, T.A. and Bostock, H. (1981) Conduction failure in demyelination: is it inevitable? In: Waxman, S.G. and Ritchie, J.M., eds. *Demyelinating Diseases: Basic and Clinical Electrophysiology*, New York: Raven Press, pp. 357–375.

Sears, T.A., Bostock, H., and Sherratt, M. (1978) The pathophysiology of demyelination and its implications for the symptomatic treatment of multiple sclerosis. *Neurology* 28:21–26.

Shrager, P. (1989) Sodium channels in single demyelinated mammalian axons. *Brain Res.* 483:149–154.

Sleeper, A.A., Cummins, T.R., Dib-Hajj, S.D., Hormuzdiar, W., Tyrrell, L., Waxman, S.G., and Black, J.A. (2000) Changes in expression of two tetrodotoxin-resistant sodium channels and their currents in dorsal root ganglion neurons after sciatic nerve injury but not rhizotomy. *J. Neurosci.* 20:7279–7289.

Smith, K.J., Blakemore, W.F., and McDonald, W.I. (1981) The restoration of conduction by central remyelination. *Brain* 104:383–404.

Smith, K.J., Blakemore, W.F., and McDonanld, W.I. (1983) Central remyelination restores secure conduction. *Nature* 280:395–396.

Smith, K.J., Bostock, H., and Hall, S.M. (1982) Saltatory conduction precedes remyelination in axons demyelinated with lysophosphatidyl choline. *J. Neurol. Sci.* 54:13–31.

Smith, K.J. and Hall, S.M. (1980) Nerve conduction during peripheral demyelination and remyelination. *J. Neurol. Sci.* 104:383–404.

Smith, K.J. and McDonald, W.I. (1980) Spontaneous and mechanically evoked activity due to central demyelinating lesions. *Nature* 286:154–155.

Smith, M.E., Kocsis, J.D., and Waxman, S.G. (1983) Myelin protein metabolism in demyelination and remyelination in sciatic nerve. *Brain Res.* 270:37–44.

Sontheimer, H., Black, J.A., Ransom, B.R., and Waxman, S.G. (1992) Ion channels in spinal cord astrocytes in vitro. I. Transient expression of high levels of Na^+ and K^+ channels. *J. Neurophysiol.* 68:985–1000.

Sontheimer, H., Fernandez-Marques, E., Ullrich, N., Pappas, C.A., and Waxman, S.G. (1994) Astrocyte Na^+ channels are required for maintenance of Na+/K(+)-ATPase activity. *J. Neurosci.* 14:2464–2475.

Sontheimer, H., Ransom, B.R., Cornell-Bell, A.H., Black, J.A., and Waxman, S.G. (1991) Na^+-current expression in rat hippocampal astrocytes in vitro: Alterations during development. *J. Neurophysiol.* 65:3–19.

Stanley, G.P. and Pender, M.P. (1991) Pathophysiology of chronic relapsing experimental allergic encephalomyelitis. *Brain* 114:1827–1853.

Tasaki, I. (1959) Conduction of the nerve impulse: In: Field, J., Magoun, H.W., and Hall, V.E., eds. *American Physiological Society Handbook of Physiology*, Sect. 1, *Neurophysiology*, Vol. 1. Washington, D.C.: American Physiological Society, pp. 75–121.

Utzschneider, D.A., Archer, D.R., Kocsis, J.D., Waxman, S.G., and Duncan, I.D. (1994) Transplantation of glial cells enhances action potential conduction of amyelinated spinal cord axons in the myelin-deficient rat. *Proc. Natl. Acad. Sci. USA* 91:53–57.

Vabnick, I. and Shrager, P. (1998) Ion channel redistribution and function during development of the myelinated axon. *J. Neurobiol.* 37:80–96.

Vollmer, T.L., Brass, L.M., and Waxman, S.G. (1991) Lhermitte's sign in a patient with herpes zoster. *J. Neurol. Sci.* 106:153–157.

Wang, H., Kunkel, D.D., Martin, T.M., Schwartkroin, P.A., and Tempel, B.L. (1993) Heteromultimeric K^+ channels in terminal juxtaparanodal regions of neurons. *Nature* 365:75–79.

Waxman, S.G. (1977) Conduction in myelinated, unmyelinated, and demyelinated fibers. *Arch. Neurol.* 34:585–590.

Waxman, S.G. (1978) Prerequisites for conduction in demyelinated fibers. *Neurology* 28:27–34.

Waxman, S.G. (1982) Membranes, myelin and the pathophysiology of multiple sclerosis. *N. Engl. J. Med.* 306:1529–1533.

Waxman, S.G. (1987) Molecular organization of the cell membrane in normal and pathological axons: relation to glial contact. In: Althaus, H. and Seifert, W., eds. *Glial-Neuronal Communication in Development and Regeneration.* Germany: Springer-Verlag, pp. 711–736.

Waxman, S.G. (1992) The perinodal astrocyte: functional and developmental considerations. In: Fedoroff, S., Doucette, R., and Juurlink, B.H., eds. *Biology and Pathobiology of Astrocyte-Neuron Interactions.* New York: Plenum Press, pp. 15–26.

Waxman, S.G. (2002) Ion channels, neuronal dysfunction and the pathophysiology of multiple sclerosis. *Arch. Neurol.* 59:1377–1380.

Waxman, S.G., and Bennett, M.V.L. (1972) Relative conduction velocities of small myelinated and non-myelinated fibers in the central nervous system. *Nat/. New Biol.* 238:217–219.

Waxman, S.G. and Black, J.A. (1984) Freeze-fracture ultrastructure of the perinodal astrocyte and associated glial junctions. *Brain Res.* 308:77–87.

Waxman, S.G., Black, J.A., Kocsis, J.A., and Ritchie, J.M. (1989) Low density of sodium channels supports conduction in axons of neonatal rat optic nerve. *Proc. Natl. Acad. Sci. USA* 86:1406–1410.

Waxman, S.G. and Brill, M.H. (1978) Conduction through demyelinated plaques in multiple sclerosis: computer simulations of facilitation by short internodes. *J. Neurol. Neurosurg. Psychiatry* 41:408–417.

Waxman, S.G., Kocsis, J.D., and Black, J.A. (1994) Type III sodium channel mRNA is expressed in embryonic but not adult spinal sensory neurons, and is reexpressed following axotomy. *J. Neurophysiol.* 72:466–470.

Waxman, S.G. and Ritchie, J.M. (1993) Molecular dissection of the myelinated axon. *Ann. Neurol.* 33:121–136.

Waxman, S.G. and Sims, T.J. (1984) Specificity in central myelination: evidence for local regulation of myelin thickness. *Brain Res.* 292:179–185.

Waxman, S.G., Sims, T.J., and Gilmore, S.A. (1988) Cytoplasmic membrane elaborations in oligodendrocytes during myelination of spinal motoneuron axons. *Glia* 1:286–291.

Waxman, S.G. and Wood, S.L. (1984) Impulse conduction in inhomogeneous axons: effects of variation in voltage-sensitive ionic conductances on invasion of demyelinated axon segments and preterminal fibers. *Brain Res.* 294:111–122.

Weber, F., Brinkmeier, H., Aulkemeyer, P., Wollinsky, K.H., and Rudel, R. (1999) A small sodium channel-blocking factor in the CSF is preferentially found in Guillain-Barre syndrome. *J. Neurol.* 246:955–960.

Weiner, L.P., Waxman, S.G., Stohlman, S.A., and Kwan, A. (1980) Remyelination following viral-induced demyelination: Ferric ion-ferrocyanide staining of nodes of Ranvier within the CNS. *Ann. Neurol.* 8:580–583.

Westenbroek, R.E., Noebels, J.L., and Catterall, W.A. (1992) Elevated expression of type II Na^+ channels in hypomyelinated axons of shiverer mouse brain. *J. Neurosci.* 12:2259–2267.

Zhou, W. and Goldin, A.L. (2002) Functional differences between the Nav1.6 and Nav1.2 sodium channels. *Soc. Neurosci. Abstr.* 834.4.

Zhou, L., Zhang, C.L., Messing, A., and Chiu, S.Y. (1998) Temperature-sensitive neuromuscular transmission in Kv1.1-null mice: role of potassium channels under the myelin in young nerves. *J. Neurosci.* 18:7200–7215.

22 Cytokine production

FRANCESCA ALOISI

Cytokines are small proteins that serve as chemical messengers between cells, regulating cell growth and differentiation, tissue homeostasis and repair, and many aspects of inflammatory and immune responses. The past two decades have witnessed a growing interest in the role of cytokines in the development, normal functioning, and pathology of the nervous system. This has led to significant advances in our understanding of the way cytokines act in the central nervous system (CNS) and peripheral nervous system (PNS), serving as key signaling and regulatory molecules that stabilize, modify, or even disrupt the neural microenvironment, and acting as links between the nervous, endocrine, and immune systems. However, owing to the fact that cytokines are pleiotropic, redundant to some degree, and induce the production of other cytokines, the specific sites and mechanisms of action of cytokines in the above processes have proved difficult to unravel. This chapter will discuss recent research on cytokines that are produced by and/or act on glial cells, focusing on those involved in the regulation of inflammatory, immune, and tissue repair processes.

CYTOKINES IN THE NERVOUS SYSTEM: GENERAL FEATURES

With few exceptions (e.g., transforming growth factor-β and some colony-stimulating factors and chemokines that are constitutively expressed or developmentally regulated), most cytokines are undetectable or expressed at low levels in the normal nervous system. Cytokine mRNAs and/or proteins are readily detected in the CNS and PNS upon alteration of tissue homeostasis by physiological and pathological stimuli. Systemic stimuli (eg., infusion of pro-inflammatory cytokines or bacterial endotoxin) preferentially induce cytokine expression in circumventricular organs, in leptomeninges, in choroid plexuses, and at the level of the blood–brain barrier. More localized stimuli (e.g., acute injury or infection by neurotropic pathogens) also induce cytokine production within the neural parenchyma, which is sustained by tissue-infiltrating inflammatory cells and/or resident tissue cells. In earlier studies, glial cells, particularly microglia and astrocytes in the CNS and Schwann cells in the PNS, have been identified as potential sources and targets of many of the currently identified cytokines (Fig. 22.1).

Most of the present knowledge regarding cytokine production in the nervous system derives from studies in primary cultures of neural cells and in animal models of severe neurological diseases. The latter include experimental autoimmune encephalomyelitis (EAE) and neuritis (EAN), models for the inflammatory, demyelinating diseases multiple sclerosis and Guillain-Barré syndrome, respectively; models of acute brain injury such as ischemia, trauma, axonal transection, and chemical and excitotoxic damage; models of chronic neurodegenerative disorders, such as Alzheimer's disease and prion disease; and experimental infections with neurotropic viruses, bacteria, and parasites. Studies using autoptic human brain material or cerebrospinal fluid (CSF) from neurological patients have also provided important clues to the source and possible role of cytokines in pathology. *In vitro* studies have often generated conflicting results on cytokine sources and targets in the CNS, owing to the fact that astrocyte cultures have variable degrees of microglia contamination and neuronal cultures are never devoid of glial cells. Due to the limits of immunohistochemical techniques, opinions also frequently differ as to the cell type(s) responsible for production of certain cytokines in the nervous tissue. Fewer *in situ* hybridization studies have allowed researchers to localize expression of cytokine transcripts in defined neural cell types, although not providing information on cytokine availability at the protein level.

Laboratory animals and *in vitro* systems have also been used to study the effects of recombinant cytokines or to block the activity of endogenous cytokines. During the past decade, the development of genetically manipulated mice, in which expression of selected cytokine genes was either targeted to the CNS under the transcriptional control of neural cell–specific promoters or disrupted by homologous recombination, has allowed us to answer more directly questions regarding specific functions and local effects of cytokines in pathophysiological conditions. In this case, results need to be carefully evaluated, as cytokine actions may differ markedly, depending on the source and levels of

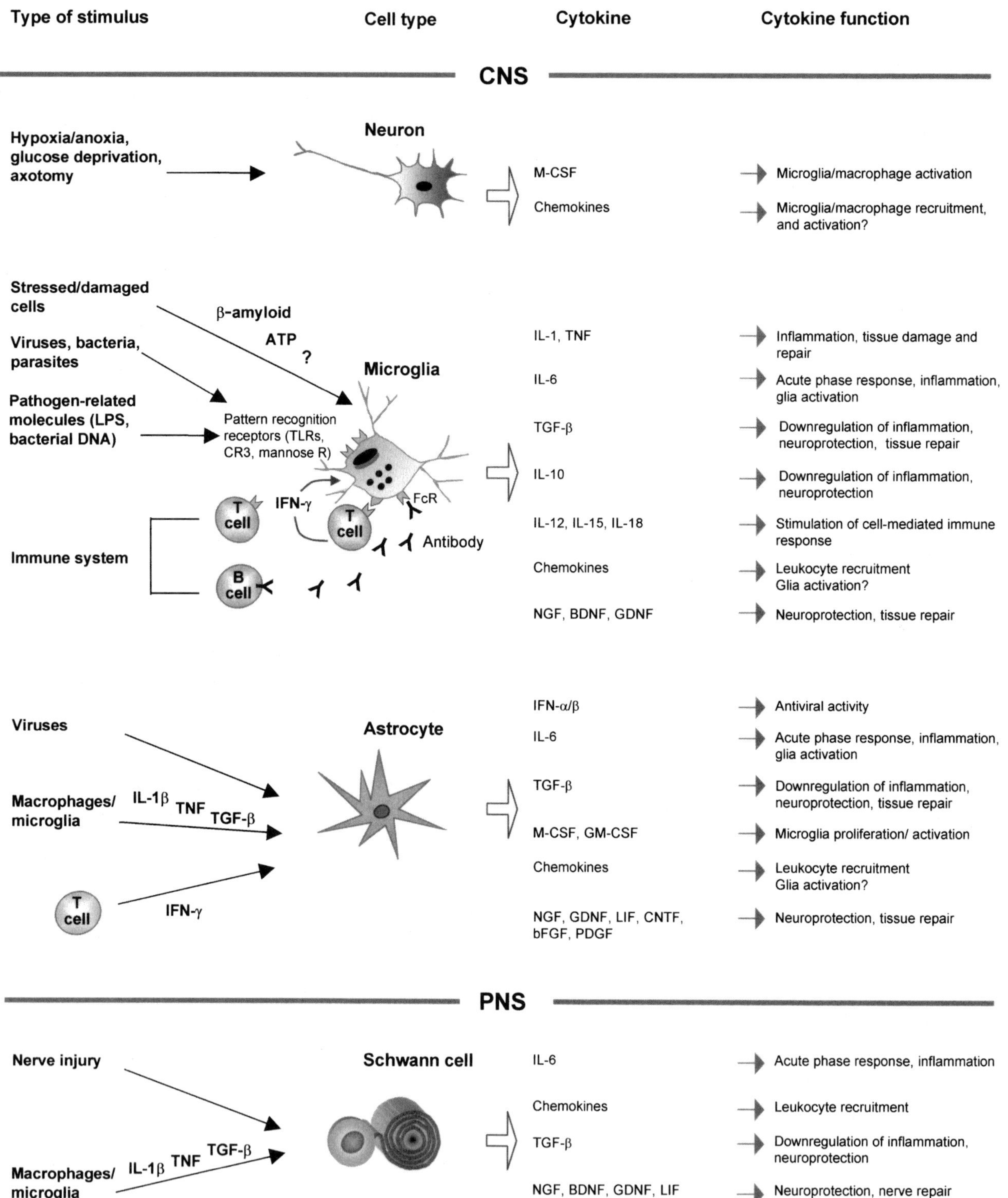

transgene expression, whereas gene deletion also has effects outside the CNS and may induce compensatory mechanisms.

Another major issue regarding the actions of cytokines in the nervous system concerns the mechanisms regulating their activity. Cytokine bioactivity is known to be regulated at the levels of transcription, translation, cleavage, and cellular release, as well as through receptor and postreceptor signaling mechanisms (see Chapter 11). The activity of some cytokines, like interleukin-1 (IL-1), IL-6, and tumor necrosis factor (TNF), is also regulated by soluble binding proteins and receptors, and by endogenous receptor antagonists, as in the case of IL-1. Recently, a new family of cytokine-

FIGURE 22.1 Schematic representation of major signals inducing cytokine production by neurons and glia and of cytokines produced by each cell population. Major cytokine-related functions in the nervous system are also listed. Damaged neurons may produce cytokines early after injury, providing the first signals for recruitment of macrophages/microglia and, together with oligodendrocytes, are vulnerable targets of cytokine actions during inflammation. Similarly to other cells of the innate immune system, microglia produce a large array of master inflammatory and immunoregulatory cytokines in response to numerous stimuli, including pathogens, signals from stressed/damaged cells, and immune-derived signals. The rapid response of microglia to infectious agents is due to the presence on the microglia plasma membrane of pattern recognition receptors [e.g., Toll-like receptors (TLRs), complement receptor 3 (CR3), mannose receptor] that interact directly with microbial structures. Microglia also express surface receptors that trigger cell activation via direct membrane interactions with T cells (see also Fig. 22.3), T cell–derived cytokines, and antibodies (Fc receptors). Astrocytes and Schwann cells respond mainly to macrophage- and T cell–derived cytokines. Both cell types produce cytokines regulating inflammation or involved in tissue repair and remodeling processes. The latter include nerve growth factor (NGF), glial cell line-derived neurotrophic factor (GDNF), leukemia inhibitory factor (LIF), ciliary neurotrophic factor (CNTF), basic fibroblast growth factor (bFGF), and platelet-derived growth factor (PDGF). GM-CSF: granulocyte/macrophage colony-stimulating factor; M-CSF: macrophage colony-stimulating factor; IFN-α/β: interferon-α/β; IL-1: interleukini-1; LPS: lipopolysaccharide; TGF-β: transforming growth factor-β; TNF: tumor necrosis factor.

inducible proteins, termed *suppressors of cytokine signaling* (SOCS), has been discovered, which function as negative regulators of signaling pathways activated by many cytokines. Investigations on the expression and role of these molecules in neural cells are just beginning, and could yield important new insights into the regulation of cytokine actions and their involvement in neurological diseases (Wang and Campbell, 2002).

Interferons

The interferons (IFNs) are a family of secreted proteins with a leading role in the host defense against pathogens and in immunoregulation. The type I IFNs, α and β (IFN-α/β), are composed of the products of multiple (up to 12) IFN-α genes and a single IFN-β gene that are produced by many cell types in response to virus or double-stranded RNA and use a common heterodimeric receptor expressed on most cells. Interferon-γ (type II IFN) is the product of a single gene, binds to a distinct receptor that is ubiquitously expressed, and is produced mainly by CD8$^+$ cytotoxic T cells, a subset of CD4$^+$ T helper cells (Th1), and natural killer (NK) cells. Interferon-α/β and IFN-γ receptor signaling is mediated through the Janus kinase–signal transducer and activator of transcription (JAK-STAT) pathway leading to the induction of partially overlapping patterns of target genes, including those encoding for cytokines.

Interferon-α/β has been detected in brain tissue and CSF from humans and experimental animals following viral infection. Synthesis of biologically active IFN-α/β has been demonstrated in glioma cells, mixed glial and purified astrocyte cultures after induction with virus, and polyribonucleotide or vasoactive intestinal peptide (VIP) (Chelbi-Alix et al., 1994). These findings suggest that glia-derived IFN-α/β may help to induce a state of antiviral resistance in CNS cells. Interferon-α immunoreactivity has also been localized in reactive microglia and astrocytes *in situ* during chronic neurodegenerative and infectious diseases (Akiyama et al., 1994; Rho et al., 1995). Transgenic expression of IFN-α1 in the CNS confers protection against lethal neurotropic viral infection and induces inflammation and neurodegeneration, supporting both a beneficial and a detrimental role for type I IFNs in the neural tissue (Wang et al., 2002). Because IFN-β is used as an immunomodulatory agent in the therapy of multiple sclerosis, many studies have analyzed its action on neural cells *in vitro* and have shown that it may affect several glial functions (Table 22.1).

Interferon-γ has a key role in enhancing protective immune responses against neurotropic pathogens, but may also contribute to amplify immunopathological alterations and tissue damage in postinfectious encephalopathies and autoimmune diseases. Strong expression of IFN-γ in the nervous system is associated with tissue infiltration by activated NK, CD8$^+$ cytotoxic, and Th1-type T cells (Owens et al., 2001). Although IFN-γ-like immunoreactivity and expression of IFN-γ mRNA have been described in CNS and PNS neurons, astrocytes, and microglia, the biological significance of these findings remains uncertain (Benveniste, 1998). Direct injection or transgenic expression of IFN-γ in the CNS induces or exacerbates inflammatory pathology, demyelination, and neurodegeneration (Owens et al., 2001; Wang et al., 2002). Interferon-γ is the best-known endogenous inducer/amplifier of the antimicrobial, cytotoxic, pro-inflammatory, and antigen-presenting functions of macrophages and microglia (Deckert-Schlüter et al., 1999; Aloisi, 2001). Binding of IFN-γ to its receptor on microglia induces trascription of many immune genes (Table 22.1), via the classical IFN-γ-induced signal transduction cascade, involving activation of the transcription factor STAT-1 and its binding to IFN-γ activation site (GAS) elements in the promoter region of IFN-γ-responsive genes (see Chapter 11). Moreover, IFN-γ potentiates or primes microglia for production of cytokines, chemokines, proteases, nitric oxide (NO), and reactive oxygen intermediates induced by stimuli that activate the transcription factor NF-kB, like lipopolysaccharide (LPS) and CD40 ligation. CD40 is a molecule belonging to the TNF receptor superfamily, binds to CD154 (or CD40 ligand) on activated T cells, and is considered a

TABLE 22.1 *Glial Cells As Sources of and Targets for Interferons*

	IFN-α/β	*IFN-γ*
Cell source:	Astrocytes, microglia (?)	Astrocytes (?), microglia (?)
Effects on microglia:	Antiviral ↑ Fc receptor ↓ or no effect on IFN-γ-induced MHC class II expression ↑ ↓ IL-1, ↑ IL-1ra ↑ Superoxide anion (O2-) ↑ Chemokine production ↓ Proliferation	↑ Antigen processing/presentation: induction of Fc receptors, cathepsin L and S, MHC class I and class II molecules, adhesion/costimulatory (CD40, ICAM-1/CD54, CD80/B7-1, CD86/B7-2) molecules ↑ Phagocytosis ↑ Fas-mediated apoptosis; ↑ Fas/Fas ligand expression; ↓ Bcl-2/Bcl-xL expression ↑ Superoxide anion (O2-) and (NO) production ↓ Proliferation ↑ TNF, IL-12 and chemokine production induced by β-amyloid, LPS, or CD40 ligation ↓ LPS-stimulated IL-10 production ↑ Gap junction formation, Ca^{2+} influx, and K^+ currents
Effects on astrocytes:	Antiviral ↑ MHC class I molecules ↓ or no effect on IFN-γ-induced MHC class II expression ↑ NGF production ↓ Proliferation	↑ MHC class I and class II and adhesion (ICAM-1/CD54, VCAM-1/CD106) molecules ↑ Complement components and regulators ↑ NO production, in combination with IL-1β ↑ Cytokine (IL-6, G-CSF) and chemokine (IP-10/CXCL10) production induced by IL-1β and TNF ↑ Fas and FasL expression ↑ Type I TNFR expression ↑ ↓ Proliferation ↑ Glutamate uptake, Na^+/K^+ exchange activity and ATP release
Effects on oligodendrocytes:	Antiviral	↑ MHC class I molecules ↑ Fas-mediated apoptosis and Fas expression ↑ Type I TNFR; ↓ Proliferation, in combination with TNF ↓ Differentiation and myelin protein synthesis, in combination with TNF
Effects on Schwann cells:		↑ MHC class I and class II molecules, ICAM-1/CD54 ↑ Apoptosis ↑ NO production, in combination with TNF ↓ Differentiation, myelin-associated glycoprotein synthesis and interactions with neurons, in combination with TNF

ICAM-1: intercellular adhesion molecule-1; G-CSF: granulocyte-colony-stimulating factor; IFN: interferon; IL: interleukin; IL-1ra: interleukin-1 receptor antagonist; LPS: lipopolysaccharide; MHC: major histocompatibility complex; NGF, nerve growth factor; NO: nitric oxide; TNF: tumor necrosis factor; TNFR: tumor necrosis factor receptor; VCAM-1: vascular cell adhesion molecule-1.

key pathway for microglia activation triggered by CNS-infiltrating T cells (Aloisi et al., 2000). Interferon-γ acts on astrocytes and Schwann cells, stimulating expression of major histocompatibility complex (MHC) and adhesion molecules and amplifying the inducing effects of IL-1β and/or TNF on the production of chemokines, cytokines, and NO. Interferon-γ may affect also basic homeostatic mechanisms in glial cells, such as membrane ionic fluxes, glutamate transport, and release of adenosine triphosphate (ATP) (Table 22.1). *In vitro* studies have revealed the particular vulnerability of Schwann cell and oligodendrocyte progenitors to IFN-γ or combinations of IFN-γ and TNF, which involves activation of cell death programs or reduced growth/differentiation (Agresti et al., 1998; Popko and Baerwald, 1999). These findings support an effector role for IFN-γ in demyelinating disorders. In apparent contrast with its predominant pro-inflammatory action, IFN-γ has been reported to alleviate EAE and to promote apoptosis of encephalitogenic T cells and microglia, which suggests that IFN-γ may also inhibit CNS inflammation (Owens et al., 2001).

Colony-Stimulating Factors

Colony-stimulating factors (CSFs) are hematopoietic cytokines that regulate the growth and differentiation of bone marrow progenitor cells. This group of cytokines includes IL-3, macrophage-CSF (M-CSF), granulocyte-macrophage CSF (GM-CSF), and granulocyte-CSF (G-CSF). Early work demonstrated that CSFs are produced by cultured glia, and in the developing and injured brain (Malipiero et al., 1990; Giulian et al., 1991).

Macrophage-CSF is produced in the CNS and PNS during infectious, autoimmune, and neurodegenerative diseases. Studies in mice lacking functional M-CSF indicate that M-CSF is important for microglia proliferation and differentiation in the developing brain and for microglia activation following brain injury (Raivich et al., 1999). Macrophage-CSF immunoreactivity has been detected in neurons early after focal brain injury and subsequently in microglia (Takeuchi et al., 2001). *In vitro*, M-CSF production is induced in astrocytes by IL-1β and TNF and in microglia by LPS.

Granulocyte-macrophage-CSF is induced in the CNS and PNS in a variety of pathological conditions, and expression of its receptor is increased in microglia following nerve injury. Granulocyte-macrophage-CSF is a potent stimulator of microglia proliferation, phagocytic capability, and antigen-presenting function (Re et al., 2002). Granulocyte-CSF is produced in the CNS during viral and bacterial meningitis and is thought to participate in neutrophil recruitment and activation. Astrocytes have been identified as a major intracerebral source of GM-CSF and G-CSF.

Interleukin-3 promotes the proliferation and maturation of pluripotent myeloid progenitor cells. *In vitro* and *in vivo* studies indicate that IL-3 supports the proliferation of microglia and may serve as a neurotrophic/neuroprotective factor. Interleukin-3 is upregulated in the CNS during EAE and in peripheral neuropathies. *In vitro*, it is produced by activated microglia. Transgenic mice expressing IL-3 under the regulatory control of the glial fibrillary acidic protein (GFAP) promoter develop a progressive motor disorder and show massive accumulation of activated macrophages/microglia, astrocytosis, blood–brain barrier alterations, and demyelination leading to neuronal damage (Wang et al., 2002). These findings highlight the importance of IL-3 in driving microglia/macrophage activation and the deleterious consequences of these events in the CNS.

Transforming Growth Factor-β Family

Members of the transforming growth factor-β (TGF-β) family, which includes TGF-βs, bone morphogenetic proteins, and activins, are widely distributed throughout the body and are potent regulators of cell proliferation, differentiation, migration, and apoptosis. The three mammalian TGF-β isoforms, TGF-β1, -β2 and -β3, are all constitutively expressed in the nervous system, and their secretion and activation are regulated by latency-associated peptides and latent TGF-β-binding proteins (Bottner et al., 2000). Transforming growth factor-β interacts with at least three cell-surface receptors; type I and type II receptors have been identified in neuronal and glial cells. Most studies addressing the role of TGF-β in the nervous system have focused on TGF-β1.

Transforming growth factor-β1 has been indicated as a key regulator of the brain's responses to injury and inflammation through its ability to modulate astrocyte proliferation and extracellular matrix synthesis, to induce vascular modifications, and to regulate macrophage/microglia activation and leukocyte recruitment. Moreover, TGF-β1 has neurotrophic activities, inhibits apoptosis in neurons, and protects neurons from a variety of insults (Krieglstein et al., 2002). Its neuroprotective effects are thought to occur through induction of neurotrophic factors in glial cells.

Transforming growth factor-β1, -2 and -3 mRNAs and/or proteins are upregulated in the CNS and PNS in infectious, autoimmune, and neurodegenerative diseases (Pratt and McPherson, 1997). All three TGF-β isoforms have been detected in macrophages/microglia and reactive astrocytes in multiple sclerosis lesions. *In situ* hybridization studies indicate that TGF-β1 mRNA is expressed predominantly in invading leukocytes and microglia after acute brain injury and in EAE (Kiefer et al., 1998). Schwann cells also upregulate TGF-β1 mRNA following peripheral nerve lesions. Increased intracerebral levels of TGF-β1 and/or TGF-β2 have been detected in Alzheimer's, Parkinson's, and prion diseases, and in acquired immune deficiency syndrome (AIDS) dementia complex. Both neuronal and glial expression have been reported. It is still unclear whether increased TGF-β synthesis during chronic neurodegenerative diseases represents a compensatory response to restore tissue homeostasis or contributes to pathology. Studies in transgenic and infusion animal models have shown that TGF-β1 increases β-amyloid production and deposition, causing damage to the brain microvasculature, but it can also prevent β-amyloid accumulation by enhancing its clearance by microglia (Wyss-Coray et al., 2001). In animal models of CNS and PNS autoimmunity, TGF-β has primarily an anti-inflammatory and neuroprotective role (Owens et al., 2001). Transforming growth factor-β produced by malignant gliomas is thought to be involved in tumor growth, angiogenesis, and suppression of anti-tumor immune surveillance (Platten et al., 2001).

In vitro, astrocytes, Schwann cells, and oligodendrocytes express RNA for all three TGF-β isoforms, whereas microglia express only TGF-β1 (Pratt and McPherson, 1997). Astrocytes secrete bioactive TGF-β2 (Benveniste, 1998). Transforming growth factor-β1 causes changes in astrocyte motility, morphology, and proliferation and enhances production of several cytokines, including IL-6, leukemia inhibitory factor (LIF), nerve growth factor (NGF), platelet-derived growth factor (PDGF), and monocyte chemoattractant protein-1 (MCP-1)/CCL2. TGF-β1 also promotes differentiation of cultured oligodendrocytes and acts as a potent suppressor of the pro-inflammatory and cytotoxic functions of microglia (Benveniste, 1998) (Fig. 22.2).

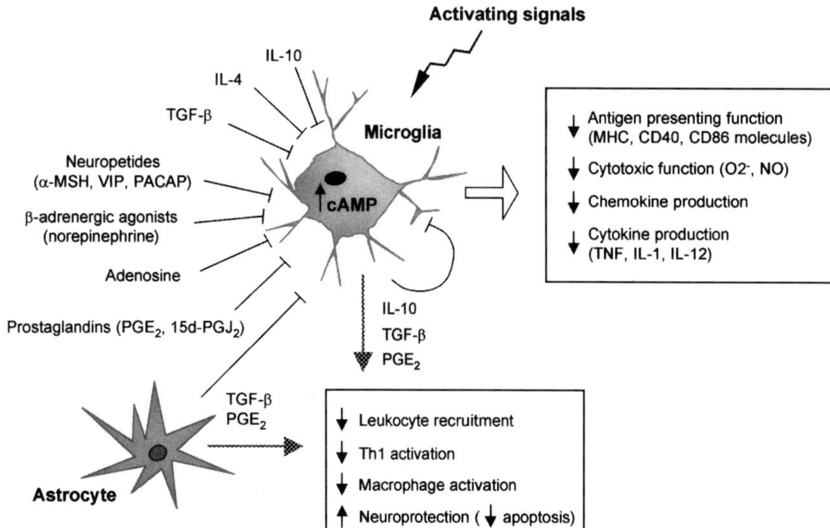

FIGURE 22.2 Anti-inflammatory cytokine circuits in the central nervous system (CNS). Substances produced in the normal and inflamed CNS, like neuropeptides, neurotransmitters, adenosine, and prostaglandins, downregulate microglia activation by increasing cyclic adenosine monophosphate (cAMP) levels. Cytokines, like interleukin (IL)-4, IL-10, and transforming growth factor-β (TGF-β) also inhibit microglia pro-inflammatory and cytotoxic functions. Upon activation, microglia and astrocytes can themselves secrete anti-inflammatory/neuroprotective mediators that may act in an autocrine and paracrine manner. MHC: major histocompatibility complex; α-MSH: α-melanocyte-stimulating hormone; NO: nitric oxide; PACAP: pituitary adenylate cyclase-activating polypeptide; PGE_2: prostaglandin E_2; 15d-PGJ_2: 15-deoxy-delta 12, 14 prostaglandin J2; VIP: vasoactive intestinal peptide.

Tumor Necrosis Factor Family

The TNF-cytokine family comprises nearly 20 members that are critically involved in the regulation of inflammation and immune responses, development of lymphoid organs, and tissue homeostasis. These are type II membrane proteins that can act in a membrane-bound form or as proteolytically processed, soluble cytokines in an autocrine, paracrine, or endocrine manner. Studies of TNF-related cytokines in the nervous system have been limited largely to TNF (also denominated TNF-α) and, to a lesser extent, to lymphotoxin-α (previously denominated TNF-β). Tumor necrosis factor is a pleiotropic cytokine produced primarily by activated macrophages and expressed as a 26 kDa transmembrane protein that can be cleaved by the enzyme TNF convertase (TACE/ADAM17) to release a 17 kDa soluble TNF form. Tumor necrosis factor binds and signals its effects through two structurally related but functionally distinct receptors, TNFR1 (p55 TNF receptor) and TNFR2 (p75 TNF receptor), that are coexpressed on most cell types, including neurons, glial cells, and cerebrovascular endothelial cells. Most of the TNF-induced biological responses are mediated by TNFR1. Tumor necrosis factor plays a crucial role in immunity and inflammation, mainly through its ability to induce synthesis of adhesion molecules and chemokines implicated in leukocyte recruitment, and in the control of cell proliferation, differentiation, and apoptosis.

Tumor necrosis factor is a key cytokine in regulating neuroinflammation. Production of TNF has been demonstrated in the CNS and PNS in numerous clinical and experimental pathologies (Table 22.2). Owing to its pro-inflammatory activity, TNF has been implicated in the pathogenesis of multiple sclerosis, EAE, and EAN (Owens et al., 2001) and is thought to contribute to early neuronal injury following acute brain damage (Allan and Rothwell, 2001). Several transgenic mice have been developed in which TNF is expressed in CNS neurons or glial cells such as oligodendrocytes and astrocytes. Depending on the source and onset of transgene expression, these mice develop no or only mild CNS pathology, spontaneous neurological disease with CNS inflammation and demyelination, or persistent disease following EAE induction (Owens et al., 2001; Probert and Akassoglou, 2001). All these studies have unraveled a role for TNF in microglia activation. Conversely, studies in TNF receptor-KO mice indicate that TNF has immunosuppressive properties, serves a neuroprotective function, and promotes remyelination (Bruce et al., 1996; Arnett et al., 2001; Wang et al., 2002). These apparently conflicting data likely reflect the complexity of TNF actions on different cellular targets, in different experimental disease models, and in different phases of the inflammatory process.

Together with brain-associated and infiltrating macrophages, microglia represent the major source of TNF in CNS autoimmune disease and following acute brain injury (Renno et al., 1995; Gregersen et al., 2000). Tumor necrosis factor synthesis in cultured microglia is readily induced by numerous stimuli (Table 22.2). Lipopolysaccharide and bacterial DNA containing motifs of unmethylated CpG dinucleotides (CpG-DNA) are the most potent stimuli for induction of TNF in microglia through binding and activation of Toll-like receptors (TLR)-4 and TLR-9, respectively (Aloisi, 2001; Dalpke et al., 2002). Toll-like receptors represent recognition and signal transducing receptors for microbial molecular components that could be implicated in microglia activation in various neuropathological conditions (Nguyen et al., 2002). Microglia-derived TNF has been shown to be part of an autocrine loop inducing synthesis of pro- and anti-inflammatory cyto-

TABLE 22.2 *Glial Cells As Sources and Targets of Master Inflammatory Cytokines IL-1, TNF and IL-6*

Cytokine	*CNS/PNS Expression*	*Implicated in*	*Major Cell Source*	*In Vitro Stimuli*	*Effects on Glial Cells*
IL-1β	Axonal injury Excitotoxic injury Ischemia Alzheimer's disease Parkinson disease Viral, bacterial and parasitic infections EAE, EAN, MS, GBS	Neuroinflammation Neurodegeneration CNS remyelination	Microglia	Gram-positive and Gram-negative bacteria LPS, CpG-DNA, T. *gondii*, HIV-1 Tat and gp120, HTLV-1 tax, HSV, CMV, MV IFN-γ + β-amyloid; prion protein SP ATP Myelin phagocytosis	↑ M-CSF, GM-CSF, G-CSF, IL-6, chemokine, LIF, CNTF, NGF, GDNF, bFGF; PDGF, PGE_2, α1-antichymotrypsin and tissue factor production in astrocytes ↑ ICAM-1/CD54, VCAM-1/CD106 in astrocytes and Schwann cells
TNF	As above	Neuroinflammation Neurodegeneration Neuroprotection CNS remyelination	Microglia	As above	As above ↑ IL-10, IL-12 production in microglia ↑ IL-6, LIF, MCP-1/CCL2 and NO production in Schwann cells ↓ Oligodendrocyte survival, proliferation and differentiation, in combination with IFN-γ ↓ Schwann cell differentiation and myelin production, in combination with IFN-γ
IL-6	As above	Antiviral protection Neuroinflammation Neurodegeneration Neuroprotection	Microglia Astrocytes Schwann cells	As above IL-1β, TNF, SP + IL-1β, adenosine, VIP, PACAP, β-adrenergic agonists, Oncostatin M TNF	↑ NGF production in astrocytes ↑ IL-10 production in microglia ↑ LIF production in Schwann cells

EAE, experimental autoimmune encephalomyelitis; EAN, experimental autoimmune encephalomyelitis; MS, multiple sclerosis; GBS, Guillain-Barré syndrome; HIV-1, human immunodeficiency virus-1; *T. gondii*, *Toxoplasma gondii*; HTLV-1, human T-lymphotropic virus type-1; HSV, herpes symplex virus; CMV, cytomegalovirus; MV, measles virus; SP, substance P; VIP, vasoactive intestinal peptide; PACAP, pituitary adenylate-activating peptide; PGE_2, prostaglandinE_2; LIF, leukemia inhibitory factor; CNTF, ciliary neurotrophic factor; NGF, nerve growth factor; GDNF, glial cell line-derived neurotrophic factor; bFGF, basic fibroblast growth factor; PDGF, platelet-derived growth factor.

kines (Becher et al., 2000). Tumor necrosis factor synthesis in microglia appears to be under strict control, as it is suppressed by numerous anti-inflammatory substances produced in the normal and pathological CNS (Aloisi, 2001; Delgado et al., 2003) (Fig. 22.2). Production of TNF, but not of TGF-β or IL-10, by microglia is inhibited during phagocytosis of apoptotic cells, suggesting that microglia engaged in the removal of damaged cells exhibit a noninflammatory phenotype (Magnus et al., 2002). In light of recent studies showing that neurons regulate microglia activation through direct cell-to-cell interactions (the CD200-CD200 receptor pathway) (Hoek et al., 2000), it would be interesting to determine whether such interactions are implicated in dysregulated cytokine production by microglia in neurodegenerative diseases.

In vitro, TNF affects axonal conduction and inhibits neurite outgrowth, is toxic to oligodendrocytes, and stimulates microglia phagocytosis and cytokine production, thus supporting an effector role for TNF in CNS tissue injury (Benveniste, 1998; Beattie et al., 2002; Neumann et al., 2002). Treatment of astrocytes and Schwann cells with TNF induces synthesis of numerous membrane-associated and soluble molecules, including cytokines (Table 22.2). The dual action (detrimental and beneficial) of TNF in the CNS makes it difficult to predict the therapeutic potential of TNF-blocking agents in neurological diseases and underscores the need to know more about the timing, source, and regulation of this cytokine and its receptors in the nervous tissue.

Similarly to TNF, lymphotoxin-α binds to TNFR1 and TNFR2 and influences tissue inflammation through induction of adhesion molecules, cytokines, and chemokines. Lymphotoxin production in the CNS has been demonstrated during autoimmune diseases, mainly in infiltrating macrophages and microglia.

Interleukin-1 Family

Interleukin 1 comprises two molecules, IL-1α and IL-1β, with similar biological effects. The expression of these molecules is regulated independently, but they share and have similar affinity for a common receptor, the type I IL-1R. Interleukin-1α and IL-1β also bind to the type II IL-1R, which does not mediate any biological signals but serves to regulate IL-1 activity. Expression of type I IL-1R has been reported on subsets of neurons, microglia, astrocytes, and Schwann cells. The IL-1 family also includes another natural regulator of IL-1, the IL-1 receptor antagonist (IL-1ra), which binds to type I IL-1R but fails to recruit the IL-1R accessory protein required for IL-1 signaling. Interleukin-1α, IL-1β, and IL-1ra are produced as precursors. Pro-IL-1β is inactive and must be cleaved by the IL-1 converting enzyme caspase-1 to generate and release biologically active IL-1β. Interleukin-1 is a master proinflammatory cytokine that is produced predominantly by cells of the monocyte/macrophage lineage and regulates various steps of the innate and adaptive immune response. Similarly to TNF, IL-1 acts as an inducer/amplifier of the inflammatory and healing responses. Many biological effects of IL-1 are known to occur through NF-κB- and AP-1-mediated mechanisms.

Interleukin-1β has been detected in the nervous system during infectious, autoimmune, and neurodegenerative disorders (Table 22.2). It is an important mediator of the inflammatory response in various forms of acute brain damage (Allan and Rothwell, 2001; Jander et al., 2001; Basu et al., 2002; Shamash et al., 2002). In these conditions, IL-1β is thought to induce expression of cell adhesion molecules and production of chemokines promoting the recruitment of leukocytes (mainly neutrophils and monocytes/macrophages) that exacerbate the primary neuronal damage through release of noxious substances like cytokines, proteases, and toxic free radicals. Although IL-1β has been proposed as a pathogenic marker of Alzheimer's disease, recent work has doubted the contribution of IL-1β to chronic neurodegenerative processes (Walsh et al., 2001). Antagonizing IL-1 protects neural cells in experimental models of stroke and multiple sclerosis. A role for IL-1 in CNS repair is supported by studies showing that mice deficient in IL-1 fail to upregulate neurotrophic factors in response to injurious stimuli and fail to remyelinate properly (Herx et al., 2000; Mason et al., 2001).

Interleukin-1β is produced mainly by activated microglia (Table 22.2), although some studies indicate that astrocytes and Schwann cells can also express IL-1 in some pathological conditions. Similarly to TNF, IL-1β acts on astrocytes and Schwann cells and, alone or in synergism with TNF and IFN-γ, induces expression of multiple inflammatory genes and neurotrophic factors in these glial cell types (Benveniste, 1998) (Table 22.2). These findings highlight the importance of cytokines produced by macrophages/microglia and T cells early after induction of brain injury in recruiting other glial cell types into the inflammatory network. Microglia are also a major intracerebral source of IL-1ra, which has an anti-inflammatory and neuroprotective role (Allan and Rothwell, 2001). Little is known about regulation of IL-1ra in microglia, except that it is inhibited by IFN-γ and potentiated by IL-4 (Liu et al., 1998).

Interleukin-4

Interleukin-4, a 20 kDa cytokine produced mainly by mature Th2 cells and cells of the mast cell and basophil lineage, has an important role in allergic diseases and in the regulation of inflammation. Interleukin-4 also has potent antitumor activity and suppresses macrophage activation. Interleukin-4 is produced in the CNS and PNS during infectious and autoimmune diseases and is proposed to play a role in preventing/reducing EAE and EAN (Owens et al., 2001). A neuroprotective role for IL-4 in the CNS is supported by its ability to inhibit production of NO and pro-inflammatory cytokines by activated microglia (Chao et al., 1993) and to stimulate NGF synthesis in cultured astrocytes (Awatsuji et al., 1993). Malignant and reactive astrocytes also express the IL-4 receptor. Neither astrocytes nor microglia have been shown to produce IL-4. Owing to the efficacy of IL-4 in the treatment of malignant gliomas (Benedetti et al., 1999) and in inhibiting inflammation when overexpressed in the CNS, the regulation and role of IL-4 in the neural tissue require further investigation.

Interleukin-6 Family

Members of the IL-6 family of cytokines comprise LIF, IL-6, IL-11, ciliary neurotrophic factor (CNTF), oncostatin M (OSM), cardiotrophin-1, and growth-promoting activity. These proteins share a four-helical bundle structure, a common signal transducer (gp130) in their receptor complexes, and, in some cases, overlapping functions. Among them, IL-6 has been the most extensively studied for its role in neuroinflammation and neurodegeneration (Gadient and Patterson, 1999).

Interleukin-6 is a pleiotropic cytokine whose functions include induction of acute-phase proteins and regulation of hematopoiesis, B cell growth, and antibody production. Interleukin-6 may also act as an anti-inflammatory cytokine, as it inhibits production of pro-inflammatory cytokines and induces IL-1ra and soluble p55 TNF receptor (TNFR) that attenuate inflammation. Expression of IL-6 is increased in the CNS and PNS in numerous pathological conditions (Table 22.2) (Van Wagoner and Benveniste, 1999). The IL-6 receptor is expressed on neurons and astrocytes and is increased during CNS inflammation. Astrocytes express IL-6 after brain ischemia and during viral and parasitic infection, and secrete substantial amounts of IL-6 in culture (Benveniste, 1998). Expression of IL-6 has also been demonstrated in microglia after cerebral ischemia and excitotoxic cell damage, and following *in vitro* activation (Table 22.2). Schwann cells express IL-6 *in situ* after sciatic nerve crush and *in vitro* (Bolin et al., 1995). Following infection, IL-6 produced in the nervous system is thought to play a protective role by activating a rapid pro-inflammatory response and favoring immune-mediated elimination of the infectious agent. Interleukin-6-deficient mice are resistant to EAE, and the available data suggest that IL-6 may promote leukocyte recruitment to the CNS (Owens et al., 2001). Transgenic mice expressing IL-6 in astrocytes develop CNS inflammation and neurodegeneration, whereas transgenic mice with neuronal expression of IL-6 display intense microgliosis and astrogliosis but no neuronal damage, indicating that the level and/or source of IL-6 expression are crucial in determining the severity of pathology in different animal models (Wang et al., 2002). Evidence has also been provided that IL-6 has neuroprotective effects, promotes nerve regeneration, and induces NGF production in astrocytes (Loddick et al., 1998; Otten et al., 2000). The notion that glial cells are a primary target for the action of IL-6 is supported by studies in IL-6-deficient mice showing reduced activation of astrocytes and microglia following axotomy or cryo-injury (Klein et al., 1997).

Leukemia inhibitory factor is a cytokine implicated in the development of central and peripheral neurons, astrocytes, and oligodendrocytes, and is a key regulator of the tissue response to neural injury. Signaling through the LIF receptor prevents oligodendrocyte apoptosis in experimental autoimmune demyelination (Butzkueven et al., 2002). Leukemia inhibitory factor is expressed predominantly in some CNS neurons and is upregulated in glial cells, mainly in astrocytes, after cortical brain injury and focal cerebral ischemia, and in Schwann cells after peripheral nerve transection (Gadient and Patterson, 1999; Tofaris et al., 2002). *In vitro*, LIF production in astrocytes is induced by IL-1β, TNF, and TGF-β_1, whereas Schwann cells produce LIF in response to TGF-β_1 and IL-6. Leukemia inhibitory factor–deficient mice show less inflammation after mechanical injury to the sciatic nerve and slower microglial and astroglial responses to cortical injury, indicating that LIF regulates the inflammatory response in the nervous system (Sugiura et al., 2000).

Oncostatin M is a pleiotropic cytokine produced by macrophages and T cells, and has been implicated in the wound-healing process and regulation of the inflammatory response. The few studies available suggest a role for OSM in glia communication and activation. Oncostatin M has been detected in reactive astrocytes and microglia in multiple sclerosis lesions (Ruprecht et al., 2001). *In vitro*, OSM is produced by microglia after stimulation with prostaglandin E_2 (PGE_2) and cyclic adenosine monophosphate (cAMP)–elevating agents, and stimulates cytokine expression in astrocytes (Repovich and Benveniste, 2002).

Ciliary neurotrophic factor is a cytokine expressed primarily by Schwann cells in the normal PNS and by reactive astrocytes following acute brain damage. It supports neuronal and glial development and survival and has been implicated in astrogliosis. Interleukin-1β is a major stimulus for CNTF production in the damaged CNS (Herx et al., 2000) and in cultured astrocytes. Studies in CNTF-deficient mice and *in vitro* indicate that CNTF regulates glial cell survival in an inflammatory context and protects oligodendrocytes from TNF-mediated injury (Linker et al., 2002).

Interleukin-10

Interleukin-10 is a 35 kDa cytokine with major immunosuppressive and anti-inflammatory activities that is produced primarily by monocytes/macrophages and subsets of T cells. Interleukin-10 downregulates cellular immunity by acting directly on T cells, but also affects T cell responses indirectly by inhibiting expression of MHC, adhesion and costimulatory molecules, cytokines, chemokines, cytokine/chemokine receptors, prostaglandins, and NO in monocytes/macrophages and other immune cell types. Stimulation of IL-10 receptors regulates numerous life- or death-signaling pathways (e.g., JAK1/STAT3, phosphatidylinositol (PI) 3-kinase, mitogen-activated protein kinase (MAPK), SOCS, and NF-κB) and ultimately promotes cell survival.

The IL-10 receptor is constitutively expressed in the brain, and IL-10 production is induced in the CNS and PNS following infection and acute injury and during autoimmunity. In all these circumstances, IL-10 is produced by both infiltrating and tissue resident cells and is thought to play a major anti-inflammatory and neuroprotective role (Strle et al., 2001). Several studies have shown that IL-10 reduces brain damage after focal stroke, trauma, and excitotoxic injury (Grilli et al., 2000; Bachis et al., 2001). Following brain trauma, local application of IL-10 decreases microglia activation, TNF production, and astrocyte reactivity (Balasingam and Yong, 1996). When overexpressed in transgenic mice, delivered into the CNS, or administered peripherally, IL-10 prevents or ameliorates EAE (Strle et al., 2001). *In vitro*, IL-10 inhibits the ability of microglia to function as antigen-presenting cells and to produce pro-inflammatory mediators (Aloisi, 2001) (Fig. 22.2). Microglia produce IL-10 in the inflamed CNS (Jander et al., 1998) and secrete IL-10 *in vitro* following infection or exposure to LPS, TNF, and IL-6 (Benveniste, 1998). Microglia-derived IL-10 acts in an autocrine manner, inhibiting microglia pro-inflammatory functions (Frei et al., 1994). In contrast to what has been observed for pro-inflammatory cytokines like TNF and IL-12, IFN-γ inhibits whereas cAMP-elevating agents [like pituitary adenylate cyclase-activating polypeptide (PACAP) isoproterenol, and PGE_2] enhance LPS-induced IL-10 production by cultured microglia, implicating differential regulation of microglia pro- and anti-inflammatory activities (Aloisi, 2001). Astrocytes and Schwann cells have been reported to display IL-10 immunoreactivity in some neuroinflammatory conditions but fail to synthesize and secrete IL-10 *in vitro*. The therapeutic potential of IL-10 in CNS and PNS diseases will certainly require a better understanding of IL-10 sources and functions in the neural tissue.

Interleukin-12 Family

The IL-12 family comprises heterodimeric cytokines that play an important role in the development of innate and adaptive immune responses and in the regulation of IFN-γ production. It includes IL-12 and the two recently discovered cytokines IL-23 and IL-27. Interleukin-12, a 70 kDa heterodimeric cytokine consisting of a p35 and a p40 subunit, promotes the differentiation of naive T cells into Th1 cells and has been implicated in the development of cell-mediated immune responses during infectious and autoimmune CNS diseases (Owens et al., 2001). Studies in transgenic mice with astrocyte-targeted expression of p35 and p40 indicate that intracerebrally produced IL-12 favors CNS inflammation and, upon induction of EAE, facilitates the recruitment and activation of encephalitogenic T cells (Wang et al., 2002). Together with CNS-infiltrating macrophages, microglia have been indicated as a potential intracerebral source of IL-12 in inflammatory conditions (Becher et al., 2000). *In vitro*, microglia express IL-12 p35 and p40 mRNAs and secrete bioactive IL-12 p70 after exposure to IFN-γ plus LPS. Ligation of the costimulatory molecule CD40 on microglia by CD154 expressed on activated Th1 cells represents another major pathway involved in the induction of microglia IL-12 production (Aloisi et al., 1999) (Fig. 22.3). Microglia also express functional IL-12 receptors whose stimulation induces production of cytokines, including IL-12 and NO, which suggests that IL-12 may also promote microglia activation.

Interleukin-23, a heterodimer composed of the IL-12 p40 subunit combined with a unique p19 subunit, has potent activities on memory-activated T cells and stimulates macrophages to produce pro-inflammatory cytokines. Interleukin-23 was recently shown to be a crucial regulator of the CNS inflammatory process following EAE induction (Cua et al., 2003). In the inflamed CNS, both microglia and CNS-infiltrating macrophages upregulate production of IL-23, whereas no specific IL-23 receptor has been detected in microglia.

Interleukin-15

Interleukin-15 is a 14–15 kDa polypeptide that belongs to the 4-alpha-helix-bundle family of cytokines and uses the signal-transducing components of the IL-2 receptor complex (IL-2/IL-15R$\beta\gamma_c$), in addition to its high-affinity private receptor subunit IL-15Rα. Interleukin-15 has a key role in the development and function of NK cells and in the expansion of $CD8^+$ cytotoxic T cells, and has been implicated in the induction of Th1 responses. Interleukin-15 and IL-15Rα mRNAs are expressed in the normal brain, and IL-15 is augmented in the CNS in autoimmune and infectious diseases. *In vitro* activated microglia and astrocytes express IL-15 mRNA and secrete IL-15. Microglia also express functional IL-15R, whose stimulation regulates cell survival and NO production (Hanisch, 2002). These findings suggest that glia-derived IL-15 could

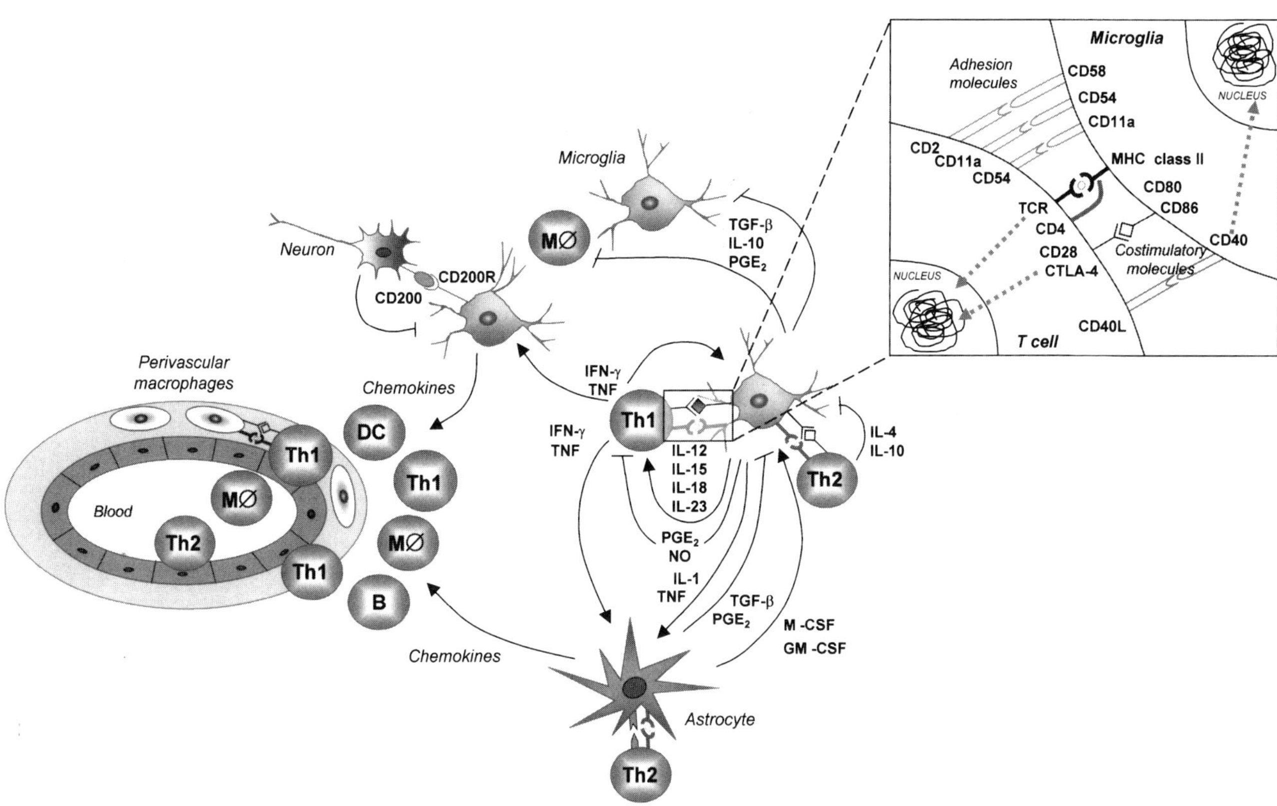

FIGURE 22.3 Intracerebral regulation of CD4$^+$ T cell responses by glia-derived cytokines. In infectious and autoimmune diseases of the central nervous system (CNS), CD4$^+$ T helper (Th) cells primed in peripheral lymphoid organs cross the blood–brain barrier and become reactivated upon recognition of the target antigen on local antigen presenting cells, most likely meningeal and perivascular macrophages (M∅), and microglia. During inflammation, microglia are the only CNS intraparenchymal cell type capable of expressing surface molecules mediating antigen-specific, adhesive, and costimulatory interactions with CD4$^+$ T cells (inset). Inhibitory signals delivered by neuronal cells, via direct cell-to-cell interactions (CD200-CD200R pathway) and/or soluble mediators such as neuropeptides, neurotrophins, neurotransmitters, may attenuate microglia activation (Aloisi, 2001). *In vitro*, microglia are able to process and present antigen and efficiently restimulate Th1 and Th2 cells. Following activation by Th1 cells and Th1-derived cytokines, microglia produce chemokines capable of attracting several types of immune cells [CD4$^+$ Th1 and Th2 cells, CD8$^+$ T cells, B cells, monocytes/macrophages, and dendritic cells (DC)] and cytokines such as interleukin (IL)-12, IL-15, IL-18, and IL-23 that promote Th1 responses and CNS inflammation. Anti-inflammatory mediators [transforming growth factor-β) (TGF-β), IL-10, prostaglandin E_2 (PGE_2)] produced by microglia may prevent further recruitment and activation of Th1 cells and macrophages/microglia. Cytokine-activated astrocytes may also contribute to the intracerebral regulation of T cell responses through secretion of chemokines, presentation of antigenic peptides to Th2 cells, and production of colony-stimulating factors [macrophage and granulocyte/macrophage colony-stimulating factors (M-CSF, GM-CSF)], promoting macrophage/microglia activation and anti-inflammatory mediators. NO: nitric oxide; TNF: tumor necrosis factor. (Slightly modified from Aloisi, 2001; *Glia*©2001 Wiley-Liss Inc.)

participate in the regulation of cell-mediated immune responses and microglia reactivity.

Interleukin-18

Interleukin-18 is related to the IL-1 family by structure, receptors, and signaling molecules. It is produced primarily by macrophages and dendritic cells and, like IL-1, is released as an inactive precursor, requiring cleavage by IL-1β-converting enzyme/caspase-1 for its maturation. Interleukin-18 induces production of IFN-γ by T and NK cells, promotes IL-12-driven Th1 responses, and has been implicated in the clearance of neurotropic viruses and in CNS autoimmunity. Expression of IL-18 mRNA and/or protein has been detected in the nervous system in normal conditions, in multiple sclerosis and EAE, and after focal brain ischemia and nerve injury, suggesting an important role for IL-18 in mediating neuroinflammation. Microglia are the primary source of IL-18 in the CNS (Hanisch, 2002; Hedtjarn et al., 2002) and express functional IL-18 receptors. Studies in IL-18-deficient mice suggest a role for IL-18 in promoting microglia activation during virus infection, possibly through induction of IFN-γ synthesis in the brain parenchyma (Mori et al., 2001).

Chemokines

Chemokines are a group of small (8-14 kDa), structurally related molecules that regulate cell migration in a variety of physiological and pathological conditions. Chemokines have been divided into four subfamilies, CXC, CC, C, and CX_3C, based on the sequence motif of conserved N-terminal cysteine residues, and act through interactions with a subset of seven-transmembrane, G-protein-coupled selective receptors expressed on target cells (Zlotnik and Yoshie, 2000).

Research on chemokines in the nervous system started in the early 1990s, focusing primarily on the role of these mediators in the recruitment of leukocytes into the injured nervous system and, recently, on novel functions such as development, homeostasis, and synaptic transmission (Asensio and Campbell, 1999). Since then, considerable evidence has accumulated that chemokines can be produced by neurons and glial cells in the CNS and PNS, and that all types of neural cells express functional chemokine receptors (Ransohoff, 1997; Hesselgesser and Horuk, 1999; Bajetto et al., 2002). Table 22.3 lists chemokines and chemokine receptors that have been shown to be expressed by glial cells *in situ* and/or *in vitro*. Because a new nomenclature for chemokines has been introduced recently (Zlotnik and Yoshie, 2000), in this chapter both the traditional and new denominations are used.

Constitutive chemokines

Chemokines that are constitutively expressed in the developing and adult nervous system include SDF-1/CXCL12 and fractalkine/CX3CL1. SDF-1/CXCL12 has three isoforms, SDF-1α, -β, and -γ, that are produced by alternative splicing from a single gene transcript and are differentially regulated during CNS and PNS development. SDF-1/CXCL12 mRNA is expressed in neurons and astrocytes *in vitro* and *in vivo*, and its levels appear to be barely influenced by disruption of nervous system homeostasis. The SDF-1/CXCL12 receptor, CXCR4, has been demonstrated in neurons, astrocytes, and microglia. Studies in mice engineered to lack SDF-1/CXCL12 or CXCR4 have unraveled a critical role for this chemokine/chemokine receptor pair in regulating neuronal precursor migration and neurogenesis in the cerebellum and hippocampus (Wang et al., 2002). Owing to its ability to stimulate proliferation of astrocytes and glioblastoma tumor cells, SDF-1/CXCL12 has been implicated in reactive gliosis and brain tumor formation (Bajetto et al., 2002).

Fractalkine/CX_3CL1 can exist as a membrane-bound protein or in a soluble form and acts by binding to CX_3CR1. Fractalkine/CX_3CL1 is expressed primarily by neurons in different brain areas, whereas CX_3CR1 appears confined to microglia and other brain-associated macrophages (Asensio and Campbell, 1999). Fractalkine/CX_3CL1 is upregulated in neurons and reactive astrocytes in pathological conditions, and in cultured activated astrocytes and microglia. Although a role for fractalkine/CX_3CL1 in the signaling from neurons to microglia has been proposed, mice deficient in either fractalkine/CX_3CL1 or the *CX_3CR1* gene show no CNS developmental abnormalities and no alterations in microglial reactivity, neuronal damage, or survival following acute brain injury (Jung et al., 2000; Wang et al., 2002). *In vitro*, fractalkine/CX_3CL1 affects microglia chemotaxis and cytokine production, and protects microglia from Fas-induced cell death.

Another chemokine expressed during CNS development in a subset of spinal cord astrocytes is GRO-α/CXCL1, which affects proliferation and migration of oligodendrocyte precursors (Tsai et al., 2002). Transgenic expression of GRO-α/CXCL1 in the CNS leads to recruitment of neutrophils and induces neurological symptoms, which could be mediated by direct effects of this chemokine on the functional activity of neuronal populations expressing the GRO-α/CXCL1 receptor CXCR2 (Asensio and Campbell, 1999).

Inducible chemokines

Inducible or inflammatory chemokines are expressed in numerous pathological conditions and play an essential role in regulating the migration of specific leukocyte subsets to the CNS and PNS (Ransohoff, 2002). A precise understanding of the role of chemokines in the injured neural tissue is, however, made difficult by the simultaneous expression of multiple chemokines with redundant and partially overlapping functions, as well as by the finding that inducible chemokines often bind more than one receptor.

Under inflammatory conditions, activated leukocytes penetrate the blood–brain barrier according to the multistep model of leukocyte-endothelial cell recognition, involving sequential interactions of adhesion molecules with their counterreceptors on activated endothelial cells and leukocytes, as well as interactions of chemokines with their receptors. Chemokines produced by endothelial cells and exposed on their luminal surface play a role in mediating firm adhesion by activating integrins on the leukocyte surface. The leukocytes are then directed by chemoattractant gradients to migrate across the endothelium and through the extracellular matrix into the tissue. Recent studies indicate that abluminal-to-luminal chemokine transcytosis and presentation by endothelial cells provides a mechanism that enables chemokines produced by intraparenchymal cells to reach the blood-endothelial interface and stimulate lymphocyte emigration (Middleton et al., 2002).

Cerebrovascular endothelial cells, brain-associated macrophages, resident neural cells, and tissue-infiltrating immune cells have all been shown to contribute to chemokine production in the inflamed nervous system. Due to the close association of astrocytes and microglia with the blood–brain barrier, chemokines produced by these cell types are thought to play an important role in regulating leukocyte migration into the CNS (Table 22.3). Evidence is also emerging that CNS and PNS neurons express chemokines that could recruit macrophages/microglia to sites of neuronal injury (Biber et al., 2002). *In vitro*, astrocytes, microglia, and, to a lesser extent, Schwann cells can produce a broad and largely overlapping panel of chemokines in response to a variety of activating stimuli (cytokines, infection, microbial components, β-amyloid), whereas the expression of chemokines *in vivo* seems to be more restricted to a given glial cell type and varies depending on the type of pathological insult (Ambrosini and Aloisi, 2004) (Table 22.3).

MCP-1/CCL2 and its receptor CCR2 represent one of the most extensively investigated chemokine/chemokine receptor pairs in neuroinflammation and have been implicated in the recruitment of monocytes/macrophages into the nervous tissue during autoimmune, infectious, and neurodegenerative diseases (Mahad and Ransohoff, 2003). Transgenic expression of MCP-1/CCL2 in the CNS leads to discrete perivascular infiltration by monocytes/macrophages, whereas mice lacking MCP-1/CCL2 or CCR2 are protected from EAE and show decreased macrophage infiltration and neuronal damage following brain ischemia or nerve transection. MCP-1/CCL2 is produced by astrocytes in various pathological conditions and by Schwann cells following nerve transection. Astrocytes also produce IP-10/CXCL10, a chemokine implicated in the recruitment of Th1 cells to the CNS during infectious and autoimmune diseases (Hesselgesser and Horuk, 1999).

MIP-1α/CCL3 and MIP-1β/CCL4, which attract T cells and monocytes/macrophages, are confined predominantly to activated microglia in HIV-1 encephalitis, multiple sclerosis, and following cerebral ischemia, whereas MIP-3α/CCL20, a chemokine acting on T cells, B cells, and dendritic cells, is produced mainly by astrocytes *in vitro* and during EAE. Thus, chemokines produced by distinct glial cell types may attract different immune cell populations and act in concert to regulate neuroinflammation. Similarly to other pro-inflammatory cytokines, chemokine synthesis by microglia is regulated by anti-inflammatory mediators (Fig. 22.2).

In addition to recruiting blood-derived leukocytes, chemokines produced during CNS inflammation may also regulate migration and activation of glial cells. Evidence is emerging that glial cells themselves express receptors for and respond to a number of inflammatory chemokines (Bajetto et al., 2002; Ambrosini and Aloisi, 2004). Microglia express CCR3 and CCR5, which are though to act as coreceptors for HIV infection, and show enhanced migration and production of proteases and cytokines in response to various CC chemokines. Astrocytes express CCR1 and CCR5, the promiscuous receptors for MIP-1α/CCL3 and RANTES/CCL5, and CCR2, the receptor for MCP-1/CCL2. *In vitro*, RANTES/CCL5 acts on astrocytes promoting growth and survival, stimulating production of chemokines and modulating chemokine receptor expression.

Chemokines are viewed as the most promising targets for inhibition of inflammatory diseases, and chemokine antagonists are currently being developed and tested for their efficacy in blocking acute and chronic neuroinflammatory processes. Such efforts will certainly benefit from a deeper understanding of the mechanisms regulating chemokine synthesis and actions in the nervous system.

SUMMARY AND PERSPECTIVES

From this chapter, a picture emerges in which maintenance of tissue homeostasis and responses to pathological stimuli in the nervous system are governed by the integrated action of multiple cytokines, most of which appear to be produced by glial cells. Although each glial cell type has the potential to express various cytokines, it is the kind of stimulus that dictates the temporal and cellular cascade of cytokine expression that is initiated under a given condition. Recent studies in transgenic and knockout mice have led to the recognition that several glia-derived cytokines, such as IL-1, TNF and IL-6, may subserve both neuroinflammatory and neuroprotective functions. The application of advanced molecular approaches that allow control of transgene expression using an inducible expression system or inactivation of gene espression in specific cell types with a conditioned gene targeting system represents a further step toward a better understanding of cytokine functions in the nervous system and of the contribution of glial cells to the cytokine network.

Cytokines are instrumental in determining the nature, magnitude, and duration of inflammatory reactions and, as such, represent ideal targets for interfering with pathogenic processes. Because dysregulated cytokine production has been detected in immunological and nonimmunological neurological diseases and because cytokines have complex effects on neural cells, it is important that the biological significance and impact of such imbalances be defined for each condition. The recent discovery of cytokine polymorphisms associated with neurological diseases (e.g., Alzheimer's disease, multiple sclerosis) strongly suggests that such associations could be relevant for disease pathogenesis and prognosis. The current challenges in cytokine research in the nervous system are to better understand the mechanisms controlling cytokine expression and activity, as well as the tissue- and cell-specific consequences of dysregulated expression of a given cytokine. Elucidation of these issues is an important and obligatory step in the development and use of cytokines as therapeutic agents for acute and chronic neurological diseases.

TABLE 22.3 *Chemokine Production and Chemokine Receptor Expression by Central Nervous System and Peripheral Nervous System Glia*

Cell Type	*Chemokine*	In Vivo *Expression*	In Vitro *Stimuli*	*Chemokine Receptors*
Astrocyte	Gro-α/KC/CXCL1	EAE[a]		CXCR3,CXCR4, CCR1, CCR2, CCR5, CX_3CR1
	IL-8/CXCL8		IL-1β, TNF, HIV-1, HIV-1 Tat, CMV	
	SDF-1α,β/CXCL12	Developing CNS	Constitutive	
	IP-10/CXCL10	Ischemia, EAE, MS, TE, experimental viral infections	IFN-γ + TNF, IFN-β, TMEV, NDV, HIV-1 Tat and gp120	
	I-TAC/CXCL11			
	I-309/CCL1		IFN-γ, IFN-β	
	MCP-1/CCL2	Trauma, ischemia, excitotoxicity, EAE, MS HIV-1, encephalitis experimental viral infections, TE, bacterial meningitis, tumor	IL-1β, TNF, TGF-β, HIV-1 Tat, CMV	
	MIP-1β/CCL4	AD, EAE, Trauma	IL-1β, TNF	
	RANTES/CCL5	EAE, MS, bacterial meningitis	IL-1β, IL-1β + IFN-γ, TNF, TMEV, HIV-1	
	MIP-3α/CCL20	EAE	IL-1β, TNF	
	MIP-3β/CCL19	EAE		
	Fractalkine/CX_3CL1	Prion disease, HIV-1-associated dementia	IL-1β, TNF	
Microglia	IL-8/CXCL8		LPS, IL-1β, β-amyloid, CMV	CXCR3, CXCR4, CCR2, CCR3, CCR5, CCR8, CX_3CR1
	IP-10/CXCL10		LPS, IFN-γ, IFN-γ + CD40 ligation, IFN-β, HSV, NDV	
	I-309/CCL1	EAE	LPS, IFN-γ, IFN-β	
	MCP-1/CCL2	Ischemia, excitotoxicity, AD, tumor	LPS, IFN-γ + CD40 ligation, IFN-β, HIV-1 Tat, β-amyloid, CMV	
	MIP-1α/CCL3	HIV-1 encephalitis, MS, ischemia	LPS, CpG-DNA, TNF, IFN-β, HIV-1 Tat, β-amyloid	
	MIP-1β/CCL4	HIV-1 encephalitis, MS	LPS, CpG-DNA, TNF, IFN-β, HIV-1 Tat, β-amyloid	
	RANTES/CCL5	EAE, bacterial meningitis, HIV-1 encephalitis, TE	LPS, IFN-β, IL-1β, TNF, HSV	
	MIP-3β/CCL19	EAE		
	MDC/CCL22	EAE	LPS, IFN-γ + CD40 ligation	
	Fractalkine/CX3CL1		LPS	
Oligodendrocyte				CXCR1, CXCR2
Schwann cell	IL-8/CXCL8	Nerve transection		
	SDF-1β/γ/CXCL12	Constitutive		
	MCP-1/CCL2	Nerve transection	TNF, LIF	
	MIP-1α/CCL3	Nerve transection		

AD: ; CNS: central nervous system; CMV: cytomegalovirus; EAE: experimental autoimmune encephalomyelitis; HIV-1: human immunodeficiency virus-1; HSV: herpes symplex virus. IFN: interferon; IL: interleukin; LPS: lipopolysaccharide; MS: multiple sclerosis; NDV: Newcastle disease virus; TE: *Toxoplasma* encephalitis; TMEV: Theiler's murine encephalomyelitis virus; TNF: tumor necrosis factor.

ACKNOWLEDGMENT

Owing to space limits, many relevant studies could not be quoted in this chapter. I thank Dr. Giulio Levi for his valuable comments and Mrs. Estella Sansonetti for her help in preparing the figures.

REFERENCES

Agresti, C., Bernardo, A., Del Russo, N., Marziali, G, Battistini, A., Aloisi, F., Levi, G., and Coccia, E.M. (1998) Synergistic stimulation of major histocompatibility complex class I and interferon regulatory factor 1 gene expression by interferon γ and tumor necrosis factor α in oligodendrocytes. *Eur. J. Neurosci.* 10:2975–2983.

Akiyama, H., Ikeda, K., Katoh, M., McGeer, E.G., and McGeer, P.L. (1994) Expression of MRP14, 27E10, interferon-alpha and leukocyte common antigen by reactive microglia in postmortem human brain tissue. *J. Neuroimmunol.* 50:195–201.

Allan, S.M. and Rothwell, N.J. (2001) Cytokines and acute neurodegeneration. *Nat. Rev. Neurosci.* 2:734–744.

Aloisi, F. (2001) Immune function of microglia. *Glia* 36:165–179.

Aloisi, F., Penna, G., Polazzi, E., Minghetti, L., and Adorini, L. (1999) CD40-CD154 interaction and IFN-γ are required for IL-12 but not prostaglandin E_2 secretion by microglia during antigen presentation to Th1 cells. *J. Immunol.* 162:1384–1391.

Aloisi, F., Ria, F., and Adorini, L. (2000) Regulation of T-cell responses by CNS antigen-presenting cells: different roles for microglia and astrocytes. *Immunol. Today* 21:141–147.

Ambrosini, E. and Aloisi, F. (2004) Glial cells and chemokines: a complex network in the central nervous system. *Neurochem. Res.* 29:1017–1038.

Arnett, H.A., Mason, J., Marino, M., Suzuki, K., Matsushima, G.K., and Ting, J.P. (2001) TNFalpha promotes proliferation of oligodendrocyte progenitors and remyelination. *Nat. Neurosci.* 4:1116–1122.

Asensio, V.C. and Campbell, I.L. (1999) Chemokines in the CNS: plurifunctional mediators in diverse states. *Trends Neurosci.* 22:504–512.

Awatsuji, H., Urukawa, Y., Hirota, M., Murakami, Y., Nii, S., Furukawa, S., and Hayashi, K. (1993) Interleukin-4 and -5 as modulators of nerve growth factor synthesis/secretion in astrocytes. *J. Neurosci. Res.* 34:539–545.

Bachis, A., Colangelo, A.M., Vicini, S., Doe, P.P., De Bernardi, M.A., Brooker, G., and Mocchetti, I. (2001) Interleukin-10 prevents glutamate-mediated cerebellar granule cell death by blocking caspase-3-like activity. *J. Neurosci.* 21:3104–3112.

Bajetto, A., Bonavia, R., Barbero, S., and Schettini, G. (2002) Characterization of chemokines and their receptors in the central nervous system: pathophysiological implications. *J. Neurochem.* 82:1311–1329.

Balasingam, V. and Yong, V.W. (1996) Attenuation of astrocglial reactivity by interleukin-10. *J. Neurosci.* 16:2945–2955.

Basu, A., Krady, J.K., O'Malley, M., Styren, S.D., Dekosky, S.T., and Levison, S. (2002) The type 1 interleukin-1 receptor is essential for the efficient activation of microglia and the induction of multiple proinflammatory mediators in response to brain injury. *J. Neurosci.* 22:6071–6082.

Beattie, E.C., Stellwagen, D., Morishita, W., Bresnahan, J.C., Ha, B.K., Von Zastrow, M., Beattie, M.S., and Malenka, R.C. (2002) Control of synaptic strength by glial TNFalpha. *Science* 295: 2282–2285.

Becher, B., Prat, A., and Antel, J.P. (2000) Brain-immune connection: immuno-regulatory properties of CNS-resident cells. *Glia* 29:293–304.

Benedetti, S., Bruzzone, M.G., Pollo, B., Di Meco, F., Magrassi, L., Pirola, B., Cirenei, N., Colombo, M.P., and Finocchiaro, G. (1999) Eradication of rat malignant gliomas by retroviral-mediated in vivo delivery of the interleukin-4 gene. *Cancer Res.* 59:645–652.

Benveniste, E.N. (1998) Cytokine actions in the central nervous system. *Cytok. Growth Factor Rev.* 9:259–275.

Biber, K., Zuurman, M.W., Dijkstra, I.M., and Boddeke, H.W. (2002) Chemokines in the brain: neuroimmunology and beyond. *Curr. Opin. Pharmacol.* 2:63–68.

Bolin, L.M., Verity, A.N., Silver, J.E., Shooter, E.M., and Abrams, J.S. (1995) Interleukin-6 production by Schwann cells and induction in sciatic nerve injury. *J. Neurochem.* 64:850–858.

Bottner, M., Krieglstein, K., and Unsicker, K. (2000) The transforming growth factor-βs: structure signaling, and roles in nervous system development and functions. *J. Neurochem.* 75:2227–2240.

Bruce, A.J., Boling, W., Kindy, M.S., Peschon, J., Kraemer, P.J., Carpenter, M.K., Holtsberg, F.W., and Mattson, M. P. (1996) Altered neuronal and microglial responses to excitotoxic and ischemic brain injury in mice lacking TNF receptors. *Nat. Med.* 2:788–794.

Butzkueven, H., Zhang, J.-G., Soilu-Hanninen, M.S., Hochrein, H., Chionh, F., Shipham, K.A., Emery, B., Turnley, A.M., Petratos, S., Ernst, M., Bartlett, P.F., and Kilpatrick, T.J. (2002) LIF receptor signaling limits immune-mediated demyelination by enhancing oligodendrocyte survival. *Nat. Med.* 8:613–619.

Chao, C.C., Molitor, T.W., and Hu, S. (1993) Neuroprotective role of IL-4 against activated microglia. *J. Immunol.* 151:1473–1481.

Chelbi-Alix, M.K., Brouard, A., Boissard, C., Pelaprat, D., Rostene, W., and Thang, M.N. (1994) Induction by vasoactive intestinal peptide of interferon alpha/beta synthesis in glial cells but not in neurons. *J. Cell. Physiol.* 158:47–54.

Cua, D.J., Sherlock, J., Chen, Y., Murphy, C.A., Joyce, B., Seymour, B., Lucian, L., To, W., Kwan, S., Churakova, T., Zurawski, S., Wiekowski, M., Lira, S.A., Kastelein, R.A., and Sedgwick, J.D. (2003) Interleukin-23 rather than interleukin-12 is the critical cytokine for autoimmune inflammation of the brain. *Nature* 421:744–748.

Dalpke, A.H., Schafer, M.K., Frey, M., Zimmermann, S., Tebbe, J., Weihe, E., and Heeg, K. (2002) Immunostimulatory CpG-DNA activates murine microglia. *J. Immunol.* 168:4854–4863.

Deckert-Schlüter, M., Bluethmann, H., Kaefer, N., Rang, A., and Schlüter, D. (1999) Interferon-gamma receptor-mediated but not tumor necrosis factor receptor type 1- or type 2-mediated signalling is crucial for the activation of cerebral blood vessel endothelial cells and microglia in murine *Toxoplasma* encephalitis. *Am. J. Pathol.* 154:1549–1561.

Delgado, M., Leceta, J., and Ganea, D. (2003) Vasoactive intestinal peptide and pituitary adenylate cyclase-activating polypeptide inhibit the production of inflammatory mediators by activated microglia. *J. Leukocyte Biol.* 73:155–164.

Frei, K., Lins, H., Schwerdel, C., and Fontana, A. (1994) Antigen presentation in the central nervous system. The inhibitory effect of IL-10 on MHC class II expression and cytokine production depends on the inducing signals and the type of cell analyzed. *J. Immunol.* 152:2720–2728.

Gadient, R.A. and Patterson, P.H. (1999) Leukemia inhibitory factor, interleukin 6, and other cytokines using the gp130 transducing receptor: roles in inflammation and injury. *Stem Cells* 17:127–137.

Giulian, D., Johnson, B., Krebs, J.F., George, J.K., and Tapscott, M. (1991) Microglial mitogens are produced in the developing and injured mammalian brain. *J. Cell Biol.* 112:323–333.

Gregersen, R., Lambertsen, K., and Finsen, B. (2000) Microglia and macrophages are the major source of tumor necrosis factor in permanent middle cerebral artery occlusion in mice. *J. Cereb. Flow Metab.* 20:53–65.

Grilli, M., Barbieri, I., Basudev, H., Brusa, R., Casati, C., Lozza, G., and Ongini, E. (2000) Interleukin-10 modulates neuronal threshold of vulnerability to ischeamic damage. *Eur. J. Neurosci.* 12: 2265–2272.

Hanisch, U.K (2002) Microglia as a source and target of cytokines. *Glia* 40:140–155.

Hedtjarn, M., Leverin, A.L., Eriksson, K., Blomgren, K., Mallard, C., and Hagberg, H. (2002) Interleukin-18 involvement in hypoxic-ischemic brain injury. *J. Neurosci.* 22:5910–5919.

Herx, L.M., Rivest, S., and Yong, W.V. (2000) Central nervous system-initiated inflammation and neurotrophism in trauma: IL-1β is required for the production of ciliary neurotrophic factor. *J. Immunol.* 165:2232–2239.

Hesselgesser, J.H. and Horuk, R. (1999) Chemokine and chemokine receptor expression in the central nervous system. *J. Neurovirol.* 5:13–26.

Hoek, R.M., Ruuls, S.R., Murphy, C.A., Wright, G.J., Goddard, R., Zurawski, S.M., Blom, B., Homola, M.E., Streit, W.J., Brown, M., Barclay, A.N. and Sedgwick, J.D. (2000) Downregulation of the macrophage lineage through interaction with OX2 (CD200) *Science* 290:1768–1771.

Jander, S., Pohl, J, D'Urso, D., Gillen, C., and Stoll, G. (1998) Time course and cellular localization of interleukin-10 mRNA and protein expression in autoimmune inflammation of the rat central nervous system. *Am. J. Pathol.* 152:975–982.

Jander, S., Schroeter, M., Peters, O., Witte, O.W., and Stoll, G. (2001) Cortical spreading depression induces proinflammatory cytokine gene expression in the rat brain. *J. Cereb. Flow Metab.* 21:218–225.

Jung, S., Aliberti, J., Graemmel, P., Sunshine, M.J., Kreutzberg, G.W., Sher, A., and Littman, D.R. (2000) Analysis of fractalkine receptor CX_3CR1 function by targeted deletion and green fluorescent reporter gene insertion. *Mol. Cell. Biol.* 20:4106–4114.

Kiefer, R., Schweitzer, T., Jung, S., Toyka, K.V., and Hartung, H.P. (1998) Sequential expression of transforming growth factor-β1 by T-cells, macrophages, and microglia in rat spinal cord during autoimmune inflammation. *J. Neuropathol. Exp. Neurol.* 57:385–395.

Klein, M.A., Moller, J.C., Jones, L.L., Bluethmann, H., Kreutzberg, G.W., and Raivich, G. (1997) Impaired neuroglial activation in interleukin-6 deficient mice. *Glia* 1997:227–233.

Krieglstein, K., Strelau, J., Schober, A., Sullivan, A., and Unsicker, K. (2002) TGF-beta and the regulation of neuron survival and death. *J. Physiol. (Paris)* 96:25–30.

Linker, R.A., Maurer, M., Gaupp, S., Martini, R., Holtmann, B., Giess, R., Rieckmann, P., Lassmann, H., Toyka, K.V., Sendtner, M., and Gold, R. (2002) CNTF is a major protective factor in demyelinating CNS disease: a neurotrophic cytokine as modulator in neuroinflammation. *Nat. Med.* 8:620–624.

Liu, J.S.H., Amaral, T.D., Brosnan, C.F., and Lee, S.C. (1998) IFNs are critical regulators of IL-1 receptor antagonist and IL-1 expression in human microglia. *J. Immunol.* 161:1989–1996.

Loddick, S.A., Turnbull, A.V., and Rothwell, N.J. (1998) Cerebral interleukin-6 is neuroprotective during permanent focal cerebral ischemia in the rat. *J. Cereb. Blood Flow Metab.* 18:176–179.

Magnus, T., Chan, A., Savill, J., Toyka, K., and Gold, R. (2002) Phagocytic removal of apoptotic, inflammatory lymphocytes in the central nervous system by microglia and its functional implications. *J. Neuroimmunol.* 130:1–9.

Mahad, D.J. and Ransohoff, R.M. (2003) The role of MCP-1 (CCL2) and CCR2 in multiple sclerosis and experimental autoimmune encephalomyelitis. *Semin. Immunol.* 15:23–32.

Malipiero, U.V., Frei, K., and Fontana, A. (1990) Production of hemopoietic colony-stimulating factors by astrocytes. *J. Immunol.* 144:3816–3821.

Mason, J.L., Suzuki, K., Chaplin, D.D., and Matsushima, G.K. (2001) Interleukin-1β promotes repair of the CNS. *J. Neurosci.* 21:7046–7052.

Middleton, J., Patterson, A.M., Gardner, L., Schmutz, C., and Ashton, B.A. (2002) Leukocyte extravasation: chemokine transport and presentation by the endothelium. *Blood* 100:3853–3860.

Mori, I., Hossain, M.J., Takeda, K., Okamura, H., Imai, Y., Kohsaka, S., and Kimura, Y. (2001) Impaired microglial activation in the brain of IL-18-gene-disrupted mice after neurovirulent influenza A virus infection. *Virology* 287:163–170.

Neumann, H., Schweigreiter, R., Yamashita, T., Rosenkranz, K., Wekerle, H., and Barde, Y.A. (2002) Tumor necrosis factor inhibits neurite outgrowth and branching of hippocampal neurons by a rho-dependent mechanism. *J. Neurosci.* 22:854–862.

Nguyen, M.D., Julien, J.P., and Rivest, S. (2002) Innate immunity: the missing link in neuroprotection and neurodegeneration? *Nat. Rev. Neurosci.* 3:216–227.

Otten, U., Marz, P., Heese, K., Hock, C., Hunz, D., and Rose-John, S. (2000) Cytokines and neurotrophins in normal and disease states. *Ann. NY Acad. Sci.* 917:322–330.

Owens, T., Wekerle, H., and Antel, J. (2001) Genetic models for CNS inflammation. *Nat. Med.* 7:161–166.

Platten, M., Wick, W., and Weller, M. (2001) Malignant glioma biology: role for TGF-β in growth, motility, angiogenesis, and immune escape. *Microsc. Res. Tech.* 52:401–410.

Popko, B. and Baerwald, K.D. (1999) Oligodendroglial response to the immune cytokine interferon-gamma. *Neurochem. Res.* 24: 331–338.

Pratt, B.M. and McPherson, J.M. (1997) TGF-β in the central nervous system: potential roles in ischemic injuries and neurogegenerative diseases. *Cytokine Growth Factor Rev.* 8:267–292.

Probert, L. and Akassoglou K. (2001) Glial expression of tumor necrosis factor in transgenic animals: how do these models reflect the "normal situation"? Glia 36:212–219.

Raivich, G., Jones, L.L., Werner, A., Bluthmann, H., Dötschmann, T., and Kreutzberg, G.W. (1999) Molecular signals for glial activation: pro- and anti-inflammatory cytokines in the injured brain. *Acta Neurochir. Suppl.* 73:21–30.

Ransohoff, R.M. (1997) Chemokines in neurological disease models: correlation between chemokine expression patterns and inflammatory pathology. *J. Leukoc. Biol.* 62:645–652.

Ransohoff, R.M (2002) The chemokine system in neuroinflammation: an update. *J. Infect. Dis.* 186:S152–S156.

Re, F., Belyanskaia, S.L., Riese, R.J., Cipriani, B., Fischer, F.R., Granucci, F., Ricciardi-Castagnoli, P., Brosnan, C., Stern, L.J., Strominger, J.L., and Santambrogio, L. (2002) Granulocyte-macrophage colony-stimulating factor induces an expression program in neonatal microglia that primes them for antigen presentation. *J. Immunol.* 169:2264–2273.

Renno, T., Krakowshi, M., Piccirillo, C., Lin, J.Y., and Owens, T. (1995) TNF-α expression by resident microglia and infiltrating leukocytes in the central nervous system of mice with experimental autoimmune encephalomyelitis. Regulation by Th1 cytokines. *J. Immunol.* 154:944–953.

Repovich, P. and Benveniste, E.N. (2002) Prostaglandin E2 is a novel inducer of oncostatin-M expression in macrophages and microglia. *J. Neurosci.* 22:5334–5343.

Rho, M.B., Wesselingh, S., Glass, J.D., McArthur, J.C., Choi, S., Griffin, J., and Tyor, W.R. (1995) A potential role for interferon-alpha in the pathogenesis of HIV-associated dementia. *Brain Behav. Immun.* 9:366–377.

Ruprecht, K., Kuhlmann, T., Seif, F., Hummel, V., Kruse, N., Bruck, W., and Rieckmann, P. (2001) Effects of oncostatin M on human cerebral endothelial cells and expression in inflammatory brain lesions. *J. Neuropathol. Exp. Neurol.* 60:1087–1098.

Shamash, S., Reichert, F., and Rotshenker, S. (2002) The cytokine network of Wallerian degeneration: tumor necrosis factor-α, interleukin-α, and interleukin-β. *J. Neurosci.* 22:3052–3060.

Strle, K., Zhou, J.H., Shen, W.H., Broussard, S.R., Johnson, R.W., Freund, G.G., Dantzer, R., and Kelley, W.K. (2001) Interleukin-10 in the brain. *Crit. Rev. Immunol.* 21:427–449.

Sugiura, S., Lahav, R., Han, J., Kou, S.-Y., Banner, L.R., De Pablo, F., and Patterson, P.H. (2000) Leukemia inhibitory factor is required for normal inflammatory responses to injury in the peripheral and central nervous systems in vivo and is chemotactic for macrophages in vitro. *Eur. J. Neurosci.* 12:457–466.

Takeuchi, A., Miyaishi, O., Ciuchi, K., and Isobe, K. (2001) Macrophage-colony-stimulating factor is expressed in neurons and microglia after focal brain injury. *J. Neurosci. Res.* 65:38–44.

Tofaris, G.K., Patterson, P.H., Jessen, K.R., and Mirsky, R. (2002) Denervated Schwann cells attract macrophages by secretion of leukemia inhibitory factor (LIF) and monocyte chemoattractant protein-1 in a process regulated by interleukin-6 and LIF. *J. Neurosci.* 22:6696–6703.

Tsai, H., Frost, E., To, V., Robinson, S., ffrench-Constant, C., Geertman, R., Ransohoff, R. and Miller, R., (2002) The chemokine receptor CXCR2 controls positioning of oligodendrocyte precursors in developing spinal cord by arresting their migration. *Cell* 110:373–383.

van Wagoner, N.J. and Benveniste, E.N. (1999) Interleukin-6 expression and regulation in astrocytes. *J. Neuroimmunol.* 100:124–139.

Walsh, D.T., Betmouni, S., and Perry, V.H. (2001) Absence of detectable IL-1β production in murine prion disease: a model of chronic neurodegeneration. *J. Neuropathol. Exp. Neurol.* 60:173–182.

Wang, J., Asensio, V.C., and Campbell, I.L. (2002) Cytokines and chemokines as mediators of protection and injury in the central nervous system assessed in transgenic mice. *Curr. Top. Microbiol. Immunol.* 265:23–48.

Wang, J. and Campbell, I.L. (2002) Cytokine signaling in the brain: putting a SOCS in it? *J. Neurosci. Res.* 67:423–427.

Wyss-Coray, T., Lin, C., Yan, F., Yu, G.Q., Rohde, M., McConlogue, L., Masliah, E., and Mucke, L. (2001) TGF-β1 promotes microglial amyloid-beta clearance and reduces plaque burden in transgenic mice. *Nat. Med.* 7:612–618.

Zlotnik, A. and Yoshie, O. (2000) Chemokines: a new classification system and their role in immunity. *Immunity* 12:121–127.

23 Interaction of glial cells with monocytes

INGO BECHMANN AND ROBERT NITSCH

The brain, the spinal cord, and their meninges are populated by both resident phagocytes (*histiocytes*) and bypassing monocytes and macrophages. Both cell types derive from the same CD45$^+$ bone marrow precursors, which give rise to antigen-presenting cells (APCs) of the monocyte/macrophage and myeloid dendritic cell lineage. Such CD45$^+$ derivates reside in virtually all tissues, where their differentiation and activation state is regulated by direct cell-cell interaction with parenchymal cells and factors such as cytokines and chemokines, which provide an organ-specific immune environment. This environment drives a local adoption of APCs affecting features such as morphological transformation, phagocytic activity, or the capacity to present antigens and/to stimulate (or downregulate!) T cells (Wilbanks and Streilein, 1992; Hailer et al., 1998; Aloisi et al., 2000; Rappert et al., 2002). Besides these phenotypic alterations, the organ-specific immune environment may also affect the motility of phagocytes, thereby modulating whether invading CD45$^+$ derivates readily enter and leave tissues or reside within an organ for long periods of time. Therefore, cells of this lineage develop differentially within tissues; thus, organ-specific phagocytes such as Kupffer cells of the liver, Hofbauer cells of the placenta, and the microglia of the central nervous system (CNS) differentiate into constitutive elements of the respective tissue.

Similarly, under inflammatory conditions or after mechanical injury, each tissue has its particular means of recruiting blood-derived monocytes and of shaping their differentiation according to the local requirements in regard to the costs and benefits of an immune response. Once the pathological signals have ceased, at least some of the invading monocytic cells remain in the tissue, where they are hardly discernible from previously present tissue phagocytes.

As a rule, organs with poor regenerative capacity strictly control the recruitment and activation state of immune-competent cells in order to minimize inflammation-induced damage. This state of *immune privilege* (Medawar, 1948; Streilein, 1996) applies particularly to the CNS, where inflammatory responses are suppressed, as the postmitotic, and thus irreplaceable, neurons require protection from inflammation-induced cell loss. Therefore, invading leukocytes are quickly adapted to the local homeostasis under normal and even under many pathological conditions.

In this chapter, we shall discuss how glial cells drive these phenotypic and functionally adaptive changes in *de novo* invading monocytic cells. As we will see, these alterations occur quickly and efficiently; therefore, such infiltrating CD45$^+$ derivates soon acquire the typical characteristics of what are regarded as resident microglia. However, not only can blood-derived CD45$^+$ cells transform into ramified microglia-like cells inside the CNS parenchyma; microglia can also be activated to a form of APC that, on the basis of its immune phenotype and morphology, is hardly discernible from activated macrophages and, under certain circumstances, from dendritic cells (Thanos et al., 1992; Bechmann and Nitsch, 1997; Aloisi et al., 2000; Fischer and Reichmann, 2001; Reichmann et al., 2002). These two faces become evident in microglial as well as in monocyte cultures: in such cultures, both cell types exhibit a round morphology. However, if they are seeded on top of astrocytes or allowed to invade organotypic brain slice cultures, both ramify and downregulate activation markers such as adhesion/costimulatory molecules (Sievers et al., 1994a, 1994b; Hailer et al., 1998). Thus, the local environment within the CNS not only affects the differentiation and activation state of infiltrating monocytes/macrophages, but obviously also shapes the intrinsic microglia. Only a recent methodological development, that is, the transplantation of bone marrow transfected with green fluorescent protein (GFP), allowed clear identification of bone marrow/blood-derived CD45$^+$ derivates as distinct from intrinsic microglia (Priller et al., 2001). Such approaches have provided evidence that all APCs in the CNS may be supplanted by hematogenous cells, yet at different turnover

See the list of abbreviations at the end of the chapter.

rates, rendering the concept of a strict distinction between resident and bypassing phagocytes untenable (Flugel et al., 2001; Priller et al., 2001). However, at least under normal conditions, this concept is still helpful in distinguishing APCs that have just invaded and thus still exhibit a blood-macrophage-like morphology, and those that have already acquired the morphology and immune phenotype typical of what are regarded as resident microglia.

Therefore, we will first give a brief overview of the different brain phagocyte populations in regard to the kinetics of their permanent supplementation by blood-derived precursors. We will then provide a timely view of how (astro)glial cells regulate the local adoption of invading APCs. Since any immune response can be regarded as a double-edged sword providing both harm and help for lesioned tissues, we will finally discuss whether the rapid deactivation of immune cells by glia is beneficial or detrimental for repair and regeneration following CNS lesion (Merrill and Benveniste, 1996; Bechmann and Nitsch, 2001). This question definitely depends on the type of lesion. In the case of infections, due to the local downregulation of immune responses within the CNS, certain viruses persist; however, this persistence is often less detrimental for the individual than the elimination of all infected neurons, reflecting only one example of the phylogenetic need to be *more tolerant* in poorly regenerative tissues such as the brain. On the other hand, after the development of axonal lesions such as those resulting from spinal cord injury, the quick adoption of invading monocytes and macrophages limits the restorative functions of the innate immune response, which may explain in part the poor capacity of central axons to regenerate (Lazarov-Spiegler et al., 1998; Rapalino et al., 1998; Moalem et al., 1999). Since (re-)stimulation of T cells by local APCs is crucial for the maintenance of their activation and the differentiation into effector, regulatory (suppressor), or anergic T lymphocytes, the local downregulation of costimulatory molecules on APCs is linked to the adaptive immune response by hindering (auto)immunity, but probably also to protection provided by T cells (Moalem et al., 1999; Schwartz et al., 1999; Bechmann et al., 2001b; Wolf et al., 2002). Therefore, boosting immune responses by overcoming local downregulating mechanisms may provide a new therapeutic avenue to enhance recovery in a variety of brain pathologies, particularly if the destructive autoimmunity and the damage of bystander cells accompanying any inflammation can be avoided. This strategy of *shaping* an immune response requires in-depth understanding of the mechanisms involved in damage and protection, but also of the cellular interactions regulating the trafficking and local integration of immunocompetent cells such as monocytes in the normal and injured CNS.

The chapter is divided into three parts:

1. Turnover of brain phagocytes
2. Interaction of astrocytes with monocytic cells: modulation of (immune) function
3. Macrophage invasion: Harmful or helpful?

TURNOVER OF BRAIN PHAGOCYTES

In regard to the microenvironment, two secluded compartments can be distinguished within the CNS: the *immune-privileged* brain and spinal cord parenchyma, in which various immune suppressive cell surface proteins such as CD200 (Hoek et al., 2000; Wright et al., 2001) and CD95L (Bechmann et al., 1999, 2000, 2002; Flugel et al., 2000; Medana et al., 2001) are expressed and in which anti-inflammatory factors are released by intrinsic cells (Hailer et al., 1998; Aloisi et al., 2000), and the *non-immune-privileged* subarachnoid, subpial, and perivascular spaces, which are filled with cerebrospinal fluid (CSF) and—under pathological conditions—may contain pro-inflammatory factors such as antibodies, complement, cytokines, and chemokines at higher concentrations than those in the parenchyma. These compartments are alienated by the astrocytes of the *glia limitans*. Their endfeet, covered by a basement membrane, build the superficial border of the parenchyma, thereby separating it from the subpial space (*lamina limitans gliae superficialis*) and the perivascular (Virchow-Robin) space (*lamina limitans gliae perivascularis*). Thus, any cell entering the CNS parenchyma from the blood must cross the *glia limitans* (see Fig. 23.3). The *glia limitans* is not only a tissue barrier for cells and molecules, but its astrocytes secrete pro- and anti-inflammatory factors, thereby actively contributing to an immunological barrier that separates the two compartments (Bechmann et al., 1999). Their particular microenvironments induce remarkable differences in the local $CD45^+$-derived phagocytes in regard to their size, morphology, and function.

Extraparenchymal phagocytes are located in the meninges, the choroid plexus, and the perivascular spaces. They exhibit broad morphological and functional heterogeneity, ranging from round macrophages to large process-bearing phagocytes (Fig. 23.1). These are the two extremes of an obvious continuum, which may reflect the degree of local adaptation. At least under some circumstances, this degree of adaptation makes it possible to estimate when bone marrow/blood-derived cells left the bloodstream to reside in the meninges and the choroid plexus. The perivascular cells, which are also known as perivascular phagocytes, perivascular macrophages, or fluorescent granular perithelial cells (Mato et al., 1980, 1985, 1996; Graeber and Streit, 1990; Angelov et al., 1998), are located

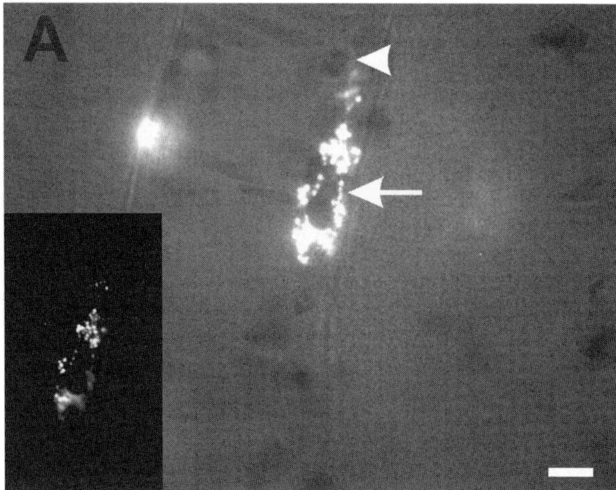

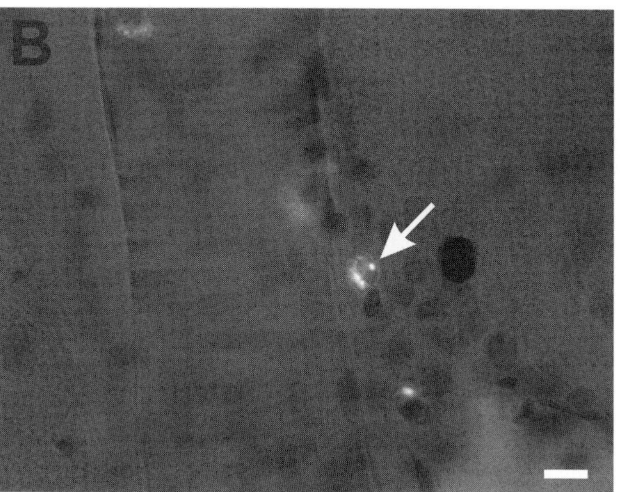

FIGURE 23.1 Morphological heterogeneity of perivascular phagocytes. *A*. Intraventricular injection of hydrophilic tracers (here: rhodamine coupled with dextranamine Mini Ruby molecular probes) leads to phagocytosis-dependent labeling of the perivascular phagocytes due to diffusion along the Virchow-Robin spaces (see Fig. 23.2). Note the remarkable difference in size between the perivascular cell (*arrow*) and a granulocyte within the lumen (*arrowhead*). Counterstained with hematoxylin-eosin. Insert: TRICT filter. *B*. Besides the long, spiny cells shown in *A*, there is a population of phagocytes that resemble monocytic cells in size and morphology. Scale bars: 10 μm.

at the interface between blood and brain within the perivascular spaces. This compartment between the basement membrane around pericytes and the membrane on top of the *glia limitans* is connected with the subarachnoid space and therefore partially filled with CSF (Fig. 23.2). This location allows (a subtype of) perivascular cells to phagocytose exogenous and endogenous particles from the CSF, leading to a bright autofluorescence that increases with age. Therefore, injection of neuroanatomical tracers into the CNS leads to a phagocytosis-dependent labeling of this population due to diffusion of the tracer along the perivascular spaces (Mato et al., 1984, 1985; Ichimura et al., 1991; Bechmann et al., 2001a; Williams et al., 2001). In rats, most of the phagocytosing perivascular cells (but not the microglia) are immune-positive for the mature macrophage marker ED-2, which recognizes the scavenger receptor CD163 (Dijkstra et al., 1985). While many studies show their continuous supplementation by blood-derived precursors (Hickey and Kimura, 1988; Bechmann et al., 2001a, 2001c), India ink injected into

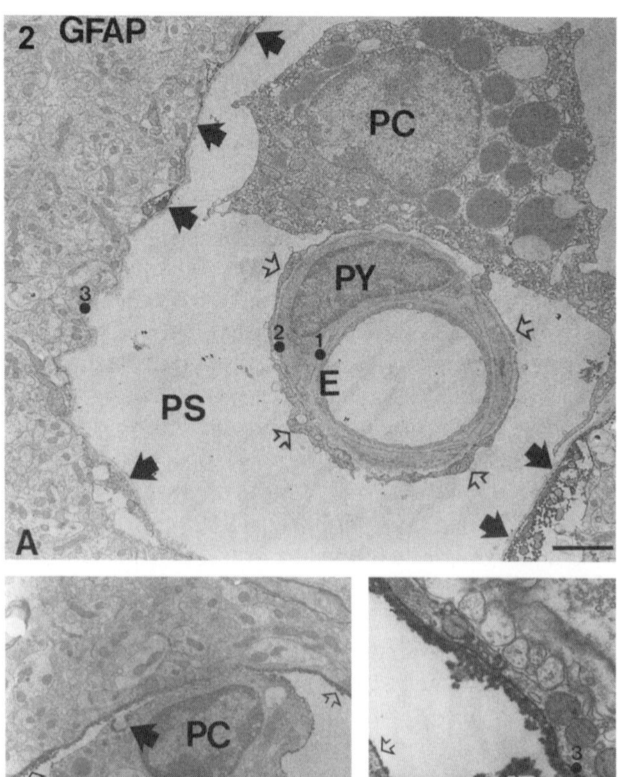

FIGURE 23.2 Brain perivascular cells in Virchow-Robin spaces *A*. Location of perivascular cells (*PC*) in the perivascular spaces (*PS*). The dots mark the basement membranes. A first basement membrane (*1*) surrounds the endothelial cell (*E*), which, in turn, is surrounded by a pericyte (*PY*) and the second basement membrane (*2*). The third basement membrane (*3*) is located on the glia limitans, which is visualized by glial fibrillary acidic protein-immunocytochemistry (*arrows*). The PC are located between the second and third basement membranes and are often found to wrap small processes (*open arrows*) around brain vessels (scale bar, 2 μm). *B*. Perivascular space after intraventricular injection of Mini Ruby (MR). The tracer can be found in the PS (*open arrows*) and is phagocytosed (*arrow*) by PC (scale bar, 1 μm). C. Mini Ruby clusters confined to the PS. Following injection of MR, the tracer remains confined to the space between the second and third basement membranes. Mini Ruby clusters are attached to the processes of PC (*open arrows*) but cannot be found within pericytes or astrocytic processes of the glia limitans (scale bar, 0.5 μm). (Reproduced with permission from Bechmann et al., 2001a, *Exp. Neurol.* 168:242–249.)

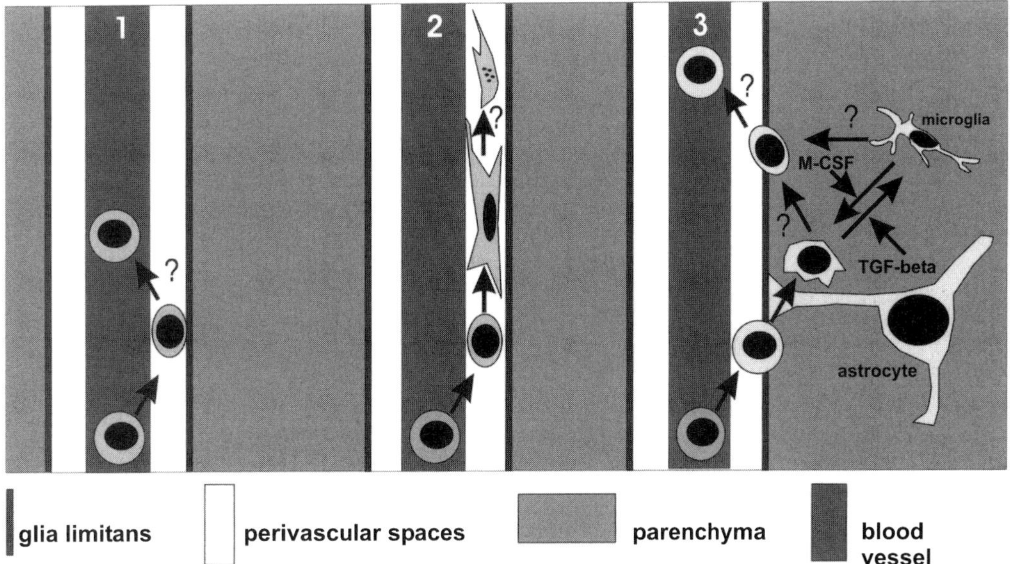

FIGURE 23.3 Possible routes of invading monoctyic cells into the central nervous system (CNS) *1*. Migration of monocytes across the vessel wall into the perivascular spaces has been shown in chimeric and normal animals. It is, however, difficult to show whether they are also able to leave this compartment to reach the lymphoid organs via the bloodstream. 2. Alternatively, invading monocytic cells may transform into the locally adopted perivascular cells shown in Figure 23.1*A*). These cells appear to be long-lived and may finally undergo apoptosis. *3*. Monocytic cells are also able to cross the glia limitans. Once inside the CNS, they transform into microglia-like cells (see Fig. 23.4) under the influence of astrocytic factors such as transforming growth factor-β (see Figs. 23.5–23.7). In turn, pro-inflammatory cytokines can trigger microglial activation to cells that are hardly distinguishable from macrophages. Thus, the differentiation state of monocytes/microglia depends on the local cytokine/chemokine environment.

the perivascular spaces is still present in perivascular cells 2 years after injection (Kida et al., 1993). Since the total number of perivascular cells does not increase remarkably during aging, the contradiction between these findings may be explained by the existence of different subpopulations (resident and bypassing APCs) or may indicate that perivascular cells die and are phagocytosed by *de novo* invading monocytic cells, which retain the label. An alternative explanation is that some perivascular cells cross the *glia limitans* (Angelov et al., 1996) and finally transform into microglia (Fig. 23.3).

Intraparenchymal phagocytes are microglia, which exhibit a fine bi- or multipolar ramification and which, by definition, are located behind the basement membrane of the *glia limitans* within the parenchyma (Fig. 23.3). Some researchers distinguish *juxtavascular microglia* adjacent to blood vessels from microglia remote from vessels within the CNS. However, what appears to be remote from vessels may turn out to be juxtavascular if single cells are reconstructed three-dimensionally. The term *perivascular microglia* is not applied consistently. Some use it for the *juxtavascular microglia*, others for the perivascular cells, although they are located clearly outside the parenchyma within the Virchow-Robin spaces. The microglia are believed to be highly resident phagocytes, which may derive from precursors in the blood, the pia, or the yolk sac (Del Rio-Hortega, 1932; Dalmau et al., 1998; Alliot et al., 1999). Once inside the parenchyma, they initially proliferate (Alliot et al., 1991) and thereafter form a highly stable population with little supplementation from blood-derived cells of the monocyte/macrophage lineage. Microglia appear to be uncommitted or immature precursors (Carson et al., 1998; Santambrogio et al., 2001) or able to trans-cross established lines of differentiation (Graf, 2002), because they can transform into cells sharing immune phenotypical and morphological features with macrophages or dendritic cells. By contrast, cultured microglial cells showing features of blood macrophages readily return to their typical delicate morphology after invasion of living brain tissue (Heppner et al., 1998). *In vitro*, macrophage colony-stimulating factor (M-CSF) drives microglia into the macrophage direction, while granulocyte/macrophage colony-stimulating factor (GM-CSF) induces transformation into dendritic cell-like APCs (Fig. 23.3) (Fischer and Reichmann, 2001; Mitrasinovic et al., 2001; Santambrogio et al., 2001; Re et al., 2002). *In vivo*, virtually any kind of brain pathology induces a process of microglial activation, which, depending on the type of lesion, may favor differentiation into either macrophages or dendritic-like cells. For example, within hours after axonal lesions in the CNS, microglia are

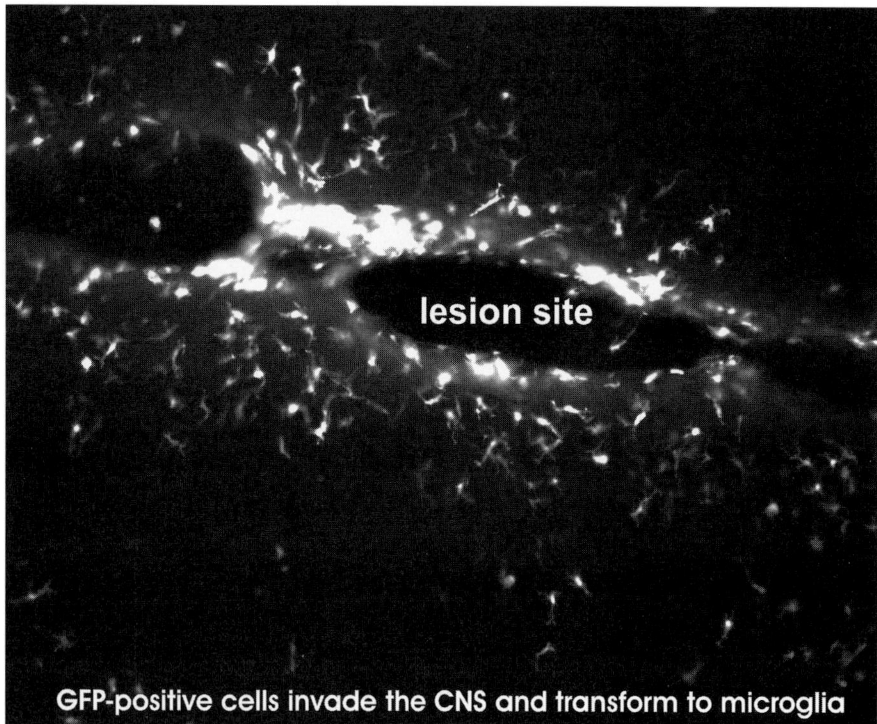

FIGURE 23.4 Transformation of monocytic cells into microglia-like cells *in vivo*. Using chimeras which received green fluorescent protein (GFP)-transfected bone-marrow transplants allows identification of blood-derived cells within the central nervous system (CNS) (Priller et al., 2001). At 72 hours after mechanical lesioning, invaded precursors exhibit the typical ramified morphology of microglia.

activated to round, amoeboid cells that phagocytose myelin debris (Bechmann and Nitsch, 1997), while the area around the zones of degeneration is depleted of microglia, indicating their capacity to sense pathology and to migrate from neighboring areas into fields of degeneration. Weeks after axonal lesioning, the microglia in these zones of axonal degeneration are ramified, as in normal brains, but still show strongly upregulated expression of major histocompatibility complex (MHC-II) complexes and adhesion molecules such as intercellular adhesion molecule-1 (ICAM-1), VLA-4, and costimulatory molecules such as lymphocyte function-associated antigen 1 (LFA-1) and CD86 (B7-2), though they lack expression of CD80 (B-7-1) (Hailer et al., 1997; Bechmann et al., 2001b). The latter costimulatory molecule is expressed only in highly activated APCs and seems crucial for the induction of autoimmune diseases, for example, against myelin [multiple sclerosis (MS) or its animal model experimental autoimmune encephalomyelitis (EAE)] (Kuchroo et al., 1995; Racke et al., 1995). Interestingly, CD80 is found in MS plaques (Windhagen et al., 1995). Thus, the differentiation/activation state of microglia differs significantly, depending on the type of pathology, and their activation state is likely to crucially impact the further development of a disease, for example, in regard to T cell responses upon their restimulation by microglia within the CNS. In turn, the infiltrating T cells also induce changes in microglia: while lymphocytes of the T helper 2 type induce strong expression of costimulatory B7-2 (CD86), only the presence of T helper 1 cells leads to B7-1 (CD80) expression (Wolf et al., 2001). Thus, a first wave of infiltrating T cells may activate the microglia to competent antigen-presenting cells (Matyszak et al., 1999).

Unfortunately, similar bidirectional regulatory loops between microglia and invading monocytes are difficult to study. Due to their common origin, there are no *in situ* markers allowing a clear-cut distinction between the two. Only *ex vivo* isolation allows distinction of a $CD45^{high}$ population, which is extraparenchymally located or—under inflammatory conditions—recently invaded, and a $CD45^{low}$ population that is regarded as resident (Carson et al., 1998). However, this approach does not allow a distinction between intra- and extraparenchymal $CD45^{+}$ derivates. Therefore, our knowledge of the infiltration of monocytes and their precursors to extra- and intraparenchymal sites of the CNS and their effects on glia cells (and vice versa) is mostly based on data from bone marrow–transplanted animals and humans. Although inflicted with artifacts due to irradiation and immune activation (Yuan et al., 2003), most studies in such chimeras revealed continuous supplementation of the perivascular and pial populations, while the turnover of microglia appeared to be relatively low. Further, there is some indication that such "new" microglia derive from early-stage myeloid precursors (Hickey and Kimura, 1988; Hickey, 1991; de Groot et al., 1992; Hickey et al., 1992; Unger et al., 1993; Krall et al., 1994; Kennedy and Abkowitz, 1997; Ono et al., 1999; Bechmann et al., 2001c; Priller et al., 2001) (Fig. 23.4).

Under pathological conditions such as transient focal ischemia, fimbria-fornix transsection, and facial nerve axotomy, infiltration of monocytic cells and their morphological transformation into microglia have been demonstrated using GFP-transfected bone marrow chimeras (Priller et al., 2001) or injection of carbon into labeled (blood) macrophages (Flugel et al., 2001). Such experiments provided the first *in vivo* evidence that blood-derived monocytic cells remain in the tissue after pathology, where they acquire the phenotype of resident microglia, supporting the view that local factors determine the microglia-like phenotype of $CD45^+$ derivates within the CNS. We will now give an overview of what is known about the molecular background of this adoptive process.

INTERACTION OF MACROPHAGES AND ASTROCYTES: MODULATION OF (IMMUNE) FUNCTION

Based on the observation that allogeneic transplants survive better in the brain than in other sites of the body, the CNS has been considered an *immune privileged* organ (Medawar, 1948; Streilein, 1996; Streilein et al., 1997; Perry 1998; Harling-Berg et al., 1999). The immune privilege in the CNS has been attributed to two morphological peculiarities: the blood–brain barrier blocking the afferent arm of the immune system and the absence of classic lymph vessels blocking its efferent arm. It was therefore believed that antigens in the CNS are largely *ignored* by the immune system. However, a study published over 50 years ago (Medawar, 1948) showed that this putative immune ignorance to antigens in the CNS is incomplete: While allogeneic skin grafts survived in brains of rabbits for prolonged periods of time, they were readily rejected when a second graft was placed into the animals' skin. Medawar concluded that grafts in the CNS "submit to but cannot elicit an immune state." Thus, immunogenic antigens appear to be tolerated in the CNS unless they are presented in an inflammatory environment outside the brain. Indeed, ovalbumin (OVA) injected into the brain induces a systemic suppression of the immune responses to OVA unless the microglial cells are activated before antigen injection by mechanical lesions (Wenkel et al., 2000). Thus, mechanisms of actively induced immune tolerance rather than immune ignorance (Kamradt and Mitchison, 2001) appear to maintain immune privilege in the brain. However, if T cells with specificity to an antigen that occurs inside and outside of the brain are activated in lymphoid organs, they readily invade the CNS. Depending on activation state, cytokine pattern, cell number, and type of pathology, they may then contribute to a microglial differentiation into mature APCs, which are capable of sufficiently (re-) stimulating T cells. Therefore, the rigorous control of APC activity must be regarded as a key instrument of immune privilege within the brain. In fact, in mice lacking CD200, a glycoprotein expressed on neurons that downregulates cells of the monocyte lineage microglial cells, appear to be activated. Strikingly, these mice exhibit an accelerated microglial response upon lesioning and are more susceptible to EAE (Hoek et al., 2000).

In fact, the local suppression of APCs is illustrated by the observation that microglial cells show little or no constitutive expression of MHC-I and -II complexes and costimulatory molecules under physiological conditions (McGeer et al., 1988; Ford et al., 1995). Only if the microglial cells are activated by a multistep transformation process involving both stimulation through cytokines [GM-CSF and interferon-gamma (IFN-gamma)] and costimulatory signaling (B7-CD28 and CD40–CD40 ligand interactions) do they differentiate to mature APCs (Matyszak et al., 1999; Aloisi et al., 2000; Fischer and Reichmann, 2001; Santambrogio et al., 2001; Kostulas et al., 2002). It is likely that the same applies to invaded monocytic cells. In the absence of such strong signals, antigen presentation by microglia may lead to the appearance of anergic/regulatory T cells, which in turn suppress APCs, for example by releasing transforming growth factor-β (TGF-β) (Chen et al., 1996). Thus, in order to block T cell restimulation, the delicate balance between (auto-)immunity and immune tolerance crucially depends on the activation state of intrinsic microglia and invading monocytes and the efficient transformation of invading APCs into a similar cell type.

This balance is endangered by pro-inflammatory signals released from infiltrating leukocytes (Perry et al., 1993; Rinner et al., 1995; Williams and Hickey, 1995). Therefore, infiltration of mononuclear cells during brain inflammation and/or damage is tightly regulated by specific molecular cues involving adhesion molecules (Rosseler et al., 1992) and members of the chemokine family (Hery et al., 1995; Mennicken et al., 1999). Still, noticeable infiltration does occur in a variety of pathological conditions. A pool of CCR1+/CCR5+ mononuclear phagocytes accumulate in the CNS in MS (Trebst et al., 2001). In human immunodeficiency virus (HIV) encephalitis, chemokine and cytokine production is presumed to control the early traffic of monocytes into the brain, a crucial phenomenon in this disease (Pulliam et al., 1997; Langford and Masliah, 2001; Williams and Hickey, 2002). *In vitro*, monocyte chemoattractant protein (MCP)-1 is able to direct the transmigration of monocytes across the blood–brain barrier (Weiss et al., 1998). Such molecules involved in attracting monocytes to the CNS may derive from cells of the blood–brain barrier itself (Carlos et al., 1991; Sasseville et al., 1994; Nottet et al., 1996; Dobrogowska et al., 1998; Boven et al., 2000) or from cells

FIGURES 23.5 TO 23.7 Transformation of macrophages into microglia-like cells *in vitro*.

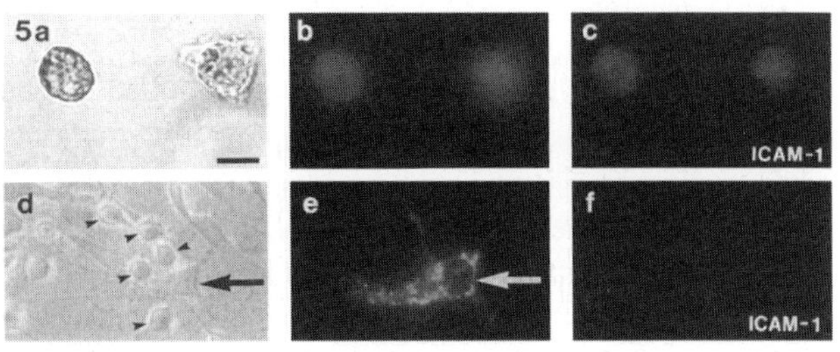

FIGURE 23.5 Morphological transformation and downregulation of intercellular adhesion molecule-1 (ICAM-1) expression of rat spleen macrophages following coculture with mixed glial cultures. *a–c*. Control experiment with fluorescent-prelabeled macrophages in isolated culture after nine divisions. *a*. Phase contrast microscopy of two ameboid macrophages. *b*. Rhodamine fluorescence of the prelabeled macrophages. *c*. Fluorescein isothiocyanate fluorescence microscopy following staining for ICAM-1. The macrophages still display spherical or ameboid morphology, and ICAM-1 is expressed. *d–f*. Macrophage coculture with mixed glial cells after nine divisions. *d*. Phase contrast microscopy showing an astrocyte monolayer, several ameboid microglial cells (*arrowheads*), and a macrophage (*arrow*). *e*. The macrophage is identified by rhodamine fluorescence microscopy, visualizing the prelabeled cell with its delicate cytoplasmic processes following morphological transformation. *f*. Fluorescein isothyocyanate fluorescence microscopy following immunostaining for ICAM-1 does not result in detectable staining of the prelabeled cell shown in *d*. and *e*. Scale bar: 10 mm for all figures. (Reproduced with permission from Hailer et al, 1998, *Brain Pathol.* 8: 459–474.)

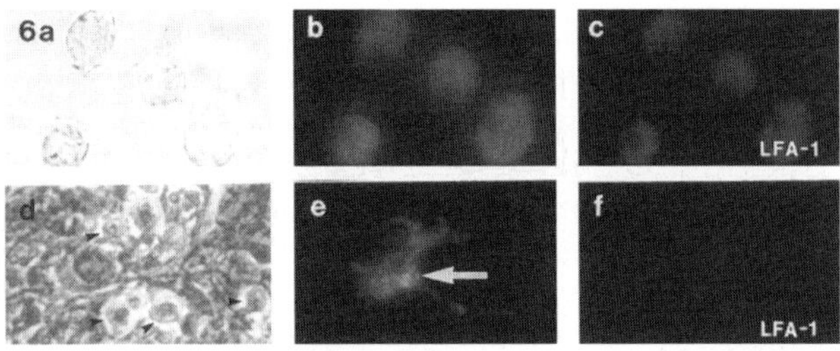

FIGURE 23.6 Morphological transformation and downregulation of lymphocyte function-associated antigen 1 (LFA-1) expression of rat spleen macrophages following coculture with mixed glial cultures. *a–c*. Control experiment showing fluorescent prelabeled macrophages after nine divisions without coculture with mixed glial cells. *a*. Phase contrast microscopy of four ameboid macrophages. *b*. Rhodamine fluorescence of the prelabeled macrophages. *c*. Fluorescein isothyanate (FITC) fluorescence microscopy after staining for LFA-1. Lymphocyte function-associated antigen 1 is expressed on the prelabeled macrophages, and no morphological transformation has occurred. *d.–f*. Macrophage coculture with mixed glial cells after nine divisions. *d*. Phase contrast microscopy shows the astrocyte monolayer with several ameboid microglial cells on its surface (*arrowheads*). *e*. The prelabeled spleen macrophage, visualized by rhodamine fluorescence microscopy, has been morphologically transformed, now showing cytoplasmic processes of fine caliber and secondary branches. *f*. Immunostaining for LFA-1 and subsequent FITC fluorescence microscopy does not result in fluorescence of the prelabeled macrophage shown in *d*. and *e*. (Reproduced with permission from Hailer et al., 1998, *Brain Pathol.* 8:459–474.)

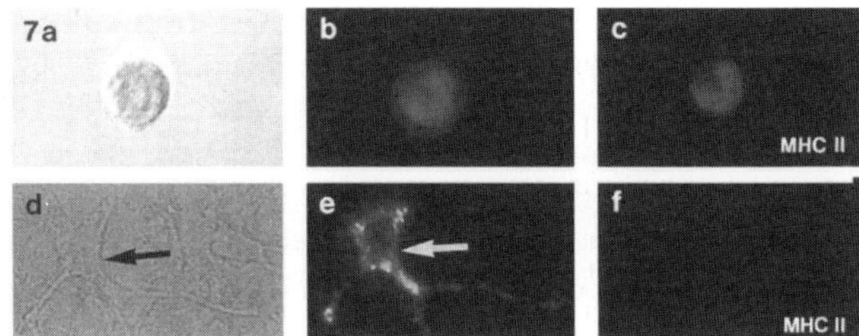

FIGURE 23.7 Morphological transformation and downregulation of major histocompatibility complex-II (MHC-II) expression of rat spleen macrophages following coculture with mixed glial cultures. *a–c*. Control experiment with fluorescent-prelabeled spleen macrophages in isolated culture after nine divisions. *a*. Phase contrast microscopy of spleen macrophage. *b*. Rhodamine fluorescence microscopy of the prelabeled cell in *a*. *c*. Fluorescein isothyanate fluorescence microscopy following staining for MHC-II shows expression of the antigen on the prelabeled macrophage. The macrophage is still spherical and has not undergone morphological transformation. *d–f*. Coculture of spleen macrophages with mixed glial cells after nine divisions. *d*. Phase contrast microscopy shows a spleen macrophage that is embedded in the astrocyte monolayer (*arrow*). *e*. The prelabeled macrophage vaguely seen in *d* is visualized by rhodamine fluorescence microscopy, showing a prelabeled cell following morphological transformation that now possesses cytoplasmic processes. *f*. Fluorescein isothyanate fluorescence microscopy following immunostaining for MHC-II does not result in detectable staining of the prelabeled cell shown in *a*. and *e*. (Reproduced with permission from Hailer et al., 1998, *Brain Pathol.* 8:459–474.)

located inside the CNS (Weiss et al., 1998, 1999; Persidsky et al., 1999), such as astrocytes, which have been identified as one source of chemokines important for monocyte infiltration into the CNS (Weiss et al., 1998; Oh et al., 1999; Andjelkovic and Pachter 2000). If a pro-inflammatory environment is further maintained during brain pathology, excessive damage of irreparable structures follows.

However, after lesions such as those resulting from axonal injury, infiltrating monocytic cells, once inside the CNS, soon acquire the phenotype of microglia (Flugel et al., 2001; Priller et al., 2001) (Fig. 23.4). The first evidence for this adoption derives from *in vitro* experiments: Sievers et al. (1994a) have shown that macrophages seeded on top of astrocytes transform into microglia-like cells in regard to electrophysiological and morphologial characteristics. In addition, such cocultures of rat spleen macrophages with mixed glial cultures induce lower expression of adhesion molecule and MHC-II complexes, thus downregulating their capacity to present antigens (Hailer et al., 1998). This effect could clearly be attributed to astrocytes since coincubation of human monocytes with CCF-STTG1 astrocytoma cells resulted in ramification and reduced adhesion molecule expression. In an attempt to clarify whether soluble or membrane-bound factors are important in driving this phenotypic alteration, rat spleen macrophages were incubated with supernatant from astrocyte cultures. These experiments showed strong downregulation of adhesion molecules (ICAM-1, LFA-1) and MHC-II complexes (Figs. 23.5–23.7). Within that supernatant, TGF-β produced by astrocytes could be detected as one crucial signal for monocyte transformation, as its blockage by antibodies diminished the modulatory effects of the supernatant (Hailer et al., 1998). This is also the case for microglial potassium channel function (Eder et al., 1999). However, there seem to be additional astrocyte-derived signals, which are provided via directed cell-cell interaction, since ramification can also be observed when microglia are seeded on fixed astrocytes (Tanaka and Maeda, 1996).

Ramification may not always reflect general downregulation, but may under certain circumstances indicate differentiation into dendritic cell-like APCs as exemplified by experiments with (G)M-CSF (Liu et al., 1994; Sievers et al., 1994b; Fujita et al., 1996; Wilms et al., 1997; Heppner et al., 1998; Fischer and Reichmann, 2001; Mitrasinovic et al., 2001; Santambrogio et al., 2001; Re et al., 2002). It is important to determine whether these phenotypic alterations of macrophages/microglia are astrocyte-specific or whether other cell types can induce similar changes. Findings of Wilms et al. (1997) suggest that epithelial but not mesenchymal cells have the capacity to induce deactivation of macrophages, as ramification of rat macrophages was observed following coculture with rat hepatoma cells (MH1C1) or with a renal epithelial cell line (NRK-52E). By contrast, coculturing with fibroblasts induced only slight morphological changes (Wilms et al., 1997). Recent data demonstrate that endotoxin-induced expression of nitric oxide synthase in microglial cells is inhibited by astrocyte-derived TGF-β, and Aloisi et al. have found that the production of IL-12 by microglial cells is inhibited in the presence of astrocytes (Aloisi et al., 1997; Vincent et al., 1997). *In vivo*, infiltration of monocytes into the CNS appears to increase substantially following forebrain stab injury in adult mice after ablation of astrocytes using a transgenic herpes simplex virus-thymidine kinase (*HSV-TK*) at the glial fibrillary acidic protein (GFAP) promotor, which allows selective killing of astrocytes with ganciclovir (Bush et al., 1999). All these experiments demonstrate an important role for astrocytes in maintaining the integrity of the blood–brain barier and the transformation of invading CD45$^+$ derivates into microglia-like cells, and identify TGF-β as a key player of this process. However, TGF-β is also expressed by microglia, for example after axonal injury (Morgan et al., 1993; McTigue et al., 2000), suggesting the existence of a feedback mechanism of microglial cells that triggers monocytes to differentiate into microglia-like cells. Since cultured microglial cells alone do not ramify and downregulate activation markers such as adhesion/costimulatory molecules *in vitro*, while they quickly undergo these phenotypic changes in the presence of astrocytes (Hailer et al., 1998), they at least seem to need astrocytic help before they can be involved in downregulating other CD45$^+$ derivates. In summary, APCs that invade the brain parenchyma are functionally modulated. In addition to neurons, which control myeloid cells via CD200/CD200L (Hoek et al., 2000; Wright et al., 2000), astrocytes were identified as key players in this process. This could be confirmed in *in vitro* experiments using coculture of macrophages or monocytes with astrocytes and in the complex microenvironment of cultered organotyoic brain tissue with its multitude of growth factors and cytokines. Thus, the CNS cytokine network seems to be carefully orchestrated, resulting in strict control over endogenous and exogenous APCs.

MACROPHAGE INVASION: HARMFUL OR HELPFUL?

As we have pointed out, the suppression of immunity within the CNS may well reflect a phylogenetic need to protect the highly vulnerable cellular networks from inflammation-induced irreparable damage. This suppression is, of course, incomplete, since immune-mediated secondary cell loss occurs under many pathological conditions in the CNS. Following spinal cord lesion, such damage was shown by studies in which the immune response was therapeutically downregulated by systemic administration of interleukin-10 (Bethea et al., 1999) or by depletion of macrophages (Popovich et al., 1999). Both strategies significantly improved hind limb motor function in open-field behavioral tests and decreased the lesion volume. In organotypic brain slice cultures, microglial cells activated through the addition of T cells began to phagocytose living myelinated fibers, providing one cellular pathway through which phagocytes are involved in secondary damage (Gimsa et al., 2000). Conversely, reduction of secondary damage was achieved by inhibition of the capacity of microglial cells to migrate to a site of neuronal injury (Ullrich et al., 2001). However, there is also a clear indication of protective and restorative functions of immune cells. *In vitro* studies suggested that neurotrophic factors released by monocytes and macrophages support neuronal survival (Hikawa and Takenaka 1996). In a series of elegant studies, Michal Schwartz's group enhanced functional recovery following axonal lesioning in the CNS by implanting macrophages prestimulated with peripheral nerve segments (Moneta et al., 1993). It was also reported that depletion of macrophages impairs oligodendrocyte remyelination following lysolecithin-induced demyelination (Kotter et al., 2001). These beneficial effects of monocytic cells may derive from their release of molecules such as neurotrophic factors, but also from stimulation of benign T cell responses (Moalem et al., 1999). Alternatively, they may simply be a result of enhanced phagocytosis of degenerated myelin, which is known to suppress axonal (re-)growth (Cadelli et al., 1992; Schwab, 2002). This exemplifies the fine line between the helpful and destructive actions of brain phagocytes: while the removal of debris is definitely an important step in regeneration, the same process may endanger intact axons in the vicinity of degenerated fibers and denervated dendrites (Eyupoglu et al., 2003). It is currently unknown how far invading leukocytes themselves influence sprouting and reactive synaptogenesis following axonal lesioning.

Intensive research over the past decade has identified many helpful and harmful molecular pathways of microglia/macrophages *in vitro* (Merrill and Benveniste, 1996) and the above-described *in vivo* experiments have corroborated this dual role of phagocytes in brain pathology (Bechmann and Nitsch, 2001). Thus, relatively nonspecific therapeutic modulation of immune responses within the CNS is always dangerous, as such strategies may support both damage and protection at the same time. While the total outcome of therapeutic interventions can be estimated in *in vivo* experiments, it remains difficult to identify the molecular and cellular pathways and to establish their contribution to help or additional damage in the course of a given disease. As part of this puzzle, we have described here how cells of the monocyte/macrophage lineage are locally adopted within the CNS environment and how glial cells drive this process of organ-specific differentiation of phagocytes. Many issues remain unresolved, and future research may identify molecular cues that allow specific shaping of the differentiation state of invading and resident monocytic cells in order to enhance their restorative functions while abrogating their harmful effects. This shift of the balance from destructive to benign immunity has become an important goal for clinical neuroscience, and we have only just begun to explore this exciting field.

ACKNOWLEDGMENTS

The authors thank Kimberly Rosegger for excellent editorial assistance. Parts of our own work reviewed here were performed in collaboration with Drs. Nils Hailer (Stockholm), Frank Heppner (Zürich), Ulrika Gimsa (Rostock) and Susanne Wolf (Bethesda). This work was supported by the Deutsche Forschungsgemeinschaft: SFB 507/B7 to R.N. and Be2272 to I.B.

ABBREVIATIONS

APC	antigen-presenting cell
CSF	cerebrospinal fluid
EAE	experimental autoimmune encephalomyelitis
GFAP	glial acidic fibrillary protein
GFP	green fluorescent protein
GM-CSF	granulocyte-macrophage colony-stimulating factor
HIV	human immunodeficiency virus
HSV-tk	Herpes simplex virus thymidine kinase
ICAM-1	intercellular adhesion molecule-1
IFN	interferon
LFA-1	lymphocyte function-associated antigen
MCP-1	monocyte chemoattractant protein-1
M-CSF	macrophage colony-stimulating factor
MHC	major histocompatibility complex
MS	multiple sclerosis
OVA	ovalbumin
PC	perivascular cells
TGF-β	transforming growth factor-β
VLA-4	very late antigen-4

REFERENCES

Alliot, F., Godin, I., and Pessac, B. (1999) Microglia derive from progenitors, originating from the yolk sac, and which proliferate in the brain. *Brain Res. Dev. Brain Res.* 117:145–152.

Alliot, F., Lecain, E., Grima, B., and Pessac, B. (1991) Microglial progenitors with a high proliferative potential in the embryonic and adult mouse brain. *Proc. Natl. Acad. Sci. USA* 88:1541–1545.

Aloisi, F., Penna, G., Cerase, J., Menendez, I.B., and Adorini, L. (1997) IL-12 production by central nervous system microglia is inhibited by astrocytes. *J. Immunol.* 159:1604–1612.

Aloisi, F., Serafini, B., and Adorini, L. (2000) Glia–T cell dialogue. *J. Neuroimmunol.* 107:111–117.

Andjelkovic, A.V. and Pachter, J.S. (2000) Characterization of binding sites for chemokines MCP-1 and MIP-1alpha on human brain microvessels. *J. Neurochem.* 75:1898–1906.

Angelov, D.N., Neiss, W.F., Streppel, M., Walther, M., Guntinas-Lichius, O., and Stennert, E. (1996) ED2-positive perivascular cells act as neuronophages during delayed neuronal loss in the facial nucleus of the rat. *Glia* 16:129–139.

Angelov, D.N., Walther, M., Streppel, M., Guntinas-Lichius, O., and Neiss, W.F. (1998) The cerebral perivascular cells. *Adv. Anat. Embryol. Cell Biol.* 147:1–87.

Bechmann, I., Kwidzinski, E., Kovac, A., Simburger, E., Horvath, T., Gimsa, U., Dirnagl, U., Priller, J., and Nitsch, R. (2001a) Turnover of rat brain perivascular cells. *Exp. Neurol.* 168:242–249.

Bechmann, I., Lossau, S., Steiner, B., Mor, G., Gimsa, U., and Nitsch, R. (2000) Reactive astrocytes upregulate Fas (CD95) and Fas ligand (CD95L) expression but do not undergo programmed cell death during the course of anterograde degeneration. *Glia* 32:25–41.

Bechmann, I., Mor, G., Nilsen, J., Eliza, M., Nitsch, R., and Naftolin, F. (1999) FasL (CD95L, Apo1L) is expressed in the normal rat and human brain: evidence for the existence of an immunological brain barrier. *Glia* 27:62–74.

Bechmann, I. and Nitsch, R. (1997) Astrocytes and microglial cells incorporate degenerating fibers following entorhinal lesion: a light, confocal, and electron microscopical study using a phagocytosis-dependent labeling technique. *Glia* 20:145–154.

Bechmann, I. and Nitsch, R. (2001) Plasticity following lesion: help and harm from the immune system. *Restor. Neurol. Neurosci.* 19:189–198.

Bechmann, I., Peter, S., Beyer, M., Gimsa, U., and Nitsch, R. (2001b) Presence of B7—2 (CD86) and lack of B7-1 (CD(80) on myelin phagocytosing MHC-II-positive rat microglia is associated with nondestructive immunity in vivo. *FASEB J.* 15:1086–1088.

Bechmann, I., Priller, J., Kovac, A., Bontert, M., Wehner, T., Klett, F.F., Bohsung, J., Stuschke, M., Dirnagl, U., and Nitsch, R. (2001c) Immune surveillance of mouse brain perivascular spaces by blood-borne macrophages. *Eur. J. Neurosci.* 14:1651–1658.

Bechmann, I., Steiner, B., Gimsa, U., Mor, G., Wolf, S., Beyer, M., Nitsch, R., and Zipp, F. (2002) Astrocyte-induced T cell elimination is CD95 ligand dependent. *J. Neuroimmunol.* 132:60–65.

Bethea, J.R., Nagashima, H., Acosta, M.C., Briceno, C., Gomez, F., Marcillo, A.E., Loor, K., Green, J., and Dietrich, W.D. (1999) Systemically administered interleukin-10 reduces tumor necrosis factor-alpha production and significantly improves functional recovery following traumatic spinal cord injury in rats. *J. Neurotrauma.* 16:851–863.

Boven, L.A., Middel, J., Verhoef, J., de Groot, C.J., and Nottet, H.S. (2000) Monocyte infiltration is highly associated with loss of the tight junction protein zonula occludens in HIV-1-associated dementia. *Neuropathol. Appl. Neurobiol.* 26:356–360.

Bush, T.G., Puvanachandra, N., Horner, C.H., Polito, A., Ostenfeld, T., Svendsen, C.N., Mucke, L., Johnson, M.H., and Sofroniew, M.V. (1999) Leukocyte infiltration, neuronal degeneration, and neurite outgrowth after ablation of scar-forming, reactive astrocytes in adult transgenic mice. *Neuron* 23:297–308.

Cadelli, D.S., Bandtlow, C.E., and Schwab, M.E. (1992) Oligodendrocyte- and myelin-associated inhibitors of neurite outgrowth: their involvement in the lack of CNS regeneration. *Exp. Neurol.* 115:189–192.

Carlos, R.Q., Seidler, F.J., Lappi, S.E., and Slotkin, T.A. (1991) Fetal dexamethasone exposure affects basal ornithine decarboxylase activity in developing rat brain regions and alters acute responses to hypoxia and maternal separation. *Biol. Neonate* 59: 69–77.

Carson, M.J., Reilly, C.R., Sutcliffe, J.G., and Lo, D. (1998) Mature microglia resemble immature antigen-presenting cells. *Glia* 22: 72–85.

Chen, Y., Inobe, J., Kuchroo, V.K., Baron, J.L., Janeway, C.A., Jr., and Weiner, H.L. (1996) Oral tolerance in myelin basic protein T-cell receptor transgenic mice: suppression of autoimmune encephalomyelitis and dose-dependent induction of regulatory cells. *Proc. Natl. Acad. Sci. USA* 93:388–391.

Dalmau, I., Finsen, B., Zimmer, J., Gonzalez, B., and Castellano, B. (1998) Development of microglia in the postnatal rat hippocampus. *Hippocampus* 8:458–474.

de Groot, C.J., Huppes, W., Sminia, T., Kraal, G., and Dijkstra, C.D. (1992) Determination of the origin and nature of brain macrophages and microglial cells in mouse central nervous system, using non-radioactive in situ hybridization and immunoperoxidase techniques. *Glia* 6:301–309.

Del Rio-Hortega (1932) *Cytology and Cellular Pathology of the Nervous System.* Vol. 2, Penfield, W., ed. New York: Paul B. Hoeber, pp. 481–534.

Dijkstra, C.D., Van Vliet, E., Dopp, E.A., van der Lelij, A.A., and Kraal, G. (1985) Marginal zone macrophages identified by a monoclonal antibody: characterization of immuno- and enzyme-histochemical properties and functional capacities. *Immunology* 55:23–30.

Dobrogowska, D.H., Lossinsky, A.S., Tarnawski, M., and Vorbrodt, A.W. (1998) Increased blood–brain barrier permeability and endothelial abnormalities induced by vascular endothelial growth factor. *J. Neurocytol.* 27:163–173.

Eder, C., Schilling, T., Heinemann, U., Haas, D., Hailer, N., and Nitsch, R. (1999) Morphological, immunophenotypical and electrophysiological properties of resting microglia in vitro. *Eur. J. Neurosci.* 11:4251–4261.

Eyupoglu, I.Y., Bechmann, I., and Nitsch, R. (2003) Modification of microglia function protects from lesion-induced neuronal alterations and promote sprouting in the hippocampus. *FASEB J.* 17(9):1110–1111.

Fischer, H.G. and Reichmann, G. (2001) Brain dendritic cells and macrophages/microglia in central nervous system inflammation. *J. Immunol.* 166:2717–2726.

Flugel, A., Bradl, M., Kreutzberg, G.W., and Graeber, M.B. (2001) Transformation of donor-derived bone marrow precursors into host microglia during autoimmune CNS inflammation and during the retrograde response to axotomy. *J. Neurosci. Res.* 66:74–82.

Flugel, A., Schwaiger, F.-W., Neumann, H., Medana, I., Willem, M., Wekerle, H., Kreutzberg, G.W., and Graeber, M.B. (2000) Neuronal FasL induces cell death of encephalitogenic T lymphocytes. *Brain Pathol.* 10:353–364.

Ford, A.L., Goodsall, A.L., Hickey, W.F., and Sedgwick, J.D. (1995) Normal adult ramified microglia separated from other central nervous system macrophages by flow cytometric sorting. Phenotypic differences defined and direct ex vivo antigen presentation to myelin basic protein-reactive CD4+ T cells compared. *J. Immunol.* 154:4309–4321.

Fujita, H., Tanaka, J., Toku, K., Tateishi, N., Suzuki, Y., Matsuda, S., Sakanaka, M., and Maeda, N. (1996) Effects of GM-CSF and ordinary supplements on the ramification of microglia in culture: a morphometrical study. *Glia* 18:269–281.

Gimsa, U., Peter, S.V.A., Lehmann, K., Bechmann, I., and Nitsch, R. (2000) Axonal damage induced by invading T cells in organotypic central nervous system tissue in vitro: involvement of microglial cells. *Brain Pathol.* 10:365–377.

Graeber, M.B. and Streit, W.J. (1990) Perivascular microglia defined. *Trends Neurosci.* 13:366.

Graf, T. (2002) Differentiation plasticity of hematopoietic cells. *Blood* 99:3089–3101.

Hailer, N.P., Bechmann, I., Heizmann, S., and Nitsch, R. (1997) Adhesion molecule expression on phagocytic microglial cells following anterograde degeneration of perforant path axons. *Hippocampus* 7:341–349.

Hailer, N.P., Heppner, F.L., Haas, D., and Nitsch, R. (1998) Astrocytic factors deactivate antigen presenting cells that invade the central nervous system. *Brain Pathol.* 8:459–474.

Harling-Berg, C.J., Park, T.J., and Knopf, P.M. (1999) Role of the cervical lymphatics in the Th2-type hierarchy of CNS immune regulation. *J. Neuroimmunol.* 101:111–127.

Heppner, F.L., Skutella, T., Hailer, N.P., Haas, D., and Nitsch, R. (1998) Activated microglial cells migrate towards sites of excitotoxic neuronal injury inside organotypic hippocampal slice cultures. *Eur. J. Neurosci.* 10:3284–3290.

Hery, C., Sebire, G., Peudenier, S., and Tardieu, M. (1995) Adhesion to human neurons and astrocytes of monocytes: the role of interaction of CR3 and ICAM-1 and modulation by cytokines. *J. Neuroimmunol.* 57:101–109.

Hickey, W.F. (1991) Migration of hematogenous cells through the blood–brain barrier and the initiation of CNS inflammation. *Brain Pathol.* 1:97–105.

Hickey, W.F. and Kimura, H. (1988) Perivascular microglial cells of the CNS are bone marrow-derived and present antigen in vivo. *Science* 239:290–292.

Hickey, W.F., Vass, K., and Lassmann, H. (1992) Bone marrow–derived elements in the central nervous system: an immunohistochemical and ultrastructural survey of rat chimeras. *J. Neuropathol. Exp. Neurol.* 51:246–256.

Hikawa, N. and Takenaka, T. (1996) Myelin-stimulated macrophages release neurotrophic factors for adult dorsal root ganglion neurons in culture. *Cell Mol. Neurobiol.* 16:517–528.

Hoek, R.M., Ruuls, S.R., Murphy, C.A., Wright, G.J., Goddard, R., Zurawski, S.M., Blom, B., Homola, M.E., Streit, W.J., Brown, M.H., Barclay, A.N., and Sedgwick, J.D. (2000) Down-regulation of the macrophage lineage through interaction with OX2 (CD200). *Science* 290:1768–1771.

Ichimura, T., Fraser, P.A., and Cserr, H.F. (1991) Distribution of extracellular tracers in perivascular spaces of the rat brain. *Brain Res.* 545:103–113.

Kamradt, T. and Mitchison, A. (2001) Tolerance and autoimmunity. *N. Engl. J. Med.* 344:655–664.

Kennedy, D.W. and Abkowitz, J.L. (1997) Kinetics of central nervous system microglial and macrophage engraftment: analysis using a transgenic bone marrow transplantation model. *Blood* 90:986–993.

Kida, S., Steart, P.V., Zhang, E.T., and Weller, R.O. (1993) Perivascular cells act as scavengers in the cerebral perivascular spaces and remain distinct from pericytes, microglia and macrophages. *Acta Neuropathol. (Berl.)* 85:646–652.

Kostulas, N., Li, H.L., Xiao, B.G., Huang, Y.M., and Kostulas, V. (2002) Dendritic cells are present in ischemic brain after permanent middle cerebral artery occlusion in the rat. *Stroke* 33:1129–1134.

Kotter, M.R., Setzu, A., Sim, F.J., van Rooijen, N., and Franklin, R.J. (2001) Macrophage depletion impairs oligodendrocyte remyelination following lysolecithin-induced demyelination. *Glia* 35:204–212.

Krall, W.J., Challita, P.M., Perlmutter, L.S., Skelton, D.C., and Kohn, D.B. (1994) Cells expressing human glucocerebrosidase from a retroviral vector repopulate macrophages and central nervous system microglia after murine bone marrow transplantation. *Blood* 83:2737–2748.

Kuchroo, V.K., Das, M.P., Brown, J.A., Ranger, A.M., Zamvil, S.S., Sobel, R.A., Weiner, H.L., Nabavi, N., and Glimcher, L.H. (1995) B7-1 and B7-2 costimulatory molecules activate differentially the Th1/Th2 developmental pathways: application to autoimmune disease therapy. *Cell* 80:707–718.

Langford, D. and Masliah, E. (2001) Crosstalk between components of the blood brain barrier and cells of the CNS in microglial activation in AIDS. *Brain Pathol.* 11:306–312.

Lazarov-Spiegler, O., Solomon, A.S., and Schwartz, M. (1998) Peripheral nerve–stimulated macrophages simulate a peripheral nerve–like regenerative response in rat transected optic nerve. *Glia* 24:329–337.

Liu, W., Brosnan, C.F., Dickson, D.W., and Lee, S.C. (1994) Macrophage colony-stimulating factor mediates astrocyte-induced microglial ramification in human fetal central nervous system culture. *Am. J. Pathol.* 145:48–53.

Mato, M., Ookawara, S., and Kurihara, K. (1980) Uptake of exogenous substances and marked infoldings of the fluorescent granularpericyte in cerebral fine vessels. *Am. J. Anat.* 157:329–332.

Mato, M., Ookawara, S., Mato, T.K., and Namiki, T. (1985) An attempt to differentiate further between microglia and fluorescent granular perithelial (FGP) cells by their capacity to incorporate exogenous protein. *Am. J. Anat.* 172:125–140.

Mato, M., Ookawara, S., Sakamoto, A., Aikawa, E., Ogawa, T., Mitsuhashi, U., Masuzawa, T., Suzuki, H., Honda, M., Yazaki, Y., Watanabe, E., Luoma, J., Yla-Herttuala, S., Fraser, I., Gordon, S., and Kodama, T. (1996) Involvement of specific macrophage-lineage cells surrounding arterioles in barrier and scavenger function in brain cortex. *Proc. Natl. Acad. Sci. USA* 93:3269–3274.

Mato, M., Ookawara, S., Sugamata, M., and Aikawa, E. (1984) Evidence for the possible function of the fluorescent granular perithelial cells in brain as scavengers of high-molecular-weight waste products. *Experientia* 40:399–402.

Matyszak, M.K., Denis-Donini, S., Citterio, S., Longhi, R., Granucci, F., and Ricciardi-Castagnoli, P. (1999) Microglia induce myelin basic protein-specific T cell anergy or T cell activation, according to their state of activation. *Eur. J. Immunol.* 29:3063–3076.

McGeer, P.L., Itagaki, S., and McGeer, E.G. (1988) Expression of the histocompatibility glycoprotein HLA-DR in neurological disease. *Acta Neuropathol. (Berl.)* 76:550–557.

McTigue, D.M., Popovich, P.G., Morgan, T.E., and Stokes, B.T. (2000) Localization of transforming growth factor-beta1 and receptor mRNA after experimental spinal cord injury. *Exp. Neurol.* 163:220–230.

Medana, I., Li, Z., Flugel, A., Tschopp, J., Wekerle, H., and Neumann, H. (2001) Fas ligand (CD95L) protects neurons against perforin-mediated T lymphocyte cytotoxicity. *J. Immunol.* 167: 674–681.

Medawar, P.B. (1948) Immunity to homologous grafted skin. III. The fate of skin homografts transplanted to the brain, to subcutaneous tissue, and to the anterior chamber of the eye. *Br. J. Exp. Pathol.* 29:58–69.

Mennicken, F., Maki, R., de Souza, E.B., and Quirion, R. (1999) Chemokines and chemokine receptors in the CNS: a possible role in neuroinflammation and patterning. *Trends Pharmacol. Sci.* 20:73–78.

Merrill, J.E. and Benveniste, E.N. (1996) Cytokines in inflammatory brain lesions: helpful and harmful. *Trends Neurosci.* 19:331–338.

Mitrasinovic, O.M., Perez, G.V., Zhao, F., Lee, Y.L., Poon, C., and Murphy, G.M. (2001) Overexpression of macrophage colony-stimulating factor receptor on microglial cells induces an inflammatory response. *J. Biol. Chem.* 276:30142–30149.

Moalem, G., Leibowitz-Amit, R., Yoles, E., Mor, F., Cohen, I.R., and Schwartz, M. (1999) Autoimmune T cells protect neurons from secondary degeneration after central nervous system axotomy. *Nat. Med.* 5:49–55.

Moneta, M.E., Gehrmann, J., Topper, R., Banati, R.B., and Kreutzberg, G.W. (1993) Cell adhesion molecule expression in the regenerating rat facial nucleus. *J. Neuroimmunol.* 45:203–206.

Morgan, T.E., Nichols, N.R., Pasinetti, G.M., and Finch, C.E. (1993) TGF-beta 1 mRNA increases in macrophage/microglial cells of the hippocampus in response to deafferentation and kainic acid-induced neurodegeneration. *Exp. Neurol.* 120:291–301.

Nottet, H.S., Persidsky, Y., Sasseville, V.G., Nukuna, A.N., Bock, P., Zhai, Q.H., Sharer, L.R., McComb, R.D., Swindells, S., Soderland, C., and Gendelman, H.E. (1996) Mechanisms for the transendothelial migration of HIV-1-infected monocytes into brain. *J. Immunol.* 156:1284–1295.

Oh, J.W., Schwiebert, L.M., and Benveniste, E.N. (1999) Cytokine regulation of CC and CXC chemokine expression by human astrocytes. *J. Neurovirol.* 5:82–94.

Ono, K., Takii, T., Onozaki, K., Ikawa, M., Okabe, M., and Sawada, M. (1999) Migration of exogenous immature hematopoietic cells into adult mouse brain parenchyma under GFP-expressing bone marrow chimera. *Biochem. Biophys. Res. Commun.* 262:610–614.

Perry, V.H. (1998) A revised view of the central nervous system microenvironment and major histocompatibility complex class II antigen presentation. *J. Neuroimmunol.* 90:113–121.

Perry, V.H., Andersson, P.B., and Gordon, S. (1993) Macrophages and inflammation in the central nervous system. *Trends Neurosci.* 16:268–273.

Persidsky, Y., Ghorpade, A., Rasmussen, J., Limoges, J., Liu, X.J., Stins, M., Fiala, M., Way, D., Kim, K.S., Witte, M.H., Weinand, M., Carhart, L., and Gendelman, H.E. (1999) Microglial and astrocyte chemokines regulate monocyte migration through the blood–brain barrier in human immunodeficiency virus-1 encephalitis. *Am. J. Pathol.* 155:1599–1611.

Popovich, P.G., Guan, Z., Wei, P., Huitinga, I., van Rooijen, N., and Stokes, B.T. (1999) Depletion of hematogenous macrophages promotes partial hindlimb recovery and neuroanatomical repair after experimental spinal cord injury. *Exp. Neurol.* 158:351–365.

Priller, J., Flugel, A., Wehner, T., Boentert, M., Haas, C.A., Prinz, M., Fernandez-Klett, F., Prass, K., Bechmann, I., deBoer, B.A., Frotscher, M., Kreutzberg, G.W., Persons, D.A., and Dirnagl, U. (2001) Targeting gene-modified hematopoietic cells to the central nervous system: use of green fluorescent protein uncovers microglial engraftment. *Nat. Med.* 7:1356–1361.

Pulliam, L., Gascon, R., Stubblebine, M., McGuire, D., and McGrath, M.S. (1997) Unique monocyte subset in patients with AIDS dementia. *Lancet* 349:692–695.

Racke, M.K., Scott, D.E., Quigley, L., Gray, G.S., Abe, R., June, C.H., and Perrin, P.J. (1995) Distinct roles for B7-1 (CD-80) and B7-2 (CD-86) in the initiation of experimental allergic encephalomyelitis. *J. Clin. Invest.* 96:2195–2203.

Rapalino, O., Lazarov-Spiegler, O., Agranov, E., Velan, G.J., Yoles, E., Fraidakis, M., Solomon, A., Gepstein, R., Katz, A., Belkin, M., Hadani, M., and Schwartz, M. (1998) Implantation of stimulated homologous macrophages results in partial recovery of paraplegic rats. *Nat. Med.* 4:814–821.

Rappert, A., Biber, K., Nolte, C., Lipp, M., Schubel, A., Lu, B., Gerard, N.P., Gerard, C., Boddeke, H.W., and Kettenmann, H. (2002) Secondary lymphoid tissue chemokine (CCL21) activates CXCR3 to trigger a Cl− current and chemotaxis in murine microglia. *J. Immunol.* 168:3221–3226.

Re, F., Belyanskaya, S.L., Riese, R.J., Cipriani, B., Fischer, F.R., Granucci, F., Ricciardi-Castagnoli, P., Brosnan, C., Stern, L.J., Strominger, J.L., and Santambrogio, L. (2002) Granulocyte-macrophage colony-stimulating factor induces an expression program in neonatal microglia that primes them for antigen presentation. *J. Immunol.* 169:2264–2273.

Reichmann, G., Schroeter, M., Jander, S., and Fischer, H.G. (2002) Dendritic cells and dendritic-like microglia in focal cortical ischemia of the mouse brain. *J. Neuroimmunol.* 129:125–132.

Rinner, W.A., Bauer, J., Schmidts, M., Lassmann, H., and Hickey, W.F. (1995) Resident microglia and hematogenous macrophages as phagocytes in adoptively transferred experimental autoimmune encephalomyelitis: an investigation using rat radiation bone marrow chimeras. *Glia* 14:257–266.

Rosseler, K., Neuchrist, C., Kitz, K., Scheiner, O., Kraft, D., and Lassmann, H. (1992) Expression of leucocyte adhesion molecules at the human blood–brain barrier (BBB). *J. Neurosci. Res.* 31: 365–374.

Santambrogio, L., Belyanskaya, S.L., Fischer, F.R., Cipriani, B., Brosnan, C.F., Ricciardi-Castagnoli, P., Stern, L.J., Strominger, J.L., and Reise, R. (2001) Developmental plasticity of CNS microglia. *Proc. Natl. Acad. Sci. USA* 98:6295–6300.

Sasseville, V.G., Newman, W., Brodie, S.J., Hesterberg, P., Pauley, D., and Ringler, D.J. (1994) Monocyte adhesion to endothelium in simian immunodeficiency virus–induced AIDS encephalitis is mediated by vascular cell adhesion molecule-1/alpha 4 beta 1 integrin interactions. *Am. J. Pathol.* 144:27–40.

Schwab, M.E. (2002) Repairing the injured spinal cord. *Science* 295:1029–1031.

Schwartz, M., Cohen, I., Lazarov-Spiegler, O., Moalem, G., and Yoles, E. (1999) The remedy may lie in ourselves: prospects for immune cell therapy in central nervous system protection and repair. *J. Mol. Med.* 77:713–717.

Sievers, J., Parwaresch, R., and Wottge, H.U. (1994a) Blood monocytes and spleen macrophages differentiate into microglia-like cells on monolayers of astrocytes: morphology. *Glia* 12:245–258.

Sievers, J., Schmidtmayer, J., and Parwaresch, R. (1994b) Blood monocytes and spleen macrophages differentiate into microglia-like cells when cultured on astrocytes. *Anat. Anz.* 176:45–51.

Streilein, J.W. (1996) Peripheral tolerance induction: lessons from immune privileged sites and tissues. *Transplant Proc.* 28:2066–2070.

Streilein, J.W., Ksander, B.R., and Taylor, A.W. (1997) Immune deviation in relation to ocular immune privilege. *J. Immunol.* 158:3557–3560.

Tanaka, J. and Maeda, N. (1996) Microglial ramification requires nondiffusible factors derived from astrocytes. *Exp. Neurol.* 137: 367–375.

Thanos, P.K., Jhamandas, K., and Beninger, R.J. (1992) *N*-methyl-D-aspartate unilaterally injected into the dorsal striatum of rats produces contralateral circling: antagonism by 2-amino-7-phosphonoheptanoic acid and cis-flupenthixol. *Brain Res.* 589:55–61.

Trebst, C., Sorensen, T.L., Kivisakk, P., Cathcart, M.K., Hesselgesser, J., Horuk, R., Sellebjerg, F., Lassmann, H., and Ransohoff, R.M. (2001) CCR1+/CCR5+ mononuclear phagocytes accumulate in the central nervous system of patients with multiple sclerosis. *Am. J. Pathol.* 159:1701–1710.

Ullrich, O., Diestel, A., Eyupoglu, I.Y., and Nitsch, R. (2001) Regulation of microglial expression of integrins by poly(ADP-ribose) polymerase-1. *Nat. Cell Biol.* 3:1035–1042.

Unger, E.R., Sung, J.H., Manivel, J.C., Chenggis, M.L., Blazar, B.R., and Krivit, W. (1993) Male donor-derived cells in the brains of female sex-mismatched bone marrow transplant recipients: a Y-chromosome specific in situ hybridization study. *J. Neuropathol. Exp. Neurol.* 52:460–470.

Vincent, V.A., Tilders, F.J., and Van Dam, A.M. (1997) Inhibition of endotoxin-induced nitric oxide synthase production in microglial cells by the presence of astroglial cells: a role for transforming growth factor beta. *Glia* 19:190–198.

Weiss, J.M., Downie, S.A., Lyman, W.D., and Berman, J.W. (1998) Astrocyte-derived monocyte-chemoattractant protein-1 directs the transmigration of leukocytes across a model of the human blood–brain barrier. *J. Immunol.* 161;6896–6903.

Weiss, J.M., Nath, A., Major, E.O., and Berman, J.W. (1999) HIV-1 Tat induces monocyte chemoattractant protein-1-mediated monocyte transmigration across a model of the human blood-brain barrier and up-regulates CCR5 expression on human monocytes. *J. Immunol.* 163:2953–2959.

Wenkel, H., Streilein, J.W., and Young, M.J. (2000) Systemic immune deviation in the brain that does not depend on the integrity of the blood-brain barrier. *J. Immunol.* 164:5125–5131.

Wilbanks, G.A. and Streilein, J.W. (1992) Fluids from immune privileged sites endow macrophages with the capacity to induce antigen-specific immune deviation via a mechanism involving transforming growth factor-beta. *Eur. J. Immunol.* 22:1031–1036.

Williams, K., Alvarez, X., and Lackner, A.A. (2001) Central nervous system perivascular cells are immunoregulatory cells that connect the CNS with the peripheral immune system. *Glia* 36:156–164.

Williams, K.C. and Hickey, W.F. (1995) Traffick of hematogenous cells through the central nervous system. In: Oldstone, M.B.A. and Vitkovic, L., eds. *HIV and Dementia*. Berlin: Springer-Verlag, pp. 221–246.

Williams, K.C. and Hickey, W.F. (2002) Central nervous system damage, monocytes and macrophages, and neurological disorders in AIDS. *Annu. Rev. Neurosci.* 25:537–562.

Wilms, H., Hartmann, D., and Sievers, J. (1997) Ramification of microglia, monocytes and macrophages in vitro: influences of various epithelial and mesenchymal cells and their conditioned media. *Cell Tissue Res.* 287:447–458.

Windhagen, A., Newcombe, J., Dangond, F., Strand, C., Woodroofe, M.N., Cuzner, M.L., and Hafler, D.A. (1995) Expression of co-stimulatory molecules B7-1 (CD80), B7-2 (CD86), and interleukin 12 cytokine in multiple sclerosis lesions. *J. Exp. Med.* 182:1985–1996.

Wolf, S.A., Fisher, J., Bechmann, I., Steiner, B., Kwidzinski, E., and Nitsch, R. (2002) Neuroprotection by T-cells depends on their subtype and activation state. *J. Neuroimmunol.* 133:72–80.

Wolf, S.A., Gimsa, U., Bechmann, I., and Nitsch, R. (2001) Differential expression of costimulatory molecules B7-1 and B7-2 on microglial cells induced by Th1 and Th2 cells in organotypic brain tissue. *Glia* 36:414–420.

Wright, G.J., Jones, M., Puklavec, M.J., Brown, M.H., and Barclay, A.N. (2001) The unusual distribution of the neuronal/lymphoid cell surface CD200 (OX2) glycoprotein is conserved in humans. *Immunology* 102:173–179.

Wright, G.J., Puklavec, M.J., Willis, A.C., Hoek, R.M., Sedgwick, J.D., Brown, M.H., and Barclay, A.N. (2000) Lymphoid/neuronal cell surface OX2 glycoprotein recognizes a novel receptor on macrophages implicated in the control of their function. *Immunity* 13:233–242.

Yuan, H., Gaber, M.W., McColgan, T., Naimark, M.D., Kiani, M.F., and Merchant, T.E. (2003) Radiation-induced permeability and leukocyte adhesion in the rat blood–brain barrier: modulation with anti-ICAM-1 antibodies. *Brain Res.* 969(1–2):59–69.

24 Antigen processing, presentation, and T cell interaction

HARALD NEUMANN

In contrast to most other organs, the central nervous system (CNS) is protected by a blood–brain barrier (BBB) designed to minimize the passage of immune cells and macromolecules into the brain parenchyma. Furthermore, in the normal CNS parenchyma antigen-presenting cells (APCs) are functionally inactivated and lack expression of major histocompatibility complex (MHC) molecules. Nevertheless, the CNS is routinely surveyed by activated T lymphocytes. Perivascular macrophages situated adjacent to the endothelium cells of the blood vessels take up and present antigens to T lymphocytes. Most cells of the brain parenchyma are immunologically quiescent in the healthy CNS, but can be stimulated to become facultative APCs that process and present antigens via their MHC molecules to T lymphocytes in neuroinflammatory diseases.

ANTIGEN-PRESENTING CELLS

Unlike most organ systems, the CNS is located in an immunologically privileged environment behind a BBB formed by tight junctions of endothelial cells (Fig. 24.1) (Huber et al., 2001). In addition, immune responses and defense from microorganisms are strictly controlled and kept to a minimum to avoid unwanted immune-mediated damage (Lowenstein, 2002). Nevertheless, during neuroinflammatory diseases such as multiple sclerosis (MS), viral or bacterial disease and brain injury genes are turned on in the CNS tissue, which allow for specific and efficient defense against dangerous pathogens and healing (Neumann and Wekerle, 1998). Antigens derived from viruses or bacteria do not stimulate T lymphocytes directly. Instead, specialized cells named *antigen-presenting cells* (APCs) process and display the antigens on their cell surface to make them recognizable by specific T lymphocytes. The T lymphocytes recognize antigen-derived peptide fragments bound to MHC molecules. T cells can be divided into two major populations: one subset carrying the T cell receptor (TCR) and the CD4 antigen that shows cognate binding to the peptide and MHC class II molecule displayed on the APC, and another subset carrying the TCR and the CD8 antigen that specifically recognize the peptide together with MHC class I on the APC. Recognition of antigens on APCs leads to physical contact between T lymphocytes and APCs, which allows for reciprocal signaling via a variety of molecules clustered at the region of contact.

See the list of abbreviations at the end of the chapter.

Professional Antigen-Presenting Cells

Cells specialized to initiate or propagate the development of antigen-specific T lymphocytes are often termed *professional antigen-presenting cells.* Professional APCs are dendritic cells, macrophages, and B lymphocytes. Dendritic cells and B lymphocytes are not detectable in the healthy CNS parenchyma, but a small subpopulation of macrophages or blood-derived monocytes, the perivascular macrophages, are situated in the perivascular space. The professional APCs effectively take up antigens from their environment, process these antigens into small peptides, and express the components in conjunction with the MHC molecules on the cell surface in a form that can be recognized by T lymphocytes. Further, the professional APCs are capable of delivering additional costimulatory signals to the T lymphocytes that support and stimulate the full activation program of naive T cells.

The dendritic cell is the prototype and the most important professional APC. Dendritic cells are present in most tissues of the body. They acquire antigens, transport them to the draining lymph nodes, and present them to the recirculating pool of naive T cells stimulating their full activation program. Further, dendritic cells are mobilized from the blood into the tissue by chemokines that are induced by inflammatory stimuli such as tumor necrosis factor-α (TNF-α) and interleukin-1β (IL-1β). As mentioned before, tissue-resident dendritic cells are not detectable in the normal CNS parenchyma, but are localized in the leptomeninges and dura mater. They migrate and accumulate in the

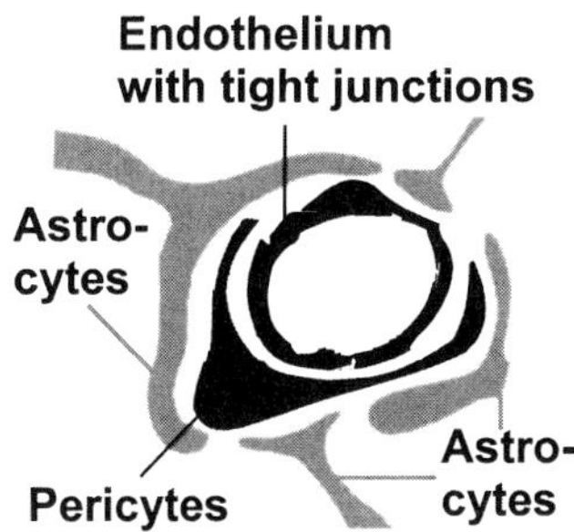

FIGURE 24.1 The blood–brain barrier (BBB). The brain endothelium with its tight junctions forms the BBB, which is covered by pericytes and astrocytic endfeets.

perivascular areas of the CNS when strong inflammatory foci develop (Fischer and Reichmann, 2001). In particular, dendritic cells are recruited into the CNS in neuroinflammatory conditions such as experimental autoimmune encephalomyelitis (EAE) (Serafini et al., 2000) and cerebral toxoplasmosis (Fischer and Reichmann, 2001).

Macrophages engulf and degrade particles and microorganisms via a process termed *phagocytosis* and present antigens via their MHC class II molecules to $CD4^+$ T cells. Macrophages home to a special area of the normal CNS, the perivascular space, termed *Virchow-Robin space*, the leptomeninges, the dura mater, and the choroid plexus. Various names have been used to describe the macrophages localized adjacent to endothelial cells in the Virchow-Robin space, including *perivascular macrophages*, *perivascular cells, perivascular microglia*, and *fluorescent granular perithelial cells*. The perivascular macrophages are bone marrow–derived and continuously enter this area of the normal brain across the intact BBB (Bechmann et al., 2001). They show low expression of MHC class II molecules, and can take up antigenic material from their local environment and present it to T lymphocytes (Ford et al., 1995). Under certain pathological conditions, including autoimmune inflammation and viral encephalitis, perivascular macrophages substantially increase in number, and either remain for long periods or stay transiently and resolve (Lassmann et al., 1993; Weller, 1998). Although it is known that there is a continuous turnover of these perivascular macrophages under normal conditions and accumulation during neuroinflammatory disease, it is still controversial whether they could return to the lymph nodes and spleen carrying materials collected from the CNS perivascular area.

B lymphocytes, another professional APC and a major effector cell type of the immune system, are responsible for the neutralization of viruses or foreign antigens and removal of toxic material. On the one hand, they produce specific antibodies, which are capable of binding directly to antigen; on the other hand, they participate as APCs in the activation of T lymphocytes and stimulation of immune responses. In contrast to perivascular macrophages, there is no evidence that B cells home to specific CNS areas, patrol the CNS, or enter the CNS under normal conditions (Hickey, 2001). Nevertheless, B cells, at least in low numbers, are capable of entering the CNS under pathological conditions when the BBB is impaired following inflammatory CNS stimulation. Furthermore, B cells can be numerous in certain inflammatory plaques of multiple sclerosis (MS) and EAE. Thus B cells, as professional APCs, are available in the CNS only during inflammatory processes, including viral or bacterial meningitis, or encephalitis or autoimmune diseases (Hickey, 2001). In such diseases, the presence of *oligoclonal bands*—immunoglobulin bands in the cerebrospinal fluid detected by protein electrophoresis—indicates the entry of B cells into the CNS, clonal expansion, differentiation into plasma cells, and secretion of antibodies (Hickey, 2001).

Nonprofessional Antigen-Presenting Cells

The nonprofessional antigen-presenting cells are a wide spectrum of tissue cells that present antigens for secondary or effector T cell function. Recognition of antigenic material presented on the cell surface of APCs permits T cells to detect an intracellular pathogen at an early stage before substantial replication of the microorganism can occur. This recognition of peptide fragments by T cells can result in direct killing of the host cells or clearance of the microorganism from the host cells by cytotoxic $CD8^+$ T lymphocyte–derived mediators. Expression of MHC class I or MHC class II molecules is a prerequisite for APCs to interact with $CD8^+$ or $CD4^+$ T lymphocytes, respectively. In most organs of the body the tissue resident cells do express MHC class I molecules, and a subpopulation of professional APCs express MHC class II molecules. Due to its immune privileged status, the CNS is exceptional in this respect. Major histocompatibility complex class I and class II molecules are not constitutively expressed on neural cells in the healthy CNS parenchyma, but can be induced during most inflammatory and degenerative CNS diseases (Neumann and Wekerle, 1998). Thus, invading cytotoxic T lymphocytes (CTLs) do not find constitutive MHC-expressing target cells that present antigens in a recognizable manner in the parenchyma proper of the healthy CNS. However, the invading CTLs release pro-inflammatory cytokines such as interferon-γ (IFN-γ) and TNF-α that have been shown to induce *de novo* expression of MHC molecules on brain cells *in vitro* (Neumann, 2001). All glial cell types, as well as neurons, are capable of expressing MHC class I and therefore fulfill the basic requirement for interaction with secondary or effector T lymphocytes (reviewed recently by Neumann, 2001). Microglial cells qualify as neural APCs expressing MHC class II (Aloisi, 2001). Although they lack expression of MHC molecules under resting conditions, microglia are readily induced by IFN-γ to express MHC class I and class II and to present antigen to specific T lymphocytes. Recently, diverse classes of MHC class I gene transcripts (including nonclassical class I genes) were observed in distinct mosaics of neurons, suggesting a role for MHC class I expression in CNS development and plasticity (Corriveau et al., 1998; Huh et al., 2000). Whether this developmental and activity-dependent regulation of MHC class I genes in neurons is involved in antigen presentation has not been firmly established.

ANTIGEN PROCESSING AND PRESENTATION TO T LYMPHOCYTES

As mentioned before, peptides bound to MHC class I are presented to CD8$^+$, mainly cytotoxic T cells, while peptides bound to MHC class II are presented to CD4$^+$ T cells. The molecular mechanisms of antigen processing and presentation by class I and class II MHC molecules are quite different.

Antigen Presentation By Major Histocompatibility Complex Class II

The specialized professional APCs use distinct mechanisms for endocytosis of antigens from the environment. Macrophages and dendritic cells take up antigens by phagocytosis and pinocytosis, while B lymphocytes use a specific receptor-bound, immunoglobulin-mediated antigen uptake.

The phagocytic pathway used by macrophages is the main mechanism of antigen uptake in the injured or inflamed CNS. Phagocytosis is initiated by binding of target structures to specific receptors on the macrophages including Fc receptors, complement receptors, acute phase protein receptors, and phosphatidyl serine receptors. The phagocytic pathway is a form of endocytosis in which particles from microorganisms, apoptotic cells, or degenerated proteins are engulfed to form an endosome and are subsequently cleaved by a number of proteases in the endocytic compartment. Peptides from endocytosed material are then loaded onto the MHC class II heterodimer.

Expression of MHC class II molecules in general is one prerequisite to activate CD4$^+$ helper T cells, resulting in humoral immune responses with the production of specific antibodies by B lymphocytes and stimulation of macrophages and CD8$^+$ T lymphocytes. Microglial cells show high and early MHC class II upregulation during most inflammatory processes in the CNS. Due to their sensitivity to microenvironmental changes, they can function as sentinels (Kreutzberg, 1996). Activated microglial cells can take up apoptotic cells, including T cells (Magnus et al., 2001), and can readily present the antigens via their MHC class II molecules to CD4$^+$ T lymphocytes. Recent data indicate that resting parenchymal microglial cells are like uncommitted myeloid progenitors (Santambrogio et al., 2001). They appear to be in an immature state of antigen presentation with "empty" class II MHC molecules and a cysteine protease (cathepsin) profile comparable to that of immature dendritic cells (Santambrogio et al., 2001).

Stimulated astrocytes are far less competent in presenting antigens than microglial cells (Aloisi et al., 2000). Although astrocytes were the first brain cell type demonstrated *in vitro* to process and present myelin antigens to CD4$^+$ T lymphocytes via MHC class II molecules, they normally do not trigger the full activation program of naive T lymphocytes due to their lack of costimulatory molecules, as discussed below (Aloisi, 2001).

Antigen Presentation By Major Histocompatibility Complex Class I

Antigens presented via MHC class I molecules are derived predominantly from intracellular proteins. The proteasome, a multisubunit proteolytic complex, is responsible for the generation of peptides from cytosolic proteins. The peptides are transported into the endoplasmic reticulum by the transporters associated with antigen processing (TAPs), where they (if they have the strict peptide length requirement of 8–11 amino acids) associate with heterodimers of MHC class I heavy chain and β2-microglobulin. The trimeric stably assembled complex is transported via the endoplasmic reticulum and the Golgi network to the cell surface. The above-described processing of intracellular proteins is the main source of MHC class I bound peptides. However, processing of exogenous antigens for presentation on class I molecules has been described and might be required for cytotoxic T lymphocytes (CTL) responses against microorganisms that do not infect the professional APCs themselves. Presentation of peptides via MHC class I could result in activation of CD8$^+$ cytotoxic T cells that either kill cells infected by pathogens or render host cells resistant to pathogen replication by secretion of cytokines such as IFN-γ or TNF-α.

All brain glial cell types including microglia, astrocytes, and oligodendrocytes have been shown to process and present antigens to CD8$^+$ T lymphocytes (Neumann et al., 2002). Neurons stimulated by the inflammatory cytokine IFN-γ do transcribe gene transcripts of the TAPs (Neumann et al., 1997), but the formal evidence that neurons indeed can process antigens for presentation to CD8$^+$ T lymphocytes is still missing. Inducibility of MHC class I in neurons is very strictly regulated (Neumann et al., 1995). In particular, cell membrane expression of MHC class I is induced only in a minority of cultured neurons by IFN-γ, but is increased after additional blockade of neuronal activity with tetrodotoxin (Neumann et al., 1997). Loading of the neuronal MHC class I binding groove with a fitting peptide does allow recognition of the neurons by $CD8^+$ T lymphocytes (Neumann et al., 2002).

MODULATION OF THE ANTIGEN-PRESENTING CAPACITY BY THE CENTRAL NERVOUS SYSTEM ENVIRONMENT

As mentioned before, the APCs in the CNS parenchyma are quiescent cells under normal conditions. They are functionally inactivated, and their expression of MHC and costimulatory molecules is downregulated. Which environmental factors in the CNS are responsible for this exceptional immunosuppressive effect? One of the major breakthroughs in this field of research was the discovery that the local CNS microenvironment, apart from the BBB, plays a key role in shaping the immunoprivileged state of the CNS (Neumann, 2001). Glial cells monitor the neuronal signals, and their immune function is under strict control of the neurochemical microenvironement (Fig. 24.2). Numerous receptors for neurotransmitters, neuropeptides, and neurotrophins normally required for neuronal signaling are expressed on glial cells. *In vitro* studies demonstrated that signals coming from normal neuronal activity counteract the immunostimulatory effects of the pro-inflammatory cytokine IFN-γ. Intact neurons counterregulate IFN-γ-mediated induction of MHC class II molecules on surrounding astrocytes and microglia (Neumann et al., 1996, 1998). The exact mechanism by which neurons influence the antigen-presenting capacity of neighboring glial cells is still not known. In principle, the local interactions between neurons and glial cells could be mediated via indirect electrical coupling due to changes in ion concentrations, cell adhesion molecules, or soluble mediators such as neurotransmitters or neuropeptides. Classical neurotransmitters and neuropeptides such as norepinephrine, α-melanocyte-stimulating hormone (α-MSH), and vasoactive intestinal peptide (VIP) counteract lipopolysaccharide (LPS)-mediated stimulation of cytokine and nitric oxide (NO) release by microglial cells (Aloisi, 2001). Further, norepinephrine and VIP act directly on cultured astrocytes and prevent IFN-γ-mediated induction of MHC class II molecules (Neumann. 2001). Astrocytes have also been shown to downregulate microglial activation and inhibit MHC class II and intercellular adhesion molecule-1 (ICAM-1) expression of microglia/ macrophages (Hailer et al., 1998), possibly via release of transforming growth factor-β (TGF-β) (Aloisi et al., 2000). It has been demonstrated that neurotrophins inhibit MHC class II inducibility in microglia (Neumann et al., 1998). In cultured brain slices, the neurotrophins nerve growth factor, brain-derived growth factor, and neurotrophin-3 are capable of downregulating the expression of MHC

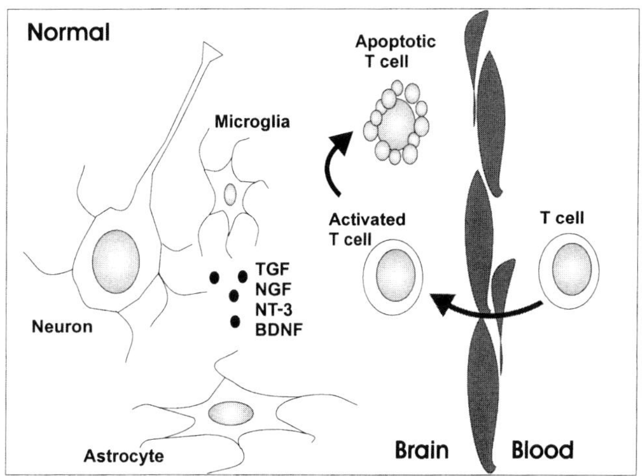

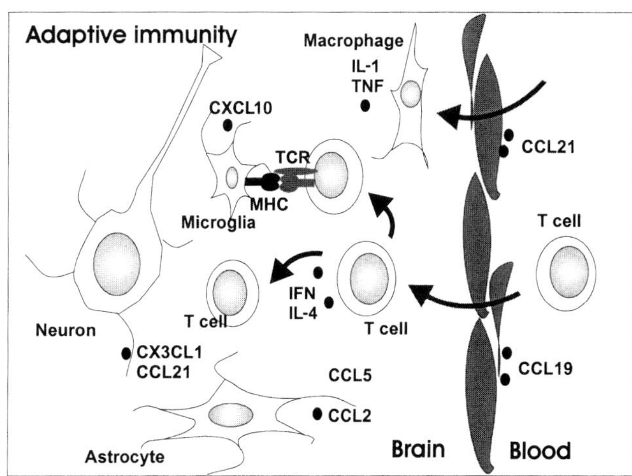

FIGURE 24.2 Central nervous system (CNS) immune surveillance by T lymphocytes. *Normal*: In the normal CNS the tissue growth factor and cytokine milieu maintain the brain cells in an immunologically quiescent state. Neurons produce neurotrophins [nerve growth factor (NGF), brain-derived neurotrophic factor (BDNF), and neurotrophin-3 (NT-3)], which have been shown to prevent expression of immunological molecules on glial cells. Astrocytes produce transforming growth factor-β (TGF-β) having immunosuppressive activity. Expression of the major histocompatibility complex (MHC) is undetectable or relative low in the normal CNS. Only activated T cells can pass the blood–brain barrier and undergo apoptosis after entering the brain tissue. *Adaptive immunity*: During inflammatory processes glial cells, neurons, and endothelium cells produce chemokines (CXCL10, CX3CL1, CCL2, CCL5, CCL19 and CCL21) and cytokines [interleukin-1β (IL-1β) and tumor necrosis factor-α (TNF-α)]. Chemokines attract the motile microglia and macrophages to the lesion sites, and promote attraction and transmigration of T lymphocytes into the CNS. Antigen-specific recognition locally stimulates T lymphocytes and facilitates their full-blown effector function, including cytotoxictiy and cytokine secretion. Major histocompatibility complex molecules are induced on brain cells by the cytokines and present antigens to the invading T cells.

class II on microglia. Nerve growth factor acts directly on microglia and inhibits the expression of MHC class II and the costimulatory molecule CD86 (Neumann et al., 1998; Wei and Jonakait, 1999).

Recently, it has been shown that a new type of receptor-ligand interaction controls microglial activation. While neurons express CD200, the corresponding receptor CD200R, a membrane glycoprotein, is detected on microglial cells (Hoek et al., 2000). Microglia of CD200-deficient mice spontaneously exhibit many features of activation, including a less ramified morphology and increased expression of CD11b and CD45. Following induction of EAE, an autoimmune CNS animal model for MS, CD200-deficient mice show increased expression of inducible nitric oxide synthase in inflammatory microglia and macrophages. These data indicate that CD200 expressed by resident CNS cells, including neurons, might silence and downregulate the immune function of microglia.

IMMUNE SURVEILLANCE BY T LYMPHOCYTES

As mentioned before, the CNS is surveyed by a mechanism that allows activated T lymphocytes to patrol the brain tissue (Fig. 24.2). However, there is no specific homing of certain antigen-specific T cells or subpopulations into the CNS, and the entry of T cells appears to be random (Flügel et al., 2001; Hickey, 2001; Cabarrocas et al., 2003). The number of T cells in the normal CNS is lower compared to other tissues, and trafficking studies demonstrate that the CNS has the smallest T cell concentrations per gram of tissue (Hickey, 2001). The number of T cells also differs in distinct brain areas. It is much lower in the cerebellum than in the spinal cord (Hickey, 2001). Although T cell entry into the CNS is not antigen specific, T cells encountering their antigen in the CNS accumulate there and can reach relatively high numbers in inflammatory foci (Flügel et al., 2001). It has been shown that pathogenic T cells, able to recognize their antigen in the CNS, accumulate (Flügel et al., 2001), while those that cannot find their antigen in the CNS possibly disappear via apoptosis (Bauer et al., 1998). The T cells, recognizing their antigen, are locally re-activated in the brain and their pathogenic potential determines the clinical outcome (Kawakami et al., 2004).

While T cells including CTLs are low in number or virtually absent in the normal CNS, the situation changes dramatically not only in the CNS infected by microbial organisms but also in the lesioned CNS (Fig. 24.1). Under these circumstances, the endothelium is activated locally and glial cells attract T lymphocytes via release of chemokines. Increased recruitment of T lymphocytes in the CNS parenchyma has been demonstrated following transection of the spinal cord (Popovich et al., 1996) and axotomy of the peripheral facial nerve (Raivich et al., 1998). After axonal injury chemokine expression is induced on glial cells that directs leukocytes to the site of damage (Babcock et al., 2003). The chemokines together with the matrix metalloproteinase-9 play a key role in leukocytes migration across the BBB (Sellebjerg et al., 2003). The matrix metalloproteinase-9 loosens the tight junctions of the endothelium cells (Sellebjerg et al., 2003).

ACTIVATION VERSUS APOPTOSIS OF T LYMPHOCYTES

The consequence of antigen presentation to T lymphocytes is influenced by environmental factors, the amount and avidity of the TCR-MHC/peptide interaction, and the presence or absence of costimulatory signals of the APCs (Fig. 24.3*A*). Additional interactions between adhesion molecules CD11a (LFA-1), CD58 (LFA-3), or CD54 (ICAM-1) on the APCs and their counterreceptors on T cells are required for optimal T cell activation. The sum of all these signals determines whether a T cell is activated or not.

Activation of T Lymphocytes By Costimulation

Expression of costimulatory molecules such as CD80 (B7-1), CD86 (B7-2), or CD40 on APCs is mandatory to stimulate the full activation program of T lymphocytes. CD80 and CD86 support TCR activation through binding to CD28 on T cells. CD40 of APCs is stimulated by CD40 ligand expressed on T cells and enhances MHC class II and CD80/ CD86 expression

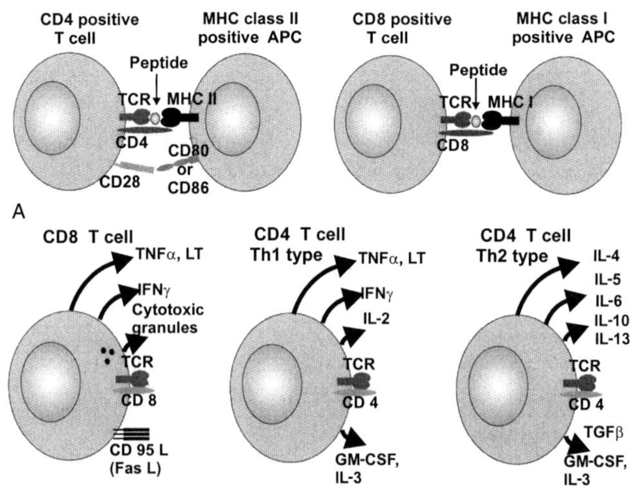

FIGURE 24.3 *A*. Interactions between the T cell receptor (TCR) and the major histocompatibility complex (MHC)-peptide complex. *B*. Effector molecules and cytokines produced by distinct T cell subtypes. APC: antigen-presenting cell; GM-CSF: granulocyte-macrophage colony-stimulating factor; IFNγ: interferon-γ; IL-2, IL-3: interleukin-2, -3; LT: lymphophotoxin; TNFd: tumor necrosis factor d; TGFβ: transforming growth factor-β.

of the APCs, which in turn promotes T cell activation. In the absence of accessory and costimulatory molecules, APCs have been shown to anergize or induce apoptosis of T cells.

In the normal CNS, expression of MHC class I and class II molecules is restricted to perivascular macrophages, which can be stimulated to express costimulatory molecules and play an important role in the induction of T cell responses against microbial and self-antigens (Ford et al., 1995). As mentioned before, microglia in their resting conditions from normal CNS behave as poor APCs and express only low levels of CD14, CD45, and Fc receptors and no costimulatory molecules. However, evidence shows that microglia readily upregulate MHC class II and adhesion molecules (CD11a and CD54) in virtually all inflammatory and neurodegenerative CNS processes (Kreutzberg, 1996). Moreover, activated microglia in inflammatory CNS lesions, including MS lesions, can acquire a macrophage-like phenotype and have been shown to express the costimulatory molecules CD80, CD86, and CD40 (Aloisi et al., 2000), and *in vitro* can stimulate the full activation program of T cells (Aloisi et al., 2000). Further, activated microglial cells in inflammatory brain lesions recruit additional immune cells via the release of chemokines, including macrophage inflammatory protein 1α (MIP-1α), and locally promote T cell responses via release of interleukin-12 (IL-12) (Aloisi et al., 2000).

In contrast to microglia and perivascular macrophages, astrocytes fail to express costimulatory molecules *in vivo*, although occasionally or under strong inflammatory conditions they can express MHC class II (Aloisi et al., 2000). It is unlikely that they function as efficient APCs for CD4$^+$ T cells *in vivo*, because they do not express costimulatory molecules and sufficient amounts of MHC class II. Although astrocytes produce and secrete chemotactic factors including monocytes chemotactic protein-1 (MCP-1) and IFN-γ-induced protein-10, which could recruit monocytes/macrophages and T cells into the affected brain tissue during inflammatory brain diseases (Ransohoff and Tani, 1998), they are mainly involved in the inhibition of T cell responses and T cell activation. They produce the anti-inflammatory mediators transforming growth factor-β (TGF-β) and interleukin-10 (IL-10) during EAE and MS (Aloisi et al., 2000). Therefore, it has been suggested that astrocytes have an important function in downregulating T cell responses in the CNS. Like astrocytes, oligodendrocytes lack the expression of costimulatory molecules and are unable to trigger the full activation program of T cells.

Apoptosis of T Lymphocytes

Normal individuals have T lymphocytes capable of reacting to CNS autoantigens such as myelin basic protein (MBP). The physiological control of autoreactive T cells in the CNS is likely to have an important role in preventing autoimmune CNS disorders such as MS. T cells that have entered the CNS parenchyma die rapidly via an apoptotic mechanism. Apoptosis of T cells has been studied mainly in the EAE model. In EAE, apoptosis of T cells is maximum during the phase of spontaneous recovery from the disease (Bauer et al., 1995). The main site of T cell apoptosis is the CNS parenchyma rather than the perivascular space (Bauer et al., 1995). T cell death is independent of antigen recognition and is not selective to T cells directed against specific CNS antigens (Bauer et al., 1998). Using T cells carrying specific genetic markers, it has been shown that both ovalbumin-specific T cells and MBP-specific T cells undergo apoptosis in the CNS during EAE. The apoptotic T cells are phagocytosed by macrophages and glia (Nguyen and Pender, 1998). Thus, there must be something inherent in the CNS environment that leads to apoptosis of T cells. T cells may interact with glial cells and neurons in the CNS and thereby receive signals that influence their susceptibility to apoptosis. Astrocytes inhibit antigen-specific proliferation of T cells and prime them for apoptosis *in vitro*. In EAE, apoptotic inflammatory cells associate more closely with astrocytes than with microglia. It has been suggested that Fas ligand/CD95 ligand constitutively expressed by astrocytes induces apoptosis of Fas/CD95-expressing T cells (Suvannavejh et al., 2000). Also, microglial cells do express CD95 ligand and can induce apoptosis by binding to the CD95 receptor of T cells. Recently, it has been demonstrated that neurons constitutively express CD95 ligand *in vitro* and *in vivo* (Flügel et al., 2000). Furthermore, autoreactive T cells rapidly undergo apoptosis in the vicinity of CD95 ligand–expressing neurons in the facial nerve axotomy model (Flügel et al., 2000). This study proposes that the CD95 ligand might be involved in apoptosis of T cells in the CNS. Other studies indicate different mechanisms (Bauer et al., 1998), including the fact that the gangliosides of the brain might be toxic to T cells (Irani, 1998).

EFFECTOR FUNCTION OF T LYMPHOCYTES

T lymphocytes can be divided into distinct, specialized subtypes. As mentioned before, CD4$^+$ T lymphocytes interact with MHC class II–expressing APCs and have mainly helper and immunoregulatory functions, while CD8$^+$ T lymphocytes interact with MHC class I–expressing APCs and have mainly a cytotoxic function (Fig. 24.3*B*).

Effects of CD4$^+$ T Lymphocytes

CD4$^+$ T cells within the CNS play an important role in regulating immune responses, exert immunoregulatory effects via secretion of soluble mediators, and ultimately trigger repair during a variety of CNS diseases. The subtypes of CD4$^+$ T lymphocytes appear as two major and distinct phenotypes due to the profiles of cytokines, which they produce. CD4$^+$ T cells of the Th1 phenotype produce interleukin-2 (IL-2), IFN-γ, TNF-α, and lymphotoxin-α (Fig. 24.3*B*). The Th1 cells stimulate inflammatory responses, activate macrophages, and induce tissue damage. They are essential in promoting the maturation of resting microglial cells into APCs that express adhesion molecules (e.g., CD54), costimulatory molecules (CD80, CD86, and CD40), pro-inflammatory cytokines (TNF-α, IL-1β), and chemokines (e.g., MIP-1α). During inflammatory CNS diseases, the CD40 ligand (CD40L/CD154) of activated Th1 cells can bind to CD40 of activated microglia and stimulate microglial production of IL-12, nitric oxide, and other cytotoxic and immunoregulatory mediators.

During viral CNS diseases, the Th1 T cells have been implicated in the clearance of neurotropic viruses and virus-induced CNS inflammation. In addition, they promote differentiation of CD8$^+$ T cells in cytotoxic effector T cells. Th1 cells have been shown to be the disease-inducing cell type in EAE. Studies with the passive transfer of T lymphocytes in Lewis rats established that CD4$^+$ T lymphocytes of the Th1 phenotype freshly activated *in vitro* by specific myelin antigens (e.g., MBP) migrate into the brain tissue and induce an autoimmune inflammatory disease in the CNS. After intravenous injection, the T lymphocytes interact with brain cells and APCs of secondary immune organs during an initial phase lasting for 3–4 days. The cells then accumulate in perivascular brain regions, leading to a second wave of T lymphocyte recruitment, monocyte brain invasion, and transient neurological deficits. The exact mechanism by which the Th1 CD4$^+$ T lymphocytes induce clinical symptoms such as hind limb paralysis in these animals is not known. It has been suggested that the Th1 cytokines TNF-α and IFN-γ released by these CD4$^+$ T lymphocytes affect oligodendrocyte and neuronal function directly (Merrill and Benveniste, 1996).

In contrast, CD4$^+$ T cells of the Th2 phenotype produce IL-4, IL-5, IL-6, IL-10, IL-13, and TGF-β (Fig. 24.3*B*), cytokines that support humoral immune responses by stimulation of the differentiation of B cells and inhibit numerous macrophage inflammatory functions. Within the CNS, Th2 cells downregulate immune responses of Th1 cells and inhibit macrophage and microglia activation (Aharoni et al., 2000). The Th2 cytokines inhibit CNS inflammation and suppress EAE (Mathisen et al., 1997). Isolated T cell clones directed against myelin proteolipid protein were transfected to overexpress the Th2 anti-inflammatory cytokine IL-10. Upon transfer, these genetically engineered T cells inhibited the onset of EAE and clinical signs of established EAE (Mathisen et al., 1997). Likewise, statins (HMG-CoA reductase inhibitors) have been shown to reverse paralysis of EAE via stimulation of Th2 and suppression of Th1 cytokines (Youssef et al., 2002).

Surprisingly, CD4$^+$ T lymphocytes, which induce a monophasic paralytic EAE after passive transfer, have been shown to protect injured neurons from secondary degeneration (Schwartz et al., 1999). Following partial lesioning of the rat optic nerve, activated CD4$^+$ T lymphocytes directed against the autoantigen MBP were transferred and accumulated at the site of the lesion (Moalem et al., 1999). Two weeks after injury, rats injected with the autoreactive myelin peptide–restricted CD4$^+$ T lymphocytes showed less secondary degeneration of the retinal ganglion neurons (Moalem et al., 1999). The exact cytokine profile of these neuroprotective T cells was not analyzed in this study. In an animal model of toxin-induced demyelination T cells were required for efficient CNS remyelination. Particularly, mice lacking or depleted of either CD4$^+$ or CD8$^+$ T lymphocytes exhibited reduced remyelination after lysolecithin-induced demyelination of the spinal cord (Bieber et al., 2003). It is not understood how the autoreactive T cells protect injured neurons from secondary degeneration, but recent data demonstrate that T lymphocytes secrete significant amounts of neurotrophic factors that might be involved in the observed neuroprotective effect (Kerschensteiner et al., 1999). Recently, a subpopulation of suppressor/regulatory CD4$^+$/CD25$^-$ T lymphocytes was described, which controlled autoimmune MBP-specific T cells via cell-cell contact and inhibited both, their activation and capacity to secrete IFN-γ (Bynoe et al., 2003). Epicutaneous immunization with autoantigenic peptides induced these T suppressor cells that prevented EAE (Bynoe et al., 2003).

Effects of CD8$^+$ T Lymphocytes

Antigen-presenting cells present peptides via MHC class I molecules to CD8$^+$ T cells, which are mainly CTLs. Following the encounter of their antigen, three major, although not mutually exclusive, pathways are triggered by the CTLs to destroy the target cells (Trapani et al., 2000). They secrete cytotoxic granules containing perforin and serine proteases, express CD95 ligand that activates CD95 on target cells, and secrete cytotoxic cytokines of the TNF family (Fig. 24.3*B*). The main CTL effector pathway is mediated via the vectoral release of cytotoxic granules. The major constituent of the granules is the lytic protein perforin, which integrates and polymerizes in the plasma membrane of cultured target cells to form a cylindrical pore 16 nm in diameter. The pore could lead to rapid entry of ions and water into the target cell, resulting in disintegration of the cell membrane. Another major constituent of the granules is granzymes (e.g., granzyme A and granzyme B), which belong to the family of serine proteases. The granzymes act by inducing apoptosis, either by activating a cell membrane receptor or by acting within the target cell, having gained access with the help of perforin (Trapani et al., 2000).

CD95 ligand expressed in the membrane of activated CTLs binds to CD95 of the target cell. Activation of the CD95 can induce the apoptotic cascade from the target cell membrane (Siegel et al., 2000). Tumor necrosis factor-α can directly kill some target cells through interaction with the TNF receptor I, which contains an intracellular death domain. Other TNF-related molecules such as TRAIL can also induce apoptosis in susceptible target cells.

Primary microglia and astrocytes prestimulated with the inflammatory cytokine IFN-γ can be lysed by MHC class I–restricted CTL lines recognizing their antigen (Bergmann et al., 1999; Medana et al., 2001a), a process that is mediated primarily via the granule release mechanism (Medana et al., 2001a). Oligodendrocytes are targets of primed CTLs and MHC class I–expressing human oligodendrocytes are lysed by alloreactive and peptide-restricted CD8$^+$ CTLs derived from blood donors (Jurewicz et al., 1998). Furthermore, cytokine-stimulated astrocytes and oligodendrocytes express CD95 and are susceptible to CD95-mediated apoptosis (Pouly et al., 2000; Medana et al., 2001a). Neurons are highly susceptible to the direct application of purified cytotoxic granules. However, neurons are partially and selectively protected against CTL attack, showing segmental disruption of neurites and signs of CD95-mediated apoptosis (Fig. 24.4) following attack by CTLs (Medana et al., 2000, 2001a, 2001b).

Cytotoxic effects of CD8$^+$ T cells have been observed in a variety of animal models and human CNS diseases. In the model of transfer EAE, the autoimmune disease induced by myelin protein–specific CD4$^+$ T cells, CD8$^+$ T lymphocytes have a dual role. First, they have a regulatory function and might be involved in the induction of disease remission (Sun et al., 1988). Second, they are involved in tissue damage (Sun et al., 2001). Following injection into the CNS or after systemic transfer, they can directly induce tissue destruction (Huseby et al., 2001). The importance of CD8$^+$ T cells in brain defense and immune surveillance has also been demonstrated in the clearance of viral infections, defense of brain tumors, and rejection of transplants (Neumann et al., 2002). In murine Theiler's virus infection, CD8$^+$ T cells are involved in the clearance of virally infected oligodendrocytes, but they also appear to be responsible for demyelination and axonal damage of the spinal cord (Murray et al., 1998; Rivera-Quinones et al., 1998). Mice deficient in β2-microglobulin, the MHC class I light chain, show impaired function of CD8$^+$ CTLs and have preservation of axons despite extensive virus-mediated deymelination (Rivera-Quinones et al., 1998). CD8$^+$ CTLs are also involved in tissue destruction of virus encephalitis and in neuronal injury of experimental cerebral malaria via a perforin-dependent mechanism (Nitcheu et al., 2003).

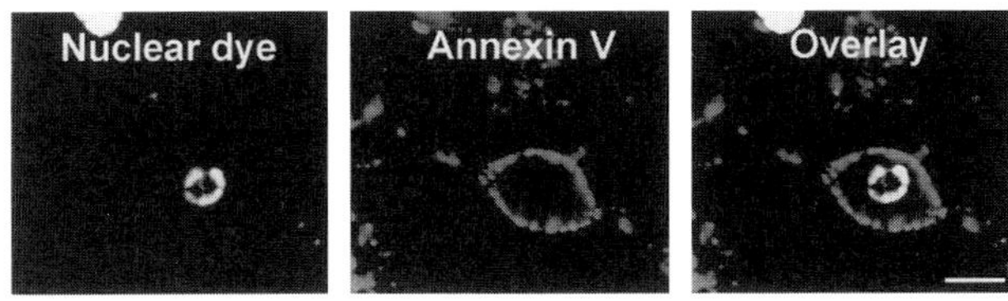

FIGURE 24.4 Cultured murine hippocampal neuron analyzed 3 hours after major histocompatibility complex (MHC) class I/peptide-specific attack by cytotoxic T cells. The neuron shows apoptotic signs with condensation of the nucleus (nuclear dye) and outer cell membrane staining with Annexin V. The neuron was pretreated with interferon-γ to stimulate expression of MHC class I molecules. Scale bar: 10 μm.

In Rasmussens's encephalitis and in patients with paraneoplastic diseases of the CNS, close apposition of CD8$^+$ CTLs to MHC class I–expressing, degenerating neurons has been observed, indicating a CTL-mediated destruction of neurons (Bien et al., 2002). In adrenoleukodystrophy, CD8$^+$ CTLs predominate in the immune cell infiltrate, and appear to be involved in tissue destruction and cytolysis of oligodendrocytes (Ito et al., 2001). These findings strongly suggest that CTLs are directly involved in the destruction of brain tissue.

PERSPECTIVE

Brain immunity is under tight control of the neural growth factor and cytokine milieu. Therefore, immune responses in the CNS are suppressed and delayed compared to those in other organs. For many years, it was believed that neurons are immunologically inert and escape immune surveillance due to their lack of MHC expression. Recently, it was established that strong interactions take place between T cells and neurons during brain immunity. Both cell types communicate via cytokines, growth factors, adhesion molecules, and cell membrane receptors. Furthermore, T cells can attack neurons expressing MHC class I *in vitro*. In the future, it must be established whether autoimmunity directed against neurons involves T cells. In particular, neuronal antigens recognized by autoantibodies were described in paraneoplastic neurological diseases, Rasmussen en-

TABLE 24.1 *Neuronal Autoantigens Recognized By Autoantibodies*

Disease	*Neuronal Autoantigen*	*Functional Impairment*	*Reference*
Paraneoplastic neurological diseases	Neuro-oncological ventral antigen 1 (NOVA1) receptor subunits	Aberrant RNA splicing of γ-aminobutyric acid (GABA) and glycine receptor subunits	Buckanovich et al. (1993)
	hu	Deficient RNA binding	Musunuru et al. (2001)
	Cerebellar degeneration–related protein 2 (Cdr2)	Disruption of cell-cycle signaling	Musunuru et al. (2001)
	Metabolotropic glutamate receptor 1 (mGluR)	Impaired plasticity	Solimena et al. (2000)
Rasmussen encephalitis	Ionotropic glutamate receptor 3 (GluR39)	Excitotoxicity	Rogers et al. (1994)
	Munc-18	Impaired synaptic function	Yang et al. (2000)
Stiff-person syndrome	Gephyrin	Impaired neurotransmission	Butler et al. (2000)
	Glutamic acid decarboxylase (GAD)	Impaired GABA synthesis	Li et al. (1994)
	Amphiphysin	Impaired presynaptic activity	De Camilli et al. (1993)

cephalitis, and stiff-person syndrome, while the identification of neuronal T cell epitopes is still missing (Table 24.1).

ACKNOWLEDGMENTS

I am grateful to Prof. Francesca Aloisi and Dr. Kazuya Takahashi for critically reading the manuscript and providing helpful comments. I thank Prof. Hartmut Wekerle for supporting our work for many years and Dr. Isabelle Medana for help with the experiments involving attack of neurons by CTLs.

ABBREVIATIONS

APCs	antigen-presenting cells
BBB	blood-brain barrier
CNS	central nervous system
CTLs	cytotoxic T lymphocytes
EAE	experimental autoimmune encephalomyelitis
GM-CSF	granulocyte-macrophage colony-stimulating factor
ICAM-1	intercellular adhesion molecule-1
IFN-γ	interferon-γ
IFN-β	interleukin-β
IL-2	interleukin-2
LPS	lipopolysaccharide
MBP	myelin basic protein
MHC	major histocompatibility complex
MIP-1α	macrophage inflammatory protein-1α
MS	multiple sclerosis
α-MSH	α-melanocyte-stimulating hormone
NO	nitric oxide
TAPs	transporters associated with antigen processing
TCR	T cell receptor
TGF-β	transforming growth factor-β
TNF-α	tumor necrosis factor-α
VIP	vasoactive intestinal peptide

REFERENCES

Aharoni, R., Teitelbaum, D., Leitner, O., Meshorer, A., Sela, M., and Arnon, R. (2000) Specific Th2 cells accumulate in the central nervous system of mice protected against experimental autoimmune encephalomyelitis by copolymer 1. *Proc. Natl. Acad. Sci. USA* 97(21):11472–11477.

Aloisi, F. (2001) Immune function of microglia. *Glia* 36(2):165–179.

Aloisi, F., Ria, F., and Adorini, L. (2000) Regulation of T-cell responses by CNS antigen-presenting cells: different roles for microglia and astrocytes. *Immunol. Today* 21(3):141–147.

Babcock, A.A., Kuziel, W.A., Rivest, S., and Owens, T. (2003) Chemokine expression by glial cells directs leukocytes to sites of axonal injury in the CNS. *J. Neurosci.* 23(21):7922–7930.

Bauer, J., Bradl, M., Hickley, W.F., Forss-Petter, S., Breitschopf, H., Linington, C., Wekerle, H., and Lassmann, H. (1998) T-cell apoptosis in inflammatory brain lesions: destruction of T cells does not depend on antigen recognition. *Am. J. Pathol.* 153(3):715–724.

Bauer, J., Wekerle, H., and Lassmann, H. (1995) Apoptosis in brain-specific autoimmune disease. *Curr. Opin. Immunol.* 7(6):839–843.

Bechmann, I., Priller, J., Kovac, A., Bontert, M., Wehner, T., Klett, F.F., Bohsung, J., Stuschke, M., Dirnagl, U., and Nitsch, R. (2001) Immune surveillance of mouse brain perivascular spaces by blood-borne macrophages. *Eur. J. Neurosci.* 14(10):1651–1658.

Bergmann, C.C., Yao, Q., and Stohlman, S.A. (1999) Microglia exhibit clonal variability in eliciting cytotoxic T lymphocyte responses independent of class I expression. *Cell Immunol.* 198(1):44–53.

Bieber, A.J., Kerr, S., and Rodriguez, M. (2003) Efficient central nervous system remyelination requires T cells. *Ann. Neurol.* 53(5):680–684.

Bien, C.G., Bauer, J., Deckwerth, T.L., Wiendl, H., Deckert, M., Wiestler, O.D., Schramm, J., Elger, C.E., and Lassmann, H. (2002) Destruction of neurons by cytotoxic T cells: a new pathogenic mechanism in Rasmussen's encephalitis. *Ann. Neurol.* 51(3):311–318.

Buckanovich, R.J., Posner, J.B., and Darnell, R.B. (1993) Nova, the paraneoplastic Ri antigen, is homologous to an RNA-binding protein and is specifically expressed in the developing motor system. *Neuron* 11(4):657–672.

Butler, M.H., Hayashi, A., Okhoshi, N., Villmann, C., Becker, C.M., Feng, G., De Camilli, P., and Solimena, M. (2000) Autoimmunity to gephyrin in Stiff-Mann syndrome. *Neuron* 26(2): 307–312.

Bynoe, M.S., Evans, J.T., Viret, C., and Janeway, C.A., Jr. (2003) Epicutaneous immunization with autoantigenic peptides induces T suppressor cells that prevent experimental allergic encephalomyelitis. *Immunity* 19(3):317–328.

Cabarrocas, J., Bauer, J., Piaggio, E., Liblau, R., and Lassmann, H. (2003) Effective and selective immune surveillance of the brain by MHC class I-restricted cytotoxic T lymphocytes. *Eur. J. Immunol.* 33(5):1174–1182.

Corriveau, R.A., Huh, G.S., and Shatz, C.J. (1998) Regulation of class I MHC gene expression in the developing and mature CNS by neural activity. *Neuron* 21(3):505–520.

De Camilli, P., Thomas, A., Cofiell, R., Folli, F., Lichte, B., Piccolo, G., Meinck, H.M., Austoni, M., Fassetta, G., Bottazzo, G., et al. (1993) The synaptic vesicle-associated protein amphiphysin is the 128-kD autoantigen of Stiff-Man syndrome with breast cancer. *J. Exp. Med.* 178(6):2219–2223.

Fischer, H.G. and Reichmann, G. (2001) Brain dendritic cells and macrophages/microglia in central nervous system inflammation. *J. Immunol.* 166(4):2717–2726.

Flügel, A., Berkowicz, T., Ritter, T., Labeur, M., Jenne, D.E., Li, Z., Ellwart, J.W., Willem, M., Lassmann, H., and Wekerle, H. (2001) Migratory activity and functional changes of green fluorescent effector cells before and during experimental autoimmune encephalomyelitis. *Immunity* 14(5):547–560.

Flügel, A., Schwaiger, F.W., Neumann, H., Medana, I., Willem, M., Wekerle, H., Kreutzberg, G.W., and Graeber, M.B. (2000) Neuronal FasL induces cell death of encephalitogenic T lymphocytes. *Brain Pathol.* 10(3):353–364.

Ford, A.L., Goodsall, A.L., Hickey, W.F., and Sedgwick, J.D. (1995) Normal adult ramified microglia separated from other central nervous system macrophages by flow cytometric sorting. Phenotypic differences defined and direct ex vivo antigen presentation to myelin basic protein-reactive CD4+ T cells compared. *J. Immunol.* 154(9):4309–4321.

Hailer, N.P., Heppner, F.L., Haas, D., and Nitsch, R. (1998) Astrocytic factors deactivate antigen presenting cells that invade the central nervous system. *Brain Pathol.* 8(3):459–474.

Hickey, W.F. (2001) Basic principles of immunological surveillance of the normal central nervous system. *Glia* 36(2):118–124.

Hoek, R.M., Ruuls, S.R., Murphy, C.A., Wright, G.J., Goddard, R., Zurawski, S.M., Blom, B., Homola, M.E., Streit, W.J., Brown, M.H., Barclay, A.N., and Sedgwick, J.D. (2000) Down-regulation of the macrophage lineage through interaction with OX2 (CD200). *Science* 290(5497):1768–1771.

Huber, J.D., Egleton, R.D., and Davis, T.P. (2001) Molecular physiology and pathophysiology of tight junctions in the blood–brain barrier. *Trends Neurosci.* 24(12):719–725.

Huh, G.S., Boulanger, L.M., Du, H., Riquelme, P.A., Brotz, T.M., and Shatz, C.J. (2000) Functional requirement for class I MHC in CNS development and plasticity. *Science* 290(5499):2155–2159.

Huseby, E.S., Liggitt, D., Brabb, T., Schnabel, B., Ohlen, C., and Goverman, J. (2001) A pathogenic role for myelin-specific CD8(+) T cells in a model for multiple sclerosis. *J. Exp. Med.* 194(5):669–676.

Irani, D.N. (1998) The susceptibility of mice to immune-mediated neurologic disease correlates with the degree to which their lymphocytes resist the effects of brain-derived gangliosides. *J. Immunol.* 161(6):2746–2752.

Ito, M., Blumberg, B.M., Mock, D.J., Goodman, A.D., Moser, A.B., Moser, H.W., Smith, K.D., and Powers, J.M. (2001) Potential environmental and host participants in the early white matter lesion of adreno-leukodystrophy: morphologic evidence for CD8 cytotoxic T cells, cytolysis of oligodendrocytes, and CD1-mediated lipid antigen presentation. *J. Neuropathol. Exp. Neurol.* 60(10): 1004–1019.

Jurewicz, A., Biddison, W.E., and Antel, J.P. (1998) MHC class I-restricted lysis of human oligodendrocytes by myelin basic protein peptide–specific CD8 T lymphocytes. *J. Immunol.* 160(6): 3056–3059.

Kawakami, N., Lassmann, S., Li, Z., Odoardi, F., Ritter, T., Ziemssen, T., Klinkert, W.E., Ellwart, J.W., Bradl, M., Krivacic, K., Lassmann, H., Ransohoff, R.M., Volk, H.D., Wekerle, H., Linington, C., and Flugel, A. (2004) The activation status of neuroantigen-specific T cells in the target organ determines the clinical outcome of autoimmune encephalomyelitis. *J. Exp. Med.* 199(2):185–197.

Kerschensteiner, M., Gallmeier, E., Behrens, L., Leal, V.V., Misgeld, T., Klinkert, W.E., Kolbeck, R., Hoppe, E., Oropeza-Wekerle, R.L., Bartke, I., Stadelmann, C., Lassmann, H., Wekerle, H., and Hohlfeld, R. (1999) Activated human T cells, B cells, and monocytes produce brain-derived neurotrophic factor in vitro and in inflammatory brain lesions: a neuroprotective role of inflammation? *J. Exp. Med.* 189(5):865–870.

Kreutzberg, G.W. (1996) Microglia: a sensor for pathological events in the CNS. *Trends Neurosci.* 19(8):312–318.

Lassmann, H., Schmied, M., Vass, K., and Hickey, W.F. (1993) Bone marrow derived elements and resident microglia in brain inflammation. *Glia* 7(1):19–24.

Li, L., Hagopian, W.A., Brashear, H.R., Daniels, T., and Lernmark, A. (1994) Identification of autoantibody epitopes of glutamic acid decarboxylase in stiff-man syndrome patients. *J. Immunol.* 152(2):930–934.

Lowenstein, P.R. (2002) Immunology of viral-vector-mediated gene transfer into the brain: an evolutionary and developmental perspective. *Trends Immunol.* 23(1):23–30.

Magnus, T., Chan, A., Grauer, O., Toyka, K.V., and Gold, R. (2001) Microglial phagocytosis of apoptotic inflammatory T cells leads to down-regulation of microglial immune activation. *J. Immunol.* 167(9):5004–5010.

Mathisen, P.M., Yu, M., Johnson, J.M., Drazba, J.A., and Tuohy, V.K. (1997) Treatment of experimental autoimmune encephalomyelitis with genetically modified memory T cells. *J. Exp. Med.* 186(1):159–164.

Medana, I.M., Gallimore, A., Oxenius, A., Martinic, M.M., Wekerle, H., and Neumann, H. (2000) MHC class I–restricted killing of neurons by virus-specific CD8+ T lymphocytes is effected through the Fas/FasL, but not the perforin pathway. *Eur. J. Immunol.* 30(12):3623–3633.

Medana, I.M., Li, Z., Flügel, A., Tschopp, J., Wekerle, H., and Neumann, H. (2001a) Fas ligand (CD95L) protects neurons against perforin-mediated T lymphocyte cytotoxicity. *J. Immunol.* 167(2):674–681.

Medana, I.M., Martinic, M.A., Wekerle, H., and Neumann, H. (2001b) Transection of major histocompatibility complex class I–induced neurites by cytotoxic T lymphocytes. *Am. J. Pathol.* 159(3):809–815.

Merrill, J.E. and Benveniste, E.N. (1996) Cytokines in inflammatory brain lesions: helpful and harmful. *Trends Neurosci.* 19(8):331–338.

Moalem, G., Leibowitz-Amit, R., Yoles, E., Mor, F., Cohen, I.R., and Schwartz, M. (1999) Autoimmune T cells protect neurons from secondary degeneration after central nervous system axotomy. *Nat. Med.* 5(1):49–55.

Monsonego, A., Zota, V., Karni, A., Krieger, J.I., Bar-Or, A., Bitan, G., Budson, A.E., Sperling, R., Selkoe, D.J., and Weiner, H.L. (2003) Increased T cell reactivity to amyloid beta protein in older humans and patients with Alzheimer disease. *J. Clin. Invest.* 112(3):415–422.

Murray, P.D., Pavelko, K.D., Leibowitz, J., Lin, X., and Rodriguez, M. (1998) CD4(+) and CD8(+) T cells make discrete contributions to demyelination and neurologic disease in a viral model of multiple sclerosis. *J. Virol.* 72(9):7320–7329.

Musunuru, K., and Darnell, R.B. (2001) Paraneoplastic neurologic disease antigens: RNA-binding proteins and signaling proteins in neuonal degeneration. *Annu. Rev. Neurosci.* 24:239–262.

Neumann, H. (2001) Control of glial immune function by neurons. *Glia* 36(2):191–199.

Neumann, H., Boucraut, J., Hahnel, C., Misgeld, T., and Wekerle, H. (1996) Neuronal control of MHC class II inducibility in rat astrocytes and microglia. *Eur. J. Neurosci.* 8(12):2582–2590.

Neumann, H., Cavalie, A., Jenne, D.E., and Wekerle, H. (1995) Induction of MHC class I genes in neurons. *Science* 269(5223): 549–552.

Neumann, H., Medana, I.M., Bauer, J., and Lassmann, H. (2002) Cytotoxic T lymphocytes in autoimmune and degenerative CNS diseases. *Trends Neurosci.* 25(6):313–319.

Neumann, H., Misgeld, T., Matsumuro, K., and Wekerle, H. (1998) Neurotrophins inhibit major histocompatibility class II inducibility of microglia: involvement of the p75 neurotrophin receptor. *Proc. Natl. Acad. Sci. USA* 95(10):5779–5784.

Neumann, H., Schmidt, H., Cavalie, A., Jenne, D., and Wekerle, H. (1997) Major histocompatibility complex (MHC) class I gene expression in single neurons of the central nervous system: differential regulation by interferon (IFN)-gamma and tumor necrosis factor (TNF)-alpha. *J. Exp. Med.* 185(2):305–316.

Neumann, H. and Wekerle, H. (1998) Neuronal control of the immune response in the central nervous system: linking brain immunity to neurodegeneration. *J. Neuropathol. Exp. Neurol.* 57(1):1–9.

Nitcheu, J., Bonduelle, O., Combadiere, C., Tefit, M., Seilhean, D., Mazier, D., and Combadiere, B. (2003) Perforin-dependent brain-infiltrating cytotoxic CD8+ T lymphocytes mediate experimental cerebral malaria pathogenesis. *J. Immunol.* 170(4):2221–2228.

Nguyen, K.B. and Pender, M.P. (1998) Phagocytosis of apoptotic lymphocytes by oligodendrocytes in experimental autoimmune encephalomyelitis. *Acta Neuropathol.* (*Berl.*), 95(1):40–46.

Popovich, P.G., Stokes, B.T., and Whitacre, C.C. (1996) Concept of autoimmunity following spinal cord injury: possible roles for T lymphocytes in the traumatized central nervous system. *J. Neurosci. Res.* 45(4):349–363.

Pouly, S., Becher, B., Blain, M., and Antel, J.P. (2000) Interferon-gamma modulates human oligodendrocyte susceptibility to Fas-mediated apoptosis. *J. Neuropathol. Exp. Neurol.* 59(4):280–286.

Raivich, G., Jones, L.L., Kloss, C.U., Werner, A., Neumann, H., and Kreutzberg, G.W. (1998) Immune surveillance in the injured nervous system: T-lymphocytes invade the axotomized mouse facial motor nucleus and aggregate around sites of neuronal degeneration. *J. Neurosci.* 18(15):5804–5816.

Ransohoff, R.M. and Tani, M. (1998) Do chemokines mediate leukocyte recruitment in post-traumatic CNS inflammation? *Trends Neurosci.* 21(4):154–159.

Rivera-Quinones, C., McGavern, D., Schmelzer, J.D., Hunter, S.F., Low, P.A., and Rodriguez, M. (1998) Absence of neurological deficits following extensive demyelination in a class I-deficient murine model of multiple sclerosis. *Nat. Med.* 4(2):187–193.

Rogers, S.W., Andrews, P.I., Gahring, L.C., Whisenand, T., Cauley, K., Crain, B., Hughes, T.E., Heinemann, S.F., and McNamara, J.O. (1994) Autoantibodies to glutamate receptor GluR3 in Rasmussen's encephalitis. *Science* 265(5172):648–651.

Santambrogio, L., Belyanskaya, S.L., Fischer, F.R., Cipriani, B., Brosnan, C.F., Ricciardi-Castagnoli, P., Stern, L.J., Strominger, J.L., and Riese, R. (2001) Developmental plasticity of CNS microglia. *Proc. Natl. Acad. Sci. USA* 98(11):6295–6300.

Schwartz, M., Moalem, G., Leibowitz-Amit, R., and Cohen, I.R. (1999) Innate and adaptive immune responses can be beneficial for CNS repair. *Trends Neurosci.* 22(7):295–299.

Sellebjerg, F., and Sorensen, T.L. (2003) Chemokines and matrix metalloproteinase-9 in leukocyte recruitment to the central nervous system. *Brain Res. Bull.* 61(3):347–355. Review.

Serafini, B., Columba-Cabezas, S., Di Rosa, F., and Aloisi, F. (2000) Intracerebral recruitment and maturation of dendritic cells in the onset and progression of experimental autoimmune encephalomyelitis. *Am. J. Pathol.* 157(6):1991–2002.

Siegel, R.M., Chan, F.K., Chun, H.J., and Lenardo, M.J. (2000) The multifaceted role of Fas signaling in immune cell homeostasis and autoimmunity. *Nat. Immunol.* 1(6):469–474.

Solimena, M., and De Camilli, P. (2000) Synaptic autoimmunity and the Salk factor. *Neuron* 28(2):309–310.

Sun, D., Qin, Y., Chluba, J., Epplen, J.T., and Wekerle, H. (1988) Suppression of experimentally induced autoimmune encephalomyelitis by cytolytic T-T cell interactions. *Nature* 332(6167): 843–845.

Sun, D., Whitaker, J.N., Huang, Z., Liu, D., Coleclough, C., Wekerle, H., and Raine, C.S. (2001) Myelin antigen-specific CD8+ T cells are encephalitogenic and produce severe disease in C57BL/6 mice. *J. Immunol.* 166(12):7579–7587.

Suvannavejh, G.C., Dal Canto, M.C., Matis, L.A., and Miller, S.D. (2000) Fas-mediated apoptosis in clinical remissions of relapsing experimental autoimmune encephalomyelitis. *J. Clin. Invest* 105(2):223–231.

Trapani, J.A., Davis, J., Sutton, V.R., and Smyth, M.J. (2000) Proapoptotic functions of cytotoxic lymphocyte granule constituents in vitro and in vivo. *Curr. Opin. Immunol.* 12(3):323–329.

Wei, R. and Jonakait, G.M. (1999) Neurotrophins and the anti-inflammatory agents interleukin-4 (IL-4), IL-10, IL-11 and transforming growth factor-beta1 (TGF-beta1) down-regulate T cell costimulatory molecules B7 and CD40 on cultured rat microglia. *J. Neuroimmunol.* 95(1–2):8–18.

Weller, R.O. (1998) Pathology of cerebrospinal fluid and interstitial fluid of the CNS: significance for Alzheimer disease, prion disorders and multiple sclerosis. *J. Neuropathol. Exp. Neurol.* 57(10): 885–894.

Yang, R., Puranam, R.S., Butler, L.S., Qian, W.H., He, X.P., Moyer, M.B., Blackburn, K., Andrews, P.I., and McNamara, J.O. (2000) Autoimmunity to munc-18 in Rasmussen's encephalitis. *Neuron* 28(2):375–383.

25 The role of glia in the formation and function of the blood–brain barrier

HANNELORE BAUER, HANS-CHRISTIAN BAUER, REINER F. HASELOFF, AND INGOLF E. BLASIG

To enable the neurons within the vertebrate brain to function normally, the internal environment of the brain must be carefully regulated to ensure constancy in the concentrations of hormones, ions, transmitters, and other substances. The local mechanisms involved in achieving such homeostasis make use of two different *barrier systems*. The blood–cerebrospinal fluid (CSF) barrier is the site between the blood in the choroid plexus and the CSF in the ventricles. It consists of a monolayer of epithelial cells without interaction with cerebral cells. The second barrier system, the blood–brain barrier (BBB), represents the boundary between the central nervous capillaries and the extracellular fluid of neurons and glia cells. The BBB is formed by brain capillary endothelial cells in close association with macroglial cells or astrocytes covering the majority of cerebral surface of the endothelium (Fig. 25.1*A*,*B*). This suggests a possible influence of astrocytes on capillary endothelial cells. This chapter focuses on the role of glial cells in the formation and function of the BBB. The blood–CSF barrier will not be dealt with further in this survey.

MORPHOLOGY OF CELLS IN THE AREA OF THE BLOOD–BRAIN BARRIER

Endothelial Cells

Although the concept of a BBB was conceived nearly 100 years ago, the role of capillary endothelial cells representing this barrier was appreciated only much later. Detailed microscopic analysis using horseradish peroxidase as a tracer revealed that the BBB is located in the cerebral endothelium (Reese and Karnovsky, 1967). Permeability studies of cerebral and noncerebral endothelium affirmed the special role of brain capillary endothelial cells, demonstrating that they undergo an additional step of differentiation that results in a specific cellular phenotype (for review see Van Deurs, 1979). The most prominent feature of cerebral endothelial cells is the occurrence of continuous tight junctions (TJs) that seal the paracellular passage for macromolecules and cells from the bloodstream (Brightman and Reese, 1969) (Fig. 25.1*B*). Other characteristics include the absence of fenestrations, a large number of pinocytotic vesicles, and a variety of transport systems in the luminal and abluminal cellular membranes (Fig. 25.1*A*). Tight junctions are a key structure in the barrier function of cerebral endothelial cells and have been a focus of intense research throughout the past decades. This has led to the elucidation of an unanticipated complexity of the molecular architecture of TJs, together with the emergence of new functional aspects of TJ-associated proteins (for review see Tsukita et al., 1999).

However, endothelial cells are not the only cell type involved in BBB function. There is sufficient experimental evidence to suggest a relationship between endothelial cells, glial cells, and neurons (Dermietzel and Krause, 1991) to create and/or support the BBB. Neurons are supposed to influence astroglial morphology, differentiation, and proliferation, while astrocytes contribute directly or indirectly to the maintenance of the BBB.

Astrocytes

Originally, astrocytes were considered to create the BBB in mammals, comparable to that in lower vertebrates like primitive fish (Bradbury, 1979). Astrocytes almost completely ensheath the capillary walls with their foot processes, thereby covering not only endothelial cells but also the intimately associated pericytes. In this way, astrocytes become the only mediators between endothelial cells and the surrounding neuronal tissue. In addition to their role in transport, astrocytes are required for structural support of the BBB—an issue discussed in more detail below.

Neurons, Pericytes, and Microglia

In the adult mammalian brain, neurons are usually not in contact with cerebral endothelial cells. However,

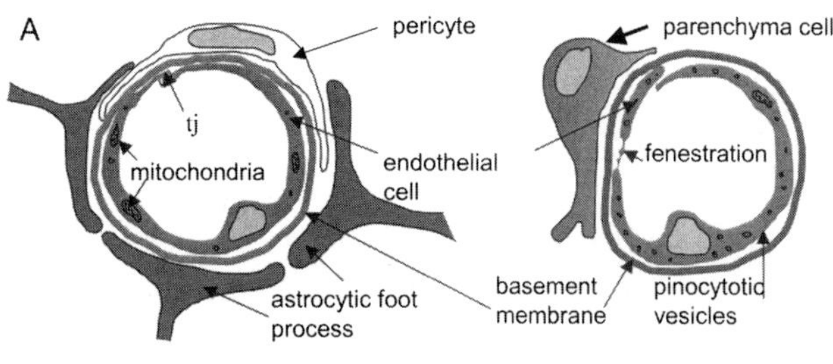

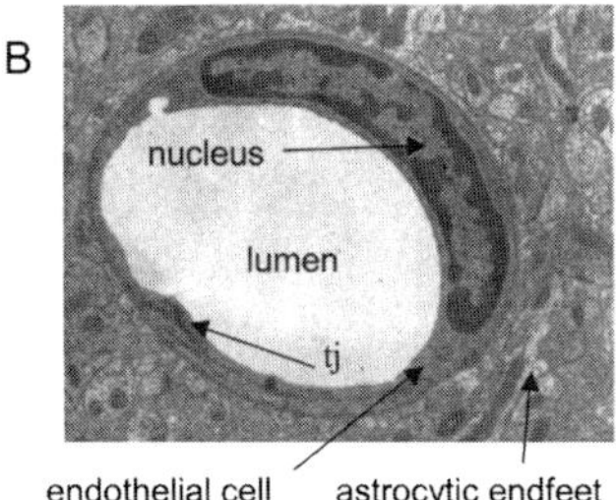

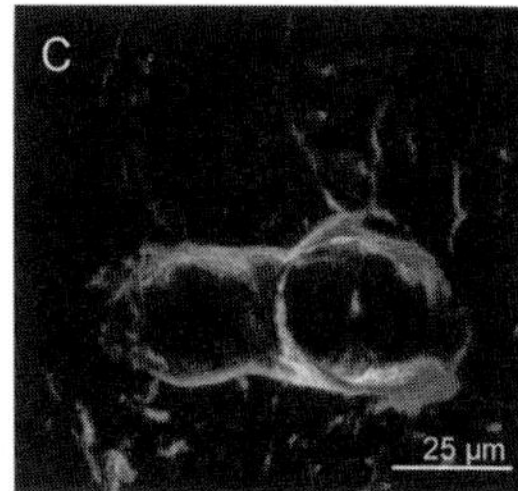

FIGURE 25.1 Brain capillary endothelial cells representing the main constituent of the blood–brain barrier. *A*. Comparison of brain capillary and peripheral capillary in a cross-sectional diagram. Morphological characteristics of brain capillary endothelial cells include the presence of tight junctions, reduced number of pinocytotic vesicles, increased number of mitochondria, and the close proximity of astrocytes compared to peripheral capillary endothelial cells. *B*. Electron microscopic picture of a cross-sectioned adult mouse brain. The region of a capillary endothelial cell is shown, ensheathed by astrocyte foot processes. C. Confocal laser scan micrograph of adult rat cortex. Immunoreactivity of glial fibrillary acidic protein, showing astrocyte endfeet covering the basal side of a brain capillary horizontally sectioned. tj: tight junction.

during early development, when astrocytes are still absent, neuroblasts and undifferentiated neurons are the only partners of endothelial cells. Thus, it is not unreasonable to suggest that early neurons may play a critical role in the initial induction of the BBB in cerebral endothelial cells. It is unclear whether there are signals from endothelial cells to neurons, and vice versa, that could be important for brain homeostasis or for neuronal function (Pardridge, 1999).

The mesoderm-derived pericytes (PCs) are located close to cerebral endothelial cells, separated from them only by a common basement membrane (Fig. 25.1*A*). Pericytes seem to comigrate with endothelial cells into the neuroepithelial cell layer during neovascularization of the developing brain. Interestingly, the number of PCs associated with cerebral barrier–forming capillaries is higher than the number of PCs found with nonbarrier capillaries. Pericytes are phagocytic cells but have also been suggested to be involved in capillary contraction, a finding that is still being debated (Nehls and Drenckhahn, 1991). The role of PCs in BBB formation and their possible interaction with perivascular astrocytic endfeet is still unknown (Balabanov and Dore-Duffy, 1998).

Microglia are blood-borne cells and are regarded as an endogenous immune cell class within the central nervous system (CNS). They apparently comigrate with endothelial cells into the expanding neuroepithelial domain, exhibiting an ameboid phenotype in the neighborhood of astrocytes and cerebral capillaries. The role of microglia in BBB function is still unclear, but there are indications that they are involved in the traffic of monocytes across the cerebral endothelium under pathological conditions (Persidsky et al., 1999). Together with PCs, microglia are involved in trapping serum-derived foreign substances that might afflict the BBB (Xu and Ling, 1994).

FUNCTIONS OF THE BLOOD–BRAIN BARRIER

Barrier Function

The general function of the BBB is to protect the homeostasis within the brain from changes arising from the vascular system and to meet the nutritional demands of the CNS. Thus, the BBB is a selective border for cells, solutes, and certain xenobiotics, and has a selective transport function for substrates and products essential to the brain (Fig. 25.2).

The BBB excludes cerebral transmitter substances such as catecholamines and cholecystokinin from the

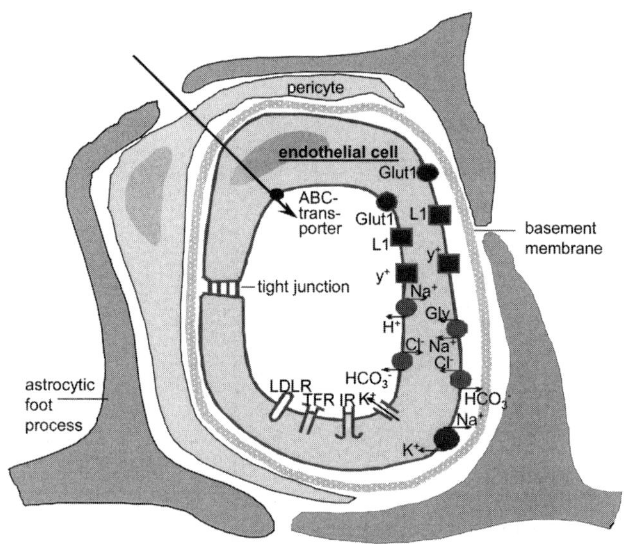

FIGURE 25.2 Scheme of brain capillary endothelial cells showing the main functional structures. Tight junctions sealing the interendothelial cleft. Adenine nucleotide-binding cassette (ABC) transporters in the luminal cell membrane excreting xenobiotics. Asymmetrically distributed membrane transporters such as glutamate transporters (Glut1); amino acid transporters (L1, y+); ion antiporters (Na^+/H^+; Cl^-/HCO_3^-); cotransporter (Gly/Na^+); Na^+,K^+-ATPase (Na^+,K^+); ion channels (K^+). Transport mechanisms are mediated via receptors, such as those of low density lipoprotein (LDLR), transferrin (TFR), or insulin (IR).

brain, neither substance having specific transporters in the cerebral microvasculature. Within the cerebral endothelial cells pinocytosis is less developed than in endothelial cells of other tissues. The barrier function is supported by adenosine triphosphate (ATP)–consuming transporters (ABC transporters) containing an adenine nucleotide-binding cassette (ABC). The ABC transporters excrete certain xenobiotics from the endothelium into the bloodstream, which results in cerebral drug resistance for several antibiotics, cytostatics, and others, such as morphine, dexamethason, vinblastin, anthracycline, and reduced glutathione (for review see Tamai and Tsuji, 2000; Lee et al., 2001). In addition, outward-directed transporters (synonyms are *P-glycoproteins*, *multidrug resistance–associated proteins*, or *multidrug resistance proteins*) are localized at the luminal plasma membrane. Although numerous studies have demonstrated that P-glycoprotein limits the brain penetration of several drug substrates, many questions concerning the physiological role of these proteins [e.g., P170 glycoprotein: 170 kDa, 10-transmembrane domains, 2 intracellular adenosine triphosphatase (ATPase) carrying domains] remain.

Structural features of the blood–brain barrier

The barrier function of brain endothelial cells relies heavily upon the TJs. This important morphological characteristic of the BBB seals the intercellular cleft between neighboring endothelial cells, blocking the para-endothelial passage even for small molecules. The exact molecular structure and regulation of the TJs are not clear, but it is assumed that they are formed by the interaction of different transmembrane and membrane-associated proteins regulated by several signal transduction cascades.

As shown in Figure 25.3, three types of transmembrane proteins act together at TJs: occludin, claudins, and junctional adhesion molecules (JAMs). *Occludin* was the first TJ-specific integral membrane protein to be described (Furuse et al., 1993). While occludin's extracellular loops are supposedly involved in the regulation of paracellular permeability and cell adhesion, interaction with peripheral junctional proteins has been found to occur via its C terminus. *Claudins*, actually a superfamily of about 24 members, are considered the major structural components of TJs (Tsukita and Furuse, 2000; Wolburg and Lippoldt, 2002). Claudins are predicted to have four transmembrane segments, with both N and C termini located in the cytoplasm, but do not show any sequence homology to occludin. Like occludin, claudins are physically involved in the formation of the tight junctional strands. The third type of TJ-related transmembrane protein is represented by *JAMs*, single-spanning transmembrane proteins with two extracellular immunoglobulin (Ig)-like domains, believed to mediate homotypic cell adhesion (Bazzoni et al., 2000). Although JAMs are concentrated around TJ strands, it is still unknown whether they are directly involved in the formation of the fibrils.

When considering the molecular interactions of occludin, claudins, and JAMs with peripheral cytoplasmic proteins, it becomes evident that all of them associate with at least one of the zonula occludens (ZO) proteins, which, in turn, establish a link between the junction site and the cytoskeleton by interacting directly with F-actin or with the actin binding proteins fodrin and spectrin (Wittchen et al., 1999; Gonzalez-Mariscal et al., 2000). The observation that ZO proteins even associate with adherens junctions and gap junctions in cells lacking TJs (Howarth and Stevenson, 1995) suggests a universal role for ZO proteins at the cytoplasmic surface of the junctional plaque.

Transport Function

The transport systems localizing at the BBB (carrier systems, transport ATPases, and receptor-mediated transport processes) (Fig. 25.2) are responsible for both the uptake of substances, mediators, and regulators essential for the brain and the release of products or factors from the brain. The tetrameric glucose transporter Glut1 55K is specific for endothelial cells and allows, together with other glucose transporters of the CNS, an enormous uptake of substrate to satisfy the aerobic energy demand of the brain (reviewed in Bauer, 1999). Specific amino acid transporters in the cerebral microvascular endothelium are L1 (large neutral Leu, Ileu, Val, Met, Phe, Trp, Tyr) and y+ (basic Arg, Lys), mainly facilitating neurotransmitter synthesis. These transporters are Na^+-independent and bidirectional, and they play a particularly important role in the uptake of those amino acids that are not synthesized in the brain, although a netto efflux is possible from the brain if excessive amounts of amino acids are formed (for review see Armer, 2000; Yudkoff et al., 2001). Sodium uptake for electrophysiological processes occurs via luminal Na^+ channels and abluminal Na^+,K^+-ATPase, which is accompanied by passive water transfer for hydrolytic brain metabolism. By contrast, potassium is excreted via basal K^+ channels and apical outward-directed K^+ channels (for review see Frelin and Vigne, 1999). Finally, hormones, metabolites, and substrates such as insulin, low density lipoprotein or transferrin are taken up by receptor-mediated transporters (Moos and Morgan, 2000) (Fig. 25.2).

ONTOGENIC DEVELOPMENT OF THE BLOOD–BRAIN BARRIER

Neovascularization of the mammalian CNS starts from a preexisting perineural plexus from which endothelial cells invade the neurectoderm (Fig. 25.4) and—by fusion and branching—establish the first vascular system in the developing neocortex (Risau, 1997). Endothelial cells of perineural vessels are fenestrated but appear to be joined by TJs (Yoshida et al., 1988). Obviously, upon contact with neuroectodermal tissue or neuroectoderm-derived soluble factors, the invading endothelial cells develop BBB characteristics. Cerebral capillary endothelial cells of the mature BBB lack fenestrations, exhibit continuous TJs, and are tightly ensheathed by astroglial foot processes (Bauer et al., 1993).

It is generally agreed that the BBB matures gradually during development. The exclusion of dyes from large parts of the embryonic and neonatal CNS is a strong indication that there is already a functional BBB, at least for proteins and macromolecules, at early stages of embryonic development (Fig. 25.5) (Risau et al., 1986; Bauer et al., 1995; for review see Saunders et al., 2000). Smaller molecules, such as inulin (5 kDa) are less rigorously excluded by the BBB in developing animals (Habgood et al., 1992), which may be explained by structural and functional differences between TJs in the developing brain and the adult brain (Stewart and Hayakawa, 1994).

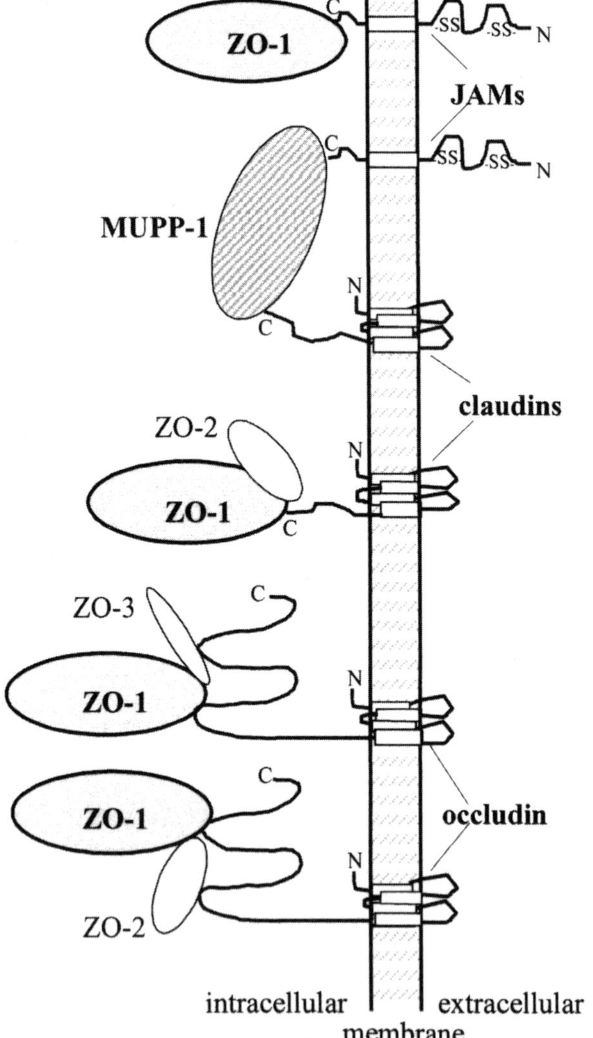

FIGURE 25.3 Scheme of known tight junction proteins localized at the inner surface of the cell membrane or in the cell membrane and potential protein-protein interactions. The transmembranal proteins are junction-associated molecules (JAMs, possibly interacting with leukocytes), claudin-1, -3, and -5 (presumably constituents of tight junction strands), and occludin (assumed to function as a regulatory tight junction protein). At the inner membrane surface one finds zonula occludens (ZO) proteins (ZO-1 especially is thought to recruit other tight junction proteins) and MUPP-1 (multi-PDZ protein 1, possibly involved in the formation of junctional strands).

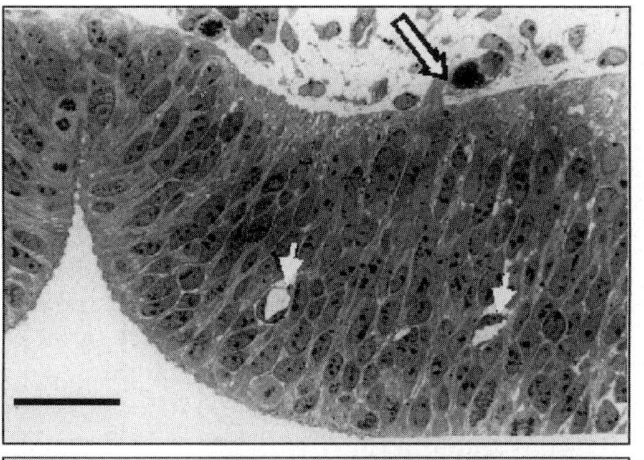

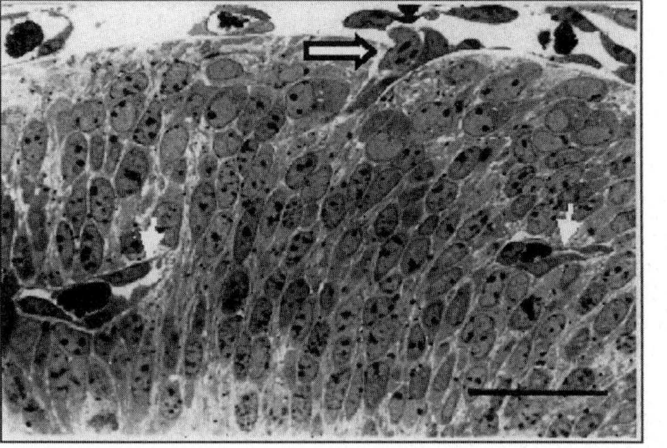

FIGURE 25.4 Microscopic images of ontogenic blood–brain barrier formation. *a,b* At embryonic day 10 (E 10) the intraneural domain is vascularized from an already existing perineural plexus. Mesenchymal cells (endothelial cells and pericytes) invade the neuroectoderm (*large arrows*). Small arrows indicate cross-sectioned blood vessels containing blood cells. Bars = 10 μm and 20 μm, resp.

ACTION OF GLIAL CELLS ON THE BLOOD–BRAIN BARRIER

Gliogenesis begins late in vertebrate development. In the embryonic brain, astrocytes are almost absent and radial glia are the only cells that have close contact with cerebral endothelial cells. Therefore, it appears unlikely that astrocytes are responsible for the initial induction of the BBB. However, a possible role for radial glia in early BBB establishment remains to be determined. Interestingly, recent work suggests that radial glia not only provide scaf-

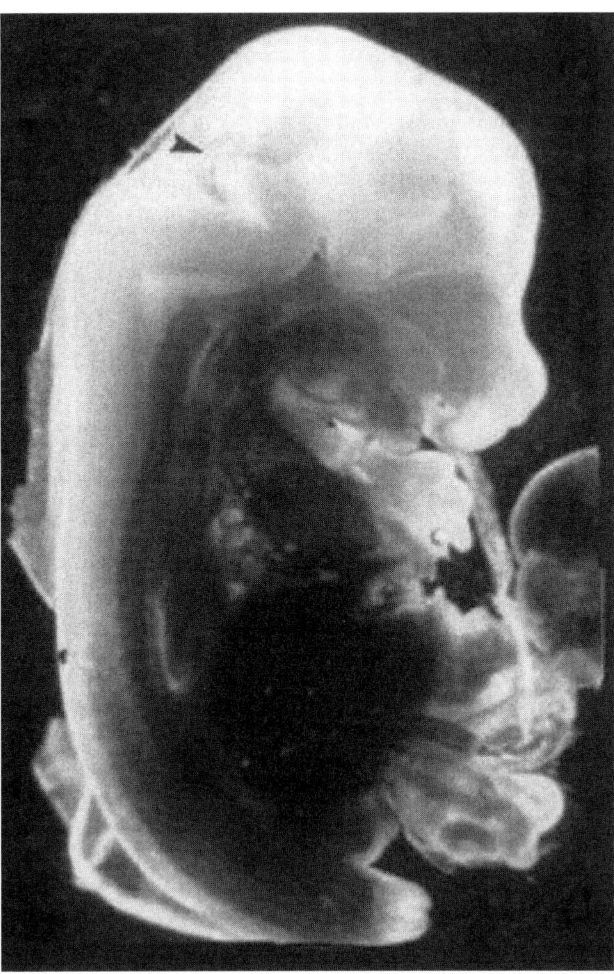

FIGURE 25.5 Medially sectioned 12-day-old mouse embryo after perfusion with 0.5% Trypan Blue solution. The dye (bound to protein) was excluded from most parts of the central nervous system. A weak staining is observed in the frontal cortex and in the area of the developing choroid plexus (*arrow*), probably reflecting gradual establishment of the blood–brain barrier.

folding for migration and placement of neurons but exhibit neurogenic properties themselves. These specialized cells represent many, if not most, of the neuronal progenitors in the developing cortex (Fishell and Kriegstein, 2003). In this light, the earlier findings by Tontsch and Bauer (1991), showing that a neuronal membrane fraction from 14-day-old mouse embryos induces BBB properties in cloned cerebral capillary endothelial cells to even a greater extent than do glial cells, may be considered an important step toward a new understanding of the mechanism(s) underlying BBB induction (for review see Bauer and Bauer, 2000). However, additional molecular and physiological studies will be needed to identify a new role for early neurons in BBB formation.

During advanced embryonic and postnatal development, astroglia become the predominant cell population in the CNS and astrocytic endfeet get intimately attached to the capillary walls. Therefore, a crucial role for glial cells in the maintenance of the mature BBB has been suggested (Davson and Oldendorf, 1967; Holash et al., 1993). In this context, astroglia-dependent induction of barrier-associated characteristics, such as an increase in BBB-related marker enzyme activities, the elevation of glucose transporter protein levels, and the enhancement of transendothelial electrical resistance (Tao-Cheng et al., 1987), as well as the increased expression of P-glycoprotein in cultured cerebral endothelial cells, has been documented (Gaillard et al., 2000). Barrier properties of the capillary brain endothelium which are influenced by astrocytes are summarized in Table 25.1.

The potential of astroglia to determine the barrier characteristics of the central nervous capillaries has strong confirmation, although the situation is more complex than was originally expected (Greenwood, 1991; Risau, 1991). When astrocyte-conditioned medium (ACM) was added to cultured cerebral endothelial cells, no stimulation of γ-glutamyl transpeptidase (γ-GT) activity was observed (Papandrikopoulou et al., 1989). In contrast, when a supplement of serum together with ACM was added, a significant increase in γ-GT activity was detectable (Maxwell et al., 1987). Several lines of evidence indicate that the induction of BBB features in cerebral endothelial cells depends on a close, long-lasting contact between astrocytes and capillary endothelium (Stewart and Wiley, 1981). Moreover, direct contact between endothelial cells and astrocytes has been found to be essential (Tontsch and Bauer, 1991). Further, the susceptibility of cerebral endothelial cells to astroglial induction of BBB enzymes was shown to depend on their proliferative state (Meyer et al., 1991). A recent investigation on the effect of the removal of astrocytes from a co-culture model of the BBB demonstrated that, although an elevated permeability of ^{3}H-inulin and ^{14}C-sucrose was found, there was no change in the molecular composition of the TJs and even in the localization, neither of TJ-related proteins such as claudin-3, claudin-5, occludin, ZO-1 or ZO-2 nor of the adherens junction-associated proteins β-catenin or p120cas (Hamm et al., 2004).

The fact that ACM replaces astrocytes in inducing junctional development emphasizes the importance of a soluble factor (Arthur et al., 1987; Rubin et al., 1991). However, despite the considerable efforts of several groups to characterize this factor, its nature is still obscure. Inhibitors of protein synthesis or trypsin were shown to prevent astrocyte-related actions on the BBB (Maxwell et al., 1987), which points to a protein or peptide as the inductive factor. Recently, src-suppressed C-kinase substrate (SSeCKs) has attracted considerable interest: this factor has been shown to stimulate astrocytic expression of angiopoietin-1 and its secretion into the cell culture medium. Treatment of brain endothelial cells with SSeCKS-conditioned medium increases the expression of TJ proteins and decreases the ^{3}H-

TABLE 25.1 *Effects of Astrocytes and Astrocyte-Derived Material On Permeability Characteristics of Cerebral Endothelial Cells*

Effector	*Increase of*	*Reference*
AC-serum supplement	γ-GT	Maxwell et al. (1987)
AC cocultivated	γ-GT	Mertsch et al. (1999)
C6 glioma cells cocultivated	γ-GT	DeBault and Cancilla (1980), Bauer et al. (1990),* Tontsch and Bauer (1991)
C6 glioma-serum supplement	γ-GT	Maxwell et al. (1987)
C6 glioma cell membranes	γ-GT	Tontsch and Bauer (1991)
AC cocultivated	Alkaline phosphatase activity	Mertsch et al. (1999), Blasig et al. (2001)
ACM	TEER	Rubin et al. (1991), Giese et al. (1995)
AC cocultivated	TEER	Giese et al. (1995)
AC cocultivated	Tight junction length, number, and complexity	Tao-Cheng et al. (1987)
C6 Glioma cells	Asymmetry of amino acid tranport	Beck et al. (1984)
AC preconditioning	Paraendothelial sucrose tightness	Pardridge et al. (1990)
AC cocultivated	Paraendothelial sucrose tightness	Mertsch et al. (1997)

*Effective in phenotype I brain capillary endothelial cells only. AC: astrocyte; ACM: astrocyte-conditioned medium; γ-GT: γ-glutamyl transpeptidase activity; TEER: transendothelial electrical resistance.

sucrose permeability (Lee et al., 2003). However, these experiments were undertaken *in vitro*, and there are results from *in vivo* experiments that contradict an active role for astrocytes on BBB function (Krum, 1996). Interestingly, BBB properties are also inducible in nonneural endothelial cells by close apposition to cocultured astrocytes (Hayashi et al., 1997).

Astrocytes themselves seem to be influenced by their interaction with endothelial cells. In this respect, astrocytes show strong polarization in adult brains, where the BBB is well differentiated, but are rather unpolarized in neonates, with a poorly developed BBB (Wolburg, 1995). The astrocytic endfeet oriented toward the blood vessel exhibit characteristically arranged particles in their cell membrane (Dermietzel, 1974). These particles could be increased by cocultivation with brain endothelial cells (Tao-Cheng et al., 1990). The antioxidative activity of astrocytes and endothelial cells kept in coculture has been reported to be significantly higher than that in monocultures of astrocytes (Schroeter et al., 1999). The endothelial factor released is a polypeptide (>50 kDa) that stimulates DNA synthesis in astrocytes; its secretion is partially inhibited by interleukin-1 (Estrada et al., 1990).

THE BLOOD–BRAIN BARRIER UNDER PATHOPHYSIOLOGICAL CONDITIONS—ROLE OF GLIAL CELLS

Lesions of the BBB are associated with different pathologies such as glioblastoma, stroke, degenerative diseases (e.g., Parkinson's disease, Alzheimer's disease), inflammatory processes (e.g., meningitis and multiple sclerosis; for review see Abbott, 2000), and mood disorders (Rubin and Staddon, 1999). Associated leakage of the BBB and activation of astrocytes have often been reported. It appears that especially in brain tumors and cerebral areas following oxidative stress, astrocytes are affected, which, in turn, may cause deterioration of endothelial and, hence, BBB functions.

Brain Tumors

The status of the BBB in glial tumors is of great therapeutic relevance and thus has attracted considerable research interest. In general, the BBB in gliomas or astrocytomas is impaired: the expression of TJ-associated proteins is decreased, the paracellular pathways are partially opened, and edema forms in the surrounding brain due to the failure to clear excess fluid. For example, the TJ-protein claudin-1 is not found in vessels of glioblastoma multiforme, and occludin expression is extremely low in brain tumors (Liebner et al., 2000; Proescholdt et al., 2001, Papadopoulos et al., 2001a). However, it is almost impossible to treat brain tumors effectively with immunotherapy because in young, small tumors (smaller than 0.25 mm in diameter) the BBB is still intact, probably due to the release of vascular endothelial growth factor (VEGF). Vascular endothelial growth factor is produced by astrocytomas, inducing proliferation of the endothelial cells and resulting in vascularization and BBB function of the tumor sufficient for its existence (Machein et al., 1999).

During advanced tumor growth, the BBB of the tumor capillaries becomes more and more permeable (Wiranowska et al., 1992; Fidler et al., 2002). Currently, it is not clear why the BBB in brain tumors, especially in gliomas, becomes defunct. Apparently, glioma or astrocytoma cells lack the signals that are necessary to maintain the BBB in cerebral endothelial cells. Moreover, it cannot be ruled out that excessive VEGF production overstimulates endothelial cell proliferation while simultaneously suppressing BBB properties (Machein et al., 1999). Capillaries of advanced tumors also show abnormalities in the composition of their basement membrane. For example, the expression of tenascin was found to accumulate in the basal lamina of tumor vessels (Rascher et al., 2002).

Blood–Brain Barrier Function During Oxidative Stress

Astrocytes have been considered to protect the BBB during ischemic and oxidative stress conditions. There are indications that cerebral endothelial cells cocultured with glial cells are less susceptible to hypoxic insult; that is, they restore membrane structures more quickly and do not exhibit hypoxia-induced paracellular permeability changes (Abbruscato and Davis, 1999; Schroeter et al., 1999; Fischer et al., 2000). Astrocytes obviously induce the expression of radical defense enzymes in endothelial cells, thereby improving the overall defense against oxidative stress (Schroeter et al., 1999, 2001).

In general, astrocytes cope more readily with hypoxic insults than do endothelial cells and neurons, since they are able to upregulate their glycolytic capacity, allowing anaerobic glycolysis to provide sufficient ATP for cell survival or glutamate uptake during hypoxic conditions. Acute traumatic injury, ischemia-hypoxia, or neurodegenerative diseases induce *reactive astrocytes*. Phenotypically, these astrocytes resemble neonatal astrocytes, for example in the expression of nestin, an intermediate filament protein, which is not normally expressed in mature astrocytes. In culture, astrocytes show higher antioxidant activity than endothelial cells (Schroeter et al., 1999). The latter are more vulnerable to oxidative stress, which results in genotoxic damage, apoptosis, and, of importance to the BBB, loss of TJ-related protein expression (Giese et al., 1995; Mark and Davis, 2002). Thus ischemia-hypoxia leads to an increased permeability that allows plasma proteins to move into the brain tissue and results in brain edema (Plateel et al., 1997; Papadopoulos et al., 2001b).

Oxidative stress may cause inflammatory reactions of cerebral endothelial cells and astrocytes. Locally secreted chemokines such as interleukin-8 and the monocyte chemoattractant protein-1 are important signals for leukocyte recruitment to an inflammatory site (Zhang et al., 1999). Using *in vitro* systems, it has also been shown that hypoxia/reoxygenation induced an increase in the release of interleukin-1β into the culture medium. Endothelial cells treated with that medium responded with a pronounced elevation of chemokine expression (Zhang et al., 2000).

DIRECTIONS FOR THE FUTURE

In this chapter we describe the structure and function of the BBB represented by brain capillary endothelial cells. Special attention is given to the influence of astrocytes and astrocytic factors. Ontogenetic development and pathological aspects of the BBB are considered.

New and important scientific developments and discoveries may be expected in the near future, especially with respect to the molecular structure, function, and regulation of TJ-related proteins and of transporters (e.g., ABC transporters). Moreover, new insights will be gained concerning BBB function in conditions of oxidative stress, inflammation, and in brain tumors.

The mechanisms of how glial cells may intervene with BBB properties of endothelial cells remain unresolved. Further efforts are required to elucidate the exact nature of the glial factor(s) responsible for the induction and/or maintenance of BBB functions of endothelial cells. For these investigations experiments in cell culture systems will be necessary, as well as validation of the results by *in vivo* studies.

REFERENCES

Abbott, N.J. (2000) Inflammatory mediaters and modulation of blood–brain barrier permeability. *Cell. Mol. Neurobiol.* 20:131–149.

Abbruscato, T.J. and Davis, T.P. (1999) Protein expression of brain endothelial cell E-cadherin after hypoxia/aglycemia: influence of astrocyte contact. *Brain Res.* 842:277–286.

Armer, R.E. (2000) Inhibitors of mammalian central nervous system selective amino acid transporters. *Curr. Med. Chem.* 7:199–209.

Arthur, F.E., Shivers, R.R., and Bowman, P.D. (1987) Astrocyte-mediated induction of tight junctions in brain capillary endothelium: an efficient in vitro model. *Dev. Brain Res.* 36:155–159.

Balabanov, R. and Dore-Duffy, P. (1998) Role of the CNS microvascular pericyte in the blood-brain barrier. *J. Neurosci. Res.* 53:637–644.

Bauer, H. (1999) Glucose transporters in mammalian brain development. In: Pardridge, W.B., ed. *Introduction to the Blood–Brain Barrier*. Cambridge: Cambridge University Press, pp. 175–187.

Bauer, H., Sonnleitner, U., Lametschwandtner, A., Steiner, M., Adam, H., and Bauer H.C. (1995) Ontogenic expression of the erythroid-type glucose transporter (GLUT1) in the telencephalon of the mouse: correlation to the tightening of the blood–brain barrier. *Dev. Brain Res.* 86:317–325.

Bauer, H.C. and Bauer, H. (2000) The blood–brain barrier: still an enigma? *Cell. Mol. Neurobiol.* 20:13–29.

Bauer, H.C., Bauer, H., Lametschwandtner, A., Amberger, A., Ruiz, P., and Steiner, M. (1993) Neovascularization and the appearance of morphological characteristics of the blood–brain barrier in the embryonic mouse central nervous system. *Dev. Brain Res.* 75:269–278.

Bauer, H.C., Tontsch, U., Amberger, A., and Bauer, H. (1990) Gamma-glutamyl transpeptidase (GGTP) and Na^+,K^+-ATPase activities in different subpopulations of cloned cerebral endothelial cells: response to glial stimulation. *Biochem. Biophys. Res. Commun.* 168:358–363.

Bazzoni, G., Martinez-Estrada, O.M., Mueller, F., Nelboeck, P., Schmid, G., Bartfai, T., Dejana, E., and Brockhaus, M. (2000) Homophilic interaction of junctional adhesion molecule. *J. Biol. Chem.* 275:30970–30976.

Beck, D.W., Vinters, H.V., Hart, M.N., and Cancilla, P.A. (1984) Glial cells influence polarity of the blood–brain barrier. *J. Neuropathol. Exp. Neurol.* 43:219–224.

Blasig, I.E., Giese, H., Schroeter, M.L., Sporbert, A., Utepbergenov, D.I., Buchwalow, I.B., Neubert, K., Schönfelder, G., Freyer, D., Schimke, I., Siems, W.-E., Paul, M., Haseloff, R.F., and Blasig, R. (2001) NO and oxy-radical metabolism in new cell lines of rat brain capillary endothelial cells forming the blood–brain barrier. *Microvasc. Res.* 62:114–127.

Bradbury, M. (1979) *The Concept of a Blood–Brain Barrier.* London: Wiley.

Brightman, M.W. and Reese, T.S. (1969) Junctions between intimately apposed cell membranes in the vertebrate brain. *J. Cell Biol.* 40:648–677.

Davson, H. and Oldendorf, W.H. (1967) Transport in the central nervous system. *Proc. R. Soc. Med.* 60:326–328.

DeBault, L.E. and Cancilla, P.A. (1980) Gamma-glutamyl transpeptidase in isolated brain endothelial cells and induction by glial cells in vitro. *Science* 207:653–655.

Dermietzel, R. (1974) Junctions in the central nervous system of the cat. III. Gap junctions and membrane-associated orthogonal particle complexes (MOPC) in astrocytic membranes. *Cell Tissue Res.* 149:121–135.

Dermietzel, R. and Krause, D. (1991) Molecular anatomy of the blood–brain barrier as defined by immunocytochemistry. *Int. Rev. Cytol.* 12:57–109.

Estrada, C., Bready, J.V., Berliner, J.A., Pardridge, W.M., and Cancilla, P.A. (1990) Astrocyte growth stimulation by a soluble factor produced by cerebral endothelial cells in vitro. *J. Neuropathol. Exp. Neurol.* 49:539–549.

Fidler, I.J., Yano, S., Zhang, R.D., Fujimaki, T., and Bucana, C.D. (2002) The seed and soil hypothesis: vascularisation and brain metastasis. *Lancet Oncol.* 3:53–57.

Fischer, S., Wobben, M., Kleinstuck, J., Renz, D., and Schaper, W. (2000) Effect of astroglial cells on hypoxia-induced permeability in PBMEC cells. *Am. J. Physiol. Cell Physiol.* 279:C935–C944.

Fishell, G. and Kriegstein, A.R. (2003) Neurons from radial glia: the consequences of asymmetric inheritance. *Curr. Opin. Neurobiol.* 13:34–41.

Frelin, C. and Vigne, P. (1999) Ion channels in endothelial cells. In: Pardridge, W.B., ed. *Introduction to the Blood–Brain Barrier.* Cambridge: Cambridge University Press, pp. 214–220.

Furuse, M., Hirase, T., Itoh, M., Nagafuchi, A., Yonemura, S., Tsukita, S., and Tsukita, S. (1993) Occludin: a novel integral membrane protein localizing at tight junctions. *J. Cell Biol.* 123:1777–1788.

Gaillard, P.J., van der Sandt, J.C., Voorwinden, L.H., Vu, D., Nielsen, J.L., de Boer, A.G., and Breimer, D.D. (2000) Astrocytes increase the funtional expression of P-glycoprotein in an in vitro model of the blood–brain barrier. *Pharm. Res.* 17:1198–1205.

Giese, H., Mertsch, K., and Blasig, I.E. (1995) Effect of MK-801 and U83836E on a porcine brain capillary endothelial cell barrier during hypoxia. *Neurosci. Lett.* 191:169–172.

Gonzalez-Mariscal, L., Betanzos, A., and Avila-Flores, A. (2000) MAGUK proteins: structure and role in the tight junction. *Cell Dev. Biol.* 11:315–324.

Greenwood, J. (1991) Astrocytes, cerebral endothelium, and cell culture. The pursuit of an in vitro blood–brain barrier. *Ann. NY Acad. Sci.* 633:424–431.

Habgood, M.D., Sedgwick, J.E.C., Dziegielewska, K.M., and Saunders, N.R. (1992) A developmentally regulated blood–cerebrospinal fluid barrier exchange during postnatal brain development in the rat. *J. Physiol.* 468:73–83.

Hamm, S., Dehouck, B., Kraus, J., Wolburg-Buchholz, K., Wolburg, H., Risau, W., Cecchelli, R., Engelhardt, B., and Dehouck, M.P. (2004) Astrocyte mediated modulation of blood–brain barrier permeability does not correlate with a loss of tight junction proteins from the cellular contacts. *Cell Tissue Res.* 315:157–166.

Hayashi, Y., Nomura, M., Yamagishi, S., Harada, S., Yamashita, J., and Yamamoto, H. (1997) Induction of various blood–brain barrier properties in non-neural endothelial cells by close apposition to co-cultured astrocytes. *Glia* 19:13–26.

Holash, J.A., Noden, D.M., and Stewart, P.A. (1993) Re-evaluation the role of astrocytes in blood–brain barrier induction. *Dev. Dynam.* 197:14–25.

Howarth, A.G. and Stevenson, B.R. (1995) Molecular environment of ZO-1 in epithelial and non-epithelial cells. *Cell Motil. Cytoskel.* 31:323–332.

Krum, J.M. (1996) Effect of astroglial degeneration on neonatal blood–brain barrier marker expression. *Exp. Neurol.* 142:29–35.

Lee, G., Dallas, S., Hong, M., and Bendayan, R. (2001) Drug transporters in the central nervous system: brain barriers and brain parenchyma considerations. *Pharmacol. Rev.* 53:569–596.

Lee, S.W., Kim, W.J., Choi, Y.K., Song, H.S., Son, M.J., Gelman, I.H., Kim, Y.J., and Kim, K.W. (2003) SSeCKS regulates angiogenesis and tight junction formation in blood–brain barrier. *Nature Med.* 9:900–906.

Liebner, S., Fischmann, A., Rascher, G., Duffner, F., Grote, E.H., Kalbacher, H., and Wolburg, H. (2000) Claudin-1 and claudin-5 expression and tight junction morphology are altered in blood vessels of human glioblastoma multiforme. *Acta Neuropathol.* 100:323–331.

Machein, M.R, Kullmer, J., Fiebich, B.L., Plate, K.H., and Warnke, P.C. (1999) Vascular endothelial growth factor expression, vascular volume, and capillary permeability in human brain tumors. *Neurosurgery* 44:732–740.

Mark, K.S. and Davis, T.P. (2002) Cerebral microvascular changes in permeability and tight junctions induced by hypoxia-reoxygenation. *Am. J. Physiol. Heart Circ. Physiol.* 282:H1485–H1494.

Maxwell, K., Berliner, J.A., and Cancilla P.A. (1987) Induction of gamma-glutamyl transpeptidase in cultured endothelial cells by a product released by astrocytes. *Brain Res.* 410:309–314.

Mertsch, K., Haseloff, R.F., and Blasig, I.E. (1997) Investigations of radical scavengers by using an in vitro model of blood–brain barrier. *Dev. Animal Vet. Sci.* 27:881–886.

Mertsch, K., Haseloff, R.F., Schroeter, M.L., and Blasig, I.E. (1999) In vitro models of the blood–brain barrier for the investigation of cerebroprotective agents. In: Carter, A.J. and Kettenmann, H., eds. *Practical Handbook of Methods.* Jülich: Forschungszentrum Jülich, pp. 99–124.

Meyer, J., Rauh, J., and Galla, H.-J. (1991) The susceptibility of cerebral endothelial cells to astroglial induction of blood–brain barrier enzymes depends on their proliferative state. *J. Neurochem.* 57:1971–1977.

Moos, T. and Morgan, E.H. (2000) Transferrin and transferrin receptor function in brain barrier systems. *Cell. Mol. Neurobiol.* 20:77–95.

Nehls, V. and Drenckhahn, D. (1991) Heterogeneity of microvascular pericytes for smooth muscle type alpha-actin. *J. Cell Biol.* 113:147–154.

Papadopoulos, M.C., Saadoun, S., Davies, D.C., and Bell, B.A. (2001b) Emerging molecular mechanisms of brain tumour oedema. *Br. J. Neurosurg.* 15:101–108.

Papadopoulos, M.C., Saadoun, S., Woodrow, C.J., Davies, D.C., Costa-Martins, P., Moss, R.F., Krishan, S., and Bell, B.A. (2001a)

Occludin expression in microvessels of neoplastic and non-neoplastic human brain. *Neuropathol. Appl. Neurobiol.* 27:384–395.

Papandrikopoulou, A., Frei, A., and Grasser, M.G. (1989) Cloning and expression of gamma-glutamyltranspeptidase from isolated porcine brain capillaries. *Eur. J. Biochem.* 183:693–698.

Pardridge, W.M. (1999) Blood–brain barrier biology and methodology. *J. Neurovirol.* 5:556–569.

Pardridge, W.M., Triguero, D., Yang, J., and Cancilla, P.A. (1990) Comparison of in vitro and in vivo models of drug transcytosis through the blood–brain barrier. *J. Pharmacol.* 253:844–891.

Persidsky, Y., Ghorpade, A., Rasmussen, J., Limoges, J., Liu, X.J., Stins, M., Fiala, M., Way, D., Kim, K.S., Witte, M.H., Weinand, M., Carhart, L., and Gendelman, H.E. (1999) Microglial and astrocyte chemokines regulate monocyte migration through the blood–brain barrier in human immnodeficiency virus-1 encephalitis. *Am. J. Pathol.* 15:1599–1611.

Plateel, M., Teisier, E., and Cecchelli, R. (1997) Hypoxia dramatically increases the nonspecific transport of blood-borne proteins to the brain. *J. Neurochem.* 68:874–877.

Proescheldt, M.A., Merill, M.J., Ikejiri, B., Walbridge, S., Akbasak, A., Jacobson, S., and Oldfield E.H. (2001) Site-specific immune response to implanted gliomas. *J. Neurosurg.* 95:1012–1019.

Rascher, G., Fischmann, A., Krüger, S., Duffner, F., Grote, E.-H., and Wolburg, H. (2002) Extracellular matrix and the blood–brain barrier in glioblastoma multiforme: spatial segregation of tenascin and agrin. *Acta Neuropathol.* 104:85–91.

Reese, T.S. and Karnovsky, M.J. (1967) Fine structural localization of a blood–brain barrier to exogenous peroxidase. *J. Cell Biol.* 34:207–217.

Risau, W. (1991) Induction of blood–brain barrier endothelial cell differentiation. *Ann. NY Acad. Sci.* 633:405–419.

Risau, W. (1997) Mechanisms of angiogenesis. *Nature* 386:671–674.

Risau, W., Halemann, R., and Albrecht, U. (1986) Differentiation-dependent expression of proteins in brain endothelium during development of the blood-brain barrier. *Dev. Biol.* 117:537–545.

Rubin, L.L., Hall, E., Porter, S., Barbu, K., Cannon, C., Horner, H.C., Janatpour, M., Liaw, C.W., Manning, K., Morales, J., et al., (1991) A cell culture model of the blood–brain barrier. *J. Cell Biol.* 115:1725–1735.

Rubin, L.L. and Staddon, J.M. (1999) The cell biology of the blood–brain barrier. *Annu. Rev. Neurosci.* 22:11–28.

Saunders, N.R., Knott, G.W., and Dziegielewska, K.M. (2000.) Barriers in the immature brain. *Cell. Mol. Neurobiol.* 20:29–41.

Schroeter, M.L., Mertsch, K., Giese, H., Müller, S., Sporbert, A., Hickel, B., and Blasig, I.E. (1999) Astrocytes enhance radical defence in capillary endothelial cells constituting the blood–brain barrier. *FEBS Lett.* 449:241–244.

Schroeter, M.L., Müller, S., Lindenau, J., Wiesner, B., Hanisch, U.K., Wolf, G., and Blasig, I.E. (2001) Astrocytes induce manganese superoxide dismutase in brain capillary endothelial cells. *NeuroReport* 8:2513–2517.

Stewart, P.A. and Hayakawa, K. (1994) Early structural changes in blood–brain barrier vessels of the rat embryo. *Dev. Brain Res.* 78:25–34.

Stewart, P.A. and Wiley, M.J. (1981) Developing nervous tissue induces formation of the blood-barrier characteristics in invading endothelial cells: a study using Quail-chick transplantation chimeras. *Dev. Biol.* 84:183–192.

Tamai, I. and Tsuji, A. (2000) Transporter-mediated permeation of drugs across the blood–brain barrier. *J. Pharm. Sci.* 89:1371–1388.

Tao-Cheng, J.-H., Nagy, Z., and Brightman, M.W. (1987) Tight junctions of brain endothelium in vitro are enhanced by astroglia. *J. Neurosci.* 7:3293–3299.

Tao-Cheng, J.-H., Nagy, Z., and Brightman, M.W. (1990) Astrocytic orthogonal arrays in intramembranous particle assemblies modulated by brain endothelial cells in vitro. *J. Neuropathol.* 19:143–153.

Tontsch, U. and Bauer, H.C. (1991) Glial cells and neurons induce blood–brain barrier related enzymes in cultured cerebral endothelial cells. *Brain Res.* 539:247–253.

Tsukita, S. and Furuse, M. (2000) Pores in the wall: claudins constitute tight junction strands containing aqueous pores. *J. Cell Biol.* 149:13–16.

Tsukita, S., Furuse, M., and Itoh, M. (1999) Structural and signalling molecules come together at tight junctions. *Curr. Opin. Cell Biol.* 11:628–633.

Van Deurs, B. (1979) Structural aspects of brain barriers, with special reference to the permeability of the cerebral endothelium and choroidal epithelium. *Int. Rev. Cytol.* 65:117–191.

Wiranowska, M., Gonzalvo, A.A., Saporta, S., Gonzalez, O.R., and Prockop, L.D. (1992) Evaluation of blood–brain barrier permeability and the effect of interferon in mouse glioma model. *J. Neurooncol.* 14:225–236.

Wittchen, E.S., Haskins, J., and Stevenson, B.R. (1999) Protein interactions at the tight junction. Actin has multiple binding partners, and ZO-1 forms independent complexes with ZO-2 and ZO-3. *J. Biol. Chem.* 274:35179–35185.

Wolburg, H. (1995) Orthogonal arrays of intramembranous particles: a review with special reference to astrocytes. *J. Hirnforsch.* 36:239–258.

Wolburg, H. and Lippoldt, A. (2002) Tight junctions of the blood–brain barrier: development, composition and regulation. *Vasc. Pharmacol.* 38:323–337.

Xu, J. and Ling, E.A. (1994) Studies of the ultrastructure and permeability of the blood–brain barrier in the developing corpus callosum in postnatal rat brain using electron dense tracers. *J. Anat.* 84:227–237.

Yoshida, Y., Yamada, M., Wakabayashi, K., and Ikuta, F. (1988) Endothelial fenestrae in the rat fetal cerebrum. *Dev. Brain Res.* 44:211–219.

Yudkoff, M., Daikhin, Y., Nissim, I., Lazarow, A., and Nissim, I. (2001) Ketogenic diet, amino acid metabolism, and seizure control. *J. Neurosci. Res.* 66:931–940.

Zhang, W., Smith, C., Howlett, C., and Stanimirovic, D. (2000) Inflammatory activation of human brain endothelial cells by hypoxic astrocytes in vitro is mediated by IL-1beta. *Cereb. Blood Flow Metab.* 20:967–978.

Zhang, W., Smith, C., Shapiro, A, Monette, R., Hutchison, J., and Stanimirovic, D.B. (1999) Increased expression of bioactive chemokines in human cerebromicrovascular endothelial cells and astrocytes subjected to simulated ischemia in vitro. *J. Neuroimmunol.* 101:148–160.

26 Extracellular potassium and pH: homeostasis and signaling

JONATHAN A. COLES AND JOACHIM W. DEITMER

INTERCELLULAR ION MOVEMENTS IN NERVOUS TISSUE

Electrical signaling in nervous systems involves considerable fluxes of ions across the neuronal membranes to carry electrical charge in and out. These ion fluxes inevitably tend to change the ion concentrations inside and outside cells, and these concentration changes, if sufficiently large, would change the functioning of cells and hence of the tissue as a whole. Usually, changes in ion concentrations are opposed by homeostatic processes and, in general, are not large enough to have radical effects on function. However, modest changes in ion concentrations during physiological activity are often observed, and some of these can be regarded as signals passing through the extracellular spaces (ECS). Ions participating in major fluxes across cell membranes include those responsible for electrical signaling (mainly Na^+, K^+, and Cl^-), and also HCO_3^-, H^+, and NH_4^+, which are linked to metabolism.

For periods of up to tens of seconds, exchange between the brain and blood is slight compared to the movements of ions between the three intraparenchymal compartments: neurons, glial cells, and ECS (Mutsaga et al., 1976). In the relatively small ECS (Box 26.1) Na^+ and Cl^- are present in high concentrations, so when these ions enter neurons during electrical activity, the decreases in their extracellular concentrations are small (and largely compensated for by shrinking of the ECS; Coles et al., 1986; Dietzel et al., 1989). The reverse is true of the extracellular K^+ concentration ($[K^+]_e$), which is low and can undergo large fractional changes. Extracellular pH (pH_e) also varies significantly. The interplay between homeostasis and signaling functions of $[K^+]_e$ and of pH_e is the theme of this chapter.

POTASSIUM

Physiological Variations in Extracellular $[K^+]$

Extracellular $[K^+]$ in most parts of rat brain is about, or less than, 2.5 mM (Moghaddam and Adams, 1987; Coles and Poulain, 1991). When electrical stimulation is used to activate entire nerve tracts, $[K^+]_e$ in mammals can rise more than 3-fold, up to a "ceiling" level of 10–12 mM (Fig. 26.1*B*). But during physiological activity, for example, in response to sensory stimulation, the changes are much smaller, typically less than 0.1 mM, with a maximum of about 0.4 mM (Fig. 26.1*A*; Singer and Lux, 1975; Sykova et al., 1980). Within the supraoptic nucleus of the lactating rat, a 70 Hz burst of synchronized firing by a group of oxytocin neurons produces a rise in $[K^+]_e$ (of about 0.22 mM) no greater than that produced by firing at 10 Hz in vasopressin neurons (Coles and Poulain, 1991). So here, the capacity for K^+ clearance appears to be locally adapted to the specific requirements of small groups of neurons.

Pathological Variations in Extracellular $[K^+]$

$[K^+]$ increases to the ceiling level of 10–12 mM during seizure activity in animal models of epilepsy (Hablitz and Heinemann, 1987). Even greater rises in $[K^+]_e$ occur in ischemia and also during spreading depression, which is a wave of electrical silence that slowly moves through cortex or retina. Spreading depression occurs in humans suffering brain trauma (Strong et al., 2002) and is also the probable cause of migraine auras (James et al., 2001). A similar phenomenon, the peri-infarct depolarization, is triggered by ischemia in animal models (Nedergaard and Hansen, 1993). In animal experiments on spreading depression, $[K^+]_e$ typically rises transiently to 55 mM (see Fig. 26.1*C*; Kraig and Nicholson, 1978; Hansen and Zeuthen, 1981). These excessive increases in $[K^+]_e$ are part of the mechanism of spreading depression and represent a failure of $[K^+]_e$ homeostasis.

Clearance of Excess K^+ from Extracellular Space

Glial cells, not inactive neurons, remove excess K^+ from extracellular clefts (Coles and Orkand, 1983; Schlue and Wuttke, 1983; Rose and Ransom, 1997). The

See the list of abbreviations at the end of the chapter.

Box 26.1 Extracellular Space as the Path for Neuroglial Interaction

A. A typical geometry of ECS in a small region of rat cortex. *B*. The main technique for investigating the macroscopic diffusional properties of ECS. A double-barreled, ion-selective microelectrode (ISM) sensitive to tetramethylammonium (TMA^+-ISM) is glued to an iontophoresis micropipette containing TMA (bent) with the tips 100–200 μm apart. Tetramethylammonium is chosen because it is not endogenous, it remains extracellular, and electrodes can be made that are very sensitive to it. The electrode assembly is illustrated with the tips in rat cortex. *C*. Tetramethylammonium was driven out of the iontophoresis pipette by passing 80 nA for 60 seconds (bar). It diffused through extracellular space and was detected by the ISM. Analysis of the amplitude and time course of arrival of TMA at the ISM determines two parameters: α, the volume of the ECS (expressed as a fraction of the total volume), and a parameter λ, which reflects mainly the tortuosity of the extracellular clefts. Under normal conditions, the values are almost always close to those found in this example (*normoxia*): an ECS fraction of 0.20 and a tortuosity factor of 1.50. If a solute has a diffusion coefficient in free solution of D, in the brain it has an apparent diffusion coefficient $D^* = 1/\lambda^2 D$ for "long" distances (>10 μm). Part C also shows the response to ejection of TMA at the same site 10 minutes after cardiac arrest. The cells have swollen so that α is much smaller. λ has also changed, becoming larger; a possible explanation is that when the extracellular matrix is compressed, it significantly obstructs diffusion. α is also reduced during normal neuronal activity and in some pathologies. (Figures modified from Nicholson and Sykova, 1988, with permission.)

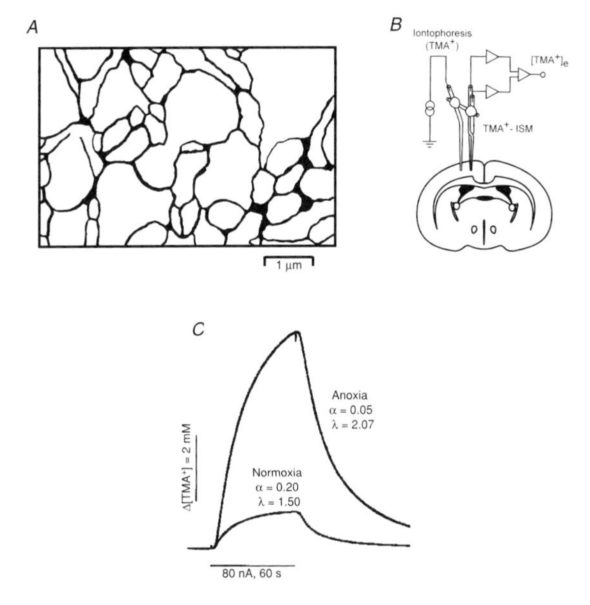

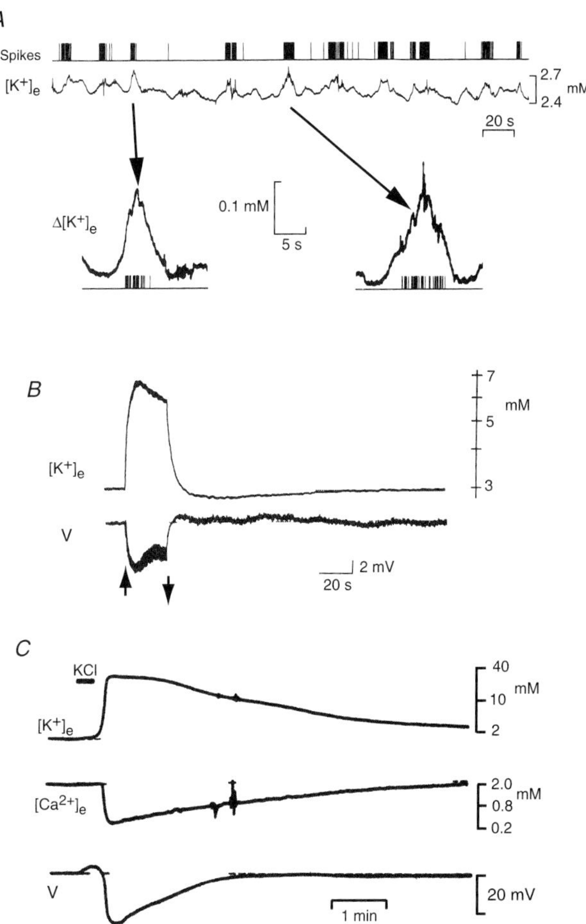

FIGURE 26.1 Physiological and nonphysiological changes in extracellular $[K^+]$. Response to a physiological stimulus (*A*), response to electrical stimulation of an entire input tract (*B*), and a massive increase in $[K^+]_e$ during spreading depression (*C*). For each recording, a double-barreled K^+-selective microelectrode, its tip located in extracellular space, recorded $[K^+]_e$ and the extracellular electrical potential. *A*. Recording from a location close to a vasopressin-secreting cell in the supraoptic nucleus of the rat. The occurrence of each action potential is shown by a line in the top trace. The phasic firing (maximum frequency about 10 Hz) had been increased by increasing the osmolarity of the blood. The fluctuations in extracellular $[K^+]$ ($[K^+]_e$) are small; they are caused partly by the activity of the recorded cell, and partly by neighboring cells. The two enlarged insets show an increase in $[K^+]_e$ occurring before the onset of a burst. (Modified from Coles and Poulain, 1991.) *B*. In the cortex of the rat, the nucleus ventroposterolateralis was stimulated for 30 seconds (between *arrows*) at 25 Hz, causing $[K^+]_e$ to more than double. After the stimulation, $[K^+]_e$ fell below baseline as K^+ uptake by the neurons exceeded the return of K^+ to this extracellular space. The extracellular potential (filtered to reduce action potentials, positive upward) shows a negative shift when $[K^+]_e$ is high. (Modified from Heinemann and Lux, 1977 with permission.) *C*. In the cerebellum of the catfish, spreading depression was initiated by microinjection of KCl at another site in the cerebellum. $[K^+]_e$ rose by a factor of 20, $[Ca^{2+}]_e$ fell to less than half (note that the ion concentration scales are nonlinear), and there was a large negative extracellular potential. (Modified from Kraig and Nicholson, 1978 with permission.)

cation conductance of glial cell membranes is highly selective for K^+ (Orkand et al., 1966; Newman, 1986) and in normal $[K^+]_e$, K^+ is at, or close to, electrochemical equilibrium across the membrane. If $[K^+]_e$ rises, the equilibrium is disturbed and K^+ enters the cell. But entry of K^+ alone is not sufficient: only a tiny fraction of the K^+ lost by a neuron would enter neighboring glial cells before the inward ion currents depolarized the membranes to the new equilibrium potential. Three processes are available to take care of the charge balance: *spatial buffering*, net uptake of K^+, with the charge balanced by uptake of Cl^-; and exchange of K^+ for Na^+ by the Na^+,K^+-ATPase (the *sodium pump*).

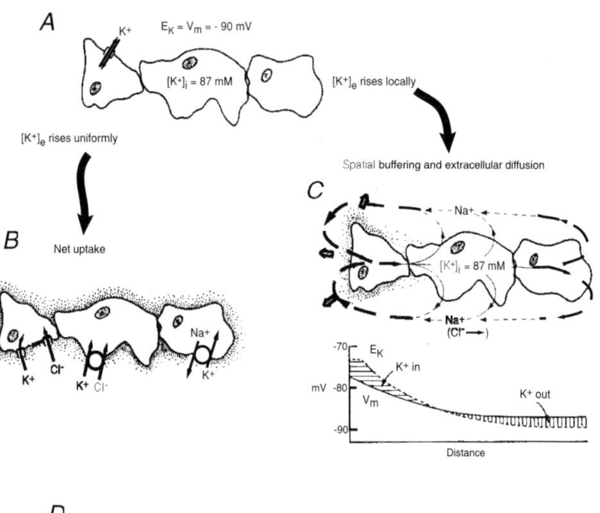

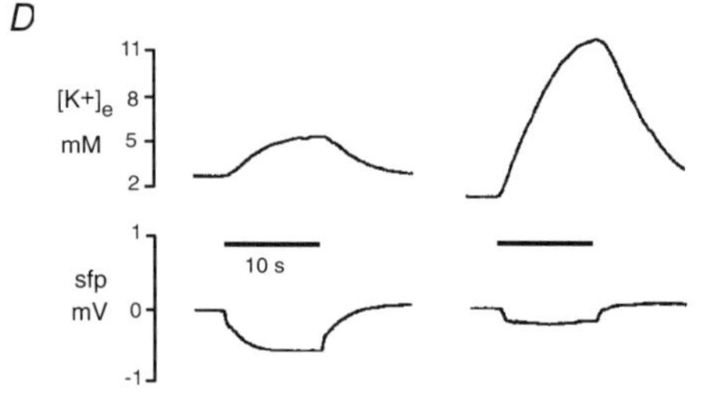

FIGURE 26.2 Routes of K^+ clearance into glial cells. *A*. Scheme showing three electrically coupled glial cells. The dominant K^+ conductance brings the membrane potential (V_m) close to the K^+ electrochemical equilibrium potential (E_K). *B*. *Net uptake*. If $[K^+]_e$ rises in the spaces all round the glial cells, then K^+ enters them (*lower left*): the charge is neutralized by entry of Cl^-. Cl^- can enter through separate ion channels or on a K,Cl cotransporter protein. In addition, K^+ may be taken up in exchange for Na^+ on the Na^+,K^+-ATPase. *C*. *Spatial buffering*. If the increase in $[K^+]_e$ is nonuniform, two "space-dependent" processes occur. The simpler one is passive diffusion of K^+ ions through the extracellular clefts (*thick white arrows*). There is also spatial buffering. Spatial buffering occurs because where $[K^+]_e$ is high, K^+ is no longer in equilibrium across the glial membrane ($E_K > V_m$). K^+ therefore enters the nearest glial cell. This entry of positive charge slightly depolarizes electrically coupled cells farther away, and this depolarization drives out K^+ ($V_m > E_K$; see graph, *bottom right*). The phenomenon is essentially electric, and its onset is in milliseconds; it does not depend on diffusion of intracellular K^+ ions down an intracellular concentration gradient. In the scheme, dashed lines represent current carried by whatever ions are available, mainly Na^+ and Cl^- in extracellular space and K^+ in intracellular space. (Scheme modified from Orkand, 1986.) *D*. Barium reduces spatial buffering. The tip of a double-barreled, K^+-selective microelectrode was in the CA1 area of a slice of human hippocampus, and $[K^+]_e$ (*upper traces*, linear scale) and slow field potentials (*lower traces*) were measured. Stimulation of the alveus at 20 Hz (*bar*) caused a rise in $[K^+]_e$ and a negative slow potential. Reducing glial K^+ conductance with Ba^{2+} impaired K^+ clearance and reduced the field potential (right-hand panel). (From Kivi et al., 2000 with permission.)

Spatial buffering and K^+ siphoning

In their groundbreaking work on the membrane properties of glial cells, Stephen Kuffler and colleagues pointed out that cells with membranes permeable only to K^+ can still remove K^+ from ECS, provided that the increase in $[K^+]_e$ is localized to only a part of the glial cell membrane, and K^+ can be dumped by *spatial buffering* into ECS farther away (Fig. 26.2). The return to the initial state occurs after the neurons have repolarized and the neuronal Na^+,K^+-ATPase removes K^+ from the ECS. Local $[K^+]_e$ is now lower than remote $[K^+]_e$, so the spatial buffering operates in the reverse direction. Arguments for a major role of spatial buffering in clearing K^+ released by neurons *in vivo* are based on detailed quantitative analysis of changes in extracellular ion concentrations (Dietzel et al., 1989) and on the effects of barium, which reduces the K^+ conductance of glial cells (Fig. 26.2D; see Chapter 9, this volume).

Since spatial buffering usually involves current flowing from one astrocyte to the next through gap junctions (Chapter 13, this volume), it is modulated when gap junction coupling is altered. Holthoff and Witte (2000) suggest that in rat cortex, activation of a group of neurons increases coupling, in a radial direction, between the astrocytes in the same region. Hence spatial buffering is increased and is directed radially.

An elegant refinement of spatial buffering was first demonstrated in the retina of *Necturus*, an Amphibian. The Müller glial cells extend through the thickness of the retina from the photoreceptor layer to the vitreal face, where they form endfeet with extensive membranes. E.A. Newman et al., (1984) isolated Müller cells and showed that when K^+ was applied at the distal end, so that K^+ entered the cell there, little K^+ leaked out of the stalk of the cell but much K^+ was rapidly driven out of the vitreal endfoot (Fig. 26.3). Such directed spatial buffering is called *siphoning*. Subsequent work has shown that astrocyte endfeet, which often ensheathe blood capillaries in the brain, have a high K^+ conductance (Newman, 1986). More recent studies of Müller cells have added details to the picture and have shown that the fine lateral processes of the cell have a high K^+ conductance. The K^+ channels are inward rectifiers, the main molecular type being Kir 4.1 (Kofuji et al., 2000).

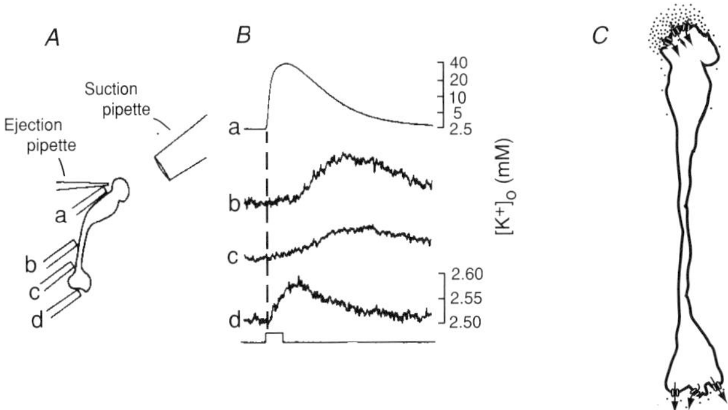

FIGURE 26.3 Potassium siphoning. *A*. The scheme shows a Müller glial cell isolated from salamander retina. An ejection pipette containing 85 mM KCl was placed near the distal end (*top*). KCl was ejected by pressure pulses, the spread of KCl being limited by the suction pipette. A K^+-sensitive electrode was placed successively at the four positions shown (*a–d*). When K^+ was ejected, a large rise was measured at position *a* (top trace in *B*). At *b* and *c* only small, slow rises were measured; these were due to extracellular diffusion of K^+. Strikingly, at *d*, near the Müller cell endfoot, the K^+ rise was fast and large. *C*. Scheme showing the mechanism underlying the result of *B*. (*A* and *B* modified from Newman et al., 1984.)

The extracellular currents associated with spatial buffering give rise to field potentials (Fig. 26.2*D*). These can be detected outside the skull, but in normal clinical practice the potentials of the electroencephalogram and the electroretinogram are high-pass filtered to leave mainly faster potentials coming from the neurons.

Net uptake of K^+

In spatial buffering, the amount of K^+ that leaves the glial cells is equal to the amount that enters (apart from the minute amount needed to charge the membrane capacitance to the new potential). However, $[K^+]_g$ (the concentration in the glial cells) has been observed to increase at the onset of neuronal activity (Coles and Orkand, 1983; Schlue and Wuttke, 1983; Ballanyi et al., 1987). The electrical charge associated with this extra K^+ has to be balanced, and this occurs mainly by entry of Cl^-. There are two main routes of Cl^- entry: through Cl^- ion channels separate from the K^+ channels (Coles et al., 1989; Ballanyi and Schlue, 1990; Munsch et al., 1995) and by uptake together with K^+ on a K,Cl cotransporter (or a Na,K,2Cl cotransporter), these latter being known mainly on cultured cells (see Amédée et al., 1997; Su et al., 2002). Net uptake of K^+ with Cl^- as a counter ion increases intracellular osmolytes and hence causes uptake of water, swelling of the cell, and shrinkage of the ECS (Dietzel et al., 1980; Ballanyi et al., 1990).

In principle, another way of balancing the charge of a net uptake of K^+ would be by extruding Na^+ in exchange for K^+ on the ubiquitous Na,K-ATPase. In intact tissues, the contribution of the Na,K-ATPase to clearance of stimulus-induced increases in $[K^+]_e$, or to modest increases of bath $[K^+]$, appears to be small (Coles and Orkand, 1985; Ballanyi et al., 1987; see Amédée et al., 1997). However, in adult rat optic nerve, when all the axons are made to fire at a high frequency (an unphysiological situation), the Na^+ pump does appear to play the major role (Ransom et al., 2000).

The Relative Importance of the Different Ways of Clearing Extracellular K^+

Extracellular diffusion, spatial buffering, and entry of K^+ in association with Cl^-, through ion channels or on a K^+,Cl^- cotransporter (but not on a $Na^+,K^+,2Cl^-$ cotransporter), all have the advantages that they require no energy from glial cells, and that they reverse when $[K^+]_e$ is reduced as a result of K^+ being taken back into the neurons. The evidence is in favor of these routes of K^+ clearance, particularly spatial buffering, being the major ones during normal physiological activity (Dietzel et al., 1989; Holthoff and Witte, 2000).

Under pathological conditions, such as ischemia or during an epileptic discharge, where the volume of tissue suffering from high $[K^+]_e$ extends well beyond a small group of cells, extracellular diffusion and spatial buffering will be less effective for clearing K^+ since these routes require sink regions of low $[K^+]_e$. Net uptake of K^+ is then expected to make a greater contribution. Uptake of K^+ with Cl^- as the counter ion does have the disadvantage that it causes swelling of the glial cells and can lead to edema (Chapter 44, this volume). Activation of the Na^+/K^+ exchange ATPase, which may account for the ceiling level of $[K^+]_e$ seen in epileptiform activity (Fig. 26.1*B*), will counteract cell swelling. In ischemia, however, activity of the Na^+/K^+-ATPase eventually fails for lack of ATP and the cells swell, this swelling being a major part of the pathology.

Changes in Extracellular $[K^+]$ as Signals

The membrane potentials of inactive neurons are only weakly sensitive to changes in $[K^+]_e$ in the small range observed physiologically, but briefly become much more sensitive to $[K^+]_e$ when K^+ conductance is increased after an action potential, notably by the activation of delayed rectifier conductances (Frankenhaeuser and Hodgkin, 1956). Also, in neurons that fire phasically, even small changes in $[K^+]_e$ may be critical in setting off a burst of repetitive firing (this may be the case in Fig. 26.1*A*). However, the contribution of changes in $[K^+]_e$ to synaptic function seems to be minor (Erulkar and Weight, 1977). An initial interest in $[K^+]_e$ in locomotor pattern generation in the lamprey brainstem–spinal cord (Wallen et al., 1984) has been overtaken by a new awareness of the importance of more specific modulation of neuronal ion channels by neurotransmitters (Grillner et al., 2001).

In contrast to the membrane potential of inactive neurons, that of glial cells is very sensitive to changes in $[K^+]_e$ (Orkand et al., 1966), and any change in membrane potential will affect all electrogenic transport. In most glial cells, an important electrogenic transporter is the Na^+,HCO_3^- cotransporter (see the section "pH Changes Related to Neuronal Activity"). If this transport is initially in a steady state, depolarizing the cell will tend to make intracellular pH more acid, and hyperpolarization will make it more alkaline. Astrocytes from most parts of the nervous system can also take up glutamate on the GLT-1 transporter, which cotransports Na^+ with a net inward movement of charge, so uptake is reduced (or even reversed) when the membrane is depolarized. A mechanism of a different kind, at present only a theoretical possibility for glial cells, is that membrane depolarization might activate G-proteins (Anis et al., 1999; Martinez-Pinna et al., 2004).

Raised $[K^+]_e$ can modify the glycogen metabolism of astrocytes, usually by stimulating degradation, but the effects are less than those of neurotransmitters, and in bee retina, application of K^+ does not mimic the signal from neurons to glial cells (Evequoz-Mercier and Tsacopoulos, 1991).

In contrast to these apparently minor effects of physiological variations in $[K^+]_e$, the much greater increases that can occur pathologically do have major effects. Neurons that are ischemic or undergoing epileptiform bursts of activity lose K^+ and raise $[K^+]_e$, which contributes to the depolarization of both neurons and glial cells. Depolarization relieves the magnesium block of *N*-methyl-D-aspartate (NMDA) receptors, making them sensitive to glutamate. Furthermore, raised $[K^+]_e$ tends to reverse the direction of glutamate transporters, partly by depolarizing membranes and partly because K^+ is normally transported outward on glutamate transporters. Hence, in raised $[K^+]_e$, cells, particularly neurons, release glutamate which, by acting on NMDA receptors, causes further depolarization and further release of K^+ (Rossi et al., 2000).

AMMONIUM

In mammalian brain, glutamate is taken up by astrocytes and converted to glutamine, which is then transferred to neurons, where it is deamidated to glutamate (Chapter 27, this volume). A corollary is that ammonium must be transferred from neurons to astrocytes (Benjamin and Quastel, 1975). In cultured rat astrocytes, ammonium enters as NH_4^+, mainly by way of Ba^{2+}-sensitive ion channels (Nagaraja and Brookes, 1998). A recent development is the discovery of transporters and channels specific for NH_4^+. Those best known to molecular biologists belong to the (Amt/MEP/Rh) superfamily, which are expressed in several tissues in mammals, including brain (Huang and Liu, 2001). Although NH_4^+ has almost the same ionic radius as K^+, it has been found, on glial cells of bee retina, that the NH_4^+ transporter transports little, if any, K^+ and the main K^+ conductance lets through little, if any, NH_4^+: the routes of uptake of these two ions are remarkably separate (Marcaggi et al., 2004).

Ammonium affects glial cell behavior by participating in reactions, notably the amidation of glutamate to glutamine. In addition, ammonium activates phosphofructokinase, a rate-limiting enzyme of glycolysis, and, conversely, inhibits the α-ketoglutarate dehydrogenase complex, a rate-limiting enzyme of the tricarboxylic acid (TCA) cycle (see Marcaggi and Coles, 2001). Poitry et al. (2000) have reported that when 0.1 mM ammonium is applied to retinal Müller glial cells in the presence of glutamate, it stimulates release of lactate, which is known to be an energy substrate for the inner segments of the photoreceptor neurons.

pH

The Extracellular Space as a Mediator of Acid/Base Transfer

Protons are chemically the most active ions. Several amino acids have proton binding sites that are intermittently occupied at physiological pHs (i.e., their pK_as are in this range), so most proteins, including ion channels and enzymes, are highly sensitive to pH. Therefore, changes in intra- and extracellular pH have a prominent role in the physiology and pathology of nervous tissue. While both intra- and extracellular pH in the steady state are regulated in a relatively narrow range, large pH changes may occur, for example, during neuronal activity. These may be initiated by augmented H^+ extrusion via carriers, or via neurotransmitter-gated ion channels, or via transmitter and metabolite uptake carriers. In particular, neurotransmission with glutamate, γ-aminobutyric acid (GABA), or glycine is associated with intra- and extracellular pH changes, which can be large and rapid. Unlike intracellular calcium changes, which rise and then recover, pH shifts can occur in two directions, acid and alkaline. Indeed, because several acid/base fluxes with different time courses may be elicited by a single stimulus (e.g., a brief train of action potentials), the pH changes, particularly in the extracellular space, may be multiphasic. These changes in extracellular pH (pH_e) may, in turn, affect the electrical and synaptic activity of neurons.

The plasma membranes of neurons and glial cells contain a variety of acid/base-transporting proteins, most of them counter- or co-transporters with sodium and/or chloride as the co- or counterion for protons and bicarbonate (Chapter 12, this volume). In general, influx or extrusion of protons or bicarbonate into or out of the cells always changes the pH_e. The magnitudes of the changes depend on four main variables: (*1*) the amount of acid/base flux across the cell membranes, (*2*) the volume of the ECS, (*3*) the buffering power of the ECS fluid, and (*4*) the removal of acid/base equivalents from the ECS.

All four of these variables affect neuronal functioning, and hence information processing, by modulating the magnitude and kinetics of the pH_e transients. For a given initial acid/base flux, the magnitude of the pH_e change is greater if the extracellular domain is small and has weak buffering power (see below), and attenuated if the effective extracellular volume is large and the buffering power is greater. The effectiveness of pH_e regulation, that is, acid/base fluxes that counteract shifts in pH_e, depends on, among other factors, the density and activity of acid/base transporters on adjacent cell membranes. Extracellular pH shifts can be rapid, lasting only for seconds, and may be signals rather than only a result of inadequate homeostatic acid/base regulation (see also Deitmer and Rose, 1996).

Changes in pH_e modify processes at the extracellular surface of the cells, resulting in the modulation of neuronal excitability, synaptic transmission, and a variety of membrane carriers. For instance, glutamate receptors of the NMDA type are highly sensitive to extracellular pH, and synaptic transmission via these receptors is suppressed if pH_e falls below 7.0 (Traynelis and Cull-Candy, 1990). Extracellular acidification may itself gate acid-sensing ion channels (ASICs, a family of Na^+ channels that contribute to synaptic plasticity in the central nervous system (Wemmie et al., 2002). Acid-sensing ion channel null mice had reduced excitatory postsynaptic potentials and NMDA receptor activation. Moreover, loss of ASICs impaired hippocampal long-term potentiation, and ASIC null mice displayed defective spatial learning. In addition, ASICs affect a range of sensory functions that includes perception of gentle touch, harsh touch, heat, sour taste, and pain (Bianchi and Driscoll, 2002). Since synaptic vesicles are acidic (pH 5.6; Miesenbock et al., 1998), a transient local fall of pH_e is associated with synaptic transmission, and such pH changes at the synapse might influence synaptic transmission. However, available techniques are inadequte to monitor the magnitude and time course of the pH changes in the small volume of synaptic domains.

Measuring pH in Cells and Tissues

In order to understand the mechanisms of the acid and alkaline transients, it is often necessary to monitor pH in all three compartments: neurons, ECSs, and glial cells. The pH shifts in the ECSs are usually approximate mirror images of intracellular pH changes. However, it is usually difficult to make an accurate quantitative inverse match, partly because the volumes and spatial distributions of the cells involved are uncertain and because H^+ ions effectively diffuse very rapidly through extracellular clefts. In addition, we still know little about intracellular handling of H^+, particularly the capacity and time courses of sequestration of H^+ by intracellular organelles (cf. Thomas, 2002).

The Distribution of Acid and Base in the Brain

The intracellular pH value (pH_i) of "resting" neurons and astrocytes is between 6.8 and 7.5, that is, between 30 and 160 nM H^+. In isolated cells and tissues, pH_i depends on whether the preparation is bathed in a solution buffered with a standard buffer, such as HEPES, or with CO_2 and HCO_3^-. Carbon dioxide, the end product of oxidative metabolism, reacts reversibly with water to release a proton: $CO_2 + H_2O \longleftrightarrow HCO_3^- + H^+$. Neurons are the main consumers of adenosine triphosphate (ATP), and therefore the main producers of CO_2 (Attwell and Laughlin, 2001). This CO_2 can leave the neuron by diffusion through the plasma membrane, and the efflux increases when the neuron is active. The link between CO_2 production and pH is the CO_2/HCO_3 buffer system, which plays a major role both intra- and extracellularly (see below).

Addition of CO_2/HCO_3^- to the milieu of neurons usually lowers their pH_i by 0.2–0.4 pH unit. In glial cells, the addition CO_2/HCO_3^- rarely lowers pH_i and indeed may raise it by up to 0.3 pH unit, as in the leech giant glial cell (Deitmer and Schlue, 1987). This is due to activation of the Na^+-HCO_3^- cotransporter (NBC, see below). The pH_e in nervous tissue is usually in the range of 7.1 to 7.3. (lower than the usual 7.4 of blood). This means that there is often only a small chemical gradient of H^+ concentration, if any, across the cell membranes of resting neurons and glial cells. The main driving force of H^+ from the ECS to the cell interior is the negative membrane potential.

Buffer Capacities of Different Compartments

Although free H^+ concentrations are in the nanomolar range, the high buffering capacity of cells provides a reservoir of acid equivalents in the millimolar range. In other words, there is a pool of protons in rapid exchange between buffer sites and free solution, some 10^5 protons being buffered for each one in solution. The chemical buffering capacity (or buffering power) of a compartment is denoted by β in mM and defined as the concentration β (in mM) of a strong acid (or base) whose addition to a system causes a pH change of 1 pH unit. The value β in cells is highly dependent on the whether CO_2/HCO_3^- is present. In experiments on isolated tissues or cells, β is usually measured either in the nominal absence of CO_2/HCO_3^- (the *intrinsic buffer capacity*, β_i) or in the presence of CO_2/HCO_3^-, providing the *total buffer capacity*, β_t. The difference between β_t and β_i gives the *bicarbonate-dependent buffer capacity*, β_{CO2}.

For neurons and glial cells, β_i has been measured as 10–40 mM, while β_{CO2}, which is approximately 2.3 times the HCO_3^- concentration (Roos and Boron, 1981), is between 14 mM (corresponding to 6 mM HCO_3^- at a pH_i of 6.8) and 40 mM (corresponding to 17 mM HCO_3 at a pH_i of 7.2) in the presence of 5% CO_2. Hence, β_t is usually between 24 and 80 mM in neural cells.

The CO_2/HCO_3^- system contributes a large part of the pH buffering in cells and tissues. Its effectiveness is dependent on the activity of carbonic anhydrase (CA), which catalyzes the reaction $CO_2 + H_2O \longleftrightarrow HCO_3^- + H^+$. In the absence of enzyme the reaction is very slow, but CA can accelerate it by a factor of 300. Within the vertebrate nervous system CA is present primarily in oligodendrocytes (Cammer, 1984; Tong et al., 2000) and astrocytes (Giacobini, 1962; Sapirstein et al., 1984). Due to the rapid conversion of CO_2 to H^+ and HCO_3^- by CA, glial cells may act as sinks for CO_2 (Newman, 1994; Deitmer and Rose, 1996), resulting in a rise of H^+ and HCO_3^-.

Little is known about the extracellular intrinsic buffer capacity; estimates range from 3 to 10 mM (Chesler et al., 1994; Deitmer and Rose, 1996). Thus, not only are the ECSs, and therefore the buffer reservoir, small, but also the buffer capacity per unit volume appears to be considerably lower than it is inside cells. These two factors render the ECS a domain of potentially much larger pH changes than the cytosol of the cells. Changes of pH_e following the addition of a weak acid or ammonium have been used to estimate the relative buffer capacity in the ECS in different buffer solutions (Fig. 26.4). In the presence of the CA inhibitor ethoxyzolamide, the increase in buffer capacity due to CO_2/HCO_3^- is greatly reduced (Fig. 26.4), indicating that CA activity enhances not only intracellular but also extracellular buffer capacity and that the buffer capacity contributed by the CO_2/HCO_3^- buffer system is largely dependent on CA activity.

On the other hand, the *recovery* from pH_e changes depends mainly on acid/base transport across the cell membranes and may therefore also reflect intracellular pH changes. Thus, the cells may sense pH_i changes in neighboring cells by the pH changes in the ECS. When trying to measure buffering power, it is often assumed that the pH changes truly reflect the H^+ binding capacity (*chemical buffering*) of a cellular or extracellular compartment. However, this may not be so, because the time course of monitoring pH is presumably slow not only in relation to chemical buffering (which is very fast), but also with respect to the transport of acid/base equivalents via the plasma membrane and across organellar membranes in the cells (*sequestration*). Hence, it must be expected that "immediate" pH changes, as are used to determine buffer capacity, are affected not only by chemical buffering but also by transport and sequestration processes. Therefore, the term *H muffling* has been introduced; it includes all fast processes that contribute to the damping of measured pH changes and is usually denoted as *physiological buffering* or *apparent buffer capacity*, to distinguish it from pure chemical buffering, which probably cannot be measured accurately in living cells and tissues (Thomas et al., 1991). In the leech central nervous system, uptake of glutamate into the glial cells (see below) was enhanced in the presence of the CO_2/HCO_3^- buffer system, presumably due to increased H^+ muffling, part of which was due to fast acid/base shuttling by the sodium-bicarbonate cotransporter (NBC) (Deitmer and Schneider, 2000). We have retained the term *buffering* here,

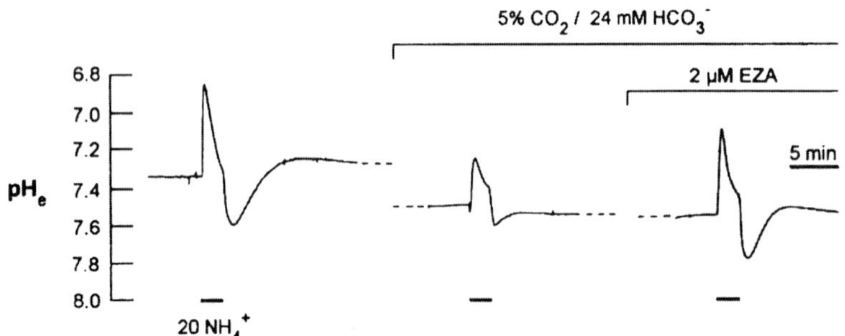

FIGURE 26.4 CO_2/HCO_3^- increases buffering capacity of extracellular space. The records show extracellular pH (acid upward) in a leech ganglion. *First panel*: In HEPES-buffered saline with no added HCO_3^-, a bath application of 20 mM NH_4Cl caused a large, rapid acidification followed by recovery. When the ammonium was removed, there was an alkaline transient. *Second panel*: When CO_2/HCO_3^- was added, the ammonium-induced changes in pH_e were buffered much more effectively. *Third panel*: Inhibition of the endogenous enzyme carbonic anhydrase by ethoxyzolamide (2 μM) reversed most of the buffering effect of CO_2/HCO_3^-. (From Deitmer, 1992.)

because it has been used so widely in physiology and cell biology. It is important to be aware, however, of the limits to measuring true chemical buffering in tissues with the tools available.

pH Changes Related to Neuronal Activity

Studies on the central nervous systems of vertebrates and invertebrates have shown that neuronal activity leads to extra- and intracellular pH changes (Fig. 26.5; Deitmer and Rose, 1996). These consist of mono- or multiphasic pH shifts indicating that they might originate from multiple sources and/or via multiple processes (Fig. 26.6). Due to the increase in extracellular potassium concentration (see the section "Changes in Extracellular [K^+] as Signals") and to excitatory neurotransmitters, glial cells may respond to the activity of neighboring neurons with a substantial depolarization of their cell membrane, accompanied by an intracellular alkalinization. In the rat cortex, the stimulus-evoked glial depolarization is accompanied by an intracellular alkalinization of astrocytes, the amplitude of which is dependent on the amplitude of the glial de-

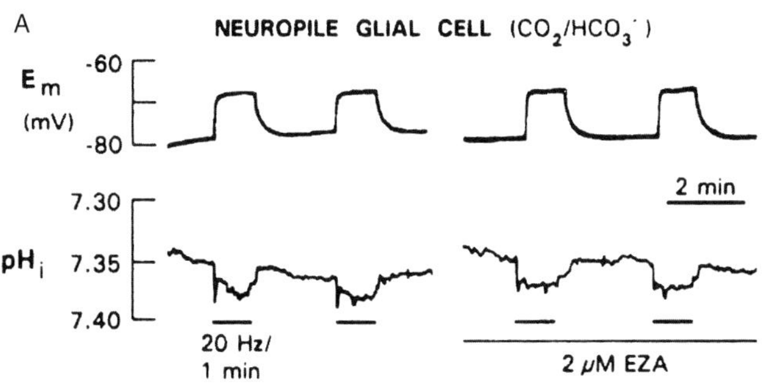

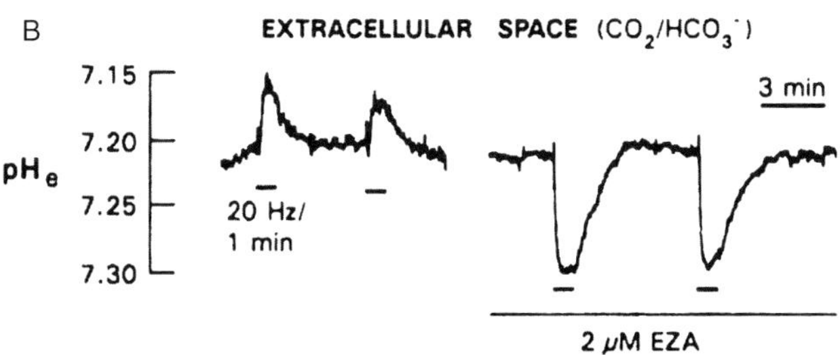

FIGURE 26.5 Intraglial and extracellular pH changes in leech ganglion following side nerve stimulation before and after inhibition of carbonic anhydrase. *A*. Membrane potential (*upper traces*) and intracellular pH (*lower traces*) were measured with a double-barreled, pH-sensitive microelectrode in a leech neuropile glial cell in saline buffered with 5% CO_2/24 mM HCO_3^-. Stimulation of a ganglionic side nerve (*bar*) caused depolarization and alkalinization. In the presence of 2 μM ethoxyzolamide (EZA) the change in pH_i was not altered. *B*. A similar experiment, but with the electrode tip in extracellular space. Ethoxyzolamide dramatically converted the stimulus-induced acid transient to a large alkalinization. (From Rose and Deitmer, 1995b.)

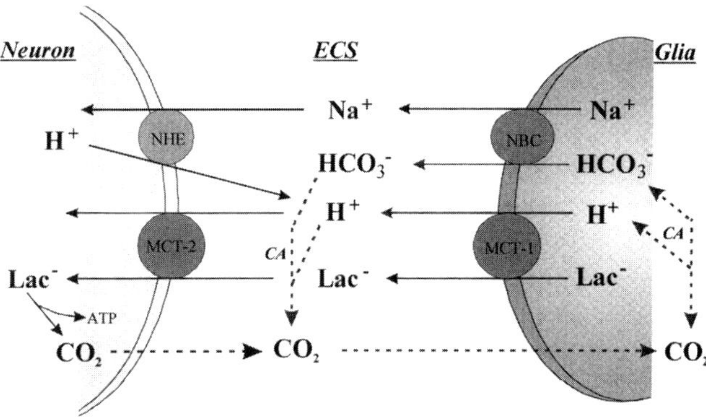

FIGURE 26.6 Scheme of acid-base transport and metabolic shuttling between neurons and glial cells. Diagram illustrating some possibly related and functionally linked acid base transporters across the cell membrane of a neuron (*left*) and a glial cell (*right*) in the brain. CO_2 diffusing out of active neurons into glial cells is converted into H^+ and HCO_3^-, catalyzed by carbonic anhydrase (CA). Intraglial protons are used to drive lactate out of the glial cell via the monocarboxylate transporter (MCT-1), and intraglial bicarbonate activates the sodium-bicarbonate cotransporter (NBC). Lactate is taken up by the neuron via MCT-2 by cotransport with a proton, which is extruded from the neuron via sodium-hydrogen exchange (NHE). In the neuron, lactate is metabolized to give adenosine triphosphate and CO_2. The possibility of CO_2 recycling is indicated by the formation of CO_2, catalyzed by CA in the extracellular space (ECS), and the subsequent diffusion of CO_2 back into the glial cell. High activity of CA would ensure rapid equilibrium of CO_2, H^+, and HCO_3^-, and hence the continuous flow of CO_2 into glial cells. This would result in net secretion of sodium and lactate from glial cells into the ECS. (From Deitmer, 2002.)

polarization (Chesler and Kraig, 1989). In leech ganglion, nerve stimulation, which elicits an intraglial alkalinization, simultaneously evokes an acid transient in the ECS (Fig. 26.5*A*,*B*). While the intraglial pH shift is unaffected by the CA inhibitor ethoxyzolamide, the extracellular acid transient is converted to a large alkaline transient following inhibition of CA activity (Fig. 26.5*A*,*B*; Rose and Deitmer, 1995b). This suggests that these pH_e changes are greatly affected by the activity of extracellular and/or intracellular CA.

Several lines of evidence suggest that the depolarization-induced alkalinization of glial cells in both vertebrate and invertebrate preparations is due to inward transport of bicarbonate via the electrogenic NBC activated by the K^+-induced membrane depolarization (Deitmer and Szatkowski, 1990; Grichtchenko and Chesler, 1994; Pappas and Ransom, 1994; Bevensee et al., 1997). The glial NBC is electrogenic and, like the mammalian renal NBC (Heyer et al., 1999), cotransports one sodium ion with two bicarbonate ions (Deitmer and Schlue, 1989; Deitmer and Schneider, 1995). The transport can operate in both directions, depending on the intra- and extracellular pH (and bicarbonate), the intracellular Na^+ concentration, and the membrane potential. *In situ* hybridization has shown expression of NBC mRNA throughout the rat central nervous system in both glial cells and neurons, (Schmitt et al., 2000; Giffard et al., 2000) but functional operation of the NBC has so far been reported only in glial cells.

In the cortex, the stimulus-induced glial alkaline shift was inhibited in Na^+-free saline and turned into a small acidification when the K^+-induced depolarization was reduced by the application of Ba^{2+} (Chesler and Kraig, 1989; Grichtchenko and Chesler, 1994). The stimulus-induced alkalinization of the leech giant glial cell was turned into an acidification by all experimental protocols suppressing the activation of the NBC: (*1*) by voltage-clamping the glial cell (Rose and Deitmer, 1994), (*2*) in the presence of the stilbene (DIDS), and (*3*) in CO_2,HCO_3^--free saline (Rose and Deitmer, 1995a, 1995b). Suppressing the glial depolarization during nerve root stimulation not only reversed the intraglial pH change but also influenced the pH_e transient (Rose and Deitmer, 1994).

Glial cells have a variety of transmitter receptors coupled to ion channels (Seifert and Steinhauser, 2001; Chapter 10, this volume). The activation of these transmitter receptors can induce pH transients in nervous systems, which either emerge directly in response to the action of the neurotransmitters themselves by both HCO_3^--dependent and -independent mechanisms or are secondary to membrane potential changes (Chesler and Kaila, 1992; Munsch and Deitmer, 1994). The majority of available data concern pH changes induced by GABA and glutamate; the effects of other transmitters, such as acetylcholine or serotonin, on extra- or intracellular pH in the nervous system have been investigated in only a few systems.

Glial Modulation of the Extracellular pH

Glial cells possess an array of mechanisms that regulate and change intraglial pH as well as the pH in the ECS (Fig. 26.6). Under normal physiological conditions, most pH_e transients are expected to be very brief (milliseconds to seconds) and local (e.g., in synaptic domains). They may be considerably larger in amplitude and faster *in vivo* compared to those recorded with invasive recording techniques such as pH microelectrodes.

Astrocyte membranes contain several transport systems, which transport protons or bicarbonate out of the cell. Bicarbonate can be removed either by a Cl^-/HCO_3^- exchanger, the classical anion exchange protein that reverses intracellular alkalinization, or by the NBC (see above), which probably has the greatest impact on regulating pH in most glial cells, equal to or even more than that of the ubiquitous sodium-hydrogen exchanger (NHE). The amiloride-sensitive NHE is the principal acid remover from most types of cell, including neurons, and, with some exceptions, glial cells. It is activated by intracellular acidosis and inhibited by extracellular acidosis, as might occur, for example, during hypoxia or ischemia (Siesjo et al., 1993; Glunde et al., 2002). Protons can also be extruded in cotransport with organic anions, such as lactate, pyruvate, and other monocarboxylates, via the monocarboxylate transporter (MCT; see Halestrap and Price, 1999). Of the different isoforms of MCT, in the mammalian brain MCT1 has been found primarily in astrocytes and MCT2 in neurons (Bröer et al., 1997, 1998). The different substrate affinities favor release of lactate/H^+ by astrocytes and uptake by neurons (Fig. 26.6). While the extrusion of lactate from astrocytes tends to acidify the ECS, this acidification would be canceled if the neurons took up the lactate. Cooperation of MCTs and NBC in the glial membrane may indeed enhance the flow from glial cells to neurons (Fig. 26.6; Deitmer, 2002; Becker et al., 2004).

The Na^+-HCO_3^- cotransporter has been described in nearly all types of macroglial cells, including astrocytes, oligodendrocytes, Schwann cells, and retinal Müller glial cells (see Deitmer and Rose, 1996), and has been summarized above (see the section "pH Changes Related to Neuronal Activity"). The glial NBC may well be one mechanism responsible for neurotransmitter-induced extracellular pH changes: due to ionotropic receptors for the excitatory neurotransmitter glutamate, glial cells would depolarize and alkalinize following depolarization-induced activation of inward-moving NBC. The same transport would remove base equivalents from the ECS and hence lower extracellular pH.

Another group of acid/base transporting glial carriers are the neurotransmitter uptake systems. In particular those for glutamate uptake [the family of excitatory amino acid transporters (EAAT) (see Danbolt, 2001)], driven mainly by the Na^+ gradient, also transport H^+ into the cell, and hence remove acid equivalents from the ECS. Two of the five EAATs, GLT-1 and the glutamate/aspartate transporter (GLAST), are expressed primarily by glial cells, in particular at astrocytic processes near synaptic domains (Chaudhry et al., 1995). Since acid equivalents pour into the synaptic cleft during the exocytosis of acidic transmitter vesicles (Miesenbock et al., 1998), the uptake of H^+ via the EAAT may attenuate or counteract an extracellular acidosis associated with synaptic transmitter release and glial NBC-mediated loss of extracellular base equivalents (see above). In addition, the inward gradient of H^+ may increase inward transport of glutamate, though much less than the three sodium ions involved in a glutamate transport cycle (Zerangue and Kavanaugh, 1996). Overall, the ion channels, ligand channels, and acid/base-coupled carriers in both glial cells and neurons, acting in combination, are probably the main determinants of the extracellular pH changes during and after neuronal activity.

ACKNOWLEDGMENTS

We thank the following copyright holders for permission to reproduce figures: Elsevier, Box 1, Figs. 26.1*B*,*C*; Blackwell Publishing, Figs. 26.2*D*, 26.6; *Journal of Physiology*, Fig. 26.1*A*; Wiley, Fig. 26.4; Nature Publishing Group, Fig. 26.3*A*,*B*; the American Physiological Society, Fig. 26.5.

ABBREVIATIONS

Amt/MEP/Rh	Ammonium transporter/ methylammonium permeases/Rhesus
ASIC	acid-sensing ion channel
CA	carbonic anhydrase
DIDS	4,4′-diisothiocyanatostilbene-2,2′-disulfonic acid
EAT	excitatory amino acid transporter
ECS	extracellular space
GABA	γ-aminobutyric acid
GLAST	glutamate/aspartate transporter
GLT-1	glutamate transporter-1
ISM	ion-selective microelectrode
MCT	monocarboxylic acid transporter
NBC	sodium-bicarbonate cotransporter
NMDA	*N*-methyl-*D*-aspartate
NHE	sodium/hydrogen exchanger
TCA	tricarboxylic acid
TMA	tetramethylammonium

Subscripts for buffering capacity

- i: intrinsic
- t: total

Subscripts for pH and [K^+]

- e: extracellular
- g: glial
- i: intracellular

REFERENCES

Amédée, T., Robert, A., and Coles, J.A. (1997) Potassium homeostasis and glial energy metabolism. *Glia* 21:46–55.

Anis, Y., Nurnberg, B., Visochek, L., Reiss, N., Naor, Z., and Cohen-Armon, M. (1999) Activation of G_o-proteins by membrane depolarization traced by in situ photoaffinity labeling of $G_{\alpha o}$-proteins with [α^{32}P]GTP-azidoanilide. *J. Biol. Chem.* 274:7431–7440.

Attwell, D. and Laughlin, S.B. (2001) An energy budget for signaling in the grey matter of the brain. *J. Cereb. Blood Flow Metab.* 21:1133–1145.

Ballanyi, K., Grafe, P., Serve, G.. and Schlue, W.R. (1990) Electrophysiological measurements of volume changes in leech neuropile glial cells. *Glia* 3:151–158.

Ballanyi, K., Grafe, P., and ten Bruggencate, G. (1987) Ion activities and potassium uptake mechanisms of glial cells in guinea-pig olfactory cortex slices. *J. Physiol.* 382:159–174.

Ballanyi, K. and Schlue, W.R. (1990) Intracellular chloride activity in glial cells of the leech central nervous system. *J. Physiol.* 420: 325–336.

Becker, H., Bröer, S., and Deitmer, J.W. (2004) Facilitated lactate transport by MCT1 when coexpressed with the sodium bicarbonate cotransporter (NBC) in Xenopus oocytes. *Biophys. J.* 86:235–247.

Benjamin, A. and Quastel, J. (1975) Metabolism of amino acids and ammonia in rat brain cortex slices in vitro: a possible role of ammonia in brain function. *J. Neurochem.* 25:197–206.

Bevensee, M.O., Apkon, M., and Boron, W.F. (1997) Intracellular pH regulation in cultured astrocytes from rat hippocampus. II. Electrogenic Na/HCO_3 cotransport. *J. Gen. Physiol.* 110:467–483.

Bianchi, L. and Driscoll, M. (2002) Protons at the gate: DEG/ENaC ion channels help us feel and remember. *Neuron* 34:337–340.

Bröer, A., Rahman, B., Pellegri, G., Pellerin, L., Martin, J.L., Verleysdonk, S., Hamprecht, B. and Magistretti, P.J. (1997) Comparison of lactate transport in astroglial cells and monocarboxylate transporter 1 (MCT 1) expressing *Xenopus laevis* oocytes. Expression of two different monocarboxylate transporters in astroglial cells and neurons. *J. Biol. Chem.* 272:30096–30102.

Bröer, S., Schneider, H.P., Bröer, A., Rahman, B., Hamprecht, B., and Deitmer, J.W. (1998) Characterization of the monocarboxylate transporter 1 expressed in *Xenopus laevis* oocytes by changes in cytosolic pH. *Biochem. J.* 333:167–174.

Cammer, W. (1984) Carbonic anhydrase in oligodendrocytes and myelin in the central nervous system. *Ann. NY Acad. Sci.* 429:494–497.

Chaudhry, F.A., Lehre, K.P., van Lookeren Campagne, M., Ottersen, O.P., Danbolt, N.C., and Storm-Mathisen, J. (1995) Glutamate transporters in glial plasma membranes: highly differentiated localizations revealed by quantitative ultrastructural immunocytochemistry. *Neuron* 15:711–720.

Chesler, M., Chen, J.C., and Kraig, R.P. (1994) Determination of extracellular bicarbonate and carbon dioxide concentrations in brain slices using carbonate and pH-selective microelectrodes. *J. Neurosci. Meth.* 53:129–136.

Chesler, M. and Kaila, K. (1992) Modulation of pH by neuronal activity. *Trends Neurosci.* 15:396–402.

Chesler, M. and Kraig, R.P. (1989) Intracellular pH transients of mammalian astrocytes. *J. Neurosci.* 9:2011–2019.

Coles, J.A. and Orkand, R.K. (1983) Modification of potassium movement through the retina of the drone (*Apis mellifera* ♂) by glial uptake. *J. Physiol.* 340:157–174.

Coles, J.A. and Orkand, R.K. (1985) Changes in sodium activity during light stimulation in photoreceptors, glia and extracellular space in drone retina. *J. Physiol.* 362:415–435.

Coles, J.A., Orkand, R.K., and Yamate, C. (1989) Chloride enters glial cells and photoreceptors in response to light stimulation in the retina of the honey bee drone. *Glia* 2:287–297.

Coles, J.A., Orkand, R.K., Yamate, C.L., and Tsacopoulos, M. (1986) Free concentrations of Na, K and Cl in the retina of the honeybee drone: stimulus-induced redistribution and homeostasis. *Ann. NY Acad. Sci.* 481:303–317.

Coles, J.A. and Poulain, D.A. (1991) Extracellular K^+ in the supraoptic nucleus of the rat during reflex bursting activity by oxytocin neurones. *J. Physiol.* 439:383–409.

Danbolt, N.C. (2001) Glutamate uptake. *Prog. Neurobiol.* 65:1–105.

Deitmer, J.W. (1992) Evidence for glial control of extracellular pH in the leech central nervous system. *Glia* 5:43–47.

Deitmer, J.W. (2002) A role for CO_2 and bicarbonate transporters in metabolic exchanges in the brain. *J. Neurochem.* 80:721–726.

Deitmer, J.W. and Rose, C. (1996) pH regulation and proton signalling by glial cells. *Prog. Neurobiol.* 48:73–103.

Deitmer, J.W. and Schlue, W.R. (1987) The regulation of intracellular pH by identified glial cells and neurones in the central nervous system of the leech. *J. Physiol.* 388:261–283.

Deitmer, J.W. and Schlue, W.R. (1989) An inwardly directed electrogenic sodium-bicarbonate co-transport in leech glial cells. *J. Physiol.* 411:179–194.

Deitmer, J.W. and Schneider, H.P. (1995) Voltage-dependent clamp of intracellular pH of identified leech glial cells. *J. Physiol.* 485:157–166.

Deitmer, J.W. and Schneider, H.P. (2000) Enhancement of glutamate uptake transport by CO_2/bicarbonate in the leech giant glial cell. *Glia* 30:392–400.

Deitmer, J.W. and Szatkowski, M. (1990) Membrane potential dependence of intracellular pH regulation by identified glial cells in the leech central nervous system. *J. Physiol.* 421:617–631.

Dietzel, I., Heinemann, U., Hofmeier, G., and Lux, H.D. (1980) Transient changes in the size of the extracellular space in the sensorimotor cortex of cats in relation to stimulus-induced changes in potassium concentration. *Exp. Brain Res.* 40:432–439.

Dietzel, I., Heinemann, U., and Lux, H.D. (1989) Relations between slow extracellular potential changes, glial potassium buffering, and electrolyte and cellular volume changes during neuronal hyperactivity in cat brain. *Glia* 2:25–44.

Erulkar, S.D. and Weight, F.F. (1977) Extracellular potassium and trasmitter release at the giant synapse of squid. *J. Physiol.* 266: 209–218.

Evequoz-Mercier, V. and Tsacopoulos, M. (1991) The light-induced increase of carbohydrate metabolism in glial cells of the honeybee retina is not mediated by K+ movement nor by cAMP. *J. Gen. Physiol.* 98:497–515.

Frankenhaeuser, B. and Hodgkin, A.L. (1956) After-effects of impulses in the giant nerve fibres of *Loligo*. *J. Physiol.* 131:341–376.

Giacobini, E. (1962) A cytochemical study of the localization of carbonic anhydrase in the nervous system. *J. Neurochem.* 9:169–177.

Giffard, R.G., Papadopoulos, M.C., van Hooft, J.A., Xu, L., Giuffrida, R., and Monyer, H. (2000) The electrogenic sodium bicarbonate cotransporter: developmental expression in rat brain and possible role in acid vulnerability. *J. Neurosci.* 20:1001–1008.

Glunde, K., Dussmann, H., Juretschke, H.P., and Leibfritz, D. (2002) Na^+/H^+ exchange subtype 1 inhibition during extracellular acidification and hypoxia in glioma cells. *J. Neurochem.* 80:36–44.

Grichtchenko, II and Chesler, M. (1994) Depolarization-induced alkalinization of astrocytes in gliotic hippocampal slices. *Neuroscience* 62:1071–1078.

Grillner, S., Wallen, P., Hill, R., Cangiano, L., and El Manira, A. (2001) Ion channels of importance for the locomotor pattern generation in the lamprey brainstem–spinal cord. *J. Physiol.* 533:23–30.

Hablitz, J.J. and Heinemann, U. (1987) Extracellular K^+ and Ca^{2+} changes during epileptiform discharges in the immature rat neocortex. *Dev. Brain Res.* 36:299–303.

Halestrap, A.P. and Price, N.T. (1999) The proton-linked monocarboxylate transporter (MCT) family: structure, function and regulation. *Biochem. J.* 343:281–299.

Hansen, A.J. and Zeuthen, T. (1981) Extracellular ion concentrations during spreading depression and ischemia in the rat brain cortex. *Acta Physiol. Scand.* 113:437–445.

Heinemann, U. and Lux, H.D. (1977) Ceiling of stimulus induced rises in extracellular potassium concentration in the cerebral cortex of cat. *Brain Res.* 120:231–249.

Heyer, M., Muller-Berger, S., Romero, M.F., Boron, W.F., and Fromter, E. (1999) Stoichiometry of the rat kidney Na^+-HCO_3^- cotransporter expressed in *Xenopus laevis* oocytes. *Pflügers Arch.* 438:322–329.

Holthoff, K. and Witte, O.W. (2000) Directed spatial potassium redistribution in rat neocortex. *Glia* 29:288–292.

Huang, C.H. and Liu, P.Z. (2001) New insights into the Rh superfamily of genes and proteins in erythroid cells and nonerythroid tissues. *Blood Cells Mol. Dis.* 27:90–101.

James, M.F., Smith, J.M., Boniface, S.J., Huang, C.L., and Leslie, R.A. (2001) Cortical spreading depression and migraine: new insights from imaging? *Trends Neurosci.* 24:266–271.

Kivi, A., Lehmann, T.N., Kovacs, R., Eilers, A., Jauch, R., Meencke, H.J., von Deimling, A., Heinemann, U., and Gabriel, S. (2000) Effects of barium on stimulus-induced rises of $[K^+]_o$ in human epileptic non-sclerotic and sclerotic hippocampal area CA1. *Eur. J. Neurosci.* 12:2039–2048.

Kofuji, P., Ceelen, P., Zahs, K.R., Surbeck, L.W., Lester, H.A., and Newman, E.A. (2000) Genetic inactivation of an inwardly rectifying potassium channel (Kir4.1 subunit) in mice: phenotypic impact in retina. *J. Neurosci.* 20:5733–5740.

Kraig, R.P. and Nicholson, C. (1978) Extracellular ionic variations during spreading depression. *Neuroscience* 3:1045–1059.

Marcaggi, P. and Coles, J.A. (2001) Ammonium in nervous tissue: transport across cell membranes and fluxes from neurons to glial cells. *Prog. Neurobiol.* 64:157–183.

Marcaggi, P., Jeanne, M., and Coles, J.A. (2004) Neuron-glial trafficking of NH_4^+ and K^+: separate routes of uptake into glial cells of bee retina. *Eur. J. Neurosci.* 19:966–976.

Martinez-Pinna, J., Tolhurst, G., Gurung, I.S., Vandenberg, J.I., and Mahaut-Smith, M.P. (2004) Sensitivity limits for voltage control of P2Y receptor-evoked Ca^{2+} mobilization in the rat megakaryocyte. *J. Physiol. (Lond.)* 555:61–70.

Miesenbock, G., De Angelis, D.A., and Rothman, J.E. (1998) Visualizing secretion and synaptic transmission with pH-sensitive green fluorescent proteins. *Nature* 394:192–195.

Moghaddam, B. and Adams, R.N. (1987) Regional differences in the resting extracellular potassium levels of rat brain. *Brain Res.* 406:337–340.

Munsch, T. and Deitmer, J.W. (1994) Sodium-bicarbonate cotransport current in identified leech glial cells. *J. Physiol.* 474:43–53.

Munsch, T., Reusch, M., and Deitmer, J.W. (1995) Intracellular chloride activity of leech neurones and glial cells in physiological, low chloride saline. *J. Comp. Physiol. A* 176:273–280.

Mutsaga, N., Schuette, W.H., and Lewis, D.V. (1976) The contribution of local blood flow to the rapid clearance of potassium from the cortical extracellular space. *Brain Res.* 406:337–340.

Nagaraja, T.N. and Brookes, N. (1998) Intracellular acidification induced by passive and active transport of ammonium ions in astrocytes. *Am. J. Physiol.* 274:C883–C891.

Nedergaard, M. and Hansen, A.J. (1993) Characterization of cortical depolarizations evoked in focal cerebral ischemia. *J. Cereb. Blood Flow Metab.* 13:568–574.

Newman, E.A. (1986) High potassium conductance in astrocyte endfeet. *Science* 233:453–454.

Newman, E.A. (1994) A physiological measure of carbonic anhydrase in Muller cells. *Glia* 11:291–299.

Newman, E.A., Frambach, D.A., and Odette, L.L. (1984) Control of extracellular potassium levels by retinal glial cell K^+ siphoning. *Science* 225:1174–1175.

Nicholson, C. and Sykova, E. (1998) Extracellular space structure revealed by diffusion analysis. *Trends Neurosci.* 21:207–215.

Orkand, R.K. (1986) Introductory remarks: glial-interstitial fluid exchange. *Ann. NY Acad. Sci.* 481:269–272.

Orkand, R.K., Nicholls, J.G., and Kuffler, S.W. (1966) Effects of nerve impulses on the membrane potential of glial cells in the central nervous system of amphibia. *J. Neurophysiol.* 29:788–806.

Pappas, C.A. and Ransom, B.R. (1994) Depolarization-induced alkalinization (DIA) in rat hippocampal astrocytes. *J. Neurophysiol.* 72:2816–2826.

Poitry, S., Poitry-Yamate, C.L., Ueberfeld, J., MacLeish, P.R., and Tsacopoulos, M. (2000) Mechanisms of glutamate metabolic signaling in retinal glial (Müller) cells. *J. Neurosci.* 20:1809–1821.

Ransom, C.B., Ransom, B.R., and Sontheimer, H. (2000) Activity-dependent extracellular K^+ accumulation in rat optic nerve: the role of glial and axonal Na^+ pumps. *J. Physiol.* 522:427–442.

Roos, A. and Boron, W.F. (1981) Intracellular pH. *Physiol. Rev.* 61:296–434.

Rose, C.R. and Deitmer, J.W. (1994) Evidence that glial cells modulate extracellular pH transients induced by neuronal activity in the leech central nervous system. *J. Physiol.* 481:1–5.

Rose, C.R. and Deitmer, J.W. (1995a) Stimulus-evoked changes of extra- and intracellular pH in the leech central nervous system. I. Bicarbonate dependence. *J. Neurophysiol.* 73:125–131.

Rose, C.R. and Deitmer, J.W. (1995b) Stimulus-evoked changes of extra- and intracellular pH in the leech central nervous system. II. Mechanisms and maintenance of pH homeostasis. *J. Neurophysiol.* 73:132–140.

Rose, C.R. and Ransom, B.R. (1997) Regulation of intracellular sodium in cultured rat hippocampal neurones. *J. Physiol.* 499:573–587.

Rossi, D.J., Oshima, T., and Attwell, D. (2000) Glutamate release in severe brain ischaemia is mainly by reversed uptake. *Nature* 403:316–321.

Sapirstein, V.S., Strocchi, P., and Gilbert, J.M. (1984) Properties and function of brain carbonic anhydrase. *Ann. NY Acad. Sci.* 429: 481–493.

Schlue, W.R. and Wuttke, W. (1983) Potassium activity in leech neuropile glial cells changes with external potassium concentration. *Brain Res.* 270:368–372.

Schmitt, B.M., Berger, U.V., Douglas, R.M., Bevensee, M.O., Hediger, M.A., Haddad, G.G., and Boron, W.F. (2000) Na/HCO_3 cotransporters in rat brain: expression in glia, neurons, and choroid plexus. *J. Neurosci.* 20:6839–6848.

Seifert, G. and Steinhauser, C. (2001) Ionotropic glutamate receptors in astrocytes. *Prog. Brain Res.* 132:287–299.

Siesjo, B.K., Katsura, K., Mellergard, P., Ekholm, A., Lundgren, J., and Smith, M.L. (1993) Acidosis-related brain damage. *Prog. Brain Res.* 96:23–48.

Singer, W. and Lux, H.D. (1975) Extracellular potassium gradients and visual receptive fields in the cat striate cortex. *Brain Res.* 96:378–383.

Strong, A.J., Fabricius, M., Boutelle, M.G., Hibbins, S.J., Hopwood, S.E., Jones, R., Parkin, M.C., and Lauritzen, M. (2002) Spreading and synchronous depressions of cortical activity in acutely injured human brain. *Stroke* 33:2738–2743.

Su, G., Kintner, D.B., and Sun, D. (2002) Contribution of Na^+-K^+-Cl^- cotransporter to high-$[K^+]_o$-induced swelling and EAA release in astrocytes. *Am. J. Physiol.* 282:C1136–C1146.

Sykova, E., Czeh, G., and Kriz, N. (1980) Potassium accumulation in the frog spinal cord induced by nociceptive stimulation of the skin. *Neurosci. Lett.* 17:253–258.

Thomas, R.C. (2002) The effects of HCl and $CaCl_2$ injections on intracellular calcium and pH in voltage-clamped snail (*Helix aspersa*) neurons. *J. Gen. Physiol.* 120:567–579.

Thomas, R.C., Coles, J.A., and Deitmer, J.W. (1991) Homeostatic muffling. *Nature* 350:564.

Tong, C.K., Brion, L.P., Suarez, C., and Chesler, M. (2000) Interstitial carbonic anhydrase (CA) activity in brain is attributable to membrane-bound CA type IV. *J. Neurosci.* 20:8247–8253.

Traynelis, S.F. and Cull-Candy, S.G. (1990) Proton inhibition of *N*-methyl-D-aspartate receptors in cerebellar neurons. *Nature* 345: 347–350.

Wallen, P., Grafe, P., and Grillner, S. (1984) Phasic variations of extracellular potassium during fictive swimming in the lamprey spinal cord in vitro. *Acta Physiol. Scand.* 120:457–463.

Wemmie, J.A., Chen, J., Askwith, C.C., Hruska-Hageman, A.M., Price, M.P., Nolan, B.C., Yoder, P.G., Lamani, E., Hoshi, T., Freeman, J.H., and Welsh, M.J. (2002) The Acid-Activated Ion Channel ASIC contributes to synaptic plasticity, learning, and memory. *Neuron* 34:463–477.

Zerangue, N. and Kavanaugh, M.P. (1996) Flux coupling in a neuronal glutamate transporter. *Nature* 383:634–637.

27 Astrocyte neurotransmitter uptake

RAYMOND A. SWANSON

The action of neurotransmitters can be terminated by cleavage, diffusion, binding, or cellular uptake. Binding and uptake are performed by neurotransmitter transporters. In many cases, reuptake occurs back into the presynaptic neurons, thereby permitting neurotransmitter recycling. In other cases, uptake is accomplished by glial cells localized at or near the synapse. It is now recognized that glial cells express a variety of neurotransmitter uptake systems and that these uptake systems play a fundamental role in both normal brain function and disease states. All types of glial cells—astrocytes, oligodendrocytes, and microglia—can express transporters for neurotransmitter uptake. Astrocytes are the most numerous glial cell type and are most closely associated with synapses. Neurotransmitter uptake by astrocytes has received intensive study in recent years, but at present very little is known about uptake by microglia and oligodendrocytes. Among the several neurotransmitter uptake systems expressed by astrocytes, the uptake systems for the amino acid neurotransmitters, namely, glutamate, gamma-aminobutyric acid (GABA), and glycine, have been best characterized. Astrocyte expression of other neurotransmitter uptake systems has thus far been studied almost exclusively in cell culture preparations, and the extent to which these systems contribute to brain function remains uncertain. This chapter will emphasize astrocyte glutamate uptake since this is the most fully characterized of the astrocyte neurotransmitter uptake systems.

ASTROCYTE GLUTAMATE UPTAKE

Glutamate is the major excitatory neurotransmitter in the mammalian central nervous system (CNS). Glutamate is also a potent neurotoxin, with glutamate excitotoxicity contributing to neuronal death in stroke, amyotrophic lateral sclerosis, epilepsy, and other neurological diseases. Clearance of glutamate from the extracellular space is accomplished primarily by the actions of Na^+-dependent glutamate transporters localized on astrocytes. The astrocyte Na^+-dependent glutamate transporters were originally cloned from rat brain and termed glutamate/aspartate transporter (GLAST) and glutamate transporter (GLT-1) (Anderson and Swanson, 2000). Human homologs of GLAST and GLT-1 are termed excitatory amino acid transporter (EAAT1) and EAAT2, respectively. Other members of this glutamate transporter gene family are EAAT3, which is present on neuronal cell bodies; EAAT4, identified in cerebellar Purkinje cells; and EAAT5, expressed in retinal photoreceptors and bipolar cells (Table 27.1).

The astrocyte glutamate transporters GLAST and GLT-1 are 65% identical at the amino acid level and have similar hydropathy plots. GLT-1 is the dominant astrocyte glutamate transporter and is expressed throughout the CNS. A splice variant of GLT-1 has been identified and termed GLT-1b (Utsunomiya-Tate et al., 1997). GLT-1b is kinetically indistinguishable from GLT-1, but GLT-1b has a different pattern of expression, including expression in some adult neuron populations (Chen et al., 2002). GLAST is also diffusely expressed, but at a lower density than GLT-1 except in Bergmann glia of the cerebellum (Rothstein et al., 1994; Schmitt et al., 1997). Astrocytes facing glutamatergic synapses express much more GLAST than those facing pia or capillaries, suggesting that GLAST is important for clearing synaptically released glutamate (Chaudhry et al., 1995). While GLAST is present in rat forebrain and cerebellum at birth, GLT-1 is undetectable in brain until postnatal week 3 and reaches adult patterns by week 5.

Astrocyte expression of both GLT-1 and GLAST is strongly influenced by neurons. Astrocytes in culture exhibit upregulation of both transporters when cultured with neurons (Swanson et al., 1997), and astrocytes *in vivo* exhibit downregulation of GLAST and especially of GLT-1 after glutamatergic denervation (Levy et al., 1995) or insults that cause neuronal death (Bruhn et al., 2000).

FUNCTIONAL PROPERTIES OF THE ASTROCYTE GLUTAMATE TRANSPORTERS

Brain extracellular glutamate concentrations are normally maintained well below 2–5 μM, while astrocyte cytosolic glutamate concentrations are estimated to be 1–10 mM (Erecinska and Silver, 1990). GLT-1 and GLAST achieve glutamate uptake against this concen-

See the list of abbreviations at the end of the chapter.

TABLE 27.1 *Cloned Neurotransmitter Transporters Expressed By Astrocytes and Neurons*

Neurotransmitter	*Transporter Subtypes expressed By Astrocytes*	*Transporter Subtypes Expressed by Neurons*
Glutamate	EAAT1 (GLAST) EAAT2 (GLT-1), (GLT-1b)	EAAT3 (EAAC1), EAAT4* EAAT5,† (GLT-1b)
GABA	GAT-3 > GAT-1, GAT-2, BGT-1‡	GAT-1 > GAT-2, GAT-3
Glycine	GlyT1	GlyT2 > GlyT1
Histamine	Not determined	Not determined
Noerepinephrine	NET, OCT3	NET
Dopamine	DAT, OCT3	DAT
Serotonin	SERT	SERT
Adenosine	ENT1, ENT2	ENT1, ENT2, CNT2

Note. Transporter expression for neurotransmitters other than glutamate, GABA, and glycine have been assessed only in cell cultures. For the glutamate transporters, parentheses denote names of originally cloned rat homologs.

*Primarily expressed by cerebellar Purkinje neurons.

†Primarily expressed by retinal neurons.

‡May function as an osmoregulator rather than as a GABA transporter.

DAT: dopamine transporter; EAAC1: excitatory amino acid carrier-1; EAAT1, 2: excitatory amino acid transporter-1, -2; ENT1, 2: equilibrative nucleoside transporter 1, 2; GABA: gamma-aminobutyric acid; GAT: GABA transporter; GLAST: glutamate/aspartate transporter; GlyT1, GlyT2: glycine transporter 1, 2; NET: norepinephrine transporter; OCT3: organic cation transporter 3; SERT: serotonin transporter.

GLT-1: glutamate transporter-1

BGT-1: betaine and GABA transporter-1

CNT-1: concentrative nucleoside transporter

tration gradient by coupling the inward movement of glutamate to the movement of Na^+ and K^+ down their respective concentration gradients (Fig. 27.1). The cell membrane potential also contributes to the driving force because of the net inward movement of two positive charges with each glutamate molecule transported into the cell (Fig. 27.1). In addition to these ion fluxes that are coupled to glutamate uptake, there is an inward anion flux that is not coupled to glutamate uptake but is gated by glutamate binding to transporters. The function of this anion influx has not yet been established, although one effect may be to diminish the membrane depolarization that results from glutamate uptake (Wadiche et al., 1995a).

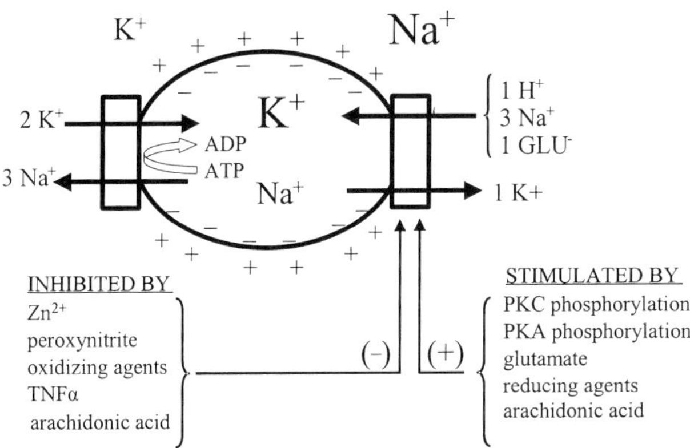

FIGURE 27.1 Schematic representation of astrocyte glutamate uptake. Uptake of glutamate (*GLU-*) (with H^+) is driven by the coupled transport of Na^+ and K^+ down their respective concentration gradients. The cell membrane potential also contributes to the uptake driving force because there is a net inward movement of positive charge with each glutamate transported. Not shown here are the anion and proton currents gated by glutamate binding to transporters. Transporter function can be regulated by several factors acting either directly or indirectly on the transporters. The specific factors modulating transporter activity differ among the different transporter subtypes (for review see Anderson and Swanson, 2000). Since the membrane potential and the transmembrane Na^+, and K^+ gradients are supported by the membrane Na^+/K^+-ATPase, uptake can also be influenced by changes in adenosine triphosphate (*ATP*) availability. The Na^+ and K^+ gradients dissipate during ATP depletion, and this leads to glutamate efflux from astrocytes by reversal of transporter-mediated uptake. ADP: adenosine diphosphate; PKA, PKC: protein kinase A, C; TNFα: tumor necrosis factor-α.

GLT-1 and GLAST appear to have similar binding affinities for glutamate, with reported K_M values ranging from 10 to 77 μM. A possible reason for this wide range is that the glutamate concentration near transporter binding sites is affected to a variable extent by transporter activity, which in turn is influenced by local transporter density and other factors. In addition to L-glutamate, both GLT-1 and GLAST can transport L-aspartate and a number of nonphysiological compounds, including D-aspartate and the competitive transporter inhibitors DL-threo-3-hydroxyaspartate (TBHA) and L-trans-2,4-pyrrolidine dicarboxylate (Anderson et al., 2001). Of note, several potent glutamate receptor excitotoxins such as *N*-methyl-D-aspartate (NMDA) and kainate are not substrates for the transporters, and the consequent slow clearance of these compounds from brain extracellular space is a major factor contributing to their neurotoxicity.

Energetics of Glutamate Uptake and Metabolism

The energetic cost of glutamate uptake is at least 1.5 adenine triphosphate (ATP) per glutamate transported, depending on the magnitude of transport-gated anion and proton currents. This expenditure has been estimated to account for a large fraction of total brain ATP turnover (Sibson et al., 1998); accordingly, one potential advantage of glutamate uptake by astrocytes is the shift in this large energy expenditure away from neurons. There has been controversy as to whether the ATP consumed by astrocyte glutamate uptake is generated selectively by glycolysis. This concept was proposed by Pellerin and Magistretti (1994), who found that glutamate uptake by cultured astrocytes induced an increase in glucose utilization and lactate production, indicative of a mismatch between rates of glycolytic and mitochondrial metabolism. However, other studies suggest that oxidative metabolism of glutamate itself provides ATP for glutamate uptake (Peng et al., 2001).

Once taken up by astrocytes, glutamate can be metabolized in several ways (Fig. 27.2), of which glutamine formation and oxidative metabolism through the tricarboxylic acid cycle are the two most important. Glutamine formation is catalyzed by glutamine synthetase, an enzyme localized to astrocytes and to a lesser extent by oligodendrocytes but absent from neurons (Martinez-Hernandez et al., 1977). A substantial portion of glutamine derived from glutamate is passively released, taken up by presynaptic neurons, and there converted back into glutamate (Broer and Brookes, 2001). Oxidative metabolism of glutamate is initiated by its conversion to 2-oxoglutarate either by glutamate dehydrogenase or by transamination. The relative fluxes through these two pathways, glutamine formation and 2-oxoglutarate formation, can vary under differing metabolic conditions. Oxidative metabolism of one glutamate molecule via 2-oxoglutarate formation and the tricarboxylic acid cycle produces more than 30 ATP, or about 15- to 20-fold more than required for glutamate uptake.

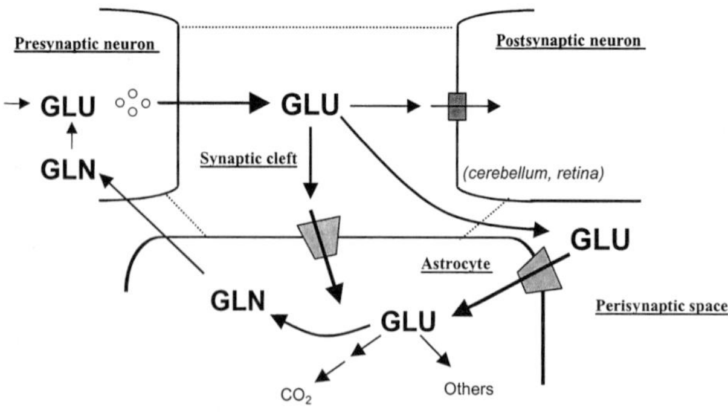

FIGURE 27.2 Fates of synaptically released glutamate. Glutamate (*GLU*) released into the synaptic cleft may be bound and taken up by astrocyte transporters within the synaptic cleft (defined here by *dotted lines*) or in the perisynaptic space. In cerebellum and retina, transporters on postsynaptic neurons also mediate a fraction of glutamate uptake. Significant uptake by presynaptic neurons has not yet been established. Glutamate taken up by astrocytes is converted in part to glutamine (*GLN*), which is cycled back to neurons for glutamate resynthesis. Glutamate may also be metabolized to CO_2 and other products.

Since glutamate transport is coupled to cotransport of 3 Na^+ plus 1 H^+ and counter-transport of 1 K^+, the equilibrium ratio of extracellular to intracellular glutamate is defined as follows: $([GLU]_e/[GLU]_i) = ([Na^+]_i/[Na^+]_e)^3 \cdot ([K^+]_e/[K^+]_i) \cdot ([H^+]_i/[H^+]_e) \exp(2VF/RT)$, where R is the gas constant, F is the Faraday constant, V is the plasma membrane potential, T is the temperature, and the subscripts i and e represent intracellular and extracellular concentrations of indicated ions, respectively. This equation indicates that a reduction in the thermodynamic driving force for uptake will result in a commensurate increase in the extracellular: intracellular glutamate ratio. Since the driving forces are all supplied by ATP hydrolysis, it follows that lowered astrocyte ATP levels will affect glutamate uptake. Studies using astrocytes in culture show that complete ATP depletion causes cessation of glutamate uptake. More moderate ATP reductions have more complex effects, in part because Na^+/K^+-ATPase activity is not a linear function of cellular ATP concentrations. Oxygen deprivation or mitochondrial inhibition, which cause only partial reductions of ATP in brain or cultured astrocytes, produce only partial reductions in glutamate transport capacity (Swanson et al., 1994). Consistent with this, brain subjected to hypoxia alone or temporary inhibition of oxidative metabolism without reduction in blood flow does not suffer excitotoxic injury (Miyamoto and Auer, 2000), suggesting that astrocyte glutamate uptake is preserved well enough to maintain extracellular glutamate below toxic levels.

The equilibrium equation also indicates that reductions in the uptake driving force result from increased extracellular K^+ or intracellular Na^+. High K^+ and low Na^+ block uptake and induce uptake reversal in whole cell patch-clamp configurations (Szatkowski et al., 1990), but surprisingly, these extracellular changes have little effect, and in some cases the opposite effect, on glutamate transport in intact astrocytes (Judd et al., 1996; Longuemare et al., 1999). This is partly because intact astrocytes respond to high K^+/low Na^+ conditions by lowering intracellular Na^+ and thereby preventing reductions in the membrane Na^+ gradient (Longuemare et al., 1999). K^+-induced alkalinization in astrocytes may also act to preserve the uptake driving force (Judd et al., 1996). However, severe ischemia and other states that cause astrocyte ATP depletion lead to elevated intracellular Na^+ levels and resultant failure of glutamate uptake (Longuemare et al., 1999).

Regulation of Astrocyte Glutamate Transporters

Astrocyte glutamate transporters are regulated by direct interaction with Zn^{2+}, arachidonic acid, and oxidants; by association with binding proteins, by phosphorylation, and by trafficking to and from the cytoplasmic membrane (Fig. 27.1). Zn^{2+} inhibits GLAST activity through interactions with histidine residues but has only weak effects on GLT-1 (Vandenberg et al., 1998). Arachidonic acid also inhibits uptake by GLAST but increases glutamate transport by GLT-1 (Zerangue et al., 1995). GLAST and GLT-1 both contain functional cysteine residues that are sensitive to oxidative formation of cystine bridges (Trotti et al., 1998). Hydrogen peroxide (H_2O_2), nitric oxide (NO), superoxide ($O_2^{-\cdot}$), and peroxynitrite can all inhibit glutamate uptake by GLT-1 and GLAST, whereas overexpression of superoxide dismutase-1 protects astrocyte glutamate transporters from inhibition by reactive oxygen species (Chen et al., 2000).

An area of increasing interest is the effect of protein-protein interactions on glutamate transporters. Proteins termed $GTRAP_{4-41}$ and $GTRAP_{4-48}$ bind to EAAT4 and activate uptake 10-fold in cotransfected cell lines. Similarly, the neuronal transporter EAAC1 is associated with $GTRAP_{18}$ and diminishes uptake by decreasing the glutamate K_M by 6-fold. A novel protein of the LIM family, Ajuba, is associated with GLT-1, and thus far represents the only such interaction for an astrocyte transporter subtype (Marie et al., 2002). Ajuba does not directly influence transport K_m or V_{max}, but may instead act as a scaffolding protein.

Both GLT-1 and GLAST have protein kinase C (PKC) phosphorylation consensus sites, but studies of PKC activation on transporter activity have yielded conflicting results (Robinson, 2002). It is likely that these differences stem in part from the fact that PKC activation has both direct and indirect effects on transporter activity. An important indirect effect is the influence of PKC activation on intracellular trafficking of glutamate transporters. Protein kinase C activation causes a rapid and large decrease in astrocyte surface expression of GLT-1 and more complex effects on GLAST (Robinson, 2002). Glutamate itself induces a rapid increase in V_{max} for glutamate uptake by initiating movement of internalized GLAST to the membrane surface (Duan et al., 1999) and surface redistribution of GLT-1 and GLAST transporters (Poitry-Yamate et al., 2002). These findings suggest that increased neuronal release of glutamate *in situ* may signal astrocytes to quickly increase local glutamate uptake capacity.

Physiological Functions of Astrocyte Glutamate Transporters

Glutamate is a potent neurotoxin, and astrocyte glutamate transporters play a critical role in maintaining brain extracellular glutamate concentrations below toxic levels. A crucial role for astrocytes is suggested by studies showing that neuronal vulnerability to glutamate is 100-fold greater in astrocyte-poor cultures than in cultures with abundant astrocytes (Rosenberg and Aizenman, 1989). The role of astrocyte transporters *in vivo* is further supported by gene knockout and antisense studies. Antisense knockdown of GLAST or GLT-1, but not of the neuronal subtype EAAC1, produces elevated extracellular glutamate levels, excitotoxic neurodegeneration, and paralysis in rats (Rothstein et al., 1996). Similarly, GLAST-deficient mice displayed motor incoordination and increased susceptibility to cerebellar injury (Watase et al., 1998). Genetic downregulation of the glial glutamate transporter GLT-1, but not of the neuronal glutamate transporter EAAC1, was shown to exacerbate ischemic neuronal damage in rat brain (Rao et al., 2001), indicating an important influence of astrocyte glutamate uptake on neuronal survival during ischemia.

Glutamate transporters can also, under conditions of ATP depletion, provide a conduit for glutamate efflux by reversal of the glutamate uptake process (Szatkowski et al., 1990). Depletion of ATP leads to dissipation of the Na^+ and K^+ gradients that maintain the steep intracellular: extracellular concentration gradient for glutamate (Fig. 27.1). Consequently, reversal of astrocyte glutamate uptake can contribute to the increase in brain extracellular glutamate and excitotoxic neuronal death that occurs during severe cerebral ischemia (Chen and Swanson, 2003).

Modulation of synaptic activity is a second established function of astrocyte glutamate transport. Glutamate released at synapses is taken up primarily by surrounding astrocyte processes (Anderson and Swanson, 2000). Immunolocalization of GLT-1 and GLAST shows these transporters to be concentrated in areas of the astrocyte membrane that face neuronal spinal processes (Chaudhry et al., 1995), and excitatory synaptic activity has been shown to activate rapid electrogenic astrocyte glutamate uptake currents (Bergles and Jahr, 1997). Synaptic glutamate is also cleared by transporters in the neighboring perisynaptic astrocyte processes, and in some brain regions, by transporters on postsynaptic neurons (Fig. 27.2). In retina and some cerebellar synapses, it is estimated that more than 20% of glutamate uptake is mediated by postsynaptic neuronal glutamate transporters (Otis et al., 1997). Significant uptake by presynaptic transporters has not yet been demonstrated.

The effects of glutamate uptake on synaptic transmission are perhaps best illustrated by the fact that glutamate uptake inhibitors prolong postsynaptic glutamate-induced transient currents (Tong and Jahr, 1994). Evidence suggests that transporters affect the amplitude and duration of postsynaptic glutamate receptor binding not only by uptake, but also by rapid binding of glutamate released into the synaptic cleft. This occurs because transporter binding to glutamate occurs far more rapidly than the translocation cycle (Wadiche et al., 1995b).

Glutamate diffusion out of the synaptic cleft may be able to stimulate neuronal glutamate receptors at neighboring synapses if synaptic glutamate concentrations are sufficiently high (Bergles et al., 1999) and if there is not extensive glial or neuronal membrane–impeding diffusion between synapses. The degree to which synapses are ensheathed by astrocyte processes varies considerably, and this may serve to regulate the extent to which diffusion of glutamate from one synapse can act on receptors at a neighboring synapse (Ventura and Harris, 1999). Moreover, the degree of ensheathment may be a dynamic, regulated process, at least in some brain regions (Oliet et al., 2001).

ASTROCYTE GAMMA-AMINOBUTYRIC ACID UPTAKE

Gamma-aminobutyric acid, the major inhibitory neurotransmitter in mammalian brain, is taken up by the high-affinity transporters GAT-1, GAT-2, GAT-3 (also termed mouse GAT4), and possibly the low-affinity transporter BGT-1. BGT-1 is also considered an osmoregulatory transporter because of its avid uptake of betaine, and its physiological function as a GABA transporter is uncertain. The GAT transporter family belongs to the superfamily of sodium- and chloride-dependent transporters (Palacin et al., 1998; Gadea and Lopez-Colome, 2001b). Like glutamate uptake, GABA uptake is electrogenic and driven primarily by the plasma membrane sodium gradient. The GAT family transporters translocate 2 Na^+ ions with each GABA translocation. Also like the glutamate transporters, GABA binding to GAT transporters gates an inward anion flux (Sonders and Amara, 1996).

The GABA transporters do not follow a specific cell-type expression pattern, as GAT-1, GAT-2, and GAT-3 can all be expressed by both neurons and glial cells (Table 27.1). GAT-2 is also expressed outside of brain and is therefore thought likely to serve a nutritive role. GAT-3, while also expressed on some neuron processes, appears to be the major astrocyte GABA transporter in most brain regions (Gadea and Lopez-Colome, 2001b). GAT-1 is localized to both presynaptic and postsynaptic membranes in GABAergic synapses as well as to glial membranes, and it is likely that most GABA released in synapses is taken up by neurons rather than by astrocytes (Schousboe, 2000). Nevertheless, pharmacological inhibitors that target astrocyte GABA uptake exhibit anticonvusant activity (Schousboe, 2000).

ASTROCYTE GLYCINE UPTAKE

Glycine acts at both excitatory and inhibitory receptors and also serves as a modulator at NMDA-type glutamate receptors. Glycine-T2 (GlyT2) is probably the dominant neuronal glycine transporter and GlyT1 is the glial dominant transporter, but the presence of GlyT1 transcripts in neurons suggests its contribution to neuronal glycine uptake as well (Zafra et al., 1995; Gadea and Lopez-Colome, 2001a). GlyT1 is expressed as three variants, GlyT1a, GlyT1b, and GlyT1c, that are transcribed from the same gene. These variants show no differences in their transport characteristics but may be regulated differently. GlyT1 expression *in vivo* correlates well with the localization of glycinergic neurons: GlyT1 is expressed at highest density in the spinal cord, brain stem, thalamus, and retina and at lower density in brain cortex.

Studies with a nontransportable GlyT1-specific antagonist suggests that for glycine, as for glutamate, astrocyte uptake is the dominant mode of clearance from the extracellular space in cerebral cortex (Herdon et al., 2001). GlyT1 expression in astrocytes is strongly influenced by neuronal factors. GlyT1 is not expressed in pure glial cultures, but it is expressed by astrocytes in mixed neuronal/glial cultures. In these mixed cultures, the glial expression of GlyT1 is down-regulated after selective elimination of the neurons (Zafra et al., 1997).

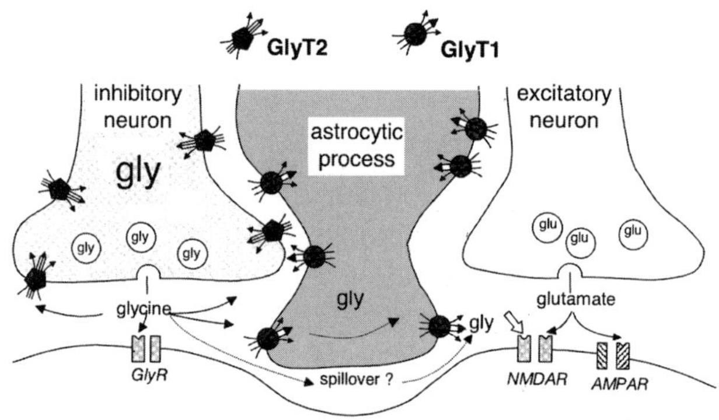

FIGURE 27.3 Possible roles of astrocyte and neuronal glycine transporters. Glycine (*gly*) uptake by the neuronal transporter GlyT2 is coupled to the inward movement of 3 Na^+ ions, whereas uptake by the predominantly astrocyte transporter GlyT1 is coupled to only 2 Na^+ ions. GlyT2 and GlyT1 both contribute to control of extracellular glycine at synapses and limit spillover to neighboring synapses. The more energetic coupling of GlyT2 maintains a high glycine concentration in presynaptic boutons, and this aids filling of synaptic vesicles. The less energetic coupling of GlyT1 may favor efflux of glycine from areas when extracellular concentrations are low or astrocyte membranes depolarize, and this efflux could facilitate transfer of glycine back to neurons. Efflux or modulated uptake at GlyT1 transporters could also influence glycine effects at NMDA receptors. AMPAR: α-amino-3-hydroxy-5-methylisoxazole-4-proprionic acid receptor; GlyR: glycine receptor; NMDA: *N*-methy-D aspartate. (Redrawn with permission of the Federation of the European Biochemical Societies from "Why glycine transporters have different stoichiometries," by S. Supplisson and M.J. Roux *FEBS Letters*, 529:93–101, 2002.)

Interestingly, the kinetic properties of the dominant astrocyte glycine transporter, GlyT1, is significantly different from those of the dominant neuronal transporter, GlyT2 (Supplisson and Roux, 2002). Glycine uptake by GlyT2 is coupled to the cotransport of 3 Na^+ and 1 Cl^-, while uptake by GlyT1 is coupled to 2 Na^+ and 1 Cl^-. This allows neurons to maintain a higher intracellular glycine concentration, a factor that may facilitate neuronal loading of glycine into synaptic vesicles (Fig. 27.3). Higher neuronal intracellular glycine concentrations are also favored by a kinetic restraint on reverse operation of the GlyT2 transporters. By contrast, astrocyte GlyT1 transporters readily function in "reverse" mode, and since these transporters operate near equilibrium, one function of astrocyte GlyT1 transporters may be to allow efflux of glycine into the extracellular space for neuronal uptake. At resting potentials, the glycine transporters are oriented with GlyT2 glycine bindings sites facing outward and GlyT1 glycine sites facing inward, an arrangement that further favors initial influx into neurons and efflux from astrocytes (Fig. 27.3).

ASTROCYTE HISTAMINE UPTAKE

High-affinity histamine uptake has been demonstrated in astrocyte cultures and astrocyte-enriched fractions of rat brain (Huszti, 1998), though the gene products responsible for uptake in brain have not yet been established. Astrocytes in culture contain high capacity for histamine metabolism, and studies using inhibitors of astrocyte metabolism suggest that astrocytes are the cell type primarily responsible for histamine uptake in brain. Histamine uptake in brain and in cultured astrocytes is sodium-dependent and, interestingly, strongly stimulated by zinc (Huszti et al., 2001).

ASTROCYTE UPTAKE OF ADENOSINE, MONOAMINES, AND SEROTONIN

Two broad types of nucleoside adenosine transporters have been characterized: equilibrative, facilitated-diffusion transporters (ENT family) and concentrative transporters that couple uptake to the plasma membrane sodium gradient (CNT family). The ENT family has two members, ENT1, which is potently inhibited by nitrobenzylthioinosine, and ENT2, which is insensitive to this inhibitor. Adenosine is a substrate for both ENT1 and ENT2 and for the concentrative nucleoside transporter, CNT2. Studies using astrocyte cultures show equilibrative transport that is both sensitive and insensitive to nitrobenzylthioinosine (Gu et al., 1996). This is presumably due to activity of ENT1 and ENT2, since these mRNAs have been demonstrated in astrocyte cultures (Anderson et al., 1999). *In situ* hybridization studies suggest that both ENT1 and ENT2, as well as the concentrative transporter CNT2, are also expressed by neurons *in situ* (Anderson, 1998). The adenosine transporters function both to regulate extracellular adenosine and to maintain intracellular nucleoside pools. At present, there is little known about the specific role of astrocyte transporters in regulating neurotransmitter actions of adenosine.

Active, high-affinity uptake of dopamine, norepinephrine, and serotonin is in each case mediated by a single transporter type: DAT, NET, and SERT, respectively (Hoffman et al., 1998). Uptake of these neurotransmitters is driven by coupled cotransport of sodium. There is in addition an uncoupled current flux through these transporters that occurs both in the presence and in the absence of their substrates (Lester et al., 1996). Dopamine transporter, NET, and SERT are expressed and functionally active in astrocyte cultures (Kimelberg and Katz, 1985; Kubota et al., 2001; Takeda et al., 2002; Inazu et al., 2003), but it remains uncertain whether these transporters are expressed or are functionally significant *in situ* (Hoffman et al., 1998; Pickel and Chan, 1999). Astrocytes in culture also express the extraneuronal monoamine transporter system (uptake2), which is a low-affinity, Na^+-independent uptake system (Kimelberg, 1986). The primary gene product responsible for this low-affinity uptake appears to be the organic cation transporter 3 (OCT3) (Wu et al., 1998; Takeda et al., 2002). The functional role of astrocyte uptake (or release) by these transporters remains to be established.

SUMMARY AND PERSPECTIVES

Neurotransmitter uptake by astrocytes does not permit direct recycling of neurotransmitters by presynaptic neurons, so the question arises: what purpose may be served by glial uptake? One potential advantage of glial uptake is that this shifts the energetic cost of neurotransmitter uptake away from the neurons. This cost can be substantial. In the case of glutamate, uptake is by far the major energy-consuming step in synaptic activity (Sibson et al., 1998). A second advantage stems from the fact that most neurotransmitter uptake systems are electrogenic, meaning that uptake results in a net inward movement of positive charge and resultant membrane depolarization. Since neuronal membrane potential is used to integrate receptor-mediated afferent input, electrogenic neurotransmitter uptake may interfere with this process. Uptake by neighboring glial cells prevents the neuronal membrane potential from influencing neurotransmitter uptake. Third, and perhaps most intriguing, a role for glia in neurotransmitter uptake may provide a mechanism for glial cells to directly influence synaptic activity and hence signal processing (Kang et al., 1998; Oliet et al., 2001). As reviewed in this chapter, there is now support for all three of these possibilities in the astrocyte glutamatergic uptake system. Important future research will involve the delineation of specific roles for other astrocyte neurotransmitter uptake systems and for neurotransmitter uptake by microglia and oligodendrocytes.

ABBREVIATIONS

ADP	adenosine diphosphate
ATP	adenosine triphosphate
BGT-1	betaine and GABA transporter-1
CNS	central nervous system
CNT	concentrative nucleoside transporter
DAT	dopamine transporter
EAAC1	excitatory amino acid carrier 1
EAT	excitatory amino acid transporter
ENT	equilibrative nucleoside transporter
GAT	GABA transporter
GLAST	glutamate/aspartate transporter
GLT	glutamate transporter
Gly	glycine
GTRAP	glutamate transporter EAAC1-associated protein
GABA	gamma-aminobutyric acid
NET	norephrine transporter
NMDA	*N*-methyl-D-aspartate
OCT3	organic cation transporter 3
PKC	protein kinase C
SERT	serotonin transporter

REFERENCES

Anderson, C.M. (1998) Distribution of nucleoside transporter subtypes in rat brain. *Pharmacol. Ther.* (Univ Manitoba) Ph.D. Thesis Dept. of Pharmacology and Therapeutics, Univ. of Manitoba.

Anderson, C.M., Bridges, R.J., Chamberlin, A.R., Shimamoto, K., Yasuda-Kamatani, Y., and Swanson, R.A. (2001) Differing effects of substrate and non-substrate transport inhibitors on glutamate uptake reversal. *J. Neurochem.* 79:1207–1216.

Anderson, C.M. and Swanson, R.A. (2000) Astrocyte glutamate transport: review of properties, regulation, and physiological functions. *Glia* 32:1–14.

Anderson, C.M., Xiong, W., Geiger, J.D., Young, J.D., Cass, C.E., Baldwin, S.A., and Parkinson, F.E. (1999) Distribution of equilibrative, nitrobenzylthioinosine-sensitive nucleoside transporters (ENT1) in brain. *J. Neurochem.* 73:867–873.

Bergles, D.E., Diamond, J.S., and Jahr, C.E. (1999) Clearance of glutamate inside the synapse and beyond. *Curr. Opin. Neurobiol.* 9:293–298.

Bergles, D.E. and Jahr, C.E. (1997) Synaptic activation of glutamate transporters in hippocampal astrocytes. *Neuron* 19:1297–1308.

Broer, S. and Brookes, N. (2001) Transfer of glutamine between astrocytes and neurons. *J. Neurochem.* 77:705–719.

Bruhn, T., Levy, L.M., Nielsen, M., Christensen, T., Johansen, F.F., and Diemer, N.H. (2000) Ischemia induced changes in expression of the astrocyte glutamate transporter GLT1 in hippocampus of the rat. *Neurochem. Int.* 37:277–285.

Chaudhry, F.A., Lehre, K.P., van Lookeren Campagne, M., Ottersen, O.P., Danbolt, N.C., and Storm-Mathisen, J. (1995) Glutamate transporters in glial plasma membranes: highly differentiated localizations revealed by quantitative ultrastructural immunocytochemistry. *Neuron* 15:711–720.

Chen, W., Aoki, C., Mahadomrongkul, V., Gruber, C.E., Wang, G.J., Blitzblau, R., Irwin, N., and Rosenberg, P.A. (2002) Expression of a variant form of the glutamate transporter GLT1 in neuronal cultures and in neurons and astrocytes in the rat brain. *J. Neurosci.* 22:2142–2152.

Chen, Y. and Swanson, R.A. (2003) Astrocytes and brain injury. *J. Cereb. Blood Flow Metab.* 23:137–149.

Chen, Y., Ying, W., Simma, V., Copin, J.C., Chan, P.H., and Swanson, R.A. (2000) Overexpression of Cu,Zn superoxide dismutase attenuates oxidative inhibition of astrocyte glutamate uptake. *J. Neurochem.* 75:939–945.

Duan, S., Anderson, C.M., Stein, B.A., and Swanson, R.A. (1999) Glutamate induces rapid upregulation of astrocyte glutamate transport and cell-surface expression of GLAST. *J. Neurosci.* 19:10193–10200.

Erecinska, M. and Silver, I.A. (1990) Metabolism and role of glutamate in mammalian brain. *Prog. Neurobiol.* 35:245–296.

Gadea, A. and Lopez-Colome, A.M. (2001a) Glial transporters for glutamate, glycine, and GABA III. Glycine transporters. *J. Neurosci. Res.* 64:218–222.

Gadea, A. and Lopez-Colome, A.M. (2001b) Glial transporters for glutamate, glycine, and GABA: II. GABA transporters. *J. Neurosci. Res.* 63:461–468.

Gu, J.G., Nath, A., and Geiger, J.D. (1996) Characterization of inhibitor-sensitive and -resistant adenosine transporters in cultured human fetal astrocytes. *J. Neurochem.* 67:972–977.

Herdon, H.J., Godfrey, F.M., Brown, A.M., Coulton, S., Evans, J.R., and Cairns, W.J. (2001) Pharmacological assessment of the role of the glycine transporter GlyT-1 in mediating high-affinity glycine uptake by rat cerebral cortex and cerebellum synaptosomes. *Neuropharmacology* 41:88–96.

Hoffman, B.J., Hansson, S.R., Mezey, E., and Palkovits, M. (1998) Localization and dynamic regulation of biogenic amine transporters in the mammalian central nervous system. *Front. Neuroendocrinol.* 19:187–231.

Huszti, Z. (1998) Carrier-mediated high affinity uptake system for histamine in astroglial and cerebral endothelial cells. *J. Neurosci. Res.* 51:551–558.

Huszti, Z., Horvath-Sziklai, A., Noszal, B., Madarasz, E., and Deli, A.M. (2001) Enhancing effect of zinc on astroglial and cerebral endothelial histamine uptake. *Biochem. Pharmacol.* 62:1491–1500.

Inazu, M., Takeda, H., and Matsumiya, T. (2003) Functional expression of the norepinephrine transporter in cultured rat astrocytes. *J. Neurochem.* 84:136–144.

Judd, M.G., Nagaraja, T.N., and Brookes, N. (1996) Potassium-induced stimulation of glutamate uptake in mouse cerebral astrocytes: the role of intracellular pH. *J. Neurochem.* 66:169–176.

Kang, J., Jiang, L., Goldman, S.A., and Nedergaard, M. (1998) Astrocyte-mediated potentiation of inhibitory synaptic transmission. *Nat. Neurosci.* 1:683–692.

Kimelberg, H.K. (1986) Occurrence and functional significance of serotonin and catecholamine uptake by astrocytes. *Biochem. Pharmacol.* 35:2273–2281.

Kimelberg, H.K. and Katz, D.M. (1985) High-affinity uptake of serotonin into immunocytochemically identified astrocytes. *Science* 228:889–891.

Kubota, N., Kiuchi, Y., Nemoto, M., Oyamada, H., Ohno, M., Funahashi, H., Shioda, S., and Oguchi, K. (2001) Regulation of serotonin transporter gene expression in human glial cells by growth factors. *Eur. J. Pharmacol.* 417:69–76.

Lester, H.A., Cao, Y., and Mager, S. (1996) Listening to neurotransmitter transporters. *Neuron* 17:807–810.

Levy, L.M., Lehre, K.P., Walaas, S.I., Storm-Mathisen, J., and Danbolt, N.C. (1995) Down-regulation of glial glutamate transporters after glutamatergic denervation in the rat brain. *Eur. J. Neurosci.* 7:2036–2041.

Longuemare, M.C., Rose, C.R., Farrell, K., Ransom, B.R., Waxman, S.G., and Swanson, R.A. (1999) K(+)-induced reversal of astrocyte glutamate uptake is limited by compensatory changes in intracellular Na+. *Neuroscience* 93:285–292.

Marie, H., Billups, D., Bedford, F.K., Dumoulin, A., Goyal, R.K., Longmore, G.D., Moss, S.J., and Attwell, D. (2002) The amino terminus of the glial glutamate transporter GLT-1 interacts with the LIM protein Ajuba. *Mol. Cell Neurosci.* 19:152–164.

Martinez-Hernandez, A., Bell, K.P., and Norenberg, M.D. (1977) Glutamine synthetase: glial localization in brain. *Science* 195: 1356–1358.

Miyamoto, O. and Auer, R.N. (2000) Hypoxia, hyperoxia, ischemia, and brain necrosis. *Neurology* 54:362–371.

Oliet, S.H., Piet, R., and Poulain, D.A. (2001) Control of glutamate clearance and synaptic efficacy by glial coverage of neurons. *Science* 292:923–926.

Otis, T.S., Kavanaugh, M.P., and Jahr, C.E. (1997) Postsynaptic glutamate transport at the climbing fiber-Purkinje cell synapse. *Science* 277:1515–1518.

Palacin, M., Estevez, R., Bertran, J., and Zorzano, A. (1998) Molecular biology of mammalian plasma membrane amino acid transporters. *Physiol. Rev.* 78:969–1054.

Pellerin, L. and Magistretti, P.J. (1994) Glutamate uptake into astrocytes stimulates aerobic glycolysis: a mechanism coupling neuronal activity to glucose utilization. *Proc. Natl. Acad. Sci. USA* 91:10625–10629.

Peng, L., Swanson, R.A., and Hertz, L. (2001) Effects of L-glutamate, D-aspartate, and monensin on glycolytic and oxidative glucose metabolism in mouse astrocyte cultures: further evidence that glutamate uptake is metabolically driven by oxidative metabolism. *Neurochem. Int.* 38:437–443.

Pickel, V.M. and Chan, J. (1999) Ultrastructural localization of the serotonin transporter in limbic and motor compartments of the nucleus accumbens. *J. Neurosci.* 19:7356–7366.

Poitry-Yamate, C.L., Vutskits, L., and Rauen, T. (2002) Neuronal-induced and glutamate-dependent activation of glial glutamate transporter function. *J. Neurochem.* 82:987–997.

Rao, V.L., Dogan, A., Todd, K.G., Bowen, K.K., Kim, B.T., Rothstein, J.D., and Dempsey, R.J. (2001) Antisense knockdown of the glial glutamate transporter GLT-1, but not the neuronal glutamate transporter EAAC1, exacerbates transient focal cerebral ischemia-induced neuronal damage in rat brain. *J. Neurosci.* 21:1876–1883.

Robinson, M.B. (2002) Regulated trafficking of neurotransmitter transporters: common notes but different melodies. *J. Neurochem.* 80:1–11.

Rosenberg, P.A. and Aizenman, E. (1989) Hundred-fold increase in neuronal vulnerability to glutamate toxicity in astrocyte-poor cultures of rat cerebral cortex [published erratum appears in Neurosci Lett 1990 Aug 24;116(3):399]. *Neurosci. Lett.* 103:162–168.

Rothstein, J.D., Dykes-Hoberg, M., Pardo, C.A., Bristol, L.A., Jin, L., Kuncl, R.W., Kanai, Y., Hediger, M.A., Wang, Y., Schielke, J.P., and Welty, D.F. (1996) Knockout of glutamate transporters reveals a major role for astroglial transport in excitotoxicity and clearance of glutamate. *Neuron* 16:675–686.

Rothstein, J.D., Martin, L., Levey, A.I., Dykes-Hoberg, M., Jin, L., Wu, D., Nash, N., and Kuncl, R.W. (1994) Localization of neuronal and glial glutamate transporters. *Neuron* 13:713–725.

Schmitt, A., Asan, E., Puschel, B., and Kugler, P. (1997) Cellular and regional distribution of the glutamate transporter GLAST in the CNS of rats: nonradioactive in situ hybridization and comparative immunocytochemistry. *J. Neurosci.* 17:1–10.

Schousboe, A. (2000) Pharmacological and functional characterization of astrocytic GABA transport: a short review. *Neurochem. Res.* 25:1241–1244.

Sibson, N.R., Dhankhar, A., Mason, G.F., Rothman, D.L., Behar, K.L., and Shulman, R.G. (1998) Stoichiometric coupling of brain glucose metabolism and glutamatergic neuronal activity. *Proc. Natl. Acad. Sci. USA* 95:316–321.

Sonders, M.S. and Amara, S.G. (1996) Channels in transporters. *Curr. Opin. Neurobiol.* 6:294–302.

Supplisson, S. and Roux, M.J. (2002) Why glycine transporters have different stoichiometries. *FEBS Lett.* 529:93–101.

Swanson, R.A., Chen, J., and Graham, S.H. (1994) Glucose can fuel glutamate uptake in ischemic brain. *J. Cereb. Blood Flow Metab.* 14:1–6.

Swanson, R.A., Liu, J., Miller, J.W., Rothstein, J.D., Farrell, K., Stein, B.A., and Longuemare, M.C. (1997) Neuronal regulation of glutamate transporter subtype expression in astrocytes. *J. Neurosci.* 17:932–940.

Szatkowski, M., Barbour, B., and Attwell, D. (1990) Non-vesicular release of glutamate from glial cells by reversed electrogenic glutamate uptake. *Nature* 348:443–446.

Takeda, H., Inazu, M., and Matsumiya, T. (2002) Astroglial dopamine transport is mediated by norepinephrine transporter. *Naunyn Schmiedebergs Arch. Pharmacol.* 366:620–623.

Tong, G. and Jahr, C.E. (1994) Block of glutamate transporters potentiates postsynaptic excitation. *Neuron* 13:1195–1203.

Trotti, D., Danbolt, N.C., and Volterra, A. (1998) Glutamate transporters are oxidant-vulnerable: a molecular link between oxidative and excitotoxic neurodegeneration? *Trends Pharmacol. Sci.* 19:328–334.

Utsunomiya-Tate, N., Endou, H., and Kanai, Y. (1997) Tissue specific variants of glutamate transporter GLT-1. *FEBS Lett.* 416: 312–316.

Vandenberg, R.J., Mitrovic, A.D., and Johnston, G.A. (1998) Molecular basis for differential inhibition of glutamate transporter subtypes by zinc ions. *Mol. Pharmacol.* 54:189–196.

Ventura, R. and Harris, K.M. (1999) Three-dimensional relationships between hippocampal synapses and astrocytes. *J. Neurosci.* 19:6897–6906.

Wadiche, J.I., Amara, S.G., and Kavanaugh, M.P. (1995a) Ion fluxes associated with excitatory amino acid transport. *Neuron* 15: 721–728.

Wadiche, J.I., Arriza, J.L., Amara, S.G., and Kavanaugh, M.P. (1995b) Kinetics of a human glutamate transporter. *Neuron* 14:1019–1027.

Watase, K., Hashimoto, K., Kano, M., Yamada, K., Watanabe, M., Inoue, Y., Okuyama, S., Sakagawa, T., Ogawa, S., Kawashima, N., Hori, S., Takimoto, M., Wada, K., and Tanaka, K. (1998)

Motor discoordination and increased susceptibility to cerebellar injury in GLAST mutant mice. *Eur. J. Neurosci.* 10:976–988.

Wu, X., Kekuda, R., Huang, W., Fei, Y.J., Leibach, F.H., Chen, J., Conway, S.J., and Ganapathy, V. (1998) Identity of the organic cation transporter OCT3 as the extraneuronal monoamine transporter (uptake2) and evidence for the expression of the transporter in the brain. *J. Biol. Chem.* 273:32776–32786.

Zafra, F., Aragon, C., Olivares, L., Danbolt, N.C., Gimenez, C., and Storm-Mathisen, J. (1995) Glycine transporters are differentially expressed among CNS cells. *J. Neurosci.* 15:3952–3969.

Zafra, F., Poyatos, I., and Gimenez, C. (1997) Neuronal dependency of the glycine transporter GLYT1 expression in glial cells. *Glia* 20:155–162.

Zerangue, N., Arriza, J.L., Amara, S.G., and Kavanaugh, M.P. (1995) Differential modulation of human glutamate transporter subtypes by arachidonic acid. *J. Biol. Chem.* 270:6433–6435.

28 Glia and synaptic transmission

ERIC A. NEWMAN

Glial cells have traditionally been viewed as passive elements in the central nervous system (CNS), providing structural and metabolic support for neurons but not actively participating in information processing. This view has been challenged in recent years as experiments have revealed robust bidirectional communication between glial cells and neurons at the synapse.

Glial cell processes envelop many synapses in the CNS and the peripheral nervous systems (PNS), often abutting the synaptic cleft. This close structural association suggests a physiological interaction between glial cells and neurons. Indeed, glial cells possess many neurotransmitter receptors and respond actively to a variety of neurotransmitters and modulators. Activated glial cells, in turn, release chemical transmitters that stimulate postsynaptic neurons and modulate transmitter release from presynaptic terminals.

These close structural and physiological interactions have led to the suggestion that glial cells function as an active partner in synaptic transmission. The importance of glial cells in synaptic function has been emphasized by the coining of the term *tripartite synapse* to stress that the third element of the synapse, the glial cell, is an essential constituent in determining synaptic function, along with the presynaptic and postsynaptic neurons (Araque et al., 1999).

This chapter reviews recent evidence defining glial-neuronal interactions at the tripartite synapse. The reader is also referred to recent reviews of glial cells and synaptic function (Araque et al., 1999; Araque et al., 2001; Vesce et al., 2001; Fields and Stevens-Graham, 2002).

STRUCTURE OF THE TRIPARTITE SYNAPSE

Glial cells ensheath some but not all synapses in the CNS, with glial processes often extending up to the edge of synaptic zones (Fig. 28.1*A*). In the hippocampus, 57% of all synapses are associated with astrocytic processes (Ventura and Harris, 1999), while in the piriform cortex, synapses are often surrounded by glial cell processes (Schikorski and Stevens, 1999). In the visual cortex, only 29% of synapses are associated with astrocytes, and many of these are not fully ensheathed by glial cells (Spacek, 1985). In the cerebellum, 67% of parallel fiber-Purkinje cells synapses and 94% of climbing fiber-Purkinje cells synapses are ensheathed by Bergmann glia (Spacek, 1985; Grosche et al., 1999; Xu-Friedman et al., 2001).

If glial cells play an essential role in synaptic transmission, why aren't all synapses ensheathed by glial cell processes? Glial cells may be associated with those synapses that release transmitter but not with those (silent) synapses that are inactive (Ventura and Harris, 1999). Selective association of glial cells with active synapses may be explained by the affinity of glial cells for neurotransmitters; astrocytes in culture extend processes toward sources of glutamate (Cornell-Bell et al., 1990b). *In situ*, glial processes may grow toward synapses that release transmitter and may withdraw from silent synapses.

One clear example of glial plasticity at the synapse is seen in the magnocellular (supraoptic and paraventricular) nuclei of the hypothalamus (Theodosis and Poulain, 2001; Hatton, 2002). In virgin female rats, most somata and dendrites of oxytocin-secreting neurons are separated by astrocytic processes. During parturition and lactation, however, glial processes withdraw from these neurons, and new excitatory and inhibitory synapses are formed. These morphological changes are reversible, with glial processes and synaptic numbers returning to the "virgin" state a month after cessation of lactation.

At the tripartite synapse, glial cell processes surround neuronal elements but normally do not form direct junctions with neighboring neurons. In the hippocampus, however, classical synapses from pyramidal cell axons onto NG2–positive, glial fibrillary acidic protein (GFAP)–negative oligodendrocyte precursor (glial) cells are observed (Bergles et al., 2000). Electrical stimulation of neurons evokes rapid, AMPA-mediated excitatory postsynaptic potentials (EPSPs) and currents (EPSCs) in the glial cells (Fig. 28.1*B*). Synapses onto these oligodendrocyte precursor cells are seen in both young and adult animals.

Gap junctional coupling between neurons and glial cells has also been observed. Coupling between astrocytes and neurons in the locus ceruleus has been demonstrated in dye coupling experiments (Alvarez-

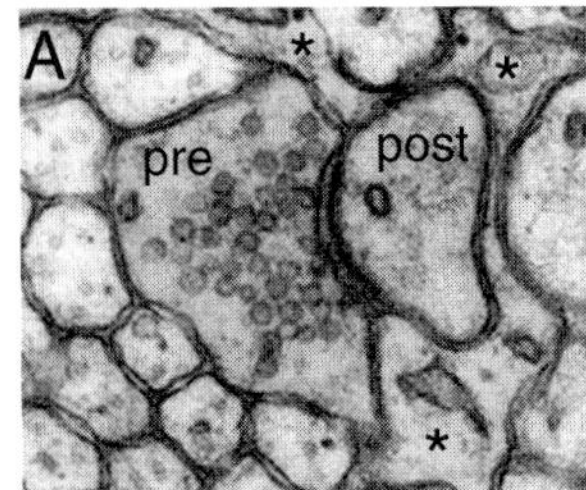

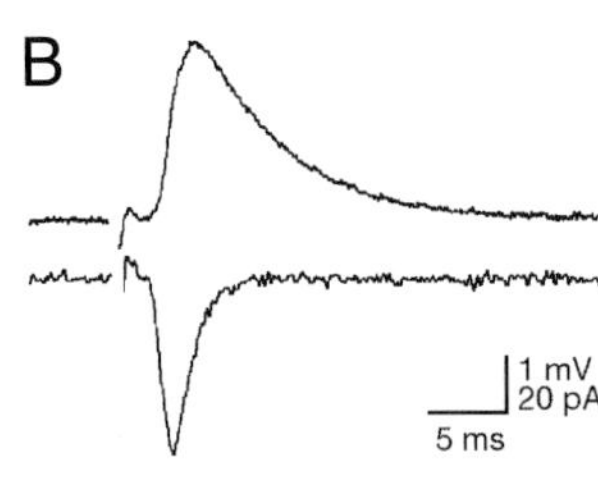

FIGURE 28.1 Glial cells at synapses. *A*. Morphology of a tripartite synapse. Electron micrograph of a synapse between a parallel fiber terminal (*pre*) and a Purkinje cell spine (*post*) in the rat cerebellum. Processes of an astrocyte (*) abut the active zone and ensheath the synapse. (From Xu-Friedman et al., 2001.) *B*. Neuron-glial synapse. Recordings from an oligodendrocyte precursor (glial) cell in the rat hippocampus. Stimulation of neurons evokes a brief EPSP (*top*) and EPSC (bottom) in the glial cell, demonstrating the presence of a classic, glutamate-mediated fast excitatory synapse onto the glial cell. (From Bergles et al., 2000.)

Maubecin et al., 2000). This coupling mediates electrical interactions between the cells, as depolarization of glial cells results in an increase in neuronal firing rate. Gap junctional coupling between astrocytes and embryonic neurons has also been observed in culture (Froes et al., 1999).

Glial cells are also associated with synapses in the PNS. At the neuromuscular junction, synapses between motor neuron terminals and muscle cells are ensheathed by perisynaptic Schwann cells, specialized Schwann cells that lack myelin. Processes of perisynaptic Schwann cells cover the presynaptic terminal over its length and periodically extend fine processes into the synaptic cleft (McMahan et al., 1972; Reist and Smith, 1992).

NEURONAL ACTIVATION OF GLIAL CELLS

Communication between neurons and glial cells at the synapse is a two-way affair. Neurons activate glial cells through the release of neurotransmitters while glial cells signal neurons through several mechanisms, including the release of chemical transmitters. This bidirectional interaction suggests that glial cells function as part of a feedback loop at the synapse (Araque et al., 1999). In examining this complex interaction, I will begin by discussing neuronal activation of glial cells.

Glial cells express many of the same neurotransmitter receptors present in neurons, including AMPA, NMDA and metabotropic glutamatergic receptors, GABAergic, adrenergic, P2X and P2Y purinergic, serotonergic, and muscarinic receptors, and a variety of peptidergic receptors (see Chapter 10, this volume; Finkbeiner, 1993; Porter and McCarthy, 1997; Verkhratsky et al., 1998). Activation of these receptors by exogenously applied neurotransmitters evokes a variety of glial responses, the most prominent of which is a rise in intracellular Ca^{2+} concentration.

Release of transmitters from neurons in intact tissue preparations also activates glial cells and evokes increases in glial Ca^{2+}. It is important to bear in mind, however, that glial Ca^{2+} increases may not always be the relevant glial cell response at the synapse. Activation of glial cells elicits other responses, including the release of ATP, which may occur in a Ca^{2+}-independent manner (Wang et al., 2000).

Neuronal Stimulation Evokes Glial Ca^{2+} Increases

In hippocampal brain slices, stimulation of neurons elicits Ca^{2+} increases in neighboring astrocytes (Fig. 28.2*A*; Porter and McCarthy, 1996; Pasti et al., 1997; Kang et al., 1998; Araque et al., 2002). These glial responses are evoked by the release of a number of different transmitters from neurons, activating glial metabotropic glutamate receptors (Porter and McCarthy, 1996), $GABA_B$ receptors (Kang et al., 1998), and muscarinic acetylcholine receptors (Araque et al., 2002). Glial Ca^{2+} increases are also evoked in cultured hippocampal slices, where electrical stimulation of glutamatergic neurons results in the initiation of intercellular glial Ca^{2+} waves (Dani et al., 1992).

Electrical stimulation of cerebellar parallel fibers evokes a nitric oxide–mediated Ca^{2+} increase in Bergmann glial cells, the astrocytes of the cerebellum (Grosche et al., 1999; Matyash et al., 2001). Moderate stimulation evokes Ca^{2+} increases in single subcellular compartments termed *microdomains*, suggesting that Bergmann glial cells are composed of hundreds of subcellular compartments that are functionally isolated from each other (Grosche et al., 2002). Electrical stimulation of neurons in the granule cell layer of the cerebellum also elicits Ca^{2+} increases in Bergmann glial cells, a response mediated by activation of α_1 adrenoreceptors (Kulik et al., 1999).

In the PNS, stimulation of motor nerves results in Ca^{2+} increases in the perisynaptic Schwann cells ensheathing the neuromuscular junction (Fig. 28.2*B*; Reist and Smith, 1992; Rochon et al., 2001; Jahromi et al., 2002). The glial response is mediated by activation of muscarinic acetylcholine receptors and A_1 adenosine receptors following release of acetylcholine and ATP from the presynaptic terminal (Rochon et al., 2001; Jahromi et al., 2002).

Sensitivity of Neuronal-Glial Signaling

Does neuron-glial signaling occur for modest rates of neuronal activity that are present *in vivo* under normal physiological conditions or is tetanic stimulation required to elicit glial responses? Experimental evidence suggests that moderate rates of activity are sufficient to

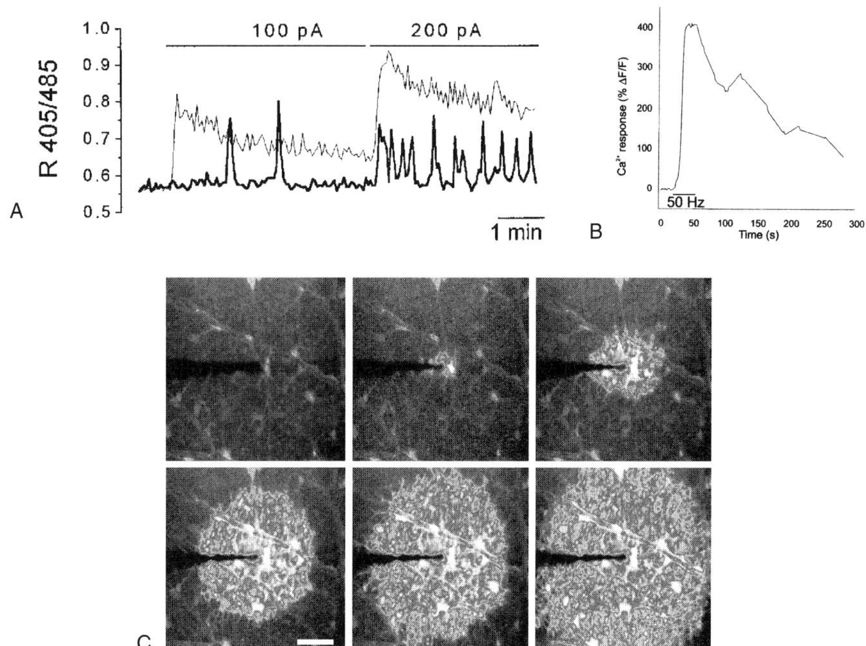

FIGURE 28.2 Calcium responses in glial cells. *A*. Electrical stimulation of neurons in the rat hippocampus evokes Ca^{2+} increases in a neuron (*thin line*) and Ca^{2+} oscillations in an adjacent astrocyte (*thick line*). Increasing the strength of the electrical stimulus (*bar at top*) elicits a higher frequency Ca^{2+} oscillation in the glial cell. (From Pasti et al., 1997.) *B*. Electrical stimulation of a motor nerve evokes a Ca^{2+} increase in a perisynaptic Schwann cell at the frog neuromuscular junction. (From Robitaille, 1998.) *C*. Mechanical stimulation of an astrocyte initiates an intercellular Ca^{2+} wave that propagates through glial cells in the rat retina. Elapsed time following stimulation: 0, 0.2, 1.5, 3.5, 5.5, 9.5 seconds. Scale bar 50 μm. (From Newman, 2001b.)

evoke small glial responses, while more intense neuronal stimulation results in larger glial Ca^{2+} increases.

Stimulation of parallel fibers in the cerebellum by single pulses evokes Ca^{2+} increases in Bergmann glial cell microdomains, while trains of 10 pulses elicit larger responses that extend into the cell soma (Matyash et al., 2001). Similarly, brief stimulation of neurons in the hippocampus evokes small Ca^{2+} increases in astrocytes, while longer-duration and higher-frequency stimulation evokes larger glial responses (Araque et al., 2002).

At the neuromuscular junction, 50 Hz stimulation of motor nerves, well within the normal activity range of spinal motorneurons, evokes large Ca^{2+} increases in perisynaptic Schwann cells (Reist and Smith, 1992; Rochon et al., 2001). Stimulation rates as low as 10 Hz evoke smaller but detectable glial Ca^{2+} increases (Rochon et al., 2001; Jahromi et al., 2002).

Afferent stimulation can also trigger long-lasting Ca^{2+} oscillations in glial cells (Pasti et al., 1997; Araque et al., 2002). In the hippocampus, both the magnitude and the frequency of these Ca^{2+} oscillations increase as the frequency of afferent stimulation is raised (Fig. 28.2*A*; Pasti et al., 1997).

Calcium Waves in Glial Cell Networks

Activation of glial cells by neurotransmitters can, in addition to evoking localized Ca^{2+} increases, initiate Ca^{2+} waves that propagate for hundreds of micrometers through glial cell networks. These intercellular Ca^{2+} waves represent a mechanism by which glial cells can signal each other independently of neuronal circuits and modulate the activity of neurons over relatively long distances. Intercellular glial Ca^{2+} waves, initiated by focal ejection of neurotransmitters or by mechanical or electrical stimulation, are observed in cultured astrocytes as well as in glial networks in intact tissue preparations (see Chapter 17, this volume; Cornell-Bell et al., 1990a; Finkbeiner, 1993; Verkhratsky et al., 1998). Activation of glial cells in the mammalian retina evokes intercellular waves that propagate through astrocytes and Müller cells, the specialized radial glial cells of the retina (Fig. 28.2*C*; Newman and Zahs, 1997; Newman, 2001a, 2001b). Glial Ca^{2+} waves are also observed in acutely isolated corpus callosum and hippocampal slices, where glial activation evokes intercellular waves in both white matter and gray matter astrocytes (Sul and Haydon, 2001; Schipke et al., 2002).

A critical unanswered question is whether intercellular glial Ca^{2+} waves occur *in vivo*. In most *in situ* systems, electrical activation of neurons evokes local nonpropagating Ca^{2+} increases in glial cells (Porter and McCarthy, 1996; Grosche et al., 1999; Kulik et al., 1999; Matyash et al., 2001; Araque et al., 2002). There are exceptions, however, indicating that normal neuronal activity may trigger propagated waves. Focal release of caged glutamate in hippocampal slices evokes propagated waves (Sul and Haydon, 2001), while spontaneous glial Ca^{2+} oscillations propagate into as many as five neighboring astrocytes in ventrobasal thalamic slices (Parri et al., 2001).

Communication between glial cells may be selective. When a single astrocyte in a hippocampal slice is activated by focal release of caged glutamate, increases in Ca^{2+} are observed in some but not all neighboring astrocytes, suggesting the existence of local glial circuits (Sul and Haydon, 2001). Selective glial cell circuits may also be present in the cerebellum, where Bergmann glial cells are coupled to each other along the parasagittal but not the transverse plane (Muller et al., 1996). Coupling between glial cells, and thus long-range communication through glial cell networks, may also be under dynamic control, as coupling is modulated by several factors, including intracellular pH and Ca^{2+} and extracellular K^+ (see Chapter 13, this volume).

Spontaneous Glial Cell Activity

In both hippocampal slices (Nett et al., 2001), and ventrobasal thalamic slices (Parri et al., 2001), astrocytes display spontaneous Ca^{2+} oscillations. Spontaneous oscillations are also observed in the mammalian retina in both astrocytes and Müller cells (Newman, 2002a). These spontaneous Ca^{2+} oscillations, if they occur *in vivo*, may permit glial cells to modulate neuronal activity without prior neuronal activation.

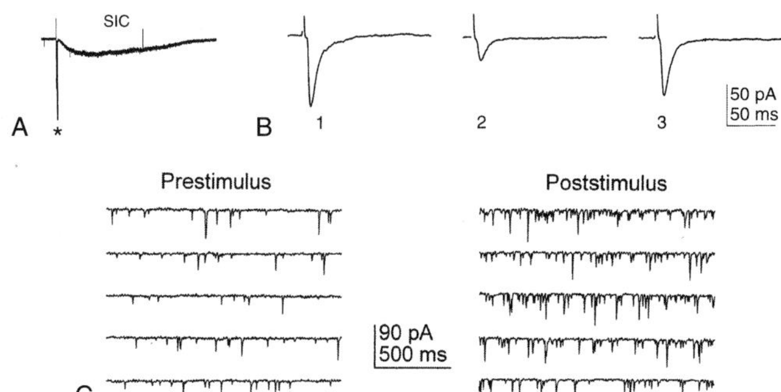

FIGURE 28.3 Glial modulation of neuronal activity in glial-neuronal cocultures. *A*. Stimulation of an astrocyte evokes a slow inward current (SIC) in a neighboring neuron. Asterisk, stimulus artifact. *B*. Stimulation of a presynaptic neuron evokes an EPSC recorded from a postsynaptic neuron (*1*). Simultaneous stimulation of an adjacent astrocyte reduces the amplitude of the EPSC (*2*). Following termination of glial stimulation, synaptic transmission recovers (*3*). (*A* and *B* from Araque et al., 1998a.) C. Spontaneous mEPSCs recorded from a neuron (prestimulus). The frequency of mEPSCs increases following stimulation of a neighboring astrocyte (poststimulus). (From Araque et al., 1998b.)

GLIAL MODULATION OF SYNAPTIC TRANSMISSION

Glial cells, in addition to responding to neuronal signals, possess several mechanisms by which they can signal back to pre- and postsynaptic neuronal elements, modulating synaptic transmission. It is convenient to divide these mechanisms into two groups: *direct* and *indirect* mechanisms of modulation. I define direct modulation as the release of chemical transmitters (glutamate, ATP) from glial cells and the subsequent stimulation of either pre- or postsynaptic neuronal elements. Indirect modulation includes all other modulatory mechanisms, including uptake of neurotransmitters by glial cells, glial release of coagonists, and glial regulation of extracellular K^+ and H^+ levels. Bear in mind that indirect mechanisms of glial modulation may be as important as direct mechanisms. For example, glial uptake of glutamate can strongly influence transmission at some synapses.

DIRECT MODULATION: GLIAL RELEASE OF CHEMICAL TRANSMITTERS

Modulation by Glutamate Release

Glial-neuronal cocultures

Glutamate-mediated modulation of synaptic transmission has been well characterized in cocultures of mammalian astrocytes and neurons, where astrocytes can be activated by electrical and mechanical stimulation and by application of peptides and prostaglandin E_2 (PGE_2; Parpura et al., 1994; Hassinger et al., 1995; Araque et al., 1998a; Bezzi et al., 1998; Sanzgiri et al., 1999). Several neuronal responses are elicited when astrocytes are activated. Excitatory currents, termed *slow inward currents*, and Ca^{2+} increases are evoked in neurons adjacent to activated astrocytes (Fig. 28.3*A*; Parpura et al., 1994; Hassinger et al., 1995; Sanzgiri et al., 1999). Synaptic transmission between cultured neurons is also modulated. Both EPSCs and inhibitory postsynaptic currents (IPSCs), evoked by electrical stimulation of presynaptic neurons, are reduced when neighboring glial cells are activated (Fig. 28.3*B*; Araque et al., 1998a; Mauch et al., 2001). The frequency of both excitatory and inhibitory miniature postsynaptic currents (mEPSCs and mIPSCs) is also increased (Fig. 28.3*C*; Araque et al., 1998b).

These neuronal responses are mediated by the release of glutamate from activated astrocytes and the subsequent stimulation of glutamate receptors on pre- and postsynaptic neuronal elements. Slow inward currents, as well as neuronal Ca^{2+} increases, are blocked by AMPA and NMDA antagonists (Parpura et al., 1994; Hassinger et al., 1995; Araque et al., 1998a; Sanzgiri et al., 1999), while inhibition of postsynaptic EPSCs and IPSCs is blocked by metabotropic glutamate receptor antagonists (mGluRs; Araque et al., 1998a). Increases in mEPSC and mIPSC frequency, in contrast, are meditated by presynaptic NMDA receptors, most likely located away from the active zone of the synapse (Araque et al., 1998b).

In situ preparations

Glutamate-mediated modulation of synaptic transmission has also been demonstrated in intact tissue prepa-

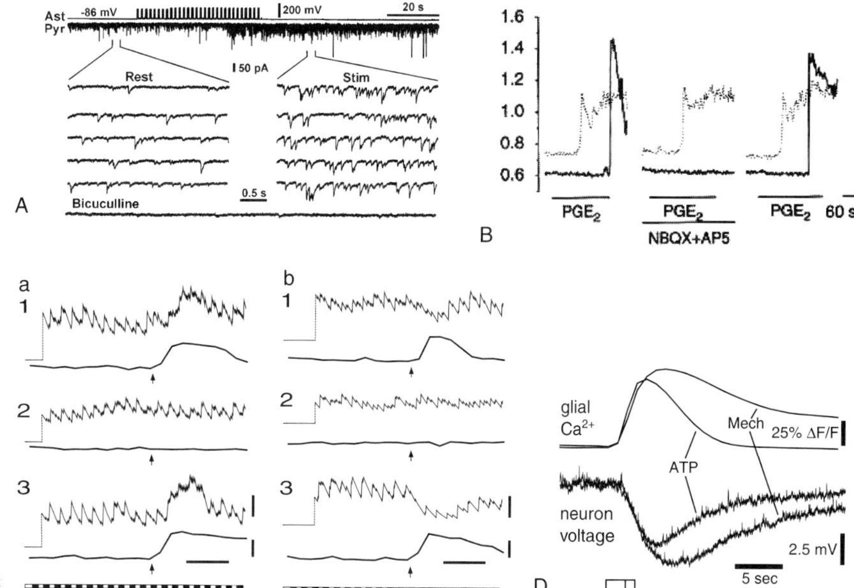

FIGURE 28.4 Glial modulation of neuronal activity in intact tissue preparations. A Spontaneous mIPSCs recorded from a pyramidal neuron in a rat hippocampal slice (Rest). Following stimulation of an astrocyte (*Ast*), the frequency of mIPSCs increases (*Stim*). The mIPSCs are blocked by the $GABA_A$ antagonist bicuculline (bottom trace). (From Kang et al., 1998.) *B*. Stimulation of astrocytes with PGE_2 in a rat hippocampal slice evokes Ca^{2+} increases in an astrocyte (*thin line*) and in an adjacent neuron (*thick line*). Addition of the glutamate antagonists NBQX and AP5 block the neuronal response but not the glial response, indicating that glial cells stimulate the neuron by release of glutamate. (From Bezzi et al., 1998.) *C*. Glial modulation of light-evoked spike activity recorded from ganglion cells in the rat retina. For each trial, a running average of neuronal spike frequency is shown in the top trace and glial Ca^{2+} in the bottom trace. (*a*) Spike frequency of a neuron increases in trials 1 and 3, when a stimulus (*arrow*) evokes a glial Ca^{2+} increase. (*b*) Spike frequency of a different neuron decreases in trials 1 and 3, when a glial Ca^{2+} increase is evoked. (From Newman and Zahs, 1998.) *D*. A retinal ganglion cell hyperpolarizes (*bottom traces*) when glial cells are stimulated by ATP ejection (*ATP*) or by mechanical stimulation (*Mech*). The amplitude and time course of the neuronal hyperpolarization closely follow the Ca^{2+} increase in neighboring glial cells (*top traces*). (From Newman, 2002b.)

rations. Electrical stimulation of astrocytes in hippocampal slices increases mIPSC frequency and raises the success rate of synaptic responses recorded from pyramidal neurons (Fig. 28.4*A*; Kang et al., 1998). This glial-mediated synaptic enhancement is responsible for the potentiation of synaptic transmission between inhibitory interneurons and pyramidal cells observed during repetitive firing of the interneurons. Potentiation arises when GABA release from the interneurons activates astrocytic $GABA_B$ receptors, evoking a Ca^{2+}-dependent release of glutamate from the glial cells. The released glutamate activates interneuron AMPA/NMDA receptors, potentiating synaptic transmission (Kang et al., 1998).

Glial modulation of neurons has been observed in thalamic slices, where spontaneous Ca^{2+} oscillations, as well as stimulated Ca^{2+} increases in astrocytes, evoke inward currents in adjacent thalamocortical neurons (Parri et al., 2001). These excitatory currents are mediated by glutamate release from astrocytes and are blocked by NMDA antagonists. Increases in neuronal Ca^{2+} are also elicited by glutamate release from astrocytes in hippocampal slices, where neuronal responses evoked by astrocyte stimulation are blocked by AMPA/NMDA antagonists (Fig. 28.4*B*; Pasti et al., 1997; Bezzi et al., 1998).

Mechanism of glutamate release from glia

The mechanism responsible for glutamate release from glial cells remains an open question, but evidence indicates that release is mediated by a Ca^{2+}-dependent exocytotic process similar to that responsible for neurotransmitter release from neurons (see Chapter 14, this volume). Stimuli that elicit Ca^{2+} increases in astrocytes result in glutamate release, while agents that block Ca^{2+} increases (thapsigargin, BAPTA, EGTA), block release (Araque et al., 1998a, 1998b; Bezzi et al., 1998; Kang et al., 1998; Sanzgiri et al., 1999; Innocenti et al., 2000; Parpura and Haydon, 2000).

It is likely that SNARE proteins, which mediate vesicular release at the presynaptic terminal, also support transmitter release from glial cells. Several SNARE proteins are expressed in astrocytes (Parpura et al., 1995;

Hepp et al., 1999; Maienschein et al., 1999) and tetanus and botulinum toxins, which cleave SNARE proteins, block transmitter release (Bezzi et al., 1998; Araque et al., 2000; Pasti et al., 2001). Bafilomycin A1, a H^+-ATPase inhibitor that blocks glutamate uptake into vesicles, also blocks release of glutamate from astrocytes (Araque et al., 2000; Pasti et al., 2001). The kinetics of glutamate release from astrocytes is extremely fast, comparable to that of vesicular release from neurons (Pasti et al., 2001).

This evidence indicates that glial cells release glutamate by a Ca^{2+}-dependent vesicular mechanism that resembles release from neurons. Important differences between glial and neuronal release exist, however. Glutamate release from glial cells occurs at a much slower rate than does release from neurons, is probably triggered by smaller increases in cytoplasmic Ca^{2+} (Parpura and Haydon, 2000), and occurs over large areas of the cell surface. It is also possible that glial cells possess additional glutamate release mechanisms, including efflux through stretch-activated channels, anion channels, or gap junctional hemichannels.

Modulation in the Retina

Glial cells modulate the activity of neurons in the mammalian retina, where the light-evoked spike activity of ganglion cells is altered by glia. When a Ca^{2+} wave is elicited in retinal glial cells, the spike activity of neighboring neurons is either enhanced or depressed (Fig. 28.4*C*; Newman and Zahs, 1998). Modulation of spike activity occurs when, and only when, a Ca^{2+} wave propagates into the glial cells adjacent to the neuron.

Glial inhibition of ganglion cells has been investigated in whole-cell recordings from neurons (Newman, 2002b). Activation of glial cells by agonist ejection or mechanical stimulation evokes a hyperpolarizing neuronal response (Fig. 28.4*D*). The inhibition is mediated by Müller glial cells rather than by astrocytes, which are not present in the synaptic layers of the retina. The inhibitory response is reduced by inhibitors of the ectoenzymes that convert ATP to adenosine and is blocked by an A_1 adenosine receptor antagonist. Thus, Müller cells inhibit neurons by release of ATP, which is converted to adenosine in the extracellular space. The adenosine subsequently activates neuronal adenosine receptors, leading to an increase in neuronal K^+ conductance (Newman, 2002b). This mechanism of glial inhibition of neurons may be widespread in the CNS, as brain astrocytes release ATP when activated (Cotrina et al., 1998; Wang et al., 2000; Newman, 2001b).

Glial cells modulate neuronal excitability in the retina by at least three different mechanisms. Glial inhibition of light-evoked spike activity is blocked by glutamate, GABA, and glycine antagonists (E.A. Newman and Zahs, 1998) and, most likely, acts presynaptically. Glia also act presynaptically to potentiate light-evoked responses (Newman, unpublished observations). Hyperpolarizing responses recorded from ganglion cells, in contrast, are unaffected by classical transmitter antagonists and are generated by direct inhibition of the postsynaptic neurons (Newman, 2002b).

Modulation at the Neuromuscular Junction

Perisynaptic Schwann cells, the glial cells that ensheath the neuromuscular junction, modulate synaptic transmission at this PNS synapse. At both the amphibian and mammalian neuromuscular junction, repetitive stimulation of motor nerves results in depression of synaptic transmission caused by a decrease in transmitter release from the presynaptic terminal. Approximately half of this depression is mediated by a complex feedback loop comprising the presynaptic terminal, the perisynaptic Schwann cell, and the postsynaptic muscle fiber.

Release of acetylcholine and ATP from the presynaptic terminal stimulates the perisynaptic Schwann cell (Reist and Smith, 1992; Rochon et al., 2001; Thomas and Robitaille, 2001; Jahromi et al., 2002), evoking release of a chemical transmitter, thought to be glutamate, from the glial cell (Pinard et al., 2002). Transmitter release stimulates the production of nitric oxide, perhaps in postsynaptic muscle fibers (Pinard et al., 2002). Nitric oxide, in turn, decreases the probability of acetylcholine release from the presynaptic terminal via a cyclic guanosine monophosphate (cGMP)-dependent mechanism (Thomas and Robitaille, 2001).

Glial cell depression of synaptic transmission is mediated by activation of G-proteins and subsequent release of the chemical transmitter from the glial cell; depression is inhibited by GDPβS and is stimulated by GTPγS injected into the perisynaptic Schwann cell (Fig. 28.5*A,B*; Robitaille, 1998). Surprisingly, depression of synaptic transmission is Ca^{2+}-independent (Castonguay and Robitaille, 2001), suggesting that the

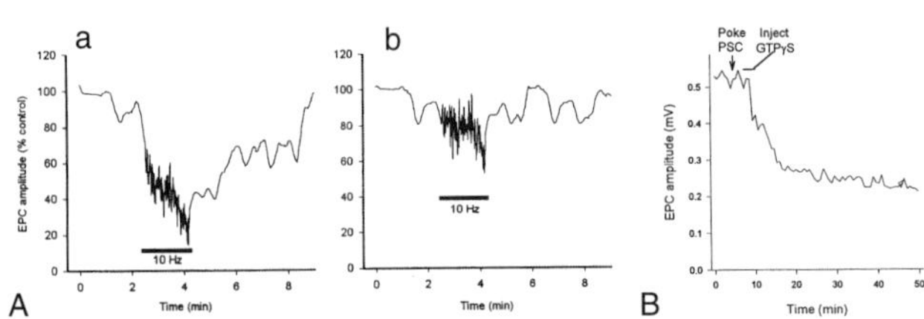

FIGURE 28.5 Glial inhibition of synaptic transmission at the frog neuromuscular junction. Plots of the amplitude of endplate current (*EPC*) recorded from a muscle fiber. *A*. (*a*) Synaptic transmission is depressed during and after a train of stimuli applied to the motor nerve. (*b*) The activity-dependent depression is blocked following GDPβS injection into the perisynaptic Schwann cell ensheathing the synapse. *B*. Injection of GTPγS into a perisynaptic Schwann cell induces depression at the synapse ensheathed by the glial cell. *A* and *B* from (Robitaille, 1998.)

mechanism of transmitter release in perisynaptic Schwann cells differs from that in astrocytes.

This mechanism of glial depression of synaptic transmission is partially counterbalanced by a second, excitatory interaction between perisynaptic Schwann cells and the presynaptic terminal. Increases in glial Ca^{2+} evoked by inositol 1,4,5-triphosphate (IP_3) injection result in a potentiation of transmitter release from the presynaptic terminal. Blocking this glial Ca^{2+} rise with BAPTA leads to a more pronounced depression of synaptic transmission induced by high-frequency afferent stimulation (Castonguay and Robitaille, 2001). These results indicate that perisynaptic Schwann cells can both enhance and depress synaptic transmission at the neuromuscular junction.

Glial-neuronal interactions at the neuromuscular junction represent the most convincing evidence to date that glial cells modulate synaptic transmission *in vivo*. Morphologically, the neuromuscular junction preparation closely reproduces conditions *in vivo*. In addition, levels of afferent stimulation that reliably evoke glial depression of synaptic transmission (10 Hz) are well within the range that occurs under normal physiological conditions *in vivo*.

INDIRECT MECHANISMS OF GLIAL MODULATION OF SYNAPTIC TRANSMISSION

Neurotransmitter Uptake by Glial Cells

Glial cells express the glutamate transporters GLAST (glutamate/aspartate transporter) and GLT-1 (glutamate transporter-1) [human homologs: excitatory amino acid transporter-1 (EAAT1) and EAAT2; see Chapter 27, this volume; Bergles et al., 1999; Anderson and Swanson, 2000]. Although glutamate transporters are also expressed in neurons, glial cells account for the bulk of glutamate uptake at the synapse (Rothstein et al., 1996; Bergles and Jahr, 1998; Rauen et al., 1998).

Despite the ubiquitous distribution of glial glutamate transporters, the effect of transport on the amplitude and time course of synaptic currents varies widely (Trussel, 1998). This variability arises for a number of reasons, including differences in neuronal glutamate receptor affinity and desensitization, variations in the duration and magnitude of glutamate release at synapses, and differences in the degree to which glutamate is cleared from the synaptic cleft by diffusion (Trussel, 1998; Bergles et al., 1999; Anderson and Swanson, 2000).

In cultured hippocampal neurons, the amplitude of mEPSCs and evoked EPSCs increases when glutamate transport is blocked (Tong and Jahr, 1994). Inhibition of glutamate transport can also prolong EPSCs (Mennerick and Zorumski, 1994) and slow the rise time of mEPSCs, indicating that the transporter modulates glutamate levels during the first few hundred microseconds of the synaptic response (Diamond and Jahr, 2002). This rapid regulation of glutamate levels arises from glutamate binding to the transporter rather than from transport into glial cells, as the transporter has a slow cycling rate (~10 msec) but rapid binding kinetics (Bergles et al., 1997; Bergles and Jahr, 1998; Anderson and Swanson, 2000).

In cerebellar slices, inhibition of glutamate transport prolongs Purkinje cell EPSCs at climbing fiber and parallel fiber synapses (Barbour et al., 1994; Takahashi et al., 2002). Similarly, blockade of glutamate transport at the caliceal synapse in the nucleus magnocellularis increases and prolongs the slowest component of the EPSC, which is generated by rebinding of glutamate at partially desensitized AMPA receptors (Otis et al., 1996). In the retina, the amplitude and duration of ganglion cell EPSCs are dramatically increased when glial glutamate transport is inhibited, although mEPSCs are not affected (Fig. 28.6*A*; Higgs and Lukasiewicz, 2002).

The glial glutamate transporter also modulates synaptic transmission in the supraoptic nucleus of the hypothalamus (Oliet et al., 2001). When GLT-1 transport is blocked, the amplitude of EPSCs decreases dramatically. This anomalous result arises because inhibition of the transporter results in an increase in glutamate concentration near the synapse and stimulation of presynaptic mGluRs, which inhibit release of transmitter. The importance of glial cells in mediating this inhibition is underscored by changes in the responses seen in lactating rats when glial processes are withdrawn from synapses and are less effective in clearing glutamate (Theodosis and Poulain, 1993, 2001); in lactating rats, transporter block produces a much smaller inhibition of evoked EPSCs (Oliet et al., 2001).

Glutamate transport can also modulate short-term synaptic plasticity. In the avian nucleus magnocellularis, repetitive neuronal stimulation produces depression of synaptic transmission. Block of glial glutamate transport augments this depression by reducing the removal of residual glutamate at the synapse (Fig. 28.6*B*; Turecek and Trussell, 2000).

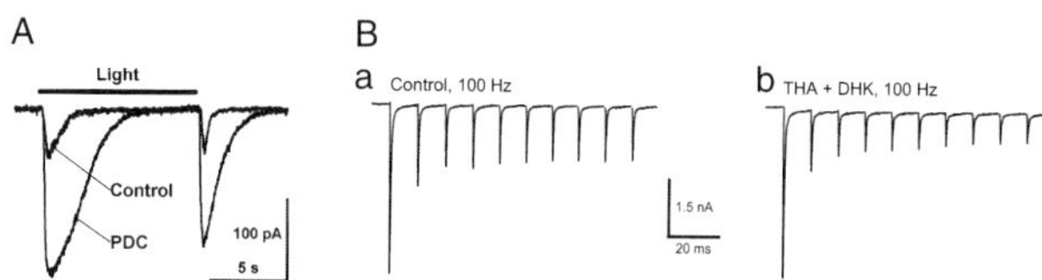

FIGURE 28.6 Glutamate transport into glial cells modulates synaptic transmission. *A*. Inhibition of the glial glutamate transporter by PDC greatly increases the amplitude and duration of a light-evoked EPSC recorded from a ganglion cell in the salamander retina. (From Higgs and Lukasiewicz, 2002.) *B*. Inhibition of the glial glutamate transporter by THA and DHK enhances synaptic depression in a neuron in the avian nucleus magnocellularis. (From Turecek and Trussell, 2000.)

Glial Release of Cofactors

Glial cells can modulate synaptic transmission by releasing cofactors. The best-studied example of this type of modulation is the glial release of D-serine, which potentiates NMDA receptor–mediated synaptic transmission (Baranano et al., 2001).

D-Serine release

The activation of neuronal NMDA receptors requires the presence of two agonists: the primary agonist glutamate and a coagonist that binds to the *glycine binding site* of the receptor. Several lines of evidence indicate that D-serine, the stereo-isomer of the common amino acid L-serine, is the endogenous agonist that activates the glycine binding site of the receptor. D-serine is up to three times more potent than glycine at activating the glycine binding site (Wolosker et al., 1999). In addition, in both hippocampal and cerebellar preparations, addition of the D-serine degrading enzyme D-amino acid oxidase attenuates NMDA receptor–mediated transmission (Mothet et al., 2000).

Glial cells are the endogenous source of D-serine in the CNS. D-Serine and the D-serine synthesizing enzyme serine racemase are localized exclusively to astrocytes in the brain (Schell et al., 1995). In addition, D-serine release from astrocytes is evoked by activation of non-NMDA glutamate receptors on glial cells (Schell et al., 1995).

Müller glial cells act to potentiate NMDA receptor–mediated transmission in the retina (Stevens et al., 2002). NMDA transmission is potentiated by exogenously applied D-serine and is attenuated by addition of D-amino acid oxidase. In addition, both D-serine and serine racemase are localized to Müller cells.

Acetylcholine-binding protein

A unique example of synaptic modulation by release of a glial cofactor occurs at the molluscan cholinergic synapse (Smit et al., 2001). In cultured molluscan cells, release of acetylcholine (ACh) from presynaptic terminals evokes the release of a soluble ACh-binding protein from adjacent glial cells. The ACh-binding protein captures ACh molecules within the synapse, depressing synaptic transmission and blocking synaptic facilitation seen at synapses without ensheathing glial cells. It is not known whether similar neurotransmitter-binding proteins are released from glial cells in vertebrates.

Glial Regulation of Extracellular Ion Levels

In addition to playing a principal role in removing glutamate from synapses, glial cells play a crucial role in regulating K^+ and H^+ in extracellular space. Potassium and H^+ levels affect neuronal excitability and can influence synaptic efficacy.

Glial regulation of K^+

Neuronal activity results in K^+ efflux from neurons and increases in extracellular K^+ levels ($[K^+]_o$) (Kelly and Van Essen, 1974; Karwoski et al., 1985). These activity-dependent $[K^+]_o$ increases are largest in synaptic layers (Karwoski et al., 1985), where they can modulate synaptic transmission by depolarizing presynaptic terminals (Raushe et al., 1990). Extracellular K^+ increases at synapses can also affect synaptic transmission by reducing glutamate transport activity, which relies on a large K^+ gradient across the glial cell membrane (see Chapter 27, this volume).

Glial cells play a dominant role in removing excess K^+ from the extracellular space (see Chapter 26, this volume). Glial cells regulate $[K^+]_o$ by several mechanisms, including active uptake mediated by a Na^+/K^+-ATPase and passive uptake by influx of K^+ and counterions through ion channels and transporters (Ballanyi et al., 1987; Walz, 1987). Glial cells also regulate $[K^+]_o$ by passively transporting excess K^+ to distant extracellular sites via current flow through glial cells, a process termed *K^+ spatial buffering* and *K^+ siphoning* (Orkand et al., 1966; Newman et al., 1984). Interfering with uptake and spatial buffering clearance mechanisms in glial cells results in much larger activity-dependent $[K^+]_o$ increases (Karwoski et al., 1989; Frishman et al., 1992).

Glial regulation of pH

Neuronal activity also results in variations in extracellular pH. Although activity-dependent pH changes are complex, the principal pH change seen in synaptic regions is a sustained alkalinization generated by synaptic transmission (Chesler and Kaila, 1992).

Extracellular alkalinization at synapses influences synaptic transmission by several mechanisms. Calcium channel conductance at the presynaptic terminal is sensitive to H^+ block, and changes in external pH result in variations in transmitter release (Prod'hom et al., 1989; Barnes and Bui, 1991). Small alkalinizations can result in large increases in the strength of synaptic transmission (Barnes et al., 1993). Also, NMDA receptor channels are blocked by H^+, and external alkalinization results in increases in NMDA-mediated synaptic transmission (Tang et al., 1990; Traynelis and Cull-Candy, 1990). In addition, glutamate transport into glial cells depends on the H^+ gradient across the glial cell membrane, and extracellular alkalinization will reduce glutamate transporter activity and thus compromise the removal of glutamate from extracellular space.

Glial cells play an important role in regulating extracellular pH and in counteracting the activity-dependent alkalinization that occurs at the synapse. Glial cells, primarily oligodendrocytes in the brain and Müller cells in the retina, express both intracellular and membrane-bound isoforms of the enzyme carbonic anhydrase (Ghandour et al., 1979; Davis et al., 1987; Newman, 1994), which catalyzes the conversion of CO_2 to HCO_3^- and contributes to the regulation of pH (Borgula et al., 1989; Chen and Chesler, 1992).

Glial cells also regulate extracellular pH via the action of an electrogenic Na^+/HCO_3^- cotransport system (Astion and Orkand, 1988; Newman, 1991). Glial depolarization evoked by neuronal activity results in a cotransport-mediated HCO_3^- influx into glial cells, generating an extracellular acidification (Ransom et al., 1988; Grichtchenko and Chesler, 1994; Newman, 1996). This acidification partially counteracts the alkalinization generated by synaptic activity, thus limiting the changes in synaptic transmission that accompany alkalinization.

Glial Modulation of Synaptogenesis

Glial cells can also modulate synaptic transmission by directly controlling synaptogenesis. Retinal ganglion cells, when cultured in the absence of glial cells, display little spontaneous synaptic activity and have a high failure rate of evoked synaptic transmission. Addition of astrocytes to these cultures substantially increases the frequency of mEPSCs, decreases the failure rate of evoked transmission, and increases the number of morphologically identified synapses (Pfrieger and Barres, 1997; Ullian et al., 2001). Glial enhancement of synapse formation is mediated, at least in part, by the release from astrocytes of cholesterol complexed to apolipoprotein-E-containing lipoproteins (Mauch et al., 2001).

CONCLUSION

Much has been learned in recent years about the interactions between glial cells and neurons at the synapse. Neurons activate glial cells by release of neurotransmitters, including glutamate, GABA, acetylcholine, ATP and nitric oxide. Glial cells, in turn, modulate synaptic transmission by a number of mechanisms. They directly activate pre- and postsynaptic neurons by release of glutamate and ATP. They also modulate synaptic efficacy by the uptake of glutamate from the synaptic cleft, by release of D-serine, and by regulating extracellular K^+ and H^+ levels.

At many synapses, glial cells have multiple effects on synaptic transmission. In culture preparations, astrocytes modulate the release of neurotransmitter from the presynaptic terminal and directly depolarize postsynaptic neurons. In the retina and at the neuromuscular junction, glial cells have both excitatory and inhibitory effects on synaptic efficacy. These glial-neuronal interactions are summarized in Figure 28.7.

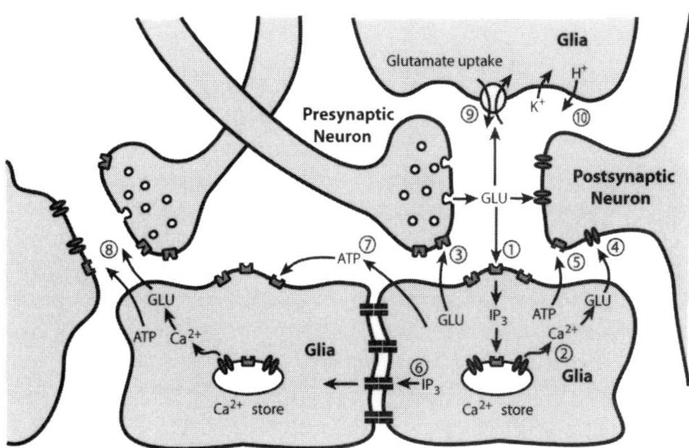

FIGURE 28.7 Summary of possible glial-neuronal interactions at the tripartite synapse. Release of glutamate from the presynaptic terminal activates glial receptors (*1*), evoking a Ca^{2+} increase (*2*) and the release of glutamate (*GLU*) from glial cells. Glutamate activation of presynaptic receptors (*3*) modulates transmitter release while activation of postsynaptic receptors (*4*) directly depolarizes neurons. Activation of glial cells also elicits the release of ATP, which inhibits postsynaptic neurons (*5*). Stimulation of glial cells at a synapse may evoke an intercellular signal which propagates between glial cells by IP_3 diffusion through gap junctions (*6*) and by release of ATP (*7*) and results in the modulation of distant synapses (*8*). Glial cells also modulate synaptic transmission by uptake of glutamate (*9*) and by regulating extracellular K^+ and H^+ levels (*10*).

Although glial-neuronal interactions have been characterized in culture as well as in intact tissue preparations, many important questions remain to be addressed. Are glial cells activated by neurons *in vivo*, as *in situ* experiments suggest? Are glial cells spontaneously active? Do glial cells modulate the release of neurotransmitters and directly stimulate neurons in vivo, as they do in culture and in intact tissue preparations? What role do glial cells play in information processing, learning, and memory? These questions must be answered before we fully understand the function of glial cells at the tripartite synapse.

ACKNOWLEDGMENTS

I thank Janice I. Gepner and Kathleen R. Zahs for helpful comments on the manuscript. Dr. Newman's research is supported by National Institutes of Health Grant EY04077.

REFERENCES

Alvarez-Maubecin, V., Garcia-Hernandez, F., Williams, J.T., and Van Bockstaele, E.J. (2000) Functional coupling between neurons and glia. *J. Neurosci.* 20(11):4091–4098.

Anderson, C.M. and Swanson, R.A. (2000) Astrocyte glutamate transport: review of properties, regulation, and physiological functions. *Glia* 32:1–14.

Araque, A., Carmignoto, G., and Haydon, P.G. (2001) Dynamic signaling between astrocytes and neurons. *Annu. Rev. Physiol.* 63: 795–813.

Araque, A., Li, N., and Haydon, P.G. (2000) SNARE protein-dependent glutamate release from astrocytes. *J. Neurosci.* 20(2): 666–673.

Araque, A., Martin, E.D., Perea, G., Arellano, J.I., and Buno, W. (2002) Synaptically released acetylcholine evokes Ca^{2+} elevations in astrocytes in hippocampal slices. *J. Neurosci.* 22(7):2443–2450.

Araque, A., Parpura, V., Sanzgiri, R.P., and Haydon, P.G. (1998a) Glutamate-dependent astrocyte modulation of synaptic transmission between cultured hippocampal neurons. *Eur. J. Neurosci.* 10:2129–2142.

Araque, A., Parpura, V., Sanzgiri, R.P., and Haydon, P.G. (1999) Tripartite synapses: glia, the unacknowledged partner. *TINS* 22: 208–215.

Araque, A., Sanzgiri, R.P., Parpura, V., and Haydon, P.G. (1998b) Calcium elevation in astrocytes causes an NMDA receptor-dependent increase in the frequency of miniature synaptic currents in cultured hippocampal neurons. *J. Neurosci.* 18:6822–6829.

Astion, M.L. and Orkand, R.K. (1988) Electrogenic Na^+/HCO_3^- cotransport in neuroglia. *Glia* 1:355–357.

Ballanyi, K., Grafe, P., and ten Bruggencate, G. (1987) Ion activities and potassium uptake mechanisms of glial cells in guinea-pig olfactory cortex slices. *J. Physiol.* 382:159–174.

Baranano, D.E., Ferris, C.D., and Snyder, S.H. (2001) Atypical neural messengers. *TINS* 24:99–106.

Barbour, B., Keller, B.U., Llano, I., and Marty, A. (1994) Prolonged presence of glutamate during excitatory synaptic transmission to cerebellar Purkinje cells. *Neuron* 12:1331–1343.

Barnes, S. and Bui, Q. (1991) Modulation of calcium-activated chloride current via pH-induced changes of calcium channel properties in cone photoreceptors. *J. Neurosci.* 11:4015–4023.

Barnes, S., Merchant, V., and Mahmud, F. (1993) Modulation of transmission gain by protons at the photoreceptor output synapse. *Proc. Natl. Acad. Sci. USA* 90:10081–10085.

Bergles, D.E., Diamond, J.S., and Jahr, C.E. (1999) Clearance of glutamate inside the synapse and beyond. *Curr. Opin. Neurobiol.* 9:293–298.

Bergles, D.E., Dzubay, J.A., and Jahr, C.E. (1997) Glutamate transporter currents in Bergmann glial cells follow the time course of extrasynaptic glutamate. *Proc. Natl. Acad. Sci. USA* 94:14821–14825.

Bergles, D.E. and Jahr, C.E. (1998) Glial contribution to glutamate uptake at Schaffer collateral-commissural synapses in the hippocampus. *J. Neurosci.* 18(19):7709–7716.

Bergles, D.E., Roberts, J.D.B., Somogyi, P., and Jahr, C.E. (2000) Glutamatergic synapses on oligodendrocyte precursor cells in the hippocampus. *Nature* 405:187–191.

Bezzi, P., Carmignoto, G., Pasti, L., Vesce, S., Rossi, D., Lodi Rizzini, B., Pozzan, T., and Volterra, A. (1998) Prostaglandins stimulate calcium-dependent glutamate release in astrocytes. *Nature* 391: 281–285.

Borgula, G.A., Karwoski, C.J., and Steinberg, R.H. (1989) Light-evoked changes in extracellular pH in frog retina. *Vision. Res.* 29:1069–1077.

Castonguay, A. and Robitaille, R. (2001) Differential regulation of transmitter release by presynaptic and glial Ca^{2+} internal stores at the neuromuscular synapse. *J. Neurosci.* 21:1911–1922.

Chen, J.C.T. and Chesler, M. (1992) pH transients evoked by excitatory synaptic transmission are increased by inhibition of extracellular carbonic anhydrase. *Proc. Natl. Acad. Sci. USA* 89:7786–7790.

Chesler, M. and Kaila, K. (1992) Modulation of pH by neuronal activity. *TINS* 15:396–402.

Cornell-Bell, A.H., Finkbeiner, S.M., Cooper, M.S., and Smith, S.J. (1990a) Glutamate induces calcium waves in cultured astrocytes: long-range glial signaling. *Science* 247:470–473.

Cornell-Bell, A.H., Thomas, P.G., and Smith, S.J. (1990b) The excitatory neurotransmitter glutamate causes filopodia formation in cultured hippocampal astrocytes. *Glia* 3:322–334.

Cotrina, M.L., Lin, J.H.C., Alves-Rodriques, A., Liu, S., Li, J., Azmi-Ghadimi, H., Kang, J., Naus, C.C.G., and Nedergaard, M. (1998) Connexins regulate calcium signaling by controlling ATP release. *Proc. Natl. Acad. Sci. USA* 95:15735–15740.

Dani, J.W., Chernjavsky, A., and Smith, S.J. (1992) Neuronal activity triggers calcium waves in hippocampal astrocyte networks. *Neuron* 8:429–440.

Davis, P.K., Carlini, W.G., Ransom, B.R., Black, J.A., and Waxman, S.G. (1987) Carbonic anhydrase activity develops postnatally in the rat optic nerve. *Dev. Brain Res.* 31:291–298.

Diamond, J.S. and Jahr, C.E. (2002) Transporters buffer synaptically released glutamate on a submillisecond time scale. *J. Neurosci.* 17(12):4672–4687.

Fields, R.D. and Stevens-Graham, B. (2002) New insights into neuron-glia communication. *Science* 298:556–562.

Finkbeiner, S.M. (1993) Glial calcium. *Glia* 9:83–104.

Frishman, L.J., Yamamoto, F., Bogucka, J., and Steinberg, R.H. (1992) Light-evoked changes in $[K^+]_o$ in proximal portion of light-adapted cat retina. J Neurophysiol 67:1201–1212.

Froes, M.M., Correia, A.H.P., Garcia-Abreu, J., Spray, D.C., Campos de Carvalho, A.C., and Moura Neto, V. (1999) Gap-junctional coupling between neurons and astrocytes in primary central nervous system cultures. *PNAS* 96:7541–7546.

Ghandour, M.S., Langley, O.K., Vincendon, G., and Gombos, G. (1979) Double labeling immunohistochemical technique provides evidence of the specificity of glial cell markers. *J. Histochem. Cytochem.* 27:1634–1637.

Grichtchenko, I.I. and and Chesler, M. (1994) Depolarization-induced acid secretion in gliotic hippocampal slices. *Neurosci.* 62:1057–1070.

Grosche, J., Kettenmann, H., and Reichenbach, A. (2002) Bergmann glial cells form distinct morphological structures to interact with cerebellar neurons. *J. Neurosci. Res.* 68:138–149.

Grosche, J., Matyash, V., Moller, T., Verkhratsky, A., Reichenbach, A., and Kettenmann, H. (1999) Microdomains for neuron-glia interaction: parallel fiber signaling to Bergmann glial cells. *Nature Neurosci.* 2(2):139–143.

Hassinger, T.D., Atkinson, P.B., Strecker, G.J., Whalen, L.R., Dudek, F.E., Kossel, A.H., and Kater, S.B. (1995) Evidence for glutamate-mediated activation of hippocampal neurons by glial calcium waves. *J. Neurobiol.* 28:159–170.

Hatton, G.I. (2002) Function-related plasticity in hypothalamus. *Annu. Rev. Neurosci.* 20:375–397.

Hepp, R., Perraut, M., Chasserot-Golaz, S., Galli, T., Aunis, D., Langley, K., and Grant, N.J. (1999) Cultured glial cells express the SNAP-25 analogue SNAP-23. *Glia* 27:181–187.

Higgs, M.H. and Lukasiewicz, P.D. (2002) Glutamate uptake limits synaptic excitation of retinal ganglion cells. *J. Neurosci.* 19(10): 3691–3700.

Innocenti, B., Parpura, V., and Haydon, P.G. (2000) Imaging extracellular waves of glutamate during calcium signaling in cultured astrocytes. *J. Neurosci.* 20(5):1800–1808.

Jahromi, B.S., Robitaille, R., and Charlton, M.P. (2002) Transmitter release increases intracellular calcium in perisynaptic Schwann cells in situ. *Neuron* 8:1069–1077.

Kang, J., Goldman, S.A., and Nedergaard, M. (1998) Astrocyte-mediated potentiation of inhibitory synaptic transmission. *Nature Neurosci.* 1(8):683–692.

Karwoski, C.J., Lu, H.-K., and Newman, E.A. (1989) Spatial buffering of light-evoked potassium increases by retinal Muller (glial) cells. *Science* 244:578–580.

Karwoski, C.J., Newman, E.A., Shimazaki, H., and Proenza, L.M. (1985) Light-evoked increases in extracellular K^+ in the plexiform layers of amphibian retinas. *J. Gen. Physiol.* 86:189–213.

Kelly, J.P. and Van Essen, D.C. (1974) Cell structure and function in the visual cortex of the cat. *J. Physiol.* 238:515–547.

Kulik, A., Haentzsch, A., Luckermann, M., Reichelt, W., and Ballanyi, K. (1999) Neuron-glia signaling via α_1 adrenoceptor-mediated Ca^{2+} release in Bergmann glial cells *in situ*. *J. Neurosci.* 19(19):8401–8408.

Maienschein, V., Marxen, M., Volknandt, W., and Zimmermann, H. (1999) A plethora of presynaptic proteins associated with ATP-storing organelles in cultured astrocytes. *Glia* 26:233–244.

Matyash, V., Filippov, V., Mohrhagen, K., and Kettenmann, H. (2001) Nitric oxide signals parallel fiber activity to Bergmann glial cells in the mouse cerebellar slice. *Mol. Cell Neurosci.* 18:664–670.

Mauch, D.H., Nagler, K., Schumacher, S., Goritz, C., Muller, E.-C., Otto, A., and Pfrieger, F.W. (2001) CNS synaptogenesis promoted by glia-derived cholesterol. *Science* 294:1354–1357.

McMahan, U.J., Spitzer, N.C., and Peper, K. (1972) Visual identification of nerve terminals in living isolated skeletal muscle. *Proc. R. Soc. Lond. B* 181:421–430.

Mennerick, S. and Zorumski, C.F. (1994) Glial contributions to excitatory neurotransmission in cultured hippocampal cells. *Nature* 368:59–62.

Mothet, J.-P., Parent, A.T., Wolosker, H., Brady, R.O., Jr., Linden, D.J., Ferris, C.D., Rogawski, M.A., and Snyder, S.H. (2000) D-serine is an endogenous ligand for the glycine site of the *N*-methyl-D-aspartate receptor. *PNAS* 97:4926–4931.

Muller, T., Moller, T., Neuhaus, J., and Kettenmann, H. (1996) Electrical coupling among Bergmann glial cells and its modulation by glutamate receptor activation. *Glia* 17:274–284.

Nett, W.J., Oloff, S.H., and McCarthy, K.D. (2001) Hippocampal astrocytes in situ exhibit calcium oscillations that occur independent of neuronal activity. *J. Neurophysiol.* 87:528–537.

Newman, E.A. (1991) Sodium-bicarbonate cotransport in retinal Muller (glial) cells of the salamander. *J. Neurosci.* 11:3972–3983.

Newman, E.A. (1994) A physiological measure of carbonic anhydrase in Muller cells. *Glia* 11:291–299.

Newman, E.A. (1996) Acid efflux from retinal glial cells generated by sodium-bicarbonate cotransport. *J. Neurosci.* 16:159–168.

Newman, E.A. (2001a) Glia of the retina. In: Ryan, S.J., ed. *Retina* St. Louis: Mosby, pp. 89–103.

Newman, E.A. (2001b) Propagation of intercellular calcium waves in retinal astrocytes and Müller cells. *J. Neurosci.* 21:2215–2223.

Newman, E.A. (2002a) Calcium signaling in retinal glial cells and its effect on neuronal activity. *Prog. Brain Res.* 132:241–254.

Newman, E.A. (2002b) Glial cell inhibition of neurons by release of ATP. *J. Neurosci.* 23:1659–1666.

Newman, E.A., Frambach, D.A., and Odette, L.L. (1984) Control of extracellular potassium levels by retinal glial cell K^+ siphoning. *Science* 225:1174–1175.

Newman, E.A. and Zahs, K.R. (1997) Calcium waves in retinal glial cells. *Science* 275:844–847.

Newman, E.A. and Zahs, K.R. (1998) Modulation of neuronal activity by glial cells in the retina. *J. Neurosci.* 18:4022–4028.

Oliet, S.H.R., Piet, R., and Poulain, D.A. (2001) Control of glutamate clearance and synaptic efficacy by glial coverage of neurons. *Science* 292:923–926.

Orkand, R.K., Nicholls, J.G., and Kuffler, S.W. (1966) Effect of nerve impulses on the membrane potential of glial cells in the central nervous system of amphibia. *J. Neurophysiol.* 29:788–806.

Otis, T.S., Wu, Y.-C., and Trussell, L.O. (1996) Delayed clearance of transmitter and the role of glutamate transporters at synapses with multiple release sites. *J. Neurosci.* 16(5):1634–1644.

Parpura, V., Basarsky, T.A., Liu, F., Jeftinija, K., Jeftinija, S., and Haydon, P.G. (1994) Glutamate-mediated astrocyte-neuron signalling. *Nature* 369:744–747.

Parpura, V., Fang, Y., Basarsky, T., Jahn, R., and Haydon, P.G. (1995) Expression of synaptobrevin II, cellubrevin and syntaxin but not SNAP-25 in cultured astrocytes. *FEBS Lett.* 377:489–492.

Parpura, V. and Haydon, P.G. (2000) Physiological astrocytic calcium levels stimulate glutamate release to modulate adjacent neurons. *Proc. Natl. Acad. Sci. USA* 97:8629–8634.

Parri, H.R., Gould, T.M., and Crunelli, V. (2001) Spontaneous astrocytic Ca^{2+} oscillations *in situ* drive NMDAR-mediated neuronal excitation. *Nat. Neurosci.* 4:803–812.

Pasti, L., Volterra, A., Pozzan, T., and Carmignoto, G. (1997) Intracellular calcium oscillations in astrocytes: a highly plastic, bidirectional form of communication between neurons and astrocytes in situ. *J. Neurosci.* 17:7817–7830.

Pasti, L., Zonta, M., Pozzan, T., Vicini, S., and Carmignoto, G. (2001) Cytosolic calcium oscillations in astrocytes may regulate exocytotic release of glutamate. *J. Neurosci.* 21(2):477–484.

Pfrieger, F.W. and Barres, B.A. (1997) Synaptic efficacy enhanced by glial cells in vitro. *Science* 277:1684–1688.

Pinard, A., Levesque, S., and Robitaille, R. (2002) NO-dependence of glutamate-mediated synaptic depression at the frog neuromuscular junction. *Soc. Neurosci. Abstr.* Program no. 838.6.

Porter, J.T. and McCarthy, K.D. (1996) Hippocampal astrocytes *in situ* respond to glutamate released from synaptic terminals. *J. Neurosci.* 16:5073–5081.

Porter, J.T. and McCarthy, K.D. (1997) Astrocytic neurotransmitter receptors *in situ* and *in vivo*. *Prog. Neurobiol.* 51:439–455.

Prod'hom, B., Pietrobon, D., and Hess, P. (1989) Interactions of protons with single open L-type calcium channels. Location of protonation site and dependence of proton-induced current fluctuations on concentration and species of permeant ion. *J. Gen. Physiol.* 94:23–42.

Ransom, B.R., Carlini, W.G., and Connors, B.W. (1988) Brain extracellular space: developmental studies in rat optic nerve. *Ann. NY Acad. Sci.* 481:87–105.

Rauen, T., Taylor, W.R., Kuhlbrodt, K., and Wiessner, M. (1998) High-affinity glutamate transporters in the rat retina: a major role of the glial glutamate transporter GLAST-1 in transmitter clearance. *Cell Tissue Res.* 291:19–31.

Raushe, G., Igelmund, P., and Heinemann, U. (1990) Effects of changes in extracellular potassium, magnesium and calcium concentration on synaptic transmission in area CA1 and the dentate gyrus of rat hippocampal slices. *Pflugers Arch.* 415:588–593.

Reist, N.E. and Smith, S.J. (1992) Neurally evoked calcium transients in terminal Schwann cells at the neuromuscular junction. *Proc. Natl. Acad. Sci. USA* 89:7625–7629.

Robitaille, R. (1998) Modulation of synaptic efficacy and synaptic depression by glial cells at the frog neuromuscular junction. *Neuron* 21:847–855.

Rochon, D., Rousse, I., and Robitaille, R. (2001) Synapse-glia interactions at the mammalian neuromuscular junction. *J. Neurosci.* 21(11):3819–3829.

Rothstein, J.D., Dykes-Hoberg, M., Pardo, C.A., Bristol, L.A., Jin, L., Kunci, R.W., Kanai, Y., Hediger, M.A., Wang, Y., Schielke, J.P., and Welty, D.F. (1996) Knockout of glutamate transporters reveals a major role for astroglial transport in excitotoxicity and clearance of glutamate. *Neuron* 16:675–686.

Sanzgiri, R.P., Araque, A., and Haydon, P.G. (1999) Prostaglandin E_2 stimulates glutamate receptor-dependent astrocyte neuromodulation in cultured hippocampal cells. *J. Neurobiol.* 41:221–229.

Schell, M.J., Molliver, M.E., and Snyder, S.H. (1995) D-serine, an endogenous synaptic modulator: Localization to astrocytes and glutamate-stimulated release. *Proc. Natl. Acad. Sci. USA* 92:3948–3952.

Schikorski, T. and Stevens, C.F. (1999) Quantitative fine-structural analysis of olfactory cortical synapses. *PNAS* 96:4107–4112.

Schipke, C.G., Boucsein, C., Ohlemeyer, C., Kirchhoff, F., and Kettenmann, H. (2002) Astrocyte Ca^{2+} waves trigger responses in microglial cells in brain slices. *FASEB* 16(2):255–257.

Smit, A.B., Syed, N.I., Schaap, D., van Minnen, J., Klumperman, J., Kits, K.S., Lodder, H., van der Schors, R.C., van Elk, R., Sorgedrager, B., Brejc, K., Sixma, T.K., and Geraerts, W.P.M. (2001)

A glia-derived acetylcholine-binding protein that modulates synaptic transmission. *Nature* 411:261–268.

Spacek, J. (1985) Three-dimensional analysis of dendritic spines. *Anat. Embryol.* 171:245–252.

Stevens, E.R., Esquerra, M., Kim, P., Newman, E.A., Snyder, S.H., Zahs, K.R., and Miller, R.F. (2002) D-serine and serine racemase are present in the vertebrate retina and contribute to the functional expression of NMDA receptors. *Proc. Natl. Acad. Sci. USA*. 100:6789–6794.

Sul, J.-Y. and Haydon, P.G. (2001) Focal photolysis of caged glutamate evokes intercellular calcium waves between astrocytes in the hippocampal slice. *Soc. Neurosci. Abstr.* Program no. 505.10.

Takahashi, M., Kovalchuk, Y., and Attwell, D. (2002) Pre- and postsynaptic determinants of EPSC waveform at cerebellar climbing fiber and parallel fiber to Purkinje cell synapses. *J. Neurosci.* 15(8):5693–5702.

Tang, C.-M., Dichter, M., and Morad, M. (1990) Modulation of the *N*-methyl-D-aspartate channel by extracellular H^+. *Proc. Natl. Acad. Sci. USA* 87:6445–6449.

Theodosis, D.T. and Poulain, D.A. (1993) Activity-dependent neuronal-glial and synaptic plasticity in the adult mammalian hypothalamus. *Neuroscience* 57:501–535.

Theodosis, D.T. and Poulain, D.A. (2001) Maternity leads to morphological synaptic plasticity in the oxytocin system. *Prog. Brain Res.* 133:49–58.

Thomas, S. and Robitaille, R. (2001) Differential frequency-dependent regulation of transmitter release by endogenous nitric oxide at the amphibian neuromuscular synapse. *J. Neurosci.* 21(4):1087–1095.

Tong, G. and Jahr, C.E. (1994) Block of glutamate transporters potentiates postsynaptic excitation. *Neuron* 13:1195–1203.

Traynelis, S.F. and Cull-Candy, S.G. (1990) Proton inhibition of N-methyl-D-aspartate receptors in cerebellar neurons. *Nature* 345: 347–350.

Trussel, L. (1998) Control of time course of glutamatergic synaptic currents. *Prog. Brain Res.* 116:59–69.

Turecek, R. and Trussell, L.O. (2000) Control of synaptic depression by glutamate transporters. *J. Neurosci.* 20(5):2054–2063.

Ullian, E.M., Sapperstein, S.K., Christopherson, K.S., and Barres, B.A. (2001) Control of synapse number by glia. *Science* 291: 657–661.

Ventura, R. and Harris, K.M. (1999) Three-dimensional relationships between hippocampal synapses and astrocytes. *J. Neurosci.* 19(16):6897–6906.

Verkhratsky, A., Orkand, R.K., and Kettenmann, H. (1998) Glial calcium: Homeostasis and signaling function. *Physiol. Rev.* 78:99–141.

Vesce, S., Bezzi, P., and Volterra, A. (2001) Synaptic transmission with the glia. *News Physiol. Sci.* 16:178–184.

Walz, W. (1987) Swelling and potassium uptake in cultured astrocytes. *Can. J. Physiol. Pharmacol.* 65:1051–1057.

Wang, Z., Haydon, P.G., and Yeung, E.S. (2000) Direct observation of calcium-independent intercellular ATP signaling in astrocytes. *Anal. Chem.* 72:2001–2007.

Wolosker, H., Blackshaw, S., and Snyder, S.H. (1999) Serine racemase: a glial enzyme synthesizing D-serine to regulate glutamate-*N*methyl-D-aspartate neurotransmission. *PNAS* 96:13409–13414.

Xu-Friedman, M.A., Harris, K.M., and Regehr, W.G. (2001) Three-dimensional comparison of ultrastructural characteristics at depressing and facilitating synapses onto cerebellar Purkinje cells. *J. Neurosci.* 21(17):6666–6672.

29 The central role of astrocytes in neuroenergetics

LUC PELLERIN AND PIERRE J. MAGISTRETTI

Astrocytes have been considered traditionally as structural elements within the central nervous system with the main function of maintaining the nervous tissue in place, hence their designation as *neuroglia* or "nerve glue." Indeed, astrocytes come in close contact with several cellular components of the brain parenchyma including blood vessels, pial surfaces, neurons, and other glial cells. It appeared that astrocytes were filling any gap between these different elements. Fortunately, recent studies have highlighted much more dynamic functions that could be played by these cells. In fact, one early argument in favor of their role in the regulation of brain energy metabolism came from morphological studies. Anatomists at the end of the nineteenth century noticed the strategic position occupied by astrocytes between neurons and blood vessels. Moreover, it was realized that astrocytes were sending specific processes, called *endfeet*, in close contact with capillaries, covering almost their entire surface, as recently documented unequivocally (Kacem et al., 1998). This arrangement suggested that astrocytes might dynamically regulate the entry and distribution of energy substrates to neurons. This hypothesis was eloquently formulated by Golgi (1886): "Dichiaro anzi che, dopo tutto, la parola nevroglia adoperata nel senso passato in uso mi sembra abbia titoli di preferenza, valendo ad indicare un tessuto, che sebbene sia connettivo, perchè connette elementi d'altra natura e alla sua volta *serve alla distribuzione del materiale nutritizio*, pure si differenzia dal connettivo comune per cararreri morfologici, chimici, e quasi certamente, come dirò in seguito, anche pel carattere fondamentale della diversa origine embrionale." Despite such an early suggestion for a role of astrocytes in metabolic control, only recently have we gained further insight into this important function.

In parallel, more recent investigations have revealed other important features of astrocytes. Morphologically, they contact neurons at different locations including the cell body and nodes of Ranvier, but also at synapses that they often ensheath (Grosche et al., 1999). It was also demonstrated that astrocytes express a large number of receptors and transporters for virtually every neurotransmitter (Hösli and Hösli, 1993). These characteristics endow astrocytes with the capacity to detect synaptic activity, react, and possibly respond to neurons by releasing neuroactive substances, as has been demonstrated already (see Chapters 16 and 28). But the same characteristics might also be necessary for astrocytes to adjust the metabolic environment of neurons to changing needs in register with their activity. The purpose of this chapter is to review these aspects of astrocyte function in the maintenance of metabolic homeostasis, which could be of critical importance for neuronal functions. In particular, the field of functional neuroenergetics, that is, the various metabolic and hemodynamic responses that occur following neuronal activation and that provide the signals for modern functional brain imaging, is particularly concerned with this metabolic role of astrocytes.

THE GLUTAMATE-GLUTAMINE CYCLE REVISITED: THE IMPORTANCE OF ASTROCYTES FOR GLUTAMATERGIC NEUROTRANSMISSION

One classical function attributed to astrocytes is the inactivation of neurotransmitters released into the synaptic cleft (for review, see Martin, 1995). This can occur through either neurotransmitter degradation by ectoenzymes outside the cell or inside the cell after its uptake. In the case of glutamate, the major excitatory neurotransmitter of the central nervous system, most of what is released synaptically is taken up by astrocytes via specific transporters identified as glutamate/aspartate transporter (GLAST) and glutamate transporter-1 (GLT-1) (Danbolt, 2001). Once inside astrocytes, glutamate can be metabolized via two major routes. It can be converted to glutamine by the enzyme glutamine synthetase, which is exclusively localized in glia (Martinez-Hernandez et al., 1977), or it can be metabolized in the tricarboxylic acid cycle following its transformation into α-ketoglutarate. This can occur via three different reactions catalyzed by either glutamate dehydrogenase (GDH), aspartate aminotransferase (AAT), or alanine aminotransferase (ALAT). In parallel, glutamate lost by neurons following synaptic activity needs to be replenished in order to maintain synaptic transmission. One mechanism by which glutamate can be regenerated in neurons is part of a process involving metabolic interactions between neurons and astrocytes known as the *glutamate/glutamine cycle* (Berl et al., 1962; Van den Berg et al., 1969; see Fig. 29.1). Thus, in addition to avidly taking up glutamate and converting it to glutamine, astrocytes release glutamine in large amounts into the extracellular space (Waniewski and Martin, 1986), which can then be taken up by neurons. In support of this view, a new group of transporters for glutamine has been described recently and located on both neurons and astrocytes (Bröer and Brookes, 2001). After its uptake into neurons, glutamine is converted to glutamate by a phosphate-activated glutaminase found predominantly in neuronal mitochondria (Kvamme et al., 1985), thus completing the cycle. Finally, synaptic vesicles are refilled with glutamate through a newly described family of vesicular glutamate transporters (Kaneko and Fujiyama, 2002), and are ready to be released again upon the invasion by action potentials of the presynaptic terminal.

In addition to the glutamate/glutamine cycle, other pathways have been proposed to replenish the neuronal glutamate pool; these mechanisms involve *de novo* synthesis of glutamate. One of these pathways is based on the ability of astrocytes to provide the carbon backbone for the synthesis of glutamate from glucose as α-ketoglurate. Then, α-ketoglutarate formed in the glial tricarboxylic acid (TCA) cyle could be converted to glutamate upon addition of an amino group. This amino group would be provided by either free ammonia brought from the circulation in a reaction catalyzed by GDH or from leucine also imported from the circulation via a transamination mediated by leucine transaminase (LT), leading to the formation of α-ketoisocaproate (α-KIC) in addition to glutamate (Yudkoff, 1997). Glutamate formed through this mechanism would simply reintegrate the glutamate/glutamine cycle via its conversion to glutamine in astrocytes and its subsequent release. Another possibility is that astrocytes could export α-ketoglutarate directly to neurons (Shank and Campbell, 1984; Peng et al., 1993). Neurons would themselves resynthesize glutamate either via a GDH-catalyzed reaction or by a transamination of alanine by ALAT. Notice that in these last two pathways, use of α-ketoglutarate generated by astrocytes to resynthesize glutamate could eventually lead to a depletion in TCA cycle intermediates. In order to avoid such a situation, it is necessary for the astrocyte to form new TCA cycle intermediates downstream of α-ketoglutarate. This is done by an anaplerotic reaction catalyzed by the enzyme pyruvate carboxylase, which is found specifically in astrocytes (Shank et al., 1985). In this reaction, CO_2 is fixed to pyruvate in order to form oxaloacetate. In this manner, a complete astrocytic TCA cycle can be maintained despite the loss of α-ketoglutarate for glutamate synthesis. Finally, neurons were also shown to have the possibility of synthesizing glutamate via TCA cycle intermediates and replenish their intermediate pool by an anaplerotic reaction of CO_2 fixation (Hassel and Brathe, 2000a).

In the past few years, Robert Shulman, Doug Rothman, and their colleagues at Yale have investigated with nuclear magnetic resonance (NMR) spectroscopy the extent/degree of glutamate recycling via the formation of glutamine by astrocytes in rats and humans (reviewed in Rothman et al., 1999). In contrast to a previous proposal suggesting the existence of a small nonmetabolic transmitter pool versus a large metabolic pool (Badar-Goffer et al., 1992; Peng et al., 1993), a high rate of glutamine synthesis was demonstrated, indicating a possible predominance of the glutamate/glutamine cycle (Gruetter et al., 1994; Mason et al., 1995). Moreover, when the participation of each pathway in neuronal glutamate replenishment was analyzed in more detail, it became clear that the glutamate/glutamine cycle was by far the major metabolic pathway of glutamate resynthesis. Thus, the glutamate/glutamine cycle with conversion of glutamate taken up by astrocytes into glutamine via glutamine synthetase was found to provide 80%–90% of all glutamine synthesized under physiological (normal ammonia levels) conditions, both in rats and in humans (Sibson et al., 1997; Shen et al., 1999; Sibson et al., 2001; Lebon et al., 2002). This observation leads to the conclusion that other pathways play minor roles in neuronal glutamate replenishment under physiological conditions, while under hyperammonemic condition they appear to be more involved in brain ammonia detoxification, as they contribute significantly to glutamine formation (Sibson et al., 1997; Shen et al., 1998). In addition, the metabolic importance of astrocytes for the maintenance of glutamatergic neurotransmission and normal brain function through glutamate recycling into glutamine has also been supported by a number of *in vitro* and *in vivo* studies (Ng et al., 1997; Hulsmann et al., 2000; Bacci et al., 2002).

Glutamatergic Neurotransmission Drives Energy Consumption in the Brain

Another important observation that was made from NMR studies is the relationship that appears to exist between glutamate/glutamine cycling and glucose oxidation. Parallel measurements made under different levels of anesthesia in the rat have shown that glucose oxidation increases with the rate of glutamate/glutamine cycling, and this is correlated with the level of brain electrical activity (Sibson et al., 1998). These data sug-

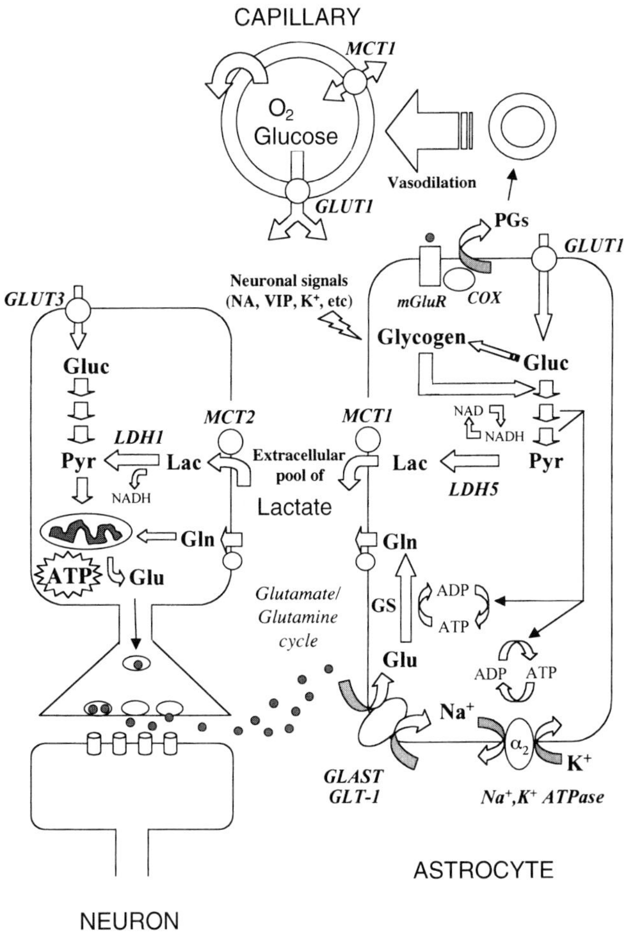

FIGURE 29.1 The central role of astrocytes in neuroenergetics. Blood-borne glucose, which is the major energy substrate for the adult brain, enters the brain parenchyma via GLUT1 (55 kd) glucose transporters located on endothelial cells forming capillaries. It is provided to both neurons and astrocytes in which it will be taken up via specific glucose transporters (GLUT3 and GLUT1, 45 kd). In astrocytes, glucose stores are present as glycogen. Due to basal conversion of glucose into lactate and its release in the extracellular space, especially by astrocytes, an extracellular lactate pool is maintained. Upon neuronal activation, three types of astrocytic responses can be evoked. First, glycogen breakdown can occur following receptor-mediated action of some neurotransmitters (NA, noradrenaline, VIP, vasoactive intestinal peptide) or by K^+ release by axons as a consequence of action potential propagation. The glucose formed will be processed glycotically into lactate, favored by the enrichment of LDH5 isofom in astrocytes. The other two responses will be specifically triggered by activity at glutamatergic synapses. Thus, the action of glutamate on postsynaptic receptors is terminated by its uptake in astrocytes via glutamate transporter-1 (GLT-1) and the glutamate/aspartate transporter (GLAST). As a consequence of cotransport with Na^+, the intracellular Na^+ concentration will increase and activate a glia-specific, Na^+/K^+-ATPase α_2 subunit. Adenosine triphosphate (ATP) consumption by the pump, but also by the glutamate-to-glutamine conversion by glutamine synthetase (GS), will activate glycolysis and the formation of lactate. Lactate will leave astrocytes by a specific monocarboxylate transporter, MCT1. Meanwhile, in addition to glucose, activated neurons will take up lactate from the extracellular pool via their own specific monocarboxylate transporter, MCT2. Lactate will be converted to pyruvate, favored by the preferential expression of LDH1 isoform in neurons, before entering the tricarboxylic acid cycle. Use of lactate by neurons in addition to glucose could have multiple purposes: it increases redox potential by providing cytoplasmic reduced nicotine adenine dinucleotide (NADH), and it can be used to generate ATP as well as enter into glutamate synthesis. Glutamine will also be taken up by neurons via their specific glutamine transporters and converted back to glutamate by glutaminase before being accumulated in synaptic vesicles via vesicular glutamate transporters, thus completing the glutamate/glutamine cycle. Finally, the third response is triggered by activation of metabotropic glutamate receptors on astrocytes that will lead to formation of prostaglandins. These substances will act on neighboring blood vessels and cause vasodilation. ADP: adenosine diphosphate; COX: cyclooxygenase; Gln: glutamine; Glu: glutamate; Gluc: glucose; GS: glutamine synthetase; Lac: lactate; mGluR: metabotropic glutamate receptor; NAD: nicotine adenine dinucleotide; PGs: prostaglandins; Pyr: pyruvate.

gest that there is somehow a particular mechanistic link between the recycling of glutamate that occurs essentially in astrocytes, and glucose metabolism that provides the energy to maintain neuronal activity. From these experiments, it was also concluded that restoration of ion gradients that occurs in parallel with glutamate/glutamine cycling as a consequence of glutamatergic neurotransmission is responsible for approximately 80% of oxidative glucose consumption under normal unanesthetized conditions. In other words, processes not involved in neurotransmission but rather in maintenance of cell structure and function, like protein and membrane turnover, account for a rather small fraction of the total energy consumption. The same can be said for other neurotransmitter systems. In the specific case of γ-aminobutyric acid (GABA), which will be included in the glutamate/glutamine cycle rate since GABA is at least partly recycled in astrocytes via glutamine synthesis by a pathway known as the *GABA shunt* (McGeer and McGeer, 1989), it was estimated that it would not account for more than 11% of the total glutamine flux in the rat (Rothman et al., 1999) or 10 times less than for glutamate in human cortex (Shen et al., 1999). The essential conclusion is that the majority of energy consumption (which consists almost entirely of glucose oxidation) is a direct reflection of the level of glutamatergic neurotransmission and its associated recycling involving astrocytes.

Interestingly, using a bottom-up approach, Attwell and Laughlin have estimated the relative energy cost of different cellular processes involved in brain activity for both rodents and primates. (Attwell and Laughlin, 2001). Indeed they concluded that the large majority of energy consumption is caused by excitatory signalling, mostly the reestablishment of ion gradients following action potential propagation and postsynaptic currents. Their value of 81%–84% of the energy cost attributed to excitatory (essentially glutamatergic) signaling is in perfect agreement with the NMR studies mentioned above. Moreover, estimation of the glial energy cost, including glutamate recycling, would account for approximately 6% of total energy usage. These data offer guidelines to assign energy consumption to specific processes and fix certain limitations as well as proportions. What they do not provide, however, is the mechanism(s) linking these energy-consuming processes to energy generation, and they do not take into account the possibility of cooperation between neurons and astrocytes.

CELLULAR MECHANISMS COUPLING NEURONAL ACTIVITY TO ENERGY METABOLISM AND BLOOD FLOW: THE ASTROCYTE AS A MISSING LINK

The preceeding NMR studies have highlighted the putative link between glutamate/glutamine cycling and glucose metabolism, although they could not give any indication of the cellular and molecular mechanisms responsible for this association. About a decade ago, it was postulated that astrocytes could play a role in coupling neuronal activity to energy metabolism (Pellerin and Magistretti, 1994). As exposed previously, astrocytes are ideally positioned between blood vessels that provide the major energy substrate for the brain, which is glucose, and neurons, which are the most important energy consumers. Astrocytic endfeet which cover the surface of capillaries express one of the glucose transporter isoforms, GLUT1, 45 kDa, on membranes facing capillaries (Morgello et al., 1995; Yu and Ding, 1998). These characteristics suggested that astrocytes might represent a privileged site of glucose uptake as it penetrates into the brain parenchyma. Combined with the aforementioned presence of receptors and transporters for most neurotransmitters and neuroactive substances on processes ensheathing synapses, the strategic position of astrocytes led to the hypothesis that they could effectively couple neuronal activity to glucose metabolism.

(Re)Emergence of a Nursing Role for Astrocytes

Experiments performed in the honeybee retina had previously suggested that a marked metabolic compartmentation occurs between glial cells and photoreceptors. Thus, it was observed that upon exposure to light, an increase in 2-deoxyglucose accumulation took place exclusively in glial cells, while an increase in oxygen consumption, indicative of increased oxidative metabolism, occurred in photoreceptors (Tsacopoulos et al., 1988). These data suggested two important points: (*1*) a neuronal signal must be released to trigger the increased glucose use in glial cells and (*2*) a substrate must be released by glial cells to serve as an oxidative fuel in photoreceptors. These issues were investigated in parallel in retinal preparations as well as in primary cultures of mouse cortical astrocytes. In cultured astrocytes, it was demonstrated that glutamate causes an increase in glucose use (Pellerin and Magistretti, 1994; Takahashi et al., 1995). The molecular mechanism reponsible for this metabolic effect was dissected out in the same preparation. First, it was shown that glutamate transport, and not glutamate receptor activation, was a key step in this process. Then, since glutamate transport is coupled to the Na^+ gradient, an increase in intracellular Na^+ concentration was seen on fluorescence microscopy (Chatton et al., 2000). As a consequence, an increase in Na^+/K^+-ATPase activity is induced that is most likely responsible for the enhancement in glucose use (Pellerin and Magistretti, 1997). Similarly, it was observed that glutamate (together with ammonia) constitutes the signal released by photoreceptors to induce the metabolic response in Müller glial cells of the retina, although the critical step in the mechanism of activation is the conversion of glutamate into glutamine by glutamine synthetase and its associated ATP consumption rather than a rise in intracellular Na^+ and an increase in Na^+/K^+-ATPase activity (Poitry et al., 2000).

In the honeybee retina, it was observed that alanine was the metabolite released by glial cells to fuel photoreceptor oxidative metabolism (Tsacopoulos et al., 1994). In contrast, it was shown that in mammals, lactate was the most likely candidate both in the retina (Poitry-Yamate et al., 1995) and in the central nervous system (Pellerin and Magistretti, 1994). Indeed, several lines of evidence indicate that lactate can constitute an adequate supplemental energy substrate for neurons (reviewed in Bouzier-Sore et al., 2002). From these observations and others, which include the particular distribution of lactate dehydrogenase (LDH) isoforms between astrocytes and neurons (Bittar et al., 1996), the existence of a mechanism that came to be known as the *astrocyte-neuron lactate shuttle* (Fig. 29.1) was postulated (Pellerin et al., 1998). In this scheme, it is proposed that astrocytes would respond to activity at glutamatergic synapses by enhancing their level of aerobic glycolysis, that is, glucose consumption and lactate production, via the aforementioned mechanism. Lactate thus produced, after its release in the extracellular space, could be taken up by active neurons and metabolized oxidatively to satisfy their energy needs. Interestingly, such a net exchange of lactate between two cell types within the same organ is not unique and has already been described in the striated muscle (Brooks, 2002) as well as in testis (Mauduit et al., 1999).

Evidence for a Concerted Mechanism of Lactate Transfer between Astrocytes and Neurons

Studies performed in cocultures of astrocytes and neurons together with NMR spectroscopy analysis have clearly demonstrated that lactate produced from glucose by astrocytes is efficiently used by neurons (Waagepetersen et al., 2000; Zwingmann et al., 2000). Further evidence *in vivo* for the existence of a coupling mechanism between neuronal activity, enhanced glycolysis in astrocytes, and lactate use by neurons was also provided in recent years. Thus, it was shown that injection of antisense oligonucleotides directed against the glial glutamate transporter GLAST reduced the accumulation of 2-deoxyglucose (2DG) in the appropriate barrel within the rat somatosensory cortex following whisker stimulation (Cholet et al., 2001). Similarly, a strong reduction in glucose use, as reflected by 2DG uptake into barrels corresponding to activated whiskers, was observed in young (postnatal day 10) knockout mice for either one or the other glial glutamate transporter, that is, GLAST or GLT-1 (Voutsinos-Porche et al., 2003). These data strongly suggest that glutamate uptake into astrocytes is intimately linked to glucose consumption *in vivo*. In *in vitro* experiments, it was observed that a specific subunit of the Na^+/K^+-ATPase, akin to the known α_2 subunit, was mobilized upon exposure of astrocytes to glutamate (Pellerin and Magistretti, 1997). It was postulated that this specific glial isoform may play a particular role in coupling glutamate uptake with glucose use in astrocytes. Based on this observation, it was inferred that this isoform must be closely associated with the glial glutamate transporter in order to play this role. A recent immunohistochemical study at both the light and electron microscopy levels demonstrated this specific distribution (Cholet et al., 2002).

Previous microdialysis experiments performed in the rat had shown the appearance of a transient lactate peak in an activated brain area in coordination of a specific behavioral task (Fellows et al., 1993; Fray et al., 1996; Demestre et al., 1997). Moreover, it was demonstrated that lactate formation under these conditions could be prevented by glutamate transporter inhibitors (Fray et al., 1996; Demestre et al., 1997), further strengthening the idea that neuronal activity triggers an increase in glial glycolysis via glutamate uptake in astrocytes. Using glucose, lactate, and O_2-sensitive microelectrodes, Hu and Wilson (1997) studied the relationship between these three parameters as a function of time in the rat hippocampus upon electrical stimulation. Their findings were consistent with an initial increase in lactate levels that paralleled glutamate release and uptake. In addition, upon repeated stimulations, a transient and parallel decline in lactate and O_2 concentrations was found, consistent with increased use of lactate during neuronal activation. Magnetic resonance spectroscopy (MRS) in humans also revealed transient increases in lactate concentration during physiological activation (Prichard et al., 1991; Sappey-Marinier et al., 1992; Frahm et al., 1996).

Investigations of lactate use in rodent brain by NMR spectroscopy have confirmed not only that it is readily used but also that it is preferentially oxidized in neurons (Bouzier et al., 2000; Hassel and Brathe, 2000b; Qu et al., 2000). To support the concept of lactate release by astrocytes and lactate use by neurons, it was necessary to demonstrate the presence of specific transporters on both cell types. A family of transporters collectively known as *monocarboxylate transporters* (MCTs) have been described. These transporters have the capacity to transport lactate, in addition to pyruvate and ketone bodies (Halestrap and Price, 1999). Three members of this family, MCT1, MCT2, and MCT4, have been found in the central nervous system. From investigations performed both *in vitro* and *in vivo*, it was shown that MCT1 was located predominantly on astrocytes, while MCT2 was the prominent neuronal transporter (Bröer et al., 1997; Gerhart et al., 1997; Hanu et al., 2000; Pierre et al., 2000, 2002; Debernardi et al., 2003). Since MCT2 has a lower K_m than MCT1 for lactate, reflecting a higher affinity, the observed distribution of these two transporters between the two cell types would be in agreement with a preferential transfer of lactate from astrocytes to neurons.

Based on calculations made by Laughlin and Attwell (2001), the proportion of energy expenditure attributed to neuronal activity would be approximatively 95%, while glial needs should not exceed 5%. Since glucose is almost the only energy substrate for the brain and its complete oxidation provides all the energy required (via oxidative phosphorylation) to support brain function, the proportion of glucose used by each cell type should be similar to the energy required. Two recent studies have evaluated the amount of glucose used by glial cells versus neurons *in vivo* and *ex vivo*. In the first case, the distribution of 2DG between neurons and astrocytes was assessed in the rat cerebral cortex by combining classical immunohistochemistry with a new autoradiographic method in order to trace back the origin of the emitted β-particles from radiolabeled 2DG (Wittendorp-Rechenmann et al., 2002). These results showed that under resting conditions, the amount of accumulated 2DG was approximately the same in neurons and in astrocytes, a major deviation from the predicted values based on energy requirements. Furthermore, distribution of 2DG, glucose, and lactate between Schwann cells and axons was determined in an isolated vagus nerve preparation under low-frequency stimulation (Véga et al., 2003). The results indicated that close to 80% of glucose use was taking place in glial cells. In addition, the results led to the conclusion that a metabolic intermediate, most likely lactate, was transferred from glial cells to axons. To reconcile the estimations of energy needs made by Attwell and Laughlin, which agreed fairly well with determinations made by NMR spectroscopy of rates of glucose oxidation and glutamate-glutamine cycling (Rothman et al., 2003), together with these new data on the distribution of glucose consumption between glial cells and neurons, it is necessary to admit that a transfer of energy substrates takes place from glial cells to neurons. It has been proposed that lactate would fulfill this role, and that the proportion of lactate transferred might vary with the level of synaptic activity, thus reducing proportionally the amount of glucose required by neurons (Pellerin and Magistretti, 2003; Fig. 29.2). Such an effect could be due to an activation of the redox switch, as previously proposed (Cruz et al., 2001), whereby consumption of lactate by neurons would reduce the levels of nicotinamide adenine dinucleotide (NAD) (via conversion of lactate to pyruvate by lactate dehydrogenase), thus slowing down glycolysis (and glucose consumption) that critically depends on the NAD/NADH (reduced NAD) ratio.

The Glycogen Enigma: What Is It For?

It has been known for a while that the brain contains small but significant amounts of glycogen and that this form of energy reserve is almost entirely found in astrocytes (Magistretti et al., 1993). Moreover, it was elegantly demonstrated in the rat brain that glycogen is mobilized upon sensory stimulation (Swanson et al., 1992) and that its turnover/restoration is slow (Choi et al., 1999; Dienel et al., 2002). Mechanisms accounting for glycogenolysis have been explored *in vitro* using slices and cultured astrocyte preparations that allowed researchers to identify a restricted set of neurotransmitters such as noradrenaline, vasoactive intestinal peptide, and adenosine as putative signals (Magistretti and Pellerin, 1996). The fate of glycosyl units mobilized from glycogen has been debated. While some groups argued that glucose could be released from astrocytes to be provided to neurons (Fillenz et al., 1999), others proposed that glucose mobilized from glycogen would be converted to lactate by astrocytes before being released for neuronal use (Dringen et al., 1993). Rather than being considered strictly as an energy reserve to be exported for neuronal use, it was recently proposed that glycogen might constitute in fact a

A

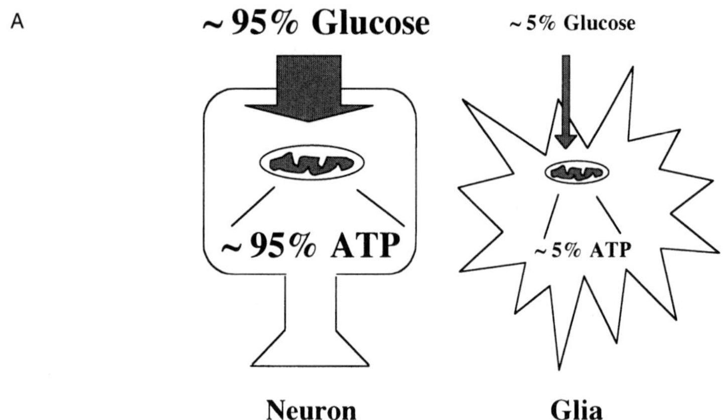

B

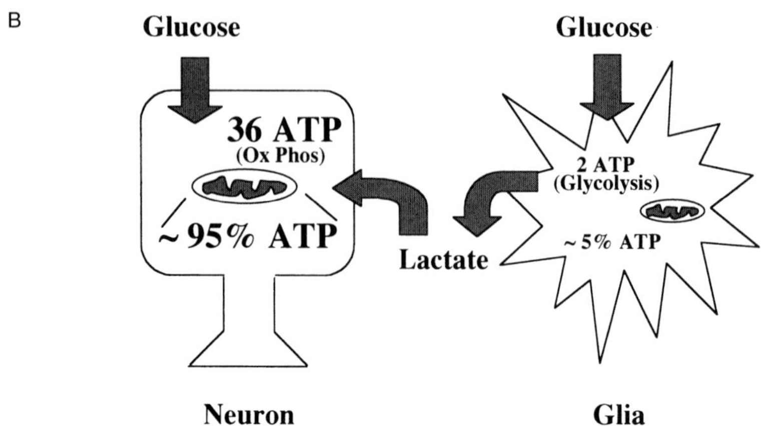

FIGURE 29.2 Lactate exchange betwen astrocytes and neurons provides an explanation for cellular glucose consumption. *A*. It is predicted, based on theoretical energy needs, that glucose use in neurons represents 95% of total consumption, while glia account for the remaining 5%. *B*. Lactate exchange between astrocytes and neurons would provide an additional energy source, thus reducing glucose consumption by neurons. The same amount of adenosine triphosphate (ATP) as in *A* (95% and 5%, respectively, for neurons and glia) could be generated in each cell type to meet their energy needs, but glucose use would be different. This glucose use ratio between astrocytes and neurons could be modulated by the level of neuronal activity. (From Pellerin and Magistretti, 2003, with permission.)

rapid source of energy for astrocytes themselves in order to meet important demands created by glutamate reuptake (Shulman et al., 2001). This hypothesis, known as the *glycogen shunt*, would help to explain the decrease in oxygen-to-glucose index occurring during certain types of stimulation, more classically referred to as the *uncoupling phenomenon* since the time of its description by Raichle and colleagues (Fox et al., 1988). Alternatively, it was proposed that the slow restoration of glycogen levels could be responsible for the nonoxidative glucose use that is sometimes observed after particularly intense sensory or motor activations (Dienel et al., 2002).

Mechanisms of long-term regulation of glycogen levels in astrocytes have begun to be uncovered *in vitro*. A protein belonging to the family of phosphoprotein phosphatase-1-associated proteins, known as *protein targeting to glycogen* (PTG), was shown to be upregulated in parallel with enhanced glycogen levels by neurotransmitters such as noradrenaline or adenosine (Allaman et al., 2000, 2003). Thus PTG could be a key effector in the control of glycogen mobilization in the central nervous system. It has been proposed that one of the functions of sleep could be the replenishment of brain glycogen stores that were depleted during waking hours (Benington and Heller, 1995). Consistent with this hypothesis, it has been observed that sleep deprivation in rodents causes both a decrease in glycogen levels (Kong et al., 2002) and an increase in PTG mRNA expression (Petit et al., 2002).Whether such long-term regulations in glycogen levels through changes in expression of PTG play other critical physiological roles in different brain functions remains to be established.

Controlling Supply: The Involvement of Astrocytes in Regulating Blood Flow

Up to now, it was assumed that blood flow regulation was mediated either by locally secreted products of metabolism, such as K^+, adenosine, lactate, or H^+ (Villringer and Dirnagl, 1995), by nitric oxide released by activated neurons (Iadecola et al., 1994), or under the direct control of nerves via neurotransmitter actions on blood vessels (Edvinsson and Hamel, 2002). This regulation is of importance not only because it allows the supply of glucose and O_2 to be precisely matched with increased neuronal activity in an activated brain area, but also because it forms the basis for the major functional brain imaging techniques in use today, that is, positron emission tomography and functional magnetic resonance imaging. Recent evidence suggests that astrocytes might be also pivotal in mediating the coupling between neuronal activity and blood flow. This concept was proposed on the basis of a series of observations showing that astrocytes stimulated by glutamate could form and release a group of vasodilator substances called *epoxyeicosatrienoic acids* (EETs) (Harder et al., 2002). It was also shown that inhibitors of P-450 epoxygenase, the enzyme responsible for EETs formation, prevented the hyperemic response in the barrel cortex caused by whisker stimulation (Harder et al., 2002). More recently, this hypothesis received further support from a study performed both *in vitro* on brain slices in *in vivo* (Zonta et al., 2003). In this work, it was found that activation of metabotropic glutamate receptors following neuronal excitation leads to Ca^{2+} oscillations in astrocytes accompanied by vasodilation of arterioles. It was further demonstrated that blockade of these astrocytic Ca^{2+} oscillations reduced vasodilation both *in vitro* and *in vivo*. Furthermore, derivatives of arachidonic acid belonging to a different family than EETs, the cyclooxygenase products called *prostaglandins*, were likely to be the vasoactive mediators released by stimulated astrocytes to act on blood vessels. These data indicate that the spectrum of astrocyte functions has been enlarged to include the possible control of the blood supply.

SUMMARY AND PERSPECTIVES

Recent findings have brought to light the fact that astrocytes may be involved in various aspects of functional neuroenergetics. As illustrated in this chapter, astrocytes play essential roles in coupling neuronal activity to energy metabolism, both through their participation in the glutamate/glutamine cycle and by providing lactate to neurons as an additional energy substrate in register with increased activity. Moreover, it appears now that astrocytes also participate in coupling neuronal activity to blood flow. Such findings are important not only for our understanding of fundamental aspects of brain functions, but also for the use of functional brain imaging techniques that rely on metabolic and vascular parameters to map cognitive processes (Magistretti and Pellerin, 1999; Bonvento et al., 2002).

REFERENCES

Allaman, I., Lengacher, S., Magistretti, P.J., and Pellerin, L. (2003) A_{2B} receptor activation promotes glycogen synthesis in astrocytes through modulation of gene expression. *Am. J. Physiol.* 284: C696–C704.

Allaman, I., Pellerin, L., and Magistretti, P.J. (2000) Protein targeting to glycogen mRNA expression is stimulated by noradrenaline in mouse cortical astrocytes. *Glia* 30:382–391.

Attwell, D. and Laughlin, S.B. (2001) An energy budget for signaling in the grey matter of the brain. *J. Cereb. Blood Flow Metab.* 21:1133–1145.

Bacci, A., Sancini, G., Verderio, C., Armano, S., Pravettoni, E., Fesce, R., Franceschetti, S., and Matteoli, M. (2002) Block of glutamate-glutamine cycle between astrocytes and neurons inhibits epileptiform activity in hippocampus. *J. Neurophysiol.* 88:2302–2310.

Badar-Goffer, R.S., Ben-Yoseph, O., Bachelard, H.S., and Morris, P.G. (1992) Neuronal-glial metabolism under depolarizing conditions. A ^{13}C-n.m.r. study. *Biochem. J.* 282:225–230.

Benington, J.H. and Heller, H.C. (1995) Restoration of brain energy metabolism as the function of sleep. *Prog. Neurobiol.* 45:347–360.

Berl, S., Takagaki, G., Clarke, D.D., and Waelsch, H. (1962) Metabolic compartments in vivo: ammonia and glutamic acid metabolism in brain and liver. *J. Biol. Chem.* 237:2562–2569.

Bittar, P.G., Charnay, Y., Pellerin, L., Bouras, C., and Magistretti, P.J. (1996) Selective distribution of lactate dehydrogenase isoenzymes in neurons and astrocytes of human brain. *J. Cereb. Blood Flow Metab.* 16:1079–1089.

Bonvento, G., Sibson, N., and Pellerin, L. (2002) Does glutamate image your thoughts? *Trends Neurosci.* 25:359–364.

Bouzier, A.K., Thiaudiere, E., Biran, M., Rouland, R., Canioni, P., and Merle, M. (2000) The metabolism of [3-(13)C]lactate in the rat brain is specific of a pyruvate carboxylase-deprived compartment. *J. Neurochem.* 75:480–486.

Bouzier-Sore, A.K., Merle, M., Magistretti, P.J., and Pellerin, L. (2002) Feeding active neurons: (re)emergence of a nursing role for astrocytes. *J. Physiol. (Paris)* 96:273–282.

Bröer, S. and Brookes, N. (2001) Transfer of glutamine between astrocytes and neurons. *J. Neurochem.* 77:705–719.

Bröer, S., Rahman, B., Pellegri, G., Pellerin, L., Martin, J.L., Verleysdonk, S., Hamprecht, B., and Magistretti, P.J. (1997) Comparison of lactate transport in astroglial cells and monocarboxylate transporter 1 (MCT 1) expressing *Xenopus laevis* oocytes. Expression of two different monocarboxylate transporters in astroglial cells and neurons. *J. Biol. Chem.* 272:30096–30102.

Brooks, G.A. (2002) Lactate shuttles in nature. *Biochem. Soc. Trans.* 30:258–264.

Chatton, J.Y., Marquet, P., and Magistretti, P.J. (2000) A quantitative analysis of L-glutamate-regulated Na^+ dynamics in mouse cortical astrocytes: implications for cellular bioenergetics. *Eur. J. Neurosci.* 12:3843–3853.

Choi, I.Y., Tkac, I., Ugurbil, K., and Gruetter, R. (1999) Noninvasive measurements of [1-(13)C]glycogen concentrations and metabolism in rat brain in vivo. *J. Neurochem.* 73:1300–1308.

Cholet, N., Pellerin, L., Magistretti, P.J., and Hamel, E. (2002) Similar perisynaptic glial localization for the Na+,K+-ATPase alpha 2 subunit and the glutamate transporters GLAST and GLT-1 in the rat somatosensory cortex. *Cereb. Cortex* 12:515–525.

Cholet, N., Pellerin, L., Welker, E., Lacombe, P., Seylaz, J., Magistretti, P., and Bonvento, G. (2001) Local injection of antisense oligonucleotides targeted to the glial glutamate transporter GLAST decreases the metabolic response to somatosensory activation. *J. Cereb. Blood Flow Metab.* 21:404–412.

Cruz, F., Villalba, M., Garcia-Espinosa, M.A., Ballesteros, P., Bogonez, E., Satrustegui, J., and Cerdan, S. (2001) Intracellular compartmentation of pyruvate in primary cultures of cortical neurons as detected by (13)C NMR spectroscopy with multiple (13)C labels. *J. Neurosci. Res.* 66:771–781.

Danbolt, N.C. (2001) Glutamate uptake. *Prog. Neurobiol.* 65:1–105.

Debernardi, R., Pierre, K., Lengacher, S., Magistretti, P.J., and Pellerin, L. (2003) Cell-specific expression pattern of monocarboxylate transporters in astrocytes and neurons observed in different mouse brain cortical cell cultures. *J. Neurosci. Res.* 73(2):141–155.

Demestre, M., Boutelle, M., and Fillenz, M. (1997) Stimulated release of lactate in freely moving rats is dependent on the uptake of glutamate. *J. Physiol. (Lond.)* 499:825–832.

Dienel, G.A., Wang, R.Y., and Cruz, N.F. (2002) Generalized sensory stimulation of conscious rats increases labeling of oxidative pathways of glucose metabolism when the brain glucose-oxygen uptake ratio rises. *J. Cereb. Blood Flow Metab.* 22:1490–1502.

Dringen, R., Gebhardt, R., and Hamprecht, B. (1993) Glycogen in astrocytes: possible function as lactate supply for neighboring cells. *Brain Res.* 623:208–214.

Edvinsson, L. and Hamel, E. (2002) Perivascular nerves in brain vessels. In: Edvinsson, L. and Krause, D.N., eds. *Cerebral Blood Flow and Metabolism*, 2nd ed. Philadelphia: Lippincott, pp. 43–67.

Fellows, L.K., Boutelle, M.G., and Fillenz, M. (1993) Physiological stimulation increases nonoxidative glucose metabolism in the brain of the freely moving rat. *J. Neurochem.* 60:1258–1263.

Fillenz, M., Lowry, J.P., Boutelle, M.G., and Fray, A.E. (1999) The role of astrocytes and noradrenaline in neuronal glucose metabolism. *Acta Physiol. Scand.* 167:275–284.

Fox, P.T., Raichle, M.E., Mintun M.A., and Dence, C. (1988) Nonoxidative glucose consumption during focal physiologic neural activity. *Science* 241:462–464.

Frahm, J., Kruger, G., Merboldt, K.D., and Kleinschmidt, A. (1996) Dynamic uncoupling and recoupling of perfusion and oxidative metabolism during focal brain activation in man. *Magn. Reson. Med.* 35:143–148.

Fray, A.E., Forsyth, R.J., Boutelle, M.G., and Fillenz, M. (1996) The mechanisms controlling physiologically stimulated changes in rat brain glucose and lactate: a microdialysis study. *J. Physiol. (Lond.)* 496:49–57.

Gerhart, D.Z., Enerson, B.E., Zhdankina, O.Y., Leino, R.L., and Drewes, L.R. (1997) Expression of monocarboxylate transporter MCT1 by brain endothelium and glia in adult and suckling rats. *Am. J. Physiol.* 273:E207–E213.

Golgi, C. (1886) *Sulla fina anatomia degli organi centrali del sistema nervosa*. Milano: Hoepli, p. 154 (footnote).

Grosche, J., Matyash, V., Moller, T., Verkhratsky, A., Reichenbach, A., and Kettenmann, H. (1999) Microdomains for neuron-glia interaction: parallel fiber signaling to Bergmann glial cells. *Nat. Neurosci.* 2:139–143.

Gruetter, R., Novotny, E.J., Boulware, S.D., Mason, G.F., Rothman, D.L., Shulman, G.I., Prichard, J.W., and Shulman, R.G. (1994) Localized ^{13}C NMR spectroscopy in the human brain of amino acid labeling from D-[1-^{13}C]glucose. *J. Neurochem.* 63:1377–1385.

Halestrap, A.P. and Price, N.T. (1999) The proton-linked monocarboxylate transporter (MCT) family: structure, function and regulation. *Biochem. J.* 343:281–299.

Hanu, R., McKenna, M., O'Neill, A., Resneck, W.G., and Bloch, R.J. (2000) Monocarboxylic acid transporters, MCT1 and MCT2, in cortical astrocytes in vitro and in vivo. *Am. J. Physiol.* 278:C921–C930.

Harder, D.R., Zhang, C., and Gebremedhin, D. (2002) Astrocytes function in matching blood flow to metabolic activity. *News Physiol. Sci.* 17:27–31.

Hassel, B. and Brathe, A. (2000a) Neuronal pyruvate carboxylation supports formation of transmitter glutamate. *J. Neurosci.* 20: 1342–1347.

Hassel, B. and Brathe, A. (2000b) Cerebral metabolism of lactate in vivo: evidence for neuronal pyruvate carboxylation. *J. Cereb. Blood Flow Metab.* 20:327–336.

Hösli, E. and Hösli, L. (1993) Receptors for neurotransmitters on astrocytes in the mammalian central nervous system. *Prog. Neurobiol.* 40:477–506.

Hu, Y. and Wilson, G.S. (1997) A temporary local energy pool coupled to neuronal activity: fluctuations of extracellular lactate levels in rat brain monitored with rapid-response enzyme-based sensor. *J. Neurochem.* 69:1484–1490.

Hülsmann, S., Oku, Y., Zhang, W., and Richter, D.W. (2000) Metabolic coupling between glia and neurons is necessary for maintaining respiratory activity in transverse medullary slices of neonatal mouse. *Eur. J. Neurosci.* 12:856–862.

Iadecola, C., Pelligrino, D.A., Moskowitz, M.A., and Lassen, N.A. (1994) Nitric oxide synthase inhibition and cerebrovascular regulation. *J. Cereb. Blood Flow Metab.* 14:175–192.

Kacem, K., Lacombe, P., Seylaz, J., and Bonvento, G. (1998) Structural organization of the perivascular astrocyte endfeet and their relationship with the endothelial glucose transporter: a confocal microscopy study. *Glia* 23:1–10.

Kaneko, T. and Fujiyama, F. (2002) Complementary distribution of vesicular glutamate transporters in the central nervous system. *Neurosci. Res.* 42:243–250.

Kong, J., Shepel, P.N., Holden, C.P., Mackiewicz, M., Pack, A.I., and Geiger, J.D. (2002) Brain glycogen decreases with increased periods of wakefulness: implications for homeostatic drive to sleep. *J. Neurosci.* 22:5581–5587.

Kvamme, E., Torgner, I.A., and Svenneby, G. (1985) Glutaminase from mammalian tissues. *Meth. Enzymol.* 113:241–256.

Lebon, V., Petersen, K.F., Cline, G.W., Shen, J., Mason, G.F., Dufour, S., Behar, K.L., Shulman, G.I., and Rothman, D.L. (2002) Astroglial contribution to brain energy metabolism in humans revealed by ^{13}C nuclear magnetic resonance spectroscopy: elucidation of the dominant pathway for neurotransmitter glutamate repletion and measurement of astrocytic oxidative metabolism. *J. Neurosci.* 22:1523–1531.

Magistretti, P.J. and Pellerin, L. (1996) Cellular bases of brain energy metabolism and their relevance to functional brain imaging: evidence for a prominent role of astrocytes. *Cereb. Cortex* 6: 50–61.

Magistretti, P.J., Pellerin, L. (1999) Cellular mechanisms of brain energy metabolism and their relevance to functional brain imaging. *Phil. Trans. R. Soc. (Lond. B Biol. Sci.)* 354:1155–1163.

Magistretti, P.J., Sorg, O., and Martin, J.-L. (1993) Regulation of glycogen metabolism in astrocytes: physiological, pharmacological, and pathological aspects. In: Murphy S., ed. *Astrocytes: Pharmacology and Function.* San Diego, CA: Academic Press, pp. 243–265.

Martin, D.L. (1995) The role of glia in the inactivation of neurotransmitters. In: Kettenmann, H. and Ransom, B.R., eds. *Neuroglia.* Oxford: Oxford University Press, pp. 732–745.

Martinez-Hernandez, A., Bell, K.P., and Norenberg, M.D. (1977) Glutamine synthetase: glial localization in brain. *Science* 195: 1356–1358.

Mason, G.F., Gruetter, R., Rothman, D.L., Behar, K.L., Shulman, R.G., and Novotny, E.J. (1995) Simultaneous determination of the rates of the TCA cycle, glucose utilization, alpha-ketoglutarate/glutamate exchange, and glutamine synthesis in human brain by NMR. *J. Cereb. Blood Flow Metab.* 15:12–25.

Mauduit, C., Chatelain, G., Magre, S., Brun, G., Benahmed, M., and Michel, D. (1999) Regulation by pH of the alternative splicing of the stem cell factor pre-mRNA in the testis. *J. Biol. Chem.* 274:770–775.

McGeer, P.L. and McGeer, E.G. (1989) Amino acid neurotransmitters. In: Siegel, G., Agranoff, B., Albers, R.W., and Molinoff, P., eds. *Basic Neurochemistry: Molecular, Cellular, and Medical Aspects*, 4th ed. New York: Raven Press, pp. 311–332.

Morgello, S., Uson, R.R., Schwartz, E.J., and Haber, R.S. (1995) The human blood-brain barrier glucose transporter (GLUT1) is a glucose transporter of gray matter astrocytes. *Glia* 14:43–54.

Ng, K.T., O'Dowd, B.S., Rickard, N.S., Robinson, S.R., Gibbs, M.E., Rainey, C., Zhao, W.Q., Sedman, G.L., and Hertz, L. (1997) Complex roles of glutamate in the Gibbs-Ng model of one-trial aversive learning in the new-born chick. *Neurosci. Biobehav. Rev.* 21:45–54.

Pellerin, L. and Magistretti, P.J. (1994) Glutamate uptake into astrocytes stimulates aerobic glycolysis: a mechanism coupling neuronal activity to glucose utilization. *Proc. Natl. Acad. Sci. USA* 91:10625–10629.

Pellerin, L. and Magistretti, P.J. (1997) Glutamate uptake stimulates Na^+,K^+-ATPase activity in astrocytes via activation of a distinct subunit highly sensitive to ouabain. *J. Neurochem.* 69: 2132–2137.

Pellerin, L. and Magistretti, P.J. (2003) How to balance the brain energy budget while spending glucose differently. *J. Physiol. (Lond)* 546:325.

Pellerin, L., Pellegri, G., Bittar, P.G., Charnay, Y., Bouras, C., Martin, J.L., Stella, N., and Magistretti, P.J. (1998) Evidence supporting the existence of an activity-dependent astrocyte-neuron lactate shuttle. *Dev. Neurosci.* 20:291–299.

Peng, L., Hertz, L., Huang, R., Sonnewald, U., Petersen, S.B., Westergaard, N., Larsson, O., and Schousboe, A. (1993) Utilization of glutamine and of TCA cycle constituents as precursors for transmitter glutamate and GABA. *Dev. Neurosci.* 15:367–377.

Petit, J.M., Tobler, I., Allaman, I., Borbely, A.A., and Magistretti, P.J. (2002) Sleep deprivation modulates brain mRNAs encoding genes of glycogen metabolism. *Eur. J. Neurosci.* 16:1163–1167.

Pierre, K., Magistretti, P.J., and Pellerin, L. (2002) MCT2 is a major neuronal monocarboxylate transporter in the adult mouse brain. *J. Cereb. Blood Flow Metab.* 22:586–595.

Pierre, K., Pellerin, L., Debernardi, R., Riederer, B.M., and Magistretti, P.J. (2000) Cell-specific localization of monocarboxylate transporters, MCT1 and MCT2, in the adult mouse brain revealed by double immunohistochemical labeling and confocal microscopy. *Neuroscience* 100:617–627.

Poitry, S., Poitry-Yamate, C.L., Ueberfeld, J., MacLeish, P.R., and Tsacopoulos, M. (2000) Mechanisms of glutamate metabolic signaling in retinal glial (Muller) cells. *J. Neurosci.* 20:1809–1821.

Poitry-Yamate, C.L., Poitry, S., and Tsacopoulos M. (1995) Lactate released by Muller glial cells is metabolized by photoreceptors from mammalian retina. *J. Neurosci.* 15:5179–5191.

Prichard, J., Rothman, D., Novotny, E., Petroff, O., Kuwabara, T., Avison, M., Howseman, A., Hanstock, C., and Shulman, R. (1991) Lactate rise detected by 1H NMR in human visual cortex during physiologic stimulation. *Proc. Natl. Acad. Sci. USA* 88:5829–5831.

Qu, H., Haberg, A., Haraldseth, O., Unsgard, G., and Sonnewald, U. (2000) (13)C MR spectroscopy study of lactate as substrate for rat brain. *Dev. Neurosci.* 22:429–436.

Rothman, D.L., Behar, K.L., Hyder, F., and Shulman, R.G. (2003) In vivo NMR studies of the glutamate neurotransmitter flux and neuroenergetics: implications for brain function. *Annu. Rev. Physiol.* 65:401–427.

Rothman, D.L., Sibson, N.R., Hyder, F., Shen, J., Behar, K.L., and Shulman, R.G. (1999) In vivo nuclear magnetic resonance spectroscopy studies of the relationship between the glutamate-glutamine neurotransmitter cycle and functional neuroenergetics. *Phil. Trans. R. Soc. (Lond. B Biol. Sci.)* 354:1165–1177.

Sappey-Marinier, D., Calabrese, G., Fein, G., Hugg, J.W., Biggins, C., and Weiner, M.W. (1992) Effect of photic stimulation on human visual cortex lactate and phosphates using ^{1}H and ^{31}P magnetic resonance spectroscopy. *J. Cereb. Blood Flow Metab.* 12:584–592.

Shank, R.P., Bennett, G.S., Freytag, S.O., and Campbell, G.L. (1985) Pyruvate carboxylase: an astrocyte-specific enzyme implicated in the replenishment of amino acid neurotransmitter pools. *Brain Res.* 329:364–367.

Shank, R.P. and Campbell, G.L. (1984) Alpha-ketoglutarate and malate uptake and metabolism by synaptosomes: further evidence for an astrocyte-to-neuron metabolic shuttle. *J. Neurochem.* 42:1153–1161.

Shen, J., Petersen, K.F., Behar, K.L., Brown, P., Nixon, T.W., Mason, G.F., Petroff, O.A., Shulman, G.I., Shulman, R.G., and Rothman, D.L. (1999) Determination of the rate of the glutamate/glutamine cycle in the human brain by in vivo ^{13}C NMR. *Proc. Natl. Acad. Sci. USA* 96:8235–8240.

Shen, J., Sibson, N.R., Cline, G., Behar, K.L., Rothman, D.L., and Shulman R.G. (1998) ^{15}N-NMR spectroscopy studies of ammonia transport and glutamine synthesis in the hyperammonemic rat brain. *Dev. Neurosci.* 20:434–443.

Shulman, R.G., Hyder, F., and Rothman, D.L. (2001) Cerebral energetics and the glycogen shunt: neurochemical basis of functional imaging. *Proc. Natl. Acad. Sci. USA* 98:6417–6422.

Sibson, N.R., Dhankhar, A., Mason, G.F., Behar, K.L., Rothman, D.L., and Shulman, R.G. (1997) In vivo ^{13}C NMR measurements of cerebral glutamine synthesis as evidence for glutamate-glutamine cycling. *Proc. Natl. Acad. Sci. USA* 94:2699–2704.

Sibson, N.R., Dhankhar, A., Mason, G.F., Rothman, D.L., Behar, K.L., and Shulman, R.G. (1998) Stoichiometric coupling of brain glucose metabolism and glutamatergic neuronal activity. *Proc. Natl. Acad. Sci. USA* 95:316–321.

Sibson, N.R., Mason, G.F., Shen, J., Cline, G.W., Herskovits, A.Z., Wall, J.E., Behar, K.L., Rothman, D.L., and Shulman, R.G. (2001) In vivo (13)C NMR measurement of neurotransmitter glutamate cycling, anaplerosis and TCA cycle flux in rat brain during [2–^{13}C] glucose infusion. *J. Neurochem.* 76:975–989.

Swanson, R.A., Morton, M.M., Sagar, S.M., and Sharp, F.R. (1992) Sensory stimulation induces local cerebral glycogenolysis: demonstration by autoradiography. *Neuroscience* 51:451–461.

Takahashi, S., Driscoll, B.F., Law, M.J., and Sokoloff, L. (1995) Role of sodium and potassium ions in regulation of glucose metabolism in cultured astroglia. *Proc. Natl. Acad. Sci. USA* 92: 4616–4620.

Tsacopoulos, M., Evequoz-Mercier, V., Perrottet, P., and Buchner, E. (1988) Honeybee retinal glial cells transform glucose and supply the neurons with metabolic substrate. *Proc. Natl. Acad. Sci. USA* 85:8727–8731.

Tsacopoulos, M., Veuthey, A.L., Saravelos, S.G., Perrottet, P., and Tsoupras, G. (1994) Glial cells transform glucose to alanine, which fuels the neurons in the honeybee retina. *J. Neurosci.* 14:1339–1351.

Van den Berg, C.J., Krzalic, L., Mela, P., and Waelsch, H. (1969) Compartmentation of glutamate metabolism in brain. Evidence for the existence of two different tricarboxylic acid cycles in brain. *Biochem. J.* 113:281–290.

Vega, C., Martiel, J.L., Drouhault, D., Burckhart, M.F., and Coles, J.A. (2003) Uptake of locally applied deoxyglucose, glucose and lactate by axons and Schwann cells of rat vagus nerve. *J. Physiol. (Lond.)* 546:551–564.

Villringer, A. and Dirnagl, U. (1995) Coupling of brain activity and cerebral blood flow: basis of functional neuroimaging. *Cereb. Brain Metab. Rev.* 7:240–276.

Voutsinos-Porche, B., Bonvento, G., Tanaka, K., Steiner, P., Welker, E., Chatton, J.Y., Magistretti, P.J., and Pellerin, L. (2003) Glial glutamate transporters mediate a functional metabolic crosstalk between neurons and astrocytes in the mouse developing cortex. *Neuron* 37:275–286.

Waagepetersen, H.S., Sonnewald, U., Larsson, O.M., and Schousboe, A. (2000) A possible role of alanine for ammonia transfer between astrocytes and glutamatergic neurons. *J. Neurochem.* 75:471–479.

Waniewski, R.A. and Martin, D.L. (1986) Exogenous glutamate is metabolized to glutamine and exported by rat primary astrocyte cultures. *J. Neurochem.* 47:304–313.

Wittendorp-Rechenmann, E., Lam, C.D., Steibel, J., Lasbennes, F., and Nehlig, A. (2002) High resolution tracer targeting combining microautoradiographic imaging by cellular ^{14}C-trajectography with immunohistochemistry: a novel protocol to demonstrate metabolism of [^{14}C]2-deoxyglucose by neurons and astrocytes. *J. Trace Microprobe Tech.* 20:505–515.

Yu, S. and Ding, W.G. (1998) The 45 kDa form of glucose transporter 1 (GLUT1) is localized in oligodendrocyte and astrocyte but not in microglia in the rat brain. *Brain Res.* 797:65–72.

Yudkoff, M. (1997) Brain metabolism of branched-chain amino acids. *Glia* 21:92–98.

Zonta, M., Angulo, M.C., Gobbo, S., Rosengarten, B., Hossmann, K.A., Pozzan, T., and Carmignoto, G. (2003) Neuron-to-astrocyte signaling is central to the dynamic control of brain microcirculation. *Nat. Neurosci.* 6:43–50.

Zwingmann, C., Richter-Landsberg, C., Brand, A., and Leibfritz, D. (2000) NMR spectroscopic study on the metabolic fate of [3-(13)C]alanine in astrocytes, neurons, and cocultures: implications for glia-neuron interactions in neurotransmitter metabolism. *Glia* 32:286–303.

30 Growth factors for neurons provided by macroglial cells

BERNHARD REUSS AND KLAUS UNSICKER

Neuronal survival and functions require bidirectional communication between neurons and glia that involves a large variety of growth factors. Neurotrophic factors are operationally defined as proteins that regulate neuron survival and differentiation. They can be synthesized by nonneuronal target cells, by neurons, and by glial cells. The focus of this chapter is neurotrophic factors secreted from macroglial cells, that is, astrocytes, oligodendrocytes, and Schwann cells, and their effects on neuronal differentiation and survival in the intact and lesioned brain and peripheral nervous system (Fig. 30.1).

EXPRESSION OF NEUROTROPHIC GROWTH FACTORS BY DIFFERENT GLIAL CELL TYPES

Schwann Cells

Neurotrophins

The neurotrophin family comprises nerve growth factor (NGF), brain-derived neurotrophic factor (BDNF), and neurotrophins 3 and 4 (NT-3, NT-4). Neurotrophins signal through the receptor tyrosine kinases trkA, -B, or -C, and a low-affinity receptor, p75. Whereas NGF binds preferably to trkA, BDNF binds specifically to the trkB receptor and NT-3 to all three trk receptors, with a preference for trkC. Neurotrophin-4 activates trkB but can also bind to trkB (Bothwell, 1998). Upon ligand binding, trk receptors dimerize and transphosphorylate each other. This event activates, via phospholipase Cγ (PLCγ), the phosphoinositol-3 (PI3)-kinase pathway, and via ras-guanosine triphosphate (GTP) the microtubule-associated (MAP)-kinase signaling pathway, resulting, among others, in the activation of early response genes, such as c-*fos* and, finally, neuronal survival and differentiation. All neurotrophins can activate p75, which, in the absence of trk activation, can induce apoptotic cell death. Via acute transforming retrovirus oncogene (AKT), the survival pathway of neurotrophins inhibits apoptotic pathways, suggesting that an appropriate balance between trk and p75 activation may determine whether a neuron survives or dies (Miller and Kaplan, 2001).

Schwann cells contain large amounts of NGF protein and mRNA *in vitro* and *in vivo* (cf. Wetmore and Olson, 1995). Neurotrophin-3 mRNA is expressed at low concentrations in cultured rat Schwann cells but is prominently upregulated upon immortalization (Watabe et al., 1995). In response to nerve injury, neurotrophins are distinctly regulated in Schwann cells. Nerve growth factor, which is expressed at low levels in the unlesioned nerve, is upregulated after injury (Heumann et al., 1987). After sciatic nerve transection, mRNAs for BDNF, NT-3, and NT-4 are also differentially expressed, with an initial increase in BDNF and NT-4 and a decrease in NT-3 (Funakoshi et al., 1993).

Neuroregulatory cytokines

Ciliary neurotrophic factor (CNTF), together with leukemia inhibitory factor (LIF), cardiotrophin, interleukin-6 (IL-6), and oncostatin-1, form a family of neuroregulatory cytokines that share, in part, receptor and signal transduction components. Ciliary neurotrophic factor binds to a complex consisting of a glycophosphatidylinositol (GPI)-anchored α receptor, the LIF receptor β (LIFRβ), and gp130. Leukemia inhibitory factor signals through a complex consisting of LIFRβ and gp130. Intracellularly, active gp130 activates the Janus kinases (JAK), which, in turn, activate a variety of intracellular signaling molecules, such as the signal transducer and activator of transcription (STAT) family of transcriptional activators.

Schwann cells in the sciatic nerve express CNTF from postnatal day 8 on, reaching adult levels at day 21 (Dobrea et al., 1992). Expression of CNTF in Schwann cells depends on axonal factors, since after axotomy CNTF expression is lost, but recovers after axon regeneration. While cultured Schwann cells express abundant LIF and CNTF mRNAs (Carroll et al, 1993; Kurek et al., 1997), myelinating Schwann cells *in vivo* display

See the list of abbreviations at the end of the chapter.

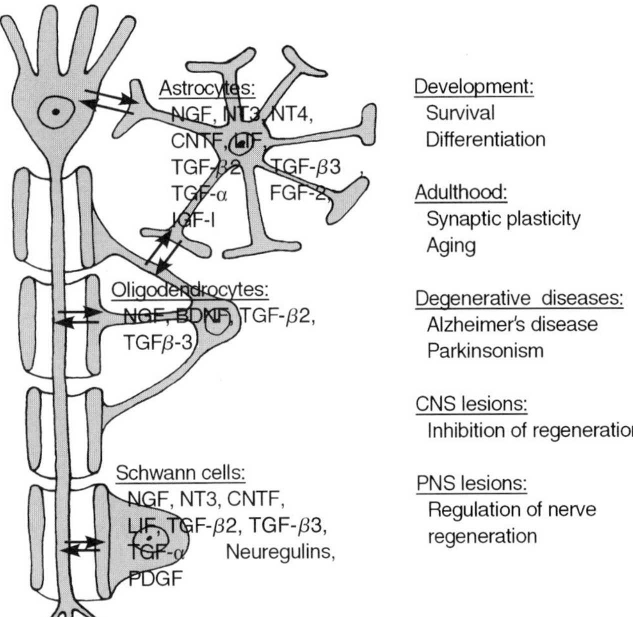

FIGURE 30.1 Schematic overview of the expression and neuronal effects of growth factors of glial origin. A tight network of bidirectional neuron-glial and interglial interactions can be found in central and peripheral nerve tissue. They are involved in cellular regulation during development and in the adult nervous system, as well as during degenerative diseases and lesioning. BDNF: brain-derived neurotrophic factor; CNS: central nervous system; CNTF: ciliary neurotrophic factor; FGF-2: fibroblast growth factor-2; IGF-I: insulin-like growth factor-1; LIF: leukemia inhibitory factor; NGF: nerve growth factor; NT3, -4: neurotrophin-3, -4; PDGF: platelet-derived growth factor; PNS: peripheral nervous system; TGF-β2, -3: transforming growth factor-β2, -3.

only CNTF (Friedman et al., 1992), whereas LIF mRNA levels are low (Kurek et al., 1997). Following nerve lesioning, retrograde transport of LIF and CNTF is increased (Neet and Campenot, 2001).

Transforming growth factors-β

Transforming growth factors-β (TGF-βs) represent a large superfamily of cytokines, with functions in morphogenesis, cell differentiation, and tissue remodeling. Transforming growth factors β1 through β3 bind to heterodimers of TGF-β receptors (TβRs) I and II. Upon ligand binding, TβR II phosphorylates and recruits TβRI into a heterotetrameric complex that activates itself as well as downstream targets, such as Smad2. Activated Smad2 dissociates from the receptor complex, dimerizes with Smad4, and accumulates in the nucleus, where it complexes with the transcription activator fas-activated serine-threonine kinase (FAST-1).

Both TGF-β2 and -β3 are expressed by Schwann cells and their precursors (Stewart et al., 1995). Following sciatic nerve transection, TGF-β1 mRNA levels increase in the distal stump, whereas TGF-β3 mRNA levels are depressed. Transforming growth factor-β1 mRNA is augmented during axon degeneration but returns to normal levels when axons regenerate. Transforming growth factor-β2 mRNA is not present in the sciatic nerve. Transforming growth factor-β1 mRNA is high in cultured Schwann cells but decreases upon mimicking axonal contact by forskolin (Scherer et al., 1993; Rufer et al., 1994) The TGF-βs in Schwann cells act primarily in an autocrine fashion (Chandross et al., 1995) but also influence Schwann cell–axon interactions during de- and remyelination (Einheber et al., 1995). They have also been shown to induce Schwann cell death (Skoff et al., 1998).

Glial cell line-derived neurotrophic factor

Together with neurturin, artemin, and persephin, glial cell line-derived neurotrophic factor (GDNF) belongs to a TGF-β subfamily that bind to GDNF receptor α (GFRα), a GPI-anchored membrane protein, forming a heterodimer with the receptor tyrosine kinase *c-ret*. This complex then activates the *ras/raf* and PI3 kinase intracellular signaling pathways. While the *ras/raf* pathway activates gene transcription via the cyclic adenosine monophosphate (cAMP) response element (CRE)-DNA binding protein, the PI3 kinase pathway acts by activation of nuclear factor κB (NFκB). While GDNF levels in normal Schwann cells and satellite cells are low, GDNF is highly upregulated after transection in the distal nerve stump as well as in satellite cells of the corresponding dorsal root ganglion (Bar et al., 1998). However, during nerve regeneration after long-term denervation, GDNF expression declines (Hoke et al., 2002).

Epidermal growth factor family

The EGF family includes epidermal growth factor (EGF), transforming growth factor (TGF)-α, amphiregulin, heparin binding (HB)-EGF, betacellulin (BTC), and epiregulin (ERG). Epidermal growth factor signals through EGF receptors, the cellular counterpart of the *v-ErbB* oncogene. Four different EGF receptors have been identified, termed ErbB1–ErbB4. Whereas EGF, TGFα, amphiregulin, HB-EGF, and BTC act through ErbB1, heregulin activates ErbB3 and ErbB4. The cognate ligand for ErbB2 has not been identified, but may also be heregulin. Activation of ErbB1 alternatively activates the JAK/STAT-pathway, the MAP-kinase pathway, and the PI3-kinase pathway. Last not least, ErbB1 leads to phosphorylation of PLCγ. Schwann cells express TGF-α and neuregulins, and also have ErbB1 on their surface (Vega et al., 1994). Neuregulins act as autocrine stimulators of Schwann cell proliferation during development (Raabe et al., 1998). In satellite cells of dorsal root ganglions (DRGs), both TGF-α and its receptor are markedly upregulated in response to nerve lesioning (Xian and Zhou, 1999).

Platelet-derived growth factor

Platelet derived growth factor (PDGF) forms homo- or heterodimers connected by disulfide bonds. It binds to tyrosine kinase receptors that upon dimerization recruit and activate SH2-like signal transducers, triggering the *ras/raf* signaling cascade. Cultured Schwann cells secrete PDGF and express PDGF receptors (Hardy et al., 1992). In neonatal rats, Schwann cells in DRG and sciatic nerve synthesize large amounts of PDGF that decrease postnatally (Eccleston et al., 1993). In the adult rat, PDGF is low in myelinating Schwann cells, but it is upregulated in nonmyelinating Schwann cells.

Oligodendrocytes

Neurotrophins

Oligodendrocytes and oligodendrocyte precursors express NGF (Gonzalez et al. 1990), BDNF. and NT-3 (Wetmore and Olson, 1995), which influence proliferation and survival of immature oligodendrocytes in an autocrine manner.

Transforming growth factors-β

The TGF-βs are important for oligodendrocyte development. Different TGF-β isoforms are expressed by O2A precursor cells (TGF-β3) and mature oligodendrocytes (TGF-β2 and -β3). Transforming growth factor-β1 released by O2A precursor cells inhibits their proliferation and maturation in an autocrine manner. All three TGF-β isoforms are produced by cultured oligodendrocytes (McKinnon et al., 1993). *In vivo*, TGF-β1 has been localized to oligodendrocytes within the human cerebral cortex (Da Cunha et al., 1993).

Astrocytes

Neurotrophins

Astrocytes have been known for a long time to synthesize NGF (Yamakuni et al., 1987). This has been confirmed by Condorelli et al. (1995), who also detected mRNA for NT-3 and NT-4, but not for BDNF, in astrocytes. Investigations *in vivo* confirmed the presence of NT-3 and NT-4 immunoreactivity at least in a subpopulation of astrocytes (Burette et al., 1998; Friedman et al., 1998).

Following central nervous system (CNS) injury, reactive astrocytes express NGF and BDNF (Goto and Furukawa, 1995). In a tissue culture model of astrogliosis, the content of NGF was significantly increased in reactive astrocytes, a process that seems to be regulated by astroglia-derived IL-1β and interferon-4 (IFN-γ) (Wu et al., 1998). This is supported by the fact that okadaic acid, an inhibitor of phosphoprotein phosphatases, increased both IL-1β and NGF in astrocytes (Pshenichkin and Wise, 1997).

Fibroblast growth factors

Astrocytes are a rich source of fibroblast growth factor-2 (FGF-2) (Sensenbrenner et al., 1987). Fibroblast growth factor-2 mRNA is found in astrocytes of cerebral cortex, hippocampus, and spinal cord, with a massive postnatal increase (Riva and Mocchetti, 1991). Fibroblast growth factor-2 binds to a group of five high-affinity transmembrane receptors (FGFR1–5), the variability of which is further enhanced by alternative splicing. Ligand binding at an immunoglobulin (Ig)-like motif is further enhanced by heparin sulfate proteoglycans (HSPGs). Ligand binding induces receptor dimerization and transphosphorylation, thereby activating intracellular signaling molecules such as protein kinase C (PKC), PLCγ, and the Ras signaling-pathway. Although FGF-2 lacks a classical signal peptide, it is released from astrocytes by a still unknown mechanism (Araujo and Cotman, 1992). However, most released FGF-2 is trapped by HSPGs in the extracellular matrix and is released only by heparitinase (Bashkin et al., 1989). Binding to the extracellular matrix (ECM) thus provides a stable long-term reservoir for FGF-2.

Neuroregulatory cytokines

Astrocytes also synthesize neuroregulatory cytokines, with CNTF mRNA being detectable in type 1 astrocytes of many brain regions including the optic nerve and olfactory bulb (Stöckli et al., 1991). Moreover, primary cultures of astrocytes contain CNTF mRNA and protein. Pronounced upregulation of CNTF has been demonstrated in different lesion paradigms, such as entorhinal cortex lesions (Lee et al., 1997), hippocampal deafferentation (Guthrie et al., 1997), and optic nerve transection (Kirsch et al., 1998), as well as after ischemia (Lin et al., 1998; Park et al., 2000).

Leukemia inhibitory factor is expressed in cultures of human fetal astrocytes (Aloisi et al., 1994), in murine cortical astrocytes (Murphy et al., 1995), and in spinal cord glial cells (Richards et al., 1997). Levels of astroglial LIF expression are increased following trauma or inflammation.

Epidermal growth factor family members

Astrocytes do not express EGF, but synthesize other members of this family, such as TGF-α and the neuregulins. Transforming growth factor-α immunoreactivity has been detected in astrocytes of corpus callosum, striatum, and globus pallidus (Fallon et al., 1990). Colocalization of TGF-α and ErbB1 in astrocytes suggests autocrine actions, a finding that is supported by the induction of astrogliosis in mice with a TGF-α transgene (Rabchevsky et al., 1998). However, after lesioning, astroglial immunoreactivity for TGF-α and ErbB1 is transiently decreased. Neuregulins are also expressed in cultured astrocytes (Francis et al., 1999) and are prominently upregulated in reactive gliosis (Tokita et al., 2001). *In vivo*, glial growth factor-2 (GGF-2) and neu differentiation factor/heregulin (NDF) have been detected in human white matter astrocytes of the spinal cord and in the cortex (Cannella et al., 1999; Tokita et al., 2001).

Insulin and insulin-like growth factors

In vitro, insulin-like growth factor-1 (IGF-1) promotes astroglial proliferation and oligodendroglial commitment of glial progenitor cells. Insulin-like growth factor-I is upregulated in astrocytes during remyelination, together with a transient induction of IGF receptor (McMorris et al., 1993). Similarly, astroglial IGF-I is increased after ischemia and possibly acts in a neuroprotective fashion (Gluckman et al., 1992). Since IGF-I stimulates proliferation of astrocytes *in vitro* (Tranque et al., 1992), a positive feedback regulation of these rescue mechanisms may exist. Expression of IGF-II in the CNS is largely restricted to the choroid plexus and leptomeninges (Hynes et al., 1988); expression by astroglial cells has not been reported.

Transforming growth factors-β

In the uninjured brain, most astrocytes can be labeled with antibodies to TGF-β2 and -β3 but do not seem to contain TGF-β1 immunoreactivity (Unsicker and Krieglstein, 2002). After injury, astrocytes respond with an upregulation of TGF-β1 (O'Brien et al., 1994), which in an autocrine loop seems to further activate TGF-β synthesis (Finch et al., 1993). Astrocytic TGF-β1 is also increased in response to EGF, NGF, IL-1α, and serotonin treatments (Lindholm et al., 1990; Da Cunha et al., 1993; Pousset et al., 1996).

Glial cell line-derived neurotrophic factor

In cultured human fetal astrocytes GDNF is expressed and induced by PKC (Moretto et al., 1996). In contrast, astroglial expression of GDNF *in vivo* can only be detected during early postnatal development (Ikeda et al., 1999). However, following brain damage, astroglial GDNF expression is highly upregulated (Wei et al., 2000). In addition, GDNF is prominently expressed in both glioma cell lines and gliomas *in situ* (Suter-Crazzolara and Unsicker, 1996; Wiesenhofer et al., 2000). Persephin, another GDNF family member, is also abundant in astrocytes (Jaszai et al., 1998).

Müller Glial Cells

Müller glial cells, the persisting radial glial cells of the retina, express a large variety of cytokines and their receptors. Expression of NGF, BDNF, and NT-3, along with neurotrophin receptors trkB and trkC, but not trkA, has been reported (Ikeda and Puro, 1994; Oku et al., 2002). Glial maturation factor β is another cytokine synthesized by Müller glia (Nishiwaki et al., 2001). Mudhar et al. (1993) have demonstrated abundant FGF-2 immunoreactivity in human Müller cells *in vivo*, with FGF-2 inducing its expression in an autocrine manner (Cao et al., 1997). In addition, FGF-2 downregulates IGF-I mRNA (Li et al., 1999). Cultured Müller cells release tumor necrosis factor-α (TNF-α) and nitric oxide (NO) upon stimulation with lipopolysaccharide (LPS) and IFN-γ (de Kozak et al., 1997). Moreover, TGF-β2 and -β3, but not TGF-β1, are expressed in Müller cells (Unsicker and Krieglstein 2002).

Glucose and pH influence expression of vascular endothelial growth factor (VEGF) in Müller cells (Brooks et al., 1998); VEGF183 has been reported as a novel splice variant specific for human Müller cells (Jingjing et al., 1999). Müller glia cells also express CNTF and FGF-2 (Walsh et al., 2001).

For an overview on expression patterns in different glial cell types, see Table 30.1.

SPECIFIC NEURAL FUNCTIONS OF GLIA-DERIVED GROWTH FACTORS

Role of Glia-Derived Growth Factors During Neural Development

Migration of neuronal progenitors

A role for glial growth factors in the migration of neuronal progenitors has been demonstrated by intraventricular injections of NT-4 (Brunstrom et al., 1997) or overexpression of BDNF (Ringstedt et al., 1998), which both lead to defects in cortical layering. Similar layering defects could also be observed in FGF-2 knockout mice (Dono et al, 1998). Moreover, glial growth factor (GGF) has been shown to promote migration of neuronal progenitors along radial glial fibers (Anton et al., 1997).

Axon pathfinding

Many growth factors can affect axonal pathfinding, as has been shown for netrin-1 from the internal capsule, which directs cortical axons to their target region (Richards et al., 1997). Netrin-1 is released from most

TABLE 30.1 *Growth Factors in Different Glial Subpopulations Under Normal Conditions and After Various Types of Nerve Lesioning*

	SC		Oli		Astro			
	norm	*les*	*norm*	*les*	*norm*	*react*	MG	BG
NGF	++	++++	+++	nd	+++	++++	++	nd
BDNF	+	+++	+++	nd	−	+++	++	nd
NT3	++	−	nd	nd	++	nd	++	nd
NT4	+	++	nd	nd	++	nd	nd	nd
CNTF	+++	+	−	−	+	+++	++	nd
LIF	+	++	nd	nd	+	+++	nd	nd
TGF-β1	−	+++	+	+++	−	+++	−	nd
TGF-β2	++	+	nd	nd	++	nd	++	nd
TGF-β3	+++	+	nd	nd	++	nd	++	nd
GDNF	+	+++	nd	nd	−	+++	nd	nd
TGF-α	++	++++	nd	nd	+	nd	nd	nd
Neuregulins	++	nd	nd	nd	++	nd	nd	nd
PDGF	++	nd	nd	nd	nd	nd	nd	nd
FGF-2	−	nd	nd	nd	+	+++	++	nd
IGF-1	nd	nd	nd	nd	nd	nd	++	nd

Astro: astrocytes; BDNF: brain-derived neurotrophic factor; BG: Bergmann glia; CNTF: ciliary neurotrophic factor; FGF-2: fibroblast growth factor-2; GDNF: glial cell line-derived neurotrophic factor; IGF-1: insulin-like growth factor-1; les: lesioned; LIF: leukemia inhibitory factor; MG: Müller glia; NGF: nerve growth factor; norm: normal; NT: neurotrophin; Oli: oligodendrocytes; PDGF: platelet-derived growth factor; react: reactive; SC: Schwann cells; TGF: transforming growth factor.

oligodendrocytes but not astrocytes (Manitt et al., 2001). Together with netrin-α, engrailed-1 also directs axons of association neurons, projecting ipsilaterally to motoneurons in the spinal cord (Saueressig et al., 1999). Consistent with this, axonal pathways are altered in netrin-1-deficient mice (Deiner and Sretavan, 1999 A number of glia-derived growth factors, such as TGF-α, have been shown to induce neuritogenesis (Zhang et al., 1990).

Ontogenetic neuron death

An important role for glia-derived growth factors is the regulation of ontogenetic neuron death. For example, FGF-2 can prevent neuron loss in the chick ciliary ganglion (Dreyer et al., 1989). Ciliary neurotrophic factor is also able to rescue motoneurons in the embryonic chick lumbar spinal cord during ontogenetic cell death (Wewetzer et al., 1990). Moreover, TGF-βs enhance survival of chick ciliary ganglionic neurons *in vitro* synergistically with different neurotrophins and CNTF. Surprisingly, immunoneutralization of TGF-βs during chick development *in vivo* enhances neuronal survival (Krieglstein et al., 2000).

Neural plasticity during puberty

A very late developmental event is puberty, during which gonadal steroids induce plastic changes in certain brain regions. In hypothalamic astrocytes this is accompanied by the production of TGF-α and neuregulins, which elicit astroglial secretion of prostaglandin E_2 (PGE_2), stimulating neuronal lutein hormone releasing hormone (LHRH) release. Hence, overexpression of TGF-α in the hypothalamus accelerates puberty, whereas blockade of TGF-α or neuregulin delays this process.

Role of Glia-Derived Growth Factors in the Adult Brain

Aging

During aging, together with astrogliosis, a continuous upregulation of TGF-β1 is observed (Pasinetti et al., 1999). In the rat dentate gyrus this goes along with a decrease in apoptotic cells (Bye et al., 2001). An age-dependent decrease in NGF levels has also been observed in specific brain regions of a senescence-accelerated mouse strain (Ohnishi et al., 1995). In mice, aging also leads to an increase in IL-6 and a decrease in IL-10 release from glial cells (Ye and Johnson, 2001).

Changes of cytokine release during senescence may also affect responses to brain injury. In the rat, enhanced glial activation and expression of IL-1β, TNF-α, and IL-6 has been observed (Kyrkanides et al., 2001). Following lysolecithin-induced demyelination, delayed remyelination and delayed induction of IGF-1, TGF-β1, and PDGF-A have been reported for aged rats (Hinks and Franklin, 2000). In the striatum of middle-aged rats, induction of astroglial fibroblast growth factor-2

(FGF-2) expression by IL-1β is more pronounced than in young animals (Ho and Blum, 1997). However, during normal aging, no changes in expression of FGF-2 and GDNF can be observed compared to young adult rats (Riva and Mocchetti, 1991; Blum and Weickert, 1995).

Neurodegenerative diseases

In Parkinson's (PD) and Alzheimer' s disease (AD), specific neuron populations degenerate by incompletely understood mechanisms. In both diseases, reactive astrogliosis is paralleled by an upregulation of glia-derived growth factors (Eddleston and Mucke 1993). However, some glial growth factors are also downregulated in the course of PD and AD, such as FGF-2 in the substantia nigra of PD patients (Tooyama et al., 1994), and NGF in the hippocampus of both PD and AD patients (Kerwin et al., 1992). Other studies support a role for glial-derived growth factors for the survival of midbrain dopaminergic neurons by FGF-2 (Otto and Unsicker, 1994), GDNF (Lin et al., 1993), CNTF (Asada et al., 1995), and BDNF (Akaneya et al., 1995).

Altered levels of glia-derived growth factors and cytokines are a common feature in postmortem AD brains. For example, β-amyloid of senile plaques induces IL-1β and FGF-2 (Araujo and Cotman, 1992), thereby contributing to self-stabilization of the disease state. The resulting reactive astrogliosis in AD brains is accompanied by a marked upregulation of FGF-1 in astrocytes surrounding senile plaques (Tooyama et al., 1991), while FGF-2 seems to be induced in astrocytes in the plaque center (Cummings et al., 1993). In addition, upregulation of other growth factors, such as endothelin-1 (Jiang et al., 1993), TGF-β2 (Flanders et al., 1995), IGF-I (Connor et al., 1997), and hepatocyte growth factor (HGF) (Fenton et al., 1998) can be observed in different astroglial subpopulations in AD. In contrast, BDNF is reduced in AD, showing a marked reduction around senile plaques (Soontornniyomkij et al., 1999). In accordance with this, exogenously applied NGF and GDNF restore the cholinergic phenotype of neurons of the basal nucleus of Meynert in organotypic slice cultures (Weis et al., 2001).

Glia-Derived Growth Factors During Neural Regeneration After Lesioning

Regeneration in the central nervous system

Early observations by Shahar et al. (1983) suggested that regeneration of neurons is enhanced by soluble proteins released from glial cells. In accordance with this suggestion, NGF prevents death and promotes fiber regrowth of transected cholinergic neurons. Whether this is an indirect effect due to the influence of NGF on oligodendrocyte maturation needs to be clarified (McMorris et al., 1993). Similarly, the release of IGF-I from astrocytes is involved in neuron regeneration after cuprizone-elicited demyelination of the CNS. Notably, IGFs are also potent regulators of remyelination following CNS damage (McMorris et al., 1993).

Glia-derived factors, the most prominent one being Nogo, also seem to be involved in the inhibition of axonal regeneration after spinal cord lesioning. Isolation of the Nogo receptor now opens an avenue to promote spinal cord regeneration by receptor inhibition (Fournier et al., 2001). Neurite outgrowth in the CNS is also inhibited by axon-repulsive molecules released from astroglial and meningeal scars such as collagen IV (Stichel and Müller, 1998).

In some brain regions, such as the olfactory system, axonal regeneration occurs throughout life. Olfactory glial cells are apparently a major factor for this capacity of sensory olfactory neurons since, when transplanted to the spinal cord, they promote regeneration of transected dorsal root axons. Whether this is due to their secretion of high levels of NGF, BDNF, GDNF, and neurturin remains to be shown (Woodhall et al., 2001).

Platelet-derived growth factor is prominently upregulated in neurons and astrocytes of the facial nucleus following facial nerve transection and seems to play an important role in neuronal regeneration (Hermanson et al., 1995). Similarly, astroglial CNTF expression is increased in fields of axonal sprouting in the deafferented hippocampus after entorhinal cortex lesioning (Guthrie et al., 1997), and BDNF and NT-3 are induced in spinal cord astrocytes and oligodendrocytes adjacent to a lesion. However, BDNF abolishes the survival effect of NT-3 in axotomized Clarke neurons (Novikova et al., 2000). Marked upregulation of astroglial GDNF adjacent to a spinal cord lesion was also reported by Widenfalk et al. (2001).

Regeneration in the peripheral nervous system

Peripheral nerve injury is followed by apoptotic death of 20%–40% of DRG neurons (Edström et al., 1996). In parallel, neurotrophins and their receptors are downregulated (Krekoski et al., 1996). Exogenously applied neurotrophins counteract these effects, improving the functioning of remaining sensory neurons (Munson et al., 1997). Schwann cells support and myelinate axons such that disruption of the neuron–Schwann cell relationship leads to a series of cellular changes depicted as Wallerian degeneration. In the distal nerve ending, morphological changes occurr during the first 3 days after injury. Axon fragmentation and shrinking gives the fragments a globular shape. By day 7, macrophages penetrate the lesion, clearing axonal debris within 15–30 days. Schwann cells undergo mitosis to fill in empty space. In the distal segment, regenerating Schwann cells form a band (von Büngner's band) that tracks regenerating axonal sprouts from the distal stump.

During regeneration, Schwann cells of the distal stump upregulate synthesis of NGF, BDNF, NT-4/5 and p75, but not NT-3 (Heumann et al., 1987; Funakoshi et al., 1993; Robertson et al., 1995). The parallel increase of NGF and p75 may also stimulate proliferation and migration of Schwann cells (Anton et al., 1994). However, neurotrophin levels are not sufficient to maintain neuron survival (Heumann et al., 1987).

In intact peripheral nerves, CNTF released from myelinating Schwann cells exerts trophic effects on adult motoneurons. Furthermore, after axotomy, CNTF mRNA decreases in the distal stump and recovers only after axons regenerate (Hiruma et al., 1997). Exogenous CNTF promotes peripheral nerve regeneration and promotes target reinnervation and intramuscular branching following motoneuron axotomy (Ulenkate et al., 1994). In addition, CNTF stimulates remyelination of regenerating axons (Sahenk et al., 1994).

Ciliary neurotrophic factor and LIF use common signaling pathways and therefore might act synergistically. Consistent with this, retrograde axonal transport of CNTF and LIF is increased after nerve injury (Curtis et al., 1993, 1994). The increase of LIF mRNA in peripheral nerve after axotomy (Sun et al., 1996) and the lack of LIF uptake by intramuscular nerve terminals (Curtis et al., 1994) suggest that, as in the case of CNTF, the main source of biologically relevant LIF may not be the target muscle but the surrounding Schwann cells. Indeed, upregulation of LIF mRNA can be induced in cultured Schwann cells (Matsuoka et al., 1997), and LIF administration to the axotomized nerve enhances nerve regeneration, myelination, muscle mass, and muscle contraction force (Tham et al., 1997). In LIF knockout mice, muscle regeneration is significantly reduced, but can be compensated for by exogenous LIF (Kurek et al., 1997).

Chronically lesioned adult rat sciatic nerve displays rapid upregulation of GDNF mRNA in Schwann cells proximal and distal to the inury site. Levels remain elevated for at least 5 months. Glial cell line-derived neurotrophic factor is also persistently increased in satellite and Schwann cells of the affected L4/L5 dorsal root ganglia, while GFRα is upregulated in the distal part of the sciatic nerve but not in proximal nerve or spinal cord. Following ventral root avulsion in adults, GDNF administration prevents motoneuron cell death (Li et al., 1995) and shows a long-term effect in reducing axotomy-induced soma atrophy (Matheson et al., 1997). In addition, in adult motoneurons GDNF prevents an axotomy-induced decrease in choline acetyltransferase (ChAT) immunoreactivity (Henderson et al., 1994).

SUMMARY AND PERSPECTIVES

This chapter has outlined the signaling and expression of principal protein growth factors and neuroregulatory cytokines in macroglial cells, that is, Schwann cells, oligodendrocytes, astrocytes, and radial glia. It has also provided an overview of the specific functions of these factors for neuronal development, maintenance, and regeneration in the mammalian peripheral and central nervous systems. It has become clear that macroglial growth factors are crucial for maintenance of neural integrity and for specific regulation of neuronal functions. Issues that will have to be dealt with in the future include more details of the involvement of macroglial growth factors in brain pathology, such as demyelinating or neurodegenerative diseases, or even for neuropsychiatric disorders like schizophrenia or manic depression. Eventually, improved knowledge of growth factor–mediated glia to neuron signaling will lead us to a better understanding of neuronal performances in the normal and diseased nervous system.

ABBREVIATIONS

AD	Alzheimer's disease
AKT	acute transforming retrovirus oncogene
BDNF	brain-derived neurotrophic factor
BTC	betacellulin
c-*fos*	cellular oncogene, transcription factor
ChAT	choline acetyltransferase
CNS	central nervous system
CNTF	ciliary neurotrophic factor
CRE	cAMP response element
c-ret	cellular-receptor tyrosine kinase
DRG	dorsal root ganglion
ECM	extracellular matrix
EGF	epidermal growth factor
EGF-R	epidermal growth factor receptor
ErbB	erythroblastosis virus B oncogene (viral homolog of the EGF receptor)
FAST	fas-activated serine/threonine kinase

FGF	fibroblast growth factor
FGFR	fibroblast growth factor receptor 1
GDNF	glial cell line-derived neurotrophic factor
GFRα	GDNF receptor α
GGF	glial growth factor
gp130	glycoprotein 130
GPI	glycophosphatidylinositol
GTP	guanosine triphosphate
HB-EGF	heparin-binding EGF
HGF	hepatocyte growth factor
HSPGs	heparan sulfate proteoglycans
IFN	interferon
Ig	immunoglobulin
IGF	insulin-like growth factor
IL	interleukin
JAK	Janus kinase
LHRH	lutein hormone releasing hormone
LIF	leukemia inhibitory factor
LIFRβ	LIF receptor β
LPS	lipopolysaccharide
MAP-kinase	microtubule-associated protein kinase
NDF	neu differentiation factor/heregulin
NFκB	nuclear factor κB
NGF	nerve growth factor
NO	nitric oxide
NT	neurotrophin
p75	protein75 (apoptosis promoter)
PD	Parkinson's disease
PDGF	platelet-derived growth factor
PGE_2	prostaglandin E_2
PI3 kinase	phosphoinositol-3 kinase
PKC	protein kinase C
PLCγ	Phospholipase Cγ
Raf	retroviral activating factor
Ras	retroviral activating sequence
SH	src homologous
Smad	mammalian homolog of the *Drosophila Mad* gene
STAT	signal transducer and activator of transcription
TGF-α	transforming growth factor α
TGF-β	transforming growth factor β
TNF-α	tumor necrosis factor α
Trk-receptors	tyrosine kinase receptors
TβR	TGF-β receptor
VEGF	vascular endothelial growth factor

REFERENCES

Akaneya, Y., Takahashi, M., and Hatanaka, H. (1995) Selective acid vulnerability of dopaminergic neurons and its recovery by brain-derived neurotrophic factor. *Brain Res.* 704:175–183.

Aloisi, F., Rosa, S., Testa, U., Bonsi, P., Russo, G., Peschle, C., and Levi, G. (1994) Regulation of leukemia inhibitory factor synthesis in cultured human astrocytes. *J. Immunol.* 152:5022–5031.

Anton, E.S., Marchionni, M.A., Lee, K.F., and Rakic, P. (1997) Role of GGF/neuregulin signaling in interactions between migrating neurons and radial glia in the developing cerebral cortex. *Development* 124:3501–3510.

Anton, E.S., Weskamp, G., Reichardt, L.F., and Matthew, W.D. (1994) Nerve growth factor and its low-affinity receptor promote Schwann cell migration. *Proc. Natl. Acad. Sci. USA* 91:2795–2799.

Araujo, D.M. and Cotman, C.W. (1992) Basic FGF in astroglial, microglial, and neuronal cultures: characterization of binding sites and modulation of release by lymphokines and trophic factors. *J. Neurosci.* 12:1668–1678.

Asada, H., Ip, N.Y., Pan, L., Razack, N., Parfitt, M.M., and Plunkett, R.J. (1995) Time course of ciliary neurotrophic factor mRNA expression is coincident with the presence of protoplasmic astrocytes in traumatized rat striatum. *J. Neurosci. Res.* 40:22–30.

Bar, K.J., Saldanha, G.J., Kennedy, A.J., Facer, P., Birch, R., Carlstedt, T., and Anand, P. (1998) GDNF and its receptor component Ret in injured human nerves and dorsal root ganglia. *NeuroReport* 9:43–47.

Bashkin, P., Doctrow, S., Klagsbrun, M., Svahn, C.M., Folkman, J., and Vlodavsky, I. (1989) Basic fibroblast growth factor binds to subendothelial extracellular matrix and is released by heparitinase and heparin-like molecules. *Biochemistry* 28:1737–1743.

Blum, M. and Weickert, C.S. (1995) GDNF mRNA expression in normal postnatal development, aging, and in Weaver mutant mice. *Neurobiol. Aging* 16:925–929.

Bothwell, M. (1998) Keeping track of neurotrophin receptors. *Cell* 65:915–918.

Brooks, S.E., Gu, X., Kaufmann, P.M., Marcus, D.M., and Caldwell, R.B. (1998) Modulation of VEGF production by pH and glucose in retinal Muller cells. *Curr. Eye Res.* 17:875–882.

Brunstrom, J.E., Gray-Swain, M.R., Osborne, P.A., and Pearlman, A.L. (1997) Neuronal heterotopias in the developing cerebral cortex produced by neurotrophin-4. *Neuron* 18:505–517.

Burette, A., Belliot, G., Albuisson, E., and Romand, R. (1998) Localization of neurotrophin-3-like immunoreactivity in the rat cochlear nucleus. *Microsc. Res. Tech.* 41:224–233.

Bye, N., Zieba, M., Wreford, N.G., and Nichols, N.R. (2001) Resistance of the dentate gyrus to induced apoptosis during ageing is associated with increases in transforming growth factor-β1 messenger RNA. *Neuroscience* 105:853–862.

Cannella, B., Pitt, D., Marchionni, M., and Raine, C.S. (1999) Neuregulin and erbB receptor expression in normal and diseased human white matter. *J. Neuroimmunol.* 100:233–242.

Cao, W., Wen, R., Li, F., Lavail, M.M., and Steinberg, R.H. (1997) Mechanical injury increases bFGF and CNTF mRNA expression in the mouse retina. *Exp. Eye Res.* 65:241–248.

Carroll, P., Sendtner, M., Meyer, M., and Thoenen, H. (1993) Rat ciliary neurotrophic factor (CNTF): gene structure and regulation of mRNA levels in glial cell cultures. *Glia* 9:176–187.

Chandross, K.J., Chanson, M., Spray, D.C., and Kessler, J.A. (1995) Transforming growth factor-β 1 and forskolin modulate gap junctional communication and cellular phenotype of cultured Schwann cells. *J. Neurosci.* 15:262–273.

Condorelli, D.F., Salin, T., Dell' Albani, P., Mudo, G., Corsaro, M., Timmusk, T., Metsis, M., and Belluardo, N. (1995) Neurotrophins and their trk-receptors in cultured cells of the glial lineage and in white matter of the central nervous system. *J. Mol. Neurosci.* 6:237–248.

Connor, B., Beilharz, E.J., Williams, C., Synek, B., Gluckman, P.D., Faull, R.L., and Dragunow, M. (1997) Insulin-like growth factor-I (IGF-I) immunoreactivity in the Alzheimer's disease temporal cortex and hippocampus. *Brain Res. Mol. Brain Res.* 49: 283–290.

Cummings, B.J., Su, J.H., and Cotman, C.W. (1993) Neuritic involvement within bFGF immunopositive plaques of Alzheimer's disease. *Exp. Neurol.* 124:315–325.

Curtis, R., Adryan, K.M., Zhu, Y., Harkness, P.J., Lindsay, R.M., and DiStefano, P.S. (1993) Retrograde axonal transport of ciliary neurotrophic factor is increased by peripheral nerve injury. *Nature* 365:253–255.

Curtis, R., Scherer, S.S., Somogyi, R., Adryan, K.M., Ip, N.Y., Zhu, Y., Lindsay, R.M., and DiStefano, P.S. (1994) Retrograde axonal transport of LIF is increased by peripheral nerve injury: correlation with increased LIF expression in distal nerve. *Neuron* 12:191–204.

Da Cunha, A., Jefferson, J.A., Jackson, R.W., and Vitkovic, L. (1993) Glial cell-specific mechanisms of TGF-β 1 induction by IL-1 in cerebral cortex. *J. Neuroimmunol.* 42:71–85.

Deiner, M.S. and Sretavan, D.W. (1999) Altered midline axon pathways and ectopic neurons in the developing hypothalamus of netrin-1- and DCC-deficient mice. *J. Neurosci.* 19:9900–99012.

De Kozak, Y., Cotinet, A., Goureau, O., Hicks, D., and Thillaye-Goldenberg, B. (1997) Tumor necrosis factor and nitric oxide production by resident retinal glial cells from rats presenting hereditary retinal degeneration. *Ocular Immunol. Inflammation* 5:85–94.

Dobrea, G.M., Unnerstall, J.R., and Rao, M.S. (1992) The expression of CNTF message and immunoreactivity in the central and peripheral nervous system of the rat. *Brain Res. Dev. Brain Res.* 66:209–219.

Dono, R., Texido, G., Dussel, R., Ehmke, H., and Zeller, R. (1998) Impaired cerebral cortex development and blood pressure regulation in FGF-2-deficient mice. *EMBO J.* 17:4213–4225.

Dreyer, D., Lagrange, A., Grothe, C., and Unsicker, K. (1989) Basic fibroblast growth factor prevents ontogenetic neuron death in vivo. *Neurosci. Lett.* 99:35–38.

Eccleston, P.A., Funa, K., and Heldin, C.H. (1993) Expression of platelet-derived growth factor (PDGF) and PDGF α- and β-receptors in the peripheral nervous system: an analysis of sciatic nerve and dorsal root ganglia. *Dev. Biol.* 155:459–470.

Eddleston, M. and Mucke, L. (1993) Molecular profile of reactive astrocytes—implications for their role in neurologic disease. *Neuroscience* 54:15–36.

Edström, A., Ekstrom, P.A., and Tonge, D. (1996) Axonal outgrowth and neuronal apoptosis in cultured adult mouse dorsal root ganglion preparations: effects of neurotrophins, of inhibition of neurotrophin actions and of prior axotomy. *Neuroscience* 75:1165–1174.

Einheber, S., Hannocks, M.J., Metz, C.N., Rifkin, D.B., and Salzer, J.L. (1995) Transforming growth factor-β 1 regulates axon/Schwann cell interactions. *J. Cell Biol.* 129:443–458.

Enomoto, H., Araki, T., Jackman, A., Heuckeroth, R.O., Snider, W.D., Johnson, E.M., Jr., and Milbrandt, J. (1998) GFR α1-deficient mice have deficits in the enteric nervous system and kidneys. *Neuron* 21:317–324.

Fallon, J.H., Annis, C.M., Gentry, L.E., Twardzik, D.R., and Loughlin, S.E. (1990) Localization of cells containing transforming growth factor-α precursor immunoreactivity in the basal ganglia of the adult rat brain. *Growth Factors* 2:241–250.

Fenton, H., Finch, P.W., Rubin, J.S., Rosenberg, J.M., Taylor, W.G., Kuo-Leblanc, V., Rodriguez-Wolf, M., Baird, A., Schipper, H.M., and Stopa, E.G. (1998) Hepatocyte growth factor (HGF/SF) in Alzheimer's disease. *Brain Res.* 779:262–270.

Finch, C.E., Laping, N.J., Morgan, T.E., Nichols, N.R., and Pasinetti, G.M. (1993) TGF-β1 is an organizer of responses to neurodegeneration. *J. Cell. Biochem.* 53:314–522.

Flanders, K.C., Lippa, C.F., Smith, T.W., Pollen, D.A., and Sporn, M.B. (1995) Altered expression of transforming growth factor-β in Alzheimer's disease. *Neurology* 45:1561–1569.

Fournier, A.E., Grand Pre, T., and Strittmatter, S.M. (2001) Identification of a receptor mediating Nogo-66 inhibition of axonal regeneration. *Nature* 409:341–346.

Francis, A., Raabe, T.D., Wen, D., and DeVries, G.H. (1999) Neuregulins and ErbB receptors in cultured neonatal astrocytes. *J. Neurosci. Res.* 57:487–494.

Friedman, B., Scherer, S.S., Rudge, J.S., Helgren, M., Morrisey, D., McClain, J., Wang, D.Y., Wiegand, S.J., Furth, M.E., and Lindsay, R.M. (1992) Regulation of ciliary neurotrophic factor expression in myelin-related Schwann cells in vivo. *Neuron* 9:295–305.

Friedman, W.J., Black, I.B., and Kaplan, D.R. (1998) Distribution of the neurotrophins brain-derived neurotrophic factor, neurotrophin-3, and neurotrophin-4/5 in the postnatal rat brain: an immunocytochemical study. *Neuroscience* 84:101–114.

Funakoshi, H., Frisen, J., Barbany, G., Timmusk, T., Zachrisson, O., Verge, V.M., and Persson, H. (1993) Differential expression of mRNAs for neurotrophins and their receptors after axotomy of the sciatic nerve. *J. Cell Biol.* 123:455–465.

Gluckman, P., Klempt, N., Guan, J., Mallard, C., Sirimanne, E., Dragunow, M., Klempt, M., Singh, K., Williams, C., and Nikolics, K. (1992) A role for IGF-1 in the rescue of CNS neurons following hypoxic-ischemic injury. *Biochem. Biophys. Res. Commun.* 182:593–599.

Gonzalez, D., Dees, W.L., Hiney, J.K., Ojeda, S.R., and Saneto, R.P. (1990) Expression of β-nerve growth factor in cultured cells derived from the hypothalamus and cerebral cortex. *Brain Res.* 511:249–258.

Goto, A. and Furukawa, S. (1995) Experimental changes in BDNF- and NT-3-like immunoreactivities in the spinal cord following its transection. *Nippon Seikeigeka Gakkai Zasshi* 69:506–516.

Griesbeck, O., Parsadanian, A.S., Sendtner, M., and Thoenen, H. (1995) Expression of neurotrophins in skeletal muscle: quantitative comparison and significance for motoneuron survival and maintenance of function. *J. Neurosci. Res.* 42:21–33.

Guthrie, K.M., Woods, A.G., Nguyen, T., and Gall, C.M. (1997) Astroglial ciliary neurotrophic factor mRNA expression is increased in fields of axonal sprouting in deafferented hippocampus. *J. Comp. Neurol.* 386:137–148.

Hardy, M., Reddy, U.R., and Pleasure, D. (1992) Platelet-derived growth factor and regulation of Schwann cell proliferation in vivo. *J. Neurosci. Res.* 31:254–262.

Henderson, C.E., Phillips, H.S., Pollock, R.A., Davies, A.M., Lemeulle, C., Armanini, M., Simmons, L., Moffet, B., Vandlen, R.A., and Simpson, L.C. (1994) GDNF: a potent survival factor for motoneurons present in peripheral nerve and muscle. *Science* 266:1062–1064.

Hermanson, M., Olsson, T., Westermark, B., and Funa, K. (1995) PDGF and its receptors following facial nerve axotomy in rats: expression in neurons and surrounding glia. *Exp. Brain Res.* 102:415–422.

Heumann, R., Korsching, S., Bandtlow, C., and Thoenen, H. (1987) Changes of nerve growth factor synthesis in nonneuronal cells in response to sciatic nerve transection. *J. Cell Biol.* 104:1623–1631.

Hinks, G.L. and Franklin, R.J. (2000) Delayed changes in growth factor gene expression during slow remyelination in the CNS of aged rats. *Mol. Cell. Neurosci.* 16:542–556.

Hiruma, S., Shimizu, T., Huruta, T., Satou, T., Hu, J., Tanji, K., and

Hashimoto, S. (1997) Ciliary neurotrophic factor immunoreactivity in rat intramuscular nerve during reinnervation through a silicone tube after severing of the rat sciatic nerve. *Exp. Mol. Pathol.* 64:23–30.

Ho, A. and Blum, M. (1997) Regulation of astroglial-derived dopaminergic neurotrophic factors by interleukin-1 β in the striatum of young and middle-aged mice. *Exp. Neurol.* 148:348–359.

Hoke, A., Gordon, T., Zochodne, D.W., and Sulaiman O.A. (2002) A decline in glial cell-line-derived neurotrophic factor expression is associated with impaired regeneration after long-term Schwann cell denervation. *Exp. Neurol.* 173:77–85.

Hynes, M.A., Brooks, P.J., Van Wyk, J.J., and Lund, P.K. (1988) Insulin-like growth factor II messenger ribonucleic acids are synthesized in the choroid plexus of the rat brain. *Mol. Endocrinol.* 2:47–54.

Ikeda, T. and Puro, D.G. (1994) Nerve growth factor: a mitogenic signal for retinal Muller glial cells. *Brain Res.* 649:260–264.

Ikeda, T., Xia, X.Y., Xia, Y.X., Ikenoue, T., and Choi, B.H. (1999) Expression of glial cell line–derived neurotrophic factor in the brain and cerebrospinal fluid of the developing rat. *Int. J. Dev. Neurosci.* 17:681–691.

Jaszai, J., Farkas, L., Galter, D., Reuss, B., Strelau, J., Unsicker, K., and Krieglstein, K. (1998) GDNF-related factor persephin is widely distributed throughout the nervous system. *J. Neurosci. Res.* 53:494–501.

Jiang, M.H., Hoog, A., Ma, K.C., Nie, X.J., Olsson, Y., and Zhang, W.W. (1993) Endothelin-1-like immunoreactivity is expressed in human reactive astrocytes. *NeuroReport* 4:935–937.

Jingjing, L., Xue, Y., Agarwal, N., and Roque, R.S. (1999) Human Muller cells express VEGF183, a novel spliced variant of vascular endothelial growth factor. *Invest. Ophthalmol. Vis. Sci.* 40: 752–759.

Kerwin, J.M., Morris, C.M., Perry, R.H., and Perry, E.K. (1992) Hippocampal nerve growth factor receptor immunoreactivity in patients with Alzheimer's and Parkinson's disease. *Neurosci. Lett.* 143:101–104.

Kirsch, M., Schneider, T., Lee, M.Y., and Hofmann, H.D. (1998) Lesion-induced changes in the expression of ciliary neurotrophic factor and its receptor in rat optic nerve. *Glia* 23:239–248.

Krekoski, C.A., Parhad, I.M., and Clark, A.W. (1996) Attenuation and recovery of nerve growth factor receptor mRNA in dorsal root ganglion neurons following axotomy. *J. Neurosci. Res.* 43:1–11.

Krieglstein, K., Richter, S., Farkas, L., Schuster, N., Dünker, N., Oppenheim, R.W., and Unsicker, K. (2000) Reduction of endogenous transforming growth factors β prevents ontogenic neuron death. *Nat. Neurosci.* 3:1085–1090.

Kurek, J.B., Bower, J.J., Romanella, M., Koentgen, F., Murphy, M., and Austin, L. (1997) The role of leukemia inhibitory factor in skeletal muscle regeneration. *Muscle Nerve* 20:815–822.

Kyrkanides, S., O'Banion, M.K., Whiteley, P.E., Daeschner, J.C., and Olschowka, J.A. (2001) Enhanced glial activation and expression of specific CNS inflammation-related molecules in aged versus young rats following cortical stab injury. *J. Neuroimmunol.* 119:269–277.

Lee, M.Y., Deller, T., Kirsch, M., Frotscher, M., and Hofmann, H.D. (1997) Differential regulation of ciliary neurotrophic factor (CNTF) and CNTF receptor α expression in astrocytes and neurons of the fascia dentata after entorhinal cortex lesion. *J. Neurosci.* 17:1137–1146.

Li, F., Cao, W., Steinberg, R.H., and LaVail, M.M. (1999) Basic FGF-induced down-regulation of IGF-I mRNA in cultured rat Muller cells. *Exp. Eye Res.* 68:19–27.

Li, L., Wu, W., Lin, L.F., Lei, M., Oppenheim, R.W., and Houenou, L.J. (1995) Rescue of adult mouse motoneurons from injury-induced cell death by glial cell line-derived neurotrophic factor. *Proc. Natl. Acad. Sci. USA* 92:9771–9775.

Lin, L.F., Doherty, D.H., Lile, J.D., Bektesh, S., and Collins, F. (1993) GDNF: a glial cell line–derived neurotrophic factor for midbrain dopaminergic neurons. *Science* 260:1130–1132.

Lin, T.N., Wang, P.Y., Chi, S.I., and Kuo, J.S. (1998) Differential regulation of ciliary neurotrophic factor (CNTF) and CNTF receptor α (CNTFR α) expression following focal cerebral ischemia. *Brain Res. Mol. Brain Res.* 55:71–80.

Lindholm, D., Hengerer, B., Zafra, F., and Thoenen, H. (1990) Transforming growth factor-beta 1 stimulates expression of nerve growth factor in the rat CNS. *NeuroReport* 1:9–12.

Manitt, C., Colicos, M.A., Thompson, K.M., Rousselle, E., Peterson, A.C., and Kennedy, T.E. (2001) Widespread expression of netrin-1 by neurons and oligodendrocytes in the adult mammalian spinal cord. *J. Neurosci.* 21:3911–3922.

Matheson, C.R., Wang, J., Collins, F.D., and Yan, Q. (1997) Long-term survival effects of GDNF on neonatal rat facial motoneurons after axotomy. *NeuroReport* 8:1739–1742.

Matsuoka, I., Nakane, A., and Kurihara, K. (1997) Induction of LIF-mRNA by TGF-β 1 in Schwann cells. *Brain Res.* 776:170–180.

McKinnon, R.D., Piras, G., Ida, J.A., Jr., and Dubois-Dalcq, M. (1993) A role for TGF-β in oligodendrocyte differentiation. *J. Cell Biol.* 121:1397–1407.

McMorris, F.A., Mozell, R.L., Carson, M.J., Shinar, Y., Meyer, R.D., and Marchetti, N. (1993) Regulation of oligodendrocyte development and central nervous system myelination by insulin-like growth factors. *Ann. NY Acad. Sci.* 692:321–334.

Miller, F.D. and Kaplan, D.R. (2001) Neurotrophin signalling pathways regulating neuronal apoptosis. *Cell. Mol. Life Sci.* 58: 1045–1053.

Moretto, G., Walker, D.G., Lanteri, P., Taioli, F., Zaffagnini, S., Xu, R.Y., and Rizzuto, N. (1996) Expression and regulation of glial-cell-line-derived neurotrophic factor (GDNF) mRNA in human astrocytes in vitro. *Cell Tissue Res.* 286:257–262.

Mudhar, H.S., Pollock, R.A., Wang, C., Stiles, C.D., and Richardson, W.D. (1993) PDGF and its receptors in the developing rodent retina and optic nerve. *Development* 118:539–552.

Munson, J.B., Shelton, D.L., and McMahon, S.B. (1997) Adult mammalian sensory and motor neurons: roles of endogenous neurotrophins and rescue by exogenous neurotrophins after axotomy. *J. Neurosci.* 17:470–476.

Murphy, G.M., Jr., Song, Y., Ong, E., Lee, Y.L., Schmidt, K.G., Bocchini, V., and Eng, L.F. (1995) Leukemia inhibitory factor mRNA is expressed in cortical astrocyte cultures but not in an immortalized microglial cell line. *Neurosci. Lett.* 184:48–51.

Neet, K.E. and Campenot, R.B. (2001) Receptor binding, internalization, and retrograde transport of neurotrophic factors. *Cell. Mol. Life Sci.* 58:1021–1035.

Nishiwaki, A., Asai, K., Tada, T., Ueda, T., Shimada, S., Ogura, Y., and Kato, T. (2001) Expression of glia maturation factor during retinal development in the rat. *Brain Res. Mol. Brain Res.* 95: 103–109.

Novikova, L.N., Novikov, L.N., and Kellerth, J.O. (2000) BDNF abolishes the survival effect of NT-3 in axotomized Clarke neurons of adult rats. *J. Comp. Neurol.* 428:671–680.

O'Brien, M.F., Lenke, L.G., Lou, J., Bridwell, K.H., and Joyce, M.E. (1994) Astrocyte response and transforming growth factor-β localization in acute spinal cord injury. *Spine* 19:2321–2329.

Ohnishi, K., Tomimoto, H., Akiguchi, I., Seriu, N., Kawamata, T., Nakamura, S., Kimura, J., Nishio, T., Higuchi, K., and Hosokawa, M. (1995) Age-related decrease of nerve growth factor-like immunoreactivity in the basal forebrain of senescence-accelerated mice. *Acta Neuropathol. (Berl.)* 90:11–16.

Oku, H., Ikeda, T., Honma, Y., Sotozono, C., Nishida, K., Nakamura, Y., Kida, T., and Kinoshita, S. (2002) Gene expression of neurotrophins and their high-affinity trk receptors in cultured human Muller cells. *Ophthal. Res.* 34:38–42.

Otto, D. and Unsicker, K. (1994) FGF-2 in the MPTP model of Parkinson's disease: effects on astroglial cells. *Glia* 11:47–56.

Park, C.K., Ju, W.K., Hofmann, H.D., Kirsch, M., Ki Kang, J., Chun, M.H., and Lee, M.Y. (2000) Differential regulation of ciliary neurotrophic factor and its receptor in the rat hippocampus following transient global ischemia. *Brain Res.* 861:345–353.

Pasinetti, G.M., Hassler, M., Stone, D., and Finch, C.E. (1999) Glial gene expression during aging in rat striatum and in long-term responses to 6-OHDA lesions. *Synapse* 31:278–284.

Pousset, F., Fournier, J., Legoux, P., Keane, P., Shire, D., and Soubrie, P. (1996) Effect of serotonin on cytokine mRNA expression in rat hippocampal astrocytes. *Brain Res. Mol. Brain Res.* 38:54–62.

Pshenichkin, S.P. and Wise, B.C. (1997) Okadaic acid stimulates nerve growth factor production via an induction of interleukin-1 in primary cultures of cortical astroglial cells. *Neurochem. Int.* 30:507–514.

Raabe, T.D., Francis, A., and DeVries, G.H. (1998) Neuregulins in glial cells. *Neurochem. Res.* 23:311–318.

Rabchevsky, A.G., Weinitz, J.M., Coulpier, M., Fages, C., Tinel, M., and Junier, M.P. (1998) A role for transforming growth factor α as an inducer of astrogliosis. *J. Neurosci.* 18:10541–10552.

Richards, L.J., Koester, S.E., Tuttle, R., and O'Leary, D.D. (1997) Directed growth of early cortical axons is influenced by a chemoattractant released from an intermediate target. *J. Neurosci.* 17:2445–2458.

Ringstedt, T., Linnarsson, S., Wagner, J., Lendahl, U., Kokaia, Z., Arenas, E., Ernfors, P., and Ibanez, C.F. (1998) BDNF regulates reelin expression and Cajal-Retzius cell development in the cerebral cortex. *Neuron* 21:305–315.

Riva, M.A. and Mocchetti, I. (1991) Developmental expression of the basic fibroblast growth factor gene in rat brain. *Brain Res. Dev. Brain Res.* 62:45–50.

Robertson, M.D., Toews, A.D., Bouldin, T.W., Weaver, J., Goines, N.D., and Morell, P. (1995) NGFR-mRNA expression in sciatic nerve: a sensitive indicator of early stages of axonopathy. *Mol. Brain Res.* 28:231–238.

Rufer, M., Flanders, K., and Unsicker, K. (1994) Presence and regulation of transforming growth factor β mRNA and protein in the normal and lesioned rat sciatic nerve. *J. Neurosci. Research* 39:412–423.

Sahenk, Z., Seharaseyon, J., and Mendell, J.R. (1994) CNTF potentiates peripheral nerve regeneration. *Brain Res.* 655:246–250.

Saueressig, H., Burrill, J., and Goulding, M. (1999) Engrailed-1 and netrin-1 regulate axon pathfinding by association interneurons that project to motor neurons. *Development* 126:4201–4212.

Scherer, S.S., Kamholz, J., and Jakowlew, S.B. (1993) Axons modulate the expression of transforming growth factor-βs in Schwann cells. *Glia* 8:265–276.

Sensenbrenner, M., Labourdette, G., Pettmann, B., Perraud, F., and Besnard, F. (1987) Neuronal-derived factors regulating glial cell proliferation and maturation. *J. Physiol. (Paris)* 82:288–290.

Shahar, A., Schupper, H., Kimhi, Y., Mizrachi, Y., and Schwartz, M. (1983) Regeneration of adult rat brain neurons in culture is enhanced by glial factor(s) *Birth Defects* 19:457–460.

Skoff, A.M., Lisak, R.P., Bealmear, B., and Benjamins, J.A. (1998) TNF-α and TGF-β act synergistically to kill Schwann cells. *J. Neurosci. Res.* 53:747–756.

Soontornniyomkij, V., Wang, G., Pittman, C.A., Hamilton, R.L., Wiley, C.A., and Achim, C.L. (1999) Absence of brain-derived neurotrophic factor and trkB receptor immunoreactivity in glia of Alzheimer's disease. *Acta Neuropathol. (Berl.)* 98:345–348.

Stewart, H.J., Rougon, G., Dong, Z., Dean, C., Jessen, K.R., and Mirsky, R. (1995) TGF-βs upregulate NCAM and L1 expression in cultured Schwann cells, suppress cyclic AMP–induced expression of O4 and galactocerebroside, and are widely expressed in cells of the Schwann cell lineage in vivo. *Glia* 15:419–436.

Stichel, C.C. and Müller, H.W. (1998) The CNS lesion scar: new vistas on an old regeneration barrier. *Cell Tissue Res.* 294:1–9.

Stöckli, K.A., Lillien, L.E., Naher-Noe, M., Breitfeld, G., Hughes, R.A., Raff, M.C., Thoenen, H., and Sendtner, M. (1991) Regional distribution, developmental changes, and cellular localization of CNTF-mRNA and protein in the rat brain. *J. Cell Biol.* 115:447–459.

Sun, Y., Landis, S.C., and Zigmond, R.E. (1996) Signals triggering the induction of leukemia inhibitory factor in sympathetic superior cervical ganglia and their nerve trunks after axonal injury. *Mol. Cell. Neurosci.* 7:152–163.

Suter-Crazzolara, C. and Unsicker, K. (1996) GDNF mRNA levels are induced by FGF-2 in rat C6 glioblastoma cells. *Brain Res. Mol. Brain Res.* 41:175–182.

Tham, S., Dowsing, B., Finkelstein, D., Donato, R., Cheema, S.S., Bartlett, P.F., and Morrison, W.A. (1997) Leukemia inhibitory factor enhances the regeneration of transected rat sciatic nerve and the function of reinnervated muscle. *J. Neurosci. Res.* 47: 208–215.

Tokita, Y., Keino, H., Matsui, F., Aono, S., Ishiguro, H., Higashiyama, S., and Oohira, A. (2001) Regulation of neuregulin expression in the injured rat brain and cultured astrocytes. *J. Neurosci.* 21:1257–1264.

Tooyama, I., Akiyama, H., McGeer, P.L., Hara, Y., Yasuhara, O., and Kimura, H. (1991) Acidic fibroblast growth factor-like immunoreactivity in brain of Alzheimer patients. *Neurosci. Lett.* 121:155–158.

Tooyama, I., McGeer, E.G., Kawamata, T., Kimura, H., and McGeer, P.L. (1994) Retention of basic fibroblast growth factor immunoreactivity in dopaminergic neurons of the substantia nigra during normal aging in humans contrasts with loss in Parkinson's disease. *Brain Res.* 656:165–168.

Tranque, P.A., Calle, R, Naftolin, F., and Robbins, R. (1992) Involvement of protein kinase-C in the mitogenic effect of insulin-like growth factor-I on rat astrocytes. *Endocrinology* 131:1948–1954.

Ulenkate, H.J., Kaal, E.C., Gispen, W.H., and Jennekens, F.G. (1994) Ciliary neurotrophic factor improves muscle fibre reinnervation after facial nerve crush in young rats. *Acta Neuropathol. (Berl.)* 88:558–564.

Unsicker, K. and Krieglstein, K. (2002) TGF-βs and their roles in the regulation of neuron survival. *Adv. Exp. Med. Biol.* 513:353–374.

Vega, J.A., Vazquez, E., Naves, F.J., Calzada, B., del Valle, M.E., and Represa, J.J. (1994) Expression of epidermal growth factor receptor (EGFr) immunoreactivity in human cutaneous nerves and sensory corpuscles. *Anat. Rec.* 240:125–130.

Walsh, N., Valter, K., and Stone, J. (2001) Cellular and subcellular patterns of expression of bFGF and CNTF in the normal and light stressed adult rat retina. *Exp. Eye Res.* 72:495–501.

Watabe, K., Fukuda, T., Tanaka, J., Honda, H., Toyohara, K., and Sakai, O. (1995) Spontaneously immortalized adult mouse Schwann cells secrete autocrine and paracrine growth-promoting activities. *J. Neurosci. Res.* 41:279–290.

Weis, C., Marksteiner, J., and Humpel, C. (2001) Nerve growth factor and glial cell line–derived neurotrophic factor restore the cholinergic neuronal phenotype in organotypic brain slices of the basal nucleus of Meynert. *Neuroscience* 102:129–138.

Wetmore, C. and Olson, L. (1995) Neuronal and nonneuronal expression of neurotrophins and their receptors in sensory and sympathetic ganglia suggest new intercellular trophic interactions. *J. Comp. Neurol.* 353:143–159.

Wewetzer, K., MacDonald, J.R., Collins, F., and Unsicker, K. (1990) CNTF rescues motoneurons from ontogenetic cell death in-vivo, but not in-vitro. *NeuroReport* 1:203–206.

Widenfalk, J., Lundstromer, K., Jubran, M., Brene, S., and Olson, L. (2001) Neurotrophic factors and receptors in the immature and adult spinal cord after mechanical injury or kainic acid. *J. Neurosci.* 21:3457–3475.

Wei, G., Wu, G., and Cao, X. (2000) Dynamic expression of glial cell line–derived neurotrophic factor after cerebral ischemia. *NeuroReport* 11:1177–1183.

Wiesenhofer, B., Stockhammer, G., Kostron, H., Maier, H., Hinterhuber, H., and Humpel, C. (2000) Glial cell line–derived neurotrophic factor (GDNF) and its receptor (GFR-α 1) are strongly expressed in human gliomas. *Acta Neuropathol. (Berl.)* 99: 131–137.

Woodhall, E., West, A.K., and Chuah, M.I. (2001) Cultured olfactory ensheathing cells express nerve growth factor, brain-derived neurotrophic factor, glia cell line–derived neurotrophic factor and their receptors. *Brain Res. Mol. Brain Res.* 88:203–213.

Wu, V.W., Nishiyama, N., and Schwartz, J.P. (1998) A culture model of reactive astrocytes: increased nerve growth factor synthesis and reexpression of cytokine responsiveness. *J. Neurochem.* 71:749–756.

Xian, C.J. and Zhou, X.F. (1999) Neuronal-glial differential expression of TGF-α and its receptor in the dorsal root ganglia in response to sciatic nerve lesion. *Exp. Neurol.* 157:317–326.

Yamakuni, T., Ozawa, F., Hishinuma, F., Kuwano, R., Takahashi, Y., and Amano, T. (1987) Expression of β-nerve growth factor mRNA in rat glioma cells and astrocytes from rat brain. *FEBS Lett.* 223:117–121.

Ye, S.M. and Johnson, R.W. (2001) An age-related decline in interleukin-10 may contribute to the increased expression of interleukin-6 in brain of aged mice. *Neuroimmunomodulation* 9:183–192.

Zhang, M.B., Woo, D.D., and Howard, B.D. (1990) Transforming growth factor α and a PC12-derived growth factor induce neurites in PC12 cells and enhance the survival of embryonic brain neurons. *Cell Regul.* 1:511–521.

Zhou, X.F., Rush, R.A., and McLachlan, E.M. (1996) Differential expression of the p75 nerve growth factor receptor in glia and neurons of the rat dorsal root ganglia after peripheral nerve transection. *J. Neurosci.* 16:2901–2911.

31 Radial glial cells: scaffolding for cortical development and evolution

PASKO RAKIC

The embryonic central nervous system consists of a variety of neuronal and nonneuronal cell lines that cooperatively build the cytoarchitectonic organization of the diverse brain structures. Among nonneuronal cell lines, none is more fascinating than the transient population of radial glial cells. They derive from the neuroepithelial cells during restricted developmental periods in most regions of the vertebrate brain. The time of this divergence, as well as their longevity and significance for guiding migrating neurons, have increased with the evolutionary expansion of the mammalian neocortex, reaching a peak in the gyrencephalic human forebrain. The phenotypic distinction of these cells from the migrating neurons initially based on morphological criteria in human has been confirmed by their ultrastructural, molecular, and physiological characteristics. In addition, modern *in vivo* and *in vitro* approaches have revealed that these cells can also generate neuronal cell lines that, either immediately or after several additional divisions, migrate along radial shafts of the mother cells that stretch across the widening cerebral wall. In most structures of the mammalian brain, with some notable exceptions, the radial glial cells transform into astrocytes or disappear during late stages of ontogenetic development. The diversity of functions and the variety of morphogenetic transformations observed in different regions and species suggest that this cell class has played a pivotal role in the expansion of the cerebral cortex during evolution. The present review is mainly concerned with the radial and Bergmann glial cells and their role in the developing mammalian cortical structures, with particular emphasis on the cerebral and cerebellar cortex in the large primate brain.

HISTORICAL PERSPECTIVE

Since their discovery in the human fetal brain at the end of the nineteenth century, radial glial cells have been considered to be a distinct cell class. Use of the Golgi silver impregnation method revealed their distinct morphology, although investigators referred to them by a variety of terms such as *epithelial cells* (Golgi, 1885; Ramón y Cajal, 1909), *radial cells* (Magini, 1888), *fetal ependymal cells* (Retzius, 1893, 1894), and *spongioblasts* (Lenhossék, 1895; Koeliker, 1896). However, the distinction between different cell phenotypes in the embryonic tissue by the Golgi method alone was difficult even for the masters of this approach. For example, in his study of the developing frog and chick embryo (e.g., Fig. 31.1*A,B*), Cajal initially thought that the *neuroepithelial* cells spanning the width of the neural tube might actually be *neuroblasts*, which contribute neurons to the spinal cord (reviewed in Rakic, 2003). Subsequently, after examining the telencephalon at more advanced stages of development in several mammalian species (Fig. 31.1*C,D*), he recognized that the cells with voluminous radial fibers studded with lamellate expansions and terminating with endfeet at both sides of the cerebral wall might be a separate class, different from the *pyriform* neuroblasts that arise from the primitive *spheroidal* cells that give rise to bipolar migrating neurons. Thus, he concluded that neuroepithelial cells gradually diverge into more specialized neuronal and glial precursors, as had been, at the time, advocated by His (1889) and Lenhossék (1895), based on examination of the human fetal telencephalon. Cajal also noticed that each radial cell has one basal endfoot (*pied ventriculere*) at the ventricular surface, whereas at the pial side their radial fiber, several branches often form, particularly at later stages, that terminate with multiple endfeet at the pial surface. His contemporary, Gustaf Retzius, described maturation of these cells from the simple bipolar shape to a more differentiated form, with branching of the outer process as the surface of the human fetal cerebrum becomes larger and more convoluted (Fig. 31.2). Finally, Cajal suggested that radial cells transform into spider-like cells that differentiate into fibrillary or protoplasmic types of astrocytes. Thus, although the methods available at the time were not adequate to provide definitive phenotypic classification, based on the morphological criteria, most investigators have classified them

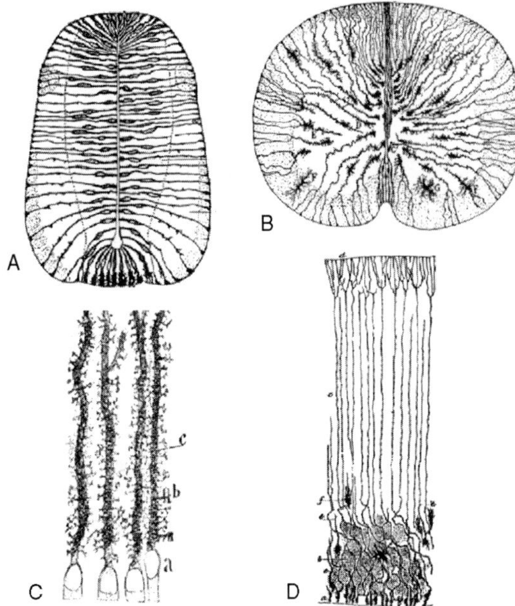

FIGURE 31.1 *A*. Primordial epithelium, including spongioblast (radial glial) cells of the spinal cord of the chick embryo—third day of incubation, when, according to Ramón y Cajal, they become stainable by the Golgi method. *B*. Epithelial (radial glial) and displaced astroglial precursors and more mature astrocytes in the spinal cord of the newborn mouse stained by the Golgi method display different phases of morphogenetic transformation of a more differentiated glial cell line. *C*. Characteristic lamellate expansion on the radial shafts of epithelial (radial glial). *D*. Epithelial (radial glial) and neuroglial cells of the cerebral cortex in neonatal rabbit stained with the Golgi method. (Assembled from Ramón y Cajal, 1909. See the text for further explanation.)

as a separate non-neuronal cell line that became known as *radial glial* (RG) cells (see the discussions in Schmechel and Rakic, 1979a; Varon and Somjen, 1979; Rickmann and Wolff, 1985; Fedoroff and Vernadakis, 1986; Rakic, 1990, 2003; Bentivoglio and Mazzarello, 1999; Nieuwenhuys et al., 1998).

PHENOTYPE AND DEFINITION

Studies using classic histological and Golgi methods indicated that RG have a distinct glia-like morphology. This notion was confirmed by electron microscopic and immunohistochemical analysis of human and nonhuman primate brains (e.g., Rakic, 1972; Choi and Lapham, 1978; Levitt and Rakic, 1980; Levitt et al., 1981, 1983; Gadisseux and Evrard, 1985; Choi, 1986; deAzevedo, 2003). The glial fibrillary acidic proteins (GFAP) that can be identified in the astrocytic glial cell types in all vertebrates studied, exclusive of cyclostomes, served as a useful marker for identification of the astrocytic phenotype, including RG cells (Onteniente et al., 1983; Dahl et al., 1985; Bignami, 1991; Zupanc, 1999). The identification of these cells as a separate cell line was also supported by their immunoreactivity to RC1, RC2, vimentin, Rat 401, and Ran-2. The problem, which has added to the confusion in the terminology, is that, unlike RG cells in primates, those in rodents are not GFAP positive until the completion of corticoneurogenesis (Dahl et al., 1981; Gadisseux et al., 1989; Cameron and Rakic, 1991). Antigenic properties of RG in rodents change during the emergence of secondary phenotypes, as indicated by a substitution in the intermediate filament protein composition from vimentin to GFAP (Bovolenta et al., 1984; Pixley and De Vellis, 1984; Rickmann et al., 1987; Hutchins and Casagrande, 1989; Voigt, 1989).

It should be emphasized that the term *radial glia* and the concept of *glial scaffolding* have been derived from

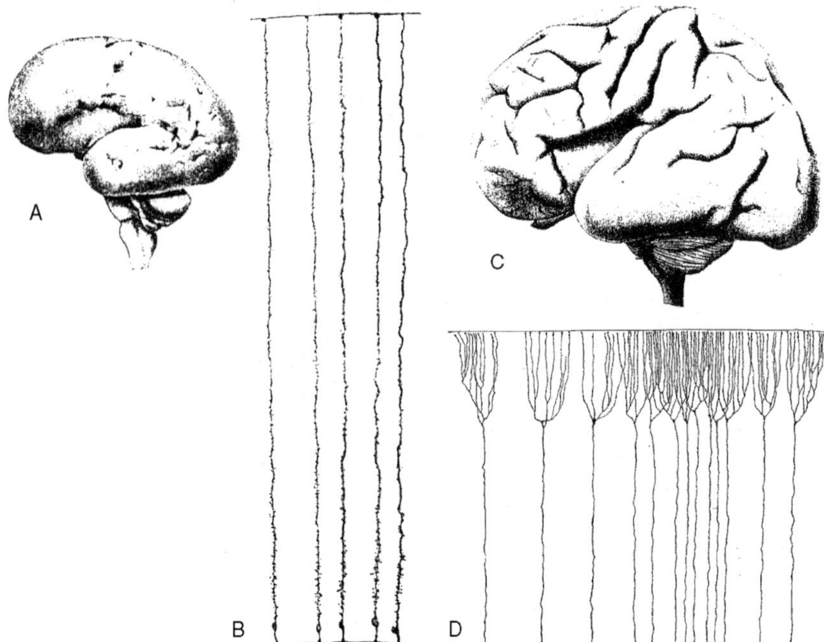

FIGURE 31.2 Drawings of the "ependymal glial cells" in the human fetal cerebrum at the age of 10 weeks (*A*,*B*) and 16 weeks (*C*,*D*) (Retzius, 1893, 1896). Note the maturation of the cells from the simple bipolar shape (*B*) to a more differentiated form in which the outer process branches within the marginal zone into several endfeet that terminate at the pial surface (*D*) as the human fetal cerebrum becomes larger and more convoluted (compare *B* and *D*).

analysis of relatively advanced developmental stages of the primate forebrain (Rakic, 1972). At these stages of corticogenesis, glial and neuronal cell lines are easily identifiable by both transmission electron microscopy (EM) and immunocytochemical methods (e.g., Levitt et al., 1981, 1983; Kadhim et al., 1988; Cameron and Rakic, 1991; deAzevedo et al., 2003). In addition to the abundance of GFAP in their cytoplasm, bipolar cells span the wide cerebral wall at late stages of corticoneurogenesis in primates and display a number of morphological and utrastructural characteristics that make them distinct from the bipolar migrating neurons with distinct leading and trailing processes (Fig. 31.3). These include lamellate expansions and cone-shaped endfeet that are interconnected by specialized intermembrane junctions, forming a continuous pial surface (glia limitans) coated with a basement membrane composed of extracellular matrix molecules (Rakic, 1971, 1972, 1995a, 1995b; Kadhim et al., 1988). In contrast, bipolar migrating neurons have a more voluminous leading process filled with a darker cytoplasm that usually terminates with pseudopodia, while the trailing process is much thinner and resembles an axon (see the discussion of reconstruction from serial EM sections in Rakic et al., 1974).

There are several morphological variations of the basic RG cell phenotype. Furthermore, some of the modified RG cells can persist after developmental periods and can assume different region-specific characteristics (e.g., *tanycytes*, *faserglia*, *Müller cells*, and *Bergmann glia*). All these cells express GFAP in their cytoplasm, and most investigators consider them to be specialized glial cells that are neither neuronal nor ubiquitous astro-, oligo-, or microglial cells. For example, as suggested by Ramón y Cajal (1909), Bergmann glial cells of the mammalian cerebellum can be considered modified RG cells. His drawing of the transformation of radial glial to Bergmann glial cells is illustrated in Fig. 31.4*A*. In primates, transformation from the RG phenotype into the Bergmann phenotype occurs between 90 and 120 embryonic days (Rakic, 1971, 1985b) and precedes a major wave of granule cell migration from the external granular layer across the molecular layer. A similar morphogenetic transformation seems to occur during the course of vertebrate evolution. Thus, in adult amphibian and reptilian cerebellum, Bergmann glial cells retain contact with both ventricular and pial surfaces and have the general spindle-shaped morphology characteristic of the transient telencephalic radial glial cell (Fig. 31.4*B*). The adult Bergmann glial cells can be induced experimentally to dedifferentiate and resume some features of the embryonic form including surface molecules needed for neuronal guidance (Sotelo et al., 1994).

As reviewed below, the term *radial glial cell* does not encompass the entire spectrum of structural and func-

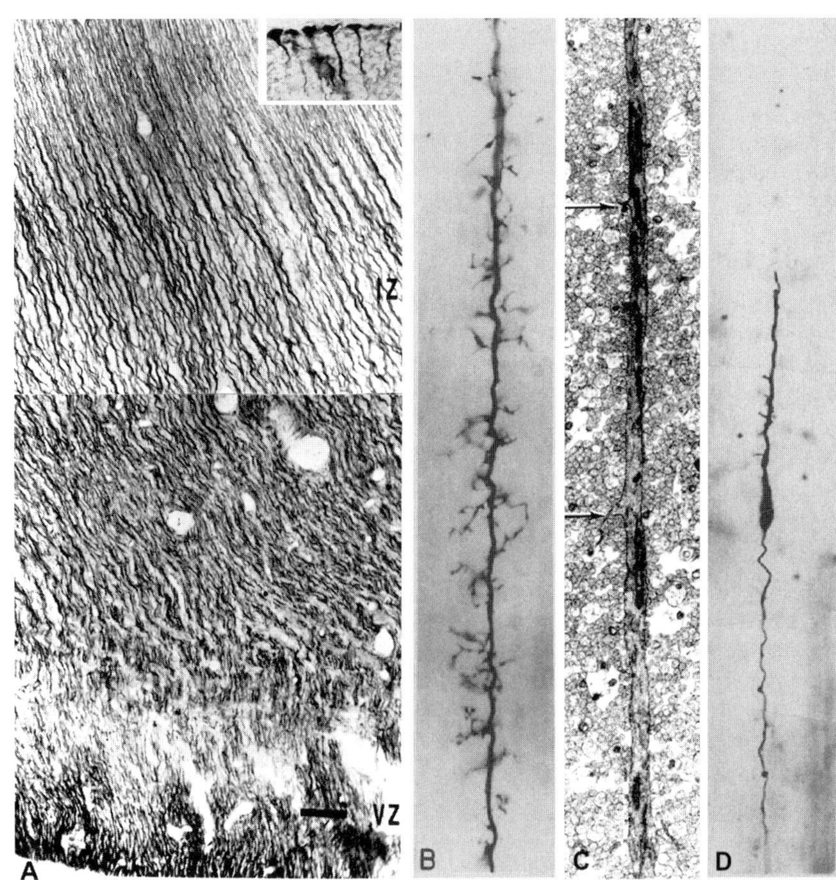

FIGURE 31.3 *A*. Photomicrograph of a portion of the fetal cerebral wall at embryonic drug 70 shows array of radial glial (RG) fibers immunostained with the antibodies to glial fibrillary acidic protein. The filed exposes the richness of the RG fiber scaffolding at the midpoint of cortical neurogenesis, with the radial fibers running from the ventricular zone (*VZ*) near the lateral cerebral ventricle (*LV*) across the intermediate zone (*IZ*) all the way to the cortical plate (not shown), where many of them terminate with the typical endfeet at the pial surface (*inset*). A radial glial cell shaft impregnated with the Golgi method (*B*) and viewed with the electron microscope (*C*) shows numerous lamellate expansions that become more prominent at later stages of corticogenesis, which make distinctions from the bipolar migrating neurons (*D*) with a relatively thick leading process and a thin trailing process. (Assembled from Levitt and Rakic, 1980; Rakic, 1972, 1984. See the text for further explanation.)

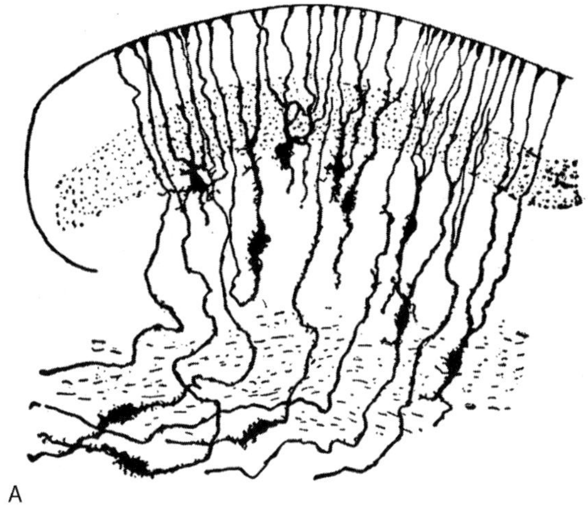

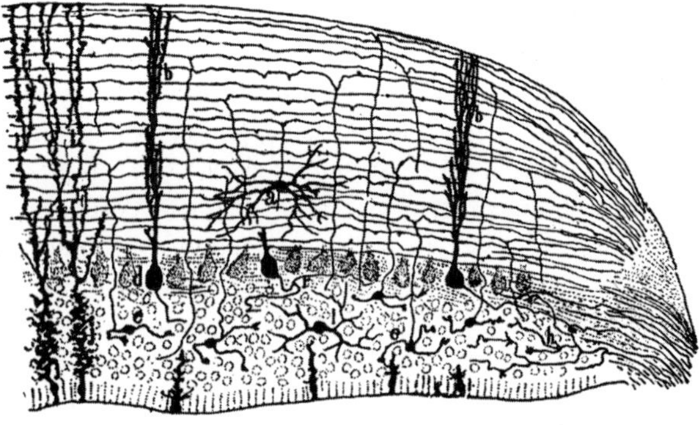

FIGURE 31.4 *A.* Sagittal section of the cerebellum of the newborn mouse stained with the Golgi method illustrates the transformation of epithelial (radial glial) cells into Bergmann glial cells. *B.* Frontal (coronal) section of the adult reptilian cerebellum stained with the Golgi method shows that in many submammalian species the cerebellum does not contain Bergmann glial cells but rather radial glial cells, which remain present throughout life. (From Ramón y Cajal, 1909.)

tional features observed in diverse species. Nevertheless, it has served a useful purpose for relating their basic phenotype during individual development to the continuity of cell morphogenetic transformation during regional and species-specific evolutionary adaptations. New discoveries about their diverse functions in the developing as well as mature brain are rapidly being made (e.g., Barres, 1991; Noctor et al., 2001; Malatesta et al, 2003; Tramontin et al., 2003) and may indicate that the term *radial glial cell* may be too narrow for this diversity. However, a similar argument can be made for most of the terms in neuroanatomy as our knowledge increases about their structure and function. Furthermore, it should be recognized that historically, the descriptive term *radial glia* was adopted in order to avoid narrow functional connotations, which inevitably change with new discoveries. This term recognizes the orientation of its elongated fiber, which persists across the mammalian species, including the large human cerebrum, as well as the other morphological, ultrastructural, and molecular characteristics that make them distinct from other, more specialized neuronal and glial cell progenitors (see below). This designation has been generally accepted in embryological and neuropathological literature (see Varon and Somjen, 1979; Rickmann and Wolff, 1985; Federoff and Verandakis, 1986; Volpe, 1987; Hatten, 1990; Hatten and Mason, 1990; Jacobson, 1991; Ketterman and Ransom, 1995; Bentivoglio and Mazzarello, 1999; Kriegstein and Parnavelas, 2003) and will be used in this chapter.

ORIGIN AND EVOLUTION

The central nervous system in all vertebrates originates as a specialization of the ectodermal epithelial cells on the dorsal surface of the embryo. As the neuronal plate transforms into a neural tube, these cells form noncommitted pseudostratifed neuroepithelium from which all brain cells, both neuronal and glial, originate. However, as development proceeds, the initially uniform epithelium becomes diversified into more restricted cell lines displaying regional differences that eventually result in the formation of species-specific size and cellular composition. This is accomplished by asymmetrical cell division that leads to differential gene expression and sequential cell specifications. Thus, the uncommitted bipolar neuroepithelial cells that initially form the embryonic cerebral vesicle serve as the stem cells from which all neuronal and nonneuronal cells, including RG, eventually emerge as more restricted and differentiated lines.

Because the Golgi methods preferentially impregnate RG cells compared to less mature migrating neurons, it has been difficult to determine the exact timing of the divergence of these cells into different types during development (Sidman and Rakic, 1973), leading to the question of whether the developing cerebral wall simultaneously contains more restricted neuronal and glial cell progenitors. The detailed analysis of the kinetics of cell division in the rodent ventricular zone using ^{3}H-thymidine autoradiography indicated the presence of two distinct populations of progenitors from the start of neurogenesis (e.g., Waechter and Jaensch, 1972; Rickmann and Wolff, 1985) without revealing their nature. However, the application of GFAP immunocytochemistry and EM revealed the coexistence of the glial and neuronal cells lines from the onset of corticoneurogenesis in the macaque monkey forebrain (Levitt at al., 1981, 1983). However, the methodological problems may be the reason that the massive waves of tangential migration of bipolar neuroblasts were less emphasized until the new experimental methods enabled detection of bipolar migrating neurons in the developing cerebral wall (e.g., Marin and Rubenstein, 2001; Letinic et al., 2002; Ang et al., 2003). Only modern higher-resolution approaches have enabled identification of several additional classes of progenitors that can produce distinct neuronal subclasses with considerable species-specific differences in their relative proportions (e.g., Letinic et al., 2002; Malatesta et al, 2003). As in other tissues, these differences are probably controlled by genes that act on the progenitor cells at or prior to their exit from their cells' mitotic cycle, generating a different outcome depending on the given evolutionary context (Bang and Goulding, 1996; Shirasaki and Pfaff, 2002).

Although the basic characteristics of RG are conserved, 100 million years of mammalian evolution have resulted in modifications of developmental programs that produce not only quantitative but also qualitative changes. There are also important structural, molecular, and functional differences between different regions within the same species, as well as between the same regions of different species (e.g., Rakic 1984, 1985a; Cooper and Steindler, 1986; Steindler et al., 1989; Hatten, 1990; Silver et al., 1993; Malatesta et al., 2003). These differences are not only of theoretical but also of biomedical significance, since many of the new traits may be particularly vulnerable to genetic and environmental factors (e.g., Steward et al., 1999; Gurwitz and Weizman, 2001; Rakic, 2002). Comparative analysis of the mouse, monkey, and human cerebrum shows that the RG cells have undergone substantial functional adaptations during mammalian evolution (Rakic, 2003).

The stability of RG scaffolding may be an essential evolutionary adaptation that enables proper allocation of neurons to the expanded and convoluted cerebral cortex (Rakic, 1995b). At this stage in the primate forebrain, many RG cells stop to divide transiently, while their shaft serves as scaffolding for a cohort of migrating neurons (Schmechel and Rakic, 1979a). At a late stage of cortical development in the human fetus, a large number of interneurons, originating from the proliferative ventricular (VZ) and the expanded subventricular (SVZ) zone of the dorsal telencephalon, migrate radially to the superficial layers of the cerebral cortex (Letinic et al., 2002). It remains to be determined if a similar population of interneurons and glial cells exists in rodents or if they are more difficult to identify due to the lack of cell, class-specific markers in these species (Tan, 2002). For example, the use of genetic labeling and *in vivo* imaging revealed the presence of ganglionic eminence–derived bipolar, tangentially migrating neurons in the intermediate and marginal zones of the rodent cerebrum (e.g., Marin and Rubenstein, 2001; Ang et al., 2003) that were apparently missed in the Golgi-stained preparations that impregnate only 1%–3% of cells.

The enormous enlargement and dramatic morphogenetic change from the smooth lysencephalic to the convoluted gyrencephalic primate cerebrum is associated with accelerated differentiation of RG cells (Sidman and Rakic, 1973; Schmechel and Rakic, 1979a; Levitt and Rakic, 1980; Levitt et al., 1981, 1983; Rakic, 1981, 1995b; Kadhim et al., 1988; deAzevedo et al., 2003). The separate neuronal and RG cell lines at these stages are easily identifiable by either EM or immunocytochemical methods in both human and monkey forebrain (Rakic, 1972; Rakic et al., 1974; Levitt and Rakic, 1980; Levitt et al., 1981, 1983; Cameron and Rakic. 1991; deAzevedo et al., 2003). The length of the RG fiber in the macaque monkey cerebrum toward the end of corticoneurogenesis may reach 3000–7000 μm, while the length of the leading process of bipolar migratory neurons, 50–200 μm (Rakic, 1972), is similar to the length observed in smaller forebrains (e.g., Misson et al., 1988) or to that of other structures such as the optic tectum or retina (e.g., Gray and Sanes, 1991; Das et al., 2003). Simple translocation of the nucleus cannot explain tangential migration of bipolar neurons. The presence of bipolar migratory cells that are distinct from RG fibers has been observed in most species but is particularly evident in large gyrencephalic brains.

PROLIFERATIVE CAPACITY

It has been recognized that the primary RG phenotype can revert to the neuroepithelial form and generate neurons (Fig. 31.5). Indeed, recent studies *in vitro* and *in vivo* provide direct evidence that RG give origin to cortical neurons (Malatesta et al., 2000, 2003; Hartfuss, et al., 2001; Noctor et al., 2001; Tamamaki et al., 2001; Alvarez-Buylla and Garcia Verdugo, 2002; Gaiano and Fishell, 2002; Tramontin et al., 2003). With the use of a retrovirus carrying the GFP reporter gene as a marker, we have confirmed that RG can both generate as well as guide the migration of cortical neurons (N. Sestan and P. Rakic, unpublished). The newly generated cells assume a bipolar shape and migrate along the radial fiber of the mother cell, which remains attached to the ventricular surface (Noctor et al., 2001; Weissman et al., 2003). Thus, in a sense, the daughter cells are guided by the radial fibers of their mother's cells to the appropriate location in the developing cortical plate (Fig. 31.5*D,F*). In the human fetal cerebrum during midgestation, a single RG fiber may simultaneously guide several generations of migrating neurons.

Studies in both human (Carpenter et al., 2001; Letinic et al., 2002; deAzevedo et al., 2003) and nonhuman primates (Levitt and Rakic, 1980; Levitt et al., 1981, 1983) show the existence of at least two stem cell lines in the VZ and a highly expanded SVZ: one glial and the other

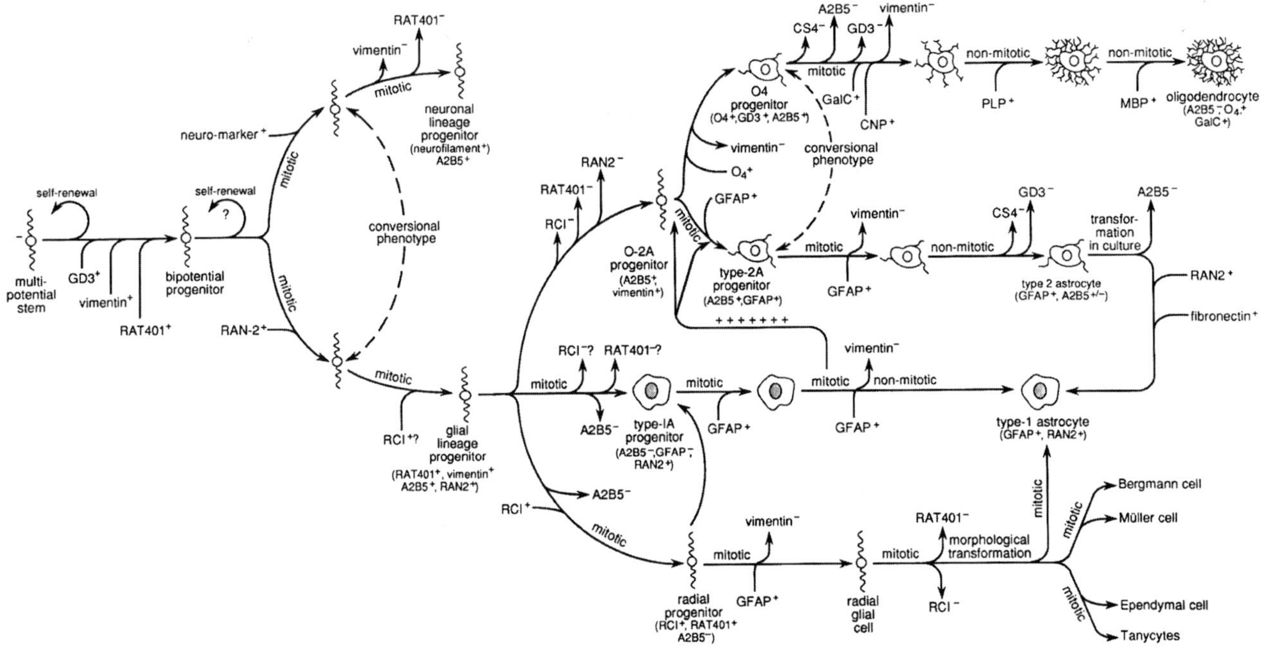

FIGURE 31.5 Schematic circuit diagram of the possible glial cell lineages that occur during the development of the cerebral cortex. In the past two decades we have witnessed the introduction of a large number of molecular markers specific for various subtypes of glial cells. The acquisition or loss of antigenic components that accompany the progressive maturation of individual cell types is indicated by arrows with (+) or (−) signs. GFAP: glial fibrillary acidic protein. (From Cameron and Rakic, 1991.)

neuronal. Unlike in rodents, cells isolated from the human VZ/SVZ, even at early stages of corticogenesis, generate separate neuron-restricted and glia-restricted precursors (Carpenter et al., 2001). The presence of GFAP(+) and GFAP(−) in the cytoplasm of mitotic figures at the ventricular surface suggested that both cell types divide (Levitt et al., 1981, 1983). Furthermore, retroviral gene transfer labeling of cell lineages in human embryonic slices shows that multiple divisions of neuronal stem cell progenitors occur in the VZ/SVZ be-

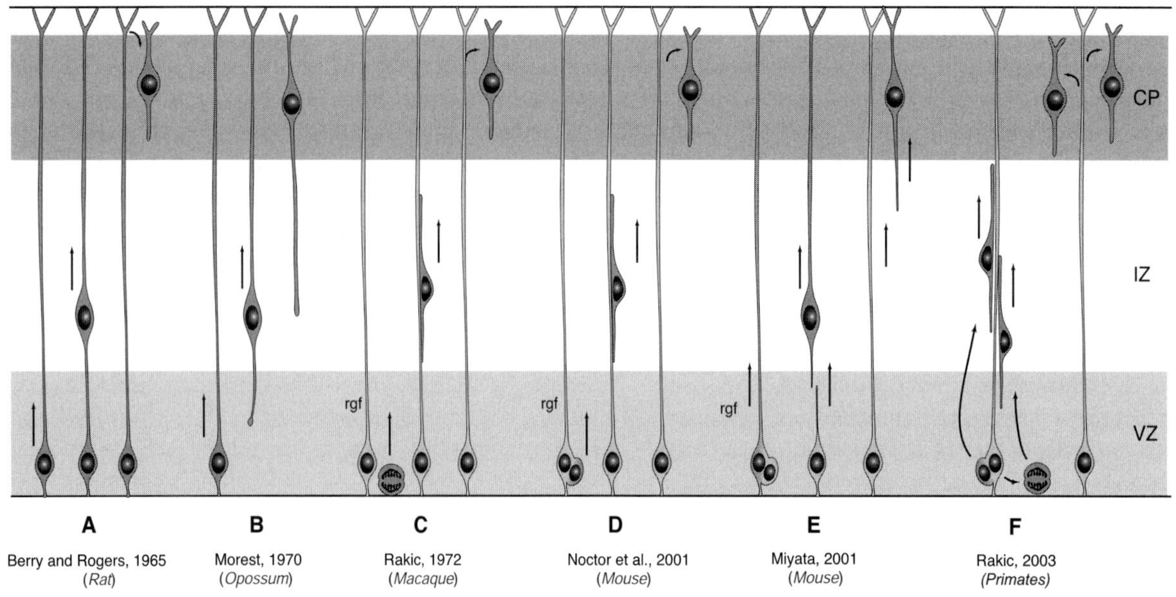

FIGURE 31.6 Schematic diagram of the evolving concepts of the relationship between radial glial cells (RG) and migrating neurons in the developing mammalian cerebral wall based on studies using increasingly sophisticated methods applied to the embryonic forebrain of species ranging from the mouse and opossum pouch young to humans and nonhumans. CP: cortical plate; IZ: intermediate zone; rgf: radial glial fiber; VZ: ventricular zone. (From Rakic, 2003.)

fore they begin radial migration to the neocortex (Letinic et al., 2002). Similarly, a diversity of progenitors may also exist in rodents, but could be overlooked because of the smaller number or lack of cell class–specific markers for their identification at early stages (e.g., McCarthy et al., 2001; Tan, 2002). There are several lines of evidence that neuron-restricted progenitors are even further specified. For example, more specialized stem cells of both glial and neuronal lineages that produce different classes of projection and local circuit neurons can be identified by retroviral labeling (Parnavelas et al., 1991; Tan et al., 1998). Likewise, heterochronous transplantation of VZ cells indicates that progenitors produce layer-specific pyramidal neurons, depending on the time when they are dissociated from the embryo (McConnell, 1988). The molecular heterogeneity of remnant stem cells in the human fetal cerebrum has also been demonstrated by molecular phenotyping of clonal neurospheres (Suslov et al., 2002).

Historically, several models of the kinetics of cellular events in the embryonic cerebral wall have been proposed (reviewed in Rakic, 2003). One major problem was that these models, illustrated graphically in Figure 31.6, were based on studies of different animal species on embryos of different ages examined by different methods of analysis. Therefore, it remains an open question whether they reflect genuine interspecies differences or technical limitations in distinguishing between cell phenotypes in rodents. The interspecies distinction appears during the evolution of the cerebral cortex as a consequence of early phenotypic differentiation and precocious expression of GFAP in the RG cells in the primate fetal telencephalon (Levitt and Rakic, 1980; Choi, 1884; Kadhim et al., 1988; deAzevedo et al., 2003), as well as the latent period in the G1 phase observed in some of these cells, while their shafts serve as transient scaffolding (Schmechel and Rakic, 1979b). The model illustrated in Figure 31.6*E* incorporates some of the data obtained in the mouse embryonic cerebrum as well as the abundant literature on RG cells in human and nonhuman primates (Rakic, 2003).

FUNCTIONAL CONSIDERATIONS

It is well established that cortical neurons in both the small lysencepalic rodents (Angevine and Sidman, 1961) and the large gyrencephalic primate cerebrum are not generated in the cortex itself (Rakic and Sidman, 1968; Sidman and Rakic, 1973). Rather, they immigrate in a precise inside-out sequence from the proliferative VZ and SVZ. This sequence, initially implied on the basis of histological observations of the distribution of mitotic figures, bipolar cells, and sequence of neuronal differentiation in the embryonic human cortex (reviewed in Sidman and Rakic, 1982), has been confirmed experimentally by ^{3}H-thymidine autoradiography in mice (Angevine and Sidman, 1961) and primates (Rakic, 1974). The short journey from the VZ to the preplate beneath the marginal zone in the small lysencephalic brain does not exceed the total length of the migrating cells and is not substantially different from the displacement of cell nuclei in other tissues, such as the optic tectum or retina (Gray and Sanes, 1991; Das et al., 2003). However, the negotiation of the long, curvilinear migratory trajectories in the large gyrencephalic cerebrum at later stages of development requires an additional strategy. The use of a combination of Golgi impregnation, ^{3}H-thymidine autoradiography, and reconstruction from EM serial sections revealed that during late stages of corticogenesis in the macaque cerebrum, cohorts of bipolar postmitotic cells originating in the same sites within the proliferative mosaic of the VZ follow a radial pathway consisting of single or, more often, multiple RG fibers, which span the expanding and increasingly convoluted cerebral wall (Rakic 1972, 1978; Fig. 31.7).

The expansion and elaboration of the neocortex is associated with an enormous increase in the size of the SVZ (Kostovic and Rakic, 1990; Smart et al., 2002). This zone in the human generates most of the cortical interneurons (Letinic et al., 2002). For example, in the wide intermediate zone of the human fetus during midgestation, as many as 30 generations of migrating neurons can be simultaneously aligned along the single radial glial shaft (Fig. 31.7; see also Sidman and Rakic, 1973, 1982). Although postmitotic neurons in the large gyrencephalic primate brain may need several weeks to reach their final destinations, clonally related cells that originate at the same spot in the VZ/SVZ follow the same guide and eventually settle within the same cortical column (Rakic, 1988a, 1995a; Kornack and Rakic, 1995). The regularity of the well-defined migratory streams (e.g., Fig. 31.7) suggests both the stability of the RG cells and the existence of a differential binding affinity mediated by heterotypic adhesion molecules present on apposing neuronal and RG cell surfaces (Rakic, 1985a; Rakic et al., 1994). In contrast, migrating cells that do not obey the glial constraints and move tangentially along axonal tracts have been considered "neurophilic" (Rakic, 1985a, 1990). Thus, with regard to pathway selection, migrating neurons fall into three major categories: (*1*) gliophilic cells, which follow elongated glial fibers and bypass neurons that may be lying within their trajectory; (*2*) neurophilic cells, which follow neuronal, particularly axonal, surfaces and bypass glial shafts; and (*3*) biphilic cells, which display temporal or regional affinities toward either glial or neuronal surfaces (Rakic, 1985a, 1990).

Migration of cerebellar granule cells can be classified as part of the biphilic category of migrating cells be-

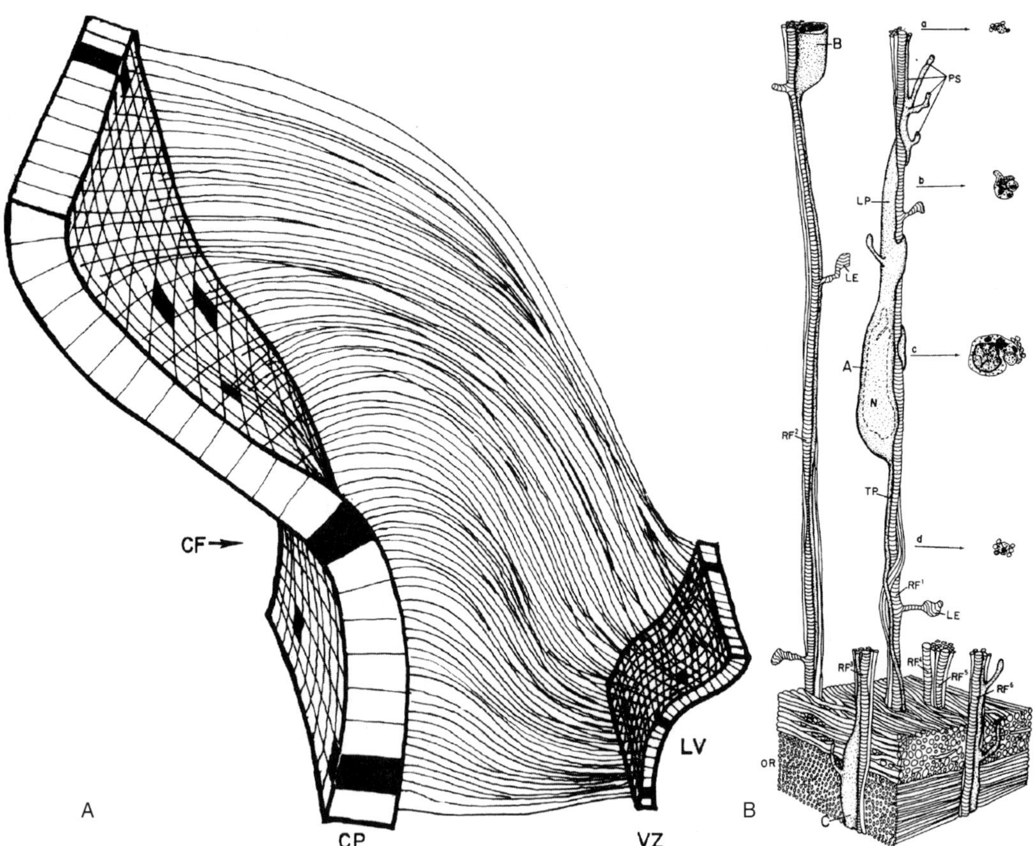

FIGURE 31.7 *A.* Schematic three-dimensional reconstruction of the portion of the medial cerebral wall at the level of the incipient calcarine fissure (*CF*) in the 80-day-old monkey fetus. The reconstruction illustrates how the corresponding points in the ventricular zone (*VZ*) are connected by the array of elongated radial glial (RG) fibers that span the full thickness of the cerebral wall to the increasingly distant cortical plate (*CP*) situated below the convoluted pial surface. LV: lateral ventricle (From Rakic, 1978.) *B.* Three-dimensional reconstruction of migrating neurons based on electron micrographs of semiserial sections of the occipital lobe of the monkey fetus. The reconstruction was made at the mid-level of the 2.5-μm-wide intermediate zone. The lower portion of the diagram contains uniform, parallel axons of the optic radiation (*OR*), while the irregularly disposed fiber systems occupying the upper part of the diagram are deleted to expose the RG fibers (*striped vertical shafts*, RF1–6) and their relations to the migrating neurons A, B, and C and other vertical processes. The soma of migrating cell A, with its nucleus (*N*) and leading process (*LP*), is situated within the reconstructed space, except for the terminal part of the attenuated trailing process (*TP*) and the tip of the vertical ascending pseudopodium. The perikaryon of cell B is cut off at the top of the reconstructed space, whereas the leading process of cell C is shown just penetrating between axons of the OR on its way across the intermediate zone. LE: lamellate expansions; PS: pseudopodia. (From Rakic, 1972.)

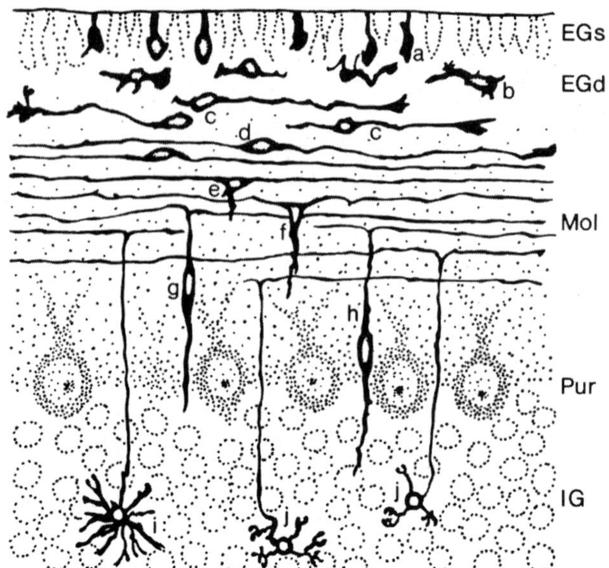

FIGURE 31.8 Morphogenetic transformation of the cerebellar granule cell as it passes from the stage of undifferentiated progenitor (*phase embrionale ou indifferente*) (*a–b*) through a horizontal bipolar shape (*phase dela bipolarite horizontale*) (*c–d*) through three-polar and finally bipolar (*phase de la bipolarite verticale*) (*e–h*) migration across the molecular and Purkinje cells layer on the way to the internal granular layer. (From Ramon y Cajal, 1909.)

cause their two horizontal neurites grow along parallel axonal fibers belonging to previously generated granule cells, while a single descending process, containing soma, follows Bergmann glial fibers (Rakic, 1971, 1973, 1985b). The cerebrellar granule cell can be considered a maverick among neurons, as it does not originate in the VZ or SVZ of the cerebellar anlage, but rather derives from the rombic lip of the brain stem and spreads over the hemispheric surface before entering the last cell division, where it starts to descend to the internal granular layer (reviewed in Rakic, 1985b). The migrating cells then pass through several morphogenetic stages, as suggested by Cajal based on the transitional forms revealed by the Golgi method (Fig. 31.8). Cajal also described transformation of the Bergmann glial cells from the RG cells (Fig. 31.4*A*), but, since the Golgi method does not stain contiguous cells, he could not observe their apposition. Only use of the EM serial section has revealed this relationship, as illustrated in the four-dimensional diagram (Fig. 31.9). Shortly after its final cell division in the external granular layer, a newly generated granule cell takes a position in the deep part of the external granular, contacting a Bergmann glial fiber (cell 1 in Fig. 31.9). It then transiently assumes a bipolar shape (cell 2) by emitting two horizontal cytoplasmic processes that run in the longitudinal plane of the cerebellar folium, at right angles to the growing Purkinje dendritic trees (Ramón y Cajal, 1909). These horizontal processes extend exclusively along the surface of parallel (axonal) fibers (Rakic, 1971). Next, the granule cell becomes tripolar by forming a third, vertical cytoplasmic process, which elongates in close apposition to the shaft of Bergmann glial cells (cell 3 in Fig. 31.8 and Fig. 31.9*A*). Examination of EM serial sections in developing macaque cerebellum shows that the leading process of granule cells grows down preferentially along the Bergmann glial shaft (Fig. 31.10*A*,*B*). When the descending process reaches the appropriate length, the nuclear part of the granule cell becomes translocated within its volume (Rakic, 1971). As a result, the entire soma passes across the complex and the synaptically interconnected molecular layer. At later stages of cerebellar development, several granule cells in succession follow the same Bergmann glial guide, as described for the developing cerebral cortex (Rakic, 1972).

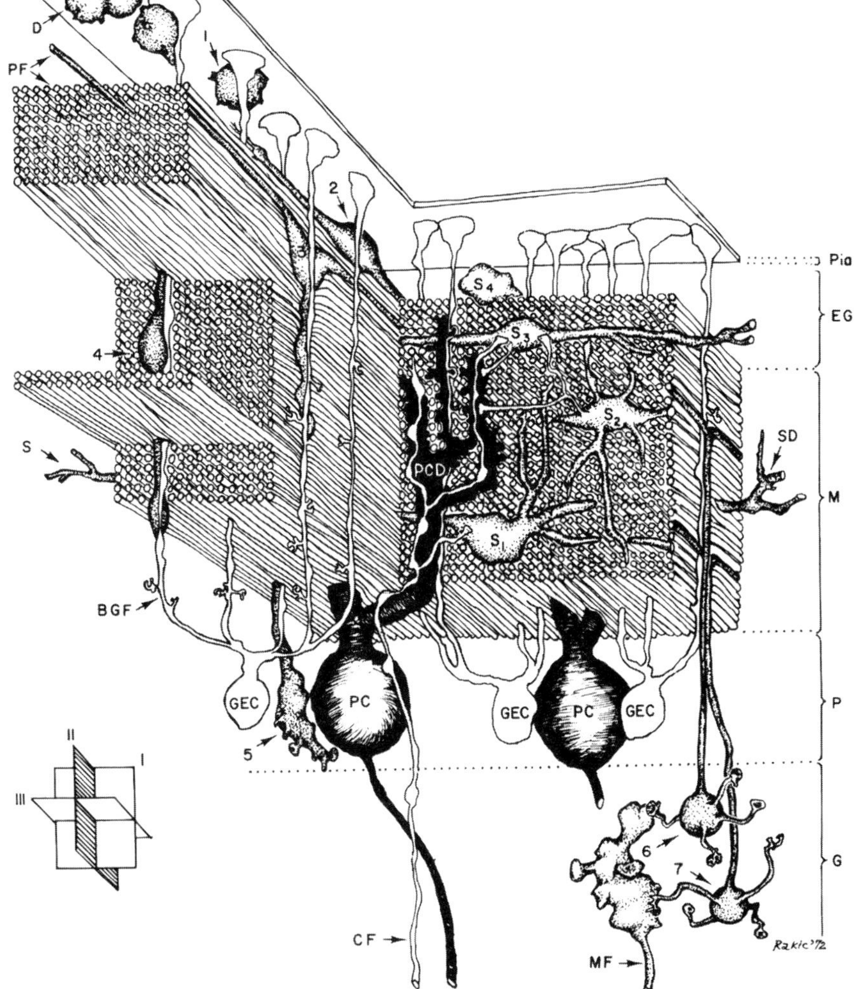

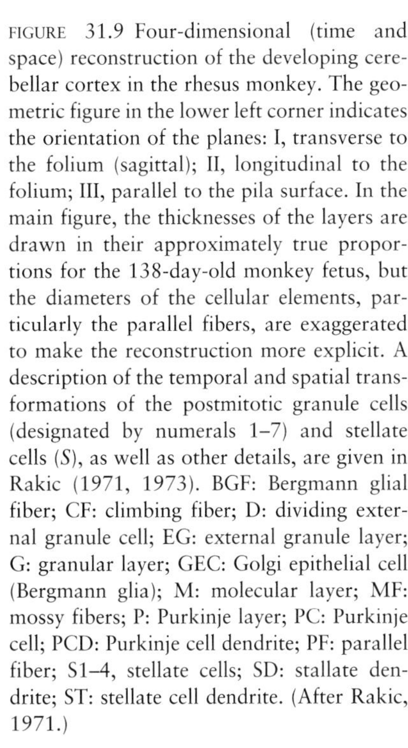

FIGURE 31.9 Four-dimensional (time and space) reconstruction of the developing cerebellar cortex in the rhesus monkey. The geometric figure in the lower left corner indicates the orientation of the planes: I, transverse to the folium (sagittal); II, longitudinal to the folium; III, parallel to the pila surface. In the main figure, the thicknesses of the layers are drawn in their approximately true proportions for the 138-day-old monkey fetus, but the diameters of the cellular elements, particularly the parallel fibers, are exaggerated to make the reconstruction more explicit. A description of the temporal and spatial transformations of the postmitotic granule cells (designated by numerals 1–7) and stellate cells (*S*), as well as other details, are given in Rakic (1971, 1973). BGF: Bergmann glial fiber; CF: climbing fiber; D: dividing external granule cell; EG: external granule layer; G: granular layer; GEC: Golgi epithelial cell (Bergmann glia); M: molecular layer; MF: mossy fibers; P: Purkinje layer; PC: Purkinje cell; PCD: Purkinje cell dendrite; PF: parallel fiber; S1–4, stellate cells; SD: stallate dendrite; ST: stellate cell dendrite. (After Rakic, 1971.)

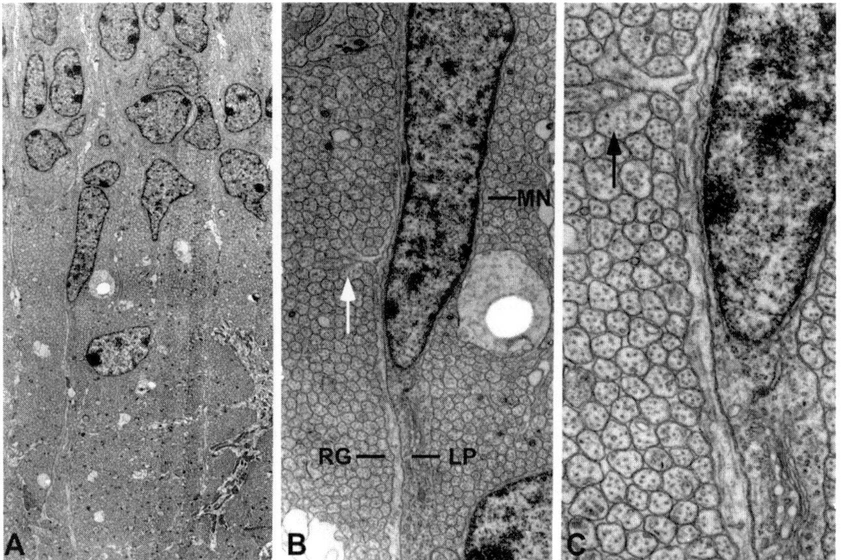

FIGURE 31.10 *A*. Low-power electron micrograph (EM) of a 135-day-old monkey fetus showing a bipolar migrating neuron descending from the external granular layer situated at the top of the field to the internal granule layer situated below. *B*. An enlargement of the migrating neuron (*MN*) selected from the EM serial section series to show that its leading process (*LP*) is closely aligned with an electron-lucent shaft of the radial Bergmann glial fiber (*RG*) with a short lamellate expansion (*white arrow*) as the cell penetrates the densely packed and already synaptically interconnected neuropile of the molecular layer. (From Rakic, 1971.) C. Higher-power EM shows the difference between darker, organelle-rich cytoplasm of the leading process of the migrating neuron and electron-lucent cytoplasm of the RG fiber from which emanates a lamellate expansion (*black arrow*). The migrating neuron remains selectively attached to the surface of the glial fiber, although it simultaneously contacts myriad axons and other cell processes.

A change in the position and shape of the cerebellar granule cells provides an example of the cooperation between neuronal and glial cells during the development of complex brain structures (Rakic, 1971). In the initial step, the horizontal and vertical segments of the cell trailing behind the nuclear region of the granule cell become the parallel fiber and vertical shaft, respectively. When the granule cell body reaches the Bergmann cell soma at the level of the Purkinje cell layer, it leaves its glial guide and takes up its permanent position in the internal granule layer (Fig. 31.9, cells 5, 6, and 7). It then emits three to five short dendrites that contact the mossy fibers originating in the brain stem. The position in the molecular layer where granule cells differentiate from round into bipolar form determines the depth of the prospective parallel fibers, so that early generated parallel fibers remain near the Purkinje cells, while those situated closest to the pial surface form the last, as evidenced by examining the position of parallel fibers belonging to cells 2, 3, 6, and 7 in Fig. 31.9.

In addition to serving as a guide for migrating neurons and possibly for axonal growth cones (e.g., Silver et al., 1982, 1993; Norris and Kalil, 1991), the large surface of elongated glial fibers may be involved in the signaling of information between proliferative zones and their distant terminations. Radial glial cells may supply trophic molecules to the surrounding cells and oxygen during embryonic stages, when visualization of the cerebral wall is absent or underdeveloped (Schmechel and Rakic, 1979a). The elongated fiber of RG cells may be involved in the transport process (Oksche, 1968) and would potentially enable these cells to transmit information from the developing cortical plate to centers of cell proliferation (Stensaas and Golson, 1972). The possibility that such information is carried by molecules within the cytoplasm of radial fibers is supported by the demonstration of vigorous retrograde transport from endfeet to RG cell bodies (Ivy and Killackey, 1978). Modulation of glial cell behavior by the interaction of their distant processes has also been suggested to occur in the newt optic tectum, where differentiation of the molecular layer by enucleation of eyes resulted in a delayed increase in the mitotic activity of RG cells situated near the ventricular surface (Gaze and Watson, 1967). There is some evidence that the glial-limiting membrane formed by terminal attachments at the pial and vascular sheeting provides a modified blood–brain barrier and a cerebrospinal fluid–brain barrier during embryonic stages (Oksche, 1968). Finally, the transient population of RG cells might also involve regulation of the voluminous extracellular fluid in loosely packed embryonic nervous tissue, a role postulated for astrocytes in adults.

MOLECULAR MECHANISMS

In the past three decades, a variety of surface molecules that might be involved in neuron-glial interaction have been identified in the leading process of migrating neurons and at the surface adjacent to the RG fibers (e.g., Fishell and Hatten, 1991; Komuro and Rakic, 1993, 1998; Cameron and Rakic, 1994; Rakic et al., 1994; Anton et al., 1996, 1997, 1999; Gongidi et al., 2004). A separate set of molecular classes may be involved in the recognition, selective adhesion, and maintenance of neuron-glial interactions during the extension of the leading process. Among the candidate molecules involved in radial migration are neuregulin, which binds to the glial surface via ErbB2 and 4 (Anton et al., 1997; Rio et al., 1997; Schmid et al., 2003), and integrins, which provide the optimal level of basic neuron-glial adhesion needed to maintain neuronal migration on the RG (Anton et al., 1999). However, a gliophilic to neurophilic switch in the preference of adhesive interactions of developing cortical neurons occurs in the absence of functional α_3 integrins (Anton et al., 1999; Schmid and Anton, 2003). In terms of the orientation and directionality of cell movement, migration can be classified into radial (proceeding from the ventricular to the pial surface) and tangential (running parallel to the brain surface; Rakic, 1990). Recently, it has been shown that many tangentially migrating neurons in both rodents and primates originate in the ganglionic eminence of the ventral telencephalon (e.g., Marin and Rubenstein, 2001; Letinic et al., 2002). Tangentially migrating neurons may use a different set of recognition molecules than those migrating radially (e.g., Denaxa et al., 2001; Wichterle et al., 2001; Marin and Rubenstein, 2002; Ang et al., 2003).

Active movement of cells to their distant locations requires not only recognition of the migratory pathway and the directed growth of the leading process, but also the displacement of the nucleus and surrounding somatic cytoplasm with its nucleus to the new location. A series of Golgi-impregnated cell images in Cajal's classical drawings have convincingly illustrated this point (Ramon y Cajal, 1909), which gained support from many subsequent studies using the same method (e.g., Morest 1970). The use of EM in the early 1970s revealed that after mitotic division the newborn neuron becomes separated from its progenitor and extends its leading process preferentially along adjacent existing glial shafts (Fig. 31.8). We found that the newly formed nucleus becomes translocated within the cytoplasmic cylinder of its own leading process (Rakic, 1971, 1972). Thus, our initial ultrastructural observations indicated that "as the nucleus moves further within the vertical cytoplasmic process, the organelles become redistributed. The cytoplasm close to the nucleus contains free ribosomes, rosettes of five to six ribosomes, smooth endoplasmic reticulum, Golgi apparatus and mitochondria, whereas further from the nucleus the cytoplasm is replete with longitudinally oriented microtubules and microfilaments" (Rakic, 1971, p. 298). The content of the cytoplasmic organelles and the membrane structure of the leading process were found to be more similar to those of the growing dendrites than to those of axonal growth cones or RG shafts (Rakic, 1972; Garcia-Segura and Rakic, 1985), the distinction also indicated by their morphology (Ramon y Cajal, 1909). Importantly, the leading process does not contain GFAP, which allows quick translocation of the nucleus within the cytoplasm of the leading process. The coordinated extension of the leading process followed by nuclear translocation is particularly prominent in the primate telencephalon at later stages of coticogenesis, when the migratory pathway substantially exceeds the length of the leading process of the migratory neuron. Thus nuclear translocation was always considered an essential component of the glia-guided migration in both cerebral and cerebellar cortex.

The cytological and molecular mechanisms of the physical translocation of the cell nucleus and perikaryal cytoplasm within the leading process of migrating neurons has only recently begun to be experimentally explored *in vivo* and *in vitro* (e.g., Komuro and Rakic, 1996, 1998; Rakic et al., 1996; Behar et al., 1999; Hirai et al., 1999; Hatten, 2002; Ang et al., in press; Nadarajah et al., 2003). Collectively, the data indicate that the combination of amplitude and frequency components of intracellular calcium ion fluctuations may provide an intracellular signal controlling the rate of neuronal cell migration (Komuro and Rakic, 1996). The time-lapse imaging of migrating neurons in slice preparations in both the cerebral and cerebellar cortex extended this mechanism by showing that the leading process extends slowly and steadily, while the nucleus moves in an intermittent, stepwise manner (Komuro and Rakic, 1995; Ang et al., 2003). Thus, the extension of the leading process and translocation of the nucleus and surrounding cytoplasm within the membrane envelope need to be orchestrated by a synchronized polymerization and disintegration of the microtubules that creates a rearrangement of the cytoskeletal scaffolding (Rivas et al., 1995; Rakic et al., 1996).

It has been suggested that defects in the assembly of microtubule protein during neuronal migration may underlie several classes of migratory defects (Reiner et al., 1993; Wynshaw-Boris and Gambello, 2001; Gleeson and Walsh, 2000). This mechanism is consistent with the finding that translocation of nuclei in the migrating neurons depends on the timing and sequence of polymerization and on depolymerization of cytoskeletal proteins (Rakic et al., 1996). Because of the much longer and curvilinear shape of RG fibers, the human brain may be particularly susceptible to defects of neuronal migration. Indeed, there appears to be a species-specific difference in the effect of the deletion of doublecortin (Dbx) mutation, which has a profound affect on neuronal migration in the human telencephalon but does not affect formation and neurogenetic gradients of the mouse cerebral cortex (Corbo et al., 2002). The modifications in the expression pattern of transcription factors in the forebrain may underlie species-specific programs for the generation of distinct lineages of cortical interneurons (Letinic et al., 2002) that may be differentially affected in genetic and acquired disorders related to neuronal migration in human (e.g., Rakic, 1988b; Jones, 1997; Gleeson and Walsh, 2000; Lewis, 2000).

TRANSFORMATION AND DISSOLUTION

As originally suggested by Ramon y Cajal, the fetal type of RG cells in most regions of the mammalian brain disappears soon after birth. Analyses of Golgi-stained and GFAP-immunolabeled sections of the monkey and human cerebra indicate that RG cells in the telencephalon become transformed into fibrillary astrocytes and/or protoplasmic astrocytes (Choi and Lapham, 1978; Rakic, 1978, 1984; Schmechel and Rakic, 1979a; Levitt and Rakic, 1980; Choi, 1986; Rickmann et al., 1987). The timetable of the disappearance of RG cells in the primate neocortex, hippocampus, and cerebellum correlates with the emergence of protoplasmic and fibrillary astrocytes (Fig. 31.11; Rakic, 1971; Schmechel and Rakic, 1979a; Eckenhoff and Rakic, 1984). The cellular or molecular events that underlie this transformation are not known. In primary cultures, neuronal cells have been shown to exert an inhibitory effect on glial cell proliferation and appear to regulate changes in the astroglial cell shape from epithelial-like to radial or stellate (Sobue and Pleasure, 1984; Hatten, 1985; Ard and Bunge, 1988; Culican et al., 1990). The morphological transformation of GFAP-positive RG cells into classical astrocytic cell forms, as well as alternative RG forms, appears to coincide with the loss of RC1, RC2, and Rat-401 antigens, which are not expressed in adulthood (Hockfield and McKay, 1985; Misson et al., 1988a, 1988b; Evrard et al., 1990). A correlative analysis of antigenic and morphologic transformation *in vivo* (Misson et al., 1991) and *in vitro* (Culican et al., 1990) demonstrates that the morphological transformation of RG cells occurs concomitantly with a gradual acquisition of GFAP immunoreactivity and a corresponding loss of RC1 immunoreactivity.

Modified RG cells may be found in some regions of the adult CNS, where a selective microenvironment may allow their maintenance (Reichenbach, 1989; Doetsch et al., 1999; Alavarez-Buylla et al, 1999; Laywell et al., 2000). In some structures of the mammalian brain, RG cells adapt to the local functional requirements and spa-

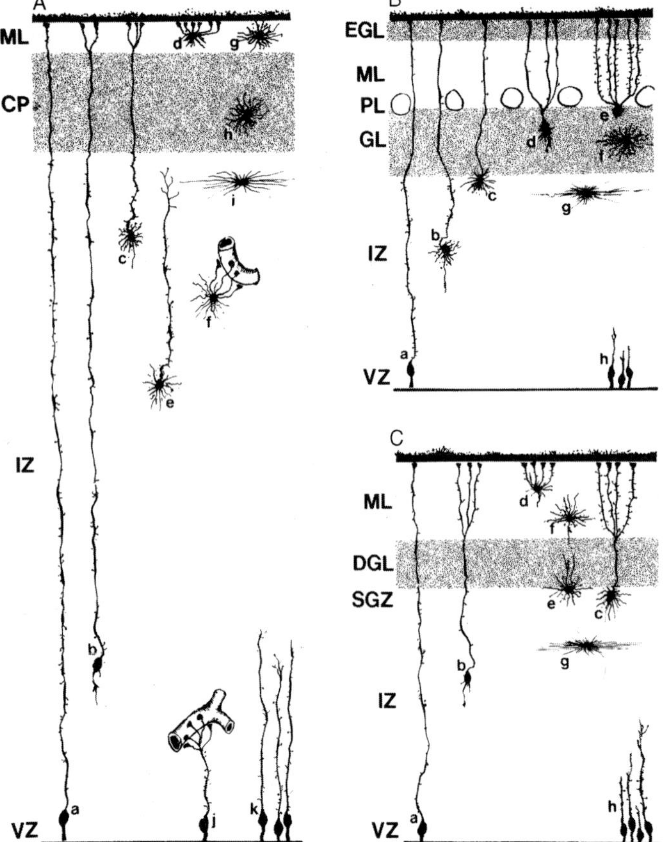

FIGURE 31.11 Semi schematic diagram illustrating the morphogenetic transformation of fetal radial glial cells into various astrocytic forms in the cerebral hemisphere (*A*), the cerebellar hemisphere (*B*), and dentate gyrus of the hippocampus (*C*). CP: cerebral cortical plate; EGL: external granule layer; DGL: dentate gyrus-granular layer of the hippocampal region; GL: granular layer (internal) of the cerebellum; IZ: intermediate zone; ML: molecular layer; PL: Purkinje cell layer; SGZ: subgranular zone of the dentate gyrus; VZ: ventricular zone. Further explanation and designation of the various transitional cell forms (*a–k*) is provided in the text. (After Rakic, 1984.)

tial conditions and transform into specialized astrocytic cell types (e.g., the Bergmann glial cells of the cerebellum, tanycytes of the hypothalamus, or Müller cells of the retina). These specialized cells retain the basic morphological, immunological, and biochemical features of RG cells that include expression of GFAP (e.g., Bartlett et al., 1981; Evrard et al., 1990; Robinson and Dreher, 1990; reviews in Craft et al., 1979; Fedoroff and Vernadakis, 1986). Thus, they may be considered genealogical, morphological, and biochemical descendants of the transient fetal RG cells. However, in some nonmammalian vertebrate species, RG cells may persist throughout the adult life span (e.g., Ramón y Cajal, 1909; King, 1966; Zupanc, 1999). The available data *in vivo* and *in vitro* indicate that the fate of the RG cells depends on the context and functional requirements, which differ between regions and between species.

It was recently discovered that the remnants of RG cells in the adult rodent forebrain are capable of transformation into neurons that can be incorporated into olfactory and hippocampal formations (e.g., Doetsch et al., 1999; Chanas-Sacre et al., 2000; Laywell et al., 2000; Gage, 2002; Tramontin et al., 2003) and/or may influence neurogenesis (Song et al., 2002). The use of the gain-of-function approach has revealed that Notch activity may be involved in cell decision making, either by promoting glial differentiation and/or by inhibiting neurogenesis (Gaiano and Fishell, 2002; Sestan and Rakic, 2002). The available data also indicate that both cell-cell interactions and cell lineages are likely to determine the fate of RG cells (Doetsch et al., 1999; Kukekov et al., 1999; Laywell et al., 2000) and indicate that the RG cell can, under certain conditions, serve as a mutipotent stem cell. Thus, while during their transient existence fetal RG cells contribute actively to brain construction, the remnant of their progeny may be involved in brain functioning in health and disease during the entire life span.

REFERENCES

Alvarez-Buylla, A. and Garcia-Verdugo, J.M. (2002) Neurogenesis in adult subventricular zone. *J. Neurosci.* 22:629–634.

Ang, E.S.B.C., Haydar, T.F., Gluncic, V., and Rakic, P. (2003) Four dimensional migratory coordinates of GABAergic neurons in the developing cerebral cortex. *J. Neurosci.* 23:5805–5815.

Angevine, J.B., Jr., and Sidman, R.L. (1961) Autoradiographic study of cell migration during histogenesis of cerebral cortex in the mouse. *Nature* 192:766–7768.

Anton, E.S., Cameron, R.S., and Rakic, P. (1996) Role of neuron–glial junctional proteins in the maintenance and termination of neuronal migration across the embryonic cerebral wall. *J. Neurosci.* 16:2283–2293.

Anton, E.S., Kreidberg, J., and Rakic, P. (1999) Distinct functions of α_3 and α_v integrin receptors in neuronal migration and laminar organization of the cerebral cortex. *Neuron* 22:227–289.

Anton, E.S., Marchionni, M.A., Lee, K-F., and Rakic, P. (1997) Role of GGF/ neuregulin signaling in interactions between migrating neurons and radial glia in the developing cerebral cortex. *Development* 124:3501–3510.

Ard, M.D. and Bunge, R.P. (1988) Heparin sulfate proteoglycan and laminin immunoreactivity on cultured astrocytes; relationship to differentiation and neurite growth. *J. Neurosci.* 8:2844–2858.

Bang, A.G. and Goulding, M.D. (1996) Regulation of vertebrate neural cell fate by transcription factors. *Curr. Opin. Neurobiol.* 6:25–32.

Barres, B.A. (1991) New role of glia. *J. Neurosci.* 11:3685–3694.

Bartlett, P.F., Noble, M.D., Pruss, R.M., Raff, M.C., Rattray, S., and Williams, C.A. (1981) Rat neural antigen 2 (RAN-2): a cell surface antigen on astrocytes, ependymal cells, Muller cells and leptomeninges defined by a monoclonal antibody. *Brain Res.* 204: 339–351.

Behar, T.N., Scott, C.A., Greene, C.L., Wen, X., Smith, S.V., Maric, D., Liu, Q.Y., Colton C.A., and Baker, J.L. (1999) Glutamate acting at NMDA receptors stimulates embryonic cortical neuronal migration. *J. Neurosci.* 19:4449–4461.

Bentivoglio, M. and Mazzarello, P. (1999) The history of radial glia. *Brain Res Bull.* 49:305–315.

Bignami, A. (1991) Glial cells in the central nervous system. *Discuss. Neurosci.* 8:1–46.

Bovolenta, P., Leim, R.K.H., and Mason, C. (1984) Development of cerebellar astroglia: transitions in form and cytoskeletal content. *Dev. Biol.* 102:248–259.

Cameron, R.S. and Rakic, P. (1991) Glial cell lineage in the cerebral cortex: review and synthesis. *Glia* 4:124–137.

Cameron, R.S. and Rakic, P. (1994) Polypeptides that comprise the plasmalemal microdomain between migrating neuronal and glial cells. *J. Neurosci.* 14:3139–3155.

Carpenter, M.K., Inokuma, M.S., Denham, J., Mujtaba, T., Chiu, C.P., and Rao, M.S. (2001) Enrichment of neurons and neural precursors from human embryonic stem cells. *Exp. Neurol.* 172:383–397.

Chanas-Sacre, G., Rogister, B., Moonen, G., and Leprince, P. (2000) Radial glia phenotype: origin, regulation, and transdifferentiation. *J. Neurosci. Res.* 61:357–363.

Choi, B.H. (1986) Glial fibrillary acid protein in radial glia of early human fetal cerebrum: A light and electron microscopic immunocytochemical study. *J. Neuropathol. Exp. Neurol.* 45:408–418.

Choi, B.H. and Lapham, L.W. (1978) Radial glia in the human fetal cerebrum: a combined Golgi, immunofluorescent and electron microscopic study. *Brain Res.* 148:295–311.

Cooper, N.G.F. and Steindler, D.A. (1986) Monoclonal antibody to glial fibrillary acidic protein reveals a parcellation of individual barrels in the early postnatal mouse somatosensory cortex. *Brain Res.* 380:341–348.

Corbo, J.C., Deuel, T.A., Long, J.M., LaPorte, P., Tsai, E., Wynshaw-Boris, A., and Walsh, C.A. (2002) Doublecortin is required in mice for lamination of the hippocampus but not the neocortex. *J. Neurosci.* 22:7548–7557.

Craft, J.L., Fulton, A.B., Silver, J., and Albart, D.M. (1979) Influence of glia on organization of developing retina. *Invest. Ophthalmol. Vis. Sci.* Suppl:43–43.

Culican, S.M., Baumrind, N.L., Yamamoto, M., and Pearlman, A.L. (1990) Cortical radial glia: identification in tissue culture and evidence for their transformation to astrocytes. *J. Neurosci.* 10: 684–692.

Dahl, D., Crosby, C.J., Sethi, J.S. and Bignami, A. (1985) Glial fibrillary acidic (GFA) protein in vertebrates: immunofluorescence and immunoblotting study with monoclonal and polyclonal antibodies. *J. Comp. Neurol.* 239:75–88.

Dahl, D., Reuger, D.C., Bignami, A., Weber, K., and Osborn, M. (1981) Vimentin, the 57000 molecular weight protein of fibroblast filament, is the major cytoskeletal protein component in immature glia. *Eur. J. Cell Biol.* 24:191–196.

Das, T., Payer, B., Cayouete, M., and Harris, W. (2003) In vivo timelapse imaging of cell divisions during neurogenesis in the developing zebrafish retina. *Neuron* 37:597–609.

DeAzevedo, L.C., Fallet, C., Moura-Neto, V., Daumas-Duport, C.,

Hedin-Pereira, C., and Lent, R. (2003) Cortical radial glial cells in human fetuses: depth-correlated transformation into astrocytes. *J. Neurobiol.* 55:288–298.

DeDiego, I., Smith-Fernandez, A., and Fairen, A. (1994) Cortical cells that migrate beyond areal boundaries: characterization of an early neuronal population in the lower intermediate zone of prenatal rats. *Eur. J. Neurosci.* 6:983–997.

Denaxa, M., Chan, C.H., Schachner, M., Parnavelas, J.G., and Karagogeos, D. (2001) The adhesion molecule TAG-1 mediates the migration of cortical interneurons from the ganglionic eminence along the corticofugal fiber system. *Development* 128:4635–4644.

Doetsch, F., Caille, I., Lim, D.A., Garcia-Verdugo, J.M., and Alvarez-Buylla, A. (1999) Subventricular zone astrocytes are neural stem cells in the adult mammalian brain. *Cell* 97:703–716.

Eckenhoff, M. and Rakic, P. (1984) Radial organization of the hippocampal dentate gyrus: a Golgi, ultrastructural and immunohistochemical analysis in the developing rhesus monkey. *J. Comp. Neurol.* 223:1–21.

Evrard, S.C., Borde, I., Marin, P., Galiana, E., Premont, J., Gros, F., and Rouget, P. (1990) Immortalization of bipotential and plastic glioneuronal precursor cells. *Proc. Natl. Acad. Sci. USA.* 87: 3026–3066.

Fedoroff, S. and Vernadakis, A. (eds.) (1986) *Astrocytes: Development, Morphology, and Regional Specialization of Astrocytes*, Vol. 1. New York: Academic Press.

Fishell, G. and Hatten, M.E. (1991) Astrotactin provides a receptor system for CNS neuronal migration. *Development* 113:755–765.

Gadisseux, J.F. and Evrard, P. (1985) Glial-neuronal relationship in the developing central nervous sytem. *Dev. Neurosci.* 7:12–32.

Gadisseux, J.F., Evrard, P., Misson, J.P., and Caviness, V.S. (1989) Dynamic structure of the radial glial fiber system of the developing murine cerebral wall: an immunocytochemical analysis. *Dev. Brain Res.* 50:55–67.

Gage, F.H. (2002) Neurogenesis in the adult brain. *J. Neurosci.* 22:612–613.

Gaiano, N. and Fishell, G. (2002) The role of notch in promoting glial and neural stem cell fates. *Annu. Rev. Neurosci.* 25:471–490.

Garcia-Segura, L.M., and Rakic, P. (1985) Differential distribution of intermembranous particles in the plasmalemma of the migrating cerebellar granule cells. *Dev. Brain Res.* 23:145–149.

Gaze, R. and Watson, W. (1967) Cell division and migration in the brain after optic nerve lesions. In: Wolstenholme, G.E.W. and O'Connor, M., eds. *Growth of the Nervous System.* Boston: Little, Brown, pp. 53-67.

Gleeson, J.G. and Walsh, C.A. (2000) Neuronal migration disorders: from genetic diseases to developmental mechanisms. *Trends Neurosci.* 23:352–359.

Golgi, C. (1885) Sulla fina anatomia degli organi centrali del sistema nervoso. I. Note preliminari sulla struttura, morfologia e vicendevoli rapporti delle cellule gangliar. *Riv. Sper. Freniat.* 8:165–195.

Gongidi, V., Ring, C., Rakic, P., and Anton, E.S. (2004) Sparc-like 1 is a radial glia-associated terminator of neuronal migration in cerebral cortex. *Neuron* 41:57–69.

Gray, G.E. and Sanes, J.R. (1991) Migratory paths and phenotypic choices of clonally related cells in the avian optic tectum. *Neuron* 6:211–225.

Gressens, P. and Evrard, P. (1993) The glial fascicle: an ontogenetic unit guiding, supplying, and distributing mammalian cortical neurons. *Dev. Brain Res.* 76:272–277.

Gurwitz, D. and Weizman, A. (2001) Animal models and human genome diversity: the pitfalls of inbred mice. *Drug Discov. Today* 6:766–768.

Hartfuss, E., Galli, R., Heins, N., and Gotz, M. (2001) Characterization of CNS precursor subtypes and radial glia. *Dev. Biol.* 229:15–30.

Hatten, M.E. (1985) Neuronal regulation of astroglial morphology and proliferation in vitro. *J. Cell Biol.* 100:384–396.

Hatten, M.E. (1990) Riding the glial monorail: a common mechanism for glial-guided neuronal migration in different regions of the developing brain. *Trends Neurosci.* 13:179–184.

Hatten, M.E. (2002) Neuroscience—new directions in neuronal migration. *Science* 297:1660–1663.

Hatten, M.E. and Mason, C.A. (1990) Mechanism of glial-guided neuronal migration in vitro and in vivo. *Experientia* 46:907–916.

Hirai, K., Yoshioka, H., Kihara, M., Hasegawa, K., Sakamoto, T., Sawada, T., Fushiki, S. (1999) Inhibition of neuronal migration by blocking NMDA receptors in the embryonic rat cerebral cortex: a tissue culture study. *Dev. Brain Res.* 114:63–67.

His, W. (1889) Die Neuroblasten und deren Entstehung im embryonalen Mark. *Abhandl. Math. Phys. Cl. Kgl. Sach. Ges. Wissensch.* 15:313–372.

Hockfield, S. and McKay, R.D.G. (1985) Identification of major classes in the developing mammalian nervous system. *J. Neurosci.* 5:5310–3238.

Hutchins, J.B. and Casagrande, V.A. (1989) Vimentin: changes in distribution during brain development. *Glia* 2:55–66.

Ivy, G.O. and Killackey, H.P. (1978) Evidence for a transient population of glial cells in the developing rat telencephalon as revealed by horseradish peroxidase. *Brain Res.* 158:213–218.

Jacobson, M. (1991) *Developmental Neurobiology.* New York: Plenum.

Jones, E.G. (1997) Cortical development and thalamic pathology in schizophrenia. *Schizophr. Bull.* 23:483–501.

Kadhim, H.J., Gadisseux, J.-F., and Evrard, P. (1988) Topographical and cytological evolution of the glial phase during prenatal development of the human brain: histochemical and electron microscopic study. *J. Neuropathol. Exp. Neurol.* 47:166–188.

Ketterman, H. and Ransom, B.R. (eds.) (1995) *Neuroglia.* New York: Oxford University Press.

King, J.S. (1966) A comparative investigation of neuroglia in representative vertebrates: a silver carbonate study. *J. Morphol.* 119: 435–466.

Koelliker, A. (1896) *Handbuch der Gewebelehre des Menschen.* Vol. 2, Nervensystem des Menshcen und der Thiere. Leipzig: W. Engelmann.

Komuro, H. and Rakic, P. (1993) Modulation of neuronal migration by NMDA receptors. *Science* 260:95–97.

Komuro, H. and Rakic, P. (1995) Dynamics of granule cell migration: a confocal microscopic study in acute cerebellar slice preparations. *J. Neurosci.* 15:1110–1120.

Komuro, H. and Rakic, P. (1996) Calcium oscillations provide signals for the saltatory movement of CNS neurons. *Neuron* 17: 257–285.

Komuro, H. and Rakic, P. (1998) Distinct modes of neuronal migration in different domains of developing cerebellar cortex. *J. Neurosci.* 15:1478–1490.

Kornack, D.R. and Rakic, P. (1995) Radial and horizontal deployment of clonally related cells in the primate neocortex: relationship to distinct mitotic lineages. *Neuron* 15:311–321.

Kostovic, I. and Rakic, P. (1990) Developmental history of the transient subplate zone in the visual and somatosensory cortex of the macaque monkey and human brain. *J. Comp. Neurol.* 297: 441–470.

Kriegstein, A.R. and Parnavelas, J.G. (2003) Changing concepts of cortical development. Special Issue. *Cereb. Cortex* 13(6).

Kukekov, V.G., Laywell, E.D., Suslov, O., Davies, K., Scheffler, B., Thomas, L.B., O'Brien, T.F., Kusakabe, M., and Steindler, D.A. (2002) Multipotent stem/progenitor cells with similar properties arise from two neurogenic regions of adult human brain. *Exp. Neurol.* 156:333–344.

Laywell, E.D., Rakic, P., Kukekov, V.G., Holland, E.C., and Steindler, D. (2000) A Identification of a multipotent astrocytic stem cell in the immature and adult mouse brain. *Proc. Natl. Acad. Sci. USA* 97:13883–13888.

Lenhossek, M. Von (1895) Centrosom and Sphäre in den Spinalganglienzellen des Frosches. *Arch. Anat.* 46:345–369.

Letinic, K, Zoncu, R, and Rakic, P. (2002) Origin of GABAegic neurons in the human neocortex. *Nature* 417:645–649.

Levitt, P., Cooper, M.L., and Rakic, P. (1981) Coexistence of neuronal and glial precursor cells in the cerebral ventricular zone of the fetal monkey: an ultrastructural immunoperoxidase analysis. *J. Neurosci.* 1:27–39.

Levitt, P., Cooper, M.L., and Rakic, P. (1983) Early divergence and changing proportions of neuronal and glial precursor cells in the primate cerebral ventricular zone. *Dev. Biol.* 96:472–484.

Levitt, P. and Rakic, P. (1980) Immunoperoxidase localization of glial fibrillary acid protein in radial glial cells and astrocytes of the developing rhesus monkey brain. *J. Comp. Neurol.* 193:815–840.

Lewis, D.A. (2000) GABAergic local circuit neurons and prefrontal cortical dysfunction in schizophrenia. *Brain Res. Rev.* 31:270–276.

Magini, G. (1888) Sur la nevroglie et les cellules nerveuses cerebrales chez les foetus. *Arch. Ital. Biol.* 9:59–60.

Malatesta, P., Hack, M.A., Hartfuss, E., Kettenmann, H., Klinkert, W., Kirchhoff, F., and Gotz, M. (2003) Neuronal or glial progeny: regional differences in radial glia fate. *Neuron* 37:751–764.

Marin, O. and Rubenstein, J.L. (2001) A long, remarkable journey: tangential migration in the telencephalon. *Nat. Rev. Neurosci.* 2:780–790.

McCarthy, M., Turnbull, D.H., Walsh, C.A., and Fishell, G. (2001) Telencephalic neural progenitors appear to be restricted to regional and glial fates before the onset of neurogenesis. *J. Neurosci.* 21:6772–6781.

McConell, S.K. (1988) Fates of visual cortical neurons in the ferret after isochronic and heterochronic transplantation. *J. Neurosci.* 8:945–974.

Misson, J.-P., Austin, C.P., Takahashi, T., Cepko, C.L., and Caviness, V.S. (1991) The alignment of migrating neural cells in relation to the murine neopallial radial glial fiber system. *Cereb. Cortex* 1:221–229.

Misson, J.-P., Edwards, M.A., Yamamoto, M., and Caviness, V.S. (1988a) Mitotic cycling of radial glial cells of the fetal murine cerebral wall: a combined autoradiographic and immunohistochemical study. *Dev. Brain Res.* 38:183–190.

Misson, J.-P., Edwards, M.A., Yamamoto, M., and Caviness, V.S. (1988b) Identification of radial glial cells within the developing murine central nervous system: studies based upon a new immunohistochemical marker. *Dev. Brain Res.* 44:95–108.

Morest, D.K. (1970) A study of neurogenesis in the forebrain of opossum pouch young. *Z. Anat. Entwickl-Gesch.* 130:265–305.

Nadarajah, B., Alifragis, P., Wang, R.O.L., and Parnavelas, J.G. (2003) Neuronal migration in the developing cerebral cortex: observations based on real-time imaging. *Cerb. Cortex* 13:607–611.

Nieuwenhuys, R., ten Donkelaar, H.J., and Nicholson, C. (1998) *The Central Nervous System of Vertebrates.* Berlin: Springer.

Noctor, S.C., Flint, A.C., Weissman, T.A., Dammerman, R.S., and Kriegstein, A.R. (2001) Neurons derived from radial glial cells establish radial units in neocortex. *Nature* 409:714–720.

Norris, C.R. and Kalil, K. (1991) Guidance of callosal axons by radial glia in developing cerebral cortex. *J. Neurosci.* 11: 3481–3492.

Nowakowski, R.S. and Rakic, P. (1979) Mode of migration of neurons to the hippocampus: a Golgi and electron microscopic analysis in fetal rhesus monkey. *J. Neurocytol.* 8:697–718.

Oksche, A. (1968) Die pränatale und vergleichende. *Entwicklungsgeschichte der Neurologia.* Suppl. IV:4–19.

Onteniente, B., Kimura, H., and Maeda, T. (1983) Comparative study of the glial fibrillary protein in vertebrates by PAP immunohistochemistry. *J. Comp. Neurol.* 215:427–436.

Parnavelas, J.G., Barfield, J.A., Franke, E., and Luskin, M.B. (1991) Separate progenitor cells give rise to pyramidal and nonpyramidal neurons in the rat telencephalon. *Cereb. Cortex* 1:463–491.

Pixley, S.K.R. and De Vellis, J. (1984) Transition between immature radial glia and mature astrocytes studied with a monoclonal antibody to vimentin. *Dev. Brain Res.* 15:201–209.

Rakic, P. (1971) Neuron-glia relationship during granule cell migration in developing cerebellar cortex. A Golgi and electronmicroscopic study in Macacus rhesus. *J. Comp. Neurol.* 141:283–312.

Rakic, P. (1972) Mode of cell migration to the superficial layers of fetal monkey neocortex. *J. Comp. Neurol.* 145:61–84.

Rakic, P. (1973) Kinetics of proliferation and latency between final cell division and onset of differentiation of cerebellar stellate and basket neurons. *J. Comp. Neurol.* 147:523–546.

Rakic, P. (1974) Neurons in the monkey visual cortex: systematic relation between time of origin and eventual disposition. *Science* 183:425–427.

Rakic, P. (1978) Neuronal migration and contact guidance in primate telencephalon. *Postgrad. Med. J.* 54:25–40.

Rakic, P. (1981) Neuronal-glial interaction during brain development. *Trends Neurosci.* 4:184–187.

Rakic, P. (1984) Emergence of neuronal and glial cell lineages in primate brain. In: Black, I., ed. *Cellular and Molecular Biology of Neural Development.* New York: Plenum: pp. 29–50.

Rakic, P. (1985a) Contact regulation of neuronal migration In: Edelman, G.M. and Thiery, J.-P., eds. *The Cell in Contact: Adhesions and Junctions as Morphogenetic Determinants.* New York: Wiley and Sons, pp. 67–91.

Rakic, P. (1985b) Mechanisms of neuronal migration in developing cerebellar cortex. In: Edelman, G.E., Cowan, W.M., and Gall, E., eds. *Molecular Basis of Neural Development.* New York: Wiley and Sons, pp. 139–160.

Rakic, P. (1988a) Defects of neuronal migration and pathogenesis of cortical malformations. *Prog. Brain Res.* 73:15–37.

Rakic, P. (1988b) Specification of cerebral cortical areas. *Science* 241:170–176.

Rakic, P. (1990) Principles of neuronal cell migration. *Experientia* 46:882–891.

Rakic, P. (1995a) Radial versus tangential migration of neuronal clones in the developing cerebral cortex *Proc. Natl. Acad. Sci. USA* 92:11323–11327.

Rakic, P. (1995b) A small step for the cell—a giant leap for mankind: a hypothesis of neocortical expansion during evolution. *Trends Neurosci.* 18:383–388.

Rakic, P. (2002) Pre and post-developmental neurogenesis in primates. *Clin. Neurosci. Res.* 2:29–39.

Rakic, P. (2003) Elusive radial glial cells: historical and evolutionary perspective. *Glia* 43:19–32.

Rakic, P. and Sidman, R.L. (1968) Supravital DNA synthesis in the developing human and mouse brain. *J. Neuropathol. Exp. Neurol.* 27:246–276.

Rakic, P., Cameron, R.S., and Komuro, H. (1994) Recognition, adhesion, transmembrane signaling, and cell motility in guided neuronal migration. *Curr. Opin. Neurobiol.* 4:63–69.

Rakic, P., Knyihar-Csillik, E., and Csillik, B. (1996) Polarity of microtubule assembly during neuronal migration. *Proc. Natl. Acad. Sci. USA* 93:9218–9222.

Rakic, P. and Sidman, R.L. (1973) Sequence of developmental abnormalities leading to granule cell deficit in cerebellar cortex of weaver mutant mice. *J. Comp. Neurol.* 152:103–132.

Rakic, P., Stensaas, L.J., Sayre, E.P., and Sidman, R.L. (1974) Computer-aided three-dimensional reconstruction and quantitative analysis of cells from serial electron microscopic montages of fetal monkey brain. *Nature* 250:31–34.

Ramon y Cajal, S. (1909) *Histologie du Système Nerveux de l'Homme et des Vertébrés.* Vol. 1. Paris: Maloine. (Reprinted in 1952 by Consejo Superior de Investigaciones Cientificas, Instituto Ramón y Cajal, Madrid.)

Reichenbach, A. (1989) Attempt to classify glial cells by means of their process specialization using the rabbit retinal Müller cell as an example of cytotopographic specialization of glial cells. *Glia* 2:250–259.

Reid, C., Liang, I., and Walsh, C. (1995) Systematic widespread clonal organization in cerebral cortex. *Neuron* 15:299–310.

Reiner, O., Carrozzo, R., Shen, Y., Wehnert, M., Faustinella, F., Dobyns, W.B., Caskey, C.T., and Ledbetter, D.H. (1993) Isolation of a Miller-Dieker lissencephaly gene containing G protein b-subunit-like repeats. *Nature* 364:717–721.

Retzius, G. (1893) Studien uber Ependym und Neuroglia. *Biol. Untersuch. (Stockh)* N.S. 5:9–26.

Retzius, G. (1894) Die Neuroglia des Gehirns deim Meuschen und fei Saugethieren. *Biol. Untersuchungen.* 6:1–24.

Retzius, G. (1896) Das Menschenhirn. Studien in der makroskopischen Morphologic. Vol 1 and 2. Stockholm: PA Norstedt & Soner.

Rickmann, M., Amaral, D.G., and Cowan, W.M. (1987) Organization of radial glial cells during the development of the rat dentate gyrus. *J. Comp. Neurol.* 264:449–479.

Rickmann, M. and Wolf, J.R. (1985) Prenatral gliogeneis in the neupalium of the rat. *Adv. Anat. Embryol. Cell Biol.* 93:1–104.

Rio, C., Rieff, H.I., Qi, P.M., and Corfas, G. (1997) Neuregulin and erbB receptors play a critical role in neuronal migration. *Neuron* 19:39–50.

Rivas, R.J. and Hatten, M.B. (1995) Motility and cytoskeletal organization of migrating cerebellar granule neurons. *J. Neurosci.* 15:981–989.

Robinson, S.R. and Dreher, Z. (1990) Muller cells in adult rabbit retinae: morphology, distribution and implications for function and development. *J. Comp. Neurol.* 292:178–192.

Schmechel, D.E. and Rakic, P. (1979a) Arrested proliferation of radial glial cells during midgestation in rhesus monkey. *Nature (Lond.)* 227:303–305.

Schmechel, D.E. and Rakic, P. (1979b) A Golgi study of radial glial cells in developing monkey telencephalon: morphogenesis and transformation in to astrocytes. *Anat. Embryol.* 156:115–152.

Schmid, R.S. and Anton, E.S. (2003) Role of integrins in the development of the cerebral cortex. *Cereb. Cortex* 13:219–224.

Schmid, R.S., McGrath, B., Berechid, B.E., Boyles, B., Marchionni, M.B., Sestan, N., and Anton, E.S. (2003) Neuregulin 1—ErbB2 signaling is required for the establishment and transformation of radial glia in cerebral cortex. *Proc. Natl. Acad. Sci. USA* 100: 4251–4256.

Sestan, N. and Rakic, P. (2002) Notch signaling in the brain: more than just a developmental story. In: Israel, A., De Stooper, B., Chechler, F., and Christen, Y., eds. *Notch from Neurodevelopment to Neurodegeneration.* Research and Perspectives in Neuroscience. Heidelberg, New York: Springer, pp. 19–40.

Shirasaki, R. and Pfaff, S.L. (2002) Transcriptional codes and the control of neuronal identity. *Annu. Rev. Neurosci.* 25:251–281.

Sidman, R.L. and Rakic, P. (1973) Neuronal migration with special reference to developing human brain: a review. *Brain Res.* 62:1–35.

Sidman, R.L. and Rakic, P. (1982) Development of the human central nervous system. In: Haymaker, W. and Adams, R.D., eds. *Histology and Histopathology of the Nervous System.* Springfield, IL: Charles C Thomas, pp. 3–145.

Silver, J., Edwards, M.A., and Levitt, P. (1993) Immunocytochemical demonstration of early appearing astroglial structures that form boundaries and pathways along axon tracts in the fetal brain. *J. Comp. Neurol.* 328:415–436.

Silver, J., Lorenz, S.E., Wahlsten, D., and Coughlin, J. (1982) Axonal guidance of the great cerebral commissures: descriptive and experimental studies, *in vivo*, on the role of preformed glial pathways. *J. Comp. Neurol.* 210:10–29.

Smart, I.H.M., Dehay, C., Giroud, P., Berland, M., and Kennedy, H. (2002) Unique morphological features of the proliferative zones and postmitotic compartments of the neural epithelium giving rise to striate and extrastriate cortex in the monkey. *Cereb. Cortex* 12:37–53.

Sobue, G. and Pleasure, D. (1984) Astroglia proliferation and phenotype are modulated by neuronal plasma membrane. *Brain Res.* 213:351–364.

Song, H., Stevens, C.F., and Gage, F.H. (2002) Astroglia induce neurogenesis from adult neural stem cells. *Nature* 417:39–44.

Sotello, C., Avalardo-Mallarat, R.-M., and Vernet, M. (1994) Molecular plasticity of adult Bergmann fibers is associated with radial migration of grafted Purkinje cells. *J. Neurosci.* 14:124–133.

Steindler, D.A., Cooper, N.G.F., Faissner, A., and Schachner, M. (1989) Boundaries defined by adhesion molecules during development of the cerebral cortex: the J1/tenascin glycoprotein in the mouse somatosensory cortical barrel field. *Dev. Biol.* 131: 243–260.

Stensaas, L.J. and Golson, B.C. (1972) Ependymal and subependymal cells of the caudatopallial junction in the lateral ventricle of the neonatal rabbit. *Z. Zellforsch*, 132:297–322.

Steward, O., Schauwecker, P.E., Guth, L., Zhang, Z., Fujiki, M., Inman, D., Wrathall, J., Kempermann, G., Gage, F.H., Saatman, K., and McIntosh, T. (1999) Genetic appaches to neurotrauma research: opportunities and potential pitfalls of murine models. *Exp. Neurol.* 157:19–42.

Suslov, O.N., Kukekov, V.G., Ignatova, T.N., and Steindler, D.A. (2002) Neural stem cell heterogeneity demonstrated by molecular phenotyping of clonal neurospheres. *Proc. Natl. Acad. Sci. USA.* 99:14506–14511.

Tamamaki, N., Nakamura, K., Okamoto, K., and Kaneko, T. (2001) Radial glia is a progenitor of neocortical neurons in the developing cerebral cortex. *Neurosci. Res.* 41:51–60.

Tan, S.S. (2002) Developmental neurobiology—Cortical liars. *Nature* 417:605–606.

Tan, S.S. and Breen, S. (1993) Radial mosaicism and tangentional cell dispersion both contribute to mouse neocortical development. *Nature* 363:638–640.

Tan, S.S., Kalloniatis, M., Sturn, K., Tam, P.P.L., Reese, B.E., and Faulkner-Jones, B. (1998) Separate progenitors for radial and tangential cell dispersion during development of the cerebral neocortex. *Neuron* 21:295–304.

Tramontin, A.D., Garcia-Verdugo, J., Lim, D.A., and Alvarez-Buylla, A. (2003) Postnatal development of radial glia and the ventricular zone (VZ): a continuum of the neural stem cell compartment. *Cerb. Cortex* 13:580–587.

Varon, S.S. and Somjen, G.G. (1979) Neuronal-glial interactions. *Neurosci. Res. Prog. Bull.* 17:27–84.

Voigt, T. (1989) Development of glial cells in the cerebral wall of ferrets: direct tracing of their transformation from radial glial into astrocytes. *J. Comp. Neurol.* 289:74–88.

Volpe, J.J. (1987) *Neurology of the Newborn*, 2nd ed. Philadelphia: W.B. Saunders.

Waecher, R. and Jaench, B. (1972) Generation times of the matrix cell during embryonic brain development: an autoradiographic study in rats. *Brain Res.* 46:235–250.

Weissman, T., Noctor, S.C., Clinton, B.K., Honig, L.S., and Kriegstein, A.R. (2003) Neurogenetic radial glial cells in reptile, rodent and human; from mitosis to migration. *Cerb. Cortex* 13:550–559

Wichterle, H., Turnbull, D.H., Nery, S., Fishell, G., and Alvarez-Buylla, A. (2001) In utero fate mapping reveals distinct migratory pathways and fates of neurons born in the mammalian basal forebrain. *Development* 128:3759–3771.

Wynshaw-Boris, A. and Gambello, M.J. (2001) LIS1 and dynein motor function in neuronal migration and development. *Genes Dev.* 15:639–651.

Zupanc, G.K.H. (1999) Neurogenesis, cell death and regeneration in gymnotiform brain. *J. Exp. Neurol.* 202:1435–1446.

32 Axon guidance

ANDREAS FAISSNER

EVIDENCE FOR CONDUCIVE FUNCTIONS OF ASTROGLIA

Astroglial Cells Constitute Axonal Growth Pathways *in Vivo*

The specialized glial cells of the retina, the so-called Müller cells, span the width of the retina and produce a specialized structure toward the inner surface of the retina, the so-called glial endfeet. After generation of the retinal ganglion cells, the axons forming the prospective optic nerve elongate along this specialized structure. The growth substrate is provided by a basal lamina that is endfeet-derived and comprises the canonical extracellular matrix (ECM) components, that is, laminin-1, collagen IV, heparan sulfate proteoglycan (HSPG), and nidogen (Halfter et al., 2000). The growth response of retinal ganglion cells to laminin-1 *in vitro* is regulated by integrins, consistent with this expression pattern. Another example of the support of axon growth by astrocytes is provided by the development of the corpus callosum. The emergence of this structure depends on the formation of a transient bridge of astrocytes that connects the left and right hemispheres of the developing telencephalon. This glial bridge, also called the *glial sling*, supports the reciprocal growth of cortical axons, and the experimental interruption of the sling leads to the formation of accalosal mice (Fig 32.1). In this situation, the cortical connecting axons roll up on either side of the cerebral midline and yield the bundles of Probst, longitudinal fascicles formed from misdirected axons. Growth promotion of cortical axons can be restored by the implantation of nitrocellulose filters covered with embryonic astrocytes or embryonic astrocyte–derived membranes, consistent with a promoting role *in vivo*. Similarly, channels outlined by astrocyte surfaces have been revealed in the developing spinal cord and have been interpreted as growth conduits for advancing corticospinal axons.

The blueprint hypothesis of axon growth states that channels walled by astrocyte surfaces might provide a mechanical growth and guidance substrate for growth cones (Jacobson, 1991). Molecular specializations of both growth cone and astrocyte surfaces might be implicated in the regulation of these interactions. The mechanistic concept of axon guidance has been modifed and geared toward an interpretation that emphasizes molecular signals in the growth environment, the readout by specific growth cone–based receptors, and integration of these influences by signal transduction cascades that eventually modulate growth cone movements (Lemke, 2001). Thus, a conduit function of astroglia based on the chemorepellent slit-2 has recently been proposed as an additional guidance principle in the corpus callosum (Shu and Richards, 2001).

Astrocytes in Culture Form a Convenient Growth Substrate for Many Neuronal Cell Types

It is well known that astrocyte monolayers constitute an excellent growth substrate for axons *in vitro*. These conducive properties are consistent with the conclusions derived from *in vivo* studies and are age- and lineage-dependent. Thus, astrocytes obtained from embryonic or perinatal central nervous system (CNS) tissues are more efficient than those obtained at later embryonic stages, exert their strongest effect after short culture periods, and tend to lose supportive properties with time in culture. So-called type I or protoplasmic astrocytes with extended surfaces are supportive, in contrast to a possibly independent lineage, the so-called rocky or cobblestone-type astrocytes that form neurite growth–inhibiting islands in monolayer cultures. This cell type can be enriched by passaging and maintains its neurite growth–reducing features. It is possible that this astroglial type represents an equivalent of so-called reactive astrocytes that are characteristically enriched in lesion areas of the CNS (see below and Chapters 33 and 37). The neurite growth–promoting properties also depend on the spatial presentation of the cells *in vitro*. Indeed, astrocytes that sustain axon growth when presented as monolayers may inhibit neurite growth when contained in a tube. In this paradigm, astrocytes are grown in a cellulose acetate tube in three dimensions and confronted to a dorsal root ganglion that is cultivated next to one end of the tube. Axons from early postnatal or perinatal dorsal root ganglions (DRGs) grow readily into tubes filled with embryonic astrocytes but less well into tubes with aged or matured astrocytes. Also, DRGs from later stages are less efficient and do not penetrate tubes with older astrocytes. This model therefore mimics properties of the dorsal root entry zone, which represents a stop zone for centripetal axons in the adult.

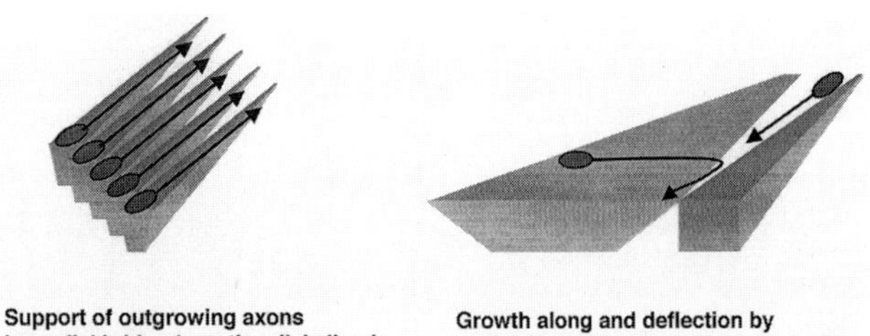

FIGURE 32.1 Axon guidance by glial surfaces. Many examples have been provided of axon guidance by astroglial cells in the developing nervous system. Both supportive properties—as shown for the developing corpus callosum—and boundary properties, for example in the rhombomeres, have been discussed.

Membrane-Based Adhesion Systems Mediate Promotion of Interactions of Neural Cell Types

Starting from aggregation experiments with dissociated sponges in the 1950s, a large body of evidence has been accumulated that suggests the regulated expression and functional significance of cell adhesion molecules (CAMs) in the nervous system. These basic types can be subdived into calcium-dependent and calcium-independent CAMs. With regard to the calcium-dependent mechanism, a growing number of cadherins has been described. The classical first cadherin found in the nervous system was N-cadherin, which mediates neuron-neuron and neuron-astrocyte interactions. This and other classical cadherins comprise five cadherin repeat motifs, calcium binding sites and a transmembrane domain that result in an overall molecular mass of about 100 kDa. Meanwhile, the number of cadherins has considerably increased, and by far the largest number of individual genes is expressed in the CNS. There, the expression patterns correlate with neuroanatomical subsystems, and recent concepts suggest a functional role in wiring and synaptogenesis within these systems. This interpretation is fostered by the fact that many classical cadherins subserve a homophilic, calcium-dependent adhesion mechanism. This mechanism is strong enough to induce sorting out of cells expressing distinct cadherin genes, and operates as early as at the blastocyst stage, as shown for E-cadherin (Takeichi, 1995). In addition to these, unconventional cadherins have been found that seem to play a role in epithelial cell junction formation or in certain tumors, for example, the gene *fat* in *Drosophila. Fat* is an atypical cadherin gene in drosophila that controls both cell growth and planar polarity. The cytoplasmic domains of classical cadherins interact with specialized proteins, the catenins. These are required for functional activation of cadherins, and the component β-catenin is involved in signal transduction to the cell nucleus (Uemura, 1998).

The other dominant family of CAMs in the nervous system consists of the immunoglobulin (Ig) superfamily. The characteristic feature of this family is the presence of at least one Ig domain, a structure consisting of 90–100 amino acids arranged as seven antiparallel beta-pleated sheets that form a globular domain (Brümmendorf and Rathjen, 1996). This domain type seems particularly well suited for the mediation of protein-protein interactions, and in numerous CAMs functional properties have been mapped to this structure. In many members, the Ig loop is combined with one or several fibronectin-type three (FNIII) domains, a structural module first discovered in the ECM glycoprotein fibronectin (see below), and a transmembrane domain. In some cases, however, CAMs of the Ig superfamily are linked to the membrane by a glycosylphosphatidylinositol (GPI) anchor that confers particular mobility within the membrane (Brümmendorf and Rathjen, 1996). These GPI-linked proteins may be associated with transmembrane glycoproteins that are involved in signal transduction processes, the paranodins. Functionally, Ig superfamily members mediate calcium-independent adhesion mechanisms of the homophilic and heterophilic types. Several neuronal adhesion molecules with strong axonal expression such as L1/Ng-CAM/neuroglian, TAG-1/axonin-1, or contactin/F11/F3 have been grouped as Ax-CAMs, referring to their prominent role in axon fasciculation. Participation of Ig CAMs in neurite growth promotion involves the activation of downstream signaling mechanisms, including modulation of intracellular calcium in the growth cone. These converge with those elicited via N-cadherin and the basic fibroblast growth factor (FGF) receptor (Walsh and Doherty, 1997). With regard to neuron-glia interactions, selected isoforms of the homophilic adhesion molecule N-CAM are expressed by astrocytes *in vitro* and mediate neuron-astrocyte adhesion (Fig. 32.2). Concerning heterophilic interactions, the small isoform of the phosphotyrosine phosphatase receptor RPTP-ζ/β is expressed by astrocytes, a transmembrane component that can interact with the neuronal adhesion molecule contactin/F11/F3 and other CAMs of the Ig superfamily. These examples illustrate the functional involvement of Ig CAMs in conducive neuron-astrocyte interactions.

The third prominent gene family of membrane-based CAMs is represented by the integrins. These are heterodimers composed of α- and β-subunits that primarily mediate the interactions of neural cells with ECM components (Fig. 32.2 and see below). In some cases, interactions between integrins and Ig superfamily members have also been reported (Dedhar and Hannigan, 1996).

ASTROGLIA AT CHOICE AND DECISION POINTS

Glial Boundaries (Subdivision of Rhombomeres, Neuromeres at the More Anterior, Rostral Central Nervous System—Thalamus)

Two extensively studied examples of segmented systems are macroanatomically visible in 3-day-old

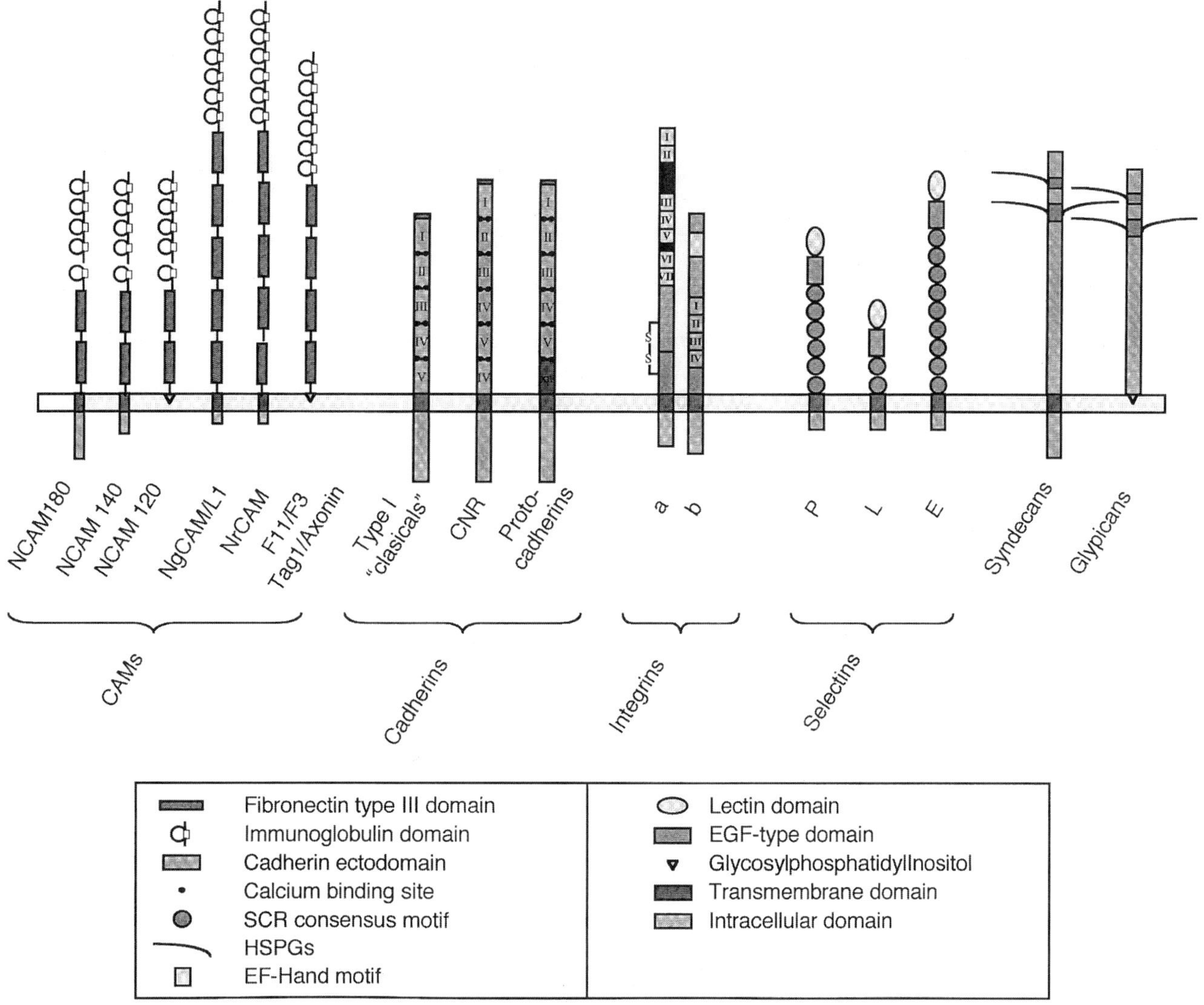

FIGURE 32.2 Structures of cell adhesion molecules (CAMs). Many molecules have been described that mediate various kinds of intercellular adhesive interactions in neural tissues. These can be grouped into large gene families according to key structural features, such as the immunoglobulin type C2 domain. EGF: epidermal growth factor; HSPG: heparan sulfate proteoglycan; SCR: serum complement-like repeat.

chicken embryos: the rhombencephalon of the brain stem, which is subdivided into rhombomeres, and the paraxial mesoderm, which is substructured into somites. The rhombomere pattern in the chick embryo hindbrain emerges between Hamburger and Hamilton stages 9 (six somites, 6s) and 12 (16s). At stage 16s the rhombomeres can be identified as a series of eight swellings along the neuraxis that are separated by grooves. Studies on axonogenesis have demonstrated that the first neurons emerge at stage 11/12s in the even-numbered rhombomeres and one stage later in the odd-numbered rhombomeres.The axons of motor neurons located in defined pairs of rhombomeres emerge from the lips to innervate specific branchial arches. For example, all the muscles derived from the first branchial arch are innervated by the trigeminal nerve, whose axons originate in rhombomeres 2 and 3 (r2 and r3) and exit in r2 at defined exit points. Also, the motor nuclei of the cranial nerves and their respective motor tracts originate from groups of cells that are generated in individual rhombomeres along the rostro-caudal axis. Lineage tracing studies have shown that the neural progeny of these nuclei display lineage restriction in individual rhombomeric segments. Thus, members of identified cellular clones do not cross from one rhombomere to another neighboring one after the anatomical boundary has formed.

This segmentation of the hindbrain is mirrored by a remarkable expression pattern of defined transcription factors. For example, on embryonic day 9.5 (E9.5), the mouse homologs of the *Drosophila* antennapedia complex of homeotic genes (e.g., the genes of the Hox-B complex) are aligned and transcribed on the mouse chromosome 2 in a 5′ to 3′ direction. The limits of expression of these genes in the mouse spinal cord progress in a caudo-rostral direction and are identical to the boundaries of rhombomeric pairs in ascending order. To illustrate the case, *Hox-a2* expression terminates at the boundary between r1 and r2, *Hox-b2* at the r2/3 boundary, and so forth. These expression boundaries coincide in many cases with those of paralogous genes of the *Hox-A* and *Hox-C* complexes, and alterations of the Hox code in the hindbrain by treatment with retinoic acid at the preheadfold stage results in homeotic transformation of rhombomeres r2/3 into rhombomeres r4/r5. These findings are consistent with the view that regional neural identities in segments are determined by transcription factor combinations such as the so-called Hox code. This concept has been extended to the more rostral parts of the CNS, where factors such as *Nkx-2.2* and two other related homeobox-containing genes, *TTF-1* and *Dlx*, correspond to neuroanatomical subdivisions. A more detailed discussion of the role of transcription factors in developing neural and other tissues is beyond the scope of this review and is available elsewhere (Pasini and Wilkinson, 2002).

The structure and modes of operation of interrhombomeric boundaries are not well understood. In boundary regions the interkinetic nuclear migration of neuroepithelial cells seems significantly reduced and intercellular adhesion is probably increased, as deduced from the finding that the polysialylated form of the neural cell adhesion molecule N-CAM is enriched within rhombomeres, while the more adhesive nonsialylated variant is expressed in the boundary. Neuroepithelial cells in this area hence presumably form a less motile and more tightly coherent group of cells 4 to 10 cell diameters wide that may constitute a barrier to the movement of epithelial cells from one rhombomere to the next. Interestingly, the cells defining the rhombencephalic interneuromeric limit display a reduced, although not completely blocked, spread of currents or diffusional dyes such as Lucifer Yellow or biocytin between themselves or from one rhombomere to the next, while the neuroepithelia within the rhombomere are extensively coupled electrically. The boundary is characterized by an increase in intercellular space compared to the intrarhombomeric compartment. The boundary cells exhibit an unusual fan-shaped array and abut with their endfeet on both the pial and ventricular surfaces. Comparably, in zebrafish, a serial arrangement of glial cells, a so-called glial curtain, has been proposed to separate individual rhombomeres. It has been envisaged that the specialized boundary cells construct a privileged pathway for outgrowing axons (Faissner and Steindler, 1995). For example, although the motor fibers emanating from the cranial nuclei traverse from the odd- to the even-numbered rhombomeres in order to reach their exit points, they preferentially elongate along boundary structures. Also, reticular axons in rhombomeres stained with neurofilament antibodies display a repetitive circumferential arrangement in register with interrhombomeric boundaries (Fig. 32.1). A directing influence of boundaries on axon pathways is supported by transplantation experiments where fiber tracts follow ectopic boundaries. The mechanism and molecular basis of hypothesized boundary functions for axon guidance are currently unknown, and differential adhesion or local inhibition concepts are being discussed.

Midline Glia at Decision Points for Growth Cones (Optic Chiasm, Roof Plate, Floor Plate, Midline Glia in *Drosophila*)

In addition to the boundaries present between rhombo- and prosomeres, a second class of boundaries associated with glial cell types has been described in the midline of developing nervous systems of vertebrates. Thus, an assembly of glial cells separates the left and right axonal projection systems at the optic chiasm. It seems that growing axons interact with this glial structure and are directed to either the ipsilateral or the contralateral cortex, as required in the context of binocular vision. Several genes have been examined as potential candidates in mediating the choice decision. Among these are the glycoproteins *L1* and *CD44*, as well as chondroitin sulfate proteoglycan(s), as visualized by the expression of chondroitin sulfate epitopes in the glial boundary territory (Chung et al., 2000; Jeffery, 2001). Analogous midline decisions are also observed in the roof and the floor plates of the developing spinal cord (Fig. 32.3). In the rat, the emerging commissural axons of the dorsal horn first migrate to the ventral half of the cord, toward the floor plate, under the influence of the chemoattractant netrin-1. Simultaneously, the dorsal midline cells of the cord express a keratan sulfate (KS) epitope that is probably carried by a proteoglycan core structure. This KS epitope delineates precisely a boundary region that is not traversed by the commissural axon fibers. When KS epitope–expressing proteoglycans are exposed as patterned substrates alternating with the glycoprotein laminin-1, various cultured neurons and their processes avoid the proteoglycan-rich regions and grow on the laminin-1 substrates. This boundary-like property *in vitro* can be neutralized by removal of the KS and chondroitin sulfate side chains using specific enzymes, or by antibodies to the proteoglycan core (Faissner and Steindler, 1995).

On the ventral side of the cord, the floor plate cells separate the left and right halves of the overall structure. The growth and decision events of the ventral side can be monitored in the so-called open book in the cul-

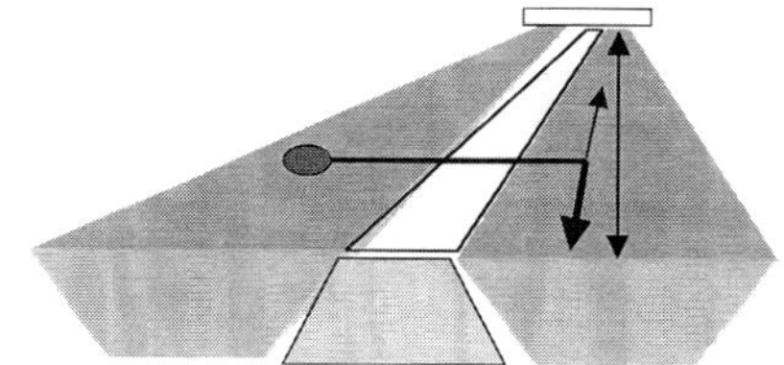

FIGURE 32.3 The open book preparation. In the developing rat spinal cord, commissural neurons send their axons toward the floor plate, following a netrin gradient. After crossing the midline at the floor plate, responsiveness to netrins is lost and substituted for by sensitivity to other types of cues. In response to these cues, the axons turn and grow along the rostrocaudal axis, fasciculating onto existing longitudinal fiber pathways. These events can partially be monitored and perturbed *in vitro* in the so-called open book preparation, an *ex-vivo* explant that is produced by cutting the developing E13 spinal cord along the midline.

ture dish, a preparation that lends itself to antibody perturbation assays (Fig. 32.3).The floor plate cells release the ECM chemoattractant netrin-1, which attracts the commissural fibers toward the midline, where they cross and subsequently turn to elongate along the rostocaudal orientation within the cord. The netrin-1 signal is decoded by the receptor DCC (deleted in colorectal cancer), an Ig superfamily member. The commissural fibers destined to cross the midline express the GPI-linked axonin-1/TAG-1, an Ig superfamily member that is downregulated after the crossing has occurred. In parallel, the Ig superfamily glycoprotein L1 appears on the longitudinally oriented fibers, an Ig-CAM involved in fasciculation.

Antibodies to the Ig superfamily member axonin-1/TAG-1 inhibit the crossing step at the midline. The latter concomitantly expresses Nr-CAM, a heterophilic axonin-1/TAG-1 ligand. Concerted interactions of these Ig superfamily members hence seem required to regulate the crossing step. Subsequently, the axons lose responsiveness to the attractant netrin-1, yet do not progress to the lateral part of the cord. This might reflect the action of selected semaphorins of the sema3 class and the complementary neuropilin receptor complexes NP1 and NP2, which seem to be involved. The recrossing of the midline is prevented by the ECM constituent slit, a repulsive chemodiffusible signal expressed by the midline that is detected by the Ig superfamily member *robo* (for *roundabout*), a component of the growth cone (Ghose and van Vactor, 2002; Fig. 32.3). Both *slit* and *robo*, which occur as several homologs in the vertebrate, were originally discovered in *Drosophila*, where the midline of the ladder-like nervous system involves the so-called midline glia. Complex genetic analysis in *Drosophila* has revealed a battery of genes that are required for midline glia generation. Upstream, the fate determination of midline cells in general is controlled by *single-minded*. Glial cells emerge under the regulatory influence of *spitz*, a *Drosophila* homolog of transforming growth factor-α (TGF-α), and the transcription factor *pointed*, which intervenes in the expression of *gcm* (glial cell missing), a further gene required for the generation of glial cells in general. Elimination of the midline glia prevents the separation of commissural fibers and eliminates the longitudinal connections of the ladder-like nervous system in *Drosophila*. The commissural fibers of the system begin to extend between the three pairs of midine glia cells, on the one hand, and the pair of MP1 neurons, on the other hand. Separation of the commissural fiber systems involves migration of the midline glia in the correct direction (Granderath and Klämbt, 1999). Recently, a genetic screen has led to the identification of a number of additional genes that control this migratory behavior, one of which, called *klötzchen*, seems to implicate the spectrin cytoskeleton of midline glia. In all cases, deficits in midline glia migration lead to errors in the separation of the connecting commissural fiber systems.

Membrane-Based Gene Families Involved in Choice Point Decisions (Eph Kinases and Ephrins, Robo and Slit, Semaphorins)

The investigation of neural cell interactions first resulted in the identification of the immunoglobulin and cadherin superfamilies, and of growth- and motility-promoting ECM constituents. But in the 1980s, it became clear that in addition to growth promotion, growth inhibitory molecules also contribute to the regulation of cell migration and growth cone movement (Goodman, 1996). In particular, the phenomenon of growth cone collapse had been described in the context of coculture models where growth cones from sympathetic neurons encounter retinal neurites in the culture dish or retinal neurites engage central myelin preparations. These interactions invariably resulted in collapse and retraction of the growth cone, which remained paralyzed for 30 to 60 minutes *in vitro* prior to resuming growth and exploratory behavior. It was realized that this inhibitory effect might also influence guidance and inhibition of regeneration. With regard to guidance, systematic analysis of the innervation of the tectum in the visual system led to the identification of RAG (retinal axon guidance molecule), a GPI-linked protein with a gradient–like distribution in the tectum (Drescher et al., 1997). It quickly became clear that RAG was homologous to a series of already described genes with no apparent functions that were subsequently renamed *ephrins*. The GPI-linked ephrins A that interact with complementary EphA-type tyrosine kinases should be distinguished from the transmembrane ephrins B that recognize the EphB-type tyrosin kinases. Both groups contain a large number of ephrin- and Eph-type kinase genes, and a certain degree of promiscuity in the mutual pairing combinations has been recorded (Klein, 2001). A salient trait of the receptor-ligand combinations is that in many cases a reciprocal gradient-like expression of the components in neural tissues has been documented. Thus, ephrin-A5 is expressed as gradient in the tectum, and so are the complemetary receptors EphA3 and EphA5 in the retinal neurons. It is believed that these complementary ligand-receptor combinations encode positional informations in the nervous system (Wilkinson, 2001). Whether the members of the pairs are expressed in neuronal and glial lineages, respectively, remains to be established. It is already clear, however, that they contribute to the emergence of the rhombomeric compartments mentioned in the previous subsection. In addition, evidence has been presented that these gene families are involved in the midline choice decision of the growing corticospinal projection. Thus, ephrin-B3 is a constituent of the midline and prevents recrossing of these axons when they enter the gray matter after migrating to the contralateral side of the spinal cord (Kullander et al., 2001).

Following the avenue of growth cone collapse induction in sympathetic neurons, the separate gene family of semaphorins has been identified, which comprises homologous members in mouse and human. Some semaphorins can induce growth cone collapse mediated by the receptor plexin and the neuropilin receptor complexes NP1 and NP2 in the growth cone membrane (Whitford and Ghosh, 2001). The signal transduction pathways downstream of receptor activation involve small guanosine triphosphate (GTP)-binding proteins such as Rho and Rac1 (Liu and Strittmatter, 2001). The contributions of these inhibitory interactions in the context of neuron-glia interactions have still to be worked out in detail. In contrast, several constituents of the myelin sheath that inhibit axon growth by inducing growth cone collapse have been identified. These include the Nogo glycoproteins; Nogo-A seems to be the principal inhibitor of growth expressed in myelin. Nogo-A contains a region that induces growth cone collapse by interacting with the comlementary Nogo receptor NgR. This receptor is GPI-anchored to the growth cone membrane and part of a receptor complex. Interestingly, two other myelin components inhibitory to axon growth have been detected, the Ig superfamily member myelin-associated glycoprotein (MAG) and oligodendrocyte-myelin glycoprotein (OMGP). Both are also able to activate the NgR complex, which suggests a common downstream pathway of myelin-dependent inhibition (McKerracher and Winton, 2002) (see Chapter 37 for a detailed discussion).

Extracellular Matrix Glycoproteins (Tenascins, Netrins, and Receptors)

The pericellular space is structured by macromolecules of the ECM, which consists of glycoproteins and proteoglycans (Garwood et al., 2001a, and see below). It was quickly realized that astrocytes *in vitro* produce many of the ECM glycoproteins originally described in other tissues, namely, fibronectin, laminin-1, vitronectin, thrombospondin, and tenascin-C. Laminin-1 is a functional component of astroglial endfeet in limiting membranes, for example in the developing retina, and forms an excellent growth substrate for axon extension of many neuronal cell types. The structurally related genes netrin-1 and netrin-2 are chemodiffusible chemoattractants that guide outgrowing commissural axons toward the floorplate of the midline in the spinal cord. This mechanism is highly conserved because it has already been evolved in the nematode where unc-5 guides circumferential axons (Tessier-Lavigne and Goodman, 1996). Fibronectin has been found in association with blood vessels, structures where astrocytes contribute to the formation of the blood–brain barrier that isolates the CNS from the bloodstream. Tenascin-C has been studied in some detail because it is transiently expressed by immature astrocytes in the developing CNS *in vivo*. There, its distribution follows functional neuroanatomical subdivisions, for example in the barrel field, where it delineates the emerging barrel field structure in layer IV. The glycoproteins of the tenascin gene family are characterized by structural motifs, which are shared by the members tenascin-C (TN-C), tenascin-R (TN-R), tenascin-X (TN-X), tenascin-Y (TN-Y), and tenascin-W (TN-W). These include a cysteine-rich amino terminus that is shared by all the different subunits, a series of egf-type repeats, a series of fibronectin type III modules, and, finally, homologies to fibrinogen-β and -γ that determine the sequence of the subunits (Garwood et al., 2001b). This basic structural organization is maintained in most members of the gene family, with the exception of a tenascin-like gene in *Drosophila*, which contains the characteristic egf-type repeats but is devoid of other structural elements. The egf-type repeats of tenascins show a particular arrangement of cysteines that has also been found in the ECM molecule reelin, which is mutated in the neuron migration-deficient mouse mutant *reeler*. This motif is distinct from the one described in other egf-type repeat modules, for example in Notch or in the laminins. The amino terminus has been shown to link tenascin monomers to multimers in some cases, for example TN-R to trimers and TN-C to hexamers under nonreducing conditions. The hexamer appears under the electron microscope as hexabrachion in rotary shadowed preparations. This typical structure has also been observed in simple organisms such as the sponge *Oscarella tuberculata*, which might indicate conservation during evolution. Downstream of the egf-type repeats the sequence is continued by fibronectin type III repeats and terminated by homologies to fibrinogen-β and -γ (Fig. 32.4).

Two isoforms that are distinguished by one FNIII motif have been described in *TN-R*, a gene that is expressed in oligodendrocytes at later stages of development. TN-C possesses an alternative splice site between the fifth and sixth FNIII modules of the basic structure. As many as six and nine additional FNIII repeats can be inserted at this position in mouse and human TN-C, respectively. These modules are highly conserved at their respective positions. Recently, a systematic analysis of mRNAs in mouse CNS has revealed up to 30 alternatively spliced variants in this segment of TN-C, about 50% of the theoretically possible number of 64 isoforms, assuming free exchange of cassettes at their respective positions (Joester and Faissner, 1999). In the human, the number might be even larger, with up to 512 possible variants on the assumption that the modules are freely exchangable. In light of this result, the glycoprotein seems suited to specify pericellular microenvironments or to distinguish glial lineages (Joester and Faissner, 2001). Furthermore, TN-C is associated with various pathological conditions including mesenchymally derived and glial tumors. It represents an interesting possibility that TN-C could serve diagnostic purposes in this context.

With regard to function, the tight association of expression with neuroanatomical boundaries, developmental events, and sites of plastic changes have motivated numerous experimental studies using *in vitro* systems. It has been shown that the glycoprotein is antiadhesive for a large variety of cell types, and deflects growth cones and neuronal cell bodies at boundaries in choice situations *in vitro* that offer a TN-C-rich environment alternating with laminin-1, a known neurite-outgrowth promoter (Faissner, 1997). On the other hand, homogeneous substrates of TN-C promote neurite outgrowth of most neuronal cell types studied so far. Using monoclonal antibodies, recombinant proteins expressed in bacteria, and chimeric Ig-Fc constructs, these divergent functions could be attributed to distinct domains of TN-C. Thus, a neurite outgrowth–promoting area could be mapped to the distal splice site surrounding cassette D, and a site interfering with the motility of oligodendrocyte precursors was located to the FNIII module pair TNfn78 (Götz et al., 1996; Fig. 32.4). Several receptors have been described, among them the Ig superfamily member F3/contactin/F11, which is involved in mediating TN-C-dependent stimulation of neurite outgrowth in embryonic hippocampal neurons (Rigato et al., 2002), and various integrins such as $\alpha v\beta 3$, $\alpha 1\beta 8$, and $\alpha 1\beta 9$ (for review see Faissner, 1997). In the ECM, TN-C interacts with proteoglycans such as phosphacan. Despite these numerous functions detected *in vitro*, knockout mice appeared viable and able to reproduce at first sight. Recent observations suggest, however, modified behaviors in re-

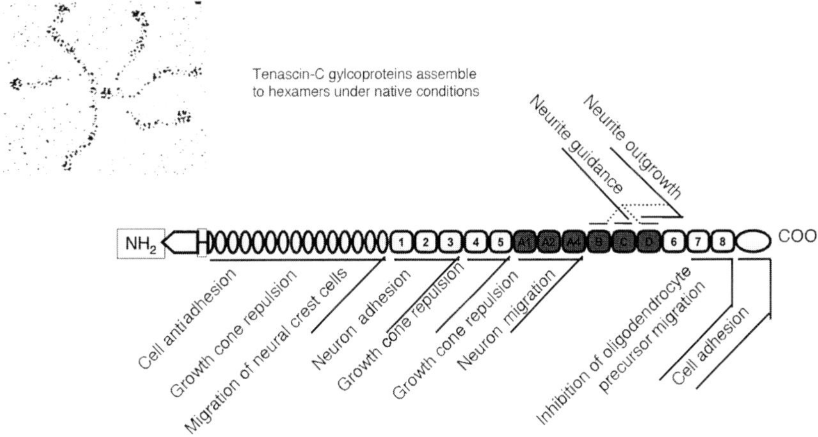

FIGURE 32.4 Structure-function model of tenascin-C glycoproteins. The scheme depicts the sructural organization of mouse tenascin-C and details functional regions that have been defined on the basis of antibody perturbation or of bioassays carried out with recombinantly expressed domains.

sponse to stress and lesions in the gene elimination mutants, and deviations in the generation and volume of neural precursor cells, suggesting both roles in the development and plasticity of mice. This and the strong association of TN-C with human pathology in CNS cancer, hippocampal sclerosis, and various types of lesion warrants further studies of this versatile multifunctional glycoprotein.

Heparan Sulfate and Chondroitin Sulfate Proteoglycans

The second class of ECM components expressed in the CNS is represented by proteoglycans (PGs). These are characterized as glycoproteins that contain at least one additional covalently linked glycosaminoglycan chain (Baudtlow and Zimmermann, 2000). Heparan sulfate, chondroitin sulfate, and keratan sulfate PGs of the CNS can be distinguished. Tissue fractionation studies performed with rat brain revealed that most HSPGs are tightly associated with cell membranes, whereas chondroitin sulfate proteoglycans (CSPGs), which constitute the major population of PGs in the CNS, are recovered in detergent-free salt extracts. In many cases the HSPGs are membrane-bound and may contribute to the signaling of growth factors such as basic fibroblast growth factor (bFGF), which binds to a specific motif in the heparan sulfate carbohydrate chain. A functional role for the transmission of wnt signals during embryogenesis has also been reported. Both members of the syndecan gene family and the GPI-linked HSPG glypican have been detected in the CNS (Yamaguchi, 2001). With regard to CSPGs, the members of the lectican family brevican, neurocan, versican, and aggrecan have been identified in the CNS (Bandtlow and Zimmermann, 2000; Yamaguchi, 2000). These CSPGs, which comprise a specific pattern of structural motifs, associate with distinct lineages. Thus, versican is expressed by mature oligodendrocytes, while neurocan and aggrecan have been found associated with neurons. Interestingly, several of the core glycoproteins carry the HNK-1 epitope, a carbohydrate structure also expressed by neural recognition molecules, or other N-linked carbohydrates, for example, of the Lewis x-type, which are recognized by specific monoclonal antibodies.

These reports indicate a substantial heterogeneity of CSPGs in the CNS. Several monoclonal antibodies (MAbs) have been described which react specifically with individual PGs, such as CAT 301, which identifies the neuronally expressed variant of aggrecan, and NG2, which recognizes the CSPG named NG2 that is expressed by oligodendrocyte precursors and in wound regions of neural tissues. Neuronal expression of CAT 301 early during spinal cord development depends on the activation of the *N*-methyl-D-aspartate (NMDA) receptor, suggesting a role for PGs in neuronal plasticity. The use of MAbs specific for epitopes on KS chains has shown that this carbohydrate polymer is transiently detectable as a boundary in the roof plate of the developing spinal cord, where it displays inhibitory properties (see the section "Midline Glia at Decision Points for Growth Cones"). Experiments performed with versican have also documented inhibitory effects on the migration of neural crest cells and of DRG axons in a laminin-1-rich territory. Finally, the neuronal CSPG neurocan, a member of the aggrecan family of PGs, binds directly to CAMs of the Ig superfamily, inhibits homophilic L1- or N-CAM-mediated cell adhesion, and interferes with both neuron adhesion to and neurite outgrowth on substrates consisting of combinations of CAMs or MAbs. In light of findings such as these, CSPGs were discussed as inhibitors of neurite outgrowth, an aspect which has caused considerable attention in the study of CNS lesions (Fawcett and Asher, 1999). On the other hand, glycosaminoglycans per se have not proven inhibitory to neurite outgrowth in every situation, and chondroitin sulfate epitopes have been found upregulated in the regenerating peripheral nerve. In some cases, chondroitin sulfate epitopes have been attributed to neurite outgrowth–stimulating properties. The functional properties for axon growth therefore need to be considered in the context of overall matrix composition and the lineage and age of the neurons involved (Oohira et al., 2000).

Phosphacan and Related Isoforms in Neuron-Glia Interactions

DSD-1-PG/phosphacan is one of the more abundant soluble CSPGs in the postnatal mouse brain and is the mouse homolog of the CSPG phosphacan from rat tissues (Faissner et al., 1994; Garwood et al., 1999). The glycosaminoglycan (GAG) composition of DSD-1-PG/phosphacan is characterized by the chondroitin sulfates CS-A and CS-C, a keratan sulfate moiety that has been detected with the MAb 3H1 and the DSD-1 epitope. The latter has been identified with the help of the MAb 473HD and requires (at least) a chain of seven disaccharides, sulfation of the carbohydrate backbone, and a significant proportion of CS-D dimers in its sequence. The DSD-1 epitope can be enriched by affinity chromatography on a column derivatized with the MAb 473HD, and displays neurite outgrowth–promoting properties for E18 hippocampal neurons (Clement et al., 1998; Garwood et al., 1999). Thus, it is an example of a glycosaminoglycan with neurite outgrowth–promoting properties.

The secreted PG phosphacan is the product of a splice variant of the transmembrane receptor protein tyrosine phosphatase beta (RPTP-ζ/β), and it corresponds to the entire extracellular region of the largest isoform of RPTP-ζ/β, which is extensively glycosylated with chondroitin sulfate glycosaminoglycan chains. The large variant and a short isoform derived therefrom possess a transmembrane domain and two phosphotyrosine phosphatase modules oriented toward the cytoplasm (see Faissner et al., 2004 for review; Fig. 32.5). Recently, a novel soluble isoform that corresponds to the carboxyterminal carboanhydrase domain has been described in the mouse, and several isoform variants have been uncovered in *Xenopus*. The different isoforms of RPTP-ζ/β display developmental regulation and lineage-restricted expression. Glial precursor cells, radial glia, Golgi cells, and astrocytes of different developmental stages and from various parts of the CNS have all been shown to express RPTP-ζ/β isoforms. For example, the large transmembrane variant is expressed in the subventricular zones of the developing and adult CNS and preferentially by oligodendrocyte precursors. The short transmembrane form is found in astrocytes, and both lineages seem to release the soluble variant phosphacan to some extent. Thus, the phosphacan mRNA at E13–E16 is largely confined to areas of active cell proliferation such as the ventricular zone of the brain and the ependymal layer surrounding the central canal of the spinal cord. Although the mRNA is mostly in the neuroepithelium of the embryonic brain and spinal cord, the protein is widely distributed in these tissues, presumably as a consequence of transport along glial processes, local secretion, and/or redistribution as a consequence of cell migration. Neuronal expression has also been observed, which may be due to the novel short phosphacan isoform (PSI), which is strongly expressed by several neuronal populations in the cortex (Garwood et al., 2003). The spatiotemporal expression pattern of the RPTP-ζ/β isoforms during the development, maintenance, and pathology of the CNS

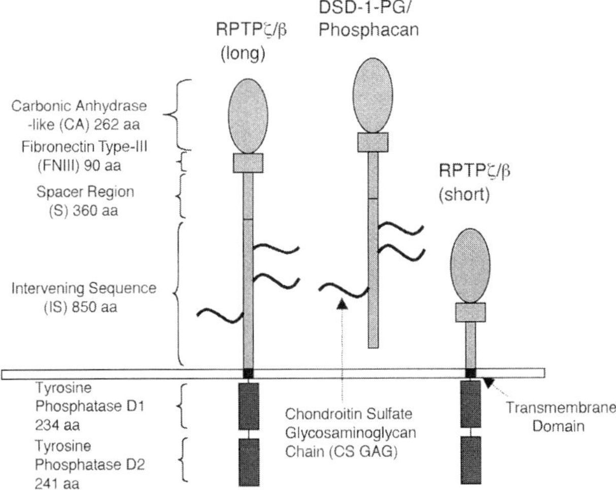

FIGURE 32.5 Structure of receptor phosphotyrosine phosphatase beta/zeta (RPTP-ζ/β). The different isoforms of the gene are shown, which occurs both as soluble proteoglycan and as transmembrane receptor.

has been correlated with a range of developmental processes that involve cell-cell signaling, including cellular proliferation, migration, differentiation, axon outgrowth, synaptogenesis, synaptic function, and tissue regeneration (reviewed in Garwood et al., 2001b; Faissner et al., 2004).

Based on the essentially glial expression of phosphacan/RPTP-ζ/β, the effects on neuronal behavior of extracellular signals presented by RPTP-ζ/β have been considered, whether as protein sequences/domains or associated with the chondroitin sulfate glycosaminoglycan (CS-GAG) chains, with which they are modified. In the adult rat brain, it has been shown that phosphacan occurs close to the surface of a selected subpopulation of neurons that express the calcium-binding protein, parvalbumin, occupying the extracellular space close to the cell body, surrounding axon terminals and glial endfeet, but not the synaptic clefts. It has been suggested that CSPGs associate with hyaluronic acid in such perineuronal nets or pericellular matrices to form a neuronal ECM structure analogous to that found in connective tissue. Different neuronal subsets display different complements of CSPGs (Celio and Blümcke, 1994) such that perineuronal CSPGs could regulate the extracellular milieu of neurons in cell type–specific ways. For example, late in development the mature ECM may be an important element in limiting synaptic plasticity (Pizzorusso et al., 2002).

Protein expression by neurons, including migrating neurons in the cerebrum and cerebellar Purkinje cells, has been difficult to interpret. One of the reasons is that phosphacan is present in the ECM surrounding certain subsets of neurons, and such an extracellular association with the neuronal surface could be of glial origin. With regard to function, phosphacan interacts with Ig superfamily members such as contactin/F3/F11, axonin-1/TAG-1, Nr-CAM, and Ng-CAM, and hence might intervene in both homophilic and heterophilic interactions of these adhesion molecules (Rios et al., 2000). Interaction of contactin/F3/F11 with the aminoterminal domains of phosphacan heterologously expressed in eukaryotic cells results in neurite outgrowth promotion (Peles et al., 1995). The transmembrane variants of RPTP-ζ/β (PTP-ζ/β) expose the same structural motifs and, therefore, also represent potential ligands of the Ig superfamily adhesion molecules. It has been proposed that the transmembrane variants expressed in glia could serve as receptors for CAMs expressed in the neuronal growth cone in the framework of neuron-glia interactions (Fig. 32.6). Because both RPTP-ζ/β and the Ig-CAMs are linked to signal transduction pathways, these interactions might involve reciprocal signaling mechanisms. These possibilities merit further investigations in light of recent reports suggesting that the intracellular phosphotyrosine-phos-

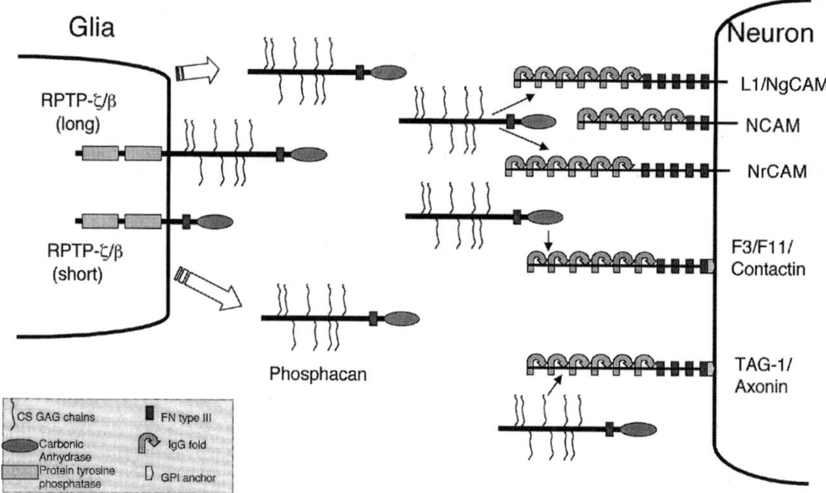

FIGURE 32.6 Receptor phosphotyrosine phosphatase beta/zeta (RPTP-ζ/β) in neuron-glia interactions. The scheme summarizes some of the studies that document interactions between phosphacan and cell adhesion membranes of the Ig superfamily. In view of the shared amino-terminal segment, the receptor forms might as well intervene in membrane-mediated interactions between neurons and astroglial surfaces. CS GAG: chondroitin sulfate glycosaminoglycan; GPI: glycophosphatidylinositol.

phatase modules of RPTP-ζ/β are involved in signal transduction pathways (Ratcliffe et al., 2000; Kawachi et al., 2001).

Within the ECM, phosphacan possesses a wealth of potential ligands, such as the ECM glycoprotein TN-C. The PG presented as a homogeneous substrate promotes neurite outgrowth by embryonic day 18 rat hippocampal and cortical neurons. In the case of hippocampal neurons, this effect can be blocked by removal of the chondroitin sulfate chains and the DSD-1-epitope, which is of crucial importance in this context. Phosphacan does not affect ougrowth of DRG neurites in an polycation-rich substrate. However, when exposed with a laminin-1 substrate, the neurite outgrowth effect of the ECM glycoprotein is abolished, suggesting that the inhibitory effect of the CSPG is context-dependent (Garwood et al., 1999). A similar result has been obtained with embryonic cortical neurons. In both cases, blockade of laminin-1-stimulated neurite growth promotion is still detectable after removal of the chondroitin sulfate chains and, therefore, is related to the ECM context and the lineage of the responsive cells (Faissner et al., 2004). The integration into ECM superstructures might explain to some extent why the elimination of the phosphacan gene does not result in serious impairment of development in mice (Harroch et al., 2000).

THE ASTROGLIAL SCAR

Scarring in Response to Lesioning, Structure of the Scar, Reactive Astrocytes, and Leptomeningeal Cells

For decades, it was believed that the regeneration of severed CNS axons is impossible. The seminal experiment by Albert Aguayo that showed that CNS neurons can extend vigorously growing axons into peripheral nerve tubes challenged this view and created considerable interest in cellular and molecular aspects of wound reactions in the CNS. In particular, the growth capacity of neurons strongly suggested that environmental factors in the lesion were responsible for the abortion of axon regrowth, and not an intrinsic lack of ability of the axon. Meanwhile, it has become well established that the inability of the CNS to regenerate is due at least in part to inhibitory factors released by glial cells into the lesion environment (Fawcett, 1998; Fawcett and Asher, 1999; Klocker and Bähr, 2001). After lesioning, microglial activation leads to the release of numerous cytokines and the removal of cellular debris. Furthermore, leptomeningeal cells often occupy wound territory, dragged into the lesion in the course of mechanical penetration or due to migration processes. This cell lineage might contribute to the release of collagen deposits into the lesion site. Concomitttantly, the astrocytes in the lesion territory change their shape, with strong star-like projections, cellular hypertrophy, and upregulation of glial fibrillary acidic protein (GFAP). The reactive astrocytes tend to form a palisade of cellular constituents destined to shield the wound from the surrounding tissue. This reactive gliosis represents a central cellular element of the scar that emerges upon lesion stimulus (Reier, 1986). Finally, myelin debris of degenerating sheaths litters the lesion zone and was discovered to conceal inhibitory constituents. Thus, one cellular lineage contributing to inhibition of regeneration is the oligodendrocyte that expresses the inhibitory protein Nogo-A, which blocks axon growth by induction of growth cone collapse in a manner dependent on calcium modulation and G-protein activation. An additional inhibitory effect is caused by MAG, an Ig superfamily member contained in adult myelin, and the oligodendrocyte/myelin protein OMPG (Fournier and Strittmater, 2001; McKerracher and Winton, 2002; see also Chapter 37).

Reactive Astrocytes Upregulate Extracellular Matrix Constituents

Independently of myelin, astrocytes also react to lesion of the CNS and form a gliotic scar (Fawcett and Asher, 1999). The reactive astrocyte inhibits neurite outgrowth *in vitro* and *in vivo*. The relevance of cellular components in CNS lesion territories is emphasized by the observation that significant regrowth of axonal connections can be obtained by implanting olfactory ensheathing and other cell types in order to foster axonal growth through lesion structures. Likewise, Schwann cells promote regeneration and are able to span bridge structures in the CNS. The molecular components that underlie the bridge properties are currently unknown, but in this regard a functional effect of ECM cannot be excluded. From this point of view, the ECM might under some circumstances exert positive effects on axon outgrowth. This ambivalence is reflected in various circumstances. Thus, upregulation of chondroitin sulfates in the peripheral nerve, which is able to regenerate, has been observed. In contrast, upregulation of chondroitin sulfate moieties in CNS structures clearly correlates with inhibition of growth in some territories. Numerous studies have emphasized that the reactive astrocytes upregulate CSPGs and keratan sulfate epitopes, and that these components are sufficient to override the beneficial influence of laminin-1, thus impeding the axon growth process. Hence, a potential role of PGs in the adult CNS relates to lesions and the impaired regeneration of axon fibers.

It has recently been proposed that neurons implanted by an atraumatic technique into the corpus callosum can regenerate long fibers in the presence of intact myelin, provided that the fibers escape a ring of reactive astrocytes emerging around the implantation site that express TN-C and CSPGs (Davies et al., 1997). In addition, TN-C is detected in stab wounds of rodent and human CNS, in the tissue of human hippocampal sclerosis, and in hippocampal structures of rodents subject to experimental seizure. Furthermore, the glycoprotein is significantly enhanced in human glial CNS tumors. In view of the numerous effects on axon growth, a functional role in scar tissue seems plausible (Faissner, 1997). These results have strongly stimulated further investigations into the molecular identity of the CSPGs expressed by reactive astrocytes. Using a cell line model system, it was shown that inhibitory activities are associated with NG2, which was identified as one important component in the inhibitory pathway (Fidler et al., 1999). The CSPG NG2 is expressed by a subclass of glial cells, is upregulated in lesions and inhibits neurite outgrowth in several *in vitro* assays (Levine et al., 2001). The functional significance of CSPGs in CNS lesions is highlighted by the observation that axon sprouting and recovery of function are enhanced following treatment with chondroitinase ABC *in vivo* (Moon et al., 2001; Bradbury et al., 2002).

The Mechanisms of Inhibition of Axon Growth May Involve Extracellular Matrix Superstructure

The mechanism of inhibition enacted by CSPGs is not well understood. One possibility is that the purified PGs by themselves have inhibitory properties. In this context, it is significant that indirect evidence for the existence of defined structural motifs in glycosaminoglycan chains of PGs has been obtained. Also, degradation of a CSPG by matrix metalloproteinase-2 neutralizes its inhibitory properties. On the other hand, several reports suggest that the core proteins of PGs as expressed in target cells are able to deter advancing growth cones. Alternatively, one might assume that inhibitory growth cone collapse–inducing components are associated with PG structures. For example, semaphorin proteins contain charged carboxyterminal ends that are well suited to interact with glycosaminoglycans in territories enriched for PGs. Evidence has been reported that netrin gene products bind to PGs, an interaction that might restrict their diffusional capacity *in vivo*. Furthermore, treatment of *ex vivo* CNS tissue slices with high-salt solutions, hyaluronidase, or chondroitinases reduced the inhibitory or antiadhesive properties of otherwise inhospitable sections. These findings are consistent with the view that the emergence of inhibitory properties might result from matrix assembly. Along these lines, recent experiments have documented that interference with basal lamina formation *in vivo* favors the regeneration of the transsected fimbria-fornix system. In this context, collagens have attracted increased attention. Indeed, collagen type IV is the major collageneous component of basal laminae, which seemed to form the obstacle to successful regeneration in that case (Stichel et al., 1999). This raises the question of whether fibrillar collagens are also upregulated by astrocytes, and whether collagen-like gene products of astroglial origin exist.

REFERENCES

Bandtlow, C.E. and Zimmermann, D.R. (2000). Proteoglycans in the developing brain: new conceptual insights for old proteins. *Phys. Rev.* 80:1267–1290.

Bradbury, E.J., Moon, L.D.F., Popat, R.J., King, V.R., Bennett, G.S., Patel, P.N., Fawcett, J.W., and McMahon, S.B. (2002). Chondroitinase ABC promotes functional recovery after spinal cord injury. *Nature* 416:636–640.

Brümmendorf, T. and Rathjen, F.G. (1996). Structure/function relationships of axon-associated adhesion receptors of the immunoglobulin superfamily. *Curr. Opin. Neurobiol.* 6:584–593.

Celio, M.R. and Blümcke, I. (1994). Perineuronal nets—a specialized form of extracellular matrix in the adult nervous system. *Brain Res. Rev.* 19:128–145.

Chung, K.Y., Taylor, J.S., Shurn, D.K., and Chan, S.O. (2000). Axon routing at the optic chiasm after enzymatic removal of chondroitin sulfate in mouse embryo. *Development* 127:2673–2683.

Clement, A.M., Nadanaka, S., Masayama, K., Mandl, C., Sugahara, K., and Faissner, A. (1998). The DSD-1 carbohydrate epitope depends on sulfation, correlates with chondroitin sulfate D motifs, and is sufficient to promote neurite outgrowth. *J. Biol. Chem.* 273:28444–28453.

Davies, S.J.A., Fitch, M.T., Memberg, S.P., Hall, A.K., Raisman, G., and Silver, J. (1997). Regeneration of axons in white matter tracts of the central nervous system. *Nature* 390:680–683.

Dedhar, S. and Hannigan, G.E. (1996). Integrin cytoplasmic interactions and bidirectional transmembrane signalling. *Curr. Opin. Cell Biol.* 8:657–669.

Drescher, U., Bonhoeffer, F., and Müller, B.K. (1997). The Eph family in retinal axon guidance. *Curr. Opin. Neurobiol.* 7:75–80.

Faissner, A. (1997). The tenascin gene family in axon growth and guidance. *Cell Tissue Res.* 290:331–341.

Faissner, A., Clement, A., Lochter, A., Streit, A., Mandl, C., and Schachner, M. (1994) Isolation of a neural chondroitin sulfate proteoglycan with neurite outgrowth promoting properties. *J. Cell Biol.* 126:783–799.

Faissner, A., Heck, N., Dobbertin, A., and Garwood, J. (2004). DSD-1-proteoglycan/phosphacan and receptor protein tyrosine phosphatase-beta isoforms during development and regeneration of neural tissues. In: M. Bähr, ed. *Brain Repair.* Kluwer Academic/ Plenum Publishers, pp. 1–29.

Faissner, A. and Steindler, D. (1995). Boundaries and inhibitory molecules in developing neural tissues. *Glia* 13:233–254.

Fawcett, J.W. (1998). Spinal cord repair: from experimental models to human application. *Spinal Cord* 36:811–817.

Fawcett, J.W. and Asher, R.A. (1999). The glial scar and central nervous system repair. *Brain Res. Bull.* 49:377–391.

Fidler, P.S., Schuette, K., Asher, R.A., Dobbertin, A., Thornton, S.R., Calle-Patino, Y., Muir, E., Levine, J.M., Geller, H.M., Rogers, J.H., Faissner, A., and Fawcett, J.W. (1999). Comparing astrocytic cell lines that are inhibitory or permissive for axon growth: the major axon-inhibitory proteoglycan is NG2. *J. Neurosci.* 19:8778–8788.

Fournier, A.E. and Strittmater, S.M. (2001). Repulsive factors and axon regeneration in the CNS. *Curr. Opin. Neurobiol.* 11:89–94.

Garwood, J., Heck, N., Rigato, F., and Faissner, A. (2001a). The extracellular matrix in neural development, plasticity and regeneration. In: Walz, W., ed. *The Neuronal Microenvironment.* Totowa, NJ: Humana Press, Inc., pp. 109–158.

Garwood, J., Rigato, F., Heck, N., and Faissner, A. (2001b). Tenascin glycoproteins and the complementary ligand DSD-1-PG/ phosphacan—structuring the neural extracellular matrix during development and repair. *Restor. Neurol. Neurosci.* 18:1–14.

Garwood, J., Heck, N., Reichardt, F., and Faissner, A. (2003) Phosphacan short isoform, a novel non-proteoglycan variant of phosphacan/RPTP-β, interacts with neuronal receptors and promotes neurite outgrowth. *J. Biol. Chem.* 278:24164–24173.

Garwood, J., Schnädelbach, O., Clement, A., Schütte, K., Bach, A., and Faissner, A. (1999). DSD-1-proteoglycan is the mouse homolog of phosphacan and displays opposing effects on neurite outgrowth dependent on neuronal lineage. *J. Neurosci.* 19:3888–3899.

Ghose, A. and Van Vactor, D. (2002). GAPs in slit-robo signaling. *BioAssays* 24:401–404.

Goodman, C.S. (1996). Mechanisms and molecules that control growth cone guidance. *Annu. Rev. Neurosci.* 19:341–377.

Götz, B., Scholze, A., Clement, A., Joester, A., Schütte, K., Wigger, F., Frank, R., Spiess, P., Ekblom, P., and Faissner, A. (1996). Tenascin-C contains distinct adhesive, anti-adhesive, and neurite outgrowth promoting sites for neurons. *J. Cell Biol.* 132:681–699.

Granderath, S. and Klämbt, C. (1999). Glia development in the embryonic CNS of *Drosophila. Curr. Opin. Neurobiol.* 5:531–536.

Halfter, W., Dong, S., Schurer, B., Osanger, A., Schneider, W., Ruegg, M., and Cole, G.J. (2000). Composition, synthesis, and assembly of the embyonic chick retinal basal lamina. *Dev. Biol.* 220:111–128.

Harroch, S., Palmeri, M., Rosenbluth, J., Custer, A., Okigaki, M., Shrager, P., Blum, M., Buxbaum, J.D., and Schlessinger, J. (2000). No obvious abnormality in mice deficient in receptor protein tyrosine phosphatase beta. *Mol. Cell. Biol.* 20:7706–7715.

Jacobson, M. (1991). *Developmental Neurobiology*, 3rd ed. New York and London: Plenum Press, pp. 1–776.

Jeffery, G. (2001). Architecture of the optic chiasm and the mechanisms that sculpt its development. *Physiol. Rev.* 81:1393–1414.

Joester, A. and Faissner, A. (1999). Evidence for combinatorial variability of tenascin-C isoforms and developmental regulation in the mouse central nervous system. *J. Biol. Chem.* 24:17144–17151.

Joester, A. and Faissner, A. (2001). Emergence of structural variability of tenascin-C: a member of the tenascin gene family expressed in the nervous system. *Matrix Biol.* 20:13–22.

Kawachi, H., Fujikawa, A., Maeda, N., and Noda, M. (2001). Identification of GIT1/Cat-1 as a substrate molecule of protein tyrosine phosphatase zeta/beta by the yeast substrate-trapping system. *Proc. Natl. Acad. Sci. USA* 98:6593–6598.

Klein, R. (2001). Excitatory Eph receptors and adhesive ephrin ligands. *Curr. Opin. Cell Biol.* 13:196–203.

Klocker, N. and Bähr, M. (2001). Brain repair—new avenues to an old dream? *Trends Neurosci.* 24:3–4.

Kullander, K., Croll, S.D., Zimmer, M., Pan, L., McClain, J., Hughes, V., Zabski, S., DeChiara, T.M., Klein, R., Yancopoulos, G.D., and Gale, N.W. (2001). Ephrin-B3 is the midline barrier that prevents corticospinal tract axons from recrossing, allowing for unilateral motor control. *Genes Dev.* 15:877–888.

Lemke, G. (2001). Glial control of neuronal development. *Annu. Rev. Neurosci.* 24:87–105.

Levine, J.M., Reynolds, R., and Fawcett, J.W. (2001). The oligodendrocyte precursor cell in health and disease. *Trends Neurosci.* 24:39–46.

Liu, B.P. and Strittmatter, S.M. (2001). Semaphorin-mediated axonal guidance via Rho-related G proteins. *Curr. Opin. Cell Biol.* 13: 619–626.

McKerracher, L. and Winton, M.J. (2002). Nogo on the Go. *Neuron* 36:345–348.

Moon L.D., Asher, R.A., Rhodes, K.E., and Fawcett, J.W. (2001). Regeneration of CNS axons back to their target following treatment of adult rat brain with chondroitinase ABC. *Nat. Neurosci.* 4:465–466.

Oohira, A., Matsui, F., Tokita, Y., and Aono, S. (2000). Molecular interactions of neural chondroitin sulfate proteoglycans in the brain development. *Arch. Biochem. Biophys.* 374:24–34.

Pasini, A. and Wilkinson, D.G. (2002). Stabilizing the regionalisation of the developing vertebrate central nervous system. *Bioassays* 24:427–438.

Peles, E., Nativ, M., Campbell, P.L., Sakurai, T., Martinez, R., Lev, S., Clary, D.O., Schilling, J., Barnea, G., Plowman, G.D., Grumet, M., and Schlessinger, J. (1995). The carbonic anhydrase domain of receptor tyrosine phosphatase beta is a functional ligand for the axonal cell recognition molecule contactin. *Cell* 82:251–260.

Pizzorusso, T., Medini, P., Berardi, N., Chierzi, S., Fawcett, J.W., and Maffei, L. (2002). Reactivation of ocular dominance plasticity in the adult visual cortex. *Science* 298:1248–1251.

Ratcliffe, C.F., Qu, Y., McCormick, K.A., Tibbs, V.C., Dixon, J.E.,

Scheuer, T., and Catterall, W.A. (2000). A sodium channel signaling complex: modulation by associated receptor protein tyrosine phosphatase beta. *Nat. Neurosci.* 3:437–444.

Reier, P.J. (1986) Gliosis following CNS injury: the anatomy of glial scars and their influences on axonal elongation. In: Federoff, S. and Vernadakis, A., eds. *Astrocytes*. New York: Academic Press, pp. 263–324.

Rigato, F., Garwood, J., Calco, V., Heck, N., Faivre-Sarrailh, C., and Faissner, A. (2002). Tenascin-C promotes neurite outgrowth of embryonic hippocampal neurons through the alternatively spliced fibronectin type III BD domains via activation of the cell adhesion molecule F3/contactin. *J. Neurosci.* 22:6596–6609.

Rios, J.C., Melendez-Vasquez, C.V., Einheber, S., Lustig, M., Grumet, M., Hemperly, J., Peles, E., and Salzer, J.L. (2000). Contactin-associated protein (Caspr) and contactin form a complex that is targeted to the paranodal junctions during myelination. *J. Neurosci.* 20:8354–8364.

Shu, T. and Richards, L.J. (2001). Cortical axon guidance by the glial wedge during the development of the corpus callosum. *J. Neurosci.* 21:2749–2758.

Stichel, C.C., Hermanns, S., Luhmann, H.J., Lausberg, F., Niermann, H., D'Urso, D., Servos, G., Hartwig, H.G., and Muller, H.W. (1999). Inhibition of collagen IV deposition promotes regeneration of injured CNS axons. *Eur. J. Neurosci.* 11:632–646.

Takeichi, M. (1995). Morphogenetic roles of classic cadherins. *Curr. Opin. Cell Biol.* 7:619–627.

Tessier-Lavigne, M. and Goodman, C.S. (1996). The molecular biology of axon guidance. *Science* 274:1123–1133.

Uemura, T. (1998). The cadherin superfamily at the synapse: more members, more missions. *Cell* 93:1095–1098.

Walsh, F.S. and Doherty, P. (1997). Neural cell adhesion molecules of the immunoglobulin superfamily: role in axon growth and guidance. *Annu. Rev. Cell Biol.* 13:425–456.

Whitford, K.L. and Ghosh, A. (2001). Plexin signaling via off-track and rho family GTPases. *Neuron* 32:1–3.

Wilkinson, D.G. (2001). Multiple roles of EPH receptors and ephrins in neural development. *Nat. Rev. Neurosci.* 2:155–164.

Yamaguchi, Y. (2000). Lecticans: organizers of the brain extracellular matrix. *Cell. Mol. Life Sci.* 57:276–289.

Yamaguchi, Y. (2001). Heparan sulfate proteoglycans in the nervous system: their diverse roles in neurogenesis, axon gidance, and synaptogenesis. *Semin. Cell Dev. Biol.* 12:99–106.

III DISEASE AND NEUROGLIAL CELLS

33 Astrocyte injury

CHRISTOPHER J. FEENEY AND PETER K. STYS

Over the past few decades, a central role for glial cells in the regulation of the extracellular ionic environment has emerged (Walz, 1989). Regulation of activity-dependent (i.e., neuronal) variations in extracellular [K^+] has been described (Newman et al., 1984; Dietzel et al., 1989). In addition, astrocytes are thought to play an essential role in the removal of excitatory amino acids from the synaptic region (Martin, 1995). Thus, glial physiology under normal and pathological states is of great importance to the functionality and stability of the central nervous system (CNS).

A general perception has emerged over the past two decades of research that astrocytes are relatively resistant to insults such as those caused by ischemia [oxygen/glucose deprivation (OGD)], and oxidative stress [e.g., reactive oxygen species (ROS)] damage (Juurlink, 1997; Wilson, 1997). Recent work, however, points to significant astrocyte dysfunction in response to these injuries (Reichert et al., 2001; Jacobson and Duchen, 2002) and to cell death (Fern, 1998). This chapter will focus on the responses of astrocytes to hypoxia/ischemia and trauma.

ASTROCYTES AND STROKE

Cytotoxicity

Numerous studies point to significant insensitivity of astrocytes (*in vitro* and *in vivo*) to stroke-like conditions (Goldberg and Choi, 1993). *In vitro*, a number of studies describe the relative insensitivity to ischemic-like insults of cultured astrocytes. These studies in general use cultured cortical astrocytes derived from fetal or early neonatal stage rodents. The absence of oxygen alone (often termed *in vitro hypoxia*) seems to be rather innocuous to the cultured astrocyte, with cells able to maintain viability for many hours (Goldberg et al., 1987; Yu et al., 1989; Sochocka et al., 1994). Prolonged oxygen deprivation (12–24 hours), however, has an without effect on the cultured astrocyte, as subsequent reoxygenation of cultures leads to pronounced ROS production (Hori et al., 1994), mitochondrial damage (Petito et al., 1991), and cell death (Sochocka et al., 1994).

In vitro studies

Cultured astrocytes can also survive many hours of OGD (often termed *in vitro ischemic* conditions) (Juurlink et al., 1992). Depending on the developmental state of the cells, no significant cell death occurs in astrocyte cultures exposed to OGD for 6–12 hours (Yager et al., 1994). Younger cultures (1 week *in vitro*) were found to be much more resistant to OGD than older astrocyte cultures (3 weeks old). Substrate withdrawal (e.g., elimination of the exogenous glucose source) also leads to relatively slow astrocyte demise. Cultured astrocytes can survive for tens of hours in the absence of glucose when oxygen is present (Yager et al., 1994). Again, immature (younger) astrocyte cultures were found to be more robust than mature (older) cultures. These findings suggest that maturational increases in metabolic rates in the developing brain *in vivo* (Corbett et al., 1993) and increases in oxidative metabolism in astrocytes *in vitro* with increasing age of the culture (Yager et al., 1994) render these cells more susceptible to hypoxic/ischemic damage.

In vivo studies

Studies using *in vivo* models of ischemia are much more varied in their conclusions of astrocyte susceptibility. A number of studies (Kindy et al., 1992; Petito et al., 1998) have shown that only minimal (if any) astrocyte cell death occurs after a transient (e.g., 10 minute) cerebral ischemic insult, an injury sufficient to produces CA1 hippocampal neuronal death by postischemic day 3, but minor or no damage to neurons in other regions (Petito et al., 1998). These studies, however, involved rather brief, transient ischemia and rather select neuronal cell death (Fern, 2001). A more profound insult, such as prolonged (2 hour; Chen et al., 1993) or permanent (Garcia et al., 1993) middle cerebral artery occlusion, leads to rapid and significant astrocyte injury within 30–60 minutes (Fern, 2001), in some cases preceding neuronal demise (Garcia et al., 1993).

See the list of abbreviations at the end of the chapter.

Acute Physiological Changes to Astrocytes in Response to Ischemia/Oxygen-Glucose Deprivation

Increased intracellular Ca^{2+}

Regardless of the ultimate fate of the astrocyte, however, significant alterations in cellular physiology do occur in this cell type in response to ischemic-like conditions. Astrocytes respond to chemical ischemia (glucose withdrawal and mitochondrial inhibition; Silver et al., 1997) and OGD (Duffy and MacVicar, 1996; Fern, 1998) with a rapid and significant increase in cytoplasmic calcium concentration ($[Ca^{2+}]_i$). In the hippocampus, a brief period of OGD causes a rapid and sustained increase in $[Ca^{2+}]_i$ (Fig. 33.1). This increase in $[Ca^{2+}]_i$ was found to be due to both voltage-gated Ca^{2+} influx and release from internal Ca^{2+} stores. Extracellular Ca^{2+} influx via voltage-gated Ca^{2+} channels has also been associated with astrocytic injury during OGD in cultured cortical astrocytes (Haun et al., 1992). Of particular interest is the fact that astrocytes *in situ* respond with a much more profound and sustained increase in $[Ca^{2+}]_i$ than isolated astrocytes from the same preparation, suggesting that neuronal responses during ischemic events can greatly affect the ability of astrocytes to regulate their own $[Ca^{2+}]_i$ adequately (Duffy and MacVicar, 1996).

In rat neonatal white matter, astrocytes appear to be remarkably sensitive to brief periods of OGD. Fern (1998) has shown that fura-2-loaded astrocytes in the very young rat optic nerve respond rapidly (5–10 minutes) with a significant increase in $[Ca^{2+}]_i$, mediated by voltage-gated T-type and L-type Ca^{2+} channel activation. In addition, there is a rapid onset of astrocytic cell death in this model with OGD, occurring as early as 10–20 minutes after the initiation of the ischemic insult (Fig. 33.2).

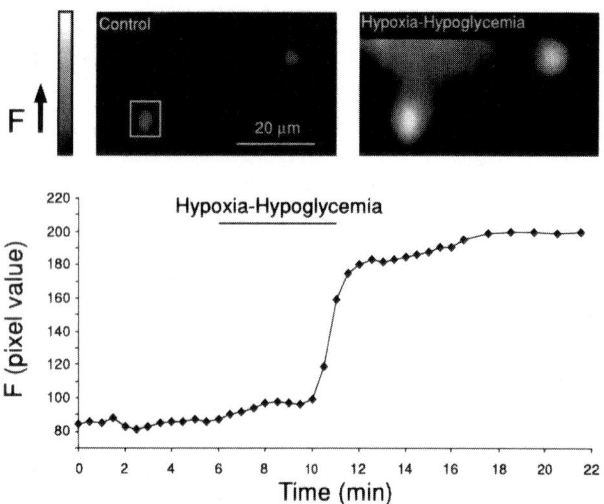

FIGURE 33.1 A brief period (5-minute) of oxygen-glucose deprivation (OGD) (here termed *hypoxia-hypoglycemia*) leads to an abrupt rise of $[Ca^{2+}]_i$ in astrocytes of hippocampal slices. Increases of fluorescence emission from the Ca^{2+}-sensitive marker calcium orange indicate an increase in $[Ca^{2+}]_i$ with OGD. (From Duffy and MacVicar, 1996, with permission. Copyright 1996 by the Society for Neuroscience.)

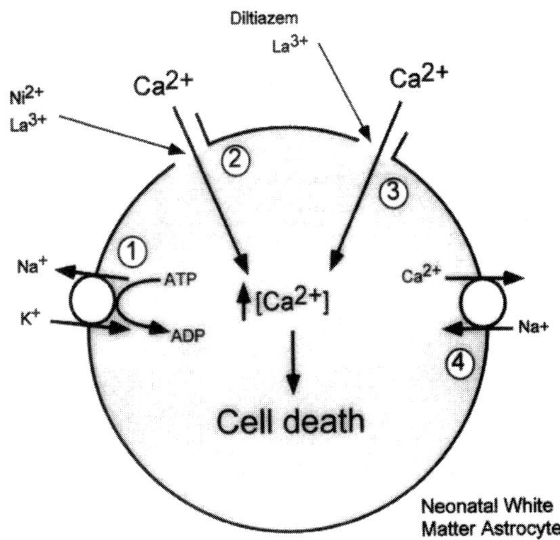

FIGURE 33.2 Oxygen-glucose deprivation leads to decreased levels of adenosine triphosphate (*ATP*) and membrane depolarization (*1*). This would lead to a transient activation of T-type Ca^{2+} channels (*2*) and then a more prolonged activation of L-type Ca^{2+} channels (*3*), leading to sustained elevation in $[Ca^{2+}]_i$ as the Na^+/Ca^{2+} exchanger's Ca extrusion activity declines (*4*). ADP: adenosine diphosphate. (From Fern, 1998, with permission. Copyright 1998 by the Society for Neuroscience.)

Cell swelling

Ischemic-type insults are also accompanied by significant astrocytic swelling. In mouse brain astrocyte cultures exposed to ischemic-like environments, the metabolically challenged cells respond to increases in extracellular K^+ with a rapid water accumulation that is preceded by an energy-independent influx of K^+, Cl^-, and HCO_3^- in response to membrane depolarization (Walz et al., 1993; see Fig. 33.3). These conditions mimic those that the *in vivo* astrocyte would be exposed to, as extracellular $[K^+]$ can rise to 80 mM due to ion released from neighboring tonically depolarized neurons (Nicholson et al., 1978). Astrocytic swelling per se is not lethal for the cells involved, as the reestablishment of normal $[K^+]_o$ results in repolarization of cell membrane. In cultured rat astrocytes the mechanisms of cell swelling may differ from those in their mouse counterparts, and likely involve lactate accumulation in addition to other mechanisms (Kempski et al., 1992).

An old term has lately been reintroduced to the field of astrocyte biology: *clasmatodendrosis*, a term coined by Cajal and first described by Alzheimer as a loss of astrocyte distal processes caused after irreversible in-

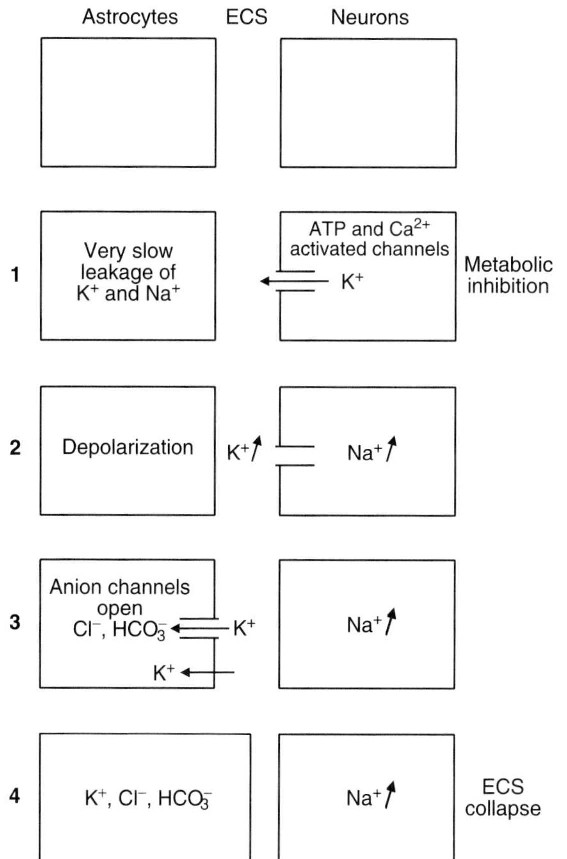

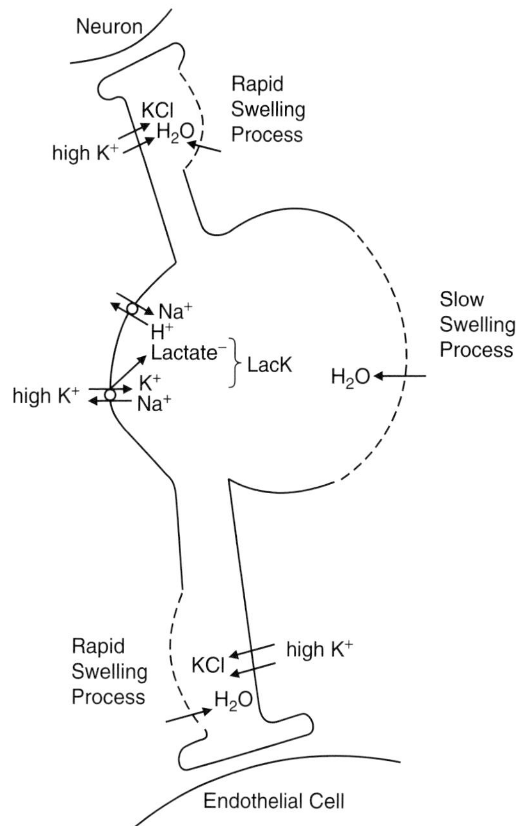

FIGURE 33.3 (*1*) Metabolic inhibition leads to K^+ efflux from neurons to equilibrium with the extracellular fluid; (*2*) increased extracellular K^+ causes astrocyte membrane depolarization, leading to (*3*) opening of anion channels and passive fluxes of K^+, Cl^-, and HCO_3^-; (*4*) finally, water accumulates in astrocytes, causing them to swell, thereby reducing the extracellular space (*ECS*). ATP: adenosine triphosphate. (From Walz et al., 1993, with permission from S. Karger AG, Basel.)

jury (Penfield, 1928). Recently, Kraig and colleagues have elucidated important mechanisms of this phenomenon whereby acidosis and mitochondrial inhibition can lead to irreversible astrocyte injury manifested by rapid process disruption (Hulse et al., 2001). Thus, in response to conditions mimicking those of ischemia/reperfusion, astrocytes can become lethally injured and will undergo clasmatodendrosis.

Glutamate uptake

Glutamate is considered the primary excitatory neurotransmitter in the mammalian CNS (Fonnum, 1984; Rothman and Olney, 1986). Excessive glutamate release, however, is undesirable and has been linked to a number of neurodegenerative processes such as epilepsy, ischemia, and trauma (Rothman and Olney, 1986; Benveniste et al., 1989; McAdoo et al., 1997). Astrocytes both *in vitro* and *in vivo* have been shown to possess high-affinity glutamate transporters, namely, (EAAT1) and EAAT2 [rat homologs glutamate/aspartate transporter (GLAST) and glutamate transporter-1 (GLT-1), respectively; Levy et al., 1993; Rothstein et al., 1994; Swanson et al., 1997], responsible for terminating the excitatory action of this transmitter at postsynaptic sites (Rothstein et al., 1996). Glutamate uptake is an electrogenic process relying on an inwardly directed Na^+ gradient maintained by Na^+/K^+-ATPase in an energy-dependent manner (Storck et al., 1992). Thus, during severe energy deprivation, for example at the core of a severe ischemic lesion or under experimental chemical ischemia induced by a combination of glycolytic (e.g., iodoacetate) and oxidative phosphorylation inhibition (e.g., azide or CN^-), these transporters cease to take up glutamate into astrocytes and may reverse their direction of transport, leading to a further increase in extracellular glutamate concentrations (Swanson, 1992; Longuemare and Swanson, 1995). This will lead to an exaggerated elevation of extracellular glutamate and further drive deleterious excitotoxic processes that have been well documented in neurons.

During sublethal ischemic conditions, the functional status of astrocytic glutamate transporters remains somewhat controversial. Some reports suggest that glutamate transporters in cultured astrocytes exposed to "incomplete" ischemia (chemical hypoxia, acidosis, and raised extracellular K^+) respond with a rapid and substantial reduction in glutamate transport activity (Yu et al., 1989; Swanson, 1992; Huang et al., 1993), even before substantial reductions in cellular adenosine triphosphate (ATP) occurs (Swanson et al., 1997). However, others have reported that experimental ischemic conditions lead to an initial *stimulation* of astrocytic glutamate uptake activity, with profound loss of this activity occurring only after 24 hours of experimental ischemia and being coincident with emerging cell death (Stanimirovic et al., 1997). As well, spinal cord astrocytes at the onset of energy failure can maintain their Na^+ gradient–dependent ion and transmitter buffering capacity by maintaining a relatively low $[Na^+]_i$, despite compromised Na^+/K^+-ATPase activity (Longuemare et al., 1999). In addition to cell type/culturing procedures, these conflicting reports may be attributed to differences in the degree of acidosis experienced by the astrocytes, with decreases in pH leading to a reduction in glutamate uptake (Swanson et al., 1995, 1997). Thus, the extent of the ischemia experienced by the astrocytes and the precise environment the cells are exposed to will likely influence the activity of their glutamate transporter activity.

Moreover, glutamate influx per se is not without deleterious consequences for astrocytes. Bender et al. (1998) showed that glutamate can induce swelling in cultured rat cortical astrocytes. The mechanism appears to involve glutamate-stimulated K^+ uptake through activation of Na^+/K^+-ATPase (Pellerin and Magistretti, 1994; Bender et al., 1998). Prolonged glutamate exposure has been shown to induce astrocytic cell death primarily through a reduction of glutathione content and subsequent oxidative stress (Chen et al., 2000).

Reactive oxygen species

Free radicals (FRs) are highly reactive physiological metabolites, the production of which is greatly increased during hypoxia-reoxygenation (Flamm et al., 1978; Perez Velazquez et al., 1997) and some neurodegenerative diseases (Beal, 1995; Dugan et al., 1995). Recent observations implicate FR-initiated oxidative stress as a key step in excitotoxic neurodegeneration, whereas excitotoxic Ca^{2+} elevations may not be toxic when FR formation is prevented (Dubinsky et al., 1995; Patel et al., 1996). Free radical formation in neurons associated with ischemic challenges has been shown to result from glutamate-dependent elevations of intracellular Ca^{2+}, leading to mitochondrial Ca^{2+} uptake (Dugan et al., 1995; Reynolds and Hastings, 1995; Perez Velazquez et al., 1997; Frantseva et al., 2001). Sustained elevation of intracellular Ca^{2+} mediated by activation of voltage-gated Ca^{2+} currents and release from intracellular stores has been demonstrated in astrocytes subjected to ischemic injury (see above; Duffy and MacVicar, 1996; Fern, 1998). Moreover, increased Ca^{2+} deposits were observed within mitochondria of astrocytes after ischemia *in vivo* (Dux et al., 1987), indicating that hypoxic $[Ca^{2+}]_i$ elevations are sufficient to load glial mitochondria with this ion, a condition that appears to be associated with excessive FR generation by neuronal mitochondria (Dugan et al., 1995; Reynolds and Hastings, 1995). Interestingly, hypoxia-induced Ca^{2+} elevation in astrocytes of the hippocampal slice were higher than that of their acutely dissociated counterparts, suggesting the possible involvement of neuronal factors in postischemic astrocyte physiology (Duffy and MacVicar, 1996). Taken together, these findings suggest that FR generation might occur in glia due to ischemia-reperfusion injury and might contribute to glial/neuronal impairment.

It is generally accepted that astrocytes are more resistant to oxidative damage than neurons. Indeed, glia were reported to contain less polyunsaturated lipids than neurons (O'Brien and Sampson, 1965) and hence are presumably less sensitive to FR-induced lipid peroxidation. Cultured astrocytes from several different species have also been found to contain high concentrations (compared to their neuronal counterparts) of antioxidants/antioxidant enzymes (vitamin E, ascorbate, glutathione) (Raps et al., 1989; Makar et al., 1994, Huang and Philbert, 1995). These observations have been interpreted as evidence that astrocytes play an important role in antioxidative processes in the brain (Makar et al., 1994). Desagher et al. (1996) have reported that astrocytes were neuroprotective against hydrogen peroxide (H_2O_2) neurotoxicity in mouse striatal cultures and are themselves highly resistant to H_2O_2-induced injury. The protective effect of astrocytes was ascribed to their ability to remove H_2O_2 from the culture medium. In addition, astrocytes have been shown to be much more resistant to oxidative stress induced by peroxynitrite (Bolanos et al., 1995) and glutamate (Oka et al., 1993) than oligodendrocytes or neurons. It is suggested that the greater resistance of cultured astrocytes to FR-induced oxidative stress derives from their low iron and high glutathione content/glutathione peroxidase activity (Huang and Philbert, 1995; Wilson, 1997; Juurlink et al., 1998).

Astrocytes are, of course, not completely invulnerable to the effects of oxidative stress, and important cellular functions have been shown to be negatively affected under these conditions. As described above, astrocytes play a pivotal role in limiting neuronal exposure to extracellular glutamate via the activity of their high-affinity glutamate transporters. Evidence suggests that oxidative stress induced by reactive oxygen species can inhibit astrocytic glutamate transporters (Volterra et al., 1994).

Astrocytes respond to oxidative stress with an increase in $[Ca^{2+}]_i$ (Robb et al., 1999) and a loss of mitochondrial membrane potential ($\Delta\Psi_M$), the principal parameter that controls oxidative phosphorylation (Feeney et al., 1998; Robb et al., 1999; Nicholls and Ward, 2000). The increase in $[Ca^{2+}]_i$ was shown not to be necessary for the occurrence of mitochondrial dysfunction, nor did its elimination (by chelation) prevent astrocytic demise (Robb et al., 1999). Recently, however, a pathological interplay between ROS production and Ca^{2+} release from internal stores has been shown in cultured astrocytes. Increases in mitochondrial ROS production were found to lead to increases in endoplasmic reticulum (ER) Ca^{2+} release, and to subsequent mitochondrial Ca^{2+} loading and dysfunction (depolarization) in adult rat astrocytes (Jacobson and Duchen, 2002). These events were found to be transient in nature and innocuous to the cells unless coupled with a background of oxidative stress, where continued ROS production and subsequent Ca^{2+} release from stores will lead to sustained mitochondrial depolarization through the induction of the mitochondrial permeability transition (MPT; Fig. 33.4). The authors suggest that very local increases in Ca^{2+} concentration, at sites of ER/mitochondrial contact shown in other cell types (Rizzuto et al., 1998), could lead to this destructive cycle of Ca^{2+} release, mitochondrial Ca^{2+} loading, and further ROS production leading to progressive mitochondrial potential collapse and necrotic cell death (Jacobson and Duchen, 2002).

Mitochondrial dysfunction

Oxygen-glucose deprivation is known to induce rapid and significant mitochondrial dysfunction in neuronal cell types. For example, in both acute hippocampal slices (Bahar et al., 2000) and hippocampal slice cultures (Perez Velazquez et al., 2000), CA1 pyramidal neurons rapidly lose their mitochondrial potential, $\Delta\Psi_M$. While prolonged exposure to oxygen and substrate deprivation must inevitably lead to mitochondrial dysfunction, conflicting evidence exists concerning the early responses (if any) of astrocytic mitochondria to OGD. Recently, Almeida et al. (2002) have shown that OGD does not induce free radical production or decrease reduced nicotine adenine dinucleotide (NADPH) (critical in the maintenance of reduced glutathione levels in the cell) in cortical astrocyte cultures, whereas the same insult does so in neuronal cultures. In addition, the authors report no loss of $\Delta\Psi_M$ or ATP depletion during a 1-hour OGD exposure of their astrocyte cultures.

Conversely, Reichert et al. (2001) have shown that *both* cultured neurons *and* astrocytes rapidly lose (45–60 minutes) their mitochondrial potential when exposed to OGD. A caveat here is that the astrocytes were cocultured with neurons, although astrocytes cultured alone

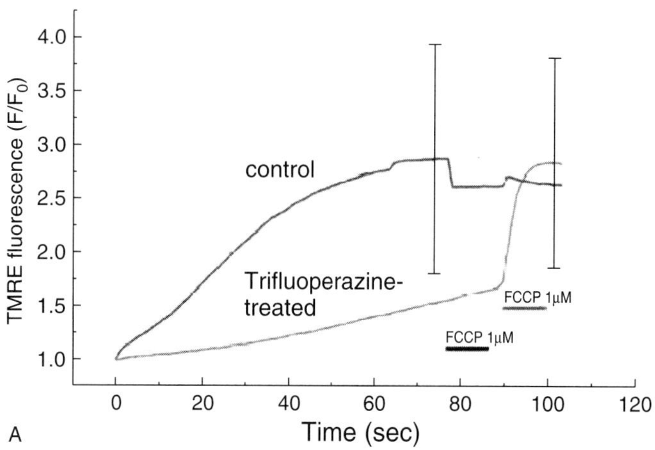

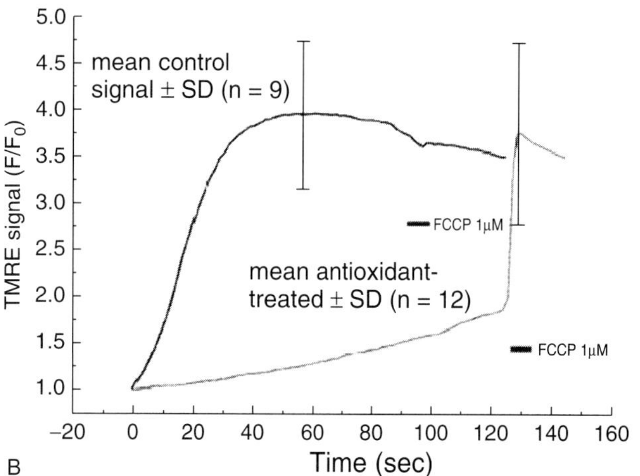

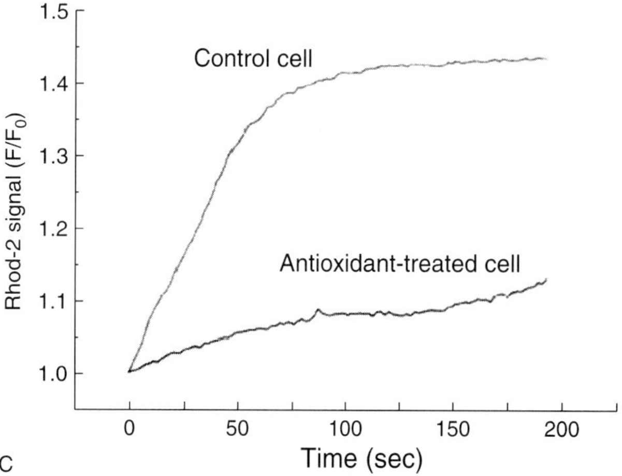

FIGURE 33.4 Astrocyte mitochondrial status followed with fluorescent dyes TMRE [mitochondrial membrane potential ($\Delta\Psi_M$); *A,B*] and rhod-2 (mitochondrial $[Ca^{2+}]$). Antioxidants (*A*, ascorbic acid, catalase, Trolox, and TEMPO) and the mitochondrial permeability transition inhibitor trifluoperazine (*B*) were both able to reduce the rate of "global" mitochondrial depolarization. (*C*) Reactive oxygen species–induced mitochondrial Ca^{2+} loading was inhibited with antioxidants. (From Jacobson and Duchen, 2002, with permission from The Company of Biologists Ltd, Cambridge.)

showed massive $\Delta\Psi_M$ loss at 90 minutes of OGD (see Fig. 33.5). This rapid mitochondrial dysfunction was found to be related to the induction of MPT, as cyclosporin A partially protected astrocytes against $\Delta\Psi_M$ loss. Likewise, Feeney et al. (1999) have also found that OGD results in a rapid loss of $\Delta\Psi_M$ in astrocytes of hippocampal slice cultures. Here, it was found that cyclosporin A completely eliminated this rapid loss of astrocytic $\Delta\Psi_M$. It is interesting that astrocytes that find themselves amid neurons (e.g., cocultures or slice cultures) respond to OGD with a more profound mitochondrial dysfunction than astrocytes in isolation.

Whether or not these differences in astrocytic response are a result of differential culturing environments, or a synergistic interaction between astrocytes and neurons leading to heightened astrocytic sensitivity, remains to be firmly established.

Astrocytes and Traumatic Injury

The proliferation and hypertrophy of astrocytes in response to a traumatic CNS injury have been well documented (Hatten et al., 1991; Norton et al., 1992). Recent work on the posttraumatic responses of astrocytes has illustrated their primary importance in the maintenance of the extracellular ionic microenvironment of the CNS. Using an *in vitro* injury to induce reactive-type astrocyte proliferation, MacFarlane and Sontheimer (1997) have shown that there is a rapid (within hours of injury) switch from inwardly rectifying to outwardly rectifying K^+ channel expression. These findings, if translatable to the *in vivo* situation, would suggest that reactive astrocytes have a diminished capacity to buffer extracellular K^+ transients effectively. These findings parallel those of D'Ambrosio et al. (1999) in an *in vivo* model of traumatic brain injury. In this study, a fluid percussion injury was followed by hippocampal isolation days later, which showed significant reactive gliosis. Here too, reactive astrocytes of the hippocampus showed significant depression of inwardly rectifying K^+ currents. Thus, reactive astrocytes might possess a significantly lower ability to passively regulate $[K^+]_o$ in the injured CNS, thereby exacerbating secondary injury processes that have been found to be associated with traumatic brain injury.

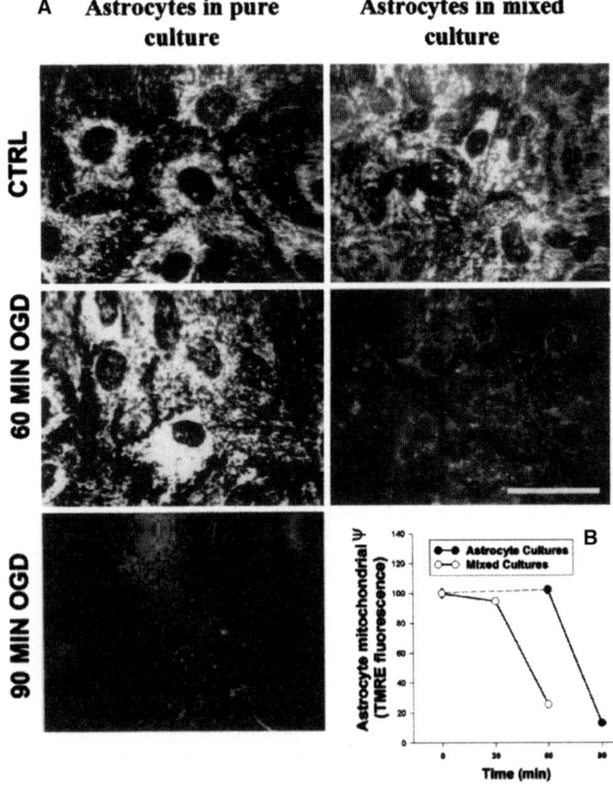

FIGURE 33.5 Cortical astrocytes in pure cultures and cocultures with neurons lose mitochondrial potential in response to oxygen-glucose deprivation (OGD). Note that here decreases in TMRE reflect loss of $\Delta\Psi_M$, as opposed to increases in TMRE fluorescence, indicating the same in Jacobson and Duchen (2002; see Fig. 33.4). This is a result of the image acquisition rate differences, and both findings are consistent with loss of mitochondrial membrane potential ($\Delta\Psi_M$). (From Reichert et al., 2001, with permission. Copyright 2001 by the Society for Neuroscience.)

Conversely, increases in the expression of L-type Ca^{2+} channels after traumatic brain injury have been noted in reactive astrocytes (Westenbroek et al., 1998). This upregulation was specific for the L-type channel, as reactive astrocytes failed to express N-type Ca^{2+} channels, and it was suggested that this increase in Ca^{2+} channel density might enhance the astrocytic Ca^{2+} buffering capacity and might also be involved in a Ca^{2+}-dependent cascade of signals leading to the release of neurotrophic factors (Vaca and Wendt, 1992; Westenbroek et al., 1998).

Plasma albumin has been shown to lead to substantial and sustained elevations of $[Ca^{2+}]_i$ in cultured astrocytes (Nadal et al., 1997). It was found that the Ca^{2+} wave initiated had a greater amplitude, and spread to coupled cells to a much greater extent, than that caused by glutamate application. Application of plasma albumin was also found to cause astrocyte mitosis *in vitro* (Nadal et al., 1995). If these findings can be extended to the *in vivo* situation, a breech in the blood–brain barrier during CNS trauma could lead to increases in Ca^{2+} of astrocyte syncytium, with implications for the extension of glial scars.

CONCLUSION

Given the importance of astrocyte functioning to the microenvironment of the CNS, it is apparent that alterations in their physiology during pathological states (such as ischemia and traumatic brain injury) could have profound implications for the progression of these insults. Future clinical interventions may address more specifically the enhancement of astrocytic viability in an effort to reduce the extent of neuropathological correlates.

ABBREVIATIONS

$\Delta\Psi_M$	mitochondrial membrane potential
CN^-	cyanide
ER	endoplasmic reticulum
FR	free radicals
H_2O_2	hydrogen peroxide
MPT	mitochondrial permeability transition
OGD	oxygen-glucose deprivation
ROS	reactive oxygen species

REFERENCES

Almeida, A., Delgado-Esteban, M., Bolanos, J.P., and Medina, J.M. (2002) Oxygen and glucose deprivation induces mitochondrial dysfunction and oxidative stress in neurones but not in astrocytes in primary culture. *J. Neurochem.* 81(2):207–217.

Bahar, S., Fayuk, D., Somjen, G.G., Aitken, P.G., and Turner, D.A. (2000) Mitochondrial and intrinsic optical signals imaged during hypoxia and spreading depression in rat hippocampal slices. *J. Neurophysiol.* 84(1):311–324.

Beal, M.F. (1995) Aging, energy and oxidative stress in neurodegenerative diseases. *Ann. Neurol.* 38:357–366.

Bender, A.S., Schousboe, A., Reichelt, W., and Norenberg, M.D. (1998) Ionic mechanisms in glutamate-induced astrocyte swelling: role of K^+ influx. *J. Neurosci. Res.* 52(3):307–321.

Benveniste, H., Jorgensen, M.B., Sandberg, M., Christensen, T., Hagberg, H., and Diemer, N.H. (1989) Ischemic damage in hippocampal CA1 is dependent on glutamate release and intact innervation from CA3. *J. Cereb. Blood Flow Metab.* 9(5): 629–639.

Bolanos, J.P., Heales, S.J., Land, J.M., and Clark, J.B. (1995) Effect of peroxynitrite on the mitochondrial respiratory chain: differential susceptibility of neurones and astrocytes in primary culture. *J. Neurochem.* 64(5):1965–1972.

Chen, C.J., Liao, S.L., and Kuo, J.S. (2000) Gliotoxic action of glutamate on cultured astrocytes. *J. Neurochem.* 75(4):1557–1565.

Chen, H., Chopp, M., Schultz, L., Bodzin, G., and Garcia, J.H. (1993) Sequential neuronal and astrocytic changes after transient middle cerebral artery occlusion in the rat. *J. Neurol. Sci.* 118(2): 109–106.

Corbett, R.J., Laptook, A.R., Garcia, D., and Ruley, J.I. (1993) Energy reserves and utilization rates in developing brain measured in vivo by ^{31}P and ^{1}H nuclear magnetic resonance spectroscopy. *J. Cereb. Blood Flow Metab.* 13(2):235–246.

D'Ambrosio, R., Maris, D.O., Grady, M.S., Winn, H.R., and Janigro, D. (1999) Impaired K^+ homeostasis and altered electrophysiological properties of post-traumatic hippocampal glia. *J. Neurosci.* 19(18):8152–8162.

Desagher, S., Glowinski, J., and Premont, J. (1996) Astrocytes protect neurons from hydrogen peroxide toxicity. *J. Neurosci.* 16(8): 2553–2562.

Dietzel, I., Heinemann, U., and Lux, H.D. (1989) Relations between slow extracellular potential changes, glial potassium buffering, and electrolyte and cellular volume changes during neuronal hyperactivity in cat brain. *Glia* 2(1):25–44.

Dubinsky, J.M., Kristal, B.S., and Elizondo-Fournier, M. (1995) An obligate role for oxygen in the early stages of glutamate-induced, delayed neuronal death. *J. Neurosci.* 15(11):7071–7078.

Duffy, S. and MacVicar, B.A. (1996) In vitro ischemia promotes calcium influx and intracellular calcium release in hippocampal astrocytes. *J. Neurosci.* 16(1):71–81.

Dugan, L.L., Sensi, S.L., Canzoniero, L.M., Handran, S.D., Rothman, S.M., Lin, T.S., Goldberg, M.P., and Choi, D.W. (1995) Mitochondrial production of reactive oxygen species in cortical neurons following exposure to *N*-methyl-D-aspartate. *J. Neurosci.* 15(10):6377–6388.

Dux, E., Mies, G., Hossmann, K.A., and Siklos, L. (1987) Calcium in the mitochondria following brief ischemia of gerbil brain. *Neurosci. Lett.* 78(3):295–300.

Feeney, C.J., Frantseva, M.V., Carlen, P.L., and Pennefather, P.S. (1998) Hydrogen peroxide induced toxicity in cultured rat hippocampal astrocytes. *Soc. Neurosci. Abstr.*

Feeney, C.J., Frantseva, M.V., Carlen, P.L., and Pennefather, P.S. (1999) Free radicals are produced in astrocytes of hippocampal slice cultures subjected to hypoxic injury. *J. Neurochem.* 73:S72.

Fern, R. (1998) Intracellular calcium and cell death during ischemia in neonatal rat white matter astrocytes in situ. *J. Neurosci.* 18(18): 7232–7243.

Fern, R. (2001) Ischemia: astrocytes show their sensitive side. *Prog. Brain Res.* 132:405–411.

Flamm, E.S., Demopoulos, H.B., Seligman, M.L., Posner, R.G., and Ranschott, J. (1978) Free radicals in cerebral ischemia. *Stroke* 9:445–447.

Fonnum, F. (1984) Glutamate: a neurotransmitter in mammalian brain. *J. Neurochem.* 42(1):1–11.

Frantseva, M.V., Carlen, P.L., and Perez Velazquez, J.L. (2001) Dynamics of intracellular calcium and free radical production during ischemia in pyramidal neurons. *Free Radical Biol. Med.* 31(10):1216–1227.

Garcia, J.H., Yoshida, Y., Chen, H., Li, Y., Zhang, Z.G., Lian, J., Chen, S., and Chopp, M. (1993) Progression from ischemic injury to infarct following middle cerebral artery occlusion in the rat. *Am. J. Pathol.* 142(2):623–635.

Goldberg, M.P. and Choi, D.W. (1993) Combined oxygen and glucose deprivation in cortical cell culture: calcium-dependent and calcium-independent mechanisms of neuronal injury. *J. Neurosci.* 13(8):3510–3524.

Goldberg, M.P., Weiss, J.H., Pham, P.C., and Choi, D.W. (1987) *N*-methyl-D-aspartate receptors mediate hypoxic neuronal injury in cortical culture. *J. Pharmacol. Exp. Ther.* 243(2):784–791.

Hatten, M.E., Liem, R.K., Shelanski, M.L., and Mason, C.A. (1991) Astroglia in CNS injury. *Glia* 4(2):233–243.

Haun, S.E., Murphy, E.J., Bates, C.M., and Horrocks, L.A. (1992) Extracellular calcium is a mediator of astroglial injury during combined glucose-oxygen deprivation. *Brain Res.* 593(1):45–50.

Hori, O., Matsumoto, M., Maeda, Y., Ueda, H., Ohtsuki, T., Stern, D.M., Kinoshita, T., Ogawa, S., and Kamada, T. (1994) Metabolic and biosynthetic alterations in cultured astrocytes exposed to hypoxia/reoxygenation. *J. Neurochem.* 62(4):1489–1495.

Huang, J. and Philbert, M.A. (1995) Distribution of glutathione and glutathione-related enzyme systems in mitochondria and cytosol of cultured cerebellar astrocytes and granule cells. *Brain Res.* 680(1–2):16–22.

Huang, R., Shuaib, A., and Hertz, L. (1993) Glutamate uptake and glutamate content in primary cultures of mouse astrocytes during anoxia, substrate deprivation and simulated ischemia under normothermic and hypothermic conditions. *Brain Res.* 618(2):346–351.

Hulse, R.E., Winterfield, J., Kunkler, P.E., and Kraig, R.P. (2001) Astrocytic clasmatodendrosis in hippocampal organ culture. *Glia* 33(2):169–179.

Jacobson, J. and Duchen, M.R. (2002) Mitochondrial oxidative stress and cell death in astrocytes—requirement for stored Ca^{2+} and sustained opening of the permeability transition pore. *J. Cell Sci.* 115:1175–1188.

Juurlink, B.H. (1997) Response of glial cells to ischemia: roles of reactive oxygen species and glutathione. *Neurosci. Biobehav. Rev.* 21(2):151–166.

Juurlink, B.H., Hertz, L., and Yager, J.Y. (1992) Astrocyte maturation and susceptibility to ischaemia or substrate deprivation. *NeuroReport* 3(12):1135–1137.

Juurlink, B.H., Thorburne, S.K., and Hertz, L. (1998) Peroxide-scavenging deficit underlies oligodendrocyte susceptibility to oxidative stress. *Glia* 22(4):371–378.

Kempski, O., Staub, F., Schneider, G.H., Weigt, H., and Baethmann, A. (1992) Swelling of C6 glioma cells and astrocytes from glutamate, high K^+ concentrations or acidosis. *Prog. Brain Res.* 94:69–75.

Kindy, M.S., Bhat, A.N., and Bhat, N.R. (1992) Transient ischemia stimulates glial fibrillary acid protein and vimentin gene expression in the gerbil neocortex, striatum and hippocampus. *Brain Res. Mol. Brain Res.* 13:199–206.

Levy, L.M., Lehre, K.P., Rolstad, B., and Danbolt, N.C. (1993) A monoclonal antibody raised against an $[Na^+ + K^+]$ coupled L-glutamate transporter purified from rat brain confirms glial cell localization. *FEBS Lett.* 317(1–2):79–84.

Longuemare, M.C., Rose, C.R., Farrell, K., Ransom, B.R., Waxman, S.G., and Swanson, R.A. (1999) K^+-induced reversal of astrocyte glutamate uptake is limited by compensatory changes in intracellular Na^+. *Neuroscience* 93(1):285–292.

Longuemare, M.C. and Swanson, R.A. (1995) Excitatory amino acid release from astrocytes during energy failure by reversal of sodium-dependent uptake. *J. Neurosci. Res.* 40(3):379–386.

MacFarlane, S.N. and Sontheimer, H. (1997) Electrophysiological changes that accompany reactive gliosis in vitro. *J. Neurosci.* 17(19):7316–7329.

Makar, T.K., Nedergaard, M., Preuss, A., Gelbard, A.S., Perumal, A.S., and Cooper, A.J.L. (1994) Vitamin E, ascorbate, glutathione disulfide, and enzymes of glutathione metabolism in cultures of chick astrocytes and neurons: evidence that astrocytes play an important role in antioxidative processes in the brain. *J. Neurochem.* 62:45–53.

Martin, D.L. (1995) The role of glia in the inactivation of neurotransmitters. In: Kettenmann, H. and Ransom, B.R., eds. *Neuroglia.* New York: Oxford University Press, pp. 732–745.

McAdoo, D.J., Hughes, M.G., Xu, G.Y., Robak, G., and de Castro, R., Jr. (1997) Microdialysis studies of the role of chemical agents in secondary damage upon spinal cord injury. *J. Neurotrauma* 14(8):507–515.

Nadal, A., Fuentes, E., Pastor, J., and McNaughton, P.A. (1995) Plasma albumin is a potent trigger of calcium signals and DNA synthesis in astrocytes. *Proc. Natl. Acad. Sci. USA* 92(5):1426–1430.

Nadal, A., Fuentes, E., Pastor, J., and McNaughton, P.A. (1997) Plasma albumin induces calcium waves in rat cortical astrocytes. *Glia* 19(4):343–351.

Newman, E.A., Frambach, D.A., and Odette, L.L. (1984) Control of extracellular potassium levels by retinal glial cell K^+ siphoning. *Science* 225(4667):1174–1175.

Nicholls, D.G. and Ward, M.W. (2000) Mitochondrial membrane potential and neuronal glutamate excitotoxicity: mortality and millivolts. *Trends Neurosci.* 23(4):166–174.

Nicholson, C., ten Bruggencate, G., Stockle, H., and Steinberg, R. (1978) Calcium and potassium changes in extracellular microenvironment of cat cerebellar cortex. *J. Neurophysiol.* 41(4):1026–1039.

Norton, W.T., Aquino, D.A., Hozumi, I., Chiu, F.C., and Brosnan, C.F. (1992) Quantitative aspects of reactive gliosis: a review. *Neurochem. Res.* 17(9):877–885.

O'Brien, J.S. and Sampson, E.L. (1965) Fatty acid and fatty aldehyde composition of the major brain lipids in normal human grey matter, white matter, and myelin. *J. Lipid Res.* 6(4):545–551.

Oka, A., Belliveau, M.J., Rosenberg, P.A., and Volpe, J.J. (1993) Vulnerability of oligodendroglia to glutamate: pharmacology, mechanisms, and prevention. *J. Neurosci.* 13(4):1441–1453.

Patel, M., Day, B.J., Crapo, J.D., Fridovich, I., and McNamara, J.O. (1996) Requirement for superoxide in excitotoxic cell death. *Neuron* 16:345–355.

Pellerin, L. and Magistretti, P.J. (1994) Glutamate uptake into astrocytes stimulates aerobic glycolysis: a mechanism coupling neuronal activity to glucose utilization. *Proc. Natl. Acad. Sci. USA* 91(22):10625–10629.

Penfield, W. (1928) Neuroglia and microglia—the interstitial tissue of the central nervous system. In: Cowdry, E.V., ed. *Special Cytology: The Form and Function of the Cell in Health and Disease.* New York: Hoeber, pp. 1033–1068.

Perez Velazquez, J.L., Frantseva, M.V., and Carlen, P.L. (1997) *In vitro* ischemia promotes glutamate-mediated free radical generation and intracellular calcium accumulation in hippocampal pyramidal neurons. *J. Neurosci.* 17(23):9085–9094.

Perez Velazquez, J.L., Frantseva, M.V., Huzar, D.V., and Carlen, P.L. (2000) Mitochondrial porin required for ischemia-induced mitochondrial dysfunction and neuronal damage. *Neuroscience* 97(2):363–369.

Petito, C.K., Juurlink, B.H., and Hertz, L. (1991) In vitro models differentiating between direct and indirect effects of ischemia on astrocytes. *Exp. Neurol.* 113(3):364–372.

Petito, C.K., Olarte, J.P., Roberts, B., Nowak, T.S. Jr., and Pulsinelli, W.A. (1998) Selective glial vulnerability following transient global ischemia in rat brain. *J. Neuropathol. Exp. Neurol.* 57(3):231–238.

Raps, S.P., Lai, J.C.K., Hertz, L., and Cooper, A.J.L. (1989) Glutathione is present in the high concentrations in cultured astrocytes, but not in cultured neurons. *Brain Res.* 493:398–401.

Reichert, S.A., Kim-Han, J.S., and Dugan, L.L. (2001) The mitochondrial permeability transition pore and nitric oxide synthase mediate early mitochondrial depolarization in astrocytes during oxygen-glucose deprivation. *J. Neurosci.* 21(17):6608–6616.

Reynolds, I.J. and Hastings, T.G. (1995) Glutamate induces the production of reactive oxygen species in cultured forebrain neurons following NMDA receptor activation. *J. Neurosci.* 15:3318–3327.

Rizzuto, R., Pinton, P., Carrington, W., Fay, F.S., Fogarty, K.E., Lifshitz, L.M., Tuft, R.A., and Pozzan, T. (1998) Close contacts with the endoplasmic reticulum as determinants of mitochondrial Ca^{2+} responses. *Science* 280(5370):1763–1766.

Robb, S.J., Robb-Gaspers, L.D., Scaduto, R.C., Jr., Thomas, A.P., and Connor, J.R. (1999) Influence of calcium and iron on cell death and mitochondrial function in oxidatively stressed astrocytes. *J. Neurosci. Res.* 55(6):674–686.

Rothman, S.M. and Olney, J.W. (1986) Glutamate and the pathophysiology of hypoxic—ischemic brain damage. *Ann. Neurol.* 19(2):105–111.

Rothstein, J.D., Dykes-Hoberg, M., Pardo, C.A., Bristol, L.A., Jin, L., Kuncl, R.W., Kanai, Y., Hediger, M.A., Wang, Y., Schielke, J.P., and Welty, D.F. (1996) Knockout of glutamate transporters reveals a major role for astroglial transport in excitotoxicity and clearance of glutamate. *Neuron* 16(3):675–686.

Rothstein, J.D., Martin, L., Levey, A.I., Dykes-Hoberg, M., Jin, L., Wu, D., Nash, N., and Kuncl, R.W. (1994) Localization of neuronal and glial glutamate transporters. *Neuron* 13(3):713–725.

Silver, I.A., Deas, J., and Erecinska, M. (1997) Ion homeostasis in brain cells: differences in intracellular ion responses to energy limitation between cultured neurons and glial cells. *Neuroscience* 78(2):589–601.

Sochocka, E., Juurlink, B.H., Code, W.E., Hertz, V., Peng, L., and Hertz, L. (1994) Cell death in primary cultures of mouse neurons and astrocytes during exposure to and "recovery" from hypoxia, substrate deprivation and simulated ischemia. *Brain Res.* 638(1–2):21–28.

Stanimirovic, D.B., Ball, R., and Durkin, J.P. (1997) Stimulation of glutamate uptake and Na,K-ATPase activity in rat astrocytes exposed to ischemia-like insults. *Glia* 19(2):123–134.

Storck, T., Schulte, S., Hofmann, K., and Stoffel, W. (1992) Structure, expression, and functional analysis of a Na(+)-dependent glutamate/aspartate transporter from rat brain. *Proc. Natl. Acad. Sci. USA* 89(22):10955–10959.

Swanson, R.A. (1992) Astrocyte glutamate uptake during chemical hypoxia in vitro. *Neurosci. Lett.* 147(2):143–146.

Swanson, R.A., Farrell, K., and Simon, R.P. (1995) Acidosis causes failure of astrocyte glutamate uptake during hypoxia. *J. Cereb. Blood Flow Metab.* 15(3):417–424.

Swanson, R.A., Farrell, K., and Stein, B.A. (1997) Astrocyte energetics, function, and death under conditions of incomplete ischemia: a mechanism of glial death in the penumbra. *Glia* 21(1): 142–153.

Vaca, K. and Wendt, E. (1992) Divergent effects of astroglial and microglial secretions on neuron growth and survival. *Exp. Neurol.* 118(1):62–72.

Volterra, A., Trotti, D., Tromba, C., Floridi, S., and Racagni, G. (1994) Glutamate uptake inhibition by oxygen free radicals in rat cortical astrocytes. *J. Neurosci.* 14:2924–2932.

Walz, W. (1989) Role of glial cells in the regulation of the brain ion microenvironment. *Prog. Neurobiol.* 33(4):309–333.

Walz, W., Klimaszewski, A., and Paterson, I.A. (1993) Glial swelling in ischemia: a hypothesis. *Dev. Neurosci.* 15:216–225.

Westenbroek, R.E., Bausch, S.B., Lin, R.C., Franck, J.E., Noebels, J.L., and Catterall, W.A. (1998) Upregulation of L-type Ca^{2+} channels in reactive astrocytes after brain injury, hypomyelination, and ischemia. *J. Neurosci.* 18(7):2321–2334.

Wilson, J.X. (1997) Antioxidant defense of the brain. a role for astrocytes. *Can. J. Physiol. Pharmcol.* 75:1149–1163.

Yager, J.Y., Kala, G., Hertz, L., and Juurlink, B.H. (1994) Correlation between content of high-energy phosphates and hypoxic-ischemic damage in immature and mature astrocytes. *Dev. Brain Res.* 82(1–2):62–68.

Yu, A.C., Gregory, G.A., and Chan, P.H. (1989) Hypoxia-induced dysfunctions and injury of astrocytes in primary cell cultures. *J. Cereb. Blood Flow Metab.* 9(1):20–28.

34 Oligodendrocyte and Schwann cell injury

JENNIFER K. NESS AND MARK P. GOLDBERG

Oligodendrocytes and Schwann cells are responsible for synthesis and maintenance of myelin in the central nervous system (CNS) and peripheral nervous system (PNS), respectively, and therefore are critical for function in health and disease. Damage to myelin is a common feature in many neurological disorders, leading to delayed or blocked axonal conduction, secondary damage to axons, and possible permanent neurological dysfunction. There is growing recognition that oligodendrocytes and Schwann cells are uniquely vulnerable to a number of injury mechanisms.

White matter injury contributes to disability in ischemic, traumatic, immune, infectious, metabolic, and hereditary disorders. Although the etiologies and pathological features of these diseases vary widely, several common injury processes have been identified in CNS and PNS white matter damage. Such cellular injury is easily established in cell culture systems. In animal disease models, whether the primary target of injury is the myelin-forming cell or the myelin itself remains an important question. This chapter reviews molecular mechanisms leading to death in oligodendrocyte and Schwann cell lineages, including pathways triggered by oxidative stress, excitotoxicity, inflammatory mediators, and trophic factor deprivation. This chapter also considers cell-cell interactions involved in white matter damage and the implications for clinical outcomes as well as potential avenues of treatment.

CLINICAL SETTINGS OF OLIGODENDROCYTE AND SCHWANN CELL INJURY

The diversity of diseases involving myelin or myelin-forming cells is impressive. Conditions such as multiple sclerosis and inherited leukodystrophies are widely considered specific for myelin, although recent evidence shows that axon cylinders are also affected. In contrast, involvement of white matter in ischemia, perinatal injury, trauma, and Alzheimer's disease typically occurs in the setting of simultaneous injury to neurons in the gray matter. Several of these conditions are described below. Our intent is not to identify every disorder that includes white matter damage, but to highlight similarities and differences among a few representative conditions.

Demyelinating Diseases

Inflammatory immune responses that target white matter are causes of demyelinating diseases including multiple sclerosis in the CNS and Guillain-Barré syndrome and variants in the PNS. Multiple sclerosis is an idiopathic disorder in which autoimmune attack causes transient or permanent loss of myelin sheaths within focal brain and spinal cord plaques (Martin et al., 1992; Noseworthy, 1999; Keegan and Noseworthy, 2002). Similar pathological patterns are observed following active or passive immunization in animal models of experimental allergic encephalomyelitis (EAE). Recent evidence makes it clear that multiple sclerosis pathology is not purely demyelinating; substantial loss of axons may also occur (Raine and Cross, 1989). Multiple sclerosis is well recognized as an autoimmune process initiated by T lymphocytes and inflammatory responses to oligodendrocyte-specific antigens, including myelin basic protein and myelin oligodendroglial glycoprotein. However, it remains to be established whether the oligodendrocyte or the myelin sheath is the primary target of injury. While active proliferation of oligodendroglia lineage cells contributes to remyelination in many active lesions, there is also considerable evidence showing dying or absent oligodendrocytes, sometimes in the same lesions (Dowling et al., 1997; Mews et al., 1998; for review see Bruck et al., 2003). Inflammatory demyelinating polyneuropathies, such as Guillain Barré syndrome, are characterized by multifocal demyelination of peripheral nerves and nerve roots (Winer, 2001). In these diseases there is also clear evidence of immune responses to peripheral myelin components. Patients with demyelinating inflammatory neuropathies have circulating antibodies to Schwann cells (Kwa et al.,

See the list of abbreviations at the end of the chapter.

2003), but it has not been determined whether Schwann cells represent primary targets for injury in these conditions. Numerous pathogenic mechanisms have been shown to contribute to injury in demyelinating diseases. Oligodendrocytes in culture and experimental models are vulnerable to apoptosis initiated by cytokine activation of cell surface death receptor signaling pathways (see below) and to injury mediated by acute toxic pathways involving reactive oxygen species or glutamate excitotoxicity.

Inherited Leukodystrophies and Neuropathies

Most leukodystrophies are inborn metabolic defects that result in destruction or failed development of central myelin (Berger et al., 2001). The pathological mechanisms and clinical progression of specific hereditary leukodystrophies can vary greatly. Metabolic storage disorders reflect deficiencies in lipid metabolism, leading to abnormal accumulation of lipids and fatty acids. For example, metachromatic leukodystrophy is an autosomal recessive disorder caused by mutation of the enzyme arylsulfatase A, leading to intralysosomal accumulation of sulfated glycolipids. Since these sphingolipids are found mainly in myelin membranes, the disease primarily affects the oligodendrocytes (Berger et al., 2001). In contrast, Pelizaeus-Merzbacher disease and X-linked spastic paraplegia type 2 constitute a range of X-linked diseases caused by mutations of the gene encoding proteolipid protein, a major structural component of myelin (Schiffmann and Boespflug-Tanguy, 2001; Koeppen and Robitaille, 2002). In human disease and animal models, these mutations result in deficiency of mature myelin and oligodendrocyte apoptosis; it is interesting that they are also associated with focal axonal swelling (Griffiths et al., 1998; Bjartmar et al., 1999). In the PNS, several different gene defects result in polyneuropathies with demyelinating features; for example, mutations in connexin 32, peripheral myelin protein 22, and myelin protein zero are all associated with various forms of Charcot-Marie-Tooth hereditary neuropathies (Snipes and Orfali, 1998). Metabolic regulation of lipids and the successful myelination of axons are essential functions of the oligodendrocyte and the Schwann cell, as mutations in the regulation of these processes lead to severe CNS dysfunction and often result in premature death.

Cerebral Ischemia

Ischemic stroke in adults has an incidence of approximately 150–400 in 100,000 with a mortality rate of approximately 25%, making it the third leading cause of death in industrialized countries (American Heart Association, 2003). Stroke is caused by a transient or permanent lack of cerebral blood flow to the affected region, resulting in energy depletion due to lack of oxygen and glucose in the tissue and disruption of glutamate and ion homeostasis. The complex series of events that evolve following an ischemic insult include brain edema, excitotoxicity, calcium overload, production of oxygen free radicals, and infiltration of inflammatory cells, all of which contribute to the initial necrosis at the ischemic core and the secondary tissue damage in the penumbra (for review see Dirnagl et al., 1999). Although the traditional view of ischemia is that it is primarily a gray matter insult of neurons, recent data indicate that oligodendrocytes can be equally vulnerable to ischemic insults *in vivo* (Pantoni et al., 1996; Petito et al., 1998). In the human, almost half of the cortical volume is white matter, and cortical strokes result in infarction of as much white as gray matter (Miller et al., 1980). It is not known why tissue hypoxia from carbon monoxide intoxication results in selective white matter injury (Ginsberg et al., 1974; Penney, 1990).

Recent evidence also indicates that mature oligodendrocytes are vulnerable to mediators of stroke damage including excitotoxicity, free radicals, and oxygen/glucose deprivation, as well as the inflammatory responses described above.

Traumatic Brain and Spinal Cord Injury

Spinal cord traumatic damage involves two stages of injury: the initial mechanical tissue destruction and secondary exacerbated tissue loss from physiological and biochemical changes, including local loss of the blood supply (for review see Young, 1993; Dumont et al., 2001). In experimental animal models, white matter damage and oligodendrocyte apoptosis occur during the initial and secondary tissue loss, while neuronal death is primarily restricted to the gross lesion area (Beattie et al., 2000). Local loss of myelin in surviving nerve fiber bundles often occurs at the site of the spinal cord lesion, leading to additional disruption of neuronal function (Schwab and Bartholdi, 1996; Kakulas, 1999). Poor myelination of axons persists long after experimental or human spinal cord injury, suggesting that prevention of secondary white matter damage and oligodendrocyte apoptosis may improve the clinical outcome (Blight, 1985; Bunge et al., 1993). Oligodendrocyte apoptosis is also found in traumatic brain injury (Raghupathi et al., 2000). An important component of the secondary tissue loss is elevation of extracellular glutamate to levels that are toxic to both oligodendrocytes and neurons (Rosenberg et al., 1999a).

Perinatal Brain Injury

White matter damage in the premature infant is the predominant form of brain injury during the perinatal period. The common pathology is termed *periventricular leukomalacia* (PVL), consisting of both focal periventricular necrosis and more diffuse cerebral white matter injury (Volpe, 1997). In addition to cerebral hypoxia-ischemia, there is a strong association with maternal intrauterine infection (Dammann and Leviton, 1997), suggesting that inflammatory or cytokine responses may contribute to the white matter pathology. While the premature brain lacks myelinated axons, immature oligodendrocytes are particularly vulnerable to damage at this stage of development (Volpe, 1997).

The selective vulnerability of pro-oligodendrobasts is a fundamental issue for the preferential white matter damage (PVL) that occurs following perinatal hypoxia-ischemia. The developmental period most vulnerable to PVL in human is 23 to 32 weeks of gestation, which coincides with the pro-oligodendrobast stage of development in the premature white matter (Back et al., 2001). In addition, developing cells in the oligodendrocyte lineage are more sensitive than mature oligodendrocytes to oxygen/glucose deprivation (Fern and Moller, 2000), kainate-induced cell death, and oxidative stress (Back et al., 1998). In animal models, preferential loss of the pro-oligodendroblast occurs during perinatal hypoxia-ischemia and during *in vitro* oxygen and glucose deprivation, which is also glutamate-dependent (Fern and Moller, 2000; Follett et al., 2000; Back et al., 2002). The developmental differences that enhance the vulnerability of premyelinating oligodendroglial cells to oxidative stress, glutamate, and potentially inflammatory mediators are not yet understood, but may provide keys to understanding oligodendrocyte sensitivity to injury in general.

COMMON INJURY PATHWAYS AND MOLECULAR MECHANISMS

Types of Oligodendrocyte Cell Death

Oligodendrocyte cell death can follow necrotic, apoptotic, or hybrid pathways. In general, features of necrotic cell death include loss of cell membrane integrity, rapid organelle swelling, mitochondrial failure, and energy depletion. Apoptotic features include nuclear condensation, intranucleosomal DNA cleavage, and membrane blebbing. Apoptotic death often follows activation of caspase-mediated cascades through the release of cytochrome c from the mitochondria and activation of caspase-9, or via death receptor–induced activation of caspase-8 that may or may not involve the mitochondria. In hybrid cell death, cells present features of both apoptosis and necrosis, which is hypothesized to result from the initiation of apoptosis followed by energy failure and necrotic mitochondrial and plasma membrane rupture (Martin et al., 1998). It is important to recognize that these cell death types are based primarily on morphological classifications that may not be helpful in understanding mechanisms of injury. Accordingly, in experiments involving oligodendrocyte lineage cells, the type of cell death observed following a given insult is often found to depend on experimental conditions, the intensity of the insult, and the oligodendrocyte maturational stage. Therefore the following discussion of the mechanisms of oligodendrocyte injury will identify common cellular and molecular pathways involved in oligodendrocyte damage without focusing on a necrotic or apoptotic structural classification.

Vulnerability to Reactive Oxygen Species

Oligodendrocytes appear to be especially sensitive to damage from reactive oxygen species (Kim and Kim, 1991; Hollensworth et al., 2000). Cellular reactive oxygen species include free radicals (such as superoxide, hydroxyl radical, nitric oxide, and peroxynitrite) and peroxides (such as hydrogen peroxide). The brain is inherently vulnerable due to its high level of oxidative metabolism; continuous production of free radicals requires specific defense pathways for detoxification. Oxidative stress is greatly increased during anaerobic respiration that occurs during ischemia and reperfusion, and is a major factor in both adult and neonatal ischemia (Bromont et al., 1989; Ikeda et al., 1999). Oxidative stress is also recognized as an important mechanism in inflammatory conditions contributing to central myelin damage (Smith et al., 1999) and peripheral nerve injury (Miinea et al., 2002; Vincent et al., 2002).

Oligodendroglial lineage cells appear to be selectively vulnerable to oxidative damage *in vitro*. Oxidative damage ensues when the cellular free radical scavenging mechanisms, which normally remove the low levels free radicals produced during normal mitochondrial respiration, fail to compensate for increased production of reactive oxygen species following damage (Fig. 34.1). During oxidative metabolism, superoxide normally produced by mitochondrial electron transport is converted to hydrogen peroxide and oxygen by superoxide dismutase. Hydrogen peroxide can be enzymatically reduced to water by catalase or by glutathione peroxidase, which requires reduced glutathione. Cellular reactive oxygen species are also reduced by nonenzymatic scavengers including reduced glutathione, α-nicotinamide adenine dinucleotide phosphate (NADPH), vitamin C, and vitamin E. When hypoxia or inflammation triggers increased levels of reactive oxygen species, overload of antioxidant defense systems leads to destructive free radical reactions including lipid peroxidation, oxidation of nucleic acids,

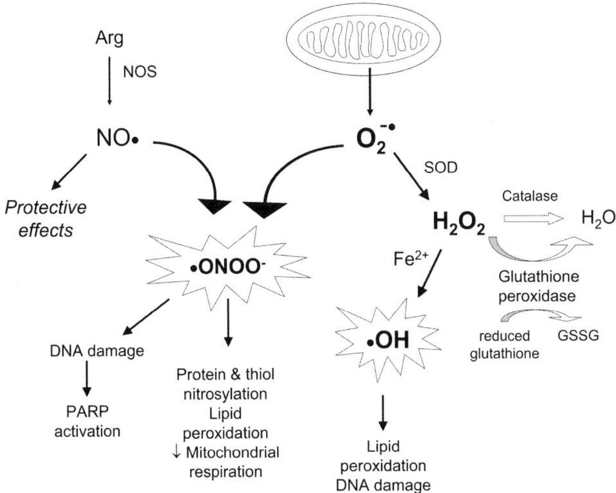

FIGURE 34.1 Schematic of the general mechanisms of reactive oxygen species production and the by-products of oxidative damage. See text for description. GSSG: oxidized glutathione; H_2O_2: hydrogen peroxide; NO: nitric oxide; NOS: nitric oxide synthase; $O_2^{\cdot -}$: superoxide; ·OH: hydroxyl radical; ·$ONOO^-$: peroxynitrate; SOD: superoxide dismutase.

and secondary production of highly toxic reactive compounds including peroxynitrate and hydroxyl radicals.

There are several reasons why oligodendroglial lineage cells may be particularly vulnerable to reactive oxygen species: lower capacity to scavenge free radicals, high iron content, and extensive lipid membranes that are a primary target of free radicals (Kim and Kim, 1991; Thorburne and Juurlink, 1996). Furthermore, production of lipids during myelination requires peroxisome activity and the generation of hydrogen peroxide, increasing the oxidative load of the cells. Comparisons of oligodendrocyte lineage cells and other glial cells have suggested that oligodendrocytes have substantially lower contents of glutathione, as well as lower enzyme activities of glutathione reductase and glutathione (Thorburne and Juurlink, 1996; Juurlink et al., 1998). On the other hand, a recent report found increased peroxide scavenging capability in mature oligodendrocytes compared other glial cells in culture (Hirrlinger et al., 2002). The extent of oligodendrocyte antioxidant defenses may depend on measurement techniques or culture conditions. Vulnerability to oxidative stress is also highly dependent on the stage of the oligodendrocyte lineage. In primary cultures, pro-oligodendroblast cells appear to be most vulnerable to depletion of intracellular glutathione and oxidative stress-induced death (Back et al., 1998).

High levels of intracellular iron in oligodendrocytes also increase their vulnerability to the conversion of hydrogen peroxide to the highly reactive hydroxyl radical by the Fenton reaction (Thorburne and Juurlink, 1996; Kress et al., 2002). Oligodendrocytes have less ability than astrocytes to repair oxidative damage of the mitochondrial DNA (Hollensworth et al., 2000) and are sensitive to the lipid peroxidation by-product 4-hydroxynonenal, which increases in the white matter following ischemia and kills oligodendrocytes *in vitro* (McCracken et al., 2000).

The role of reactive nitrogen species in damage to oligodendrocytes is less clear, as nitric oxide can have both damaging and beneficial effects on cells. Nitric oxide is produced from L-arginine by the family of nitric oxide synthases (Fig. 34.1). Although not highly toxic alone, nitric oxide can react rapidly with superoxide, forming the reactive species peroxynitrite. Peroxynitrite can nitrosylate thiols and proteins, induce lipid peroxidation, and inhibit enzymes such as protein kinase C and enzymes involved in mitochondrial respiration, as well as antioxidant enzymes including catalase and glutathione peroxidase. Peroxynitrite can also cause DNA single-strand breaks and activate poly(ADP-ribose polymerase (PARP), which depletes adenosine 5′-triphosphate (ATP) stores in the cell. On the other hand, nitric oxide can have beneficial effects, including the ability to block chain radical reactions and anti-inflammatory effects on immune cells. The beneficial effects of nitric oxide are evident in the increased severity of demyelination in experimental allergic encephalomyelitis (EAE) models with mice lacking inducible nitric oxygen synthase (iNOS) (Arnett et al., 2002).

Production of nitric oxide in the nervous system in response to inflammation is primarily due to the induction of iNOS expression, which is upregulated in astrocytes, microglia, and inflammatory cells in part by pro-inflammatory cytokines. Cytokine induction of iNOS activity has also been identified in an oligodendrocyte cell line, but the expression of the NOS family in primary oligodendroglial cells is conflicting (Bhat et al., 1999; Hewett et al., 1999). The cytokines tumor necrosis factor-α (TNF-α) and interferon-γ (IFN-γ) also induce nitric oxide production in an immortal Schwann cell clone (Nagano et al., 2001). While nitric oxide can be toxic to cultured oligodendrocytes and axons in isolated optic nerve, nitric oxide also has protective effects that are dependent on the redox state of the cell (Mitrovic et al., 1995; Rosenberg et al., 1999b; Garthwaite et al., 2002). Microglial-induced lysis of oligodendrocytes is associated with increased nitric oxide production (Merrill et al., 1993). Increased nitric oxide is also associated with demyelination in EAE and experimental allergic neuritis (EAN) animals, and protein nitrosylation is evident in the plaques of multiple sclerosis patients, suggesting that reactive nitrogen species are also involved in oligodendrocyte damage *in vivo*. Overall, the beneficial or detrimental impact of nitric oxide in the course of disease progression appears to depend on the site of action, that is, inflammatory cells versus oligodendrocytes, and production of toxic by-products such as peroxynitrate (Willenborg et al., 1999).

Therapies designed to prevent oxidative and nitrative damage in ischemia and the demyelinating EAE model have produced beneficial effects, although the direct effects of antioxidant therapies on oligodendrocyte survival are difficult to ascertain. Intravenous administration of the antioxidant ebselen reduced damage to oligodendrocytes following ischemia (Imai et al., 2001). In the EAE and EAN demyelinating models for the CNS and PNS, respectively, reduction of superoxide and nitric oxide formation reduces the clinical symptoms of the disease (for review see Smith et al., 1999). In addition, uric acid, which is a scavenger of peroxynitrite and other reactive species, reduced clinical symptoms of EAE (Hooper et al., 1998). Importantly, the beneficial effects of antioxidant therapies may be dependent on maturational differences in the endogenous antioxidant mechanisms of the CNS. Although overexpression of superoxide dismutase provides neuroprotection from ischemia in adults, in neonatal animals overexpression may exacerbate the damage (Ferriero, 2001). Further *in vivo* studies on oligodendroglial survival following antioxidant therapies are needed to determine the direct effects of oxidative damage to oligodendroglial cells during CNS injury.

Excitotoxicity

Cell death mediated by overactivation of glutamate receptors, or excitotoxicity, is a well-defined mechanism contributing to neuronal death in many acute and chronic disorders. Recent evident indicates that excitotoxic mechanisms can also contribute to oligodendrocyte injury. Oligodendrocytes in culture and *in vivo* express functional subunits of the 2-amino-3-(3-hydroxymethylisoxazole-4-yl)propionic acid (AMPA) and kainate classes of glutamate receptor (for review see Gallo and Ghiani, 2000). Initial cell culture studies defining oligodendrocyte sensitivity to glutamate demonstrated that glutamate-mediated cell death of oligodendrocyte lineage cells is elicited by activation of either AMPA or kainate receptors, but not by *N*-methyl-D-aspartic acid (NMDA) or metabotropic glutamate receptors, in a dose-dependent manner (Fig. 34.2) (Yoshioka et al., 1995; Matute et al., 1997; McDonald et al., 1998). Furthermore, AMPA receptor blockade prevents hypoxic injury of oligodendrocytes in cell culture (McDonald et al., 1998; Fern and Moller, 2000; Yoshioka et al., 2000) and in CNS slice preparations (Li and Stys, 2000; Tekkök and Goldberg, 2001), indicating that excitotoxicity represents an endogenous mechanism of oligodendrocyte death. Excitotoxicity plays a significant role in oligodendrocyte death *in vivo* as well. Administration of AMPA receptor antagonists reduces white matter injury in models of spinal cord trauma (Wrathall et al., 1994; Rosenberg et al., 1999a), EAE (Pitt et al., 2000; Smith et al., 2000), spinal ischemia (Kanellopoulos et al., 2000), and focal cerebral ischemia in mature (McCracken et al., 2002) and in neonatal animals (Follett et al., 2000).

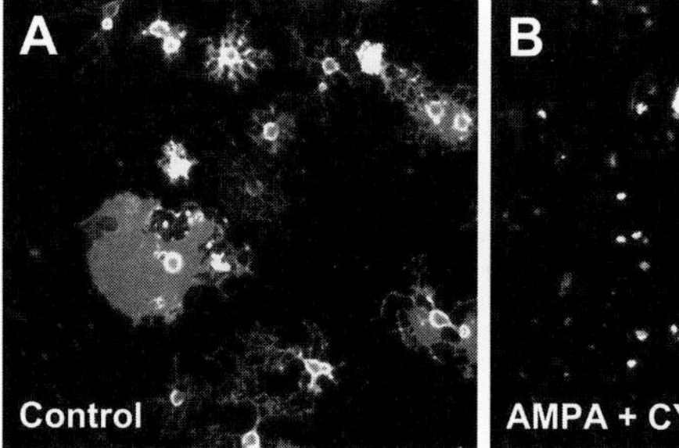

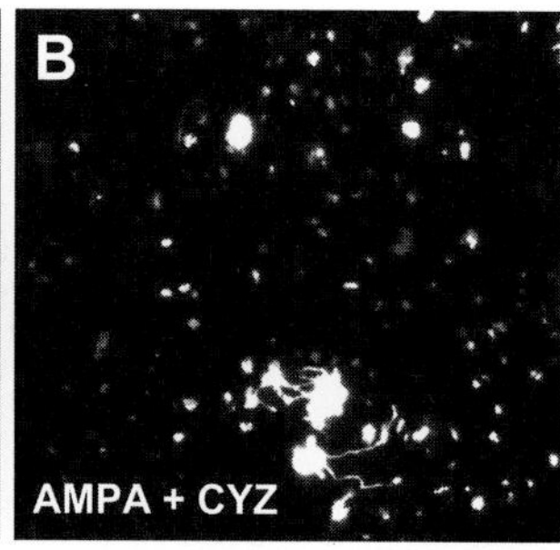

FIGURE 34.2 Excitatory amino acid–induced toxicity in mature oligodendrocytes. Mixed glial cultures were exposed to control conditions (*A*) or to glutamate receptor activation (*B*) 300 μM AMPA, with addition of 30 μM cyclothiazide (*CYZ*) to block AMPA receptor desensitization) for 2 hours followed by 22 hours of recovery. Oligodendrocytes are identified by immunofluorescence with the O1 antibody. (Contributed by Suzanne Underhill.)

Glutamate toxicity of oligodendrocyte lineage cells is mediated by Ca^{2+} influx. Removal of calcium from the media greatly reduces the cell death from both AMPA and kainate toxicity (Matute et al., 1997; Sanchez-Gomez and Matute, 1999), and calcium imaging studies show consistent $[Ca^{2+}]_i$ elevation upon AMPA or kainate exposure (Holzwarth et al., 1994; McDonald et al., 1998). Further demonstration of the essential role of Ca^{2+} influx in glutamate-mediated toxicity in oligodendrocyte lineage cells was provided by studies showing that cyclic adenosine monophosphate (cAMP)–elevating agents prevent kainate excitotoxicity by decreasing Ca^{2+} influx through the non-NMDA glutamate receptors (Yoshioka et al., 1998). There are several potential routes of calcium entry into oligodendrocytes following glutamate receptor activation (Fig. 34.3). Both the plasma membrane Na^+-Ca^{2+} exchanger and voltage-gated Ca^{2+} channels contribute to the total amplitude of Ca^{2+} current triggered by activation of the respective glutamate receptors, but Ca^{2+} influx through AMPA or kainate receptors alone is sufficient to initiate cell death in oligodendrocytes (Alberdi et al., 2002).

The intracellular mechanisms of oligodendroglial cell death from excitotoxicity are not fully identified. Death of cultured oligodendrocytes has been measured by lactic dehydrogenase (LDH) release, DNA fragmentation, and caspase-3 activation (Yoshioka et al., 1995, 1998; McDonald et al., 1998; Ness and Wood, 2002), and mitochondrial dysfunction and generation of ROS has also been identified (Sanchez-Gomez, et al., 2003). Comparison of AMPA sensitivity in immature oligo-

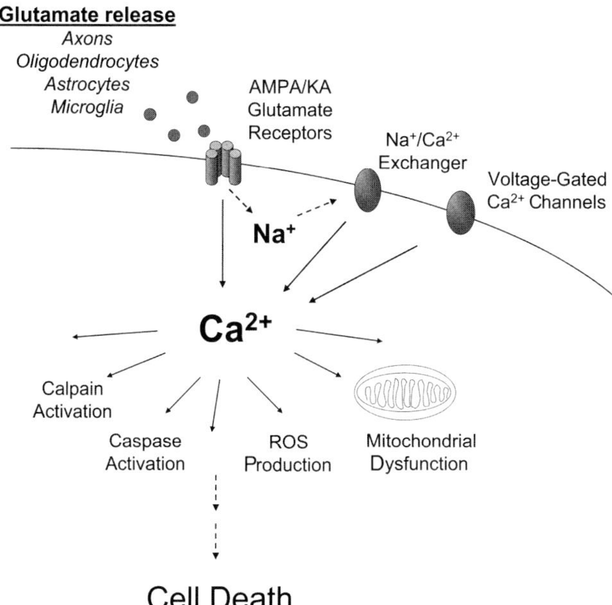

FIGURE 34.3 Schematic of glutamate-induced calcium influx and potential mediators of damage in oligodendroglial cells. See text for description. AMPA: α amino-3-hydroxy-5-methylisoxazole-4-propionic acid; KA: kainic acid; ROS: reactive oxygen species.

dendrocytes relative to the early progenitors demonstrated a greater influx of Ca^{2+} and a prolonged elevation of $[Ca^{2+}]_i$ in immature oligodendrocytes, followed by an earlier collapse of the mitochondrial membrane potential (Itoh et al., 2000). These data suggest that compromised mitochondria and a reduced capacity to buffer calcium may increase vulnerability to excitotoxicity in oligodendroglial cells. Furthermore, oligodendrocyte death by excitotoxicity can be mediated by caspase-dependent and -independent mechanisms, indicating that multiple death pathways may be initiated following glutamate receptor activation (Sanchez-Gomez, et al., 2003).

Immune-Mediated Injury

Myelin damage in the CNS and PNS is frequently associated with immune and inflammatory disorders. Oligodendrocyte and Schwann cell injury may be mediated by cytokines, antibody, complement, or specific activation of death receptors Immune cells, microglia, and reactive astrocytes are all sources of cytokines in the damaged CNS. The direct roles of immune mediators in the death of oligodendrocytes are complex, since the sensitivity of oligodendrocytes to immune-mediated damage may be dependent on the maturational stage of oligodendrocytes, and on the concentrations and interactions between cytotoxic mediators (Table 34.1). Studies on animal models increase in complexity due to the multiple effects immune mediators have on the effector inflammatory cells as well as the target oligodendrocytes. For example, effects of the cytokine TNF-α on oligodendrocytes in culture have been reported to induce apoptosis (Louis et al., 1993; Hisahara et al., 1997), necrosis (Selmaj and Raine, 1988), sublethal injury, or no effect at all (Merrill and Benveniste, 1996). Other groups determined that TNF-α can induce death of mature, but not immature, oligodendrocytes at high concentrations (Cammer and Zhang, 1999). Also, TNF-α may have a regenerative role following white matter damage (Arnett et al., 2001). The discrepancy between the destructive and protective actions of TNF-α may be due to the expression and activity of receptor subtypes. Tumor ne-

TABLE 34.1 *Summary of Data on Inflammatory Mediators of Oligodendrocytes and Schwann Cell Damage*

	Effects on Oligodendrocytes	*Effects on Schwann Cells*	*References*
TNF-α	+/−	+/−	Cammer and Zhang (1999), D'Souza et al. (1995), Gold et al. (1995), Louis et al. (1993), Mithen et al. (1990), Robbins et al. (1987), Selmaj and Raine (1988)
IFN-γ	+/−	+	Baerwald and Popko (1998), Conti et al. (2002), Gold et al. (1995), Pouly et al. (2000b)
Fas	+	−	Casha et al. (2001), Li et al. (2002), Wohlleben et al. (2000)
NGF (via p75)	+/−	+/−	Beattie et al. (2002), Casaccia-Bonnefil et al. (1996), Cosgaya et al. (2002), Hirata et al. (2001), Ladiwala et al. (1998)
NO	+/−	+/−	Gold et al. (1996), Merrill et al. (1993), Mitrovic et al. (1994), (1995), Nagano et al. (2001)
Antibody/Complement	++	+/−	Dashiell et al. (2000), Johns and Bernard (1997), Piddlesden and Morgan (1993), Sawant-Mane et al. (1994), Scolding et al. (1989)
Perforin	++	o	Scolding et al. (1990), Zeine et al. (1998)

Most data are obtained in cell culture models. ++, consistent evidence of toxicity; +, damage but not death; +/−, results range from death to no/positive effect; −, not involved in toxicity; 0, unknown effects.

IFN-γ: interferon-γ; NGF: nerve growth factor; NO: nitric oxide; TNF-α: tumor necrosis factor-α.

crosis factor receptor-1 (TNFR-1) is believed to mediate cell death, while TNFR-2 activation promotes cell growth and proliferation (Ashkenazi and Dixit, 1999; Weiss et al., 1998).

Interferon-γ (IFN-γ) is potentially cytotoxic to oligodendrocytes, especially in combination with other immune mediators. The effects of IFN-γ on oligodendrocytes in culture are similar to those of TNF-α, and can cause apoptosis in oligodendrocyte progenitors but necrosis in mature cells (Baerwald and Popko, 1998). Tumor necrosis factor-α is capable of potentiating the effects of IFN-γ, and IFN-γ can upregulate TNF receptor expression (Andrews et al., 1998). In addition, IFN-γ upregulates Fas on the cell surface, which can be activated by Fas ligand expressed by immune cells (Pouly et al., 2000b). Fas upregulation in oligodendrocytes is seen in multiple sclerosis plaques and following spinal cord injury, which coincides with Fas ligand upregulation on microglia and macrophages, potentially increasing the vulnerability to Fas-mediated apoptosis (Pouly et al., 2000a; Casha et al., 2001).

Other members of the TNF-α death receptor family also induce death in oligodendroglial cells. Activation of the low-affinity nerve growth factor (NGF) receptor p75 was shown to induce apoptosis in mature rodent oligodendrocytes, which could be prevented by the survival signaling induced by coexpression of TrkA, the high-affinity receptor for NGF (Casaccia-Bonnefil et al., 1996). ProNGF induced p75-mediated apoptosis in cultured oligodendrocytes, and absence of p75 reduced the number of apoptotic oligodendrocytes following spinal cord injury (Beattie et al., 2002). However, activation of p75 by NGF did not induce death in cultures of human (Ladiwala et al., 1998). Another death receptor, tumor necrosis factor–related apoptosis-inducing ligand (TRAIL), was recently identified to induce apoptosis in human oligodendrocytes in culture, which was enhanced by pretreatment with IFN-γ (Matysiak et al., 2002).

Complement and antibody damage myelin and mediate oligodendrocyte injury and lysis *in vitro*. Oligodendrocytes are especially susceptible to complement membrane attack complexes due to the lack of expression of the complement inhibitor CD59 on the cell surface and direct activation of complement through binding to the cell surface protein myelin oligodendrocyte glycoprotein (MOG) (Piddlesden and Morgan, 1993; Johns and Bernard, 1997). Antibody and complement also have sublytic effects on oligodendrocytes including changes in calcium influx and effects on cell surfaces membranes (Scolding et al., 1989; Dyer and Benjamins, 1990). In addition, the binding of antibody and complement to oligodendrocytes activates the classical opsonizing function that induces phagocytosis of the cells by macrophages (Scolding and Compston, 1991). *In vivo*, complement and antibody-mediated damage to the myelin unit are implicated in the destruction of myelin in demyelinating diseases, as these complexes are found deposited on myelin in multiple sclerosis plaques (Genain et al., 1999). The effects of complement/antibody myelin damage on the ultimate survival of the oligodendrocyte and its ability to remyelinate are complex, since loss of myelin also changes axonal function and interactions with the oligodendrocyte.

Trophic Factor Deprivation

Oligodendrocyte apoptosis is a prominent feature of normal CNS development. In the developing rodent optic nerve, approximately 50% of newly generated oligodendrocyte progenitors are eliminated; in the rat brain, 37% of premyelinating oligodendrocytes are lost in the first month of development (Barres et al., 1992; Trapp et al., 1997). This high rate of developmental oligodendrocyte death probably serves to match the number of maturing oligodendrocyte lineage cells to the number of axons requiring myelination (Raff et al., 1993), and may be mediated by competition for target-derived (axonal) trophic factors.

Multiple trophic factors have been identified for oligodendrocytes and Schwann cells (Table 34.2). Platelet-derived growth factor (PDGF) is a predominant survival factor for early oligodendrocyte progenitors (Grinspan, 2002). Additional trophic factor families that promote the survival of oligodendrocytes *in vitro* and *in vivo* include the insulin-like growth factors (IGF), interleukin-6-like (IL-6) family members including ciliary neurotrophic factor (CNTF), neurotrophin-3 (NT-3), and the neuregulins (Barres et al., 1993; Canoll et al., 1996). Overexpression of oligodendroglial trophic factors reduces the normal develop-

TABLE 34.2 *Survival Factors for Myelinating Cells*

	Oligodendrocytes	*Schwann cells*
PDGF	++	++
IGF-I	++	++
NT-3	++	++
CNTF	++	?
LIF	++	?
FGF-2	+	?
Neuregulins	++	+/−
TGF-β	?	+

Most data are obtained in cell culture models. ++, mediates cell survival; +, limited survival effects; +/−, some reports of survival effects; ?, survival effects unknown.

PDGF: platelet-derived growth factor; IGF-I: insulin like growth factor-I; NT-3: neurotrophin-3; CNTF: ciliary neurotrophic factor; LIF: leukemia inhibitory factor; FGF-2: fibroblast growth factor-2; TGF-β: transforming growth factor-β.

Sources. Barres et al. (1992), Canoll et al. (1996), McMorris and McKinnon (1996), Barres and Raff (1999), Delaney et al. (1999), Meier et al. (1999), Casaccia-Bonnefil (2000), Lobsiger et al. (2000), Butzkueven et al. (2002), Grinspan (2002), McLennan and Koishi (2002).

mental apoptosis of oligodendrocyte precursors (Barres et al., 1992; Raff et al., 1993; Calver et al., 1998). Prior to axonal contact, it is hypothesized that oligodendrocyte progenitors depend on astrocyte-derived trophic signals and contact with the extracellular matrix (Barres and Raff, 1999). While transgenic and knockout animal studies have shown that initial numbers of oligodendrocyte progenitors can be manipulated by overexpression or lack of individual trophic factors, adult animals ultimately develop normal numbers of oligodendrocytes and myelination, suggesting that axonal myelination and oligodendrocyte survival is regulated by multiple interacting signals (Barres et al., 1996; Calver et al., 1998; Ye et al., 2002).

Diseases that produce white matter damage may disrupt the normal trophic support that sustains oligodendrocyte survival or induce cell death by directly initiating apoptotic pathways. Ciliary neurotrophic factor, NT-3, IGF-I, and neuregulin prevent oligodendroglial cell death from various insults by inducing intrinsic survival pathways. Treatment of cultured adult rat and human oligodendrocytes with CNTF prevented TNF-α-induced death (Louis et al., 1993; D'Souza et al., 1996). Nerve growth factor, although not a common trophic factor for oligodendrocytes, also protected oligodendrocytes from TNF-α (Takano et al., 2000). Insulin-like growth factor I protects oligodendroglial cells from TNF-α-mediated damage, which includes disruption of myelin sheets and increased DNA fragmentation (Ye and D'Ercole, 1999; Takano et al., 2000). Both IGF-I and NT-3 can prevent glutamate excitotoxicity in cultured oligodendroglial cells, but only IGF-I can provide long-term protection against glutamate-induced apoptosis (Kavanaugh et al., 2000; Ness and Wood, 2002). Trophic factors have additive effects on survival when combined with antioxidants such as *N*-acetyl-cysteine, suggesting that trophic factor signaling may work in independent pathways (Mayer and Noble, 1994).

Trophic factors may reduce oligodendrocyte apoptosis through activation of several signaling pathways. Activation of the phosphatidylinositol 3′-kinase (PI3K)/Akt signaling pathway appears to be a prominent mechanism by which trophic factors mediate survival in oligodendroglial cells. For example, neuregulin inhibits death from trophic factor deprivation by activating the PI3K/Akt signaling pathway (Flores et al., 2000). Survival effects of IGF-I, NT-3, and NGF are also PI3K-dependent and involve the activation of Akt (Takano et al., 2000; Ness and Wood, 2002). Sustained activation of Akt is associated with IGF-I-induced long-term survival in pro-oligodendroblasts (Ness and Wood, 2002). Similarly, IGF-I mediates survival of Schwann cells through the PI3K/Akt pathway, and not the mitogen-activated kinase (MAPK) pathway (Campana et al., 1999). Additional pathways in oligodendrocyte lineage cells may also contribute to survival. For example, both PDGF and CNTF activate Janus kinase/signal transducer and activator of transcription (JAK/STAT), and NT-3 activates the Ras-MAPK pathway in oligodendrocyte progenitors (Cohen et al., 1996; Dell'Albani et al., 1998; Kumar et al., 1998).

SUMMARY AND PERSPECTIVES

In developing therapeutic strategies for white matter disease, the major goals are to protect oligodendrocytes or Schwann cells from damage, to prevent the spread of damage, and to repair damage that has already occurred. Development of protective strategies for myelinating cells can proceed by understanding the cellular and molecular mechanisms of injury. Damage in different disease models may be prevented by interruption of pathways involving reactive oxygen species, excitatory amino acids, cytokines, and inflammatory mediators. While immunomodulatory therapies are widely used to control inflammatory-mediated damage in multiple sclerosis, their direct effects on the protection of oligodendrocytes and axons are yet to be defined (Rieckmann and Maurer, 2002). Potassium channel blockers, such as 4-aminopyridine (4-AP), may enhance axonal conduction in demyelinated fibers and are being tested to improve function in clinical trials for spinal cord injury and multiple sclerosis. More novel approaches are directed to enhancing repair of damaged white matter. For example, remyelination may be promoted by increasing the proliferative and myelinating capacity of endogenous oligodendrocyte precursors (Fawcett and Asher, 1999; Chari and Blakemore, 2002) or by transplantation of stem cells or oligodendrocytes precursors following spinal cord injury or demyelinating diseases (Brustle et al., 1999; Liu et al., 2000; Stangel and Hartung 2002; Windrem et al., 2002; Pluchino et al., 2003).

Myelinating cells appear to be uniquely vulnerable to an array of acute and chronic insults. Understanding the mechanisms of cell death of oligodendrocyte and Schwann cells, and their interactions with axons, may help direct therapies to reduce cellular injury, prevent myelin loss, and preserve neurological function.

ACKNOWLEDGMENTS
The authors thank Suzanne Underhill for providing the photomicrographs shown in Figure 34.2.

ABBREVIATIONS

AMPA	2-amino-3-(3-hydroxymethylisoxazole-4-yl)propionic acid
4-AP	4-aminopyridine
ATP	adenosine 5′-triphosphate
cAMP	cyclic adenosine monophosphate

CNS	central nervous system
CNTF	ciliary neurotrophic factor
EAE	experimental allergic encephalomyelitis
EAN	experimental allergic neuritis
IFN-γ	interferon-γ
IGF	insulin-like growth factor
IL-6	interleukin-6
iNOS	inducible nitric oxide synthase
JAK/STAT	Janus kinase/signal transducer and activator of transcription
LDH	lactic dehydrogenase
MAPK	mitogen-activated kinase
MOG	myelin oligodendrocyte glycoprotein
NADPH	α-nicotinamide adenine dinucleotide phosphate
NGF	nerve growth factor
NMDA	*N*-methyl-D-aspartic acid
NT-3	neurotrophin-3
PARP	poly(ADP-ribose) polymerase
PDGF	platelet-derived growth factor
PI3K	phosphtidylinositol 3′-kinase
PNS	peripheral nervous system
PVL	periventricular leukomalacia
TNFα	tumor necrosis factor-α
TNFR	tumor necrosis factor receptor

REFERENCES

Alberdi, E., Sanchez-Gomez, M.V., Marino, A., and Matute, C. (2002) Ca(2+) influx through AMPA or kainate receptors alone is sufficient to initiate excitotoxicity in cultured oligodendrocytes. *Neurobiol. Dis.* 9:234–243.

American Heart Association (2003) *Heart Disease and Stroke Statistics—2003 Update.* Dallas: American Heart Association.

Andrews, T., Zhang, P., and Bhat, N.R. (1998) TNFalpha potentiates IFNgamma-induced cell death in oligodendrocyte progenitors. *J. Neurosci. Res.* 54:574–583.

Arnett, H.A., Hellendall, R.P., Matsushima, G.K., Suzuki, K., Laubach, V.E., Sherman, P., and Ting, J.P. (2002) The protective role of nitric oxide in a neurotoxicant-induced demyelinating model. *J. Immunol.* 168:427–433.

Arnett, H.A., Mason, J., Marino, M., Suzuki, K., Matsushima, G.K., and Ting, J.P. (2001) TNF alpha promotes proliferation of oligodendrocyte progenitors and remyelination. *Nat. Neurosci.* 4: 1116–1122.

Ashkenazi, A. and Dixit, V.M. (1999) Apoptosis control by death and decoy receptors. *Curr. Opin. Cell Biol.* 11:255–260.

Back, S.A., Gan, X., Li, Y., Rosenberg, P.A., and Volpe, J.J. (1998) Maturation-dependent vulnerability of oligodendrocytes to oxidative stress-induced death caused by glutathione depletion. *J. Neurosci.* 18:6241–6253.

Back, S.A., Han, B.H., Luo, N.L., Chricton, C.A., Xanthoudakis, S., Tam, J., Arvin, K.L., and Holtzman, D.M. (2002) Selective vulnerability of late oligodendrocyte progenitors to hypoxia-ischemia. *J. Neurosci.* 22:455–463.

Back, S.A., Luo, N.L., Borenstein, N.S., Levine, J.M., Volpe, J.J., and Kinney, H.C. (2001) Late oligodendrocyte progenitors coincide with the developmental window of vulnerability for human perinatal white matter injury. *J. Neurosci.* 21:1302–1312.

Baerwald, K.D. and Popko, B. (1998) Developing and mature oligodendrocytes respond differently to the immune cytokine interferon-gamma. *J. Neurosci. Res.* 52:230–239.

Barres, B.A., Burne, J.F., Holtmann, B., Thoenen, H., Sendtner, M., and Raff, M.C. (1996) Ciliary neurotrophic factor enhances the rate of oligodendrocyte generation. *Mol. Cell. Neurosc.* 8:146–156.

Barres, B.A., Hart, I.K., Coles, H.S., Burne, J.F., Voyvodic, J.T., Richardson, W.D., and Raff, M.C. (1992) Cell death and control of cell survival in the oligodendrocyte lineage. *Cell* 70:31–46.

Barres, B.A. and Raff, M.C. (1999) Axonal control of oligodendrocyte development. *J. Cell Biol.* 147:1123–1128.

Barres, B.A., Schmid, R., Sendnter, M., and Raff, M.C. (1993) Multiple extracellular signals are required for long-term oligodendrocyte survival. *Development* 118:283–295.

Beattie, M.S., Farooqui, A.A., and Bresnahan, J.C. (2000) Review of current evidence for apoptosis after spinal cord injury. *J. Neurotrauma.* 17:915–925.

Beattie, M.S., Harrington, A.W., Lee, R., Kim, J.Y., Boyce, S.L., Longo, F.M., Bresnahan, J.C., Hempstead, B.L., and Yoon, S.O. (2002) ProNGF induces p75-mediated death of oligodendrocytes following spinal cord injury. *Neuron* 36:375–386.

Berger, J., Moser, H.W., and Forss-Petter, S. (2001) Leukodystrophies: recent developments in genetics, molecular biology, pathogenesis and treatment. *Curr. Opin. Neurol.* 14:305–312.

Bhat, N.R., Zhang, P., and Bhat, A.N. (1999) Cytokine induction of inducible nitric oxide synthase in an oligodendrocyte cell line: role of p38 mitogen-activated protein kinase activation. *J. Neurochem.* 72:472–478.

Bjartmar, C., Yin, X., and Trapp, B.D. (1999) Axonal pathology in myelin disorders. *J. Neurocytol.* 28:383–395.

Blight, A.R. (1985) Delayed demyelination and macrophage invasion: a candidate for secondary cell damage in spinal cord injury. *Cent. Nerv. Syst. Trauma* 2:299–315.

Bromont, C., Marie, C., and Bralet, J. (1989) Increased lipid peroxidation in vulnerable brain regions after transient forebrain ischemia in rats. *Stroke* 20:918–924.

Bruck, W., Kuhlmann, T., and Stadelmann, C. (2003) Remyelination in multiple sclerosis. *J. Neurol. Sci.* 206:181–185.

Brustle, O., Jones, K.N., Learish, R.D., Karram, K., Choudhary, K., Wiestler, O.D., Duncan, I.D., and McKay, R.D. (1999) Embryonic stem cell–derived glial precursors: a source of myelinating transplants. *Science* 285:754–756.

Bunge, R.P., Puckett, W.R., Becerra, J.L., Marcillo, A., and Quencer, R.M. (1993) Observations on the pathology of human spinal cord injury: a review and classification of 22 new cases with details from a case of chronic cord compression with extensive focal demyelination. *Adv. Neurol.* 59:75–89.

Butzkueven, H., Zhang, J.G., Soilu-Hanninen, M., Hochrein, H., Chionh, F., Shipham, K.A., Emery, B., Turnley, A.M., Petratos, S., Ernst, M., Bartlett, P.F., and Kilpatrick, T.J. (2002) LIF receptor signaling limits immune-mediated demyelination by enhancing oligodendrocyte survival. *Nat. Med.* 8:613–619.

Calver, A.R., Hall, A.C., Yu, W.P., Walsh, F.S., Heath, J.K., Betsholtz, C., and Richardson, W.D. (1998) Oligodendrocyte population dynamics and the role of PDGF in vivo. *Neuron* 20:869–882.

Cammer, W. and Zhang, H. (1999) Maturation of oligodendrocytes is more sensitive to TNF alpha than is survival of precursors and immature oligodendrocytes. *J. Neuroimmunol.* 97:37–42.

Campana, W.M., Darin, S.J., and O'Brien, J.S. (1999) Phosphatidylinositol 3-kinase and akt protein kinase mediate IGF-I-and prosaptide-induced survival in Schwann cells. *J. Neurosci. Res.* 57:332–341.

Canoll, P.D., Musacchio, J.M., Hardy, R., Reynolds, R., Marchionni, M.A., and Salzer, J.L. (1996) GGF/neuregulin is a neuronal signal that promotes the proliferation and survival and inhibits the differentiation of oligodendrocyte progenitors. *Neuron* 17:229–243.

Casaccia-Bonnefil, P. (2000) Cell death in the oligodendrocyte lineage: a molecular perspective of life/death decisions in development and disease. *Glia* 29:124–135.

Casaccia-Bonnefil, P., Carter, B.D., Dobrowsky, R.T., and Chao, M.V. (1996) Death of oligodendrocytes mediated by the interaction of nerve growth factor with its receptor p75. *Nature* 383:716–719.

Casha, S., Yu, W.R., and Fehlings, M.G. (2001) Oligodendroglial apoptosis occurs along degenerating axons and is associated with FAS and p75 expression following spinal cord injury in the rat. *Neuroscience* 103:203–218.

Chari, D.M. and Blakemore, W.F. (2002) New insights into remyelination failure in multiple sclerosis: implications for glial cell transplantation. *Multiple Sclerosis* 8:271–277.

Cohen, R.I., Marmur, R., Norton, W.T., Mehler, M.F., and Kessler, J.A. (1996) Nerve growth factor and neurotrophin-3 differentially regulate the proliferation and survival of developing rat brain oligodendrocytes. *J. Neurosci.* 16:6433–6442.

Conti, G., De Pol, A., Scarpini, E., Vaccina, F., De Riz, M., Baron, P., Tiriticco, M., and Scarlato, G. (2002) Interleukin-1beta and interferon-gamma induce proliferation and apoptosis in cultured Schwann cells. *J. Neuroimmunol.* 124:29–35.

Cosgaya, J.M., Chan, J.R., and Shooter, E.M. (2002) The neurotrophin receptor p75NTR as a positive modulator of myelination. *Science* 298:1245–1248.

Dammann, O. and Leviton, A. (1997) Maternal intrauterine infection, cytokines, and brain damage in the preterm newborn. *Pediatr. Res.* 42:1–8.

Dashiell, S.M., Rus, H., and Koski, C.L. (2000) Terminal complement complexes concomitantly stimulate proliferation and rescue of Schwann cells from apoptosis. *Glia* 30:187–198.

Delaney, C.L., Cheng, H.L., and Feldman, E.L. (1999) Insulin-like growth factor-I prevents caspase-mediated apoptosis in Schwann cells. *J. Neurobiol.* 41:540–548.

Dell'Albani, P., Kahn, M.A., Cole, R., Condorelli, D.F., Giuffrida-Stella, A.M., and de Vellis, J. (1998) Oligodendroglial survival factors, PDGF-AA and CNTF, activate similar JAK/STAT signaling pathways. *J. Neurosci. Res.* 54:191–205.

Dirnagl, U., Iadecola, C., and Moskowtiz, M. (1999) Pathobiology of ischaemic stroke: an integrated view. *Trends Neurosci.* 22: 391–397.

Dowling, P., Husar, W., Menonna, J., Donnenfeld, H., Cook, S., and Sidhu, M. (1997) Cell death and birth in multiple sclerosis brain. *J. Neurol. Sci.* 149:1–11.

D'Souza, S.D., Alinauskas, K.A., and Antel, J.P. (1996) Ciliary neurotrophic factor selectively protects human oligodendrocytes from tumor necrosis factor–mediated injury. *J. Neurosci. Res.* 43: 289–298.

D'Souza, S.D., Alinauskas, K.A., McCrea, E., Goodyer, C., and Antel, J.P. (1995) Differential susceptibility of human CNS-derived cell populations to TNF-dependent and independent immune-mediated injury. *J. Neurosci.* 15:7293–7300.

Dumont, R.J., Okonkwo, D.O., Verma, S., Hurlbert, R.J., Boulos, P.T., Ellegala, D.B., and Dumont, A.S. (2001) Acute spinal cord injury, part I: pathophysiologic mechanisms. *Clin. Neuropharmacol.* 24:254–264.

Dyer, C.A. and Benjamins, J.A. (1990) Glycolipids and transmembrane signaling: antibodies to galactocerebroside cause an influx of calcium in oligodendrocytes. *J. Cell Biol.* 111:625–633.

Fawcett, J.W. and Asher, R.A. (1999) The glial scar and central nervous system repair. *Brain Res. Bull.* 49:377–391.

Fern, R. and Moller, T. (2000) Rapid ischemic cell death in immature oligodendrocytes: a fatal glutamate release feedback loop. *J. Neurosci.* 20:34–42.

Ferriero, D.M. (2001) Oxidant mechanisms in neonatal hypoxia-ischemia. *Dev. Neurosci.* 23:198–202.

Flores, A.I., Mallon, B.S., Matsui, T., Ogawa, W., Rosenzweig, A., Okamoto, T., and Macklin, W.B. (2000) Akt-mediated survival of oligodendrocytes induced by neuregulins. *J. Neurosci.* 20: 7622–7630.

Follett, P.L., Rosenberg, P.A., Volpe, J.J., and Jensen, F.E. (2000) NBQX attenuates excitotoxic injury in developing white matter. *J. Neurosci.* 20:9235–9241.

Gallo, V. and Ghiani, C.A. (2000) Glutamate receptors in glia: new cells, new inputs and new functions. *Trends Pharmacol. Sci.* 21:252–258.

Garthwaite, G., Goodwin, D.A., Batchelor, A.M., Leeming, K., and Garthwaite, J. (2002) Nitric oxide toxicity in CNS white matter: an in vitro study using rat optic nerve. *Neuroscience* 109: 145–155.

Genain, C.P., Cannella, B., Hauser, S.L., and Raine, C.S. (1999) Identification of autoantibodies associated with myelin damage in multiple sclerosis. *Nat. Med.* 5:170–175.

Ginsberg, M.D., Myers, R.E., and McDonagh, B.F. (1974) Experimental carbon monoxide encephalopathy in the primate. II. Clinical aspects, neuropathology, and physiologic correlation. *Arch. Neurol.* 30:209–216.

Gold, R., Toyka, K.V., and Hartung, H.P. (1995) Synergistic effect of Ifn-gamma and Tnf-alpha on expression of immune molecules and antigen presentation by Schwann cells. *Cell. Immunol.* 165:65–70.

Gold, R., Zielasek, J., Kiefer, R., Toyka, K.V., and Hartung, H.P. (1996) Secretion of nitrite by Schwann cells and its effect on T-cell activation in vitro. *Cell. Immunol.* 168:69–77.

Griffiths, I., Klugmann, M., Anderson, T., Yool, D., Thomson, C., Schwab, M.H., Schneider, A., Zimmermann, F., McCulloch, M., Nadon, N., and Nave, K.A. (1998) Axonal swellings and degeneration in mice lacking the major proteolipid of myelin. *Science* 280:1610–1613.

Grinspan, J. (2002) Cells and signaling in oligodendrocyte development. *J. Neuropathol. Exp. Neurol.* 61:297–306.

Hewett, J.A., Hewett, S.J., Winkler, S., and Pfeiffer, S.E. (1999) Inducible nitric oxide synthase expression in cultures enriched for mature oligodendrocytes is due to microglia. *J. Neurosci. Res.* 56:189–198.

Hirata, H., Hibasami, H., Yoshida, T., Ogawa, M., Matsumoto, M., Morita, A., and Uchida, A. (2001) Nerve growth factor signaling of p75 induces differentiation and ceramide-mediated apoptosis in schwann cells cultured from degenerating nerves. *Glia* 36:245–258.

Hirrlinger, J., Resch, A., Gutterer, J.M., and Dringen, R. (2002) Oligodendroglial cells in culture effectively dispose of exogenous hydrogen peroxide: comparison with cultured neurones, astroglial and microglial cells. *J. Neurochem.* 82:635–644.

Hisahara, S., Shoji, S., Okano, H., and Miura, M. (1997) ICE/CED-3 family executes oligodendrocyte apoptosis by tumor necrosis factor. *J. Neurochem.* 69:10–20.

Hollensworth, S.B., Shen, C., Sim, J.E., Spitz, D.R., Wilson, G.L., and LeDoux, S.P. (2000) Glial cell type–specific responses to menadione-induced oxidative stress. *Free Radical Biol. Med.* 28:1161–1174.

Holzwarth, J.A., Gibbons, S.J., Brorson, J.R., Philipson, L.H., and Miller, R.J. (1994) Glutamate receptor agonists stimulate diverse calcium responses in different types of cultured rat cortical glial cells. *J. Neurosci.* 14:1879–1891.

Hooper, D.C., Spitsin, S., Kean, R.B., Champion, J.M., Dickson, G.M., Chaudhry, I., and Koprowski, H. (1998) Uric acid, a natural scavenger of peroxynitrite, in experimental allergic encephalomyelitis and multiple sclerosis. *Proc. Natl. Acad. Sci. USA* 95:675–680.

Ikeda, T., Choi, B.H., Yee, S., Murata, Y., and Quilligan, E.J. (1999) Oxidative stress, brain white matter damage and intrauterine asphyxia in fetal lambs. *Int. J. Dev. Neurosci.* 17:1–14.

Imai, H., Masayasu, H., Dewar, D., Graham, D.I., and Macrae, I.M. (2001) Ebselen protects both gray and white matter in a rodent model of focal cerebral ischemia. *Stroke* 32:2149–2154.

Itoh, T., Reddy, U., Stern, J., Chen, M., Itoh, A., and Pleasure, D. (2000) Diminished calcium homeostasis and increased susceptibility to excitotoxicity of JS 3/16 progenitor cells after differentiation to oligodendroglia. *Glia* 31:165–180.

Johns, T.G. and Bernard, C.C. (1997) Binding of complement component Clq to myelin oligodendrocyte glycoprotein: a novel mechanism for regulating CNS inflammation. *Mol. Immunol.* 34:33–38.

Juurlink, B.H., Thorburne, S.K., and Hertz, L. (1998) Peroxide-scavenging deficit underlies oligodendrocyte susceptibility to oxidative stress. *Glia* 22:371–378.

Kakulas, B.A. (1999) A review of the neuropathology of human spinal cord injury with emphasis on special features. *J. Spinal Cord Med.* 22:119–124.

Kanellopoulos, G.K., Xu, X.M., Hsu, C.Y., Lu, X., Sundt, T.M., and Kouchoukos, N.T. (2000) White matter injury in spinal cord ischemia: protection by AMPA/kainate glutamate receptor antagonism. *Stroke* 31:1945–1952.

Kavanaugh, B., Beesley, J., Itoh, T., Itoh, A., Grinspan, J., and Pleasure, D. (2000) Neurotrophin-3 (NT-3) diminishes susceptibility of the oligodendroglial lineage to AMPA glutamate receptor–mediated excitotoxicity. *J. Neurosci. Res.* 60:725–732.

Keegan, B.M. and Noseworthy, J.H. (2002) Multiple sclerosis. *Annu. Rev. Med.* 53:285–302.

Kim, Y.S. and Kim, S.U. (1991) Oligodendroglial cell death induced by oxygen radicals and its protection by catalase. *J. Neurosci. Res.* 29:100–106.

Koeppen, A.H. and Robitaille, Y. (2002) Pelizaeus-Merzbacher disease. *J. Neuropathol. Exp. Neurol.* 61:747–759.

Kress, G.J., Dineley, K.E., and Reynolds, I.J. (2002) The relationship between intracellular free iron and cell injury in cultured neurons, astrocytes, and oligodendrocytes. *J. Neurosci.* 22:5848–5855.

Kumar, S., Kahn, M.A., Dinh, L., and de Vellis, J. (1998) NT-3-mediated TrkC receptor activation promotes proliferation and cell survival of rodent progenitor oligodendrocyte cells in vitro and in vivo. *J. Neurosci. Res.* 54:754–765.

Kwa, M.S., van Schaik, I.N., De Jonge, R.R., Brand, A., Kalaydjieva, L., van Belzen, N., Vermeulen, M., and Baas, F. (2003) Autoimmunoreactivity to Schwann cells in patients with inflammatory neuropathies. *Brain* 126:361–375.

Ladiwala, U., Lachance, C., Simoneau, S.J., Bhakar, A., Barker, P.A., and Antel, J.P. (1998) p75 neurotrophin receptor expression on adult human oligodendrocytes: signaling without cell death in response to NGF. *J. Neurosci.* 18:1297–1304.

Li, S. and Stys, P.K. (2000) Mechanisms of ionotropic glutamate receptor–mediated excitotoxicity in isolated spinal cord white matter. *J. Neurosci.* 20:1190–1198.

Li, W.P., Maeda, Y., Ming, X., Cook, S., Chapin, J., Husar, W., and Dowling, P. (2002) Apoptotic death following Fas activation in human oligodendrocyte hybrid cultures. *J. Neurosci. Res.* 69:189–196.

Liu, S., Qu, Y., Stewart, T.J., Howard, M.J., Chakrabortty, S., Holekamp, T.F., and McDonald, J.W. (2000) Embryonic stem cells differentiate into oligodendrocytes and myelinate in culture and after spinal cord transplantation. *Proc. Natl. Acad. Sci. USA* 97:6126–6131.

Lobsiger, C.S., Schweitzer, B., Taylor, V., and Suter, U. (2000) Platelet-derived growth factor-BB supports the survival of cultured rat Schwann cell precursors in synergy with neurotrophin-3. *Glia* 30:290–300.

Louis, J.C., Magal, E., Takayama, S., and Varon, S. (1993) CNTF protection of oligodendrocytes against natural and tumor necrosis factor-induced death. *Science* 259:689–692.

Martin, L.J., Al Abdulla, N.A., Brambrink, A.M., Kirsch, J.R., Sieber, F.E., and Portera-Cailliau, C. (1998) Neurodegeneration in excitotoxicity, global cerebral ischemia, and target deprivation: a perspective on the contributions of apoptosis and necrosis. *Brain Res. Bull.* 46:281–309.

Martin, R., McFarland, H.F., and McFarland, D.E. (1992) Immunological aspects of demyelinating diseases. *Annu. Rev. Immunol.* 10:153–187.

Matute, C., Sanchez-Gomez, M.V., Martinez-Millan, L., and Miledi, R. (1997) Glutamate receptor–mediated toxicity in optic nerve oligodendrocytes. *Proc. Natl. Acad. Sci. USA* 94:8830–8835.

Matysiak, M., Jurewicz, A., Jaskolski, D., and Selmaj, K. (2002) TRAIL induces death of human oligodendrocytes isolated from adult brain. *Brain* 125:2469–2480.

Mayer, M. and Noble, M. (1994) *N*-acetyl-L-cysteine is a pluripotent protector against cell death and enhancer of trophic factor-mediated cell survival in vitro. *Proc. Natl. Acad. Sci. USA* 91: 7496–7500.

McCracken, E., Fowler, J.H., Dewar, D., Morrison, S., and McCulloch, J. (2002) Grey matter and white matter ischemic damage is reduced by the competitive AMPA receptor antagonist, SPD 502. *J. Cereb. Blood Flow Metab.* 22:1090–1097.

McCracken, E., Valeriani, V., Simpson, C., Jover, T., McCulloch, J., and Dewar, D. (2000) The lipid peroxidation by-product 4-hydroxynonenal is toxic to axons and oligodendrocytes. *J. Cereb. Blood Flow Metab.* 20:1529–1536.

McDonald, J.W., Althomsons, S.P., Hyrc, K.L., Choi, D.W., and Goldberg, M.P. (1998) Oligodendrocytes from forebrain are highly vulnerable to AMPA/kainate receptor–mediated excitotoxicity. *Nat. Med.* 4:291–297.

McLennan, I.S. and Koishi, K. (2002) The transforming growth factor-betas: multifaceted regulators of the development and maintenance of skeletal muscles, motoneurons and Schwann cells. *Int. J. Dev. Biol.* 46:559–567.

McMorris, F.A. and McKinnon, R.D. (1996) Regulation of oligodendrocyte development and CNS myelination by growth factors: prospects for therapy of demyelinating disease. *Brain Pathol.* 6:313–329.

Meier, C., Parmantier, E., Brennan, A., Mirsky, R., and Jessen, K.R. (1999) Developing Schwann cells acquire the ability to survive without axons by establishing an autocrine circuit involving insulin-like growth factor, neurotrophin-3, and platelet-derived growth factor-BB. *J. Neurosci.* 19:3847–3859.

Merrill, J.E. and Benveniste, E.N. (1996) Cytokines in inflammatory brain lesions: helpful and harmful. *Trends Neurosci.* 19:331–338.

Merrill, J.E., Ignarro, L.J., Sherman, M.P., Melinek, J., and Lane, T.E. (1993) Microglial cell cytotoxicity of oligodendrocytes is mediated through nitric oxide. *J. Immunol.* 151:2132–2141.

Mews, I., Bergmann, M., Bunkowski, S., Gullotta, F., and Bruck, W. (1998) Oligodendrocyte and axon pathology in clinically silent multiple sclerosis lesions. *Multiple Sclerosis* 4:55–62.

Miinea, C., Kuruvilla, R., Merrikh, H., and Eichberg, J. (2002) Altered arachidonic acid biosynthesis and antioxidant protection mechanisms in Schwann cells grown in elevated glucose. *J. Neurochem.* 81:1253–1262.

Miller, A.K., Alston, R.L., and Corsellis, J.A. (1980) Variation with age in the volumes of grey and white matter in the cerebral hemispheres of man: measurements with an image analyser. *Neuropathol. Appl. Neurobiol.* 6:119–132.

Mithen, F.A., Colburn, S., and Birchem, R. (1990) Human alpha-tumor necrosis factor does not damage cultures containing rat Schwann cells and sensory neurons. *Neurosci. Res.* 9:59–63.

Mitrovic, B., Ignarro, L.J., Montestruque, S., Smoll, A., and Merrill, J.E. (1994) Nitric oxide as a potential pathological mechanism in demyelination—its differential effects on primary glial cells in vitro. *Neuroscience* 61:575–585.

Mitrovic, B., Ignarro, L.J., Vinters, H.V., Akers, M.A., Schmid, I., Uittenbogaart, C., and Merrill, J.E. (1995) Nitric oxide induces necrotic but not apoptotic cell death in oligodendrocytes. *Neuroscience* 65:531–539.

Nagano, S., Takeda, M., Ma, L., and Soliven, B. (2001) Cytokine-induced cell death in immortalized Schwann cells: roles of nitric oxide and cyclic AMP. *J. Neurochem.* 77:1486–1495.

Ness, J.K. and Wood, T.L. (2002) Insulin-like growth factor I, but not neurotrophin-3, sustains Akt activation and provides long-term protection of immature oligodendrocytes from glutamate-mediated apoptosis. *Mol. Cell. Neurosci.* 20:476–488.

Noseworthy, J.H. (1999) Progress in determining the causes and treatment of multiple sclerosis. *Nature* 399:A40–A47.

Pantoni, L., Garcia, J.H., and Gutierrez, J.A. (1996) Cerebral white matter is highly vulnerable to ischemia. *Stroke* 27:1641–1646.

Penney, D.G. (1990) Acute carbon monoxide poisoning: animal models: a review. *Toxicology* 62:123–160.

Petito, C.K., Olarte, J.P., Roberts, B., Nowak, T.S., Jr., and Pulsinelli, W.A. (1998) Selective glial vulnerability following transient global ischemia in rat brain. *J. Neuropathol. Exp. Neurol.* 57:231–238.

Piddlesden, S.J. and Morgan, B.P. (1993) Killing of rat glial cells by complement: deficiency of the rat analogue of CD59 is the cause of oligodendrocyte susceptibility to lysis. *J. Neuroimmunol.* 48:169–175.

Pitt, D., Werner, P., and Raine, C.S. (2000) Glutamate excitotoxicity in a model of multiple sclerosis. *Nat. Med.* 6:67–70.

Pluchino, S., Quattrini, A., Brambilla, E., Gritti, A., Salani, G., Dina, G., Galli, R., Del Carro, U., Amadio, S., Bergami, A., Furlan, R., Comi, G., Vescovi, A.L., and Martino, G. (2003) Injection of adult neurospheres induces recovery in a chronic model of multiple sclerosis. *Nature* 422:688–694.

Pouly, S., Antel, J.P., Ladiwala, U., Nalbantoglu, J., and Becher, B. (2000a) Mechanisms of tissue injury in multiple sclerosis: opportunities for neuroprotective therapy. *J. Neural Transm. Suppl.* 58:193–203.

Pouly, S., Becher, B., Blain, M., and Antel, J.P. (2000b) Interferon-gamma modulates human oligodendrocyte susceptibility to Fas-mediated apoptosis. *J. Neuropathol. Exp. Neurol.* 59:280–286.

Raff, M.C., Barres, B.A., Burne, J.F., Coles, H.S., Ishizaki, Y., and Jacobson, M.D. (1993) Programmed cell death and the control of cell survival: lessons from the nervous system. *Science* 262: 695–700.

Raghupathi, R., Graham, D.I., and McIntosh, T.K. (2000) Apoptosis after traumatic brain injury. *J. Neurotrauma* 17:927–938.

Raine, C.S. and Cross, A.H. (1989) Axonal dystrophy as a consequence of long-term demyelination. *Lab Invest.* 60:714–725.

Rieckmann, P. and Maurer, M. (2002) Anti-inflammatory strategies to prevent axonal injury in multiple sclerosis. *Curr. Opin. Neurol.* 15:361–370.

Robbins, D.S., Shirazi, Y., Drysdale, B.E., Lieberman, A., Shin, H.S., and Shin, M.L. (1987). Production of cytotoxic factor for oligodendrocytes by stimulated astrocytes. *J. Immunol.* 139: 2593–2597.

Rosenberg, L.J., Teng, Y.D., and Wrathall, J.R. (1999a) 2,3-Dihydroxy-6-nitro-7-sulfamoyl-benzo(f)quinoxaline reduces glial loss and acute white matter pathology after experimental spinal cord contusion. *J. Neurosci.* 19:464–475.

Rosenberg, P.A., Li, Y., Ali, S., Altiok, N., Back, S.A., and Volpe, J.J. (1999b) Intracellular redox state determines whether nitric oxide is toxic or protective to rat oligodendrocytes in culture. *J. Neurochem.* 73:476–484.

Sanchez-Gomez, M.V. and Matute, C. (1999) AMPA and kainate receptors each mediate excitotoxicity in oligodendroglial cultures. *Neurobiol. Dis.* 6:475–485.

Sanchez-Gomez, M.V., Alberdi, E., Ibarretxe, G., Torre, I., and Matute, C. (2003) Caspase-dependent and caspase-independent oligodendrocyte death mediated by AMPA and kainate receptors. *J. Neurosci.* 23:9159–9528.

Sawant-Mane, S., Estep, A., III, and Koski, C.L. (1994) Antibody of patients with Guillain-Barré syndrome mediates complement-dependent cytolysis of rat Schwann cells: susceptibility to cytolysis reflects Schwann cell phenotype. *J. Neuroimmunol.* 49: 145–152.

Schiffmann, R. and Boespflug-Tanguy, O. (2001) An update on the leukodsytrophies. *Curr. Opin. Neurol.* 14:789–794.

Schwab, M.E. and Bartholdi, D. (1996) Degeneration and regeneration of axons in the lesioned spinal cord. *Physiol. Rev.* 76: 319–370.

Scolding, N.J. and Compston, D.A. (1991) Oligodendrocyte-macrophage interactions in vitro triggered by specific antibodies. *Immunology* 72:127–132.

Scolding, N.J., Houston, W.A., Morgan, B.P., Campbell, A.K., and Compston, D.A. (1989) Reversible injury of cultured rat oligodendrocytes by complement. *Immunology* 67:441–446.

Scolding, N.J., Jones, J., Compston, D.A., and Morgan, B.P. (1990) Oligodendrocyte susceptibility to injury by T-cell perforin. *Immunology* 70:6–10.

Selmaj, K.W. and Raine, C.S. (1988) Tumor necrosis factor mediates myelin and oligodendrocyte damage in vitro. *Ann. Neurol.* 23:339–346.

Smith, K.J., Kapoor, R., and Felts, P.A. (1999) Demyelination: the role of reactive oxygen and nitrogen species. *Brain Pathol.* 9:69–92.

Smith, T., Groom, A., Zhu, B., and Turski, L. (2000) Autoimmune encephalomyelitis ameliorated by AMPA antagonists. *Nat. Med.* 6:62–66.

Snipes, G.J. and Orfali, W. (1998) Common themes in peripheral neuropathy disease genes. *Cell Biol. Int.* 22:815–835.

Stangel, M. and Hartung, H.P. (2002) Remyelinating strategies for the treatment of multiple sclerosis. *Prog. Neurobiol.* 68:361–376.

Takano, R., Hisahara, S., Namikawa, K., Kiyama, H., Okano, H., and Miura, M. (2000) Nerve growth factor protects oligodendrocytes from tumor necrosis factor-alpha-induced injury through Akt-mediated signaling mechanisms. *J. Biol. Chem.* 275:16360–16365.

Tekkök, S.B. and Goldberg, M.P. (2001) AMPA/kainate receptor activation mediates hypoxic oligodendrocyte death and axonal injury in cerebral white matter. *J. Neurosci.* 21:4237–4248.

Thorburne, S.K. and Juurlink, B.H. (1996) Low glutathione and high iron govern the susceptibility of oligodendroglial precursors to oxidative stress. *J. Neurochem.* 67:1014–1022.

Trapp, B.D., Nishiyama, A., Cheng, D., and Macklin, W. (1997) Differentiation and death of premyelinating oligodendrocytes in developing rodent brain. *J. Cell Biol.* 137:459–468.

Vincent, A.M., Brownlee, M., and Russell, J.W. (2002) Oxidative stress and programmed cell death in diabetic neuropathy. *Ann. NY Acad. Sci.* 959:368–383.

Volpe, J. (1997) Brain injury in the premature infant—from pathogenesis to prevention. *Brain Dev.* 19:519–534.

Weiss, T., Grell, M., Siemienski, K., Muhlenbeck, F., Durkop, H., Pfizenmaier, K., Scheurich, P., and Wajant, H. (1998) TNFR80-dependent enhancement of TNFR60-induced cell death is mediated by TNFR-associated factor 2 and is specific for TNFR60. *J. Immunol.* 161:3136–3142.

Willenborg, D.O., Staykova, M.A., and Cowden, W.B. (1999) Our shifting understanding of the role of nitric oxide in autoimmune encephalomyelitis: a review. *J. Neuroimmunol.* 100:21–35.

Windrem, M.S., Roy, N.S., Wang, J., Nunes, M., Benraiss, A., Goodman, R., McKhann, G.M., and Goldman, S.A. (2002) Progenitor cells derived from the adult human subcortical white matter disperse and differentiate as oligodendrocytes within demyelinated lesions of the rat brain. *J. Neurosci. Res.* 69:966–975.

Winer, J.B. (2001) Guillain-Barré syndrome. *Mol. Pathol.* 54: 381–385.

Wohlleben, G., Ibrahim, S.M., Schmidt, J., Toyka, K.V., Hartung, H.P., and Gold, R. (2000) Regulation of Fas and FasL expression on rat Schwann cells. *Glia* 30:373–381.

Wrathall, J.R., Choiniere, D., and Teng, Y.D. (1994) Dose-dependent reduction of tissue loss and functional impairment after spinal cord trauma with the AMPA/kainate antagonist NBQX. *J. Neurosci.* 14:6598–6607.

Ye, P. and D'Ercole, A.J. (1999) Insulin-like growth factor I protects oligodendrocytes from tumor necrosis factor-alpha-induced injury. *Endocrinology* 140:3063–3072.

Ye, P., Li, L., Richards, G., DiAugustine, R.P., and D'Ercole, A.J. (2002) Myelination is altered in insulin-like growth factor-I null mutant mice. *J. Neurosci.* 22:6041–6051.

Yoshioka, A., Hardy, M., Younkin, D.P., Grinspan, J.B., Stern, J.L., and Pleasure, D. (1995) Alpha-amino-3-hydroxy-5-methyl-4-isoxazolepropionate (AMPA) receptors mediate excitotoxicity in the oligodendroglial lineage. *J. Neurochem.* 64:2442–2448.

Yoshioka, A., Shimizu, Y., Hirose, G., Kitasato, H., and Pleasure, D. (1998) Cyclic AMP-elevating agents prevent oligodendroglial excitotoxicity. *J. Neurochem.* 70:2416–2423.

Yoshioka, A., Yamaya, Y., Saiki, S., Kanemoto, M., Hirose, G., Beesley, J., and Pleasure, D. (2000) Non-*N*-methyl-D-aspartate glutamate receptors mediate oxygen—glucose deprivation-induced oligodendroglial injury. *Brain Res.* 854:207–215.

Young, W. (1993) Secondary injury mechanisms in acute spinal cord injury. *J. Emerg. Med.* 1:13–22.

Zeine, R., Pon, R., Ladiwala, U., Antel, J.P., Filion, L.G., and Freedman, M.S. (1998) Mechanism of gammadelta T cell–induced human oligodendrocyte cytotoxicity: relevance to multiple sclerosis. *J. Neuroimmunol.* 87:49–61.

35 Response of microglia to brain injury

KAZUYUKI NAKAJIMA AND SHINICHI KOHSAKA

Del Rio-Hortega (1932), who first distinguished microglia from other glial cells in the central nervous system (CNS), reported that microglia transform from a ramified type into a nonramified type in response to brain injuries. Since then, there have been numerous studies investigating the molecules responsible for the activation of microglia, the quality of microglial alteration, and the intracellular mechanism of microglial activation, as well as studies on the pathological significance of activated microglia. Although these issues have not yet been completely resolved, the accumulated results and information regarding the microglial activation are summarized herein.

CELLULAR CHANGES OF MICROGLIA IN THE PATHOLOGICAL BRAIN

In the normal adult brain, microglia are present with regular spacing as process-bearing forms (ramified microglia). These cells are functionally inactive or in a resting state and comprise approximately 5%–20% of all glial cells in the normal adult brain (Lawson et al., 1992) (Fig. 35.1). As long as the brain remains healthy, the cell density and morphology of the ramified microglia are sustained.

Morphological Change of Microglia

When the brain is injured or diseased, the ramified microglia change their morphology, retract their processes, and increase their volume. This form is known as *normally activated microglia* or *reactive microglia* (Fig. 35.1). Since this microglial transformation is thought to be mediated by specific signal(s), the molecules responsible for the morphological change have been explored mainly in *in vitro* studies. However, the molecules remain largely elusive. Because microglia themselves often induce activated morphology, depending on the culture condition without any specific factors. However, it has been inferred that some soluble factors, including plasma proteins, certain growth factors and amino acids, and glial extracellular matrix (ECM) proteins modulate the morphological changes of microglia.

See the abbreviations at the end of the chapter.

On the other hand, the molecules that transform ameboid microglia into ramified microglia have been determined *in vitro*. Ameboid microglia transform into ramified cells when cultured with astrocytic-conditioned medium or with astrocytes (Wilms et al., 1997). Astrocyte-derived cytokines, including transforming growth factor β (TGFβ), macrophage colony stimulating factor (M-CSF), and granulocyte macrophage colony-stimulating factor (GM-CSF) (Schilling et al., 2001), glial substrata such as fibronectin and laminin, and astrocyte-derived insoluble factor (Tanaka et al., 1999) cause morphological ramification. Dimethylsulfoxide (DMSO) and retinoic acid (Giulian and Baker, 1986), adenosine triphosphate (ATP) and adenosine (Wollmer et al., 2001), amino acids, and vitamin E (Heppner et al., 1998) also induce ramification. These molecules may be related to the maintenance of the ramified morphology or the return of activated microglia to the ramified form in the regenerative processes of the CNS. Adenylate cyclase, calcium, phosphatase, and Gi-protein are involved in the regulation of the ramification (Kalla et al., 2003).

These results suggest that some soluble factors and/or the architecture of the astrocytic surface in extracellular spaces are important for determining microglial morphology.

Immunophenotypical Change of Microglia

A number of immunohistochemical studies have demonstrated that numerous proteins—including surface antigens, receptors, and ECM protein—are induced or upregulated in activated microglia at the site of brain injury or pathology (Fig. 35.1).

Among these antigens, major histocompatibility complex (MHC) classes I and II, complement receptor-3 (CR-3), and Fc receptor are immune-related mole-

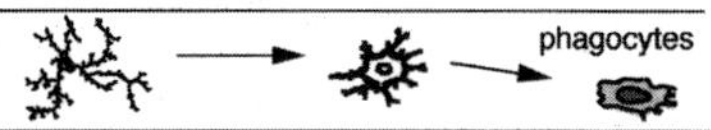

Molecules	Resting microglia	Activated microglia	phagocytes
Immune-related proteins			
MHC class I	−	++	
MHC class II	−	++	+++
CR-3 receptor	+	+++	+++
Fc receptor	−	++	
ED-1	−	−	+++
F4/80	+	++	
Cytoskeltal proteins			
Vimentin	−	++	
ECM proteins			
LFA-1	−	++	
Thrombospondin	+	++	
Ca-binding protein			
Iba1/MRF-1	+	+++	+++
IsolectinB4-recognizing molecule			
α-D galactose	+	++	
Enzymes			
5'-nucleotidase	+	++	

FIGURE 35.1 Molecules induced or enhanced in activated microglia. Microglia are activated in response to extracellular signals, and result in the increase or induction of various antigens. Activated microglia are further transformed to phagocytes in response to the signals from dying cells. CR-3: complement receptor-3; Iba1/MRF-1: ionized calcium binding adapter molecule/microglial response factor-1; LFA: leukocyte function-associated antigen; MHC: major histocompatibility complex.

cules. These molecules are upregulated in many pathological brains. For example, MHC class 1 is upregulated in microglia following CNS injury. Major histocompatibility complex class I and II have been found in brain microglia of patients with Alzheimer's disease, multiple sclerosis (MS), experimental allergic encephalomyelitis (EAE), ischemia brain, and the axotomized peripheral nucleus. Complement receptor-3 is upregulated in a variety of pathological states, including axotomized facial nucleus.

Ionized calcium binding adapter molecule 1 (Iba1) can stain microglia specifically in the CNS (Graeber et al., 1998) and is upregulated in activated microglia in various pathological states, including transient focal ischemia. Microglia are labeled with the F4/80 antibody that recognizes macrophage-specific plasma membrane protein. The staining is upregulated in activated microglia. Cell adhesion protein, leukocyte function-associated antigen-1 (LFA-1) (Moneta et al., 1993), and the ECM protein thrombospondin (Moller et al., 1996) are upregulated in activated microglia. These molecules may be associated with cellular contact or cellular recognition. One of the lectins, isolectin B4 (Griffonia simplicifolia isolectin B4), can label microglia in a wide range of species (Streit et al., 1988). The binding increases in activated microglia.

Activated microglia show high rates of certain enzyme activities, including 5′-nucleotidase, acid phosphatase, cathepsins, and thiamin pyrophosphatase activities. 5′-Nucleotidase immunoreactivity is upregulated in activated microglia in facial nerve axotomy (Schoen et al., 1992). Increase in these enzymes may play a role in the activated function of the cell membrane.

ED-1 is a marker of phagocytic cells, and the staining is induced when the activated microglia are transformed to phagocytes. The receptors for chemokines are also enhanced in activated microglia (Gebike-Haerter et al., 2001).

The upregulation or induction of the immune-related antigens, lectin-binding, ECM proteins, and chemokine receptor, generally appear to reflect the role of immune cells, particularly in chronic inflammatory conditions. However, in acute injury, the upregulation of MHC classes I and II and CR-3 is not necessarily related to immune reaction, but rather plays a role in cellular recognition.

In addition, activated microglia have been shown to highly express glutamate transporter-1 (GLT-1) around the injured motoneuron cell body in the axotomized facial nucleus (Lopez-Redondo et al., 2000). These cells seem to play a role in the elimination of glutamate (Glu).

Change of Microglia to the Proliferative State

The increase in cell number as well as morphological change can be observed in many pathological conditions. The proliferative activity of microglia contributes mainly to the increase in cell number in and around the injured sites.

The mitogenic characteristics of microglia have been demonstrated by both *in vitro* and *in vivo* studies. Microglia proliferate in response to colony-stimulating factors such as M-CSF, GM-CSF, and multi-CSF [interleukin-3 (IL-3)] *in vitro* (Giulian and Ingeman,1988). Macrophage-CSF was identified as a main factor in microglial proliferation by analyzing the osteopetrotic mouse (op/op) in which active M-CSF cannot be produced. The M-CSF-deficient mouse failed to accumulate microglial cells in the axotomized facial nucleus (Raivich et al., 1994), indicating that M-CSF plays a crucial role in microglial proliferation. In addition, M-CSF and GM-CSF were found to bind specifically to the axotomized facial nucleus of the normal adult rat (Raivich et al., 1991), suggesting the direct association of these factors with microglial proliferation via the specific receptors for M-CSF and GM-CSF.

Giulian et al. (1991) have isolated microglial mitogens (MM) from the neonatal rat brain by observing the phenomena in which microglia increase in number in the late embryonic to postnatal stage or in response to brain injury. Microglial mitogen-1 (MM1), with a molecular weight of 50 kDa and pI 6.8, showed GM-CSF-like activity. Microglial mitogen-2 (MM2), with a molecular weight of 22 kDa and pI of 5.2, showed characteristics different from those of IL-3 and was secreted from cultured astrocytes. Both factors are induced in the injured brain, but not in the normal adult brain, and have an ability to proliferate ameboid microglia, but not macroglia or monocytes and peritoneal macrophages.

Furthermore, IL-1, tumor necrosis factor-α (TNFα), IL-3, IL-4, IL-5, and IL-10 have been reported as additional mitogenic factors for microglia. However, among these factors, TNFα, IL-4, and IL-10 can inhibit microglial proliferation on astrocyte monolayers (Kloss et al., 1997).

Mobility of Microglia

The motile activity of microglia has been inferred in the axotomized facial nucleus (Streit et al., 1988), where activated microglia gather around the cell body of injured motoneurons, and in chronic inflammations such as MS in which activated microglia phagocytose distructed myelin and dead cells. These observations suggest the presence and action of a chemoattractant which is released from the injured motoneuron cell body, injured myelin, or dead cells.

Microglia have been shown to express the chemokine receptors CCR1, CCR2, CCR3, CCR5, CXCR4, and CX3CR1. Of these receptors, CCR2 and CX3CR1 were present on activated microglia in the axotomized facial nucleus, and their ligand chemokines, monocyte chemoattractant protein-1 (MCP1) and fractalkine, were produced by axotomized facial motoneurons (Harrison et al., 1998). This observation suggested that the vicinity of injured neurons and activated microglia is mediated by chemokines and the specific receptors. However, a knockout experiment with the receptors revealed that the fractalkine/MCP1–CCR2/CX3CR1 system is not a substantial mediator (Jung et al., 2000). Other systems might be included.

After focal ischemia, a large number of macrophages have been observed at the infarct core. It has been proposed that this phenomenon is due to local induction of chemokine MCP-1, which in turn induces the gathering of activated microglia and macrophages that express CCR2.

Adenosine triphosphate (ATP) has the ability to attract microglia *in vitro* (Honda et al., 2001), strongly suggesting that ATP released in response to injury is a possible chemoattractant of microglia *in vivo*.

Transformation of Microglia to Phagocytes

If cell death occurs in the CNS, activated microglia transform into phagocytes and engulf the dead and dying cells (Fig. 35.1). The phagocytosing cells have been observed in various pathological brains, such as those affected by Alzheimer's disease, Parkinson's disease, MS, ischemia, infectious diseases, toxin-injected brains, and trauma. The phagocytes are usually derived from activated microglia and macrophages/monocytes *in vivo*.

For example, in transient global cerebral ischemia, CA1 pyramidal neurons in the hippocampus selectively die after a delay of 3–4 days. These dead neurons are engulfed by phagocytes, which are transformed from resident microglia and infiltrated macrophages. This phenomenon occurs in many chronic diseases.

On the other hand, the transformation of resident microglia to macrophages *in vivo* has been clearly shown in the ricin-injected facial nucleus, in which motoneurons undergo cell death and are phagocytosed by macrophages transformed from activated microglia (Streit and Kreutzberg, 1988). The phagocytic microglia are characterized by staining with ED-1 monoclonal antibody. In this context, it should be noticed that activated microglia are not always phagocytes.

Cell Death of Activated Microglia

In the case of a peripheral nerve injury such as sciatic and hypoglossal nerve transection, microglial proliferation occurs at the early phase after transection, but afterward, many activated microglia have been found to undergo apoptosis with DNA fragmentation (Gehrmann and Banati, 1995). This may be a regulatory system that serves to maintain the microglial cell density at an appropriate level in a injured site.

Adenosine triphosphate has been shown to induce cell death in microglia via P2X7 purinergic receptor (Brough et al., 2002). Microglia might undergo cell death locally in response to ATP that is released from injured sites.

Induction of Cytotoxic Molecules in Activated Microglia

Many studies have reported that activated microglia are associated with the progression of pathological states by producing deleterious features (Chao et al., 1992; Banati et al., 1993; Giulian et al., 1993; Aschner et al., 1999; Yrjanheikki et al., 1999; Gao et al., 2002). In fact, the microglia can produce and secrete a variety of deleterious factors *in vitro* (Fig. 35.2).

Reactive oxygen species (ROS), including superoxide anion, hydroxy radicals, and hydrogen peroxide, are generally hazardous, particularly to myelin and oligodendrocytes, owing to their ability to induce lipid peroxidation. Nitrogen oxides, such as nitric oxide (NO), are highly reactive free-radicals. Nitric oxide reacts with superoxide anion to produce peroxinitrite, which shows a very strong toxicity. These radicals are believed to inhibit respiratory enzymes, oxidize the SH group of proteins, and enhance DNA injury, finally resulting in neuronal cell death. β-Amyloid can stimulate

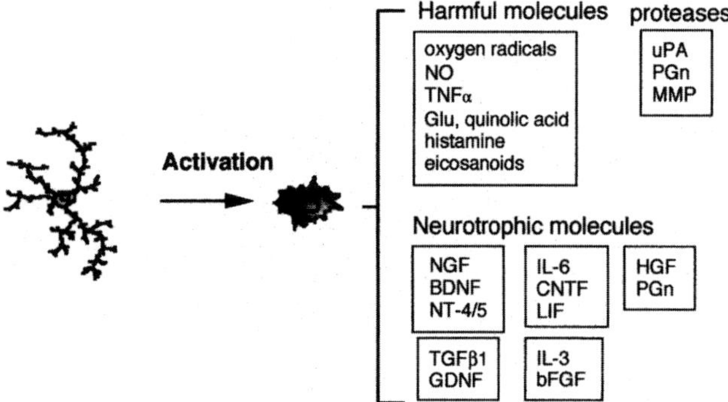

FIGURE 35.2 Ability of microglia to produce biologically active molecules. Microglia may have the ability to produce a variety of biologically active molecules, including harmful factors, neurotrophic factors, and proteases. BDNF: brain-derived neurotrophic factor; bFGF: basic fibroblast growth factor; CNTF: ciliary neurotrophic factor; GDNF: glial cell line-derived neurotrophic factor; Glu: glutamic acid; HGC: hepatocyte growth factor; IL-3, IL-6: interleukin-3, -6; LIF: leukemia inhibitory factor; MMP: matrix metalloproteinase; NGF: nerve growth factor; NO: nitric oxide; NT-4/5: neurotrophin-4/5; PGn: plasminogen; TGFβ1: transforming growth factor-β1.

NO production from microglia. The β-amyloid, in the presence of interferon-γ (INFγ), synergistically stimulates the production of NO and TNFα in microglia. Tumor necrosis factor-α causes cell death of CNS cells such as oligodendrocytes, myelin, and some neurons *in vitro*. Although activated microglia-derived TNFα has been suspected to cause inflammation in MS and acquired immunodeficiency syndrome (AIDS) dementia, it has been demonstrated by gene knockout of TNFα that this cytokine is not essential for the initiation and/or exacerbation of inflammation (Liu et al., 1998). Thus, TNFα itself is not necessarily neurotoxic but may exert cytotoxicity in the presence of another factor. In addition, microglia-derived excitotoxin Glu, eicosanoids, and vasoactive histamine may promote the degenerative processes and inflammation by themselves or in conjunction with other factors. It seems likely that the cooperative action of these microglia-derived, potentially cytotoxic molecules would severely damage neurons in pathological states *in vivo*.

Secretion of Neuroprotective Molecules from Activated Microglia

In contrast to their neurotoxic role, microglia have also been suggested to play a protective role in the pathological brain, such as in the human immunodeficiency virus-1 (HIV-1) infected striatum (Soontornniyomkij et al., 1998), in spinal cord injuries (Dougherty et al., 2000), in compression injuries (Ikeda et al., 2001), and in ischemia (Lee et al., 2002). These activated microglia have been shown to produce neuroprotective factors and cytokines (Fig. 35.2).

Neurotrophins are a family of protein factors that have strong neurotrophic effects on various types of neurons in the CNS and the peripheral nervous system (PNS). Nerve growth factor (NGF), brain-derived neurotrophic factor (BDNF), neurotrophin-3 (NT-3), and NT-4/5 are expressed in the brain of mammals, and gene knockout experiments have shown that each of these neurotrophins plays an important role in neuronal survival and development. Although the neurotrophins were initially thought to be produced in neurons, they were later shown to be produced in glial cells *in vivo*. Brain-derived neurotrophic factor has been identified in activated microglia in HIV-1 encephalitis (Soontornniyomkij et al., 1998), in the injured striatum (Batchelor et al., 1999), and in the injured spinal cord (Dougherty et al., 2000). The expression of the mRNAs and proteins of these neurotrophins was also confirmed *in vitro* (Elkabes et al., 1996; Nakajima et al., 2001). The BDNF produced in pathological situations may play a role in neuroprotection. On the other hand, microglia-derived NGF was shown to cause apoptosis of neuroepithelia (Frade and Barde, 1999).

The TGFβ family is widely expressed in various CNS cells. One of the TGFβ isoforms, TGFβ1, is expressed in activated microglia at the axotomized facial nucleus (Kiefer et al., 1993b) and in reactive microglia during experimental allergic neuritis (EAN) (Kiefer et al., 1993a). Transforming growth factor-β1 may contribute to the recovery and survival of injured motoneurons. Glial cell line-derived neurotrophic factor (GDNF), which belongs to the TGFβ superfamily, is expressed in the microglia of the injured striatum (Batchelor et al., 1999). Glial cell line-derived neurotrophic factor can protect against neuronal cell death in both the CNS and PNS. Thus, microglia might serve as neuroprotective cells by producing GDNF in the pathological CNS.

Interleukin-6 (IL-6), ciliary neurotrophic factor (CNTF), and leukemia inhibitory factor (LIF) are grouped within the same family, since these cytokines share a common receptor component (gp 130) in their signal transduction. Interleukin-6 (Ye and Johnson, 1999), CNTF (Rudge et al., 1994) and LIF are produced by activated microglia, as well as by astrocytes. Interleukin-6 exerts a neurotrophic effect on septal cholinergic neurons. Ciliary neurotrophic factor can serve as a potent neuroprotective factor in striatal neurons in the CNS (Mittoux et al., 2002). Leukemia inhibitory factor may play a role as an injury factor at the injured site. Therefore, these factors could affect neuronal survival if secreted from activated microglia or released from ruptured microglia.

In addition to these factors, fibroblast growth factor 2 (FGF2: bFGF), insulin-like growth factor-I (IGF-I), IGF-II, and hepatocyte growth factor (HGF) have been demonstrated to be expressed or produced in activated microglia. These factors can promote neuronal survival in various types of neurons in pathological conditions. Interleukin-3 produced from activated microglia can exert neurotrophic effects on cortical neurons and cholinergic neurons. Thus, activated microglia can produce various kinds of neuroprotective molecules in addition to harmful factors.

TRIGGER OF MICROGLIAL ACTIVATION

As described above, various changes, including phenotypical, immunohistochemical, and biochemical changes, are caused in activated microglia. One of the important things that remains to be determined is what kinds of specific signals from what kinds of cell types result in an induction of microglial activation *in vivo*. However, since the signals for the activation of microglia are suspected to be largely distinct in such situations as chronic and acute injuries, it will be important to clarify the cellular and molecular mechanisms.

In chronic inflammatory diseases such as Alzheimer's disease, MS, and AIDS, it is difficult to detect signals for microglial activation and observe the responses solely of resident microglia. This is because blood-derived cells including monocytes and macrophages infiltrate into the affected brain parenchyma, and these infiltrated cells and resident microglia may be stimulated by various kinds of molecules, including disease-related proteins, viruses, serum-derived proteins, and immune cell-derived factors, resulting in complicated, long-lasting reactions. Thus, the complex series of events common to these chronic injuries make it difficult to identify the trigger signal for microglia activation.

In contrast, acute and transient injury such as peripheral nerve axotomy has been shown to cause microglial activation around the neuronal cell body. In this case, the primary stimulus for microglial activation must arise from the injured neurons. As distinct from chronic degenerative diseases, the blood–brain barrier (BBB) is preserved normally, and blood-derived cells do not infiltrate into the brain parenchyma. Thus, the peripheral nerve transection model appears to be suitable for the study of trigger signals for microglial activation.

Microglia in Models of Acute Neuronal Injury

The pronounced efficacy of facial nerve axotomy and its detailed analysis have been described by Kreutzberg and colleagues (Streit et al., 1988; Kreutzberg, 1996). The most important finding of this research is that neuronal injury is performed outside the brain stem, at the stylomastoid foramen, which does not lead to the infiltration or accumulation of monocytes/macrophages in the brain parenchyma. This advantage makes it possible to examine the changes or responses of resident microglia in tissue.

Transection of the facial nerve causes activation of microglia around surviving motoneurons in the axotomized facial nucleus (Fig. 35.3). The activated microglia locate around the motoneuronal cell body and have been shown to upregulate CR-3, MHC class II, and Iba1, although they do not exhibit phagocytic properties (Graeber et al., 1998). The process of activation proceeds through a series of gradated steps (Raivich et al., 1999). Later, activated microglia become quiescent and the cell number is reduced, along with the neuronal regeneration.

Astrocytes are also activated in the axotomized facial nucleus, thereby enhancing the expression of glial fibrillary acidic protein. This activation proceeds for a long period of time after microglial activation (Graeber and Kreutzberg, 1988).

This facial nerve axotomy model allows us to predict the presence of intercellular interaction between injured motoneurons and glial cells in the facial nucleus (Fig. 35.3). The primary incident described by this model is the injury of motoneurons. Therefore, certain signals from injured motoneurons are strongly suggested to be released as triggers of microglial activation.

Neuron-Derived Signals Responsible for Microglial Activation

Axotomy of the facial nerve induces the upregulation of glucose metabolite enzyme, neuropeptide, and cytoskeletal proteins, as well as the downregulation of neurotransmitters and neurofilaments in motoneurons.

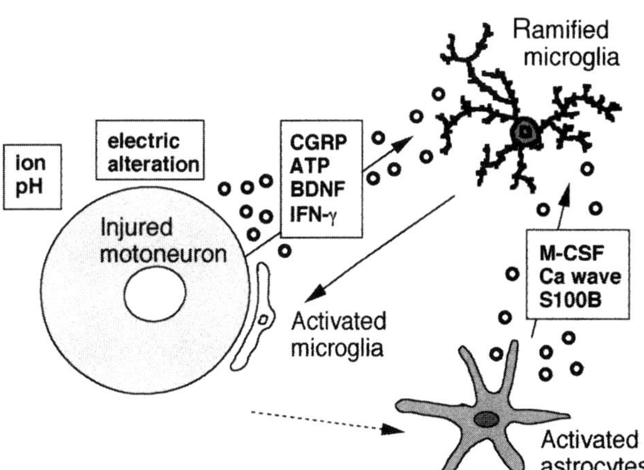

FIGURE 35.3 Putative molecules for activating microglia *in vivo*. Some putative stimulators derived from neurons and astrocytes are listed. ATP: adenosine triphosphate; BDNF: brain-derived neurotrophic factor; CGRP: calcitonin gene-related peptide; IFN-γ: interferon-γ; M-CSF: macrophage colony-stimulating factor.

In the early stages after transection, three immediate early genes, *c-jun*, *Jun-B*, and *TIS11*, have been shown to be induced in injured motoneurons (Haas et al., 1993), and this induction presumably represents a neuronal response and alterations. Certain biochemical changes subsequently occur in motoneurons, causing certain signals to activate microglia.

To date, various molecules, including ions, nucleotides, neuropeptides, chemokines, cytokines, growth factors, and neurotransmitters, have been suggested as candidates for injured motoneuron-derived signals (Fig. 35.3).

Plausible candidates are the calcitonin gene-related peptide (CGRP) and ATP. Calcitonin gene-related peptide (CGRP) is a neuropeptide whose production is enhanced in motoneurons in the axotomized facial nucleus (Streit et al., 1987). Adenosien triphosphate is known to be released from neurons in an activity-dependent manner, or the amounts are increased in the extracellular space during inflammation. Indeed, CGRP and ATP have been shown to induce immediate early gene mRNA in microglia (Priller et al., 1995). Adenosine triphosphate was found to induce an inward potassium current and increase the membrane conductance in microglia (Kettenmann et al., 1990). The ATP effect is thought to provide a sufficient stimulation for microglial activation. Furthermore, ATP stimulates the release of IL-1β (Ferrari et al., 1997a), plasminogen (PGn) (Inoue et al., 1998), and TNFα (Hide et al., 2001), whose actions are mediated by a specific receptor, P2X7. Adenosine triphosphate was also able to activate a transcription factor, nuclear factor κB (NFκB), in microglia (Ferrari et al., 1997b). The chemoattractive action of ATP for microglia has been demonstrated *in vitro* (Honda et al., 2001). Further, microglia undergo cell death by treatment with ATP (Brough et al., 2002). It is likely that ATP derived from injured neurons is at least partially associated with the activation, secretion, motility, and cell death of microglia in vivo.

The expression of BDNF has been immunohistochemically recognized in facial motoneurons, and the amounts of protein increased in response to axotomy (Kobayashi et al., 1996), suggesting that BDNF may activate microglia after its release. Neurotrophins, including BDNF, may activate microglia to enhance the release of PGn and urokinase-type plasminogen activator (uPA), and to suppress NO production *in vitro* (Nakajima et al., 1998). High concentrations of BDNF have been shown to activate NFκB in microglia. It is possible that neuron-derived BDNF, when released extracellularly (Gartner and Staiger, 2002), acts on microglia and changes their function.

Humoral factors such as cytokines are also candidates for neuron-derived activation factors for microglia. Interferon-γ is a possible cytokine that may be produced in neurons (Bentivoglio et al., 1994). This cytokine can induce the production of oxygen radicals and NO in microglia by itself or in cooperation with other factor *in vitro*. Low molecular weight molecules such as peptides are also candidates for trigger molecules from neurons.

Other than the above molecules, injured motoneuron-derived electrical change may be associated with microglial activation. Changes of ionic concentration—such as potassium or pH—in extracellular spaces may be prime candidates. Taken together, these results indicate that different types of neuronally derived signals may cooperate with more than one factor to contribute to the activation of microglia (Fig. 35.3).

In addition to the signals of living neurons, dead or dying neurons probably send certain signals to microglia for a second activation. This situation corresponds to ricin-induced neuronal cell death in the facial nucleus, in which dead neurons are phagocytosed by macrophages transformed from resident microglia (Streit and Kreutzberg, 1988). The mechanism by which dead neurons are recognized by activated microglia is poorly understood. However, there is accumulating evidence that dying cells release a chemoattractant such as phosphatidylserine or lysophosphatidylcholine to stimulate the attraction of phagocytes (Witting et al., 2000; Lauber et al., 2003). This suggests that phagocytes come in close proximity to the dying cells in response to the chemoattractant, and further engulf the cells after receiving a "consume me" signal (Lauber et al., 2003). It is speculated that the activated microglia transform into phagocytes upon receiving the "consume me" signal in the vicinity of dying neurons (Fig. 35.1).

Reactive Astrocyte-Derived Factor for Microglial Activation

The results of a study using a rat facial nerve transection model have highlighted colony stimulating factors as a prime activation factor for microglia (Raivich et al., 1994). Activated astrocytes are thought to be responsible for the production of CSFs such as M-CSF and GM-CSF. Analysis of M-CSF-deficient mice (op/op mice) revealed a reduction in the expression of activation markers of microglia (Kalla et al., 2001), suggesting that M-CSF may be a factor for the priming of activation as well as proliferation in microglia (Fig. 35.3). Astrocytic calcium waves (Schipke et al., 2002) and astrocyte-derived S-100B (Petrova et al., 2000) are possible sources of microglial activation.

DIVERSITY OF MICROGLIAL ACTIVATION

Generally, the morphological changes of microglia observed in injured or pathologically affected sites of the brain have been uniformly referred to as *activation*. However, the question arises as to whether or not the contents or qualities of such activation are always the same. Although microglia stimulated by distinct signals

stimulator / production	—	ATP	BDNF	M-CSF	GDNF	LPS
NGF	ND	ND	ND	ND	ND	↗
BDNF	+	↗	→	→	→	↗
NO	ND	→	↘	↘	↘	↗
TNFα	ND	↗	ND	ND	ND	↗
IL-1β	ND	↗	ND	ND	ND	↗
uPA	+	→	↗	↘	↘	→
plasminogen	+	↗	↗	↗	↘	↗

— : nonstimulated microglia (control)
ND : not detected
+ : limited amounts

FIGURE 35.4 Response of microglia to putative activators *in vivo*. The secretory products produced by microglia in response to ATP, BDNF, M-CSF, GDNF, and LPS are summarized. ATP: adenosine triphosphate; BDNF: brain-derived neurotrophic factor; GDNF: glial cell line-derived neurotrophic factor; IL-1β: interleukin-1β; LPS: lipopolysaccharide; M-CSF: macrophage colony-stimulating factor; NGF: nerve growth factor; NO: nitric oxide; TNFα: tumor necrosis factor-α; uPA: urokinase-type plasminogen activator.

may display different features, evidence for this possibility is not conclusive.

As described above, some molecules have been considered plausible activators for microglia. The possible responses of microglia to such molecules as stimulators have been compared *in vitro* using secretory products as parameters (Fig. 35.4).

The nonstimulated microglia as a control produced a limited amount of BDNF and uPA, but did not produce harmful factors such as TNFα, IL-1β, or NO. Adenosine triphosphate and BDNF are putative activation molecules that are released from neurons as described above. Macrophage-CSF, which is produced mainly in astrocytes, is also a candidate molecule for activation. Glial cell line-derived neurotrophic factor and lipopolysaccharide (LPS) were also included in the comparison. Glial cell line-derived neurotrophic factor is a cytokine produced in astrocytes and has been speculated to be a quiescent factor against activated microglia. Lipopolysaccharide was used as a model of bacterial infection.

The results summarized in Figure 35.4 show that the qualities of microglial responses showed specific differences among stimulators, indicating stimulator-specific responses. We speculate that activated microglia play a different role in different pathological states by managing a specific combination of secretory products.

SIGNALING MOLECULES RELATED TO THE ACTIVATION OF MICROGLIA

Figure 35.5 shows the signaling molecules associated with the microglial activation induced by each of the potential stimulators.

Nonstimulated microglia *in vitro* showed relatively high-level activation of protein kinase Cα (PKCα), but mitogen-activated protein kinases (MAPKs) including extracellular signal regulated kinase (ERK), p38, c-Jun N-terminal kinase (JNK), and transcription factors including cAMP-response element binding protein (CREB) and NFκB activation were not initiated. These microglia can be regarded as existing in a nonactivated state.

Adenosine triphosphate induced PGn, IL-1β, TNFα, and NO release from microglia via the P2X7 purinoceptor, and these releases were dependent on Ca^{2+} influx, p38, ERK, and, presumably, NFκB activation, while the chemoattraction of ATP for microglia was again shown to be mediated by the P2Y purinergic receptor and G protein. Thus, ATP can induce the secretion and mobility of microglia, and these effects are mediated by P2X and P2Y purinoceptors.

Brain-derived neurotrophic factor stimulated microglia to increase the production/release of uPA and PGn and to reduce NO production. Microglia expressed a high-affinity receptor for the neurotrophins Trk A, Trk B, and Trk C and a low-affinity receptor, p75. The inhibitor experiment showed that the production/release of PGn is mediated by Trks and suggested that uPA release occurs via p75. No activation of p38 or JNK was observed. Activation of NFκB (degradation of IκBα and IκBβ) was induced only by high concentrations of BDNF, suggesting the mediation of p75. If BDNF is released from injured neurons, it could activate microglia to promote the release of uPA and PGn and to reduce NO release via Trks and/or p75 receptors.

Macrophage-CSF is a putative prime factor for microglial activation. Macrophage-CSF stimulation does not enhance the production of neurotrophins and

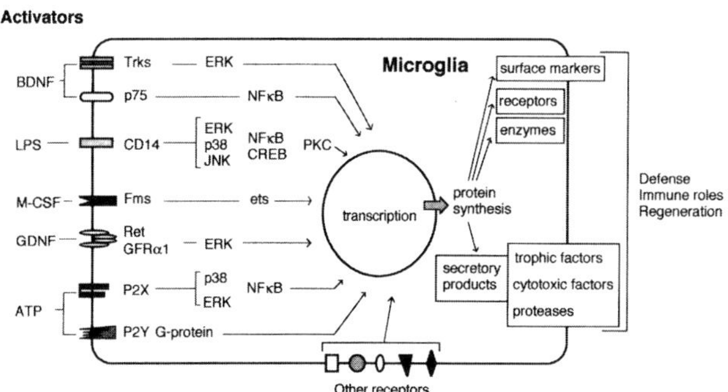

FIGURE 35.5 Summary of microglial response to various stimulators. The receptor and signaling molecules in responses to putative stimulators for microglia are summarized. ATP: adenosine triphosphate; BDNF: brain-derived neurotrophic factor; CREB: cyclic adenosine monophosphate-response element binding protein; ERK: extracellular signal related kinase; GDNF: glial cell line-derived neurotrophic factor; GFRα1: GDNF receptor α1; JNK: c-Jun N-terminal kinase; LPS: lipopolysaccharide; M-CSF: macrophage colony-stimulating factor; NFκB: nuclear factor κB: PKC: protein kinase C.

TNFα in microglia and reduces the secretion of NO and uPA. Macrophage-CSF binds to the specific receptor, c-Fms, on the microglial membrane. C-Fms is phosphorylated and transduces the signal downstream (Fig. 35.5). A transcription factor, ets1, was upregulated, and Rac was activated during M-CSF treatment. Thus, these reactions may be associated with the event of microglial activation as well as the early stages of proliferation.

The stimulation of microglia with GDNF resulted in the suppression of PGn, uPA, and NO release. Microglia express the GDNF receptor complexes, Ret and GFRα-1 (Honda et al., 1999). The Ret protein is phosphorylated by GDNF application. Shortly after GDNF stimulation, one of the MAPKs, ERK, was phosphorylated in microglia. This signaling would lead to the suppression of PGn, uPA, and NO release.

Lipopolysaccharide induced the production of TNFα, IL-1β, inducible NO, and NGF, and promoted the secretion of BDNF and NT-4/5 in microglia. Lipopolysaccharide binds to the specific receptor, CD14, in microglia, and the signal is transduced to PKC, MAPKs including ERK, p38, and JNK, and transcription factors including CREB and NFκB. These signaling molecules may be associated with the production/secretion of a variety of molecules.

Thus, the response of microglia to each of the predicted stimulators was found to be mediated by a specific signal transduction cascade, which subsequently leads to a specific combination of secretory products (Fig. 35.5).

SUMMARY

Microglia are activated to induce various cellular changes, including morphology, immunohistochemical properties, proliferative activity, chemotactic mobility, biochemical change, secretion, and phagocytosis, in response to the signal(s) produced in the extracellular milieu of the pathological brain. Some putative or plausible signals from injured neurons or activated astrocytes have been predicted based on an acute injury model. In response to these candidate molecules, the microglia produce a specific combination of secretory molecules through a specific signal transduction cascade. Thus, the activated microglia might play different roles according to the type of pathology. However, the specific signal(s) for microglial activation *in vivo* remain to be identified, and further studies will be needed to analyze the intracellular signaling cascade leading to microglia activation. Such research would help to clarify the mystery of microglial activation, as well as the pathophysiological significance of such activation in the brain.

ABBREVIATIONS

AIDS	acquired immunodeficiency syndrome
ATP	adenosine triphosphate
BBB	blood–brain barrier
BDNF	brain-derived neurotrophic factor
CGRP	calcitonin gene–related peptide
CNS	central nervous system
CNTF	ciliary neurotrophic factor
CR-3	complement receptor-3
CREB	cyclic AMP-response element binding protein
CSF	cerebrospinal fluid
DMSO	dimethylsulfoxide
EAE	experimental allergic encephalomyelitis
EAN	experimental allergic neuritis
ECM	extracellular matrix
ERK	extracellular signal-regulated kinase
FGF	fibroblast growth factor
GDNF	glial cell line-derived neurotrophic factor
GLT-1	glutamate transporter-1
Glu	glutamic acid
GM-CSF	granulocyte/macrophage-colony stimulating factor
HGF	hepatocyte growth factor
HIV-1	human immunodeficiency virus-1
Iba1	ionized calcium binding adapter molecule 1
IFN-γ	interferon-γ
IGF-1	insulin-like growth factor-1
IL	interleukin
JNK	c-Jun N-terminal kinase
LFA-1	leukocyte function-associated antigen-1
LIF	leukemia inhibitory factor
LPS	lipopolysaccharide
MAPK	mitogen-activated protein kinase
MCP1	monocyte chemoattractant protein-1
M-CSF	macrophage colony-stimulating factor
MHC	major histocompatibility complex

MM	microglial mitogen
MS	multiple sclerosis
NFκB	nuclear factor κB
NGF	nerve growth factor
NO	nitric oxide
NT-3	neurotrophin-3
PGn	plasminogen
PKC	protein kinase C
PNS	peripheral nervous system
ROS	reactive oxygen species
TGFβ	transforming growth factor β
TNFα	tumor necrosis factor-α
uPA	urokinase-type plasminogen activator

REFERENCES

Aschner, M., Allen, J.W., Kimelberg, H.K., LoPachin, R.M., and Streit, W.J. (1999) Glial cells in neurotoxicity development. *Annu. Rev. Pharmacol. Toxicol.* 39:151–173.

Banati, R.B., Gehrmann, J., Schubert, P., and Kreutzberg, G.W. (1993) Cytotoxicity of microglia. *Glia* 7:111–118.

Batchelor, P.E., Liberatore, G.T., Wong, J.Y., Porritt, M.J., Frerichs, F., Donnan, G.A., and Howells, D.W. (1999) Activated macrophages and microglia induce dopaminergic sprouting in the injured striatum and express brain-derived neurotrophic factor and glial cell line–derived neurotrophic factor. *J. Neurosci.* 19:1708–1716.

Bentivoglio, M., Florenzano, F., Peng, Z.C., and Kristensson, K. (1994) Neuronal IFN-γ in tuberomammillary neurones. *NeuroReport* 5:2413–2416.

Brough, D., Le Feuvre, R.A., Iwakura, Y., and Rothwell, N.J. (2002) Purinergic (P2X7) receptor activation of microglia induces cell death via an interleukin-1-independent mechanism. *Mol. Cell. Neurosci.* 19:272–280.

Chao, C.C., Hu, S., Molitor, T.W., Shaskan, E.G., and Peterson, P.K. (1992) Activated microglia mediate neuronal cell injury via a nitric oxide mechanism. *J. Immunol.* 149:2736–2741.

del Rio-Hortega, P. (1932) Microglia. In: Penfield, W., ed. *Cytology and Cellular Pathology of the Nervous System*, Vol. 2. New York: Hocker, pp. 481–534.

Dougherty, K.D., Dreyfus, C.F., and Black, I.B. (2000) Brain-derived neurotrophic factor in astrocytes, oligodendrocytes, and microglia/macrophages after spinal cord injury. *Neurobiol. Dis.* 7:574–585.

Elkabes, S., DiCicco-Bloom, E.M., and Black, I.B. (1996) Brain microglia/macrophages express neurotrophins that selectively regulate microglial proliferation and function. *J. Neurosci.* 16: 2508–2521.

Ferrari, D., Chiozzi, P., Falzoni, S., Hanau, S., and Di Virgilio, F. (1997a) Purinergic modulation of interleukin-1β release from microglial cells stimulated with bacterial endotoxin. *J. Exp. Med.* 185:579–582.

Ferrari, D., Wesselborg, S., Bauer, M.K., and Schulze-Osthoff, K. (1997b) Extracellular ATP activates transcription factor NF-κB through the P2Z purinoreceptor by selectively targeting NF-κB p65. *J. Cell Biol.* 139:1635–1643.

Frade, J.M. and Barde, Y.A. (1999) Genetic evidence for cell death mediated by nerve growth factor and the neurotrophin receptor p75 in the developing mouse retina and spinal cord. *Development* 126:683–690.

Gao, H.M., Jiang, J., Wilson, B., Zhang, W., Hong, J.S., and Liu, B. (2002) Microglial activation-mediated delayed and progressive degeneration of rat nigral dopaminergic neurons: relevance to Parkinson's disease. *J. Neurochem.* 81:1285–1297.

Gartner, A. and Staiger, V. (2002) Neurotrophin secretion from hippocampal neurons evoked by long-term-potentiation-inducing electrical stimulation patterns. *Proc. Natl. Acad. Sci. USA* 99: 6386–6391.

Gebicke-Haerter, P.J., Spleiss, O., Ren, L.Q., Li, H., Dichmann, S., Norgauer, J., and Boddeke, H.W. (2001) Microglial chemokines and chemokine receptors. *Prog. Brain Res.* 132:525–532.

Gehrmann, J. and Banati, R.B. (1995) Microglial turnover in the injured CNS: activated microglia undergo delayed DNA fragmentation following peripheral nerve injury. *J. Neuropathol. Exp. Neurol.* 54:680–688.

Giulian, D. and Baker, T.J. (1986) Characterization of ameboid microglia isolated from developing mammalian brain. *J. Neurosci.* 6:2163–2178.

Giulian, D., Corpuz, M., Chapman, S., Mansouri, M., and Robertson, C. (1993) Reactive mononuclear phagocytes release neurotoxins after ischemic and traumatic injury to the central nervous system. *J. Neurosci. Res.* 36:681–693.

Giulian, D. and Ingeman, J.E. (1988) Colony-stimulating factors as promoter of ameboid microglia. *J. Neurosci.* 8:4707–4717.

Giulian, D., Johnson, B., Krebs, J.F., George, J.K., and Tapscott, M. (1991) Microglial mitogens are produced in the developing and injured mammalian brain. *J. Cell Biol.* 112:323–333.

Graeber, M.B. and Kreutzberg, G.W. (1988) Delayed astrocyte reaction following facial nerve axotomy. *J. Neurocytol.* 17: 209–220.

Graeber, M.B., Lopez-Redondo, F., Ikoma, E., Ishikawa, M., Imai, Y., Nakajima, K., Kreutzberg, G.W., and Kohsaka, S. (1998) The microglia/macrophage response in the neonatal rat facial nucleus following axotomy. *Brain Res.* 813:241–253.

Haas, C.A., Donath, C., and Kreutzberg, G.W. (1993) Differential expression of immediate early genes after transection of the facial nerve. *Neuroscience* 53:91–99.

Harrison, J.K., Jiang, Y., Chen, S., Xia, Y., Maciejewski, D., McNamara, R.K., Streit, W.J., Salafranca, M.N., Adhikari, S., Thompson, D.A., Botti, P., Bacon, K.B., and Feng, L. (1998) Role for neuronally derived fractalkine in mediating interactions between neurons and CX3CR1-expressing microglia. *Proc. Natl. Acad. Sci. USA* 95:10896–10901.

Heppner, F.L., Roth, K., Nitsch, R., and Hailer, N.P. (1998) Vitamin E induces ramification and downregulation of adhesion molecules in cultured microglial cells. *Glia* 22:180–188.

Hide, I., Tanaka, M., Inoue, A., Nakajima, K., Kohsaka, S., Inoue, K., and Nakata, Y. (2001) Extracellular ATP triggers tumor necrosis factor-α release from rat microglia. *J. Neurochem.* 75:965–972.

Honda, S., Nakajima, K., Nakamura, Y., Imai, Y., and Kohsaka, S. (1999) Rat primary cultured microglia express glial cell line-derived neurotrophic factor receptors. *Neurosci. Lett.* 275: 203–206.

Honda, S., Sasaki, Y., Ohsawa, K., Imai, Y., Nakamura, Y., Inoue, K., and Kohsaka, S. (2001) Extracellular ATP or ADP induce chemotaxis of cultured microglia through Gi/o-coupled P2Y receptors. *J. Neurosci.* 21:1975–1982.

Ikeda, O., Murakami, M., Ito, H., Yamazaki, M., Nemoto, T., Koda, M., Nakayama, C., and Moriya, H. (2001) Acute up-regulation of brain-derived neurotrophic factor expression resulting from experimentally induced injury in the rat spinal cord. *Acta Neuropathol.* 102:239–245.

Inoue, K., Nakajima, K., Morimoto, T., Kikuchi, Y., Koizumi, S., Illes, P., and Kohsaka, S. (1998) ATP stimulation of Ca^{2+}-dependent plasminogen release from cultured microglia. *Br. J. Pharmacol.* 123:1304–1310.

Jung, S., Aliberti, J., Graemmel, P., Sunshine, M.J., Kreutzberg, G.W., Sher, A., and Littman, D.R. (2000) Analysis of fractalkine receptor CX(3)CR1 function by targeted deletion and green fluorescent protein reporter gene insertion. *Mol. Cell. Biol.* 20: 4106–4114.

Kalla, R., Bohatschek, M., Kloss, C.U., Krol, J., Von Maltzan, X., and Raivich, G. (2003) Loss of microglial ramification in microglia-astrocyte cocultures: involvement of adenylate cyclase, calcium, phosphatase, and Gi-protein systems. *Glia* 41:50–63.

Kalla, R., Liu, Z., Xu, S., Koppius, A., Imai, Y,. Kloss, C.U., Kohsaka, S., Gschwendtner, A., Moller, J.C., Werner, A., and Raivich, G. (2001) Microglia and the early phase of immune surveillance in the axotomized facial motor nucleus: impaired microglial activation and lymphocyte recruitment but no effect on neuronal survival or axonal regeneration in macrophage-colony stimulating factor–deficient mice. *J. Comp. Neurol.* 436:182–201.

Kettenmann, H., Hoppe, D., Gottmann, K., Banati, R., and Kreutzberg, G.W. (1990) Cultured microglial cells have a distinct pattern of membrane channels different from peritoneal macrophages. *J. Neurosci. Res.* 26:278–287.

Kiefer, R., Gold, R., Gehrmann, J., Lindholm, D., Wekerle, H., and Kreutzberg, G.W. (1993a) Transforming growth factor β expression in reactive spinal cord microglia and meningeal inflammatory cells during experimental allergic neuritis. *J. Neurosci. Res.* 36:391–398.

Kiefer, R., Lindholm, D., and Kreutzberg, G.W. (1993b) Interleukin-6 and transforming growth factor-β1 mRNAs are induced in rat facial nucleus following motoneuron axotomy. *Eur. J. Neurosci.* 5:775–781.

Kloss, C.U., Kreutzberg, G.W., and Raivich, G. (1997) Proliferation of ramified microglia on an astrocyte monolayer: characterization of stimulatory and inhibitory cytokines. *J. Neurosci. Res.* 49:248–254.

Kobayashi, N.R., Bedard, A.M., Hincke, M.T., and Tetzlaff, W. (1996) Increased expression of BDNF and trkB mRNA in rat facial motoneurons after axotomy. *Eur. J. Neurosci.* 8:1018–1029.

Kreutzberg, G.W. (1996) Microglia: a sensor for pathological events in the CNS. *Trends Neurosci.* 19:312–318.

Lauber, K., Bohn, E., Krober, S.M., Xiao, Y., Blumenthal, S.G., Lindemann, R.K., Marini, P., Wiedig, C., Zobywalski, A., Baksh, S., Xu, Y., Autenrieth, I.B., Schulze-Osthoff, K., Belka, C., Stuhler, G., and Wesselborg, S. (2003) Apoptotic cells induce migration of phagocytes via caspase-3-mediated release of a lipid attraction signal. *Cell* 113:717–730.

Lawson, L.J., Perry, V.H., and Gordon, S. (1992) Turnover of resident microglia in the normal adult mouse brain. *Neuroscience* 48:405–415.

Lee, T.H., Kato, H., Chen, S.T., Kogure, K., and Itoyama, Y. (2002) Expression disparity of brain-derived neurotrophic factor immunoreactivity and mRNA in ischemic hippocampal neurons. *NeuroReport* 13:2271–2275.

Liu, J,, Marino, M.W., Wong, G., Grail, D., Dunn, A., Bettadapura, J., Slavin, A.J., Old, L., and Bernard, C.C. (1998) TNF is a potent anti-inflammatory cytokine in autoimmune-mediated demyelination. *Nat. Med.* 4:78–83.

Lopez-Redondo, F., Nakajima, K., Honda, S., and Kohsaka, S. (2000) Glutamate transporter GLT-1 is highly expressed in activated microglia following facial nerve axotomy. *Mol. Brain Res.* 76:429–435.

Mittoux, V., Ouary, S., Monville, C., Lisovoski, F., Poyot, T., Conde, F., Escartin, C., Robichon, R., Brouillet, E., Peschanski, M., and Hantraya, P. (2002) Corticostriatopallidal neuroprotection by adenovirus-mediated ciliary neurotrophic factor gene transfer in a rat model of progressive striatal degeneration. *J. Neurosci.* 22:4478–4486.

Moller, J.C., Klein, M.A., Haas, S., Jones, L.L., Kreutzberg, G.W., and Raivich, G. (1996) Regulation of thrombospondin in the regenerating mouse facial motor nucleus. *Glia* 17:121–132.

Moneta, M.E., Gehrmann, J., Topper, R., Banati, R.B., and Kreutzberg, G.W. (1993) Cell adhesion molecule expression in the regenerating rat facial nucleus. *J. Neuroimmunol.* 45: 203–206.

Nakajima, K., Honda, S., Tohyama, Y., Imai, Y., Kohsaka, S., and Kurihara, T. (2001) Neurotrophin secretion from cultured microglia. *J. Neurosci. Res.* 65:322–331.

Nakajima, K., Kikuchi, Y., Ikoma, E., Honda, S., Ishikawa, M., Liu, Y.M., and Kohsaka, S. (1998) Neurotrophins regulate the function of cultured microglia. *Glia* 24:272–289.

Petrova, T.V., Hu, J., and Van Eldik, L.J. (2000) Modulation of glial activation by astrocyte-derived protein S100B: differential responses of astrocyte and microglial cultures. *Brain Res.* 853:74–80.

Priller, J., Haas, C.A., Reddington, M., and Kreutzberg, G.W. (1995) Calcitonin gene-related peptide and ATP induce immediate early gene expression in cultured rat microglial cells. *Glia* 15:447–457.

Raivich, G., Bohatschek, M., Kloss, U.A., Werner, A., Jones, L.L., and Kreutzberg, G.W. (1999) Neuroglial activation repertoire in the injured brain: graded response, molecular mechanisms and cues to physiological function. *Brain Res. Rev.* 30:77–105.

Raivich, G., Gehrmann, J., and Kreutzberg, G.W. (1991) Increase of macrophage colony-stimulating factor and granulocyte-macrophage colony-stimulating factor receptors in the regenerating rat facial nucleus. *J. Neurosci. Res.* 30:682–686.

Raivich, G., Moreno-Flores, M.T., Moller, J.C., and Kreutzberg, G.W. (1994) Inhibition of posttraumatic microglial proliferation in a genetic model of macrophage colony-stimulating factor deficiency in the mouse. *Eur. J. Neurosci.* 6:1615–1658.

Rudge, J.S., Morrissey, D., Lindsay, R.M., and Pasnikowski, E.M. (1994) Regulation of ciliary neurotrophic factor in cultured rat hippocampal astrocytes. *Eur. J. Neurosci.* 6:218–229.

Schilling, T., Nitsch, R., Heinemann, U., Haas, D., and Eder, C. (2001) Astrocyte-released cytokines induce ramification and outward K^+ channel expression in microglia via distinct signaling pathways. *Eur. J. Neurosci.* 14:463–473.

Schipke, C.G., Boucsein, C., Ohlemeyer, C., Kirchhoff, F., and Kettenmann, H. (2002) Astrocyte Ca2+ waves trigger responses in microglial cells in brain slice. *FASEB J.* 16:255–257.

Schoen, S.W., Graeber, M.B., and Kreutzberg, G.W. (1992) 5′-Nucleotidase immunoreactivity of perineuronal microglia responding to rat facial nerve axotomy. *Glia* 6:314–317.

Soontornniyomkij, V., Wang, G., Pittman, C.A., Wiley, C.A., and Achim, C.L. (1998) Expression of brain-derived neurotrophic factor protein in activated microglia of human immunodeficiency virus type 1encephalitis. *Neuropathol. Appl. Neurobiol.* 24:453–460.

Streit, W.J., Dumoulin, F.L., Raivich, G., and Kreutzberg, G.W. (1987) Calcitonin gene–related peptide increases in rat facial motoneurons after peripheral nerve transection. *Neurosci. Lett.* 101: 143–148.

Streit, W.J., Graeber, M.B., and Kreutzberg, G.W. (1988), Functional plasticity of microglia: a review. *Glia* 1:301–307.

Streit, W.J. and Kreutzberg, G.W. (1988) Response of endogenous glial cells to motor neuron degeneration induced by toxic ricin. *J. Comp. Neurol.* 268:248–263.

Tanaka, J., Toku, K., Sakanaka, M., and Maeda, N. (1999) Morphological differentiation of microglial cells in culture: involvement of insoluble factors derived from astrocytes. *Neurosci. Res.* 34:207–215.

Wilms, H., Hartmann, D., and Sievers, J. (1997) Ramification of microglia, monocytes and macrophages in vitro: influences of various epithelial and mesenchymal cells and their conditioned media. *Cell Tissue Res.* 287:447–458.

Witting, A., Muller, P., Herrmann, A., Kettenmann, H., and Nolte, C. (2000) Phagocytic clearance of apoptotic neurons by microglia/brain macrophages in vitro: involvement of lectin-, integrin-, and phosphatidylserine-mediated recognition. *J. Neurochem.* 75:1060–1070.

Wollmer, M.A., Lucius, R., Wilms, H., Held-Feindt, J., Sievers, J., and Mentlein, R. (2001) ATP and adenosine induce ramification of microglia in vitro. *J. Neuroimmunol.* 115:19–27.

Ye, S.M. and Johnson, R.W. (1999) Increased interleukin-6 expression by microglia from brain of aged mice. *J. Neuroimmunol.* 93:139–148.

Yrjanheikki, J., Tikka, T., Keinanen, R., Goldsteins, G., Chan, P.H. and Koistinaho, J. (1999) A tetracycline derivative, minocycline, reduces inflammation and protects against focal cerebral ischemia with a wide therapeutic window. *Proc. Natl. Acad. Sci. USA* 96:13496–13500.

36 Axonal regeneration in the peripheral nervous system of mammals

OLAWALE A.R. SULAIMAN, J. GORDON BOYD, AND TESSA GORDON

The capacity for injured neurons to regenerate axons and remake functional connections with target organs distinguishes the peripheral from the central nervous system. This unique characteristic of the peripheral nervous system stems from the ability of the Schwann cells (SCs) as opposed to the inability of the oligodendrocytes in the central nervous system to support axonal regeneration (see Chapter 37). In consequence, return of function after peripheral nerve injuries contrasts with permanent deficits associated with central nerve injuries. Yet, functional recovery after nerve injuries in humans is generally poor, despite the capacity of injured peripheral nerves to regenerate their axons. Minimal or no recovery may be the outcome for injuries that sever the peripheral nerve far from the target and that incur substantial delays before target reinnervation, regardless of considerable advances made in microsurgical repair of the injured nerves (Sunderland, 1978; Fu and Gordon, 1997). The processes of axonal regeneration and target reinnervation involve many factors that pertain to the injured neuron, the growth environment of the distal nerve stumps, and denervated targets. The neurons must survive the injuries to mount a regenerative response, regenerate their axons within the growth environment of the denervated distal nerve stump, and reinnervate the appropriate targets to restore function. In this chapter, we review the response of SCs to peripheral nerve injury in animal models. This information will provide insight into why functional recovery is often so poor despite the regenerative capacity of the peripheral nervous system and will provide the rationale for experimental approaches to improve axonal regeneration and, in turn, functional recovery.

CELLULAR RESPONSES TO PERIPHERAL NERVE INJURY

Neurons that incur axonal disruption or axotomy may succumb to cell death, depending on the age of the animal and proximity of the injury to the cell body (Fu and Gordon, 1997). Adult motoneurons and the majority of sensory neurons normally survive the injury; the axotomized neurons undergo characteristic morphological or "chromatolytic" changes that underlie a marked increase in mRNA synthesis and a change in gene expression that converts the neurons from the normally *transmitting* to the *growth* mode (reviewed by Gordon, 1983; Fu and Gordon, 1997). The specific changes that occur in peripheral neurons following axotomy have been reviewed elsewhere (Fu and Gordon, 1997; Boyd and Gordon, 2003). Thus the remainder of this section will focus on the injury-induced changes that occur in the SCs of the distal nerve sheath.

Wallerian Degeneration and Initiation of Axonal Regeneration

In 1850, Waller established that the cell nucleus is critical for survival of the axon, noting the degeneration of the axons that were physically separated from the neuronal cell body after nerve injury. This degeneration was thereafter referred to as *Wallerian degeneration* (reviewed by Vrbova et al., 1995; Fu and Gordon, 1997). The nerve stump proximal to the lesion also shows signs of traumatic degeneration or *die back*, usually up to the first node of Ranvier in association with calcium influx and activation of calcium-associated proteases that mediate the axonal and myelin breakdown (Ramon y Cajal, 1928; reviewed by Bisby, 1995; Vrbova et al., 1995; Fu and Gordon, 1997). During the first days of Wallerian degeneration, SCs play the major role in the degradation and phagocytosis of the axonal and myelin debris. Thereafter, macrophages that are recruited at the injury site and throughout the distal nerve stump cooperate with SCs over a relatively prolonged period of up to a month to complete the removal of the debris by active phagocytosis (You et al., 1997).

Schwann cells secrete chemoattractive factors that recruit macrophages into the denervated nerve stumps; these include cytokines such as interleukin-1β, leukemia inhibitory factor, and monocyte chemoattractant protein-1 (Tofaris et al., 2002; reviewed by Fu and Gordon, 1997; Kury et al., 2001). Cytokines that derive from the SCs as well as from the macrophages that enter the nerve have been implicated in both the enhancement (e.g. interleukin-1β and tumor necrosis factor-α) and the curtailment (transforming growth factor-β, TGF-β) of phagocytosis and, hence, in the regulation of the process of Wallerian degeneration (Shamash et al., 2002). In turn, the release of cytokines is associated with the expression of the nonmyelinating, dedifferentiated, *denervated* phenotype of the SCs that proliferate, form the bands of Bungner, and guide regenerating axons within the distal nerve stump [see the sections "Schwann Cells Promote Axonal Regeneration (Elongation)" and "Process of Axonal Regeneration"].

The critical dependence of Wallerian degeneration and axonal regeneration on both SCs and macrophages is evident from the severe retardation of Wallerian degeneration in Ola mutant mice where macrophage invasion of the injured nerve is severely curtailed (reviewed by Perry and Brown, 1992) and from the failure of axonal regeneration in the absence of SCs (Hall, 1986). The retarded regeneration of axons in Ola mice is consistent with the view that the intact myelin, possibly in association with glycoproteins such as myelin-associated glycoprotein, is inhibitory to axonal growth (see Chapter 37).

The Denervated Schwann Cell Phenotype

Just as a mature neuron switches from a transmitting to growth mode after nerve injury, SCs in the distal nerve stump switch their mode from myelination of electrically active axons to growth support for regenerating axons (Mirsky and Jessen, 1999; Scherer and Salzer, 2001; see Chapters 7 and 20). Denervated SCs proliferate and switch their pattern of gene expression to convert from the myelinating and nonmyelinating phenotype associated with intact axons into a dedifferentiated denervated SC phenotype in the absence of axonal contact. The phenotype of the *growth-supportive* denervated SCs is similar to that of the nonmyelinating SCs that normally surround several unmyelinated axons and that do not form myelin (Guenard et. al., 1996). However, the growth-supportive SCs express higher levels of GAP-43 and lower levels of the glycolipids, galactocerebroside, and sulfatide (Scherer and Salzer, 1996). They also extend long processes that express the p75 neurotrophin receptor (p75NTR) and that interact with the growth cones of regenerating axons (Ide, 1996; You et al., 1997). The switch in SC phenotype is associated with downregulation of myelin-associated genes and upregulation of several growth-associated genes. The myelin-associated proteins that are downregulated include P_0, myelin basic protein, myelin-associated glycoprotein, peripheral myelin protein 22 kDa (PMP22), connexin 32, and periaxin, as well as transcription factors such as Krox-20 and Oct-6 (see Chapters 7 and 20). The genes that are upregulated include several neurotrophic factors, truncated neurotrophin tyrosine kinase (trk) receptors, p75NTR, glial fibrillar acidic protein (GFAP), GAP-43, netrin-1, and the transcription factor, Krox-24 (Scherer and Salzer, 1996; Fu and Gordon, 1997).

Synthesis and release of growth factors and cytokines from both SCs and macrophages play important contributing roles in the proliferation of SCs and their conversion to the growth-supportive phenotype. Proliferative capacity of SCs in the initial stage of Wallerian degeneration, prior to the entry of macrophages and contact with regenerating axons, has been associated with the autocrine capacity of the denervated SCs to synthesize and express the neuregulins and their erbB receptors (Raabe et al., 1998). Macrophages that enter denervated distal nerve stumps secrete numerous growth factors that also enhance SC proliferation. These factors include nerve growth factor (NGF), platelet-derived growth factor, epithelial growth factor, and acidic and basic fibroblast growth factors (reviewed by Fu and Gordon, 1997). When regenerating axons contact SCs, neuregulins from the growth cones bind to erbB receptors on the SC membranes to mediate, via the formation of erbB2:erbB3 heterodimers, a second phase of SC proliferation (Rahmatullah et al., 1998).

Several interleukins, including interleukins-1α and -1β, -6, and -10, are released in the distal nerve stumps after nerve injury (Shamash et al., 2002) and have been implicated in the production of growth factors by the denervated SCs (Bolin et al., 1995; Gillen et al., 1998). Interleukin-1β induces NGF in fibroblasts and has been implicated in maintaining NGF in SCs (Lindholm et al., 1987). The cytokine TGF-β, secreted by both macrophages and SCs, induces NGF synthesis in SCs; this effect is augmented by elevated intracellular cyclic adenosine monophosphate (cAMP) levels as well as by growth factors such as platelet-derived and basic fibroblast growth factors (Ridley et al., 1989; Meyer et al., 1992). This cytokine has also been shown to be essential for the neurotrophic effect of several neurotrophic factors including glial-derived neurotrophic factor (GDNF) (reviewed by Unsicker and Kreiglstein, 2000). However, the effects of TGF-β on SCs are phenotype-dependent, as they are in other cells (Einheber et al., 1995).

Schwann Cells Promote Axonal Regeneration (Elongation)

Strands of proliferating denervated SCs within the basal lamina tube, the SC column or the *bands of*

Bungner (Bungner, 1891), are essential for guiding regenerating axons to their denervated targets (Ramon y Cajal, 1928). Axonal regeneration fails when the distal nerve stumps either lack the SCs or basal lamina (Hall, 1986; reviewed by Fu and Gordon, 1997). Regenerating axons extend along the surface of SCs and/or the inner surface of the basal lamina of the SC column, and use a variety of adhesion molecules on the cellular surfaces and basal lamina for attachment and growth (for review see Ide, 1996). Denervated SCs upregulate neural cell adhesion molecules, L1, and N-cadherin (Martini and Schachner, 1988), and basement membrane components that include laminin (Bunge and Bunge, 1983; Chernousov and Carey, 2000). The adhesion molecules mediate attachment of regenerating axons to the long processes of the SCs and the basal lamina for extension and, in turn, myelination of the axons. Growth inhibitory molecules such as chondroitin sulfate proteoglycan, which is expressed in the endoneurium and the surrounding nerve sheaths, may serve to confine regenerating axons to the growth-supportive SC–basal lamina conduits (Zuo et al., 1998). In addition to the synthesis and upregulation of basal lamina constituents, SCs synthesize and release myriad neurotrophic molecules that have been demonstrated to be critical for the survival of injured neurons and are also likely contribute to the process of axon regeneration (for review see Fu and Gordon, 1997; Boyd and Gordon, 2003).

PROCESS OF AXONAL REGENERATION

Wallerian degeneration and the *die back* degeneration of the proximal stump up to the first node of Ranvier are followed by the emergence of the growth cone (Ramon y Cajal, 1928; Vrbova et al., 1995; reviewed by Fu and Gordon, 1997). *In vitro* and *in vivo* evidence has demonstrated that growth cone formation may occur in the absence of the cell body, extension of the growth cone relying on cytoskeletal materials locally available in the proximal nerve stumps (McQuarrie, 1985). These preexisting cytoskeletal elements are transported along the microtubules into the daughter axons emerging from the parent proximal nerve stump, thereby providing the required materials for the initial stage of axonal growth (Miller et al., 1987). However, the cytoskeletal materials available at the growth cone are quickly exhausted and are not replenished by the limited protein synthesis in the axons. Hence, continued growth and axonal elongation are dependent on the capacity of injured neurons to upregulate the cytoskeletal proteins, actin and tubulin, as the neurons transform into the *regenerative mode* (see the section "Wallerian Degeneration and Initiation of Axonal Regeneration").

Sprouting, Elongation of Axons, and Reformation of Target Connections

Parent axons in the proximal stump of injured peripheral nerve elaborate multiple growth cones and produce many daughter axons. The fate of these branches depends on the availability of a neural "guiding" structure distal to the injury site. In the absence of a neural guiding structure such as the distal nerve stump, regenerating axons form a neuroma that is a mixture of immature nerve fibers and connective tissue (Sunderland, 1978; reviewed by Vrbova et al., 1995; Fu and Gordon, 1997). When numerous fine nerve fibers emanate from the parent axon, cross the injury site, and grow within the supportive environment of the distal nerve stump, an average of five daughter axonal sprouts per parent axon start to regenerate and compete for a limited number of SC-lined endoneurial pathways in the distal nerve stump (Aitken et al., 1947; Toft et al., 1988). Axonal sprouts that advance distally from an axon within the proximal nerve stump comprise a *regenerating unit* (Morris et al., 1972; Fu and Gordon, 1997). These multiple axonal sprouts remain in the distal nerve stumps unless axons make target connections (Aitken et al., 1947). Once target connections are made, all but one daughter axon are gradually withdrawn, the process taking months and even years (Aitken et al., 1947; Mackinnon et al., 1991). The final diameter of the daughter axon that makes a functional connection is dependent on the size of the parent axon, the thickness of the myelin sheath formed around the axon (i.e., local interaction with the myelinating SCs), and, importantly, the size of target reinnervated.

Axonal size is regulated by both the level of neurofilament expression and the phosphorylation of the lysine-serine-proline (KSP) repeats of the medium (NF-M) and heavy (NF-H) molecular weight isoforms of the protein (reviewed by Bisby and Tetzlaff, 1992). Neurofilament expression is downregulated after axotomy and recovers if regeneration is permitted. However, some recovery of neurofilament synthesis begins before axons reach their targets (Tetzlaff et al., 1988), suggesting that endoneurial factors within the distal nerve stump regulate neurofilament expression in the neurons. Phosphorylation of NF-M and NF-H is locally regulated by myelinating SCs such that axonal diameters are larger at internodal as compared with nodal areas (Carden et al., 1985; Hsieh et al., 1994).

While neurofilament expression and phosphorylation are linked to myelination in central axons (Brady et al., 1999), neurofilament expression in peripheral axons, unlike phosphorylation, does not depend on myelination but strongly depends on target reconnection (de Waegh et al., 1992). For example, target connection completely reverses the decline in axonal diameter of axotomized motoneurons (Gordon and Stein, 1982) consistent with normalization of the level of neurofilament expression after target reinnervation (Tetzlaff et al., 1988). Likewise, increasing the size of the innervated target increases the size and myelination of the axons (Voyvodic, 1989). Furthermore, exogenous application of GDNF increases nerve fiber conduction velocity in axotomized motoneurons (Munson and McMahon, 1997). These findings suggest that GDNF and possibly other neurotrophic factors may act as the target- or SC-derived factors that regulate axonal diameter. Therefore, it seems that the primary influence on the diameter of regenerated nerve fibers is the size of the muscle target they reinnervate. These regenerated nerve fibers are able to induce SC myelination, and their ultimate size is probably determined by the axon-SC cross-talk by way of the influence of SC myelination on phosphorylation of neurofilament proteins in the axons.

The specialized nonmyelinating perisynaptic SCs at the neuromuscular junction that normally respond to released transmitters from the intact presynaptic terminals become reactive, extend processes after denervation (Reynolds and Woolf, 1992; Georgiou et al., 1999; Rochon et al., 2001), and guide both sprouting and regenerating axons back to the denervated endplates to reinnervate muscle (Son and Thompson, 1995a, 1995b; Son et al., 1996). These reactive perisynaptic SCs resemble denervated SCs in the distal nerve stumps with respect to their process formation. They differ from them in being GFAP positive after denervation and demonstrating strong neuregulin dependence during early neonatal life. They succumb to apoptosis after nerve crush injury shortly after birth unless neuregulin is exogenously applied (Trachtenberg and Thompson, 1996). Poor muscle reinnervation during early neonatal life provides evidence for a critical role of these perisynaptic SCs in guiding regenerating axons back to the denervated endplates. The perisynaptic SCs and the basal lamina of the adult endplate appear to be sufficient to guide regenerating axons back to the endplate region. This has been demonstrated elegantly in experiments in which nerves were shown to regenerate to the endplate even after ablation of the denervated muscle (Dunaevsky and Connor, 1998).

THE BASIS FOR POOR FUNCTIONAL RECOVERY AFTER PERIPHERAL NERVE INJURIES

Unfortunately, recovery of function may be dismal after injuries that require long periods of time for axons to regenerate and reinnervate denervated targets. At a rate of 1 mm/day for axonal regeneration in humans, periods of more than a year may be required for neurons to regenerate their axons and reinnervate targets (Fig. 36.1). Generally, dismal functional recovery has

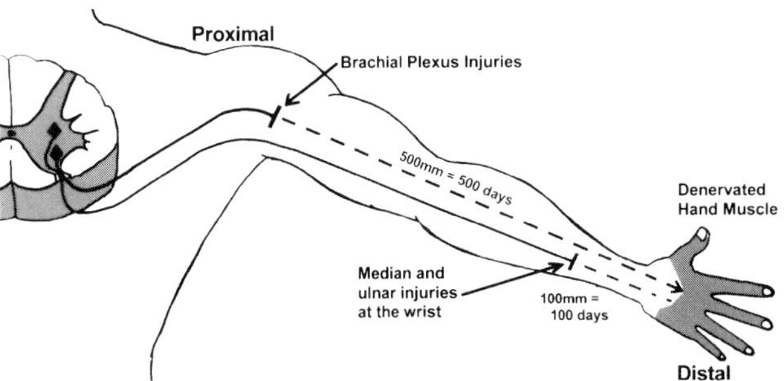

FIGURE 36.1 Schematic illustration of proximal nerve injuries that require prolonged times for the regenerating axons to traverse lengthy distances to reinnervate distant targets such as the muscles in the hand. (Adapted from Gordon, Sulaiman and Boyd, 2003.)

been attributed to irreversible denervation atrophy of the muscles and sense organs but not to the failure of the chronically axotomized neurons to regenerate axons or chronically denervated SCs to support axonal regeneration (reviewed by Fu and Gordon, 1997). Contrary to a long-held assumption, the progressive failure to recover function after peripheral nerve injuries is *not* a failure of chronically denervated muscle to accept reinnervation and develop muscle force (Fu and Gordon, 1995b). Rather, there are at least four factors that limit long-distance axonal regeneration in the peripheral nervous system: (*1*) axotomized neurons progressively lose their ability to regenerate their axons with time; (*2*) prolonged denervation of the distal nerve stump progressively reduces the capacity of the resident SCs to support axonal regeneration; (*3*) many neurons that do regenerate their axons do so much more slowly than was originally believed; and (*4*) many regenerating axons are misdirected to reinnervate inappropriate targets. The specific contibution of each of these factors to the poor functional recovery after peripheral nerve injury is described in this section.

Prolonged Axotomy of Neurons Reduces Their Regenerative Capacity

The ability of peripheral neurons to regenerate their axons following injury has been largely attributed to the permissive environment provided by the SCs of the distal nerve stump. However, the inherent ability of axotomized neurons to regenerate axons spontaneously is not sustained over long periods of time. This was demonstrated in rat experiments in which the period of motoneuronal axotomy was experimentally prolonged for up to a year prior to determining both the number of motoneurons that regenerated axons and the number of motoneurons that made functional contacts with denervated target muscles (Fu and Gordon, 1995a; Boyd and Gordon, 2001, 2002, 2003; Gordon et al., 2003). Only one-third of the chronically axotomized motoneurons succeeded in regenerating their axons if they were chronically axotomized for periods of more than 4 months prior to cross-suture to promote axonal regeneration (Fu and Gordon, 1995a). This dramatic effect of prolonged axotomy in reducing the regenerative capacity of motoneurons was not detected by the measurements of muscle force or by muscle and muscle fiber cross-sectional areas because the 3-fold enlargement of motor units fully compensated for the poor axonal regeneration (cf. Rafuse and Gordon, 1996a, 1996b). Thus, chronic axotomy impairs the ability of motoneurons to regenerate their axons but does not impair the capacity of the smaller number of regenerated motor axons to make functional connections with denervated muscles. Decline in the regenerative capacity of the chronically axotomized motoneurons was accompanied by reduced expression of regeneration-associated genes, tubulin, actin, and GAP-43 (Tetzlaff et al., 1996).

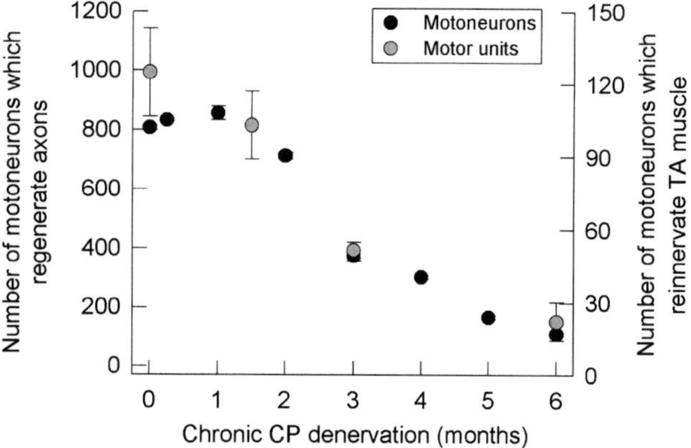

FIGURE 36.2 The number of freshly axotomized tibial motoneurons that had regenerated their axons through chronically denervated common peroneal (*CP*) nerve stumps within 3 months (black circles) and the number that reinnervated denervated tibialis anterior (*TA*) muscle within 4–9 months after cross-suture of tibial and common peroneal nerves (gray circles) progressively fall as a function of how long the common peroneal nerve was chronically denervated prior to the cross-suture. (Adapted from Fu and Gordon, 1995b; Sulaiman and Gordon, 2002.)

Prolonged Denervation Reduces the Number and the Capacity of Denervated Schwann Cells to Support Axonal Regeneration

The early finding that neither the rate of outgrowth nor the number of regenerating axons was affected if nerve repair was delayed was the basis for the enduring view that it is the irreversible atrophy of denervated targets and their replacement by connective tissue and fat that is the prime basis for poor functional recovery after nerve repair (Holmes and Young, 1942; Gutmann and Young, 1944). However, counts of axons that regenerated into the distal nerve stumps severely overestimate the number of neurons that regenerate their axons, especially when regenerated axons are counted prior to target reinnervation. This is because each parent axon gives rise to an average of five daughter sprouts (see the section "Sprouting, Elongation of Axons, and Reformation of Target Connections"). Moreover, the axonal counts made just distal to the repair site may not represent the number of axons that regenerate as far as the denervated muscle targets because of the progressive loss of the capacity of chronically denervated SCs to support axonal regeneration. We tested the latter possibility in experiments in which we enumerated both the number of freshly axotomized motoneurons that regenerated their axons into chronically denervated nerve stumps and the number of reinnervated motor units in the target muscle after cross-suture of a freshly axotomized nerve to a chronically denervated distal nerve stump (Fu and Gordon, 1995b; Sulaiman and Gordon, 2000). Predegeneration of distal nerve stumps for periods of up to a month prior to nerve repair did not affect the regenerative capacity of the motoneurons (Fig. 36.2). This was in line with evidence that the denervated SCs sustain their growth-supportive phenotype for periods of up to 2 months (Li et al., 1997; You et al., 1997). However, for longer periods of chronic denervation of the SCs prior to nerve repair, the number of freshly axotomized motoneurons that regenerated their axons and that reinnervated denervated muscles via the chronically denervated nerve stumps declined in parallel to a value of ~10% (Fig. 36.2; Fu and Gordon, 1995b; Sulaiman and Gordon, 2000).

These findings provide strong evidence that poor axonal regeneration is due to the progressive failure of axons to regenerate in the atrophic nerve stumps and *not* an inability of chronically denervated muscle fibers to accept reinnervation after long delays. In fact, wet weights of reinnervated muscles, which are directly related to their isometric forces, demonstrated a very sluggish rate of muscle atrophy compared to a drastic loss of the trophic environment of the distal nerve stumps after long-term denervation (Sulaiman and Gordon, 2000). The motoneurons that regenerated their axons formed maximally enlarged motor units to compensate for the reduced number of motoneurons that succeeded in regenerated their axons (Fu and Gordon, 1995b). The sustained capacity of denervated muscles to accept reinnervation was also demonstrated by the parallel recovery of both muscle weight and isometric force. However, a failure of the reinnervated muscle fibers to fully recover their former size suggests that limited numbers of satellite cells are incorporated into each atrophic muscle fiber to recover the muscle fiber cross-sectional area (Mussini et al., 1987; Schmalbruch et al., 1991). Hence, progressive deterioration of the growth-supportive capacity of SCs in the distal nerve stumps plays a primary role in poor functional recovery after nerve injury, and the role of muscle atrophy is secondary.

It was striking that the long-term chronically denervated SCs maintained their capacity to remyelinate the fewer axons that regenerated (Fig. 36.3) (Sulaiman and Gordon, 2000), particularly in view of the progressive regression of the capacity of the denervated SCs to sustain their growth-permissive phenotype (Li et al., 1997; You et al., 1997) and the progressive decline in the number of growth-supportive SCs in the chronically denervated distal nerve stumps (Dedkov et al., 2002).

Axonal Regeneration Across the Site Is Staggered

Axons in the proximal nerve stump do not regenerate across the suture site in a synchronous manner. Rather, regenerating axons cross the suture site surprisingly slowly, and they do so at very different rates. The progressive increase in the number of motoneurons that regenerated their axons over long (25 mm) and very short (1.5 mm) distances as a function of time after nerve repair revealed the very dramatic *staggering* of the regenerating axons across the site of surgical apposition of sectioned nerve stumps (Fig. 36.4*A–D*) (Al-Majed et al., 2000b; Brushart et al., 2002). The regeneration rates of 1–4 mm/day determined by the widely used *pinch test* reflect only the regeneration of the fastest-growing sensory neurons (reviewed in Grafstein and McQuarrie, 1978). Likewise, calculation of the regeneration rate via detection of peak radioactivity in segments of regenerating axons after radiolabeling of motoneuron pools or sensory dorsal root ganglia only reflects the regeneration of the fastest-growing axons. Also, the patterns of radioactivity detected in segments of the regenerating axons clearly indicated different rates of regeneration of the various classes of axons (Forman and Berenberg, 1978).

A

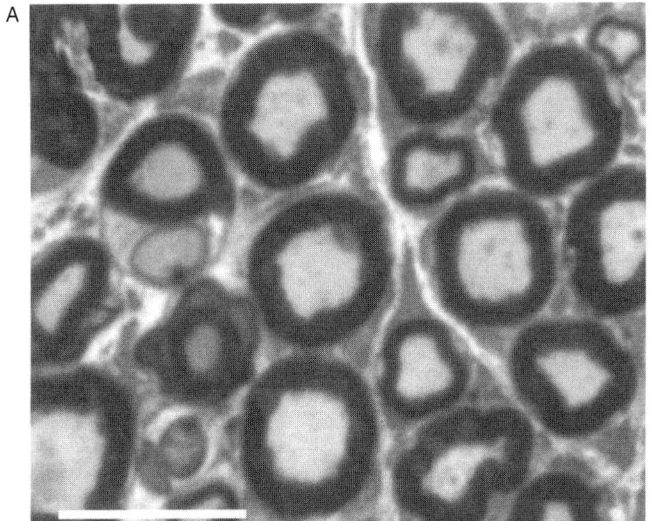

C

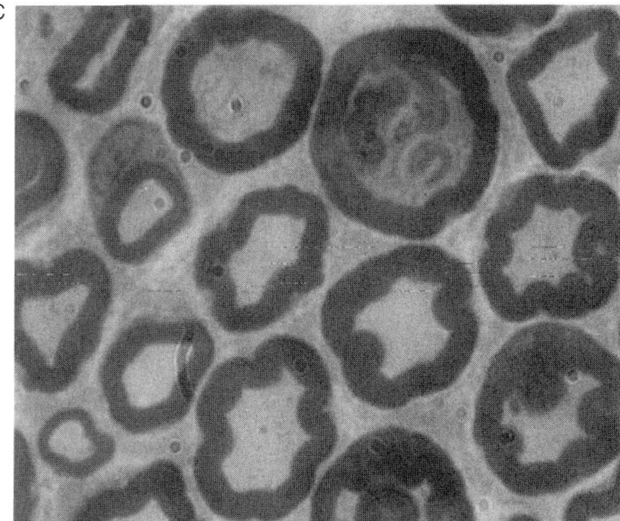

B

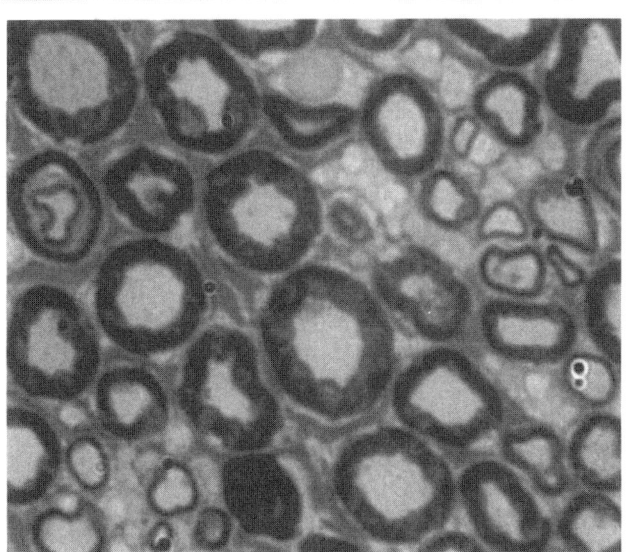

FIGURE 36.3 Light micrographs of (*A*) contralateral control tibial nerve and of regenerated tibial nerve 12 months after (*B*) 4-week short-term and (*C*) 12-week long-term chronic denervation of the distal common peroneal nerve stumps. Schwann cells were able to form elaborate myelin sheaths around regenerated axons, independent of the duration of chronic denervation. Note that the myelin thickness is decreased in *B* and increased in *C* compared to the contralateral control nerve. Also, there are more small nerve fibers in *B*, in contrast to the predominantly large nerve fibers in *C*. Scale bars = 12 μm. (Adapted from Sulaiman and Gordon, 2000.)

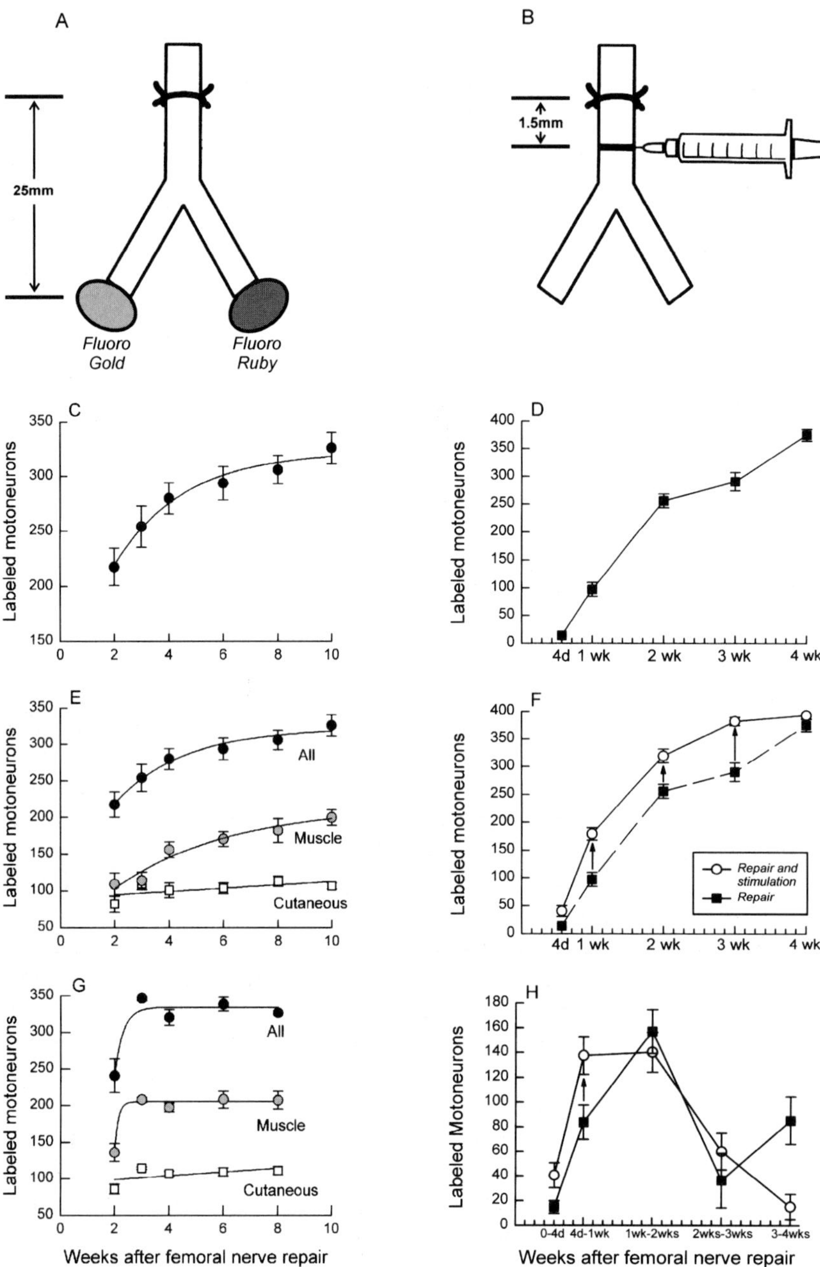

FIGURE 36.4 Counting the number of backlabeled femoral motoneurons that regenerated their axons after transection and microsurgical repair, 20 mm from the branch point of the muscle and cutaneous nerve branches and the effects of 1 hour of electrical stimulation. Each nerve branch was backlabeled with either Fluorogold or Fluororuby (*A*) or Fluororuby was injected into the femoral nerve, 1.5 mm from the site of surgical repair (*B*). Staggered motor axonal regeneration into the femoral nerve branches (*C*) and across the suture site (*D*) results in preferential motor reinnervation of the appropriate muscle branch over time (*E*). Electrical stimulation accelerates regeneration of axons across the suture site (*F,H*) and into the appropriate muscle branch (*G*). The cumulative reinnervation of the distal nerve stump, 1.5 mm distal to the femoral nerve site, shows that significantly more motoneurons regenerate their axons across the repair site when the femoral nerve is stimulated for 1 hour after repair (*F*). The accelerated regeneration of axons across the repair site, especially during the first week, can be visualized in the plot of "new crossing events" obtained by subtracting the mean number of motoneurons labeled at the beginning of a time interval from the mean number labeled at the end of an interval for both stimulated and nonstimulated groups (*G*). (Adapted from Al-Majed et al., 2000b; Brushart et al., 2002.)

Regenerating Axons Are Misdirected to Inappropriate Targets

Functional outcomes after axonal injuries are best after nerve crush injuries in which the endoneurium remains anatomically intact all the way to the target and axonal sprouts of the regenerating unit are contained within the original endoneurium such that the regenerating axons are "led" back to their original targets (Sunderland, 1978). With time, reinnervated muscle fibers display the normal mosaic distribution of muscle fiber types, motor unit and muscle isometric forces recover fully, the original number of functional motor units is restored, and the number and diameter of the myelinated nerve fibers return to normal (reviewed by Gordon and Pattullo, 1993).

The number of axons that regenerate into distal nerve stumps and successfully remake target connection is far more variable for injuries such as transection injuries that disrupt endoneurial tubes. Axonal sprouts emanating from the proximal nerve stump may enter several different endoneurial tubes with target destinations that they did not formerly supply, as in the case of motor axons that regenerate within pathways leading to the skin rather than to muscles (Brushart, 1993). Reduced populations of axons that regenerate and reach denervated muscles reinnervate up to a maximum of five to eight times their normal number of muscle fibers to compensate, at least partially, for poor axonal regeneration (Rafuse et al., 1996a, 1996b). Even so, functional recovery is often disappointing after these transection injuries, especially for the nerve injuries that occur far from their target organs (Sunderland, 1978). Regenerating axons fail to find their original targets, especially when large nerve trunks are damaged and require surgical repair.

Despite considerable improvements in microsurgical nerve repair, available evidence from both animal and human studies reveals considerable misdirection of regenerating axons. Following microsurgical repair of severed nerves to the human hand, voluntary recruitment of the reinnervated motor units revealed the random reinnervation of several muscles across the hand by the motoneurons that had previously supplied only one muscle; the random distribution of regenerating axons to different muscles essentially negated any fine control of hand movement (Thomas et al., 1987). Animal studies of motor axonal regeneration also revealed random reinnervation of muscles after surgical repair of transected nerves. Gillespie et al. (1986, 1987) demonstrated random distribution of slow and fast motor units in reinnervated soleus and lateral gastrocnemius rat muscles after surgical repair of the common LGS nerve to the two muscles. These studies demonstrate the inability of transected motor axons to "find" their original endoneurial tubes leading to the appropriate muscles. Experiments that applied retrograde dyes to regenerated axons of transected sciatic and facial nerves in rats directly demonstrated misdirection of regenerating motor axons from several different motoneuron pools to muscles that the motoneurons did not formerly supply (Brushart and Mesulam, 1980; Streppel et al., 2002). In cases where the nerves supplied muscles with antagonistic actions, axonal misdirection was associated with inappropriate movements, quite consistent with findings that flexor and extensor motoneurons sustain their normal but inappropriate pattern of firing when they are directed to inappropriately reinnervate extensor and flexor muscles, respectively (Gordon et al., 1986).

There is, however, evidence for preferential motor reinnervation of distal nerve stumps that supply skeletal muscles rather than distal nerve stumps that normally contain only cutaneous sensory axons to the skin (Brushart, 1993; Brushart et al., 1998, 2002; Al-Majed et al., 2000b). There are several peripheral nerve trunks whose branches innervate skeletal muscles and sense organs in the skin and the joints. Examples include the femoral nerve that branches into two separate branches, one muscle branch containing motor and sensory nerves to the quadriceps muscle and the other pure sensory branch, the saphenous nerve, which supplies the cutaneous innervation to the skin (Brushart, 1993). Although reinnervation of motor and sensory nerve branches is initially random, the motoneurons that progressively regenerate their axons across the suture site send their axons specifically into the appropriate motor branch (Brushart, 1993; Al-Majed et al., 2000b). This *preferential motor reinnervation* emerged in parallel with the progressive or staggered regeneration of the motor axons into the distal nerve stumps (Fig. 36.4*E,F*) (Al-Majed et al., 2000b). An unusual acidic glycan that is recognized by a monoclonal antibody L2/HNK-1 in mice was shown to be associated with the myelin profiles of motor axons but not sensory axons and to be the preferred substrate for neurite outgrowth from motoneurons (Martini et al., 1992, 1994). These findings suggest that this carbohydrate moiety of the protein backbones of such proteins as myelin-associated glycoprotein may be one molecular determinant that underlies preferential motor reinnervation.

STRATEGIES TO PROMOTE AXONAL REGENERATION

In light of the long delays incurred during axonal regeneration consequence to staggered and slow rate of axonal regeneration, neurons often remain chronically axotomized for long periods and regenerate in progressively more chronically denervated distal nerve stumps. Furthermore, regenerating sprouts entering endoneurial tubes that lead them to inappropriate targets exacerbate the declining number of axotomized neurons that regenerate their axons as far as the denervated targets. In order to counter these barriers to axonal regeneration after peripheral nerve injuries, strategies must be developed to accelerate axonal regeneration to counter the detrimental effects of chronic axotomy and chronic denervation and to promote preferential reinnervation of appropriate targets. We have developed several experimental strategies that include (*1*) electrical stimulation of the proximal nerve stump to synchronize the staggered axonal regeneration across the site of surgical apposition of proximal and distal nerve stumps; (*2*) application of exogenous growth factors to chronically axotomized nerves to reverse the effects of axotomy and, in turn, to optimize the number of axons that regenerate into the distal nerve stump; (*3*) intraperitoneal injection of the immunosuppressant drug FK406 to accelerate the outgrowth of regenerating axons; and (*4*) the incubation of chronically denervated SCs with the cytokine TGF-β to reverse the detrimental effects of chronic denervation on the SCs and thereby to promote axonal regeneration.

A Role of Electrical Activity in Accelerating Regeneration of Axons Across the Repair Site of Cut Nerves

Several attempts have been made to accelerate the relatively slow rate of axonal regeneration to optimize the recovery of function after nerve injuries. Of the many attempts made, only the conditioning crush lesion of the intact nerve prior to a more proximal test crush lesion was found to significantly increase the rate of axonal regeneration (reviewed by Grafstein and McQuarrie, 1978). A conditioning crush lesion that precedes the test lesion elevates mRNA expression of cytoskeletal proteins such as actin and tubulin and reduces the level of neurofilament expression even further than normal in association with more rapid transport of these cytoskeletal proteins (Tetzlaff et al., 1996). The parallel increase in the rate of slow component b (SCb) of axonal transport of the actin and tubulin cytoskeletal proteins and the rate of axonal regeneration in neurons after the conditioning lesion provided further evidence for a direct causal link between the rates (Hoffman and Lasek, 1980; Jacob and McQuarrie, 1991). The more rapid transport of the cytoskeletal proteins into the growth cones prevents their collapse (Jacob and McQuarrie, 1991; McQuarrie and Jacob, 1991).

Both the outgrowth of regenerating axons that normally occurs within hours of the injury and the migration of SCs from the proximal stump that follows after ~2 days are accelerated by the conditioning lesion, arguing for a role of both the neurons and the SCs in the accelerated axonal regeneration rate after a conditioning lesion (Torigoe et al., 1999). It has not yet been ascertained whether the conditioning lesion that so effectively accelerates axonal outgrowth *and* the regeneration rate is also effective in synchronizing the staggered axonal outgrowth that normally delays the process of axonal regeneration by many weeks (Fig. 36.4*C*,*D*). The conditioning lesion is nevertheless the only technique that has been demonstrated to accelerate the rate of regeneration. However, the conditioning lesion must precede the test injury by a maximum of 21days to be effective (Jacob and McQuarrie, 1993), thereby largely negating this lesion as a clinically viable technique to promote axonal regeneration in human patients.

Early promising studies reported that neuromuscular activity accelerates muscle reinnervation (e.g., Nix and Hopf, 1983; Pockett and Gavin, 1985). Recently, we found that suprathreshold low-frequency stimulation immediately after the surgical repair of transected nerve accelerated the regeneration of axons from all the axotomized motoneurons, whether the pulses were delivered continuously for the 2-week period during which motoneurons normally regenerate their axons randomly into appropriate and inappropriate pathways or for progressively shorter periods (Fig. 36.4*G*) (Al-Majed et al., 2000b). Just 1 hour's stimulation was as effective in accelerating motor axonal regeneration as longer periods (Fig. 36.4) (Brushart et al., 2002), the effect being mediated, at least in part, via the cell body and being independent of the rate of axonal transport that was not altered by the stimulation (Al-Majed et al., 2000b; Brushart et al., 2002). The effect of the stimulation is to synchronize the growth of axons across the surgical suture line by accelerating the outgrowth of axons from the proximal nerve stump (Fig. 36.4*F*–*H*) (Brushart et al., 2002). The effectiveness of the brief electrical stimulation in accelerating axonal outgrowth resembles the effectiveness of a double crush lesion to the nerve *prior* to the more distal nerve section and surgical reunion of the nerve stumps (Brushart et al., 1998). However, the effect of these proximal conditioning crush lesions in promoting axonal regeneration was attributed to positive effects of predegeneration of the distal nerve stump rather than to the priming of the injured femoral motoneurons (Brushart et al., 1998).

The effect of electrical stimulation on accelerating axonal growth across a suture site is associated with an accelerated and augmented upregulation of brain-derived neurotrophic factor (BDNF) and trkB followed shortly afterward by elevated expression of regeneration associated genes (Al-Majed et al., 2000a, 2004). This is particularly interesting because activity-induced calcium influx regulates gene expression by multiple diverse mechanisms (reviewed by Finkbeiner and Greenberg, 1998). These include initiation of gene transcription and translation via calcium-response elements, the best known of which is the calcium response element (CRE) within the c-*fos* promotor. One of two elements found within the BDNF promotor III gene that are required for calcium to induce the transcription of the BDNF gene bears a close sequence homology to a CRE and requires a CRE binding protein (CREB) or a closely related family member to mediate BDNF transcription (Tao et al., 1998; reviewed by Finkbeiner and Greenberg, 1998). Adjacent to this CRE is a newly identified element, BDNF Ca^{2+} response element (BCARE), that has close sequence homology to a CRE that also mediates BDNF transcription.

Strong links have also been made between activity-induced elevations in BDNF, intracellular calcium, and intracellular cAMP that in, turn, promote neurite outgrowth and axonal regeneration on both permissive and nonpermissive substrates *in vitro* and *in vivo* (Qui et al., 2000, 2002). Elevated BDNF in motoneurons has also been shown to sustain choline acetyltransferase levels in axotomized motoneurons (Friedman et al., 1995) to allow release of acetylcholine from growth cones (Poo et al., 1985). Stimulation of sensory neurons also releases transmitters that include adenosine triphosphate (ATP) (Stevens and Fields, 2000). The possibility that growth cones interact with denervated SCs via their neurotransmitters follows from evidence that the SCs respond to neurotransmitters via membrane receptors to elevate intracellular calcium levels and, in turn, activate cAMP-dependent CREB (Georgiou et al., 1999; Stevens and Fields, 2000). Neurotransmitter-mediated calcium influx initiates retraction of long processes of denervated perisynaptic SCs (Georgiou et al., 1999; Rochon et al., 2001). This suggests the possibility that transmitter-evoked calcium influx in the denervated SCs in the distal nerve stumps may play a role in the retraction of their long processes and the transformation of these SCs from the denervated growth-supportive phenotype to the mature myelinating phenotype as they initiate remyelination of the regenerated axons.

Counteracting the Negative Effects of Chronic Axotomy

In addition to the ability of neurotrophic factors such as BDNF and GDNF to counteract the negative effects of chronic axotomy (reviewed by Boyd and Gordon, 2003; Gordon et al., 2003), another strategy to sustain axonal regeneration for extended periods of time was suggested by the strong regeneration-promoting effects of the immunophilin ligand FK506 (Gold et al., 1995). The regeneration-promoting effects are independent of the potent immunosuppressive effects for which the drug had been used extensively for preventing the rejection of transplanted organs (Lee et al., 2000). FK506 not only enhanced neurite outgrowth *in vitro* but also accelerated the rate of regeneration after crush or section and immediate resuture (Gold et al., 1995). The effects were mediated via FKBP-52, a chaperone component of mature steroid receptor complexes, independent of the FK506-binding protein-12 that mediates the immunosuppressive effects (Gold et al., 1999). More recently, FK-506 was found to be very effective in counteracting the negative effects of chronic axotomy on axonal regeneration: twice as many chronically axotomized motoneurons regenerated their axons after 3-week daily subcutaneous injection in association with a corresponding increase in the number of regenerated axons (Sulaiman et al., 2002). The evidence of the increased number of regenerated axons and the more rapid progression of axon myelination indicated that the FK-506 also accelerated the rate of axon outgrowth, the effect being mediated on both motor and sensory neurons.

Counteracting the Effects of Prolonged Denervation of the Distal Nerve Stumps

A possible role of the cytokine TGF-β in counteracting the deleterious effects of chronic denervation was suggested by several *in vitro* studies showing that the cytokine plays a role in maintaining the growth-promoting denervated SC phenotype in addition to having mitogenic effects on the SCs (reviewed by Unsicker and Strelau, 2000; see the section "The Denervated Schwann Cell Phenotype"). Transforming growth factor-β increased SC proliferation within 2 days *in vitro*; forskolin, augmented the effects of TGF-β, presumably by increasing intracellular levels of cAMP. Hence, we removed chronically denervated SCs from the distal nerve stump and reactivated the cells *in vitro* with TGF-β and forskolin for 2 days. Thereafter these reactivated SCs were placed within a silastic cuff between proximal and distal nerve stumps *in vivo* to assess their capacity to support axonal growth. The effect was dramatic. The TGF-β- and forskolin-treated SCs increased the regeneration of axons through the silastic cuff by a factor of 4 compared to the number of motoneurons that regenerated axons into chronically denervated distal nerve stumps without pretreatment. Moreover, the regenerated nerve fibers were larger and were better myelinated than the fibers that regenerated through the untreated nerve explants (Sulaiman and Gordon, 2002). These findings are consistent with previous reports that chronically denervated SCs sustain their capacity to undergo proliferation and to remyelinate regenerated axons (Wood et al., 1998; Sulaiman and Gordon, 2000). They provide an indication that the reduced number of SCs that remain in chronically denervated nerve stumps can be reactivated by exposure to cytokines that are normally released during the process of Wallerian degeneration. The reinstated growth-supportive phenotype of the SCs is sufficient to support axonal regeneration.

CONCLUSIONS

The contributions of injured neurons, SCs, and macrophages to the regenerative process in the peripheral nervous system appear to be interlinked such that there is a window of opportunity during which the growth potential of the neurons translates into outgrowth and extension of regenerating axons. This window of opportunity is closely linked to the period during which there is active Wallerian degeneration when macrophages interact with SCs to provide the permissive growth environment. The progressive but slow advancement of regenerating axons from the proximal nerve across the site of nerve transection and repair severely slows the progress of axonal growth into the distal nerve stumps. This delay further reduces the regenerative capacity of neurons as a result of prolonged axotomy and denervation. As we begin to understand the limitations of peripheral nerve regeneration, we can begin to devise effective interventions to prolong the window of opportunity for axonal regeneration and to promote recovery of function after nerve injuries. These interventions include (*1*) electrical stimulation to accelerate axonal outgrowth across the surgical site of nerve reunion or FK506 subcutaneous injection to accelerate axonal outgrowth and the rate of regeneration,

(2) application of exogenous neurotrophic factors to compensate for suboptimal levels of endogenous neurotrophic factors from chronically denervated SCs, and (3) chemical methods to reinstate the growth-permissive SC phenotype to support axonal regeneration.

ACKNOWLEDGMENTS

Grateful thanks to the Alberta Heritage Foundation for Medical Research, the Canadian Institutes for Health Research, and the Rick Hansen Legacy Fund for their generous support, and to Dr. Rajiv Midha and Ms Karen Gordon for their critical reading of the manuscript during its preparation.

REFERENCES

Aitken, J.T., Sharman, M., and Young, J.Z. (1947) Maturation of peripheral nerve fibres with various peripheral connections. *J. Anat.* 81:1–22.

Al-Majed, A.A., Brushart, T.M., and Gordon, T. (2000a) Electrical stimulation accelerates and increases expression of BDNF and trkB mRNA in regenerating rat femoral motoneurons. *Eur. J. Neurosci.* 12:4381–4390.

Al-Majed, A.A., Tam, S.L., and Gordon, T. (2004) Electrical stimulation accelerates and enhances the altered gene expression of regeneration associated genes in regenerating rat femoral motoneurons. *J. Cell Mol. Neurobiol.* 24:379–402.

Al-Majed, A.A., Neumann, C.M., Brushart, T.M., and Gordon, T. (2000b) Brief electrical stimulation promotes the speed and accuracy of motor axonal regeneration. *J. Neurosci.* 20:2602–2608.

Bisby, M.A. (1995) Regeneration of peripheral nervous system axons. In: Waxman, S.G., Kocsis, J.D., and Stys, P.K., eds. *The Axon: Structure, Function and Pathophysiology.* New York and Oxford: Oxford University of Press, pp. 553–578.

Bisby, M.A. and Tetzlaff, W. (1992) Changes in cytoskeletal protein synthesis following axon injury and during axon regeneration. *Mol. Neurobiol.* 6:107–123.

Bolin, L.M, Verity, A.N., Silver, J.E., Shooter, E.M., and Abrams, J.S. (1995) Interleukin-6 production by Schwann cells and induction in sciatic nerve injury. *J. Neurochem.* 64:850–858.

Boyd, J.G. and Gordon, T. (2001) The neurotrophin receptors, trkB and p75, differentially regulate motor axonal regeneration. *J. Neurobiol.* 49:314–325.

Boyd, J.G. and Gordon, T. (2002) A dose-dependent facilitation and inhibition of peripheral nerve regeneration by brain-derived neurotrophic factor. *Eur. J. Neurosci.* 15:613–626.

Boyd, J.G. and Gordon, T. (2003) Signalling and function of neurotrophic factors in the normal and injured peripheral nervous system. Invited review. *Mol. Neurobiol.* 27:277–324.

Brady, S.T., Witt, A.S., Kirkpatrick, L.L., de Waegh, S.M., Readhead, C., Tu, P.H., and Lee, V.M. (1999) Formation of compact myelin is required for maturation of the axonal cytoskeleton. *J. Neurosci.* 19:7278–7288.

Brushart, T.M. (1993) Motor axons preferentially reinnervate motor pathways. *J. Neurosci.* 13:2730–2738.

Brushart, T.M., Gerber, J., Kessens, P., Chen, Y.G., and Royall, R.M. (1998) Contributions of pathway and neuron to preferential motor reinnervation. *J. Neurosci.* 18:8674–8681.

Brushart, T.M., Hoffman, P.N., Royall, R.M., Murinson, B.B., Witzel, C., and Gordon, T. (2002) Electrical stimulation promotes motoneuron regeneration without increasing its speed or conditioning the neuron. *J. Neurosci.* 22:6631–6638.

Brushart, T.M. and Mesulam, M.M. (1980) Alteration in connections between muscle and anterior horn motoneurons after peripheral nerve repair. *Science* 208:603–605.

Bunge, R.P. and Bunge, M.B. (1983) Interrelationship between Schwann cell function and extracellular matrix production. *Trends Neurosci.* 6:499–505.

Bungner, O.V. (1891) Uber die Degenerations- und Regenerationsvorgange am Nerven nach Verletzungen. Beitr. *Pathol. Anat.* 10:321–387.

Carden, M.J., Schlaepfer, W.W. and Lee, V.M. (1985) The structure, biochemical properties, and immunogenicity of neurofilament peripheral regions are determined by phosphorylation state. *J. Biol. Chem.* 260:9805–9817.

Chernousov, M.A. and Carey, D.J. (2000) Schwann cell extracellular matrix molecules and their receptors. *Histol. Histopathol.* 15:593–601.

de Waegh, S.M., Lee, V.M., and Brady, S.T. (1992) Local modulation of neurofilament phosphorylation, axonal caliber, and slow axonal transport by myelinating Schwann cells. *Cell* 68:451–463.

Dedkov, E.I., Kostrominova, T.Y., Borisov, A.B., and Carlson, B.M. (2002) Survival of Schwann cells in chronically denervated skeletal muscles. *Acta Neuropathol. (Berl.)* 103:565–574.

Dunaevsky, A. and Connor, E.A. (1998) Stability of frog motor nerve terminals in the absence of target muscle fibers. *Dev. Biol.* 194:61–71.

Einheber, S., Hannocks, M.J., Metz, C.N., Rifkin, D.B., and Salzer, J.L. (1995) Transforming growth factor-beta 1 regulates axon/Schwann cell interactions. *J. Cell Biol.* 129:443–458.

Finkbeiner, S. and Greenberg, M.E. (1998) Ca^{2+} channel-regulated neuronal gene expression. *J. Neurobiol.* 37:171–189.

Forman, D.S. and Berenberg, R.A. (1978) Regeneration of motor axons in the rat sciatic nerve studied by labelling with axonally transported radioactive proteins. *Brain Res.* 156:213–225.

Friedman, B., Kleinfeld, D., Ip, N.Y., Verge, V.M.K., Moulton, R., Boland, P., Zlotchenko, E., Lindsay, R.M., and Liu, L. (1995) BDNF and NT-4/5 exert neurotrophic influences on injured adult spinal motor neurons. *J. Neurosci.* 15:1044–1056.

Fu, S.Y. and Gordon, T. (1995a) Contributing factors to poor functional recovery after delayed nerve repair: prolonged axotomy. *J. Neurosci.* 15:3876–3885.

Fu, S.Y. and Gordon, T. (1995b) Contributing factors to poor functional recovery after delayed nerve repair: prolonged denervation. *J. Neurosci.* 5:3886–3895.

Fu, S.Y. and Gordon, T. (1997) The cellular and molecular basis of peripheral nerve regeneration. *Mol. Neurobiol.* 14:67–116.

Georgiou, J., Robitaille, R., and Charlton, M. P. (1999) Muscarinic control of cytoskeleton in perisynaptic glia. *J. Neurosci.* 19:3836–3846.

Gillen, C., Jander, S., and Stoll, G. (1998) Sequential expression of mRNA for proinflammatory cytokines and interleukin-10 in the rat peripheral nervous system: comparison between immune-mediated demyelination and Wallerian degeneration. *J. Neurosci. Res.* 51:489–496.

Gillespie, M.J., Gordon, T., and Murphy, P.R. (1986) Reinnervation of the lateral gastrocnemius and soleus muscles in the rat by their common nerve. *J. Physiol.* 372:485–500.

Gillespie, M.J., Gordon, T., and Murphy, P.R. (1987) Motor units and histochemistry in rat lateral gastrocnemius and soleus muscles: evidence for dissociation of physiological and histochemical properties after reinnervation. *J. Neurophysiol.* 57: 921–937.

Gold, B.G., Densmore, V., Shou, W., Matzuk, M.M., and Gordon, H.S. (1999) Immunophilin FK506-binding protein 52 (not FK506-binding protein 12) mediates the neurotrophic action of FK506. *J. Pharmacol. Exp. Ther.* 289:1202–1210.

Gold, B.G., Katoh, K., and Storm-Dickerson, T. (1995) The immunosuppressant FK506 increases the rate of axonal regeneration in rat sciatic nerve. *J. Neurosci.* 15:7509–7516.

Gordon, T. (1983) The dependence of peripheral nerves on their target organs. In: Burnstock, G., Vrbova, G., and O'Brien, R., eds.

Somatic and Autonomic Nerve-Muscle Interactions. New York: Elsevier, pp. 289–325.

Gordon, T. and Pattullo, M.C. (1993) Plasticity of muscle fiber and motor unit types. *Exerc. Sport Sci. Rev.* 21:331–362.

Gordon, T. and Stein, R.B. (1982) Reorganization of motor-unit properties in reinnervated muscles of the cat. *J. Neurophysiol.* 48: 1175–1190.

Gordon, T., Stein, R.B., and Thomas, C.K. (1986) Organization of motor units following cross-reinnervation of antagonistic muscles in the cat hind limb. *J. Physiol.* 374:443–456.

Gordon, T., Sulaiman, O., and Boyd, J.G. (2003) Experimental strategies to promote functional recovery after peripheral nerve injuries. *J. Periph. Nerv. Syst.* 8:236–250.

Grafstein, B. and McQuarrie, I.G. (1978) Role of the nerve cell body in axonal regeneration. In: Cotman, C.W., ed. *Neuronal Plasticity*. New York: Raven Press, pp. 155–196.

Guenard, V., Montag, D., Schachner, M., and Martini, R. (1996) Onion bulb cells in mice deficient for myelin genes share molecular properties with immature, differentiated non-myelinating, and denervated Schwann cells. *Glia* 18:27–38.

Gutmann, E. and Young, J.Z. (1944) The re-innervation of muscle after various periods of atrophy. *J. Anat.* 78:15–44.

Hall, S.M. (1986) The effect of inhibiting Schwann cell mitosis on the reinnervation of acellular autografts in the peripheral nervous system of the mouse. *Neuropathol. Appl. Neurobiol.* 12:401–414.

Hoffman, P.N. and Lasek, R.J. (1980) Axonal transport of the cytoskeleton in regenerating motor neurons: constancy and change. *Brain Res.* 202:317–333.

Holmes, W. and Young, J.Z. (1942) Nerve regeneration after immediate and delayed suture. *J. Anat.* 77:63–108.

Hsieh, S.T., Kidd, G.J., Crawford, T.O., Xu, Z., Lin, W.M., Trapp, B.D., Cleveland, D.W., and Griffin, J.W. (1994) Regional modulation of neurofilament organization by myelination in normal axons. *J. Neurosci.* 14:6392–6401.

Ide, C. (1996) Peripheral nerve regeneration. *Neurosci. Res.* 25:101–121.

Jacob, J.M. and McQuarrie, I.G. (1991) Axotomy accelerates slow component b of axonal transport. *J. Neurobiol.* 22:570–582.

Jacob, J.M. and McQuarrie, I.G. (1993) Acceleration of axonal outgrowth in rat sciatic nerve at one week after axotomy. *J. Neurobiol.* 24:356–367.

Kury, P., Stoll, G., and Muller, H.W. (2001) Molecular mechanisms of cellular interactions in peripheral nerve regeneration. *Curr. Opin. Neurol.* 14:635–639.

Lee, M., Doolabh, V.B., Mackinnon, S.E., and Jost, S. (2000) FK506 promotes functional recovery in crushed rat sciatic nerve. *Muscle Nerve* 23:633–640.

Li, H., Terenghi, G., and Hall, S.M. (1997) Effects of delayed reinnervation on the expression of c-erbB receptors by chronically denervated rat Schwann cells in vivo. *Glia* 20:333–347.

Lindholm, D., Heumann, R., Meyer, M., and Thoenen, H. (1987) Interleukin-1 regulates synthesis of nerve growth factor in nonneuronal cells of rat sciatic nerve. *Nature* 330:658–659.

Mackinnon, S.E., Dellon, A.L., and O'Brien, J.P. (1991) Changes in nerve fiber numbers distal to a nerve repair in the rat sciatic nerve model. *Muscle Nerve* 14:1116–1122.

Martini, R. and Schachner, M. (1988) Immunoelectron microscopic localization of neural cell adhesion molecules (L1, N-CAM, and myelin-associated glycoprotein) in regenerating adult mouse sciatic nerve. *J. Cell Biol.* 106:1735–1746.

Martini, R., Schachner, M., and Brushart, T.M. (1994) The L2/HNK-1 carbohydrate is preferentially expressed by previously motor axon-associated Schwann cells in reinnervated peripheral nerves. *J. Neurosci.* 14:7180–7191.

Martini, R., Xin, Y., Schmitz, B., and Schachner, M. (1992) The L2/HNK-1 carbohydrate epitope is involved in the preferential outgrowth of motor neurons on ventral roots and motor nerves. *Eur. J. Neurosci.* 4:628–639.

McQuarrie, I.G. (1985) Effect of conditioning lesion on axonal sprout formation at nodes of Ranvier. *J. Comp. Neurol.* 231:239–249.

McQuarrie, I.G. and Jacob, J.M. (1991) Conditioning nerve crush accelerates cytoskeletal protein transport in sprouts that form after a subsequent crush. *J. Comp. Neurol.* 305:139–147.

Meyer, M., Matsuoka, I., Wetmore, C., Olson, L., and Thoenen, H. (1992) Enhanced synthesis of brain-derived neurotrophic factor in the lesioned peripheral nerve: different mechanisms are responsible for the regulation of BDNF and NGF mRNA. *J. Cell Biol.* 119:45–54.

Miller, F.D., Naus, C.C., Durand, M., Bloom, F.E., and Milner, R.J. (1987) Isotypes of alpha-tubulin are differentially regulated during neuronal maturation. *J. Cell Biol.* 105:3065–3073.

Mirsky, R. and Jessen, K.R. (1999) The neurobiology of Schwann cells. *Brain Pathol.* 9:293–311.

Morris, J.H., Hudson, A.R., and Weddell, G. (1972) A study of degeneration and regeneration in the divided rat sciatic nerve based on electron microscopy. II. The development of the "regenerating unit." *Anatomy* 124:103–130.

Munson, J.B. and McMahon, S.B. (1997) Effects of GDNF on axotomized sensory and motor neurons in adult rats. *Eur. J. Neurosci.* 9:1126–1129.

Mussini, I., Favaro, G., and Carraro, U. (1987) Maturation, dystrophic changes and the continuous production of fibers in skeletal muscle regenerating in the absence of nerve. *J. Neuropathol. Exp. Neurol.* 46:315–331.

Nix, W.A. and Hopf, H.C. (1983) Electrical stimulation of regenerating nerve and its effect on motor recovery. *Brain Res.* 272: 21–25.

Perry, V.H. and Brown, M.C. (1992) Macrophages and nerve regeneration. *Curr. Opin. Neurobiol.* 2:679–682.

Pockett, S. and Gavin, R.M. (1985) Acceleration of peripheral nerve regeneration after crush injury in rat. *Neurosci. Lett.* 59:221–224.

Poo, M.M., Sun, Y.A., and Young, S.H. (1985) Three types of transmitter release from embryonic neurons. *J. Physiol. (Paris)* 80:283–289.

Qui, J., Cai, D., Dai, H., McAtee, M., Hoffman, P.N., Bregman B.S., and Filbin, M.T. (2002) Spinal axon regeneration induced by elevation of cyclic AMP. *Neuron* 34:895–903.

Qui, J., Cai, D., and Filbin, M.T. (2000) Glial inhibition of nerve regeneration in the mature CNS. *Glia* 29:166–174.

Raabe, T.D., Francis, A., and DeVries, G.H. (1998) Neuregulins in glial cells. *Neurochem. Res.* 23:311–318.

Rafuse, V.F. and Gordon, T. (1996a) Self-reinnervated cat medial gastrocnemius muscles. I. Comparisons of the capacity of regenerating nerves to form enlarged motor units after extensive peripheral nerve injuries. *J. Neurophysiol.* 75:268–281.

Rafuse, V.F. and Gordon, T. (1996b) Self-reinnervated cat medial gastrocnemius muscles. II. Analysis of the mechanisms and significance of fiber type grouping in reinnervated muscles. *J. Neurophysiol.* 75:282–297.

Rahmatullah, M., Schroering, A., Rothblum, K., Stahl, R.C., Urban, B., and Carey, D.J. (1998) Synergistic regulation of Schwann cell proliferation by heregulin and forskolin. *Mol. Cell Biol.* 18:6245–6252.

Ramon y Cajal, S. (1928) *Degeneration and Regeneration of the Nervous System* (May, R.M., trans.). Oxford: Oxford University Press, 66–69.

Reynolds, M.L. and Woolf, C.J. (1992) Terminal Schwann cells elaborate extensive processes following denervation of the motor endplate. *J. Neurocytol.* 21:50–66.

Ridley, A.J., Davis, J.B., Stroobant, P., and Land, H. (1989) Transforming growth factors-beta 1 and beta 2 are mitogens for rat Schwann cells. *J. Cell Biol.* 109:3419–3424.

Rochon, D., Rousse, I., and Robitaille, R. (2001) Synapse-glia interactions at the mammalian neuromuscular junction. *J. Neurosci.* 21:3819–3829.

Scherer, S.S. and Salzer, J.L. (1996) Axon–Schwann cell interactions during peripheral nerve degeneration and regeneration. In: Jessen, K.R. and Richardson, W.D., eds. *Glial Cell Development: Basic Principles and Clinical Relevance* Oxford University Press; pp. 299–330.

Schmalbruch, H., Al-Amood, W.S., and Lewis, D.M. (1991) Morphology of long-term denervated rat soleus muscle and the effect of chronic electrical stimulation. *J. Physiol.* 441:233–241.

Shamash, S., Reichert, F., and Rotshenker, S. (2002) The cytokine network of Wallerian degeneration: tumor necrosis factor-α, interleukin-1α, and interleukin-1β. *J. Neurosci.* 22:3052–3060.

Son, Y.J. and Thompson, W.J. (1995a) Nerve sprouting in muscle is induced and guided by processes extended by Schwann cells. *Neuron* 14:133–141.

Son, Y.J. and Thompson, W.J. (1995b) Schwann cell processes guide regeneration of peripheral axons. *Neuron* 14:125–132.

Son, Y.J., Trahtenberg, J.T., and Thompson, W.J. (1996) Schwann cells induce and guide sprouting and reinnervation of neuromuscular junctions. *Trends Neurosci.* 19:280–285.

Stevens, B. and Fields, R.D. (2000) Response of Schwann cells to action potentials in development. *Science* 287:2267–2271.

Streppel, M., Azzolin, N., Dohm, S., Guntinas-Lichius, O., Haas, C., Grothe, C., Wevers, A., Neiss, W.F., and Angelov, D.N. (2002) Focal application of neutralizing antibodies to soluble neurotrophic factors reduces collateral axonal branching after peripheral nerve lesion. *Eur. J. Neurosci.* 15:1327–1342.

Sulaiman, O.A. and Gordon, T. (2000) Effects of short- and long-term Schwann cell denervation on peripheral nerve regeneration, myelination, and size. *Glia* 32:234–246.

Sulaiman, O.A. and Gordon, T. (2002) Transforming growth factor-beta and forskolin attenuate the adverse effects of long-term Schwann cell denervation on peripheral nerve regeneration in vivo. *Glia* 37:206–218.

Sulaiman, O.A., Voda, J., Gold, B.G., and Gordon, T. (2002) FK506 increases peripheral nerve regeneration after chronic axotomy but not after chronic Schwann cell denervation. *Exp. Neurol.* 175:127–137.

Sunderland, S. (1978) *Nerves and Nerve Injuries 2nd Edition.* Edinburgh: Livingstone.

Tao, X., Finkbeiner, S., Arnold, D.B., Shaywitz, A.J., and Greenberg, M.E. (1998) Ca^{2+} influx regulates BDNF transcription by a CREB family transcription factor-dependent mechanism. *Neuron* 20:709–726.

Tetzlaff, W., Bisby, M.A., and Kreutzberg, G.W. (1988) Changes in cytoskeletal proteins in the rat facial nucleus following axotomy. *J. Neurosci.* 8:3181–3189.

Tetzlaff, W., Leonard, C., Krekoski, C.A., Parhad, I.M., and Bisby, M.A. (1996) Reductions in motoneuronal neurofilament synthesis by successive axotomies: a possible explanation for the conditioning lesion effect on axon regeneration. *Exp. Neurol.* 139: 95–106.

Thomas, C.K., Stein, R.B., Gordon, T., Lee, R.G., and Elleker, M.G. (1987) Patterns of reinnervation and motor unit recruitment in human hand muscles after complete ulnar and median nerve section and resuture. *J. Neurol. Neurosurg. Psychiatry* 50:259–268.

Tofaris, G.K., Patterson, P.H., Jessen, K.R., and Mirsky, R. (2002) Denervated Schwann cells attract macrophages by secretion of leukemia inhibitory factor (LIF) and monocyte chemattractant protein-1 in a process regulated by interleukin-6 and LIF. *J. Neurosci.* 22:6696–6703.

Toft, P.B., Fugleholm, K., and Schmalbruch, H. (1988) Axonal branching following crush lesions of peripheral nerves of rat. *Muscle Nerve* 11:880–889.

Torigoe, K., Hashimoto, K., and Lundborg, G. (1999) A role of migratory Schwann cells in a conditioning effect of peripheral nerve regeneration. *Exp. Neurol.* 160:99–108.

Trachtenberg, J.T. and Thompson, W. J. (1996) Schwann cell apoptosis at developing neuromuscular junctions is regulated by glial growth factor. *Nature* 379:174–177.

Unsicker, K. and Krieglstein, K. (2000) Co-activation of TGF-β and cytokine signalling pathways are required for neurotrophic functions. *Cytokine Growth Factor Rev.* 11:97–102.

Unsicker, K. and Strelau, J. (2000) Functions of transforming growth factor-β isoforms in the nervous system. Cues based on localization and experimental *in vitro* and *in vivo* evidence. *Eur. J. Biochem.* 267:6972–6975.

Voyvodic, J.T. (1989) Target size regulates calibre and myelination of sympathetic axons. *Nature* 342:430–433.

Vrbova, G., Gordon, T., and Jones, R. (1995) *Nerve-Muscle Interaction*, 3rd ed. London: Chapman and Hall.

Wood, P.M., Cuervo, E.F., Bunge, R.P., and Gordon, T. (1998) Functional capacities of long-term denervated Schwann cells. *Soc. Neurosci.* 24:690.8.

You, S., Petrov, T., Chung, P.H., and Gordon, T. (1997) The expression of the low affinity nerve growth factor receptor in long-term denervated Schwann cells. *Glia* 20:87–100.

Zuo, J., Hernandez, Y.J., and Muir, D. (1998) Chondroitin sulfate proteoglycan with neurite-inhibiting activity is up-regulated following peripheral nerve injury. *J. Neurobiol.* 34:41–54.

37 Axonal regeneration in the central nervous system of mammals

ISABEL KLUSMAN AND MARTIN E. SCHWAB

In contrast to the situation in the peripheral nervous system (PNS), where injured axons often regenerate successfully over long distances, axonal regeneration is minimal or absent in the adult mammalian central nervous system (CNS). Therefore, CNS trauma often results in severe and permanent deficits. It is now well accepted that the inability of CNS axons to regenerate is crucially influenced by the presence of nonneuronal inhibitory factors in the axonal environment.

HISTORY

Until the early 1980s, it was not clear if the absence of regenerative growth resulted from the lack of growth stimulatory factors in the adult CNS tissue or if it was the result of an intrinsic inability of the adult neurons to reactivate their growth program. Albert Aguayo and his group showed that axonal growth of different kinds of adult CNS neurons occurred when transplants of peripheral nerve from adult rats were grafted into the spinal cord, brain stem, or retina (David and Aguayo, 1981; Richardson et al., 1984). These results invalidated the hypothesis that adult CNS neurons are unable to reactivate their intrinsic growth program. To test the theory that a lack of trophic support is the main factor responsible for the inability of CNS axons to regenerate within CNS tissue, cocultures of explants of adult optic nerves and sciatic nerves with dissociated newborn rat sympathetic or sensory neurons in the presence of nerve growth factor were performed (Schwab and Thoenen, 1985). The results showed an abundant growth of axons into the sciatic nerves. No axons were observed growing into the optic nerve explants, suggesting that in contrast to PNS tissue, CNS tissue contains factors that can exert an inhibitory effect on neurite growth that cannot be overcome by addition of growth-promoting factors. Potent inhibitory factors were found to be present in oligodendrocytes and CNS myelin (Caroni and Schwab, 1988a; Caroni and Schwab, 1988b; Schwab and Caroni, 1988; Bandtlow and Schwab, 2000; Qui et al., 2000). Overall, the regenerative capacity of CNS neurons probably reflects a balance between the occurrence of growth-enhancing and -inhibiting factors in the axonal environment.

In contrast to the situation in mammals, in fish and in certain amphibians spontaneous recovery is seen after injury to the adult CNS. After a complete transection of the spinal cord in sea lamprey, sprouting and regenerating axons can be seen growing into the caudal spinal cord, where they form functional synapses. Spinal cord–injured animals show coordinated swimming behavior 10 weeks after lesioning (Lurie and Selzer, 1991). Similar observations were made in goldfish (for review see Bernhardt, 1999). Results from *in vitro* experiments suggest that goldfish retinal axons are sensitive to neurite growth inhibitory molecules present on mammalian oligodendrocytes or CNS myelin, but fish optic nerve oligodendrocyte-like cells and fish CNS myelin lack these inhibitory properties (Bastmeyer et al., 1991). After metamorphosis in frogs, neurite growth inhibitors are present in the hindbrain/spinal cord region but not in the optic nerve/tectum, where retinal axons are able to regenerate after undergoing injury (Lang et al., 1995).

When a lesion occurs during development or shortly after birth, regenerative nerve growth and plasticity can also take place in the mammalian CNS. Large amounts of the growth-associated protein GAP 43, which is produced in large quantities during growth and synapse formation, are present in the developing CNS. GAP-43 expression decreases during postnatal development, and in the adult CNS the protein is found in only a few specific regions. The decrease in GAP-43 expression correlates well with the myelination of the CNS (Kapfhammer and Schwab, 1994). Sprouting after a lesion in the adult is typically seen in brain areas that are only lightly myelinated and show high GAP-43 expression.

See the list of abbreviations at the end of the chapter.

CELL CULTURE EXPERIMENTS WITH PERIPHERAL AND CENTRAL NERVOUS SYSTEM TISSUE: ROLE OF THE CENTRAL NERVOUS SYSTEM MICROENVIRONMENT

In the initial experiments that Aguayo and colleagues performed in the 1980s (Aguayo et al., 1981), CNS glia were transplanted into peripheral nerves. Peripheral nerves, which are usually able to regenerate spontaneously, did not grow into the CNS glia transplant but circumvented the area of CNS tissue. In a follow-up experiment the setup was reversed; grafts of peripheral nerve were transplanted into a transected spinal cord. The CNS neurites interacted with the transplanted Schwann cells and elongated through the grafts for distances of up to several centimeters (David and Aguayo, 1981).

The properties of adult CNS tissue and cells have been studied extensively. After it was postulated that specific neurite growth inhibitory factors occurred in the adult CNS (Schwab and Thoenen, 1985; Schwab and Caroni, 1988), a number of inhibitory factors were characterized by *in vitro* assays. After a lesion develops, the CNS environment contains different cell types that could be involved in the expression of such inhibitory molecules: oligodendrocytes, astrocytes, activated microglia, and fibroblasts. All of these cell types have now been shown to express or produce inhibitory factors that can influence axonal outgrowth.

NEURITE GROWTH INHIBITORS IN THE DAMAGED CENTRAL NERVOUS SYSTEM

Myelin and scars seem to be the main structures exerting an inhibitory effect on axonal regeneration in the adult CNS. Oligodendrocytes, white matter, and myelin from intact adult CNS were shown to be nonpermissive substrates for growing neurites and to induce growth cone collapse (Schwab and Caroni, 1988; Bandtlow et al., 1993). Several molecules are currently known to be involved in these processes.

Nogo-A

Characterization of the inhibitory constituents of CNS tissue revealed that the inhibitory activities found to be present in oligodendrocytes and in CNS myelin resided in specific protein fractions. These neurite growth inhibitory protein fractions of 35 kDa (NI-35, only in rat) and 250 kDa (NI-250 in rat, NI-220 in bovine and human spinal cord) were highly nonpermissive substrates *in vitro* (Caroni and Schwab, 1988b; Spillmann et al., 1998). A monoclonal antibody (mAb IN-1) raised against NI-250 was able to reduce the inhibitory activity of CNS myelin *in vitro*, enabling fibroblast spread and neurite outgrowth (Caroni and Schwab, 1988a). Application of the mAb IN-1 *in vivo* to adult spinal cord–injured rats permitted regeneration of injured nerve fibers over long distances (Schnell and Schwab, 1990). Functional recovery after antibody treatment can be assessed by a number of behavioral tests, such as narrow beam crossing (Fig. 37.1).

The high molecular weight protein NI-220/250 was fully purified and sequenced (Spillmann et al., 1998), and the corresponding cDNA, now called Nogo-A, was cloned (Chen et al., 2000; GrandPre et al., 2000; Prinjha et al., 2000). Three splice variants (Nogo-A, -B, and -C) are produced due to alternative promotor usage. The largest of the three variants, Nogo-A, is present in the innermost adaxonal and outermost myelin membrane but not in compact myelin of the adult CNS (Huber et al., 2002). The Nogo-A protein is synthesized by oligodendrocytes but is also expressed by subpopulations of neurons. Nogo-B is present in both CNS and PNS neurons, but it is also seen in a number of tissues outside of the nervous system. Nogo-C is mainly expressed in the skeletal muscle. Nogo-A has more than one membrane topology and contains two main active sites, one in the Nogo-A-specific part (Oertle et al., (2003) and the other in the loop between the two hydrophobic regions (Fournier et al., 2001). This loop, called Nogo-66, is situated in the C-terminal region that is common to all the Nogo proteins. Both inhibitory regions are exposed to the extracellular milieu on living oligodendrocytes (Oertle et al., 2003). They probably interact with different receptors or subunits of a receptor complex. Nogo-66 is responsible for inhibition of neurite outgrowth by binding to the axonal, GPI-linked Nogo-66 receptor, NgR (Fournier et al., 2001). Two other myelin-associated neurite outgrowth inhibitors, MAG and OMgp, also act through NgR and its receptor complex, suggesting redundancy in myelin

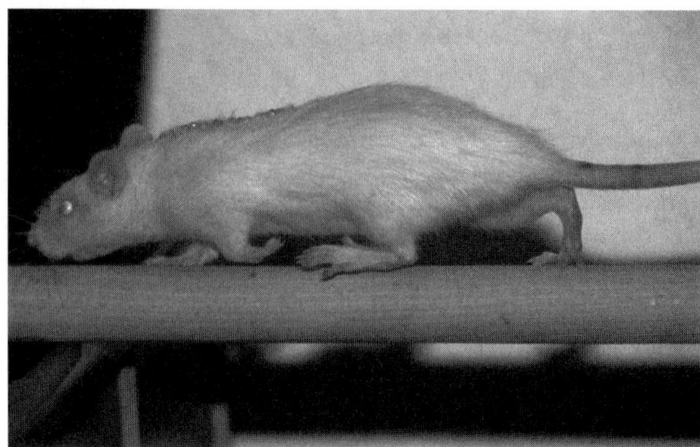

FIGURE 37.1 After treatment with the monoclonal antibody IN-1, spinal cord–injured rats showed normalization of locomotor functions evaluated by a number of behavioral tests, such as narrow beam crossing.

inhibitors in the CNS (Domeniconi et al., 2002; Liu et al., 2002; Wang et al., 2002).

Myelin-Associaetd Glycoprotein

Myelin-associated glycoprotein (MAG) is a member of the immunoglobulin superfamily and is present as a transmembrane protein in both CNS and PNS myelin. It was identified as an inhibitory protein in CNS myelin (McKerracher et al., 1994) that can, however, also promote neurite outgrowth, depending on the age of the neurons (Mukhopadhyay et al., 1994). Mice deficient in MAG did not show major effects on axonal regeneration after optic nerve or spinal cord lesioning (Bartsch et al., 1995) The MAG protein can inhibit axonal regeneration after a peripheral nerve injury *in vivo* (Schafer et al., 1996). It seems to inhibit axonal regeneration by directly binding with high affinity to NgR (Domeniconi et al., 2002; Liu et al., 2002; Wang et al., 2002). This binding is glycophosphatidylinositol (GPI) dependent and sialic acid independent (Domeniconi et al., 2002).

Oligodendrocyte-Myelin Glycoprotein

Oligodendrocyte-myelin glycoprotein (OMgp) is a GPI-linked membrane protein of oligodendrocytes and CNS myelin. It is a highly glycosylated protein that is confined to the CNS, where its developmental expression is region specific and parallels myelination (Mikol and Stefansson, 1988). Oligodendrocyte-myelin glycoprotein has been shown to be a potent inhibitor of neurite outgrowth *in vitro* that, like Nogo-66 and MAG, also binds with high affinity to NgR (Wang et al., 2002).

Proteoglycans

Proteoglycans, in particular versican V2 and brevican, are also found in adult CNS white matter (Niederöst et al., 1999; Chen et al., 2002). Their contribution to the regenerative capacity of CNS nerve fibers will be discussed below.

For a long time, scars that formed at lesion sites were recognized as potential barriers to regeneration (for review see Fawcett and Asher, 1999). It is now clear that specific biochemical components of the scar tissue rather than or in addition to mechanical effects also play a crucial role in the process of regeneration.

Chondroitin sulfate proteoglycans (CS-PGs) are expressed around the CNS injury site a few days after lesioning, and their expression in the glial scar persists for several weeks (for review see Fawcett and Asher, 1999). Axons growing out from transplanted dorsal root ganglion (DRG) cells stop at the site of CS-PG expression, suggesting that CS-PGs exert an inhibitory effect on regenerating axons *in vivo* (Davies et al., 1999). *In vitro*, CS-PGs are poor substrates for growing neurites (Snow et al., 1990). Several CS-PGs, including neurocan, brevican, phosphacan, and NG2, are expressed by astrocytes and other CNS glia and inhibit axonal growth in a number of *in vitro* assays (Niederöst et al., 1999). Application of chondroitinase ABC, a bacterial enzyme, degrades chondroitin sulfate-glycosaminoglycan after brain or spinal cord injury and promotes regeneration of nigrostriatal or corticospinal tract axons (Moon et al., 2001; Bradbury et al., 2002).

NG2

NG2 is a very potent proteoglycan produced mainly by oligodendrocyte precursors that are recruited to CNS injury sites. The growth of both sensory and cerebellar axons is inhibited by purified NG2 *in vitro* (Dou and Levine, 1994; Chen et al., 2002). Astrocytic cell lines that inhibit axon growth produce NG2, which can be neutralized by a blocking antibody that removes most of the inhibitory activity (Fidler et al., 1999).

Phosphacan

Phosphacan, which is also produced by oligodendrocyte precursor cells (Chen et al., 2002), has been shown to block axonal growth through interactions with a number of growth-promoting molecules, such as contactin, neural cell adhesion molecule (N-CAM), L1, axonin-1, and tenascin (Milev et al., 1996). Depending on the type of phosphacan, which exists in two transmembrane forms, either as the receptor tyrosine phosphatase (RPTP-β) or as the truncated secreted molecule [dermatan sulfate-dependent (DSD-1/phosphacan)], and on its glycosylation, it can have opposite modes of action on different neurons (Garwood et al., 1999). In cell culture, phosphacan is produced by oligodendrocyte precursor cells that have not yet differentiated into mature oligodendrocytes or type 2 astrocytes.

Neurocan

Neurocan is present in the normal CNS but is upregulated around the CNS injury site. It is probably the most important inhibitory proteoglycan produced by astrocytes, and its production is strongly regulated by cytokines (Asher et al., 2000). Like phosphacan, neurocan also interacts with growth-promoting molecules to inhibit axonal growth.

Versican

Versican belongs to the hyalunorate-binding CS-PGs. It is highly expressed in white matter tracts, and its expression in rats is closely correlated to myelination (Bignami et al., 1993). *In vitro* studies show that versican is a product of the oligodendrocyte lineage cells. Bovine spinal cord–derived versican inhibits axonal growth *in vitro* (Niederöst et al., 1999). *In vivo*, versican is upregulated in response to CNS injury (Asher et al., 2002).

Brevican

Brevican is a CNS-specific proteoglycan that is expressed at low levels during development, but expression is increased in the adult brain. It is primarily synthesized by astrocytes and is one of the most abundant intracellular matrix proteins in the adult brain (Yamada et al., 1997). After CNS lesioning, brevican is upregulated in areas of brain damage as well as in the denervated region (Thon et al., 2000).

ADDITIONAL POTENTIAL INHIBITORY FACTORS

Evidence is emerging that in addition to the neurite growth inhibitory factors mentioned above, proteins regulating axonal guidance during development can also contribute to the failure of mature CNS neurons to regenerate after injury. Among these proteins are netrin, tenascins, semaphorins, and ephrins. Interestingly, some of these guidance cues, which are important during development, are still expressed in the mature CNS of rodents and humans. Damage to the CNS can induce changes in the expression of these developmental factors.

Netrins

Netrins belong to a small family of guidance cues that exert attractive as well as repellent properties (for review see Tessier-Lavigne and Goodman, 1996). During development netrins play an important role in guiding axons toward the CNS midline. In this phase they can, however, also act as repellents, influencing certain motor axons to grow away from the midline (Varela-Echavarria et al., 1997). Peripheral nerve regeneration leads to a large increase in netrin-1 mRNA levels, suggesting that this protein can influence axonal regeneration in adult peripheral nerve (Madison et al., 2000). The function of netrins in the adult CNS is still completely unclear. Netrin-1 and the netrin receptors (deleted in colorectal cancer [DCC] and UNC-5H2) are expressed by nonlesioned adult retinal ganglion cells. After axotomy, both receptors were downregulated while netrin-1 remained present. Netrin and its receptors may therefore help to regulate the regenerative capacity of adult retinal ganglion cells after injury to the optic nerve (Ellezam et al., 2001).

Tenascins

Tenascins constitute a family of extracellular matrix glycoproteins that are also expressed during nervous system development (for review see Joester and Faissner, 2001). Tenascin-R is found in the CNS at later stages of development as well, and its expression is restricted mainly to oligodendrocytes. Tenascin-R is inhibitory for the outgrowth of retinal ganglion cells *in vitro*, and its expression in the optic nerve persists after injury (Becker at al., 2000). It is therefore suggested that tenascin-R contributes to the inhibition of axonal regeneration. In addition to their growth inhibitory action, tenascins have binding sites for most of the inhibitory CS-PGs.

Semaphorin 3A

Semaphorin 3A, which belongs to a large family of secreted, membrane-associated proteins, is chemorepulsive and suppresses axonal growth during embryogenesis. In the course of development semaphorin 3A expression declines, but injury to the mature CNS can induce its reexpression (for review see Pasterkamp and Verhaagen, 2001; De Winter et al., 2002). Such injury-induced reexpression also holds true for several extracellular matrix molecules, such as tenascin-C, and for a number of proteoglycans. Semaphorin 3 is not present in peripheral nerve after injury, and both facial and spinal motor neurons downregulate their semaphorin 3 mRNA expression after injury (for review see Pasterkamp and Verhaagen, 2001). This injury-induced downregulation coincides with the period of axonal regrowth.

Eph Receptors and Ephrin Ligands

Eph receptors and their ephrin ligands belong to another family of membrane molecules that play a major role in axonal pathfinding and target recognition during CNS development (for review see Orioli and Klein, 1997). These molecules may also contribute to the outcome of CNS trauma in the adult. In adult rats subjected to a spinal cord contusion lesion, marked upregulation of Eph B3 mRNA was observed in different areas around the site of injury (Miranda et al., 1999). Failure of the adult CNS to regenerate thus seems to depend on an interplay between a number of different factors that contribute to the inhibitory environment of CNS tissue.

OVERCOMING CENTRAL NERVOUS SYSTEM INHIBITION

A number of different strategies have been applied to invalidate or neutralize factors that contribute to the inhibitory nature of the CNS environment and restrain neurite outgrowth after injury.

Neutralization of Inhibitory Myelin Constituents

Prevention of myelin formation in the rat spinal cord (Savio and Schwab, 1990) or immunolysis of myelin (Dyer et al., 1998) led to a massive enhancement of regeneration after a spinal cord injury.

Administration of the monoclonal antibody IN-1 to rats suffering from a spinal cord lesion promoted regeneration of corticospinal tract (CST) fibers (Schnell and Schwab, 1990) and induced partial functional recovery (Bregman et al., 1995). Application of the same antibody to rats undergoing unilateral lesioning of the CST at the level of the brain stem enhanced collateral sprouting and structural plasticity of the unlesioned fiber tract. This phenomenon was again associated with an impressive functional recovery of the animals (Thallmair et al., 1998; Z'Graggen et al., 1998). A similar enhancement of axonal sprouting responses was seen when myelin formation was prevented (Vanek et al., 1998).

Current approaches strive to neutralize the inhibitory action of Nogo-A by administration of purified anti-Nogo-A-antibodies via miniosmotic, subcutaneously implanted pumps that deliver the antibody directly into the cerebrospinal fluid. An important future approach to neutralize the action of growth inhibitory molecules including Nogo-A, MAG, and OMgp is the administration of receptor antagonists or antibodies.

Manipulation of Downstream Signaling Pathways

Manipulating the downstream signaling pathways of inhibitory factors is another promising strategy to enhance regeneration. The intrinsic state of the neuron and growth cone influences its response to guidance cues, neurotrophic factors, and myelin-associated inhibitors. In young DRG neurons, in which axonal growth is not inhibited by myelin and myelin-associated proteins, endogenous levels of the cyclic nucleotide cyclic adenosine monophosphate (cAMP) are severalfold higher than in similar neurons at an adult stage (Cai et al., 2001). Elevating the neuronal cAMP levels can overcome inhibition by myelin and myelin inhibitors *in vitro* (Cai et al., 2001) and *in vivo*: ascending tract axons elongated more after dorsal column lesioning when cAMP was elevated in corresponding DRGs by injection of dibutyryl cAMP (Qui et al., 2002). Other signaling pathways are also thought to play a role in the inhibitory process.

Growth cone collapse is associated with a large increase in intracellular Ca^{2+} levels, and preventing this Ca^{2+} rise avoided growth cone collapse (Bandtlow et al., 1993). During neurite extension and retraction, the growth cone cytoskeleton is regulated by members of the Rho family of small guanosine triphosphatases (GTPases) (Rho, Rac, Cdc42). Rho A is activated by Nogo-A, MAG, and myelin (Lehmann et al., 1999). Inhibition of Rho or Rho-kinase activation blunts inhibitory responses *in vitro* and enhances regeneration of CST axons in the lesioned spinal cord *in vivo* (Dergham et al., 2002). When a neuron is exposed to inhibitory factors, the balance of intracellular proteins, such as cyclic nucleotides or Rho family GTPases, may define the growth response of the cell.

Vaccine Approach to Block Myelin-Associated Inhibitors

A vaccine was also applied to spinal cord–injured mice to block the myelin-associated inhibitors and promote regeneration of CST axons (Huang et al., 1999). Mice were immunized with CNS myelin or spinal cord homogenate before receiving a spinal cord lesion. Labeling of the CST fibers showed long-distance regeneration of a substantial number of axons, as well as some recovery of certain hind limb motor functions. Passive immunization of spinal cord–injured mice with anti-myelin mouse antiserum also led to long-distance regeneration of CST axons, although the results were less impressive than those after active immunization (Huang et al., 1999).

Beneficial Effects of the Immune System

Increasing evidence suggests that immune activity, which was considered to be harmful after CNS trauma, can exert beneficial effects after CNS damage. Stimulated macrophages implanted into a transected rat spinal cord were reported to increase tissue repair and partial recovery of motor functions (Rapalino et al., 1998). T cells reacting to myelin basic protein or to Nogo-A are reported to induce neuroprotective effects (Hauben et al., 2000), but these phenomena are probably complex and could also turn into a destructive reaction.

Degradation of the Proteoglycans

To degrade CS-PGs that are present in and around the scar tissue and to inhibit axonal regeneration after a spinal cord injury in the adult mammalian CNS, chondroitinase ABC was delivered to rats intrathecally. This treatment degraded CS-PG immunoreactivity at the injury site and promoted regeneration of ascending sensory projections and descending CST axons (Bradbury et al., 2002). In addition, functional recovery of locomotor and proprioceptive behaviors was promoted. After unilateral nigrostriatal axotomy lesioning, similar results were obtained for ascending dopaminergic projections growing back to their targets (Moon et al., 2001).

Neurotrophic Factors

Neurotrophic factors can enhance nerve fiber outgrowth during embryonic development. Applying neurotrophic factors such as neurotrophin-3 (NT-3), NT-4, or brain derived neurotrophic factor (BDNF) to the adult lesioned spinal cord promotes sprouting and in some cases induces long-distance regeneration of lesioned fibers (Schnell et al., 1994; for review see Blesch et al., 2002). In addition, atrophy or retrograde cell death in response to axotomy can be prevented (Giehl and Tetzlaff, 1996; Kwon et al., 2002). Only a few of the neurotrophic factors have been investigated in animal models of spinal cord lesions. The specificity of a given factor for neuronal subtypes, on the one hand, and the often broad spectrum of effects of these factors, on the other hand, complicate their application. However, new methods of application include engineered cells that secrete the factors directly into the lesion site or gene therapy with viral constructs producing the factors of interest where they are needed (Blesch et al., 2002).

Bridges

The axonal environment can be changed from a hostile surrounding to a growth-permissive milieu by adding bridges. These bridges can consist of peripheral nerve grafts, Schwann cells, olfactory ensheathing glia, fetal tissue, stem cells, or neuronal precursor cells (for review see Bunge, 2001). When peripheral nerve is used as a bridge, axons grow into and through the bridge. The growth into the CNS environment caudal of the bridge is, however, very limited (Aguayo et al., 1981; David and Aguayo, 1981). Adult rats subjected to a complete spinal cord transection and implanted with a bundle of peripheral nerve grafts were evaluated for recovery of locomotion patterns 3 and 4 months after surgery (Cheng et al., 1997). Transplanted rats used their hind limbs for 25%–30% of their movements and regained several of the specific limb movement patterns used by normal nonlesioned rats (Cheng et al., 1997).

Schwann cells and olfactory ensheathing glial cells have also served as a supportive substrate for axonal regeneration in spinal cord lesions (Ramon-Cueto et al., 1998; Bunge, 2001). Regenerating spinal axons that grew into the Schwann cell graft were often myelinated or ensheathed by the transplanted cells. Transplantation of olfactory ensheathing glial cells may be one of the most promising strategies for bridging spinal cord lesion sites. In contrast to Schwann cells, olfactory ensheathing glia migrate extensively along white matter tracts and guide regenerating axons to pass through the lesion (Ramon-Cueto et al., 1998). They synthesize and secrete cell adhesion molecules and neurotrophic growth factors that support axonal elongation and extension. At present the extensive, uncontrolled migration of these cells in the host spinal cord clearly restricts their use in animal experiments.

Embryonic spinal cord transplants have also been used to replace damaged neuronal populations and to restore some degree of anatomical continuity of the injured spinal cord. This approach has been very successful in newborn lesions but less so in adults (Bregman et al., 1993; Coumans et al., 2001). The use of other cell types as bridges is currently being explored. Possible cells include marrow stromal cells, which were reported to differentiate into neuron-like cells, neural progenitor cells, and stem cells (Hofstetter et al., 2002; for review see Cao et al., 2002).

FUNCTIONAL RECOVERY AFTER CENTRAL NERVOUS SYSTEM REGENERATION

Once the growth inhibition of the CNS is overcome, the growing axons have to recognize functionally correct targets and form synapses. This target finding can be facilitated by (re-)expression of axonal guidance cues and target recognition signals. Almost nothing is known about these molecular processes in the injured adult CNS (Bareyre et al., 2002). Functionally meaningful connections are probably stabilized by activity.

Spinal cord–injured rats or rats subjected to a middle cerebral artery occlusion showed a significant degree of functional recovery after treatment with the mAb IN-1 (Bergman et al., 1995; Merkler et al., 2001; Papadopoulos et al., 2002). Spinal cord–injured rats exhibited recovery of specific reflex and locomotor functions, while rats suffering from an ischemic stroke demonstrated functional recovery in a forelimb reaching task. Significant improvements were also seen in the electromyographic pattern of hind limb muscle activation (Merkler et al., 2001). In IN-1-treated rats but not in control antibody-treated animals, normalization of locomotor function and hind limb weight support was seen (Fig. 37.2*A,B*), in addition to the reduction of cocontractions and spasticity-like activation patterns (Merkler et al., 2001). In mice immunized with myelin or spinal cord extract, anatomical regeneration led to recovery of certain hind limb motor functions (Huang et al., 1999). Postsynaptic activity below the lesion site after electrical stimulation of corticospinal neurons was restored in spinal cord–injured rats treated with chondroitinase ABC. This treatment also promoted functional recovery of locomotor and proprioceptive behavior (Bradbury et al., 2002).

Before and shortly after birth, compensatory sprouting or circuit plasticity, that is, the ability of healthy nerve fibers to take over the role of injured axons, is pronounced; this process is much less prominent in the adult CNS. The functional recovery that occurs fol-

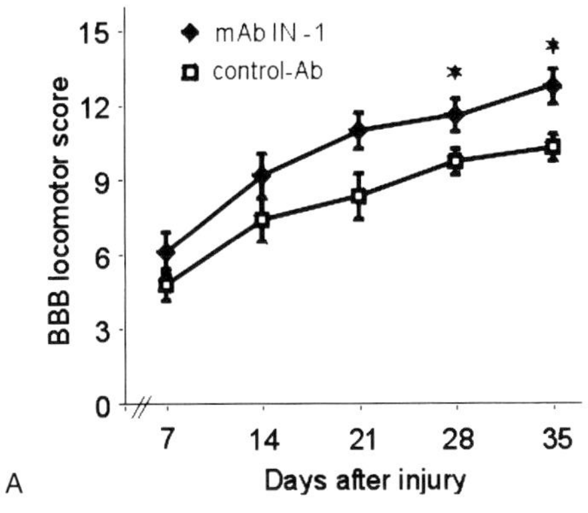

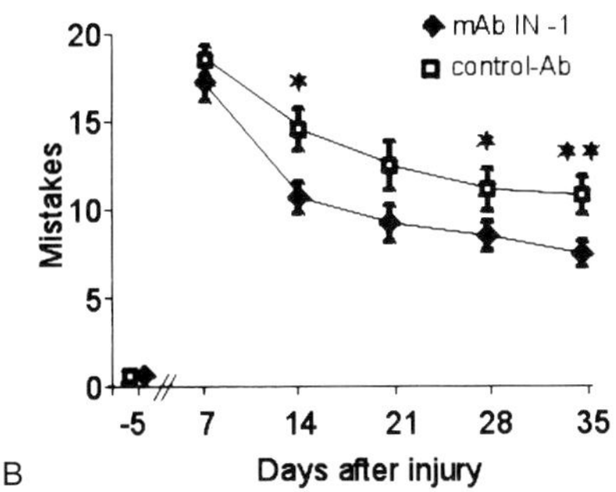

FIGURE 37.2 *A*. Functional recovery monitored with the (BBB) open-field locomotor score, which quantifies multiple aspects of spontaneous open-field, over-ground locomotion. Preoperated animals attain a maximum score of 21 points. Time course of the recovery in monoclonal (mAb) IN-1-treated and control antibody (Ab)-treated rats (n = 17 per group). At 35 days after injury, the IN-1-treated rats attained a BBB score that was significantly higher than that of the control Ab-treated group. *B*. Functional recovery depicted as the number of mistakes made in the grid walk. The number of foot-placing errors was counted while rats walked over a horizontal runway of irregularly placed metal grid bars. Over a period of 5 weeks, significantly fewer mistakes were made by the mAb IN-1-treated animals compared to control Ab-treated rats (n = 17 per group). (*A* and *B* from Merkler et al., 2001, *J. Neuroscience* 21:3665–3673 (2001), with permission.)

lowing an adult CNS injury such as a stroke is probably largely due to plasticity, for example, adjacent cortical areas taking over the function of damaged areas or utilization of alternative motor pathways (for review see Raineteau and Schwab, 2001). Some of the strategies that promote regeneration of damaged nerve fibers may also increase the compensatory growth of nonlesioned fibers. Thus, in the rat after a CST lesion or a stroke, compensatory sprouting was enhanced by the mAb IN-1. These rats tested in the food pellet reaching paradigm demonstrated a restoration of fine paw movements (Thallmair et al., 1998; Z'Graggen et al., 1998; Raineteau et al., 2001; Papadopoulos et al., 2002).

In the absence of neuronal regeneration, animals with a complete spinal cord transection can acquire the ability to generate hind limb stepping movements by treadmill training (de Leon et al., 1998). Rehabilitative locomotor training in spinal cord–injured patients with incomplete lesions has been shown to play a crucial role in inducing spared spinal pathways to control and generate locomotion and respond appropriately to sensory feedback (for review see Dietz, 2001). These results show that the adult mammalian spinal cord has plastic potentials that can be enhanced by appropriate treatments.

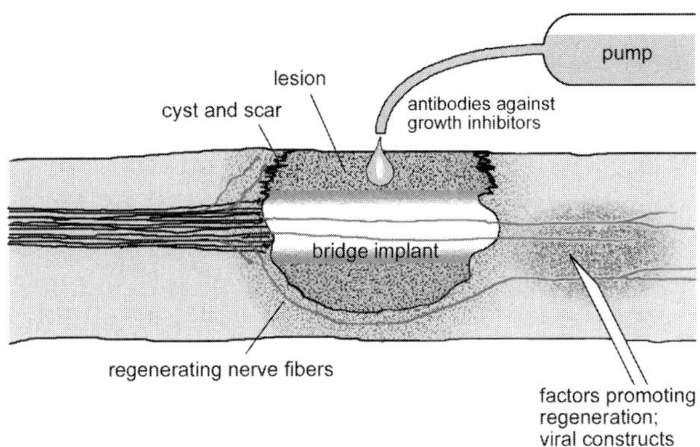

FIGURE 37.3 A number of different strategies may be required to repair the injured spinal cord. These strategies include grafts that bridge the cyst, antibodies or other agents that neutralize the effects of neurite growth inhibitory factors directly or via their receptors, and neurite growth-promoting molecules. [From *Science* 295:1029–1031 (2002). Copyright 2002 American Association for Advancement of Science. Reprinted with permission.]

SUMMARY AND PERSPECTIVES

A major element and focus of current research on CNS axonal regeneration is the inhibitory proteins and molecules that suppress or limit spontaneous regeneration, plasticity, and functional repair. Several of these proteins (Nogo-A, MAG, OMgp) are associated with oligodendrocytes, while others (CS-PGs) are mainly present in the scar tissue that forms after injury. Significant axonal regeneration in the adult mammalian CNS after injury is possible after inactivation of some of these inhibitory factors. Along with regeneration and compensatory sprouting, some degree of functional recovery is often observed. Axonal growth-enhancing strategies can therefore be applied to restore lost functions after CNS damage. Combinations of treatments (inactivation of growth inhibitors or their receptors or downstream signaling, trophic factors, bridges, rehabilitative training) may be required to deal with the full complexity of CNS injury (Fig. 37.3).

ACKNOWLEDGMENTS

We would like to thank the *Journal of Neuroscience* and the American Association for the Advancement of Science for their permission to reproduce published material in this chapter.

ABBREVIATIONS

BDNF	brain-derived neurotrophic factor
cAMP	cyclic adenosine monophosphate
CNS	central nervous system
CS-PG	chondroitin sulfate proteoglycan
CST	corticospinal tract
DRG	dorsal root ganglion
DSD-1	dermatan sulfate dependent-1
GAP-43	growth associated protein 43
GPI	glycophosphatidylinositol
GTPase	guanosine triphosphatase
mAb	monoclonal antibody
MAG	myelin associated glycoprotein
N-CAM	neural cell adhesion molecule
NgR	Nogo-66 receptor
NT-3	neurotrophin-3
NT-4	neurotrophin-4
OMpg	oligodendrocyte-myelin glycoprotein
PNS	peripheral nervous system
RPTP	receptor tyrosine phosphatase

REFERENCES

Aguayo, A.J., David, S., and Bray, G.M. (1981) Influences of the glial environment on the elongation of axons after injury: transplantation studies in adult rodents. *J. Exp. Biol.* 95:231–240.

Asher, R.A., Morgenstern, D.A., Fidler, P.S., Adcock, K.H., Oohira, A., Braistead, J.E., Levine, J.M., Margolis, R.U., Rogers, J.H., and Fawcett, J.W. (2000) Neurocan is upregulated in injured brain and in cytokine-treated astrocytes. *J. Neurosci.* 20: 2427–2438.

Asher, R.A., Morgenstern, D.A., Shearer, M.C., Adcock, K.H., Pesheva, P., and Fawcett, J.W. (2002) Versican is upregulated in CNS injury and is a product of oligodendrocyte lineage cells. *J. Neurosci.* 22:2225–2236.

Bandtlow, C.E., Schmidt, M.F., Hassinger, T.D., Schwab, M.E., and Kater, S.B. (1993) Role of intracellular calcium in NI-35-evoked collapse of neuronal growth cones. *Science* 259:80–83.

Bandtlow, C.E. and Schwab, M.E. (2000) NI-35/250/nogo-a: a neurite growth inhibitor restricting structural plasticity and regeneration of nerve fibers in the adult vertebrate CNS. *Glia* 29:175–181.

Bareyre, F.M., Haudenschild, B., and Schwab, M.E. (2002) Long-lasting sprouting and gene expression changes induced by the monoclonal antibody IN-1 in the adult spinal cord. *J. Neurosci.* 22:7097–7110.

Bartsch, U., Bandtlow, C.E., Schnell, L., Bartsch, S., Spillmann, A.A., Rubin, B.P., Hillenbrand, R., Montag, D., Schwab, M.E., and Schachner, M. (1995) Lack of evidence that myelin-associated glycoprotein is a major inhibitor of axonal regeneration in the CNS. *Neuron* 15:1375–1381.

Bastmeyer, M., Beckmann, M., Schwab, M.E., and Stuermer, C.A. (1991) Growth of regenerating goldfish axons is inhibited by rat oligodendrocytes and CNS myelin but not but not by goldfish optic nerve tract oligodendrocytelike cells and fish CNS myelin. *J. Neurosci.* 11:626–640.

Becker, T., Anliker, B., Becker, C.G., Taylor, J., Schachner, M., Meyer, R.L., and Bartsch, U. (2000) Tenascin-R inhibits regrowth of optic fibers in vitro and persists in the optic nerve of mice after injury. *Glia* 29:330–346.

Bernhardt, R.R. (1999) Cellular and molecular bases of axonal regeneration in the fish central nervous system. *Exp. Neurol.* 157: 223–240.

Bignami, A., Perides, G., and Rahemtulla, F. (1993) Versican, a hyaluronate-binding proteoglycan of embryonal precartilaginous mesenchyma, is mainly expressed postnatally in rat brain. *J. Neurosci. Res.* 34:97–106.

Blesch, A., Lu, P., and Tuszynski, M.H. (2002) Neurotrophic factors, gene therapy, and neural stem cells for spinal cord repair. *Brain Res. Bull.* 57:833–838.

Bradbury, E.J., Moon, L.D., Popat, R.J., King, V.R., Bennett, G.S., Patel, P.N., Fawcett, J.W., and McMahon, S.B. (2002) Chondroitinase ABC promotes functional recovery after spinal cord injury. *Nature* 416:636–640.

Bregman, B.S., Kunkel-Bagden, E., Reier, P.J., Dai, H.N., McAtee, M., and Gao, D. (1993) Recovery of function after spinal cord injury: mechanisms underlying transplant-mediated recovery of function differ after spinal cord injury in newborn and adult rats. *Exp. Neurol.* 123:3–16.

Bregman, B.S., Kunkel-Bagden, E., Schnell, L., Dai, H.N., Gao, D., and Schwab, M.E. (1995) Recovery from spinal cord injury mediated by antibodies to neurite growth inhibitors. *Nature* 378: 498–501.

Bunge, M.B. (2001) Bridging areas of injury in the spinal cord. *Neuroscientist* 7:325–339.

Cai, D., Qiu, J., Cao, Z., McAtee, M., Bregman, B.S., and Filbin, M.T. (2001) Neuronal cyclic AMP controls the developmental loss in ability of axons to regenerate. *J. Neurosci.* 21:4731–4739.

Cao, Q., Benton, R.L., and Whittemore, S.R. (2002) Stem cell repair of central nervous system injury. *J. Neurosci. Res.* 68:501–510.

Caroni, P. and Schwab, M.E. (1988a) Antibody against myelin-associated inhibitor of neurite growth neutralizes nonpermissive substrate properties of CNS white matter. *Neuron* 1:85–96.

Caroni, P. and Schwab, M.E. (1988b) Two membrane protein fractions from rat central myelin with inhibitory properties for neurite growth and fibroblast spreading. *J. Cell. Biol.* 106: 1281–1288.

Chen, M.S., Huber, A.B., van der Haar, M.E., Frank, M., Schnell, L., Spillmann, A.A., Christ, F., and Schwab, M.E. (2000) Nogo-A is a myelin-associated neurite outgrowth inhibitor and an antigen for monoclonal antibody IN-1. *Nature* 403:434–439.

Chen, Z.J., Ughrin, Y., and Levine, J.M. (2002) Inhibition of axon growth by oligodendrocyte precursor cells. *Mol. Cell. Neurosci.* 20:125–139.

Cheng, H., Almstrom, S., Gimenez-Llort, L., Chang, R., Ove Ogren, S., Hoffer, B., and Olson, L. (1997) Gait analysis of adult paraplegic rats after spinal cord repair. *Exp. Neurol.* 148:544–557.

Coumans, J.V., Lin, T.T., Dai, H.N., MacArthur, L., McAtee, M., Nash, C., and Bregman, B.S. (2001) Axonal regeneration and functional recovery after complete spinal cord transection in rats by delayed treatment with transplants and neurotrophins. *J. Neurosci.* 21:9334–9344.

David, S. and Aguayo, A.J. (1981) Axonal elongation into peripheral nervous system "bridges" after central nervous system injury in adult rats. *Science* 214:931–933.

Davies, S.J., Goucher, D.R., Doller, C., and Silver, J. (1999) Robust regeneration of adult sensory axons in degenerating white matter of the adult rat spinal cord. *J. Neurosci.* 19:5810–5822.

Dergham, P., Ellezam, B., Essagian, C., Avedissian, H., Lubell, W.D., and McKerracher, L. (2002) Rho signaling pathway targeted to promote spinal cord repair. *J. Neurosci.* 22:6570–6577.

de Leon, R.D., Hodgson, J.A., Roy, R.R., and Edgerton, V.R. (1998) Locomotor capacity attributable to step training versus spontaneous recovery after spinalization in adult cats. *J. Neurophysiol.* 79:1329–1340.

De Winter, F., Oudega, M., Lankhorst, A.J., Hamers, F.P., Blits, B., Ruitenberg, M.J., Pasterkamp, R.J., Gispen, W.H., and Verhaagen, J. (2002) Injury-induced class 3 semaphorin expression in the rat spinal cord. *Exp. Neurol.* 175:61–75.

Dietz, V. (2001) Spinal cord lesion: effects of and perspectives for treatment. *Neural. Plast.* 8:83–90.

Domeniconi, M., Cao, Z., Spencer, T., Sivasankaran, R., Wang, K.C., Nikulina, E., Kimura, N., Cai, H., Deng, K., Gao, Y., He, Z., and Filbin, M.T. (2002) Myelin-associated glycoprotein interacts with the Nogo66 receptor to inhibit neurite outgrowth. *Neuron* 35:283–290.

Dou, C.L. and Levine, J.M. (1994) Inhibition of neurite growth by the NG2 chondroitin sulfate proteoglycan. *J. Neurosci.* 14:7616–7628.

Dyer, J.K., Bourque, J.A., and Steeves, J.D. (1998) Regeneration of brainstem-spinal axons after lesion and immunological disruption of myelin in adult rat. *Exp. Neurol.* 154:12–22.

Ellezam, B., Selles-Navarro, I., Manitt, C., Kennedy, T.E., and McKerracher, L. (2001) Expression of netrin-1 and its receptors DCC and UNC-5H2 after axotomy and during regeneration of adult rat retinal ganglion cells. *Exp. Neurol.* 168:105–115.

Fawcett, J.W. and Asher, R.A. (1999) The glial scar and central nervous system repair. *Brain Res. Bull.* 49:377–391.

Fidler, P.S., Schuette, K., Asher, R.A., Dobbertin, A., Thornton, S.R., Calle-Patino, Y., Muir, E., Levine, J.M., Geller, H.M., Rogers, J.H., Faissner, A., and Fawcett, J.W. (1999) Comparing astrocytic cell lines that are inhibitory or permissive for axon growth: the major axon-inhibitory proteoglycan is NG2. *J. Neurosci.* 19:8778–8788.

Fournier, A.E., GrandPre, T., and Strittmatter, S.M. (2001) Identification of a receptor mediating Nogo-66 inhibition of axonal regeneration. *Nature* 409:341–346.

Garwood, J., Schnadelbach, O., Clement, A., Schutte, K., Bach, A., and Faissner, A. (1999) DSD-1-proteoglycan is the mouse homolog of phosphacan and displays opposing effects on neurite outgrowth dependent on neuronal lineage. *J. Neurosci.* 19: 3888–3899.

Giehl, K.M. and Tetzlaff, W. (1996) BDNF and NT-3, but not NGF, prevent axotomy-induced death of rat corticospinal neurons in vivo. *Eur. J. Neurosci.* 8:1167–1175.

GrandPre, T., Nakamura, F., Vartanian, T., and Strittmatter, S.M. (2000) Identification of the Nogo inhibitor of axon regeneration as a Reticulon protein. *Nature* 403:439–344.

Hauben, E., Butovsky, O., Nevo, U., Yoles, E., Moalem, G., Agranov, E., Mor, F., Leibowitz-Amit, R., Pevsner, E., Akselrod, S., Neeman, M., Cohen, I.R., and Schwartz, M. (2000) Passive or active immunization with myelin basic protein promotes recovery from spinal cord contusion. *J. Neurosci.* 20:6421–6430.

Hofstetter, C.P., Schwarz, E.J., Hess, D., Widenfalk, J., El Manira, A., Prockop, D.J., and Olson, L. (2002) Marrow stromal cells form guiding strands in the injured spinal cord and promote recovery. *Proc. Natl. Acad. Sci. USA* 99:2199–2204.

Huang, D.W., McKerracher, L., Braun, P.E., and David, S. (1999) A therapeutic vaccine approach to stimulate axon regeneration in the adult mammalian spinal cord. *Neuron* 24:639–647.

Huber, A.B., Weinmann, O., Brösamle, C., Oertle, T., and Schwab, M.E. (2002) Patterns of Nogo mRNA and protein expression in the developing and adult rat and after CNS lesions. *J. Neurosci.* 22:3553–3567.

Joester, A. and Faissner, A. (2001) The structure and function of tenascins in the nervous system. *Matrix Biol.* 20:13–22.

Kapfhammer, J.P. and Schwab, M.E. (1994) Inverse patterns of myelination and GAP-43 expression in the adult CNS: neurite growth inhibitors as regulators of neuronal plasticity? *J. Comp. Neurol.* 340:194–206.

Kwon, B.K., Liu, J., Messerer, C., Kobayashi, N.R., McGraw, J., Oschipok, L., and Tetzlaff, W. (2002) Survival and regeneration of rubrospinal neurons 1 year after spinal cord injury. *Proc. Natl. Acad. Sci. USA* 99:3246–3251.

Lang, D.M., Rubin, B.P., Schwab, M.E., and Stuermer, C.A. (1995) CNS myelin and oligodendrocytes of the *Xenopus* spinal cord—but not optic nerve—are nonpermissive for axon growth. *J. Neurosci.* 15:99–109.

Lehmann, M., Fournier, A., Selles-Navarro, I., Dergham, P., Sebok, A., Leclerc, N., Tigyi, G., and McKerracher, L. (1999) Inactivation of Rho signaling pathway promotes CNS axon regeneration. *J. Neurosci.* 19:7537–7547.

Liu, B.P., Fournier, A., GrandPre, T., and Strittmatter, S.M. (2002) Myelin-associated glycoprotein as a functional ligand for the Nogo-66 receptor. *Science* 297:1190–1193.

Lurie, D.I. and Selzer, M.E. (1991) Axonal regeneration in the adult lamprey spinal cord. *J. Comp. Neurol.* 306:409–416.

Madison, R.D., Zomorodi, A., and Robinson, G.A. (2000) Netrin-1 and peripheral nerve regeneration in the adult rat. *Exp. Neurol.* 161:563–570.

McKerracher, L., David, S., Jackson, D.L., Kottis, V., Dunn, R.J., and Braun, P.E. (1994) Identification of myelin-associated glycoprotein as a major myelin-derived inhibitor of neurite growth. *Neuron* 13:805–811.

Merkler, D., Metz, G.A., Raineteau, O., Dietz, V., Schwab, M.E., and Fouad, K. (2001) Locomotor recovery in spinal cord–injured rats treated with an antibody neutralizing the myelin-associated neurite growth inhibitor Nogo-A. *J. Neurosci.* 21:3665–3673.

Mikol, D.D., and Stefansson, K. (1988) A phosphatidylinositol-linked peanut agglutinin-binding glycoprotein in central nervous system myelin and on oligodendrocytes. *J. Cell. Biol.* 106:1273–1279.

Milev, P., Maurel, P., Haring, M., Margolis, R.K., and Margolis, R.U. (1996) TAG-1/axonin-1 is a high-affinity ligand of neurocan, phosphacan/protein-tyrosine phosphatase-zeta/beta, and N-CAM. *J. Biol. Chem.* 271:15716–15723.

Miranda, J.D., White, L.A., Marcillo, A.E., Willson, C.A., Jagid, J., and Whittemore, S.R. (1999) Induction of Eph B3 after spinal cord injury. *Exp. Neurol.* 156:218–222.

Moon, L.D., Asher, R.A., Rhodes, K.E., and Fawcett, J.W. (2001) Regeneration of CNS axons back to their target following treatment of adult rat brain with chondroitinase ABC. *Nat. Neurosci.* 4:465–466.

Mukhopadhyay, G., Doherty, P., Walsh, F.S., Crocker, P.R., and Filbin, M.T. (1994) A novel role for myelin-associated glycoprotein as an inhibitor of axonal regeneration. *Neuron* 13:757–767.

Niederöst, B.P., Zimmermann,D.R., Schwab, M.E., and Bandtlow, C.E. (1999) Bovine CNS myelin contains neurite growth-inhibitory activity associated with chondroitin sulfate proteoglycans. *J. Neurosci.* 19:8979–8989.

Oertle, T., van der Haar, M.E., Bandtlow, C.E., Robeva, A., Burfeind, P., Huber, A.B., Simonen, M., Schnell, L., Broesamle, C., Kaupmann, K., Vallon, R., and Schwab, M.E. (2003) Nogo-A: a molecule with three active sites and two membrane topologies. *J. Neurosci.* 23:5393–5406.

Orioli, D., and Klein, R. (1997) The Eph receptor family: axonal guidance by contact repulsion. *Trends Genet.* 13:354–359.

Papadopoulos, C.M., Tsai, S.Y., Alsbiei, T., O'Brien, T.E., Schwab, M.E., and Kartje, G.L. (2002) Functional recovery and neuroanatomical plasticity following middle cerebral artery occlusion and IN-1 antibody treatment in the adult rat. *Ann. Neurol.* 51:433–441.

Pasterkamp, R.J. and Verhaagen, J. (2001) Emerging roles for semaphorins in neural regeneration. *Brain Res. Brain Res. Rev.* 35: 36–54.

Prinjha, R., Moore, S.E., Vinson, M., Blake, S., Morrow, R., Christie, G., Michalovich, D., Simmons, D.L., and Walsh, F.S. (2000) Inhibitor of neurite outgrowth in humans. *Nature* 403:383–384.

Qiu, J., Cai, D., Dai, H., McAtee, M., Hoffman, P.N., Bregman, B.S., and Filbin, M.T. (2002) Spinal axon regeneration induced by elevation of cyclic AMP. *Neuron* 34:895–903.

Qiu, J., Cai, D., and Filbin, M.T. (2000) Glial inhibition of nerve regeneration in the mature mammalian CNS. *Glia* 29:166–174.

Raineteau, O., Fouad, K., Noth, P., Thallmair, M., and Schwab, M.E. (2001) Functional switch between motor tracts in the presence of the mAb IN-1 in the adult rat. *Proc. Natl. Acad. Sci. USA* 98:6929–6934.

Raineteau, O. and Schwab, M.E. (2001) Plasticity of motor systems after incomplete spinal cord injury. *Nat. Rev. Neurosci.* 2:263–273.

Ramon-Cueto, A., Plant, G.W., Avila, J., and Bunge, M.B. (1998) Long-distance axonal regeneration in the transected adult rat spinal cord is promoted by olfactory ensheathing glia transplants. *J. Neurosci.* 18:3803–3815.

Rapalino, O., Lazarov-Spiegler, O., Agranov, E., Velan, G.J., Yoles, E., Fraidakis, M., Solomon, A., Gepstein, R., Katz, A., Belkin, M., Hadani, M., and Schwartz, M. (1998) Implantation of stimulated homologous macrophages results in partial recovery of paraplegic rats. *Nat. Med.* 4:814–821.

Richardson, P.M., Issa, V.M., and Aguayo, A.J. (1984) Regeneration of long spinal axons in the rat. *J. Neurocytol.* 13:165–182.

Savio, T. and Schwab, M.E. (1990) Lesioned corticospinal tract axons regenerate in myelin-free rat spinal cord. *Proc. Natl. Acad. Sci. USA* 87:4130–4133.

Schafer, M., Fruttiger, M., Montag, D., Schachner, M., and Martini, R. (1996) Disruption of the gene for the myelin-associated glycoprotein improves axonal regrowth along myelin in C57BL/Wlds mice. *Neuron* 16:1107–1113.

Schnell, L., Schneider, R., Kolbeck, R., Barde, Y.A., and Schwab, M.E. (1994) Neurotrophin-3 enhances sprouting of corticospinal tract during development and after adult spinal cord lesion. *Nature* 367:170–173.

Schnell, L. and Schwab, M.E. (1990) Axonal regeneration in the rat spinal cord produced by an antibody against myelin-associated neurite growth inhibitors. *Nature* 343:269–272.

Schwab, M.E. and Caroni, P. (1988) Oligodendrocytes and CNS myelin are nonpermissive substrates for neurite growth and fibroblast spreading in vitro. *J. Neurosci.* 8:2381–2393.

Schwab, M.E. and Thoenen, H. (1985) Dissociated neurons regenerate into sciatic but not optic nerve explants in culture irrespective of neurotrophic factors. *J. Neurosci.* 5:2415–2423.

Snow, D.M., Lemmon, V., Carrino, D.A., Caplan, A.I., and Silver, J. (1990) Sulfated proteoglycans in astroglial barriers inhibit neurite outgrowth in vitro. *Exp. Neurol.* 109:111–130.

Spillmann, A.A., Bandtlow, C.E., Lottspeich, F., Keller, F., and Schwab, M.E. (1998) Identification and characterization of a bovine neurite growth inhibitor (bNI-220). *J. Biol. Chem.* 273:19283–19293.

Tessier-Lavigne, M., and Goodman, C.S. (1996) The molecular biology of axon guidance. *Science* 274:1123–1133.

Thallmair, M., Metz, G.A.S., Z'Graggen, W.J., Raineteau, O., Kartje, W.L., and Schwab, M.E. (1998) Neurite growth inhibitors restrict plasticity and functional recovery following corticospinal tract lesions. *Nat. Neurosci.* 1:124–131.

Thon, N., Haas, C.A., Rauch, U., Merten, T., Fassler, R., Frotscher, M., and Deller, T. (2000) The chondroitin sulphate proteoglycan brevican is upregulated by astrocytes after entorhinal cortex lesions in adult rats. *Eur. J. Neurosci.* 12:2547–2558.

Vanek, P., Thallmair, M., Schwab, M.E., and Kapfhammer, J.P. (1998) Increased lesion induced sprouting of corticospinal fibers in the myelin-free rat spinal cord. *Eur. J. Neurosci.* 10:45–56.

Varela-Echavarria, A., Tucker, A., Puschel, A.W., and Guthrie, S. (1997) Motor axon subpopulations respond differentially to the chemorepellents netrin-1 and semaphorin D. *Neuron* 18:193–207.

Wang, K.C., Koprivica, V., Kim, J.A., Sivasankaran, R., Guo, Y., Neve, R.L., and He, Z. (2002) Oligodendrocyte-myelin glycoprotein is a Nogo receptor ligand that inhibits neurite outgrowth. *Nature* 417:941–944.

Yamada, H., Fredette, B., Shitara, K., Hagihara, K., Miura, R., Ranscht, B., Stallcup, W.B., and Yamaguchi, Y. (1997) The brain chondroitin sulfate proteoglycan brevican associates with astrocytes ensheathing cerebellar glomeruli and inhibits neurite outgrowth from granule neurons. *J. Neurosci.* 17:7784–7795.

Z'Graggen, W.J., Metz, G.A.S., Kartje, G.L., Thallmair, M., and Schwab, M.E. (1998) Functional recovery and enhanced corticofugal plasticity after unilateral pyramidal tract lesion and blockade of myelin-associated neurite growth inhibitors in adult rats. *J. Neurosci.* 15:4744–4757.

38 Transplantation of myelin-forming cells

WILLIAM F. BLAKEMORE AND ROBIN J.M. FRANKLIN

Glial cell transplantation, in the form of peripheral nerve grafting, was carried out by Santiago Ramon y Cajal and Francisco Tello in the early twentieth century. However, it was the introduction of glial cell culture techniques, and the consequent increase in our understanding of glial cell lineages, that brought a new dimension to this experimental approach, which has seen considerable expansion in recent years. All glial cell types have been transplanted into a wide range of recipient environments in developing, adult, and pathological central nervous system (CNS). The purpose of these studies is equally broad. Sometimes glial cell transplantation studies have been undertaken to address a specific biological question; on other occasions, the technique has been used with a direct therapeutic purpose in mind. Although many areas of glial cell biology and CNS pathology (including traumatic injury and neurodegeneration) employ this approach, this chapter will focus on transplantation of myelin-forming cells (primarily oligodendrocyte lineage cells and Schwann cells) in the context of *myelination* and *remyelination* in the CNS, and will mainly consider astrocyte transplantation, where it has a bearing on these two processes. The chapter is divided into two sections. The first will explore methodological and conceptual issues that are important when designing and interpreting glial cell transplantation studies. The second will address issues concerned with the potential therapeutic use of glial cell transplantation in situations where remyelination failure leads to prolonged loss of function.

METHODOLOGICAL ASPECTS OF GLIAL CELL TRANSPLANTATION

The Transplanted Cells

Oligodendrocytes and Schwann cells are the myelin-forming (myelinogenic) cells of the central and peripheral nervous systems, respectively and both are able to form myelin sheaths following transplantation into the CNS. A third cell type, the olfactory ensheathing cell (OEC), although not normally myelinogenic when associated with the small-diameter axons of the olfactory system, assume a myelinating phenotype similar to that of a Schwann cell when transplanted into tissue containing large-diameter demyelinated axons.

Oligodendrocyte lineage cells

Although intuitively one might imagine that the most appropriate cell to transplant in order to achieve oligodendrocyte remyelination would be a mature oligodendrocyte, this cell has a very poor myelinogenic capacity following transplantation, especially if it has already formed a complement of myelin internodes. Oligodendrocyte precursor cells (OPCs), on the other hand, show a much greater propensity for myelination following transplantation that increases the further back in the lineage one precedes while still remaining committed to oligodendrocyte differentiation. The increasing range of phenotypes of the oligodendrocyte lineage available for transplantation is a product of the unraveling of neural cell lineages that has occurred over the past decade or so. Similarly, advances in cell culture techniques for obtaining large numbers of relatively pure populations of different stages of the lineage have enabled increasingly precise questions to be addressed by transplantation.

In early glial cell transplantation studies, donor cells were provided in the form of tissue fragments or suspensions of acutely dissociated tissue (Fig. 38.1). The precise composition of these grafts was unclear, and this limited the interpretation of the transplant experiments to the fact that the graft contained some cell that would generate myelin sheaths. Growing cells in tissue culture enables a more precise characterization of the transplant and provides the experimenter with control over the composition of the transplant by using techniques such as fluorescence-activated cell (FAC) sorting, immunopanning, and immunocytolysis. Large

See the list of abbreviations at the end of the chapter.

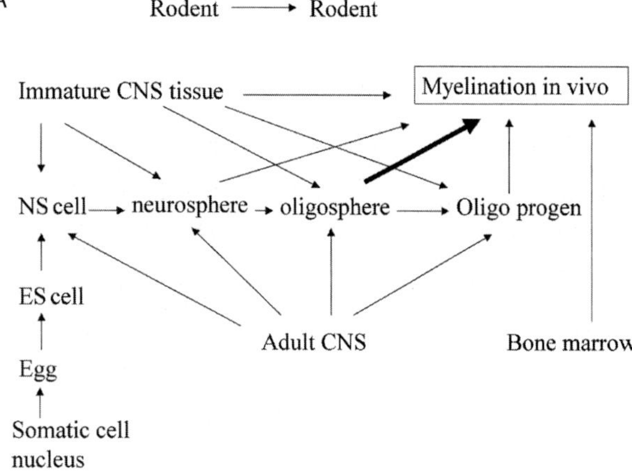

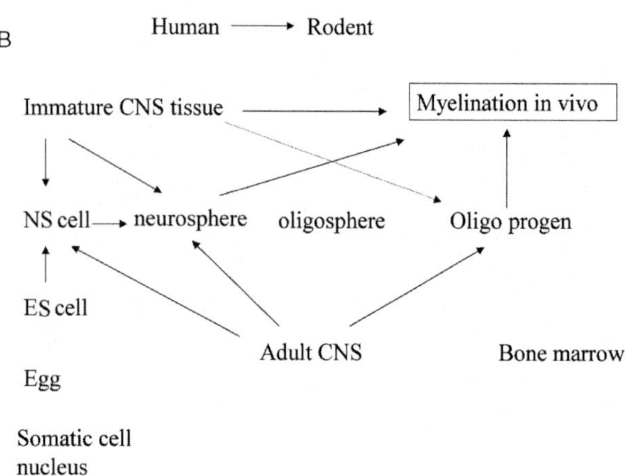

FIGURE 38.1 The relationship between the starting material and the type of cell preparation from which oligodendrocyte myelination has been achieved in rodents following transplantation of rodent cells (*A*) or human cells (*B*). Using rodent cells, the most extensive myelination is achieved following the introduction of oligosphere preparations. At present, it is not possible to produce this preparation with human cells. CNS: central nervous system; ES: embryonic stem cell; NS: neural stem cell; oligo progen: oligodendrocyte progenitor cells.

numbers of A2B5+ precursor cells can be obtained *in vitro* by growing neonatal CNS cultures in the presence of both platelet-derived growth factor (PDGF) and fibroblast growth factor-2 (FGF-2) or PDGF and neurotrophin-3 (NT3) following the selection of the A2B5+ population. Another application of growth factors for obtaining large numbers of precursors has been the use of FGF and epidermal growth factor (EGF) or media conditioned by cell lines that produce various growth factors to generate spheres of precursor cells that are either pluripotential (*neurospheres*) (Hammang et al., 1997) or committed to the oligodendrocyte lineage (*oligospheres*) (Avellana-Adalid et al., 1996). Oligodendrocytes can be generated from adult and neonatal neural stem cells, from embryonic stem (ES) cells (Brustle et al., 1999), and from stem cells present in nonneural tissue in adult animals (Bonilla et al., 2002). Although these techniques have been successfully used in rodents and dogs, the neuro- and oligosphere approaches have not yet been able to yield large numbers of oligodendrocyte lineage cells from human tissue.

An alternative source of large numbers of purified populations of oligodendrocyte lineage cells is cell lines. These can be created by the introduction of immortalizing oncogenes such as simian virus 40 (SV40) large T, the temperature-sensitive mutant of which is especially useful since the gene product, active at 32°C, is inactivated at the normal body temperature of the recipient host (Trotter et al., 1993). Cell lines may also arise spontaneously, such as the widely used CG4 line. This cell line most closely follows the behavior of primary oligodendrocyte precursor cells of the rat CNS. Although cell lines provide a user-friendly source of large numbers of defined phenotypes that are free of contaminants, their behavior is unlikely to mimic precisely that of the primary cell.

Schwann cells

Schwann cells can be obtained relatively easily from neonatal and adult peripheral nerve of most species, including humans, and expanded in tissue culture by exposure to mitogens such as neuregulin. The principal contaminants in primary cultures are cells of the connective tissue component of peripheral nerve, although techniques exist for reducing their presence, such as immunocytolysis using anti-thy-1 antibodies and complement or by positive selection using p75 antibodies. Cell lines of both Schwann cells and Schwann cell precursors have also been transplanted into areas of CNS demyelination (Jung et al., 1994; Lobsiger et al., 2001).

Olfactory ensheathing cells

Olfactory ensheathing cells (OECs) produce myelin sheaths that are anatomically indistinguishable from those made by Schwann cells and appear to use similar regulatory mechanisms (Franklin, 2003). However, OECs are slighter harder to culture because of the relative inaccessibility of the peripheral olfactory system compared to peripheral nerve. Nevertheless, OECs have been obtained from the lamina propria of the olfactory mucosa, the olfactory nerve, and the nerve fiber layer of the olfactory bulb, and their remyelination potential has been demonstrated for rat-, dog-, and human-derived cells (Franklin, 2003). Cells are transplanted either as unpurified olfactory bulb preparations, as cells selected according to distinctive antigenic markers, or as clonal cell lines, a variety of approaches that confounds the identification and interpretation of OEC behavior following transplantation.

Tracking the Fate of Transplanted Cells and Distinguishing Them from Host Cell

Various strategies have been used to distinguish transplanted cells from host cells; nearly all impose limitations on the types of studies that can be undertaken. These strategies consist either of direct identification of individual cells in order to study migration and integration into normal tissue or adopting an experimental approach that allows identification of the consequence of transplantation in such a manner that the observed results occur only in association with transplantation. Transplanted cells can be labeled *in vitro* prior to transplantation (exogenous labeling) using vital dyes such as fast-blue and bisbenzimide (Hoechst dyes 33258 and 33342) or fluorochrome-conjugated lectins for subsequent identification using fluorescence microscopy. Recent advances have been made in labeling cells with superparamagnetic iron oxide, which allows cells to be detected by magnetic resonance imaging (MRI) (Bulte et al., 1999; Franklin et al., 1999). These labels, like tritiated thymidine and BrdU, suffer the disadvantage of dilution by repeated division of cells, but more important, some dyes, such as the Hoechst dyes 33258 and 33342, are readily taken up by host cells even after careful pretransplantation washing of cells (Iwashita et al., 2000a). In addition to direct labeling of host cells at the time of implantation, there can be transfer to host cells, especially macrophages, when cells die. It has been shown that transfer of label is not a problem with tritiated thymidine and BrdU.

A strategy that overcomes the dilution and transfer problems associated with *in vitro* labeling of transplanted cells is the use of genetic markers (endogenous labels). This may take the form of introduced genes such as that for green fluorescent protein (GFP) or bacterial *Lac-Z*, or may use inherent genetic mismatches between the grafted cells and host cells. Such systems are male to female transplantation using repeat sequences on the Y chromosome as the marker and the use of cross-species transplantation involving species-specific markers to identify the transplanted cells, or, when examining oligodendrocyte differentiation, the introduction of cells from normal animals into the myelin mutants. These mutant animals include the myelin basic protein (MBP)-deficient *shiverer* mouse and the various myelin proteolipid protein (PLP) mutants: the myelin-deficient rat, the *jimpy* mouse, and the *shaking* pup. All the PLP mutants show such severe hypomyelination that any myelin formation observed following transplantation can be related to transplanted cells (Fig. 38.2). Immunostaining for PLP can, if necessary, be used to distinguish host PLP-deficient myelin from the PLP-positive myelin produced by transplanted cells. Myelin basic protein–positive normal myelin is easily recognized in the *shiverer* mouse either by immunocytochemistry or by electron microscopy. The transgenic approach has and will result in the availability of further hypomyelinated animals that can be used as transplant recipients. An example is the myelin-associated glycoprotein (MAG) and *Fyn* knockout mouse. These animals have a normal life span, and oligodendrocyte-axon interactions established by transplant-derived cells can be demonstrated by MAG immunohistochenistry (Ader et al., 2001), although the presence of MAG does not always imply myelin sheath formation (Targett et al., 1996).

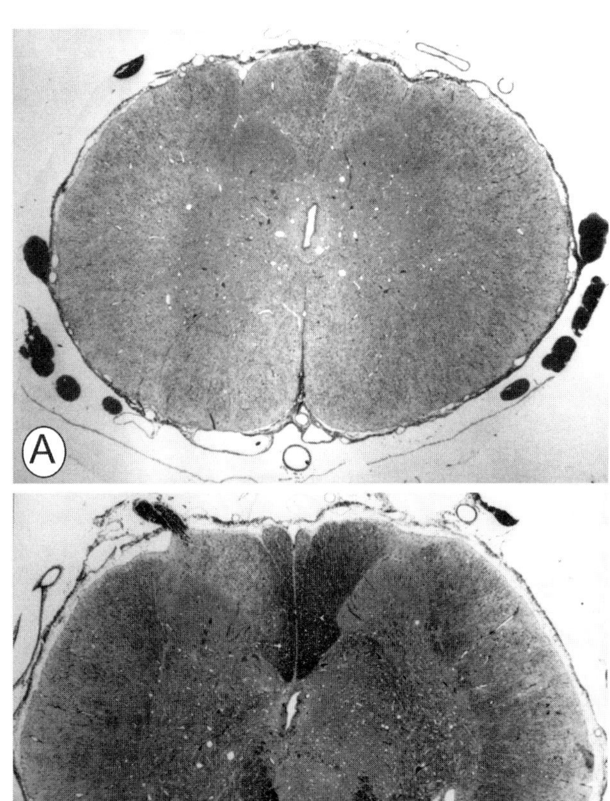

FIGURE 38.2 Spinal cord segments from a 9-week-old *shaking* pup transplanted at 1 week of age with a fetal glial cell suspension derived from an embryonic day 45 (E45) canine fetal brain. *A*. Several segments away from the transplant site, the white matter has almost no perceptible myelin. *B*. At the transplant site, the dorsal and ventral columns are totally myelinated by transplanted cells, with myelination also of the deep tracts of the right lateral column. Bar = 1 mm. (We are grateful for Ian Duncan for supplying this figure.)

An alternative strategy to the use of markers to identify transplanted cells that can be adopted in adult animals is to induce demyelination and then remove the repair capacity of the tissue into which cells are to be introduced. Abolishing the repair capacity of tissue can be achieved by X-irradiating tissue. A single dose of 40 Gy of X-irradiation depletes rat tissue of its endogenous oligodendrocyte progenitor cell (OPC) population (Hinks et al., 2001). Thus, when demyelinating lesions are made in tissue exposed to 40 Gy of X-irradiation, there is no remyelination. The nonrepairing nature of demyelinating lesions made in the middle of a 4-cm-long length of X-irradiated tissue can be rigorously tested by showing that the injection of cell preparations shown to recruit cells in normal animals fails to recruit cells from the host when injected into X-irradiated lesions. Furthermore, there is a direct correlation between the nature of the repair observed and the composition of the cells introduced into this environment, and when xenogeneic cells are injected, remyelination is seen only when animals receive immunosuppression. The X-irradiated ethidium bromide (X-EB) lesion therefore provides an ideal system for assessing the differentiation potential of cell preparations without the need to resort to the use of cell markers to identify transplanted cells (Groves et al., 1993; Franklin et al., 1995; Akiyama et al., 2001; Sasaki et al., 2001) (Fig. 38.3).

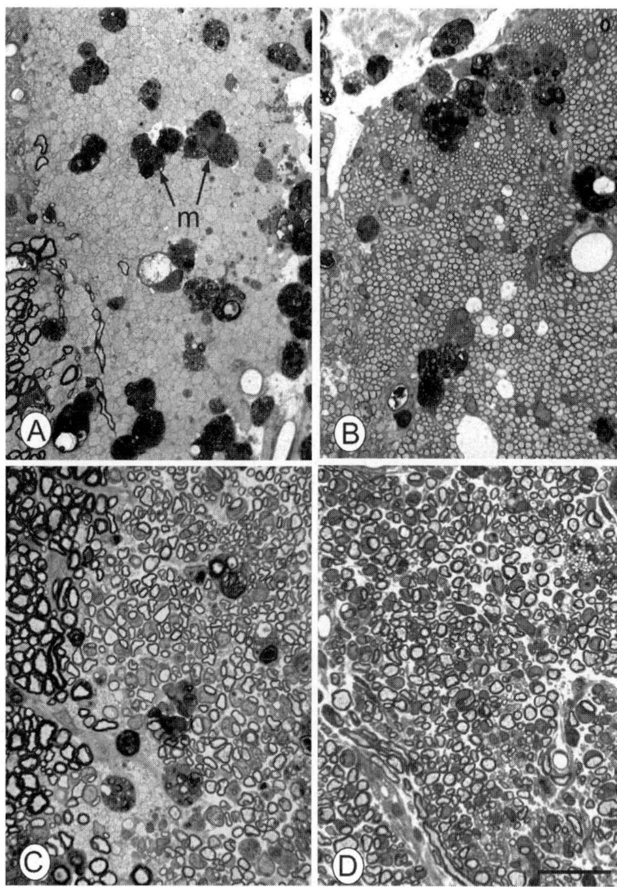

FIGURE 38.3 Injections of ethidium bromide into white matter results in the death of oligodendrocytes, astrocytes, and oligodendrocyte progenitor cells. When injected into tissue exposed to 40 Gy of X-irradiation, endogenous remyelination is totally abolished, provided that a long length (usually 4 cm) of spinal cord in exposed to X-irradiation. In this lesion, the remyelinating potential of transplanted cells can be rapidly evaluated without the need to use identification markers for the transplanted cells. One-micron toluidine blue–stained resin sections provide a useful way of identifying and distinguishing between oligodendrocyte and Schwann cell remyelination and assessing the extent of remyelination. The appearance of X-irradiated ethidium bromide lesions without transplantation (*A*) and 4 weeks following the injection of neonatal rat oligodendrocyte precursors (*B*), neonatal rat Schwann cells (*C*) and neonatal olfactory ensheathing cells (OEC) purified by immunopanning with p75 antibodies and transplanted together with cultured meningeal cells (70% OEC/30% meingeal cells) 4 weeks previously (*D*) (see Lakatos et al., 2002). In *A*. there is no remyelination, and the demyelinated axons are clumped together in a glial-free environment. The only cells present are myelin debris–filled macrophages (*m*). In *B*. the demyelinated axons are remyelinated by oligodendrocytes. This form of remyelination can be distinguished from normal central nervous system myelination because the myelin sheaths that surround the axons are thinner than normal. In *C*. the demyelinated axons are remyelinated by Schwann cells. This form of myelination can be distinguished from oligodendrocyte myelination because the axons are not as closely packed, and often a nucleus can be detected next to the myelin sheath. Some demyelinated axons are still present. In *D*. the demyelinated axons are remyelinated by OECs. The remyelination of these cells is indistinguishable from Schwann cell remyelination. Bar = 40 μm.

Areas of the CNS that are not normally myelinated, such as the retina, also provide a situation where the presence of myelination following transplantation can be related to transplant derived cells (Huang et al., 1991; Laeng et al., 1996; Setzu et al., 2004) (Fig. 38.4).

Transplantation provides a powerful way of studying the migration of glial cells, a prime example being its use to demonstrate the role of FGF in OPC migration following transplantation of wild-type OPCs and those expressing a dominant negative FGF receptor (Osterhout et al., 1997). There are many other examples, but here we consider a number of methodological issues. Primarily, it is very important to take account of the extent of passive spread of cells that occurs as a result of simply injecting a cell suspension. Even when small volumes of cells are injected into white matter, cells can be spread over a distance of 2–3 mm, the exact distance being determined by the speed of injection. When large volumes are introduced, the spread will be greater. Considerable distribution of cells can be expected when cells are introduced into the cerebrospinal fluid (CSF) compartments. Because of this passive spread, claims of cell migration can be substantiated only if a comparison is be made between the distribution of cells at two different times following injection. It is also useful to mark the injection point by, for example, mixing charcoal with the injected cell suspension. A further point that has to be considered when reporting experiments that result in the presence of cells

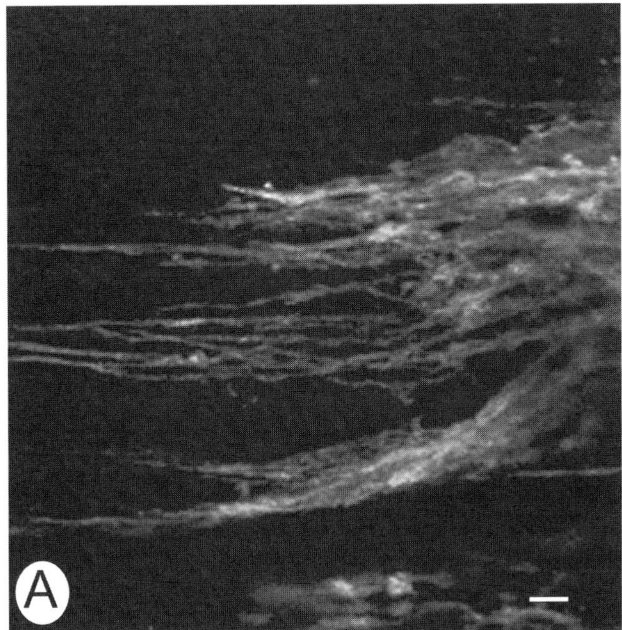

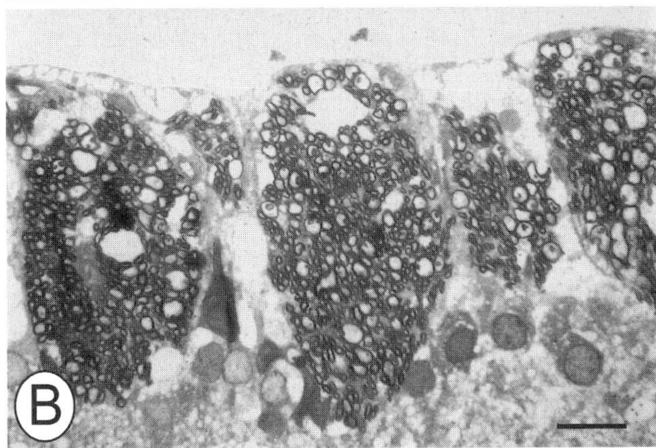

FIGURE 38.4 The retina is not normally myelinated and thus provides a suitable site at which to examining the remyelinating potential of cells in an environment that contains astrocytes. These figures show myelination in the adult retina after injection of a suspension of neonatal primary oligodendrocyte progenitors into the adult rat retina. *A*. Flat-mounted retina stained with anti-myelin basic protein antibodies after 4 weeks and *B*. bundles of myelinated retinal ganglion cell axons as visualized in resin sections 8 weeks after transplantation. Bar = 15 μm (see Setzu et al., 2004).

at some distance from their point of implantation is that it may not be possible to distinguish between an increased distribution of cells that is a consequence of proliferation and survival and that which is dependent on migration of individual transplanted cells. This is not to say that one cannot examine whether some cells have migratory potential while others do not. However, when this has been done, a close correlation has been found between the mitotic potential of the cells introduced and the distribution over which the progeny of the transplanted cells are dispersed. Thus, when neonatal OPCs were transplanted into OPC-depleted adult spinal cord, the cells progressively colonized the OPC-depleted tissue as an expanding population of cells rather than as widely dispersed single migrating cells (Blakemore et al., 2002). Unless the distinction between migration and proliferation is clearly established, it is generally better to report finding in terms of colonization by, rather than as a migration of, transplanted cells.

Recipient Environments

The recipient environment plays a significant role in determining the outcome of transplantation experiments because it not only determines whether cells can survive but also influences their differentiation. During development and in pathological tissue, transplanted cells are introduced into an environment in which cell generation is occurring in order to either create new tissue or repair lost tissue. There are therefore opportunities for the transplanted cells to survive and integrate. However, in normal mature tissue, cell numbers are stable and strictly controlled; therefore, the introduced cells will be supernumerary and surplus to requirement.

Developing central nervous system

In rodents most CNS axons are myelinated during the first 2 weeks of life; therefore, the CNS of neonatal animals provides an ideal environment in which to assess the myelinogenic potential of transplanted cells. The transplanted cells will be exposed to an environment containing signals involved in oligodendrogliogenesis. Cells can be transplanted into the CNS of animals either *in utero* or in the first few days of life. Studies can be undertaken either in the myelin mutants or in normal animals, provided that cell markers are used. When cells capable of generating oligodendrocytes are introduced into the developing CNS, extensive colonization and myelin sheath formation are generally observed. The distribution and amount of myelin produced can be related to the types of cells transplanted. The experiments of Warrington and coworkers used the neonatal *shiverer* mouse to demonstrate that the extent of myelin produced following transplantation could be directly related to the *in vitro* mitotic and migratory potential of the introduced cells (Warrington et al., 1993). Following introduction of cells into the ventricles or into the cisterna magna, a very extensive distribution of transplant derived myelination can occur (Learish et al., 1999; Mitome et al., 2001).

Normal adult tissue

The normal adult CNS is not a receptive environment for transplanted oligodendrocytes or their progenitors, neither of which survive well. This is because the normal complement of these cells in adults is regulated by the availability of axons of an appropriate diameter for myelination and by survival factors. Addition of new cells by transplantation exceeds the capacity of the tissue to permit their survival. Although new oligodendrocytes may be required to myelinate new axons that arise through plasticity and neurogenesis in the adult CNS, there is little evidence that oligodendrocytes turn over; thus, the possibility of establishing transplant derived oligodendrocytes will be minimal. In the normal adult CNS, OPCs turn over, yet the number of these cells remains constant and is regulated by the availability of survival factors such as PDGF (van Heyningen et al., 2001). When OPCs are injected into normal white matter, these cells fail to survive, and there is no evidence of cell migration such as has been extensively documented following their introduction into neonatal and embryonic CNS. This is because the number of OPCs that the availability of survival factor will allow is already accounted for by endogenous cells. Only if the endogenous cells are depleted (by, for example, X-irradiation) or if the availability of survival factors increases (as in pathology) will the tissue support transplanted OPCs. Thus, if endogenous OPCs are removed by exposing tissue to 40 Gy of X-irradiation, then transplanted OPCs will repopulate the depleted tissue (Franklin et al., 1996; Blakemore et al., 2002). The repopulation restores OPC numbers to those approaching the normal density, indicating that the implanted cells are strongly influenced by the factors that control the number and distribution of endogenous cells. The adult retina is an unusual adult tissue because, in contrast to other areas of the CNS where axons are myelinated, it will support transplanted OPCs without the need to deplete endogenous cells or increase the availability of survival factor (Setzu et al., 2004).

Embryo-derived cells behave differently from neonatal OPCs when introduced into the adult CNS in that following the introduction of neurospheres (Svendsen et al., 1997), embryonic CNS (Isacson et al., 1995), or glial restricted precursor (GRP) cells (Herrera et al., 2001) into normal tissue, cells have been observed to migrate considerable distances and differentiate into astrocytes. Extensive migration and differentiation of cells into oligodendrocytes has been reported following the introduction of certain cell lines (Yandava et al., 1999; Espinosa de los Monteros et al., 2001). Although the cell lines used have been shown capable of differentiating into oligodendrocytes *in vitro* and *in vivo*, it is still unclear how such results relate to the behavior of normal cells.

Pathological environments

The problem of survival presented by normal adult tissue does not arise in acute pathological states, since there is generally an increase in the availability of survival factors associated with the inflammatory response. This favorable situation for the survival of transplanted oligodendrocyte lineage cells may even be augmented by a deficiency of endogenous cells that would otherwise be competing for survival factors. This situation can arise to a greater or lesser degree in animals that show defective myelination due to genetic defects (myelin mutants) during development. The myelin mutants generally carry a defective gene encoding for one of the major myelin proteins, which results in a CNS containing axons that are either hypomyelinated (MBP mutants; oligodendrocytes are present but some axons are not myelinated, while other axons are enclosed by oligodendrocyte processes but normal myelin sheaths are not formed) or are largely unmyelinated (PLP mutants; oligodendrocytes are largely absent because they die in association with expression of myelin proteins). The first of these mutants to be used was the *shiverer* mouse, which contains a deletion in the MBP gene (Gumpel et al., 1983). Subsequently, a number of other mutants (PLP mutants), the *jimpy* mouse (Lachapelle et al., 1994), the myelin-deficient rat (Duncan et al., 1988), and the *shaking* pup (Archer et al., 1997), have been used that all share defects in the X-linked PLP gene and therefore resemble the human Pelizaeus-Merzbacher disease. These mutants are generally short-lived, so most experiments have involved transplantation into a neonatal or immature CNS and the transplanted cells have short survival times. However, with careful management some mutants, such as the *shaking* pup and Long Evans *shaker* rat, can survive into adulthood. Together with longer-lived mutants such as the *taiep* rat, these animals provide opportunities to examine the interactions between transplanted cells and long-term unmyelinated or demyelinated axons, which are usually surrounded by a dense network of hypertrophied astrocyte processes and thereby resemble the environment of the chronic demyelinated plaques of multiple sclerosis (MS). The number of studies using these mature animals is limited, and those that have been undertaken indicate that the extent of myelination that can be achieved is poor (Zhang et al., 2003; W.F. Blakemore, unpublished observations).

A second major recipient environment for transplantation is that provided by the gliotoxin models of demyelination. These models involve inducing foci of demyelination in the adult CNS by direct injection of chemicals such as lysolecithin or EB that are injurious to oligodendrocytes. The areas of demyelination created by gliotoxin injection undergo spontaneous remyelination, although this can be a slow process taking months in old animals. Thus, when glia are transplanted into such lesions, they compete with recruited host cells in repairing the lesion. In this situation, transplantation can be used to modify the glial composition of lesion repair, thereby providing insights into the roles and interactions of astrocytes, Schwann cells, and oligodendrocyte lineage cells during CNS remyelination (Franklin and Blakemore, 1999). The ability of transplanted neonatal cells to outcompete the endogenous repair response has been demonstrated (Blakemore et al., 2000, 2002) and was used to show the long-term survival of transplant-mediated remyelination in adult animals (O'Leary and Blakemore, 1997). As discussed in an earlier section, gliotoxin-induced lesions may be modified (using 40 Gy of X-irradiation) to prevent repopulation of the lesion by host cells.

Given the availability of immune-mediated models of demyelination such as experimental allergic encephalomyelitis (EAE) that more closely resemble MS, a major target disease for potential transplant-based therapy, it is somewhat surprising how infrequently EAE has been used as a recipient environment for transplantation studies. This is partly because the anatomical location of lesions is not always apparent, making direct transplantation difficult. Nevertheless, several studies have employed EAE lesions as a recipient environment and have found that transplanted cells integrate into areas of damage but not into normal tissue (Tourbah et al., 1997; Ben-Hur et al., 2003).

GLIAL CELL TRANSPLANTATION AS A THERAPEUTIC STRATEGY FOR REMYELINATION

Glial cell transplantation has been advocated as a therapy for chronic demyelinating diseases. However, few studies suggest that this would lead to functional recovery. Failure to obtain these behavioral data is largely a consequence of an absence of models in which such data could be obtained. The ideal model should have sufficient persistent myelin loss to show chronic functional impairment. Thus, although areas of acute demyelination and the myelin-deficient (MD) rat can be used to show transplant-mediated myelination of axons by oligodendrocytes, Schwann cells, and olfactory glia results in establishment of conduction properties associated with myelinated axons (Utzschneider et al., 1994; Honmou et al., 1996; Imaizumi et al., 1998). Such findings alone do not indicate that transplant-mediated remyelination will result in restoration of function lost as a consequence of demyelination. That successful remyelination can restore function lost through demyelination has been evaluated in the rat using focal demyelinating lesions of the corticospinal tract (Jeffery and Blakemore, 1997). In this model, demyelinating lesions were made in the cervical region of the spinal cord, and hind foot placement was evaluated as the animals crossed a narrow beam. Lesions were made in X-irradiated and normal tissue, and the functional consequences of remyelination and failure of remyelination were compared. Both groups lost function, as indicated by an increase in foot placement errors, and while the remyelinated animals showed a return to normal scores the X-irradiated animals showed incomplete recovery, a result indicating that remyelination was associated with functional recovery. In subsequent experiments, it was shown that transplantation of oligodendrocyte progenitor–rich cultures resulted in restoration of function in both non-X-irradiated and X-irradiated animals (Jeffery et al., 1999).

A degree of functional improvement has been reported following the transplantation of neural precursors into newborn *shiverer* mice (Yandava et al., 1999). However, a subsequent study in which extensive myelination was achieved following introduction of a neurosphere preparation recorded no obvious functional improvement (Mitome et al., 2001). The life span of *twitcher* mice (which have a lysosomal storage disease involving degeneration of oligodendrocytes) was increased following bone marrow and embryonic neural tissue transplantation to a greater degree than in those that just received bone marrow transplantation (Huppes et al., 1992). Transplant-derived oligodendrocytes were demonstrated, but it is likely that it was the introduction of other enzyme-secreting cells, rather than the establishment of oligodendrocytes, that caused the increased survival.

Which Cell Type Should Be Transplanted?

Oligodendrocyte precursors

Although myelination can result from transplantation of cells at an earlier (multipotent neural precursors) or later stage of differentiation (A2B5-expanded oligodendrocyte progenitors), the greatest extent of myelin formation follows the introduction of oligodendrocyte lineage–committed glial progenitors at the preoligodendrocyte progenitor stage (Zhang et al., 1998; Keirstead et al., 1999; Vitry et al., 2001) (Fig. 38.1). These cells are expanded *in vitro* as floating spheres (oligospheres) either using B104-conditioned medium or under the influence of FGF-2. They represent pre-oligodendrocyte progenitors, expressing polysialylated neural cell adhesion molecule (PSA-NCAM), platelet-derived growth factor receptor alpha (PDGFRα), and nestin, with low numbers of cells expressing GD3 or A2B5. When propagated in B104-conditioned medium, the number of cells expressing GD3 increases (Vitry et al., 2001). All cells become A2B5 positive on leaving the spheres, and removal of B104 or FGF2 results in oligodendrocyte or astrocyte differentiation, depending on whether cells are maintained in a low- or high-serum medium. A recent study compared the behavior of PSA-

NCAM- and GD3-expressing cells following transplantation into the neonatal mouse brain and found that cells at the earlier stage formed neurons, showed greater migration ability, and were able to integrate into the rostral migratory stream, unlike cells at the later stage of development (Vitry et al., 2001). This study also noted that the PSA-NCAM cells tended to show chain migration, while the GD3 cells migrated as individual cells.

Multipotent neural precursors

Although neural stem cells can generate myelinating oligodendrocytes (Hammang et al., 1997; Yandava et al., 1999; Brustle et al., 1999) when introduced into the developing CNS, a need for commitment to the oligodendrocyte lineage becomes more apparent when cells are introduced into acute demyelinating lesions in adult animals. Cell preparations that produce neurons, astrocytes, and some oligodendrocytes *in vitro* and form myelin when introduced into the developing CNS fail to generate oligodendrocytes when introduced into areas of acute demyelination (Smith and Blakemore, 2000) or spinal damage (Cao et al., 2001). The behavior of these cells in noninflammatory situations is still incompletely understood, but there are indications that there can be progressive myelination following their introduction into the immature CNS of the long-lived myelin mutants (Yandava et al., 1999; Ader et al., 2001; Mitome et al., 2001).

Schwann cells

Demyelinated CNS can be myelinated by transplanted Schwann cells or OECs, which restores function lost as a consequence of demyelination. Cross-species transplantation is possible, which allows assessment of the consequences of cryopreservation (Kohama et al., 2001), immortalization (Baron-Van Evercooren et al., 1992), and preparative procedures on the myelinating efficiency of cells (Avellana-Adalid et al., 1998; Brierley et al., 2001; Lakatos et al., 2002). The extent of remyelination achieved is related to the number of cells introduced (Iwashita and Blakemore, 2000). There is some controversy concerning the ability of transplanted Schwann cells to survive long-term when implanted into normal tissue (Brook et al., 1993; Raisman et al., 1993; Li and Raisman, 1997), and although some studies indicate that Schwann cells are attracted to areas of demyelination (Baron-Van Evercooren et al., 1992, 1993, 1996), others fail to confirm this (Iwashita et al., 2000b). Schwann cell transplant–mediated myelination is most successful in demyelinating lesions where the endogenous remyelinating cells would normally be Schwann cells (Franklin and Blakemore, 1993). These are demyelinating lesions, like those produced by EB, in which astrocytes are lost throughout the area of demyelination. The close association between astrocyte loss and Schwann cell remyelination (Shields et al., 2000), and the demonstration in transplantation experiments that the presence or reconstruction of an astrocyte environment by the cotransplantation of astrocytes, limits Schwann cell remyelination of demyelinated axons, indicate that astrocytes and Schwann cells are mutually exclusive cells.

Until recently, it was proposed that the presence of astrocytes inhibited Schwann cells originating from peripheral nerves or present with a transplanted cell suspension from accessing demyelinated CNS axons (Franklin and Blakemore, 1993). However, it is now apparent from both *in vitro* and *in vivo* studies that Schwann cells can also be generated from neural precursors. *In vitro*, cloned CNS neural precursors can be shown to give rise to both oligodendrocytes and Schwann cells (Mujtaba et al., 1998). Transplantation studies using the X-irradiated EB lesion have revealed that the introduction of glial-restricted CNS precursors results in both Schwann cell and oligodendrocyte remyelination (Keirstead et al., 1999), while introduction of cloned human neural precursors isolated from the adult human brain resulted in predominantly Schwann cell remyelination (Akiyama et al., 2001). Thus, rather than astrocytes acting as barrier that prevents differentiated Schwann cells from associating with demyelinated CNS axons, their presence or absence may determine the differentiation fate of CNS precursors that enter areas of demyelination. In the presence of astrocytes they differentiate into oligodendrocytes, while in their absence they come under the influence of factors that induce Schwann cell differentiation. Whatever the precise nature of the relationship between Schwann cells and astrocytes, whether astrocytes prevent Schwann cell differentiation from precursors or prevent their entry from peripheral sources, it is unlikely that Schwann cell remyelination will be extensive following the introduction of either Schwann cells or CNS precursors into astrocyte-containing areas of demyelination.

Olfactory ensheathing cells

Transplanted OECs are also capable of remyelinating demyelinated CNS axons, producing a peripheral-type myelin sheath ultrastructurally indistinguishable from and generated using regulatory mechanisms similar to those of Schwann cells (Franklin, 2003). Moreover, OEC-mediated remyelination leads to functional recovery (Imaizumi et al., 1998). Their remyelinating capacity has been demonstrated using cells from human, porcine, and canine tissue, and this property is retained following cryopreservation. The remyelinating properties of OECs are very similar to those of Schwann cells. In tissue culture they have greater astrocyte compatibility than Schwann cells (Lakatos et al., 2000), but whether this is true in the context of transplant-mediated remyelination remains to be firmly established.

Is It Possible to Predict the Outcome?

Multiple sclerosis is characterized by multiple areas of demyelination with axons set within an astrocytic environment, while in the leukodystrophies there is widespread loss of myelin throughout the neuraxis. Thus, if extensive remyelination, a requirement for restoration of function, is to be achieved, implanted cells will have to colonize widely if sufficient numbers of axons are to be remyelinated. To date, most transplantation studies have been conducted either in developing animals or using models of acute demyelination in which the area available for myelination by the transplanted cells was small (approximately 1–2 mm^3). Therefore, at present, it is very difficult to predict the outcome of introducing large numbers of oligodendrocyte progenitors into the human brain in the context of chronically demyelinated brain and large numbers of disseminated large areas of demyelination.

As discussed earlier, it is clear from our own work and that of others that OPCs behave very differently when introduced into the adult CNS compared to the developing CNS—a major factor being the presence of OPCs within the tissue. Therefore, if these cells are to be used, they will have to be injected into areas of demyelination. However, it has recently become apparent that many areas of chronic demyelination contain OPCs and even premyelinating oligodendrocytes (Chang et al., 2002). Such observations suggest that the establishment of further OPCs may not be possible and perhaps, more important, the environment may not support remyelination. The key to successful implementation of transplantation-based remyelination for chronic lesions therefore lies in obtaining a clearer understanding of why remyelination fails and a knowledge of the basic biological principles that underlie the remyelinating process so that it can be reactivated. On the other hand, acute lesions would be amenable to transplantation, since experimental studies indicate that in such lesions transplanted neonatal OPC have a considerable therapeutic advantage over endogenous cells and that transplanted cells can be established in the face of autoimmune-induced demyelination. The key to undertaking such therapy therefore will be (*1*) the ability to obtain large numbers of human OPCs for transplantation, (*2*) a greater understanding of whether the ongoing disease process would result in destruction of the transplanted cells and their progeny, and (*3*) an appreciation of how closely the transplanted cells would have to be tissue matched to the host to avoid rejection.

ABBREVIATIONS

A2B5	antibody epitope expressed on oligodendrocyte progenitors and neurons
B104	neuroblastoma cell line
CNS	central nervous system
CSF	cerebrospinal fluid
CG4	a spontaneously occurring oligoden drocyte progenitor cell line
EAE	experimental allergic encephalomyelitis
EB	ethidium bromide
EGF	epidermal growth factor
ES	embryonic stem cells
FAC	fluorescence-activated cell sorter
FGF	fibroblast growth factor
Fyn	a Src family protein kinase
GD3	a ganglioside
GFP	green fluorescent protein
GRP	glial-restricted precursor
Lac-Z	gene for bacterial β-galactosidase
MAG	myelin-associated glycoprotein
MBP	myelin basic protein
MD	myelin-deficient
MRI	magnetic resonance imaging
MS	multiple sclerosis
NT3	neurotrophin-3
OEC	olfactory ensheathing cell
OPC	oligodendrocyte progenitor cell
p75	low-affinity neurotrophin receptor
PDGF	platelet-derived growth factor
PDGFRα	platelet-derived growth factor receptor alpha
PLP	myelin proteolipid protein
PSA-NCAM	polysialylated neural cell adhesion molecule
SV40	simian virus 40
T	transforming protein
Thy-1	a glycoprotein

REFERENCES

Ader, M., Schachner, M., and Bartsch, U. (2001) Transplantation of neural precursor cells into the dysmyelinated CNS mutant mice deficient in the myelin-associated glycoprotein and Fyn trosine kinase. *Eur. J. Neurosci.* 14:561–566.

Akiyama, Y., Honmou, O., Kato, T., Uede, T., Hashi, K., and Kocsis, J.D. (2001) Transplantation of clonal neural precursor cells derived from adult human brain establishes functional peripheral myelin in the rat spinal cord. *Exp. Neurol.* 167:27–39.

Archer, D.R., Cuddon, P.A., Lipsitz, D., and Duncan, I.D. (1997) Myelination of the canine central nervous system by glial cell transplantation: a model for repair of human myelin disease. *Nat. Med.* 3:54–59.

Avellana-Adalid, V., Bachelin, C., Lachapelle, F., Escriou, C., Ratzkin, B., and Baron-Van Evercooren, A. (1998) In vitro and in vivo behaviour of NDF-expanded monkey Schwann cells. *Eur. J. Neurosci.* 10:291–300.

Avellana-Adalid, V., Nait-Oumesmar, B., Lachapelle, F., and Baron-Van Evercooren, A. (1996) Expansion of rat oligodendrocyte progenitors into proliferative "oligospheres" that retain differentiation potential. *J. Neurosci. Res.* 45, 558–570.

Baron-Van Evercooren, A., Avellana-Adalid, V., Ben Younes-Chennoufi, A., Gansmuller, A., Nait-Oumesmar, B., and Vignais, L. (1996) Cell-cell interactions during the migration of myelin-forming cells transplanted in the demyelinated spinal cord. *Glia* 16:147–164.

Baron-Van Evercooren, A., Duhamel-Clerin, E., Boutry, J.M., Hauw, J.J., and Gumpel, M. (1993) Pathways of migration of transplanted Schwann cells in the demyelinated mouse spinal cord. *J. Neurosci. Res.* 35:428–438.

Baron-Van Evercooren, A., Gansmuller, A., Duhamel, E., Pascal, F., and Gumpel, M. (1992) Repair of a myelin lesion by Schwann cells transplanted in the adult mouse spinal cord. *J. Neuroimmunol.* 40:235–242.

Ben-Hur, T., Einstein, O., Mizrachi-Kol, R., Ben-Menachem, O., Reinhartz, E., Karussis, D., and Abramsky, O. (2003) Transplanted multipotential neural precursor cells migrate into inflamed white matter in response to experimental autoimmune encephalomyelitis. *Glia* 41:73–80.

Blakemore, W.F., Chari, D.M., Gilson, J.M., and Crang, A.J. (2002) Modelling large areas of demyelination in the rat reveals the potential and possible limitations of transplanted glial cells for remyelination in the CNS. *Glia* 38:155–168.

Blakemore, W.F., Gilson, J.M., and Crang A.J. (2000) Transplanted cells migrate over a greater distance and remyelinate demyelinated lesions more rapidly than endogenous remyelinating cells. *J. Neurosci. Res.* 61:288–294.

Bonilla, S., Alarcon, P., Villaverde, R., Aparicio, P., Silva, A., and Martinez, S. (2002) Haematopoietic progenitor cells from adult bone marrow differentiate into cells that express oligodendroglial antigens in the neonatal mouse brain. *Eur. J. Neurosci.* 15:575–582.

Brierley, C.M.H., Crang, A.J., Iwashita, Y., Gilson, J.M., Scolding, N.J., Compston, D.A.S., and Blakemore, W.F. (2001) Remyelination of demyelinated CNS axons by transplanted human Schwann cells: the deleterious effects of contaminating fibroblasts. *Cell Transplant.* 10:305–315.

Brook, G.A., Lawrence, J.M., and Raisman, G. (1993). Morphology and migration of cultured Schwann cells transplanted into the fimbria and hippocampus in adult rats. *Glia* 9:292–304.

Brustle, O., Jones, K.N., Learish, R.D., Karram, K., Choudhary, K., Wiestler, O.D., Duncan, I.D., and McKay, R.D.G. (1999) Embryonic stem cell–derived glial precursors: a source of myelinating transplants. *Science* 285:754–756.

Bulte, J.W., Zhang, S.C., Van Gelderen, P., Herynek, V., Jordan, E.K., Duncan, I.D., and Frank, J.A. (1999) Neurotransplantation of magnetically labeled oligodendrocyte progenitors: magnetic resonance tracking of cell migration and myelination. *Proc. Natl. Acad. Sci. USA* 96:15256–15261.

Cao, Q.L., Zhang, Y.P., Howard, R.M., Walters, W.M., Tsoulfas, P., and Whittemore, S.R. (2001) Pluripotent stem cells engrafted into the normal or lesioned adult rat spinal cord are restricted to a glial lineage. *Exp. Neurol.* 167:48–58.

Chang, A., Tourtellotte, W.W., Rudick, R., and Trapp, B.D. (2002) Premyelinating oligodendrocytes in chronic lesions of multiple sclerosis. *N. Engl. J. Med.* 346:165–173.

Duncan, I.D., Hammang, J.P., Jackson, K.F., Wood, P.M., Bunge, R.P., and Langford, L. (1988) Transplantation of oligodendrocytes and Schwann cells into the spinal cord of the myelin deficent rat. *J. Neurocytol.* 17:351–360.

Espinosa de los Monteros, A., Baba, H., Zhao, P.M., Pan, T., Chang, R., de Vellis, J., and Ikenaka, K. (2001) Remyelination of the adult demyelinated mouse brain by grafted oligodendrocyte progenitors and the effect of B-104 cografts. *Neurochem. Res.* 26:673–682.

Franklin, R.J.M. (2003) Remyelination by transplanted olfactory ensheathing cells. *Anat. Rec.* 271B:71–76.

Franklin, R.J.M., Bayley, S.A., and Blakemore, W.F. (1996) Transplanted CG4 cells (an oligodendrocyte progenitor cell line) survive, migrate and contribute to repair of areas of demyelination in X-irradiated and damaged spinal cord, but not in normal spinal cord. *Exp. Neurol.* 137:263–276.

Franklin, R.J.M., Bayley, S.A., Milner, R., ffrench-Constant, C., and Blakemore, W.F. (1995) Differentiation of the O-2A progenitor cell line CG-4 into oligodendrocytes and astrocytes following transplantation into glia-deficent areas of CNS white matter. *Glia* 13:39–44.

Franklin, R.J.M. and Blakemore, W.F. (1993) Requirements for Schwann cell migration within CNS environments: a viewpoint. *Int. J. Dev. Neurosci.* 11:641–649.

Franklin, R.J.M. and Blakemore, W.F. (1999) Transplantation of myelinogenic cells into the central nervous system. In: Dunnett, S.B., Boulton, A.A., and Baker, G.B., eds. *Neural Transplantation Methods.* Totowa, NJ: Humana Press, pp. 305–317.

Groves, A.K., Barnett, S.C., Franklin, R.J.M., Crang, A.J., Mayer, M., Blakemore, W.F., and Noble, M. (1993) Repair of demyelinated lesions by transplantation of purified O-2A progenitor cells. *Nature* 362:453–455.

Franklin, R.J.M., Blaschuk, K.L., Bearchell, M.C., Prestoz, L.L., Setzu, A., Brindle, K.M., and ffrench-Constant, C. (1999) Magnetic resonance imaging of transplanted oligodendrocyte precursors in the rat brain. *NeuroReport* 10:3961–3965.

Gumpel, M., Baumann, N., Raoul, M., and Jacque, C. (1983) Survival and differentiation of oligodendrocytes from neural tissue transplanted into new-born mouse brain. *Neurosci. Lett.* 37:307–311.

Hammang, J.P., Archer, D.R., and Duncan, I.D. (1997) Myelination following transplantation of EGF-responsive neural stem cells into a myelin-deficient environment. *Exp. Neurol.* 147:84–95.

Herrera, J., Yang, H., Zhang, S.-C., Pröschel, C., Tresco, P., Duncan, I.D., Luskin, M.B., and Mayer-Proschel, M. (2001) Embryonic-derived glial-restricted precursor cells (GRP cells) can differentiate into astrocytes and oligodendrocytes in vivo. *Exp. Neurol.* 171:11–21.

Hinks, G.L., Chari, D.M., O'Leary, M.T., Zhao, C., Keirstead, H.S., Blakemore, W.F., and Franklin, R.J.M. (2001) Depletion of endogenous oligodendrocyte progenitors rather than increased availability of survival factors is a likely explanation for the enhanced survival of transplanted oligodendrocyte progenitors in X-irradiated compared to normal CNS. *Neuropathol. Appl. Neurobiol.* 27:59–67.

Honmou, O., Felts, P.A., Waxman, S.G., and Kocsis, J.D. (1996) Restoration of normal conduction properties in demyelinated spinal cord axons in the adult rat by transplantation of exogenous Schwann cells. *J. Neurosci.* 16:3199–3208.

Huang, P.P., Alliquant, B., Carmel, P.W., and Friedman, E.D. (1991) Myelination of the rat retina by transplantation of oligodendrocytes into four-day-old hosts. *Exp. Neurol.* 113:291–300.

Huppes, W., Degroot, C.J.A., Ostendorf, R.H., Bauman, J.G.J., Gossen, J.A., Smit, V., Vijg, J., and Dijkstra, C.D. (1992) Detection of migrated allogeneic oligodendrocytes throughout the central nervous system of the galactocerebrosidase-deficient *twitcher* mouse. *J. Neurocytol.* 21:129–136.

Imaizumi, T., Lankford, K.L., Waxman, S.G., Greer, C.A., and Kocsis, J.D. (1998) Transplanted olfactory ensheathing cells remyelinate and enhance axonal conduction in the demyelinated dorsal columns of the rat spinal cord. *J. Neurosci.* 18:6176–6185.

Isacson, O., Deacon, T.W., Pakzaban, P., Galpern, W.R., Dinsmore, J., and Burns, L.H. (1995) Transplanted xenogeneic neural cells in neurodegenerative disease models exhibit remarkable axonal target specificity and distinct growth patterns of glial and axonal fibres. *Nat. Med.* 1:1189–1194.

Iwashita, Y. and Blakemore, W.F. (2000) Areas of demyelination do not attract significant numbers of Schwann cells transplanted into normal white matter. *Glia* 31, 232–240.

Iwashita, Y., Crang, A.J., and Blakemore, W.F. (2000a) Redistribution of bisbenzimide Hoechst 33342 flurochrome from transplanted cells to host cells. *NeuroReport* 11:1013–1016.

Iwashita, Y., Fawcett, J.W., Crang, A.J., Franklin, R.J.M., and Blakemore, W.F. (2000b) Schwann cells transplanted into normal and x-irradiated adult white matter do not migrate extensively and show poor long-term survival. *Exp. Neurol.* 164:280–302.

Jeffery, N.D. and Blakemore, W.F. (1997) Locomotor deficits induced by experimental spinal cord demyelination are abolished by spontaneous remyelination. *Brain* 120:27–37.

Jeffery, N.D., Crang, A.J., O'Leary, M.T., Hodge, S.J., and Blakemore, W.F. (1999) Behavioural consequences of oligodendrocyte progenitor cell transplantation into experimental demyelinating lesions in rat spinal cord. *Eur. J. Neurosci.* 11:1508–1514.

Jung, M., Crang, A.J., Blakemore, W.F., Hoppe, D., Kettenmann, H., and Trotter, J. (1994) In vitro and in vivo characterisation of glial cells immortalised with a temperature sensitive oncogene mutant of the SV40 T antigen-containing retrovirus. *J. Neurosci. Res.* 37:182–196.

Keirstead, H.S., Ben-Hur, T., Rogister, B., O'Leary, M.T., Dubois-Dalcq, M., and Blakemore, W.F. (1999) PSA-NCAM positive CNS precursors generate both oligodendrocytes and Schwann cells to remyelinate the CNS following transplantation. *J. Neurosci.* 19:7529–7536.

Kohama, I., Lankford, K.L., Preiningerova, J., White, F.A., Vollmer, T.L., and Kocsis, J.D. (2001) Transplantation of cryopreserved adult human Schwann cells enhances axonal conduction in demyelinated spinal cord. *J. Neurosci.* 21:944–950.

Lachapelle, F., Gumpel, M., and Baumann, N. (1994) Contribution of transplantations to the understanding of the role of the PLP gene. *Neurochem. Res.* 19:1083–1090.

Laeng, P., Molthagen, M., Yu, E.G.X., and Bartsch, U. (1996) Transplantation of oligodendrocyte progenitor cells into the rat retina: extensive myelination of retinal ganglion cell axons. *Glia* 20: 200–210.

Lakatos, A., Franklin, R.J.M., and Barnett, S.C. (2000) Olfactory ensheathing cells and Schwann cells differ in their in vitro interactions with astrocytes. *Glia* 32:214–225.

Lakatos, A., Smith, P.M., Barnett, S.C., and Franklin, R.J.M. (2002) Meningeal cells enhance limited CNS remyelination by transplanted olfactory ensheathing cells. *Brain* 126:598–609.

Learish, R.D., Brüstle, O., Zhang, S.C., and Duncan, I.D. (1999) Intraventricular transplantation of oligodendrocyte progenitors into a fetal myelin mutant results in widespread formation of myelin. *Ann. Neurol.* 46:716–722.

Li, Y. and Raisman, G. (1997) Integration of transplanted cultured Schwann cells into the long myelinated fiber tracts of the adult spinal cord. *Exp. Neurol.* 145:397–411.

Lobsiger, C.S., Smith, P.M., Buchstaller, J., Schweitzer, B., Franklin, R.J.M., Suter, U., and Taylor, V. (2001) SpL201: a conditionally immortalized Schwann cell precursor line that generates myelin. *Glia* 36:31–47.

Mitome, M., Low, H.P., Van den Pol, A., Nunnari, J.J., Wolf, M.K., Billings-Gagliardi, S., and Schwartz, W. J. (2001) Towards the reconstruction of central nervous system white matter using neural precursor cells. *Brain* 124:2147–2161.

Mujtaba, T., Mayer-Proschel, M., and Rao, M.S. (1998) A common neural progenitor for the CNS and PNS. *Dev. Biol.* 200:1–15.

O'Leary, M.T. and Blakemore, W.F. (1997) Use of a rat Y-chromosome probe to determine the long term fate of glial cells transplanted into areas of central nervous system demyelination. *J. Neurocytol.* 26:191–206.

Osterhout, D.J., Ebner, S., Xu, J.S., Ornitz, D.M., Zazanis, G.A., and Mckinnon, R.D. (1997) Transplanted oligodendrocyte progenitor cells expressing a dominant-negative FGF receptor transgene fail to migrate *in vivo*. *J. Neurosci.* 17:9122–9132.

Raisman, G., Lawrence, J.M., and Brook, G.A. (1993) Schwann cells transplanted into the CNS. *Int. J. Dev. Neurosci.* 11:651–669.

Sasaki, M., Honmou, O., Akiyama, Y., Uede, T., Hashi, K., and Kocsis, J.D. (2001) Transplantation of an acutely isolated bone marrow fraction repairs demyelinated adult rat spinal cord axons. *Glia* 35:26–34.

Setzu, A., ffrench-Constant, C., and Franklin, R.J.M. (2004) CNS axons retain their competence for myelination throughout life. *Glia* 45:307–311.

Shields, S.A., Blakemore, W.F., and Franklin, R.J.M. (2000) Schwann cell remyelination is restricted to astrocyte-deficient areas following transplantation into demyelinated rat brain. *J. Neurosci. Res.* 60:571–578.

Smith, P.M. and Blakemore, W.F. (2000) Porcine neural progenitors require commitment to the oligodendrocyte lineage prior to transplantation in order to achieve significant remyelination of demyelinated lesions in the adult CNS. *Eur. J. Neurosci.* 12:2414–2425.

Svendsen, C.N., Caldwell, M.A., ter-Borg, M.G., Rosser, A.E., Tyers, P., Karmiol, S., and Dunnett, S.B. (1997) Long-term survival of human central nervous sytem progenitor cells transplanted into a rat model of Parkinson's disease. *Exp. Neurol.* 148: 135–146.

Targett, M.P., Sussman, J., O'Leary, M.T., Compston, D.A.S., and Blakemore, W.F. (1996) Failure to achieve remyelination of demyelinated rat axons following transplantation of glial cells obtained from the adult human brain. *Neuropathol. Appl. Neurobiol.* 22:199–206.

Tourbah, A., Linnington, C., Bachelin, C., Avellana-Adalid, V., Wekerle, H., and Baron-Van Evercooren, A. (1997) Inflammation promotes survival and migration of the CG4 oligodendrocyte progenitors transplanted in the spinal cord of both inflammatory and demyelinated EAE rats. *J. Neurosci. Res.* 50:853–861.

Trotter, J., Crang, A.J., Schachner, M., and Blakemore, W.F. (1993) Lines of glial precursor cells immortalised with a temperature-sensitive oncogene give rise to astrocytes and myelin-forming oligodendrocytes on transplantation into demyelinated lesions in the central nervous system. *Glia* 9:25–40.

Utzschneider, D.A., Archer, D.R., Kocsis, J.D., Waxman, S.G., and Duncan, I.D. (1994) Transplantation of glial cells enhances action potential conduction of amyelinated spinal cord axons in the myelin-deficient rat. *Proc. Natl. Acad. Sci. USA* 91:53–57.

van Heyningen, P., Calver, A.R., and Richardson, W.D. (2001) Control of progenitor cell number by mitogen supply and demand. *Curr. Biol.* 11:232–241.

Vitry, S., Avellana-Adalid, V., Lachapelle, F., and Baron-Van Evercooren, A. (2001) Migration and multipotentiality of PSA-

NCAM+ neural precursors transplanted in the developing brain. *Mol. Cell. Neurosci.* 17:983–1000.

Warrington, A.E., Barbarese, E., and Pfeiffer, S.E. (1993) Differential myelinogenic capacity of specific developmental stages of the oligodendrocyte lineage upon transplantation into hypomyelinating hosts. *J. Neurosci. Res.* 34:1–13.

Yandava, B.D., Billinghurst, L.L., and Snyder, E.Y. (1999) "Global" cell replacement is feasible via neural stem cell transplantation: evidence from the dysmyelinated *shiverer* mouse brain. *Proc. Natl. Acad. Sci.* USA 96:7029–7034.

Zhang, S.-C., Goetz, B.D., and Duncan, I.D. (2003) Suppression of activated microglia promotes survival and function of transplanted oligodendrocyte precursors. *Glia* 41:191–198.

Zhang, S.-C., Lundberg, C., Lipsitz, D., O'Connor, L.T., and Duncan, I.D. (1998) Generation of oligodendroglial progenitors from neural stem cells. *J. Neurocytol.* 27:475–489.

39 Multiple sclerosis

JACK ANTEL AND DOUGLAS ARNOLD

The clinical and pathological features of multiple sclerosis (MS) began to be described in the mid-1800s and by the 1870s had been synthesized into a recognizable entity by Charcot and colleagues (Murray, 2000). Vulpian had introduced the term *sclerose en plaque disseminata* in 1867. Hammond referred to the entity as *cerebro-spinal sclerosis* to distinguish it from a wide array of disorders resulting from trauma, infection, or unknown causes that contained the term *sclerosis*, referring to the scarring observed at different anatomical sites within the central nervous system (CNS) (Hammond, 1871). Charcot emphasized the loss of the myelin sheath with relative, but not absolute, preservation of axons. He referred to the observation by Reinfleisch in 1863 of inflammation around a vessel in the center of MS plaques; this can be viewed as the beginning of the continuing debate of the relative contributions of immune-mediated versus neurodegenerative processes as a basis for the disease pathology (Charcot, 1877).

The occurrence of a neuroparalytic disorder, now termed *postvaccination* or *acute disseminated encephalomyelitis* (ADEM), as a complication of immunization with neural tissue containing rabies vaccine introduced by Pasteur in the 1880s demonstrated that the CNS, and myelin in particular, could be the target of an immune-mediated attack. This disorder has been reproduced in animals by both active immunization with neural tissue and adoptive transfer of autoreactive T cells and is termed *experimental autoimmune encephalomyelitis* (EAE). To date, in contrast to other organ-specific immune disorders such as diabetes, there is no naturally occurring animal model of MS.

CLINICAL-PATHOLOGIC FEATURES OF MULTIPLE SCLEROSIS

This section describes observations made from the study of patients and their tissues that need to be accounted for when considering the biological mechanisms underlying the MS disease process.

Natural History

The initial descriptions of MS outlined a disease course characterized by recurrent relapses, most often beginning at a young adult age and occurring more frequently in women than in men. Relapses in MS have been empirically defined as the appearance or reappearance of one or more neurological abnormalities persisting for at least 24–48 hours and occurring 30 days or more after any previous relapse. The requirement that the symptoms or signs persist for at least 1–2 days is used to distinguish new pathological events from the transient physiological dysfunction that often occurs in previously damaged tissue. The interval of a month is an arbitrary attempt to define whether repeated events belong to one ongoing relapse or to different relapses. Common neurological symptoms and signs include those derived from lesions of the optic nerve [unilateral visual loss (optic neuritis)], brain stem and cerebellum (diplopia, trigeminal neuralgia, dysequilibrium), and spinal cord (motor and/or sensory dysfunction of limbs, Lhermitte's phenomenon, bladder dysfunction). In some cases, multiple levels of dysfunction occur within a single relapse. The relapse is followed by complete or partial recovery, usually over subsequent several weeks or months. This initial phase of the disease is referred to as *relapsing-remitting* (RR).

Long-term natural history data (>25 years) on MS have been derived from patients serially followed in the pretherapeutic and pre–magnetic resonance imaging era (Paty and Ebers, 1997). The natural history data sets indicate that approximately 50%–60% of RR patients will evolve into a secondary progressive (SP) phase of the disease after 10–15 years. This proportion increases even further if patients are followed for 25 years. Features of the SP phase of the disease include dysfunction at all levels of the neuraxis, including cognitive impairment. Impaired ability to walk [expanded disability status scale (EDSS > 4)] correlates most closely with spinal cord involvement. In approximately 10%–15% of cases the disease is progressive from the onset, with or without intercurrent relapses. These disease forms are referred to as *primary progressive* (PP) and *progressive relapsing* (PR). Conversely, the natural history studies indicate that 10%–15% of cases will follow a relatively benign course, that is, will have little or no neurological disability after 15 years. Predictors of a more severe disease course include the frequency of initial relapses, relapses associated with motor dysfunction, older age at disease onset, and male gender.

Para-Clinical Measures

Para-clinical tests are now being used both to expand the clinical criteria used for diagnosis and to provide insight into the course and pathogenesis of the disease.

Cerebrospinal Fluid

Increased levels of immunoglobulin (Ig), reflecting intrathecal production, have been noted in the cerebrospinal fluid (CSF) of MS patients for more than 50 years. The Ig is of restricted heterogeneity, as observed by electrophoresis techniques. This restricted heterogeneity is clinically referred to as *oligoclonal bands* (OCBs). Analysis of antigen-reactive Ig sequences encoded by mRNA derived from B cells recovered from the CSF confirms the restricted heterogeneity pattern (Qin et al., 1998). Immunoglobulin production rates do not correlate with disease activity. An ongoing question is whether the Ig in the CNS contains disease-relevant specific antibody intermixed with the presence of nonspecific antibody. Detectable titers of antibodies can be measured by enzyme-linked immunosorbent assay (ELISA)–based assays to an array of myelin proteins and microbial antigens.

Evoked Responses

Evoked responses that use averaging techniques to record the electrical signal in the brain or spinal cord associated with visual, sensory, or auditory stimulation were often used in the past to help document disruption of electrical transmission consistent with multifocal demyelination and axonal injury. None of the pivotal clinical trials leading to drug approval has used these measures.

Magnetic Resonance Imaging

The exquisite sensitivity of magnetic resonance imaging (MRI) to the pathology of MS has led to its superseding all other imaging modalities for MS. Magnetic resonance imaging provides both ease of serial studies and quantitative measurements. The widespread use of MRI has reversed patients' previous concern that physicians often withheld the diagnosis of MS, often for a number of years, into a concern that the diagnosis is being made too early, that is, after the initial clinical event. Natural history studies indicate that individuals with an initial clinical episode of neurological dysfunction consistent with CNS demyelinating disease, commonly referred to as a *clinically isolated syndrome* (CIS), and who have associated multifocal abnormalities (see below) on MRI, have an 80%–95% probability of developing recurrent clinical disease within the next 5–15 years. This compares to a 5%–20% risk in the patient whose MRI scan is normal (Brex et al., 2002).

The conventional MRI techniques used to study MS patients produce images that reflect the physicochemical state of protons that are present mainly in the water contained within the tissues that are being imaged. Contrast in such images is derived primarily from tissue-specific differences in (*1*) spin-spin relaxation time (i.e., the time constant for the decay of magnetization in the plane perpendicular to the magnetic field, referred to as *T2*) and (*2*) spin-lattice relaxation time (i.e., the time constant for the recovery of magnetization in the direction of the magnetic field, referred to as *T1*). (For a review of MRI theory and applications see Gadian, 1996.)

Conventional MRI techniques include (*1*) T2-weighted imaging, (*2*) proton density weighted imaging, (*3*) fluid-attenuated inversion-recovery imaging, (*4*) standard T1-weighted imaging, and (*5*) gadolinium-enhanced, T1-weighted imaging (Figs. 39.1, 39.2).

T2-weighted MRI scans show high sensitivity to MS lesions but lack pathological specificity in that edema, demyelination, gliosis, and axonal loss all produce a similar hyperintense signal. There is a very weak correlation between T2 lesion volume and neurological

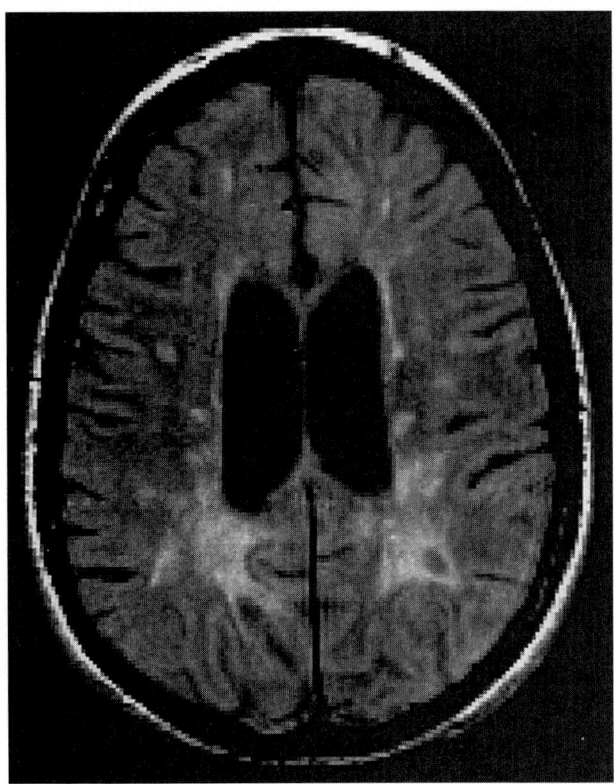

FIGURE 39.1 Cross section through the lateral ventricles of a patient with multiple sclerosis as seen on a proton density (*PD*)-weighted image. Of note are the large, hyperintense periventricular lesions that are easily discriminated from the neighboring cerebrospinal fluid.

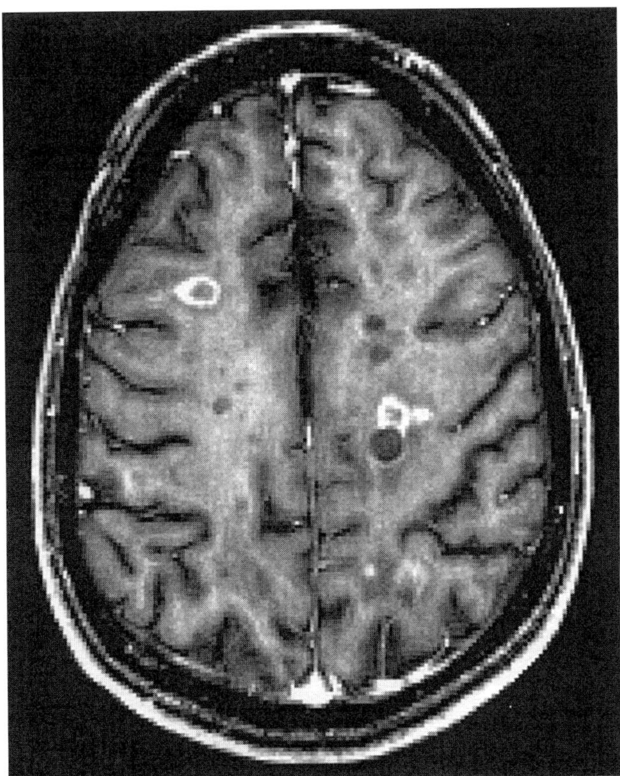

FIGURE 39.2 Cross section through the centrum semiovale of a patient with multiple sclerosis as seen on a gadolinium (*Gd*)-enhanced, T1-weighted image. Of note are the numerous hypointense lesions, two of which are still active and inflammatory (as evidenced by the ring-like Gd enhancement).

disability. T1-weighted images provide excellent anatomical detail and are used to determine quantitative measures of brain volume. Persistent T1-defined lesions reflect tissue destruction more specifically and show a stronger correlation with clinical disability. Newly appearing T2 lesions or T1 lesions that enhance when the paramagnetic contrast agent gadolinium is injected intravenously are associated with acute inflammation and thus can provide a surrogate for disease activity. Unfortunately, it is not possible on the basis of a single MRI scan to conclude reliably that some lesions are new and others are old, a requirement necessary to satisfy the diagnostic criteria for dissemination of the disease in time (>3 months) (Miller et al., 1998; McDonald et al., 2001). Follow-up scans can provide such information. The above MRI techniques have been used as primary and secondary outcome measures in clinical trials to determine the efficacy of immune-directed therapies.

Magnetic resonance imaging can provide a variety of additional techniques for visualizing the CNS that are sensitive to different aspects of pathological change (Caramanos et al., 2002). By integration of data from multiple MR techniques, a more comprehensive view of the disease emerges. The techniques described below, which are more commonly used for research rather than clinical purposes, have proved useful in this regard.

Magnetization transfer (MT) images are created by selectively saturating the MR signal from protons in macromolecules that are not normally visualized by conventional MRI and then observing the transfer of this saturation to bulk water that is normally visualized by MRI by means of the decrease that this magnetization transfer produces in the signal from bulk water. The extent of the effect can be quantified simply as the magnetization transfer ratio (MTR)—the ratio of the signal intensity before and after selectively saturating the macromolecular-associated water. A greater magnetization transfer between macromolecules and associated water implies a greater relative macromolecular pool of protons that interacts with bulk water (Fig. 39.3). Loss of macromolecular structure (as occurs with demyelination) reduces the MTR. As conventionally applied, the MTR does not specifically probe any particular class of macromolecules. However, because the relative abundance of myelin proteins in the brain is so high, changes in myelin content dominate MTR changes in MS.

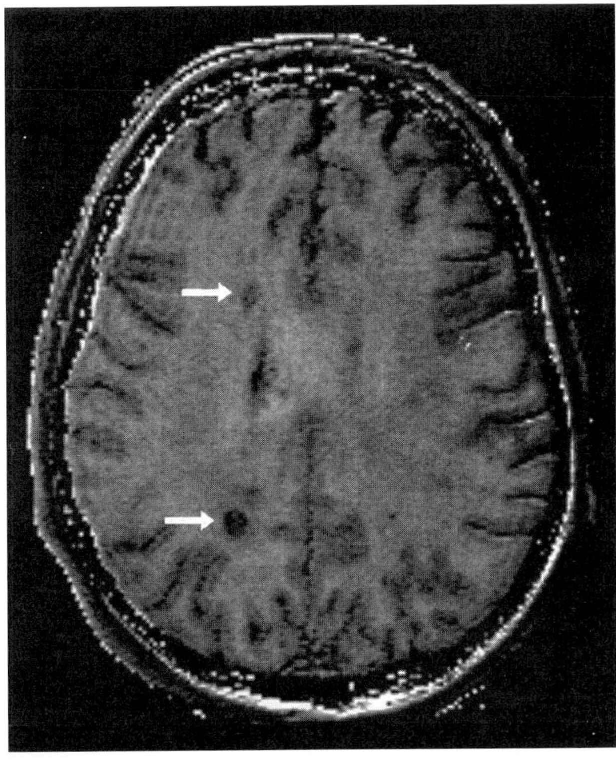

FIGURE 39.3 Magnetization transfer ratio (*MTr*) image from a patient with multiple sclerosis. Images are obtained both with (Mt_{on}) and without (MT_{off}) the presence of a saturation pulse, and pixel-by-pixel MTr values are calculated as $[1 - (MT_{on}/MT_{off})] \times 100$. Arrows indicate two lesions with differing extent of demyelination and associated change in MTr.

Magnetic Resonance Spectroscopy and Spectroscopic Imaging

Magnetic resonance spectroscopy (MRS) is fundamentally different from the water-proton-based MRI techniques described above in that it records signals that arise from protons in metabolites that are present in brain. Because the concentration of such tissue metabolites is approximately one-thousandth that of tissue water, the signal-to-noise ratio and the image resolution that is possible for these metabolite-based images are much lower than those for water-based images. However, the resulting metabolite images provide chemicopathological specificity that is not possible with conventional water-based images.

As shown in Figure 39.4, the water-suppressed, localized proton MRS spectrum of the normal human brain that is recorded at relatively long echo times (i.e., TE of 136 or 272 ms) reveals three major resonance peaks [the locations of which are expressed as the difference in parts per million (ppm) between the resonance frequency of the compound of interest and that of a standard compound (i.e., tetramethylsilane)], which are ascribed to choline (Cho), creatine (Cr), and *N*-acetylaspartate (NAA). The Cho peak at 3.2 ppm arises from tetramethyl amines, which are mainly found in Cho-containing phospholipids that participate in membrane (predominantly myelin) synthesis and degradation. The Cr peak, which resonantes at 3.0 ppm, arises from creatine and phosphocreatine (Cr). The NAA resonance at 2.0 ppm originates from *N*-acetyl (NA) groups, which are found in the brain primarily in the neuronally localized compound NAA. The resonance from NAA is arguably the most important proton MRS signal in the characterization of MS pathology because NAA is localized exclusively within neurons and neuronal processes such as axons and dendrites in the adult human brain. (Simmons et al., 1991; Bjartmar et al., 2002).

Magnetic resonance spectroscopy studies have documented that axonal injury occurs early in the course of MS, and not only within lesions but also in normal-appearing white matter (NAWM) defined by conventional MRI. Such findings could reflect microscopic lesions, distal effects of cytokines released from sites of inflammation, degeneration of axons transected within the lesions, and/or the proximal effects of axonal injury.

Magnetic resonance spectroscopy acquisitions at short TE can reveal signals from mobile macromolecules (which arise mainly from lipids) that become MRS visible due to increases in mobility associated with myelin degradation generated by demyelination. Focal increases in Cho can also be found preceding the development of new T2 lesions. This suggests that low-grade focal myelin pathology may precede the devel-

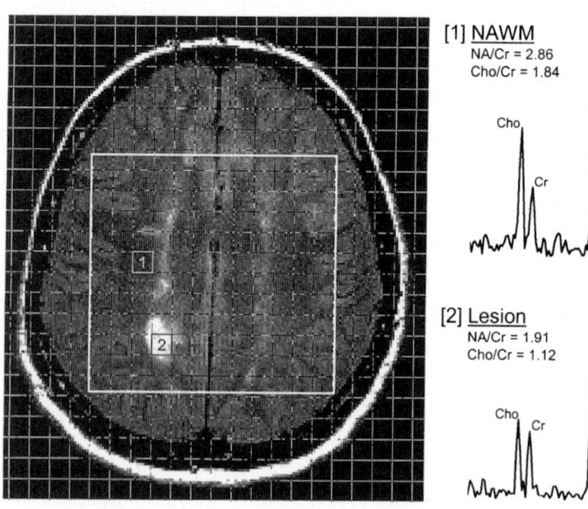

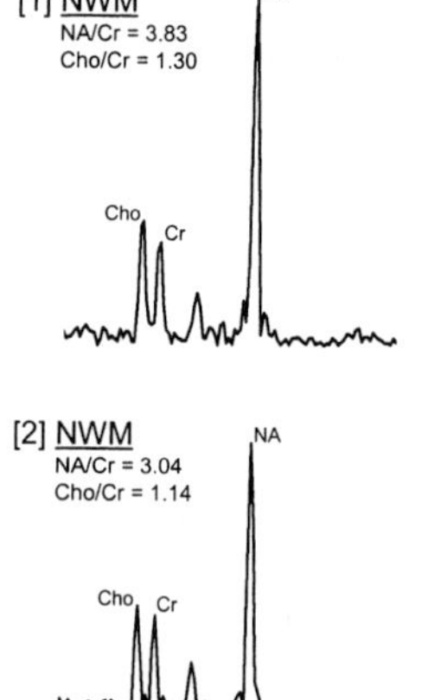

FIGURE 39.4 Proton-density-weighted magnetic resonance images through the centrum semiovale and two voxels from the proton magnetic resonance spectroscopic image (*MRSI*) from a patient with multiple sclerosis (*MS*), as well as from the homologous spatial locations in the normal white matter (*NWM*) of a normal control subject. The grid in each image shows the individual MRSI voxels, and the large, thick white box shows the volume of interest examined. The smaller numbered boxes represent voxels of normal appearing white matter (*NAWM*) and lesional brain tissue in the patient. The MRSI spectra from within each of these voxels is shown to the right of each image. The areas under the *N*-acetyl (*NA*) and choline (*Cho*) peaks [normalized to creatine (*Cr*)] are shown above each spectrum. The spectra have been scaled so that the Cr peak in each of them has the same height. Note (*1*) the decrease in NA/Cr values from the patient's NAWM voxel relative to the NWM voxels in the control subject, (*2*) the even greater decrease in lesional NA/Cr, and (*3*) the increased Cho/Cr value in the patient's NAWM voxel, which may be predictive of a soon-to-appear lesion in that location.

opment of acute, severe inflammation. Focal MTR changes also can occur prior to the appearance of T2-hyperintense lesions.

Currently, there is no specific marker associated with astrocyte reactivity (gliosis), although it has been suggested that the signal from myo-inositol, another resonance in the MR spectrum that is best seen at short TE, has some specificity for astrocytic gliosis (see Table 39.1).

EPIDEMIOLOGY OF MULTIPLE SCLEROSIS

Epidemiological studies support the contributions of both genetic and environmental factors to disease development. Population-based studies indicate that MS has an uneven geographic distribution (Paty and Ebers, 1997). Its high frequency in regions with Caucasian populations of European descent and its low frequency in black African and Oriental groups indicate a genetic contribution. The apparent north-south gradient in disease prevalence observed in Australia and North America has not, however, been explained by racial (genetic) differences alone. Migration data, although impacted by multiple variables related to opportunity and the basis for migration, suggest that individuals retain their initial risk of the region of origin if relocation occurs after the preteen age years. Molecular genetic screening surveys suggest that MS patients may share susceptibility genes with individuals who have other autoimmune disorders (Maas et al., 2002). Except for thyroid disease, however, there seems to be little association of MS with other autoimmune disorders.

Family studies indicate that the concordance rate among monozygotic female twins in Canada is about 30% compared to 2% in dizygotic twins. There is no increased risk among adopted siblings. Ebers and Sadovnick (Paty and Ebers, 1997) conclude that " familial aggregation is determined by genes and that population risk is strongly influenced by environment." The putative environmental factor is one that would affect the whole population. This could be either the presence of a risk factor such as an infectious agent or the absence of a protective factor. As regards infection, no specific agent has been identified. An aberrant host response to a ubiquitous agent such as Epstein-Barr or herpes viruses cannot be excluded. The current models for genetic susceptibility to MS invoke contributions by multiple genes, with the human leukocyte antigen (HLA) region being the most clearly defined one. Genetic factors can not only influence susceptibility but also modify the disease course. Individuals lacking the gene encoding the chemokine receptor CCR5 have a more benign disease course, whereas those lacking ciliary neurotrophic factor (CNTF) have a more severe course (Giess et al., 2002; Schreiber et al., 2002).

TREATMENT

Recombinant interferon β (IFNβ) was the first drug approved for clinical use in MS. Initial studies using IFNβ-1b were performed on patients with clinically definite MS (i.e., two or more attacks) and RR disease (reviewed in O'Connor et al., 2001). These showed a reduction in relapse frequency of about 30%–35% and an even larger decrease in MRI activity as assessed by the frequency of new lesion formation. Similar results have been obtained using IFNβ-1a. Subsequent trials of these agents in patients with SP MS have revealed little if any beneficial effect on clinical disease progression. Results of MRI in SP MS further indicate a dissociation between the effects of IFNβ therapy on new inflammatory lesion formation (reduced frequency of gadolinium-enhancing lesions) and disease progression (continued increase in T2-weighted lesion volume). This phase of disease is also resistant even to intense immunosuppressive therapy, suggesting that the mechanism of progression may no longer be directly related to ongoing inflammation. Conversely, results of trials with IFNβ given to patients with their first clinical ep-

TABLE 39.1 *Pathological Specificity of Magnetic Resonance Imaging Modalities*

MRI Modality		*Pathological Specificity in White Matter*
T2-weighted lesions		Nonspecific
T1-weighted lesions	Acute	Edema + tissue destruction
T1-weighted lesions	chronic	Tissue destruction
Magnetization transfer		Macromolecules (myelin)
Short T2 imaging		Myelin water (trapped in lamellae)
MRS	NAA	Neuronal/axonal integrity
	Cho	Membrane (myelin) breakdown
	Lipid	Membrane (myelin) breakdown

Cho: choline; MRI: magnetic resonance imaging; MRS: magnetic resonance spectroscopy; NAA: *N*-acetylaspartate.

isode (CIS) suggestive of MS and multifocal MRI abnormalities indicate an even greater response than that observed in patients with clinically definite RR MS. Follow-up is still insufficient to determine the effect of very early treatment on the long-term evolution of the disease, although natural history studies suggest that the long-term prognosis is inversely related to the initial lesion frequency and the clinical attack rate. The differences in therapeutic responses at different stages of the disease highlight the need to understand the link between inflammation and subsequent tissue destruction.

The effects of IFNβ on MS likely reflect its actions on immune cells. Interferon β is administered either subcutaneously or intramuscularly and has a very short half-life, with little or no direct entry into the CNS. Sustained IFNβ therapy downregulates the activity of antigen-presenting cells (APCs) and favors induction of anti-inflammatory cytokines, especially interleukin (IL)-10 (Yong, 2002). Interferon β inhibits passage of immune cells across a model blood–brain barrier (BBB), reflecting its capacity to inhibit matrix metalloproteinase (MMP) production by inflammatory cells (Prat et al., 2002). These effects would be consistent with the rapid reduction of inflammatory lesion activity on gadolinium-enhanced MRI scans.

Glatiramer acetate (GA) was the second category of agent approved for therapy in MS. This random copolymer of four amino acids exerts its clinical effects in RR MS after a delay of several months of therapy, with overall results on relapse rate and subsequent disease course being comparable to those achieved with IFNβ. To date there is no documentation of efficacy in the SP form of MS. This therapy also acts via modulation of the immune system, binding to a wide repertoire of T cell receptors (Neuhaus et al., 2001). Therapy results in the generation of GA-reactive T cells that are polarized in a Th2 direction. Such cells and their soluble products (cytokines) are postulated to inhibit the activity of pro-inflammatory disease-mediating cells either directly (a process termed *bystander suppression*) or indirectly by modifying the properties of APCs. Such actions could occur within the systemic compartment, within the CNS, or both. In an experimental acute trauma model, GA-reactive T cells, mainly of the Th1 phenotype, generated by short-term drug administration, accelerated recovery from injury (Schwartz and Kipnis, 2001).

PATHOLOGY

The characteristic features of actively demyelinating lesions include a reduced density of myelinated fibers, inflammatory infiltrates composed of T cells and macrophages, and the presence of myelin breakdown products in macrophages/microglia. Recent reports suggest that there is heterogeneity among cases of MS with regard to both the primary target of injury and the mediators of the injury. Two patterns of lesions described by Lucchinetti et al. (2000) feature perivenous myelin destruction with relative preservation of oligodendrocytes (OGC), cell bodies, and ongoing remyelination. These patterns resemble the lesions seen in EAE, a disorder initiated by autoreactive T cells. Pattern 2 features Ig deposition, indicating a role for autoantibodies in lesion formation. Activated macrophage products are implicated as mediators in pattern 1. Patterns 3 and 4 may be considered oligodendrogliopathies, with the primary disease insult being directed at the OGC cell body. Both of these patterns lack remyelination. In pattern 3, there is a selective loss of myelin-associated glycoprotein (MAG), a glycoprotein expressed at the most distal end (adaxonal region) of the myelin sheath, suggesting a dying back phenomenon equivalent to that seen in distal axons in metabolic neuropathies. Such OGC pathology could reflect initial infectious or toxic insults. Unlike other patterns (and unlike EAE), there is sparing of perivenous myelin. The pattern 3 cases, although mainly described in biopsy material, have not yet shown clinical features distinct from those of patterns 1 and 2. Pattern 4 cases, all of which have a primary progressive course, feature loss of all myelin proteins in addition to the cell bodies.

In chronic lesions, macrophages dominate the lesion rather than lymphocytes, with significant loss of OGC and a reduction in the extent of ongoing remyelination. Axonal transaction and loss is prominent in the chronic lesions. Axonal pathology may prevent putative myelin progenitor cells from carrying out their remyelination program (Chang et al., 2002). Although astrocytosis (gliosis) is a prominent feature in early and chronic lesions, the significance of these responses to tissue injury and repair processes and to physiological functioning of demyelinated axons remains to be defined.

BIOLOGICAL BASIS UNDERLYING THE CLINICAL-PATHOLOGICAL FEATURES OF MULTIPLE SCLEROSIS

Initiation of the Multiple Sclerosis Disease Process

The currently favored postulate is that MS is triggered by immune responses directed against myelin or its cell of origin, the OGC. Observations from both clinical disorders and experimental models indicate that the initial events leading to immune-mediated CNS demyelination can take place either within the systemic compartment or within the CNS (Fig. 39.5). An example of events in the systemic compartment initiating central demyelination is the previously mentioned compli-

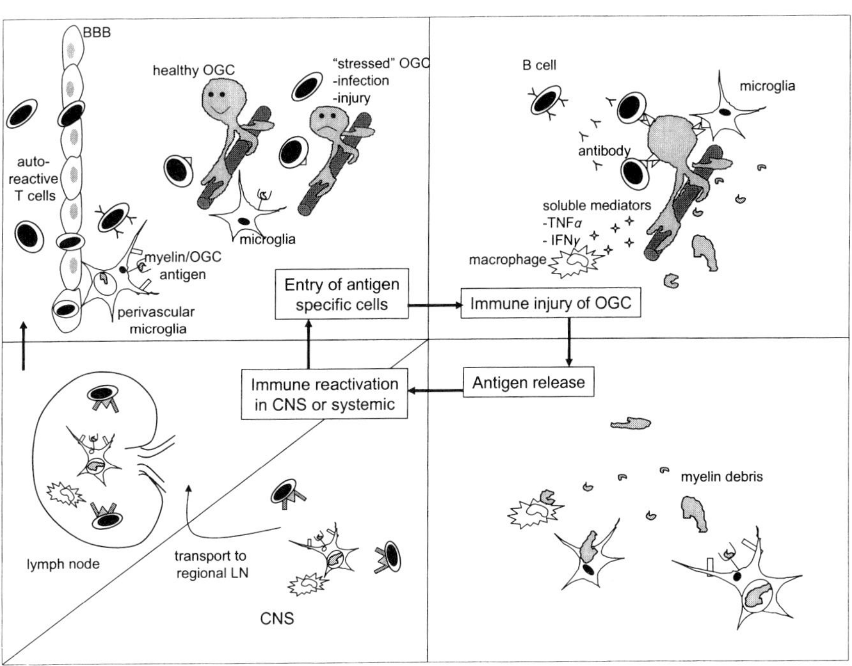

FIGURE 39.5 Model of the biological basis for the clinical-pathological features of multiple sclerosis. Illustrated are a sequence of immune–central nervous system (*CNS*) interactions that could underlie development of a target-specific recurrent or chronic immune-mediated disease: (*1*) initiation of a myelin/oligodendrocyte (*OGC*)-directed inflammatory process in the CNS; (*2*) actual mechanisms contributing to lethal or sublethal myelin/OGC injury; (*3*) release and microglia/macrophage uptake of an expanded array of antigens from damaged cells; and (*4*) presentation of the antigens to lymphocytes circulating within the CNS or in regional lymph nodes, resulting in reactivation and expansion (epitope spreading) of the disease-relevant immune response. LN: lymph node.

cation of ADEM. It should be noted that ADEM, unlike MS, is usually a uniphasic rather than a recurrent disorder. The animal disease EAE has now been induced with peptide sequences from infectious agents that share structural homology with myelin components, an occurrence referred to as *molecular mimicry* (Sung et al., 2002). The recognition that initiation of a T cell response results from contact between only one or two amino acids of a peptide contained within the major histocompatibility complex (MHC) groove and the T cell receptor predicts that a wide array of exogenous agents may share homology with autoantigens. This would seem to increase the probability that molecular mimicry may underlie the association between recent infection and relapses of MS.

Experimental models have been established in which persistent intracerebral viral infections can initiate chronic immune-mediated CNS demyelinating disease. The neurological dysfunction produced by persistent infection of the CNS with strains of mouse corona (JHEM) virus and Theiler murine encephalomyelitis virus (TMEV) is shown to be mediated by T cells sensitized to myelin antigens, presumably released as a result of initial viral-induced tissue injury (Talbot et al., 2001). Immune surveillance is an ongoing process within the CNS under physiological conditions, providing a source of lymphocytes that could respond to antigens presented by competent APCs within the CNS (Brabb et al., 2000). Myelin peptides have been recovered from microglia isolated from the CNS of TMEV-infected animals (Katz-Levy et al., 1999). The demonstration that antigens can be transported from the CNS to regional lymph nodes indicates that recurrent immune responses could be generated in the systemic compartment, as well as in the CNS, in response to events in the CNS.

T cells reactive to an array of myelin antigens can be recovered from the systemic circulation of MS patients and from normal individuals. The presence of these T cells in the normal population raises the question of whether failure of systemic immune regulatory mechanisms contributes to the development of disease in MS. The apparent increase in the number of autoreactive T cells with a memory phenotype found in the circulation of MS patients suggests prior exposure to myelin antigens or their molecular mimics (reviewed in Bieganowska et al., 1997). Most such cells demonstrate a pro-inflammatory phenotype, as defined by their bias toward secretion of Th1 cytokines. This T cell phenotype is the one most frequently used to adoptively transfer EAE.

Putative autoreactive CNS disease-mediating T cells generated in the systemic compartment need to transverse the BBB in order to reach their target sites. The cell migration process involves active molecular interactions between the immune cells and the constituents of the BBB including the specialized endothelial cells that line the brain microvessels and the astrocytes and microglia whose foot processes make physical contact with the barrier (Prat et al., 2001). The molecular mechanisms involved in immune cells crossing the BBB include adhesion, chemoattraction, and enzymatic digestion of the extracellular matrix mediated mainly by MMPs. Perivascular glial cell–derived molecules can modulate the permeability properties of the barrier by enhancing the BBB properties of endothelial cells *in vitro* (Prat et al., 2001; Chishty et al., 2002) and serving as sources of chemoattractants and MMPs involved in regulating migration of inflammatory cells. Conversely, activated microglia and astrocytes can produce molecules such as tumor necrosis factor (TNF) that enhance permeability.

Antibodies to adhesion molecules inter-cellular adhesion molecule-1 (ICAM-1) (CD54) and chemokines (CCL2) present at the BBB have been shown to inhibit the development or the subsequent course of EAE. Antibody (Antegren) directed against very late antigen-4 (VLA-4) inhibits EAE and reduces the frequency of lesion formation in MS (Miller et al., 2003). The functional ligand for VLA-4 at the BBB appears to be the connecting segment CS-1 fragment of fibronectin, a component of the extracellular matrix, rather than vascular cell adhesion molecule (VCAM). Pro-inflammatory cytokines expand the array of adhesion molecules and chemokines expressed at the BBB. Such expansion could limit the efficacy of therapies targeted at specific molecules. This concern again favors introduction of therapy as early as possible in the course of MS.

Although lymphocyte transmigration per se is not antigen or MHC restricted, persistence of the inflammatory response within the perivascular region is dependent on MHC-compatible antigen presentation (reviewed in Becher et al., 2000). Myelin-reactive T cells are more abundant in the CNS than in the systemic compartment in EAE and likely in MS, and their heterogeneity is more restricted. There is speculation regarding the sources of myelin antigen presented to the autoreactive T cells that initially enter the CNS. These could be released from cells of the OGC lineage, as part of a natural turnover rate or in response to injury or infection.

The process of competent antigen presentation requires two signals. The first involves antigen presentation to the antigen receptor on the T cells in the context of MHC molecules. For CD4 T cells, MHC class II is the required molecule. CD8 T cells recognize MHC class I. The second signals required for full T cell activation involves costimulatory molecules, prominent among which are CD80/86 interaction with CD28/CTLA-4 and CD40 interaction with CD154. Drugs that interrupt these critical signaling pathways are the subject of current clinical trials in MS. In the absence of these signals, T cells are likely to undergo apoptosis or acquire a noninflammatory (Th2) phenotype.

With regard to the APC capacities of the cellular constituents of the BBB components, human adult brain–derived endothelial cells can be induced to express the MHC and costimulatory molecules *in vitro*. Functional studies, however, indicate that interaction of such cells with nonprimed antigen-reactive T cells favor development of anergy rather than proliferation. The antigen-presenting capacity of adult human astrocytes also seems limited (Dong and Benveniste, 2001). Astrocytes do serve as potential sources of an array of immune regulatory and effector molecules, including cytokines, chemokines, and nitric oxide. The perivascular microglia are the cell type that *in situ* most prominently express both MHC and costimulatory molecules and *in vitro* are highly competent APCs. In the context of MS, monocytes, B cells, and activated T cells, all of which are prominent components of the inflammatory response, can also serve as APCs.

Within the adult human CNS parenchyma, microglia express MHC class II and costimulatory molecules even under apparently basal conditions. *In vitro* studies demonstrate that these cells can both process and present myelin antigens. The immune regulatory properties of microglia are themselves subject to regulation by molecular signals that can be derived from infiltrating immune cells or that result from disease or injury within the CNS, including to neuron/axons (Flugel et al., 2001; Nguyen et al., 2002). Microglia/macrophage uptake of myelin debris, especially if complexed with Ig, results in their activation. In contrast, phagocytosis of dead or dying cells (OGCs, lymphocytes) can result in down-regulation of activity (Chan et al., 2001).

Basis of Selective Oligodendrocyte/Myelin Injury in Multiple Sclerosis

The pathological hallmark of the early MS lesion is active demyelination associated with inflammation. As previously mentioned, there is heterogeneity among patients with regard to whether the primary injury is directed at the myelin per se or at its cell of origin, the OGC. The basis for this relatively selective OGC/myelin injury could reflect either the properties of the effector mechanisms that mediate the injury or the properties of the targets. Furthermore, one needs to consider that injury may be either lethal or sublethal.

Effector-Determined Selectivity

The working hypothesis in MS continues to be that components of the immune system constitute the effector arm of the disease process. The immune system can be considered in terms of adaptive and innate constituents. The B and T cells of the adaptive immune system have receptors with a high degree of diversity consequent to the process of rearrangement of the genes that contribute to their structure. This diversity allows for recognition of a vast array of target-specific determinants.

Antibody-Mediated Immune Responses

The long-recognized feature of intrathecal Ig production in MS, as measured by CSF analyses, and the more recent documentation of Ig deposition in the lesions of at least a subset of MS patients, indicate a humoral immune contribution to the disease process. For B cells, the Ig molecule itself serves as the antigen receptor. Myelin and OGC-directed antibodies have been detected in the serum and CSF of MS patients, although similar antibodies (e.g., antimyelin oligodendrocyte glycoprotein [MOG]) are also detected in a proportion of controls (Egg et al., 2001). Anti-MOG antibodies have also been detected within active MS lesion sites (Genain et al., 1999). Antibodies, directed at OGC progenitor cells have also been described (Niehaus et al., 2000). The determinants recognized can be protein, carbohydrate, or lipids. *In vitro* studies of OGC have not yet, however, shown that serum or CSF from MS patients selectively and specifically induces injury to these cells.

Antibodies can also provide a link whereby members of the innate immune system that are present in the inflammatory environment of MS lesions could be directed to a specific target. Members of the innate immune system include $\gamma\delta$ T cells, natural killer (NK) cells, and microglia/macrophages. These cells can all effect tissue injury by releasing an array of mediators, but due to their limited receptor heterogeneity, they would not be expected to recognize targets with the specificity of the adaptive immune system constituents. Recruitment of these nonspecific effectors to a specific target could, however, result from antibody binding to the specific target via the variable regions of the Ig molecule and to the Fc receptors that are expressed on the nonspecific effectors via the Fc portion of the molecule. This process is referred to as *antibody-dependent cell cytotoxicity* (ADCC).

$\alpha\beta$ CD4 and CD8 T Cell–Mediated Responses

As mentioned, myelin-reactive CD4 $\alpha\beta$ T cells, particularly those with a Th1 phenotype, are the cell type usually used to adoptively transfer EAE. Most current data suggest that OGCs do not express MHC class II molecules and are not susceptible to MHC class II–restricted lysis by myelin-reactive CD4 T cells. Such T cells can mediate non-MHC-restricted lysis if they upregulate the NK cell–associated surface antigen CD56 (Vergelli et al., 1996). Upregulation can be achieved *in vitro* by exposing T cell lines to cytokines (IL-2) expected to be present in an inflammatory milieu. CD8 T cells are the classic cytotoxic cell population and are prominent in the parenchyma in both MS and EAE lesions. Oligodendrocytes derived from the adult human CNS express MHC class I molecules that can be recognized by CD8 T cells. Our studies using CD8 T cells reactive to a specific peptide sequence of myelin basic protein (MBP) indicated that such cells could induce MHC class 1–restricted cytotoxicity of OGC (Jurewicz et al., 1998). Neurons whose electrical activity is interrupted can also become susceptible to cytotoxic T cell injury as a result of upregulation of MHC class I molecules on their surfaces (Neumann et al., 2002).

Target-Determined Selectivity

Relatively selective target injury, as observed in MS, in response to nonspecific effector cells and soluble molecules, could still result if a given cell target was differentially susceptible to such mediators. The potential contribution to OGC/myelin injury by molecules signaling through a number of receptors belonging to the TNF receptor (TNF-R) superfamily provide a prototype of target-determined selectivity of injury related to differential receptor expression or signaling. These receptors and their corresponding ligands include the fas-fas ligand, DR4/5 TNF-related apoptosis-inducing ligand (TRAIL), and TNF-R. All of the receptors discussed below and their ligands have been detected in the inflammatory environment of MS and/or EAE lesions.

We have observed that human OGCs, especially when exposed to IFNγ, express fas and undergo caspase-dependent cell death within 4–6 hours following exposure to fas ligand or activating anti-fas antibody (Pouly and Antel, 1999). We did not observe such injury using fetal human cortical neurons as targets. We attributed this differential cell-type injury to lack of fas expression on the neurons. Fetal human CNS-derived astrocytes express fas even under basal culture conditions but fail to activate the caspase cascade in response to fas and do not undergo programmed cell death (Wosik et al., 2001). Studies using hippocampal slice cultures demonstrate that TRAIL-mediated signaling can induce tissue injury in the CNS, although the selectivity of cell type injury remains to be defined (Nitsch et al., 2000). *In vitro* human OGCs are susceptible to TRAIL-mediated cell death only if exposed to protein synthesis inhibitors (Matysiak et al., 2002).

In contrast to the significant cell death of mature human OGCs that occurs within several hours of exposure to fas ligand, the injury effects of TNF require prolonged (several days) exposure to high concentrations of this cytokine (Ladiwala et al., 1999). Tumor necrosis factor does induce rapid activation of a number of intracellular signaling pathways, raising the question of whether the net functional effect represents the balance of injury and protective signaling pathways. *In situ* studies based largely on the use of transgenic overexpression or deletion of TNF or its receptors further indicate the dual potential effects (protection vs. injury) of this molecule (reviewed in (Finsen, 2002).

The concept of differential cell type susceptibility to nonspecific immune-to-injury mediators based on receptor expression or cell signaling variables could be extended to a wide array of cells and molecules implicated in the MS tissue injury process. $\gamma\delta$ T cells and

NK cells are highly cytotoxic to human OGC (reviewed in Pouly and Antel, 1999). Members of the heat shock protein family remain candidates as the recognition molecules for $\gamma\delta$ T cells; one such member, $\alpha\beta$ crystallin, is considered a putative autoantigen in MS. Selectivity for NK cell–mediated injury could also be conferred by the presence or absence of molecules on target cells that promote or inhibit effector-target interaction. The extent of and basis for relative susceptibility of the myelin/OGC complex to excitotoxins, pro-inflammatory cytokines, and protease-mediated injury remains under active study.

BASIS FOR RECOVERY

The recovery process from relapse in MS involves both cessation of the injury process and functional recovery of the injured tissue. The former could result from a relatively passive process in which the infiltrating disease-relevant immune cells can no longer sustain their activation state. The process may also be impacted by active immune regulatory mechanisms that can involve phenotypically specific cell subsets acting via cell-cell contact and release of anti-inflammatory cytokines. Recovery also reflects remyelination presumably mediated by progenitor cells, as discussed later, and by restoration of axonal function. The latter is mediated at least in part by redistribution of sodium channels on demyelinated nerve segments.

Perpetuation of the Disease Process

A number of immune-related mechanisms related to immune–neural cell interactions could contribute to the recurrent/chronic course of the MS disease process (Fig. 39.5). A hallmark of the active MS lesion is the presence of microglia and macrophages that contain myelin debris, indicating that these cells can take up released myelin products. Such products could then be processed, transported in conjunction with MHC molecules to the cell surface, and presented to lymphocytes in the inflammatory milieu. This sequence of events could lead to an expansion of the array of myelin antigens to which the immune system is sensitized, a phenomenon referred to as *determinant spreading*. Determinant spreading has been well documented in the chronic disease models EAE and TMEV, and can be dependent on antigen presentation inside and outside the CNS.

Initial immune and non-immune-mediated insults to OGCs could induce a series of sublethal injury responses that could render the cells susceptible to subsequent immune-mediated injury. We have found that low levels of p53 overexpression, insufficient to result in cell death, result in upregulation of fas and TRAIL receptors, making the OGC susceptible to injury by the ligands for these receptors (Wosik et al., 2003). P53 overexpression can be observed *in situ* in MS cases featuring early OGC loss. Among neural cells, OGCs seem especially likely to upregulate expression of inducible stress proteins (inducible heat shock proteins) in response to sublethal injury (reviewed in Pouly and Antel, 1999).

Protection and Repair in Multiple Sclerosis

Neural-immune interaction can also contribute to the processes of protection and repair. Human astrocytes appear to be poor APCs and thus might downregulate the activity of effector cells with which they may interact. Astrocytes have the capacity to take up a number of potential OGC/myelin injury-mediating molecules including reactive oxygen species and glutamate. Glial cells and immune cells can be sources of neurotrophin molecules that may exert a neuroprotective effect (Villoslada et al., 2000).

Histological and MR-based studies document that remyelination does occur in the early inflammation-dominated MS lesions. Antibodies are described that can promote myelin formation or regeneration. Most tend to be of germline origin rather than having undergone Ig gene rearrangement (Warrington et al., 2001). Most experimental data suggest that remyelination in the CNS is derived from progenitor cells that enter the lesion site and mature into myelin-forming cells. Multipotential and glial-restricted progenitor cells have been detected in the adult human CNS, including in the region of MS lesions (Chang et al., 2002). The process of progenitor cell activation and differentiation is dependent on specific molecular growth factor signals. To be determined is the extent to which these can be derived both from the glial environment and from infiltrating inflammatory cells in MS. Conversely, one needs to consider whether progenitor cells are more or less susceptible to the injury processes that affect the mature OGC/myelin complex.

Axon injury and transection are well recognized in MS lesions and are demonstrated to contribute significantly to neurological dysfunction. Central nervous system myelin has been shown to inhibit axonal outgrowth. Immunization of animals with myelin and administration of specific myelin component–directed antibodies are being used to improve recovery in spinal cord injured experimental animals (Huang et al., 1999). The capacity of microglia/macrophages to clear myelin debris could thus be viewed as contributing to the repair process. Axonal recovery in CNS injury models has also been observed following local or systemic injection of myelin-reactive T cells (Schwartz and Kipnis, 2001). The latter observations raise the challenge of how to predict beneficial versus harmful immune-mediated responses in the outbred human population.

CONCLUSION

The MS disease process continues to be viewed as one in which the interaction between the immune system and the nervous system contributes to both the injury and recovery components. The clinical experience with systemic immune therapy raises the concern that such therapy, even if initiated early on, will not be sufficient to completely control the cascade of events within the CNS that result in fixed tissue injury and persistent clinical deficits. Further understanding of the molecular mechanisms involved in these processes will hopefully lead to new therapeutic interventions that can promote protection and repair of the CNS.

REFERENCES

Becher, B., Prat, A., and Antel, J.P. (2000) Brain-immune connection: immuno-regulatory properties of CNS-resident cells. *Glia* 29:293–304.

Bieganowska, K.D., Ausubel, L.J., Modabber, Y., Slovik, E., Messersmith, W., and Hafler, D.A. (1997) Direct ex vivo analysis of activated, Fas-sensitive autoreactive T cells in human autoimmune disease. *J. Exp. Med.* 185:1585–1594.

Bjartmar, C., Battistuta, J., Terada, N., Dupree, E., and Trapp, B.D. (2002) N-acetylaspartate is an axon-specific marker of mature white matter in vivo: a biochemical and immunohistochemical study on the rat optic nerve. *Ann. Neurol.* 51:51–58.

Brabb, T., von Dassow, P., Ordonez, N., Schnabel, B., Duke, B., and Goverman, J. (2000) In situ tolerance within the central nervous system as a mechanism for preventing autoimmunity. *J. Exp. Med.* 192:871–880.

Brex, P.A., Ciccarelli, O., O'Riordan, J.I., Sailer, M., Thompson, A.J., and Miller, D.H. (2002) A longitudinal study of abnormalities on MRI and disability from multiple sclerosis. *N. Engl. J. Med.* 346:158–164.

Caramanos, Z., Santos, A.C., and Arnold, D.L. (2002) Magnetic resonance imaging and spectroscopy: Insights into the pathology and pathophysiology of multiple sclerosis. In: McDonald, W.I. and Noseworthy, J.H., eds. *Multiple Sclerosis.* Butterworth-Heinemann, pp. 139–167.

Chan, A., Magnus, T., and Gold, R. (2001) Phagocytosis of apoptotic inflammatory cells by microglia and modulation by different cytokines: mechanism for removal of apoptotic cells in the inflamed nervous system. *Glia* 33:87–95.

Chang, A., Tourtellotte, W.W., Rudick, R., and Trapp, B.D. (2002) Premyelinating oligodendrocytes in chronic lesions of multiple sclerosis. *N. Engl. J. Med.* 346:165–173.

Charcot, J.M. (1877) *Lectures on Diseases of the Nervous System*, Sigerson, G., ed. and trans. London: The New Sydenham Society, pp. 158–222.

Chishty, M., Reichel, A., Begley, D.J., and Abbott, N.J. (2002) Glial induction of blood–brain barrier-like L-system amino acid transport in the ECV304 cell line. *Glia* 39:99–104.

Dong, Y. and Benveniste, E.N. (2001) Immune function of astrocytes. *Glia* 36:180–190.

Egg, R., Reindl, M., Deisenhammer, F., Linington, C., and Berger, T. (2001) Anti-MOG and anti-MBP antibody subclasses in multiple sclerosis. *Mult. Scler.* 7:285–289.

Finsen, B., Antel, J., and Owens, T. (2002) TNF alpha: kill or cure for demyelinating disease? *Mol. Psychiatry* 7:820–821.

Flugel, A., Bradl, M., Kreutzberg, G.W., and Graeber, M.B. (2001) Transformation of donor-derived bone marrow precursors into host microglia during autoimmune CNS inflammation and during the retrograde response to axotomy. *J. Neurosci. Res.* 66: 74–82.

Gadian, D.G. (1996) *NMR and Its Applications to Living Systems*, 2nd ed. Oxford: Oxford University Press.

Genain, C.P., Cannella, B., Hauser, S.L., and Raine, C.S. (1999) Identification of autoantibodies associated with myelin damage in multiple sclerosis. *Nat. Med.* 5:170–175.

Giess, R., Maurer, M., Linker, R., Gold, R., Warmuth-Metz, M., Toyka, K.V., Sendtner, M., and Rieckmann, P. (2002) Association of a null mutation in the CNTF gene with early onset of multiple sclerosis. *Arch. Neurol.* 59:407–409.

Hammond, W.A. (1871) *A Treatise on Diseases of the Nervous System.* New York: D. Appleton.

Huang, D.W., McKerracher, L., Braun, P.E., and David, S. (1999) A therapeutic vaccine approach to stimulate axon regeneration in the adult mammalian spinal cord. *Neuron* 24:639–647.

Jurewicz, A., Biddison, W.E., and Antel, J.P. (1998) MHC class I-restricted lysis of human oligodendrocytes by myelin basic protein peptide-specific CD8 T lymphocytes. *J. Immunol.* 160: 3056–3059.

Katz-Levy, Y., Neville, K.L., Girvin, A.M., Vanderlugt, C.L., Pope, J.G., Tan, L.J., and Miller, S.D. (1999) Endogenous presentation of self myelin epitopes by CNS-resident APCs in Theiler's virus-infected mice. *J. Clin. Invest.* 104:599–610.

Ladiwala, U., Li, H., Antel, J.P., and Nalbantoglu, J. (1999) p53 induction by tumor necrosis factor-alpha and involvement of p53 in cell death of human oligodendrocytes. *J. Neurochem.* 73: 605–611.

Lucchinetti, C., Bruck, W., Parisi, J., Scheithauer, B., Rodriguez, M., and Lassmann, H. (2000) Heterogeneity of multiple sclerosis lesions: implications for the pathogenesis of demyelination. *Ann. Neurol.* 47:707–717.

Maas, K., Chan, S., Parker, J., Slater, A., Moore, J., Olsen, N., and Aune, T.M. (2002) Cutting edge: molecular portrait of human autoimmune disease. *J. Immunol.* 169:5–9.

Matysiak, M., Jurewicz, A., Jaskolski, D., and Selma, J.K. (2002) TRAIL induces death of human oligodendrocytes isolated from adult brain. *Brain* 125:2469–2480.

McDonald, W.I., Compston, A., Edan, G., Goodkin, D., Hartung, H.P., Lublin, F.D., McFarland, H.F., Paty, D.W., Polman, C.H., Reingold, S.C., Sandberg-Wollheim, M., Sibley, W., Thompson, A., van den, N.S., Weinshenker, B.Y., and Wolinsky, J.S. (2001) Recommended diagnostic criteria for multiple sclerosis: guidelines from the International Panel on the diagnosis of multiple sclerosis. *Ann. Neurol.* 50:121–127.

Miller, D.H., Grossman, R.I., Reingold, S.C., and McFarland, H.F. (1998) The role of magnetic resonance techniques in understanding and managing multiple sclerosis. *Brain* 121 (Pt 1):3–24.

Miller, D.H., Khan, O.A., Sheremata, W.A., Blumhardt, L.D., Rice, G.P., Libonati, M.A., Willmer-Hulme, A.J., Dalton, C.M., Miszkiel, K.A., and O'Connor, P.W. (2003) A controlled trial of natalizumab for relapsing multiple sclerosis. *N. Engl. J Med.* 348:15–23.

Murray, T.J. (2000) The history of multiple sclerosis. In: Burks, J.S. and Johnson, K.P., eds. *Multiple Sclerosis: Diagnosis, Medical Management, and Rehabilitation.* New York: Demos Medical, pp. 1–34.

Neuhaus, O., Farina, C., Wekerle, H., and Hohlfeld, R. (2001) Mechanisms of action of glatiramer acetate in multiple sclerosis. *Neurology* 56:702–708.

Neumann, H., Medana, I.M., Bauer, J., and Lassmann, H. (2002) Cytotoxic T lymphocytes in autoimmune and degenerative CNS diseases. *Trends Neurosci.* 25:313–319.

Nguyen, M.D., Julien, J.P., and Rivest, S. (2002) Innate immunity: the missing link in neuroprotection and neurodegeneration? *Nat. Rev. Neurosci.* 3:216–227.

Niehaus, A., Shi, J., Grzenkowski, M., Diers-Fenger, M., Archelos, J., Hartung, H.P., Toyka, K., Bruck, W., and Trotter, J. (2000) Patients with active relapsing-remitting multiple sclerosis synthesize antibodies recognizing oligodendrocyte progenitor cell surface protein: implications for remyelination. *Ann. Neurol.* 48:362–371.

Nitsch, R., Bechmann, I., Deisz, R.A., Haas, D., Lehmann, T.N., Wendling, U., and Zipp, F. (2000) Human brain-cell death induced by tumour-necrosis-factor-related apoptosis-inducing ligand (TRAIL). *Lancet* 356:827–828.

O'Connor, K.C., Bar-Or, A., and Hafler, D.A. (2001) The neuroimmunology of multiple sclerosis: possible roles of T and B lymphocytes in immunopathogenesis. *J. Clin. Immunol.* 21:81–92.

Paty, D. and Ebers, G.C. (1997) *Multiple Sclerosis*. Philadelphia: F.A. Davis.

Pouly, S. and Antel, J.P. (1999) Multiple sclerosis and central nervous system demyelination. *J. Autoimmun.* 13:297–306.

Prat, A., Biernacki, K., Lavoie, J.F., Poirier, J., Duquette, P., and Antel, J.P. (2002) Migration of multiple sclerosis lymphocytes through brain endothelium. *Arch. Neurol.* 59:391–397.

Prat, A., Biernacki, K., Wosik, K., and Antel, J.P. (2001) Glial cell influence on the human blood–brain barrier. *Glia* 36:145–155.

Qin, Y., Duquette, P., Zhang, Y., Talbot, P., Poole, R., and Antel, J. (1998) Clonal expansion and somatic hypermutation of V(H) genes of B cells from cerebrospinal fluid in multiple sclerosis. *J. Clin. Invest* 102:1045–1050.

Schreiber, K., Otura, A.B., Ryder, L.P., Madsen, H.O., Jorgensen, O.S., Svejgaard, A., and Sorensen, P.S. (2002) Disease severity in Danish multiple sclerosis patients evaluated by MRI and three genetic markers (HLA-DRB1*1501, CCR5 deletion mutation, apolipoprotein E). *Mult. Scler.* 8:295–298.

Schwartz, M. and Kipnis, J. (2001) Protective autoimmunity: regulation and prospects for vaccination after brain and spinal cord injuries. *Trends Mol. Med.* 7:252–258.

Simmons, M.L., Frondoza, C.G., and Coyle, J.T. (1991) Immunocytochemical localization of *N*-acetyl-aspartate with monoclonal antibodies. *Neuroscience* 45:37–45.

Sung, M.H., Zhao, Y., Martin, R., and Simon, R. (2002) T-cell epitope prediction with combinatorial peptide libraries. *J. Comput. Biol.* 9:527–539.

Talbot, P.J., Arnold, D., and Antel, J.P. (2001) Virus-induced autoimmune reactions in the CNS. *Curr. Top. Microbiol. Immunol.* 253:247–271.

Vergelli, M., Le, H., van Noort, J.M., Dhib-Jalbut, S., McFarland, H., and Martin, R. (1996) A novel population of CD4+CD56+ myelin-reactive T cells lyses target cells expressing CD56/neural cell adhesion molecule. *J Immunol.* 157:679–688.

Villoslada, P., Hauser, S.L., Bartke, I., Unger, J., Heald, N., Rosenberg, D., Cheung, S.W., Mobley, W.C., Fisher, S., and Genain, C.P. (2000) Human nerve growth factor protects common marmosets against autoimmune encephalomyelitis by switching the balance of T helper cell type 1 and 2 cytokines within the central nervous system. *J. Exp. Med.* 191:1799–1806.

Warrington, A.E., Bieber, A.J., Ciric, B., Van, K.V., Pease, L.R., Mitsunaga, Y., Paz Soldan, M.M., and Rodriguez, M. (2001) Immunoglobulin-mediated CNS repair. *J. Allergy Clin. Immunol.* 108:S121–S125.

Wosik, K., Antel, J., Kuhlmann, T., Bruck, W., Massie, B., and Nalbantoglu, J. (2003) Oligodendrocyte injury in multiple sclerosis: a role for p53. *J Neurochem* 85:635–644.

Wosik, K., Becher, B., Ezman, A., Nalbantoglu, J., and Antel, J.P. (2001) Caspase 8 expression and signaling in Fas injury-resistant human fetal astrocytes. *Glia* 33:217–224.

Yong, V.W. (2002) Differential mechanisms of action of interferon-beta and glatiramer aetate in MS. *Neurology* 59:802–808.

40 Human immunodeficiency virus infection of the central nervous system

ELENA RYZHOVA, DENNIS L. KOLSON, AND FRANCISCO GONZÁLEZ-SCARANO

A significant proportion of individuals with human immunodeficiency virus (HIV) infection develop a neurological syndrome consisting of psychomotor retardation, dementia, and associated findings that was initially termed the *acquired immunodeficiency syndrome (AIDS) dementia complex*. The name of this syndrome has undergone several revisions as new clinical and pathological information has become available, and it is now commonly known as *HIV-associated dementia* (HAD). The pathological entity that is associated with the clinical syndrome is usually referred to as *HIV encephalitis* (HIVE). Because, as we will discuss later, there is no strict concordance between the clinical and pathological syndromes, and because, depending on the specific series, not all patients have both clinical and pathological features, the terms should not be used interchangeably.

CLINICAL AND PATHOLOGICAL FEATURES OF HUMAN IMMUNODEFICIENCY VIRUS–ASSOCIATED DEMENTIA

Patients with HAD initially complain of minor memory defects and may require help with activities requiring complex recall. Whether otherwise asymptomatic individuals with HIV infection have any subtle evidence of cognitive impairment has been the subject of considerable research. The preponderant view is that although there may be some physiological and neuropsychological differences between infected individuals and appropriate control subjects, there are no significant functional deficits in patients with otherwise asymptomatic early HIV disease (Goethe et al., 1989). Progression to full HAD takes the form of motor and psychomotor retardation, with gait disorders, ataxia, and clumsiness of fine finger movements (Sacktor et al., 2002). In the most severe cases, these may eventually lead to deterioration to a nearly vegetative state.

Neuropsychological testing is widely used as a screening and research tool for studies of HIV effects on the central nervous system (CNS), but there are no other laboratory tests with sufficient sensitivity and specificity that help in the diagnosis of HAD, except by excluding other entities. Nevertheless, high cerebrospinal fluid (CSF) levels of HIV RNA can be related to the development of HAD and other neurological symptoms (Tambussi et al., 2000), and quantitative magnetic resonance imaging (MRI) analysis has shown the development of cerebral atrophy (Bencherif and Rottenberg, 1998), as well as biochemical abnormalities associated with glial activation and astrocytosis (Ernst et al., 2000). Some patients with HAD have areas of high signal intensity and other changes in the periventricular white matter seen in conventional MRI; these have been attributed to leakage of the blood–brain barrier (Power et al., 1993). The CSF of many HIV-infected patients may also have a mild inflammatory component, particularly during the early stages after infection, and some patients may have full-blown meningitis, even at the time of primary infection with HIV.

Prior to the widespread use of highly active antiretroviral therapy (HAART), the prevalence of HAD among male patients with HIV infection was estimated to be up to 20 per 100 person-years, depending on the stage of immunodeficiency. Epidemiological studies in women came later, but have in general confirmed equal susceptibility of both sexes to the effects of HIV in the CNS. The use of antiretroviral therapy has dramatically reduced the incidence of HAD. Although there are relatively few large-scale studies with which to update

See the list of abbreviations at the end of the chapter.

this number, in 1998 the incidence rate was down to fewer than 5 per 100 person-years (Sacktor et al., 2002). A less severe form of the disease, HIV-associated mild neurocognitive impairment, has been recognized in some patients who are undergoing effective therapy, and some have postulated that this less severe disorder could be just as common as HAD. However, a small study indicated that the patients on HAART are less likely to have even this mild form of HIV disease of the CNS. Nevertheless, as these individuals will presumably live longer than those with fully developed HAD because of immunological improvement, the overall prevalence of HIV-related neurological disease, albeit of a milder form, could remain steady.

Pathological Findings

The neuropathological findings in HAD are not only a cardinal feature of the disease that helps define its pathophysiology, but are arguably the most consistently accepted findings among investigators of this syndrome. As expected from the primarily neuronal manifestations of HAD, the brains of individuals with the disease have decreased numbers of neurons (Everall et al., 1993). Recent studies have demonstrated that the neuronal loss is associated with various signatures associated with apoptosis, such as DNA fragmentation and electron micrographic changes (for review see Kaul et al., 2001). Careful studies have demonstrated that the basal ganglia are most affected by HIV-induced neuronal apoptosis (D.L. Kolson et al., unpublished), a finding consistent with the higher prevalence of other changes in these areas (Fig. 40.1).

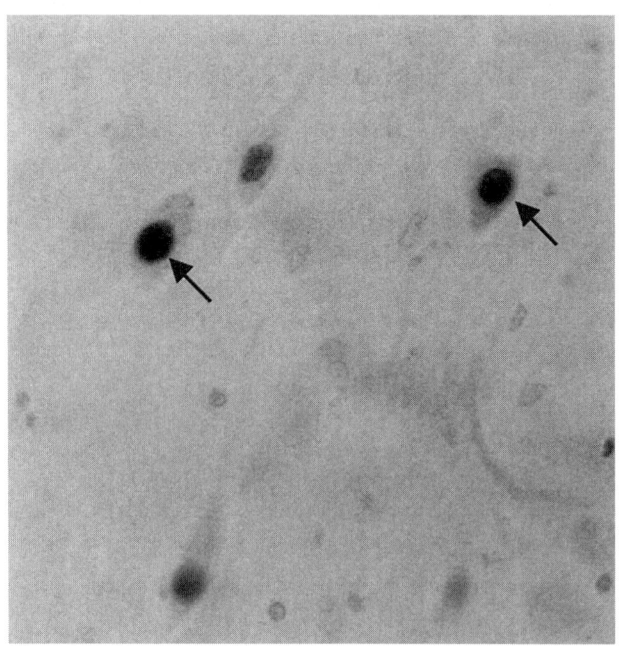

FIGURE 40.1 Neuronal apoptosis in the frontal cortex in an individual with acquired immune deficiency syndrome dementia. Terminal dUTP nick and labeling assay (TUNEL) was performed on a formalin-fixed, paraffin-embedded section of frontal cortex, demonstrating apoptotic nuclei in pyramidal neurons (*arrows*).

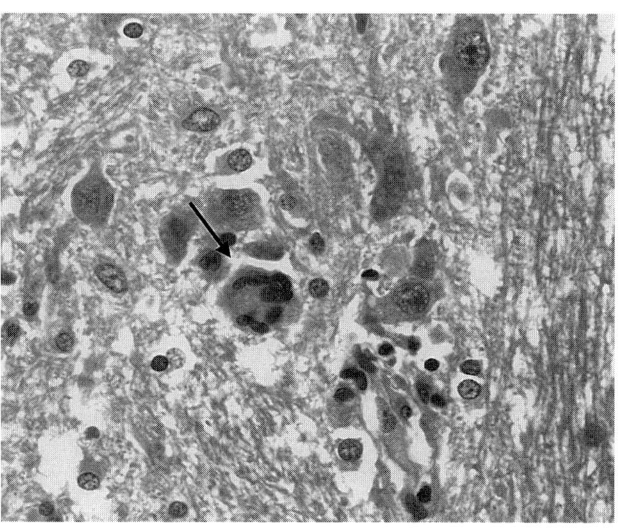

FIGURE 40.2 Multinucleated giant cell. The brain of an individual with human immunodeficiency virus encephalitis shows prominent syncytia (*arrow*). These syncytia are formed by the fusion of infected and uninfected cells that is mediated by the interaction between the viral glycoproteins, gp120 and gp41, and the cellular receptors, CD4 and CCR5. The life span of multinucleated giant cells is unknown. (Photomicrograph courtesy of Dr. Ehud Lavi, University of Pennsylvania Dept. of Pathology and Laboratory Medicine.)

However, the most specific finding in HIVE is the presence of multinucleated giant cells—which essentially define this entity. The formation of syncytia is a characteristic of HIV infection of many cell types *in vitro*, and the brain is one of two principal sites where this cytopathology can be visualized *in vivo*. Figure 40.2 demonstrates giant cell formation in a perivascular region of the brain of an individual with HIVE.

Based on extensive studies *in vitro*, the formation of giant cells is thought to be the result of the interaction between the two HIV viral glycoproteins, gp120 and gp41, and the cellular surface proteins that serve as receptors for the virus: CD4 and one of a number of chemokine receptors that have been adopted by the virus as their mechanism of cellular entry. For microglia, the principal chemokine receptor used for HIV entry is CCR5 (Albright et al., 1999), normally the receptor for macrophage inflammatory protein (MIP) 1-α and MIP 1-β. As microglia and other brain macrophages are the only cells in the CNS that express both CD4 and CCR5, they are the principal cells infected by HIV and the only cells that routinely demonstrate evidence of infection, whether they are examined for the expression of proteins or message RNA (Takahashi et al., 1996). Strains of HIV also vary somewhat in their use of receptors; some strains preferentially use another chemokine receptor, CXCR4, normally the receptor for stromal-derived factor-1 (SDF-1). CXCR4 and SDF-1 have an important role in neuronal migration, currently being studied extensively (Zou et al., 1998), and CXCR4 is expressed in many cells within the CNS, including subpopulations of neurons and astrocytes (Lavi et al., 1997; van der Meer et al., 2000). Under some circumstances, it is conceivable that HIV could enter some cells through the use of a single receptor, namely, either CCR5 or CXCR4, and such a scenario would explain occasional reports of HIV infection of neurons and other cells that do not express CD4. However, most HIV strains recovered from the CNS use CCR5 as their receptor, so the potential for significant infection of neurons via this CD4-independent pathway is relatively limited.

In vitro infection of primary astrocytes and astrocyte-derived cell lines has been widely reported in studies of HIV infection. Infection of astrocytes *in situ* is less common, however. *In situ* hybridization studies have indeed demonstrated that some astrocytes harbor and express HIV sequences (Saito et al., 1994; Tornatore et al., 1994), and one study correlated the presence of HAD with astrocytic apoptosis (Thompson et al., 2001). As much as quantitative comparisons can be made of qualitative neuropathological data, in terms of their contribution to the viral load in the CNS, astrocytes are minor players. Regarding the role of astrocytic apoptosis in mediating the clinical changes of HAD, while it is intuitively more likely that neuronal apopotosis is of greater importance, astrocytes may influence neuronal damage through their effects on glutamate uptake (see following sections).

PATHOPHYSIOLOGY OF HUMAN IMMUNODEFICIENCY VIRUS–ASSOCIATED DEMENTIA

Role of Monocytes and Lymphocytes in the Entry of Human Immunodeficiency Virus into the Central Nervous System

Certain viral isolates and specific tropisms are associated with the development of HAD (Strizki et al., 1996; Martin et al., 2001; Gorry et al., 2002). First of all, those strains that use CCR5 predominate among the brain isolates, as indicated previously. Strains that use CCR5 are typically associated with specific tropism for macrophage and macrophage-like cells such as microglia (Albright et al., 1999), reinforcing the key role of this cell type in neuropathogenesis.

Macrophages residing in the perivascular regions are the principal cells expressing virus; those cells have a relatively high turnover in comparison to parenchymal microglia, which are long-lived (Lassmann et al., 1993). These findings support a dynamic process of viral entry and replacement mediated by circulating monocytes and perivascular macrophages. At the same time, multiple studies have documented that HIV strains compartmentalize within the brain (discussed below), indicating that their presence in the CNS is long-standing. This suggests that parenchymal microglia must be involved at some steps in the viral cycle, as they imply long-term viral residence within the neuraxis. We propose a model whereby infected circulating monocytes penetrate the brain and infect the first susceptible cell available: the perivascular macrophage and, less frequently, parenchymal microglia, which when infected may not express virus as robustly. Whereas the perivascular macrophages circulate out of the CNS, and therefore could not sustain the long-term infection that is necessary for independent viral evolution, parenchymal microglia may sustain a lower-level but longer-term infection. Ultimately, the formation of multinucleated giant cells (MNGCs) is a function of both subtypes of brain macrophages.

Viral Adaptation within the Central Nervous System

Many investigators have documented that HIV strains may compartmentalize into specific tissues, and genetic analyses of HIV variants in the CNS have been particularly consistent. This is potentially the result of the specific isolation of the CNS given the blood–brain barrier, as well as the brain-specific immunological milieu. As indicated previously, brain isolates generally use CCR5 as their coreceptor, consistent with the predominance of brain macrophages and microglia as the cellular hosts within the CNS. Furthermore, regardless of the gene analyzed (*pol* or *env* have been most common), investigators have routinely found genetic differences between viral genetic material obtained from the brain parenchyma and material from other tissues, particularly the spleen and blood (Hughes et al., 1997; Wong et al., 1997) (Fig. 40.3). The CSF behaves as at least a partially separate compartment, and strains from the choroid plexus appear to be related to those from both blood and brain parenchyma (Chen et al., 2000). Some investigators have therefore suggested that the choroid plexus is a major site for HIV entry.

Although the genetic evidence is quite consistent, there is considerably less understanding of the force driving these changes. One possibility is that they are a reflection of the HIV molecular clock, which has been estimated at 0.19 substitutions/base pair/year, in an isolated population of cells with a low turnover. Alternatively, strain variability may reflect selection for replication in the brain (either robust or controlled, whichever is more advantageous to the virus in the CNS).

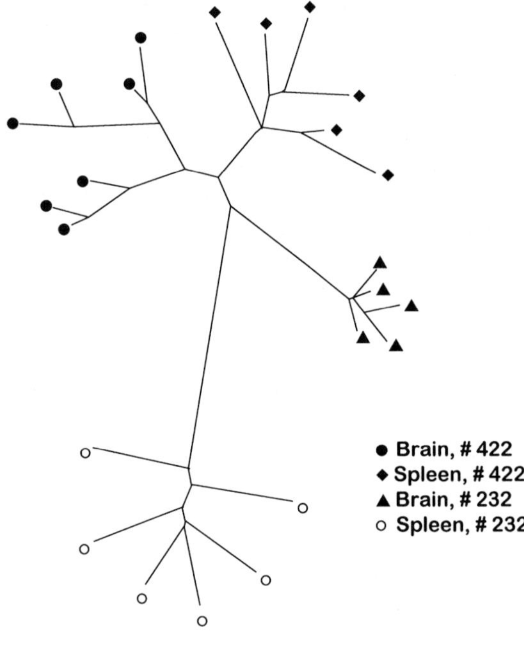

FIGURE 40.3 Genetic relationship between viral sequences obtained from the brain and splenic tissue of animals with simian immunodeficiency virus infection. Phylogenetic analysis of full-length *env* genes obtained from spleen and brain of two rhesus macaques (#422 and #232). The unrooted phylogram depicts the strict segregation of brain viral sequences from those from the periphery. The scale bar shows the genetic distance estimated by the Neighbor-Joining evolutionary model (see Ryzhova et al., 2002, for details).

Dynamics of Human Immunodeficiency Virus Evolution in the Central Nervous System

Neuroinvasion, the ability to enter the CNS after peripheral infection, is thought to be a common feature of all of the lentiviruses. However, despite ample documentation that HIV can enter the brain at early points after infection, primary viral seeding does not seem to result in productive infection, and neither viral RNA nor antigens are present in the brain in large quantities during the asymptomatic phase of AIDS. Clearance of the virus from the CNS during primary infection may be orchestrated by a small fraction of activated microglia/brain macrophages and T lymphocytes patrolling the brain under normal conditions (reviewed in Hickey, 2001) and participating in immune surveillance. Nevertheless, productive and robust viral replication is commonly found in the CNS during terminal AIDS, coincident with the onset of immunosuppression. Similar dynamics of viral turnover were observed in the rhesus macaque simian AIDS model (SAIDS). Simian immunodeficiency virus (SIV) replication, which was detected as early as days 7–10 after infection in the brain of infected macaques, was suppressed to an undetectable level by day 21, although there was persistent viral DNA. Examination of necropsy tissue samples after the onset of SAIDS showed that viral replication recrudesced later in the course of infection, particularly in those animals that progressed to SIV-associated encephalitis (Williams et al., 2001; Clements et al., 2002).

The fluctuation of virus production within the CNS can be explained by a number of potential mechanisms. First of all, the initial seeding could be composed of a viral quasi-species that is poorly adapted to the CNS; viral evolution that would be expected to increase fitness for the new environment is terminated by the immune-mediated response. Subsequent immunological failure facilitates the widespread growth of viral variants with increased ability to replicate in nonlymphoid tissues, including the CNS. The addition of this population, possibly through several waves of neuroinvasion, may result in successful evolution in the brain and lead to the emergence of viral strains that are particularly capable of efficient replication within CNS cells, specifically microglia.

Another possibility is that the strains responsible for the initial seeding escape immune-mediated clearance and establish a latent reservoir in the relatively long-living microglia. Occasional activation of these quiescently infected cells may provide low levels of ongoing replication, supporting the adaptive evolution in the brain over years of infection. These potential scenarios are not mutually exclusive, and data recently accumulating in our laboratory, as well as others, have demonstrated that late neuroinvasion and activation of a latent reservoir may contribute to the viral evolution within the brain (Wang et al., 2001; Clements et al., 2002; Lui et al., 2002; Ryzhova et al., 2002).

Perivascular macrophages and parenchymal microglia are the principal target cells for HIV in the brain. Thus, macrophage tropism (M-tropism), the ability to productively infect macrophage-lineage cells, is a prerequisite for the neurotropic phenotype. Indeed, the SIV strains associated with CNS disease, and most HIV strains isolated from the brain, also exhibit M-tropism (Mankowski et al., 1997; Gorry et al., 2002). Not surprisingly, the viral populations detected in brain autopsy samples are genetically linked to those in peripheral samples isolated from tissues where macrohages are abundant, such as the lung and colon. In fact, quasi-species from these two organs showed the closest relation to the brain variants (Wang et al., 2001), indicating that viral populations in these anatomical sites had a common precursor. The shared evolutionary history can be used to determine the time of divergence of these populations using a molecular clock hypothesis. Estimates for two cases of SIV encephalitis showed that these two populations are segregated during the last quarter of the course of the disease (E. Ryzhova, unpublished data). Furthermore, division into several subgroups was evident within the brain-specific population, possibly as a result of discrete episodes of neuroinvasions occurring during the terminal phase of AIDS.

To conclude, these data suggest that peripheral M-tropic strains invade the CNS, possibly on a regular basis, when HIV infection is advanced enough to lead to immunodeficiency. Having seeded the brain, the M-tropic founder strains further evolve, resulting in the compartmentalized brain-specific population identified in autopsy samples. These brain quasi-species may arise because of genetic drift of a relatively isolated population or may be due to selection for the variants that are particularly fit for replication in the CNS.

Recent observations that the brain populations from independent cases of HIV dementia as well as SIV encephalitis may converge to a similar genotype (Power et al., 1998; Ryzhova et al., 2002) argue for adaptive selection. Indeed, M-tropism, being a requirement for productive replication in the CNS, is insufficient for complete manifestation of the neurotropic phenotype; accordingly, infection of experimental animals with the SIV M-tropic strain does not necessarily result in the development of encephalitis (Flaherty et al., 1997). In addition to macrophage tropism, some neurotropic viruses isolated from both human and monkey brains exhibit some relaxation of the dependence on CD4, enhanced affinity for CCR5, and neutralization sensitivity—closely related features that are possibly acquired through the adaptation to the low CD4 content of microglia (Gorry et al., 2002; Puffer et al., 2002; Ryzhova et al., 2002). They also have increased fusogenic capacity and an increased propensity to induce neuronal death in some assays (Power et al., 1998; Gorry et al., 2002). Importantly, similar phenotypic characteristics were reproduced in an HIV strain obtained via the adaptation of the parental M-tropic strain to robust replication in adult microglia (Strizki et al., 1996). Furthermore, the similarity between naturally evolved neuropathogenic HIV and SIV isolates and laboratory strains adapted to microglia is not restricted to the phenotypic resemblance, but in some cases includes shared nucleotide variations in the envelope protein, particularly the loss of a potential glycosylation site in the stem of the V1/V2 loop (Martin et al., 2001; Shieh et al., 2000). These striking similarities point to adaptive selection for the microglia-tropic phenotype as a possible force driving the evolution of the viral population in the brain.

Microglia as a Cellular Reservoir for Latent Infection in the Central Nervous System

The CNS has long been suggested to be a potential anatomical site for a latent viral infection due to its relative immunological sequestration. Resident microglia represent a stable cell pool with slow turnover, and as such, microglia were hypothesized to be a likely cellular compartment for latent infection in the brain. One validation of this hypothesis comes from an *in vitro* model where nonactivated primary human adult microglia have been infected with HIV and preserve the integrated virus for close to 3 months, which is the life span of cultured microglia. Subsequent activation of the quiescently infected cells resulted in efficient viral production (Albright et al., 2000; A.V. Albright et al., unpublished).

In vivo evidence supporting a model where microglia serve as a reservoir for latent HIV infection was recently obtained from analysis of viral transcripts expressed in single MNGCs in SIV encephalitis (SIVE) (Ryzhova et al., 2002). In this study, individual MNGCs were dissected from brain sections collected at necropsy from an animal that had been infected with an SIV molecular clone of known sequence (Fig. 40.4*A*). The majority of the viral transcripts detected in the single cells represented a brain-specific population that had been identified by analysis of SIV proviral DNA obtained from larger regions of the brain. This population was significantly divergent both from the initial inoculum and from viral sequences prevalent in the periphery, reflecting evolution in the brain. But several MNGCs expressed minor groups of sequences that were closely related or identical to the initial inoculum in the region analyzed (Fig. 40.4*B*). This indicates that viral variants entering the brain during primary infection were not eradicated completely, but rather escaped immune surveillance by establishing a latent infection, presumably in long-lived microglia (although possibly in other brain macrophages). It is also possible that a subset of latently infected microglia may undergo continuous and gradually accelerating activation in response to brain inflammation over the course of the disease, supporting a low rate but ongoing expression of a latent viral pool.

ROLE OF MICROGLIA IN MEDIATING NEURONAL INJURY IN HUMAN IMMUNODEFICIENCY VIRUS INFECTION

Human immunodeficiency virus–associated dementia is distinguished from almost all other viral diseases of the nervous system by its chronicity and other clinical features, but its most important distinction is in its pathophysiology. In spite of severe cognitive and motor deterioration, abnormalities usually attributed to neuronal deterioration, there is in fact little evidence of infection of neurons in HAD or HIVE. The level of viral replication is also qualitatively low in comparison with conventional CNS infections by other viruses such as herpes simplex virus or arboviruses (difficult as those

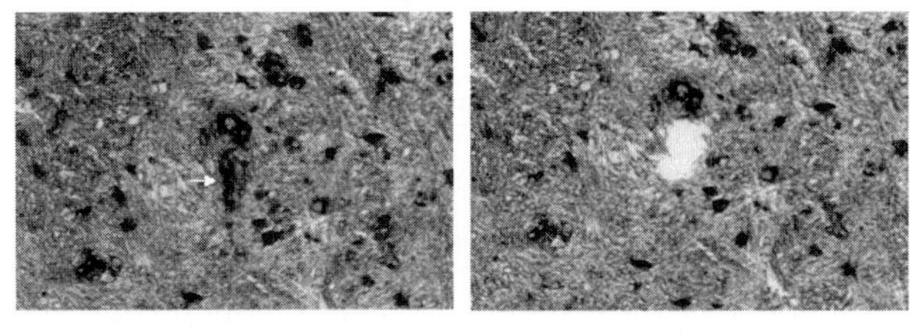

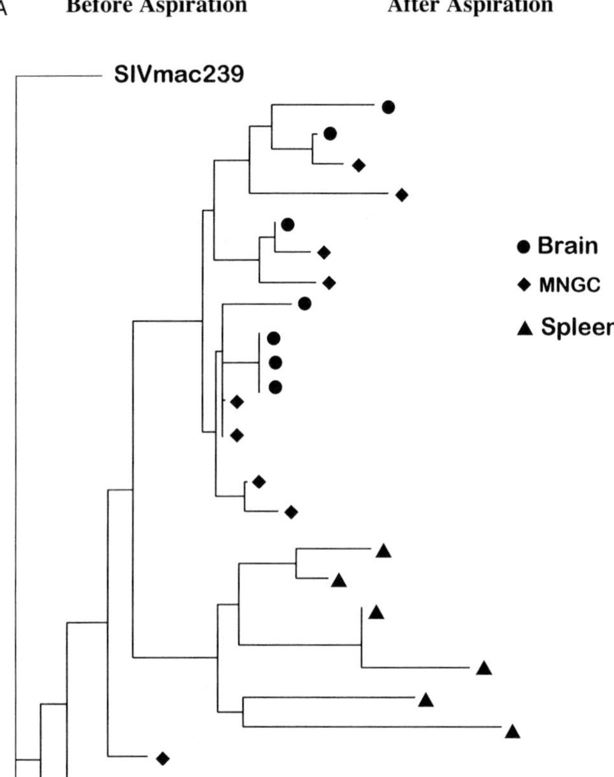

FIGURE 40.4 Single cell aspiration and genetic analysis in simian immunodeficiency virus (SIV) encephalitis. *A.* A brain section of a rhesus macaque with SIV infection was stained with RCA120 to identify syncytia formed by SIV-infected cells of macrophage lineage. The cytoplasm from a multinucleated giant cell was then aspirated from the stained section by a light microscopy microdissection technique, and any expressed SIV *env* sequences were amplified by a modified reverse transcriptase–polymerase chain reaction technique. The stained section before (left panel) and after (right panel) dissection is shown. (Adapted from Ryzhova et al., 2002.) *B.* Phylogenetic analysis of relatedness between viruses from spleen, brain tissue samples, and single multinucleated giant cell identified archival sequences that were close or identical to the initial inoculum, molecularly cloned strain SIVmac239. This is consistent with long-term preservation of the original virus inoculum in long-lived microglial cells.

comparisons may be). In general, assays for viral RNA in the CSF show some correlation with the development of HAD, and a similar correlation holds in the best animal model for this disease, SIV infection of rhesus macaques. In fact, there is general agreement that an *amplification factor*—something other than conventional viral cytopathology—is critical for the development of the clinical syndrome, and that the brain macrophage is likely to be the source of such a factor (Fig. 40.5). A number of potential secretion products have been proposed as the key mediators of neurotoxicity in HAD, categorized into two main groups: viral proteins and endogenous macrophage products (Table 40.1). Among the viral proteins, gp120, one of the two viral glycoproteins responsible for binding and entry, and *tat*, a viral transactivator, have received the widest attention.

The role of gp120 in neurodegeneration was first proposed following the observation of the toxic effect of gp120 on rat hyppocampal neurons *in vitro* (Brenneman et al., 1988). Subsequently, this suggestion was confirmed by *in vivo* studies demonstrating that injection of gp120 into rat hippocampus resulted in the death of neurons in the area of injection (Barks et al., 1997). The hypothesis was further supported by the observation that transgenic mice expressing gp120 in astrocytes displayed a pattern of neuropathological changes similar to those seen in the brains of HIV-infected individuals. Furthermore, the severity of the pathology was regionally correlated with the level of gp120 expression. The neurotoxicity of gp120 may re-

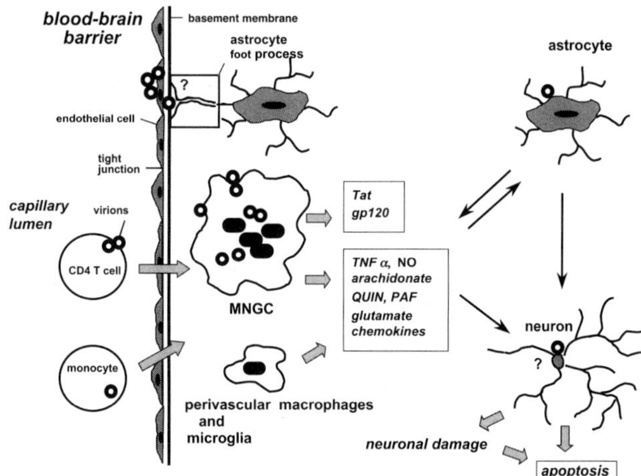

FIGURE 40.5 Neuropathogenesis of central nervous system human immunodeficiency virus (HIV) infection. Human immunodeficiency virus may enter the central nervous system through transendothelial migration of infected CD4-positive cells (T lymphocytes, monocytes), and possibly through infection of CD4-negative cells (endothelia, astrocytes). Infection in brain macrophages results in formation of multinucleated giant cells (MNGCs), which may release neurotoxic metabolites and viral proteins. In addition, activated macrophages and microglia may also release nonviral neurotoxins, any or all of which may injure neurons directly or through inhibition of supportive functions of astrocytes. Structural and functional alterations in neurons may ultimately lead to neuronal apoptosis, which is commonly found in the HIV-infected brain. NO: nitric oxide; PAF: platelet activating factor; QUIN: quinolinic acid; TNFα: tumor necrosis factor alpha.

TABLE 40.1 *Macrophage/Microglia Secretion Products Implicated in the Pathophysiology of HAD*

Tumor necrosis factor alpha
Platelet activating factor
Nitric oxide
Viral proteins: gp120 and Tat
Chemokines (MIP-1α, MIP-1β, RANTES)
Macrophage chemoattractant protein-1

HAD: human immunodeficiency virus–associated dementia; MIP-1α, -1β: macrophage inflammatory protein-1α, -1β; RANTES: regulated on activation, normal T cells expressed and secreted.

sult from a direct interaction with neurons or indirectly, via activation of macrophages/microglia, leading to the alteration of their secretory functions and subsequent release of toxic products. Both direct and indirect mechanisms are centered on the dysregulation of neuronal calcium homeostasis (reviewed in Haughey and Mattson, 2002).

Human immunodeficiency virus doesn't establish productive infection in neurons, and in all likelihood is not able to infect neurons at all, but gp120 may bind CXCR4, whose expression on neuronal cells is well documented (Lavi et al., 1997; van der Meer et al., 2000). Moreover, interaction of gp120 with neuronal CXCR4 induces activation of the receptor and intracellular calcium signaling and, in some instances, apoptotic neuronal death. Interestingly, the authentic CXCR4 ligand, SDF-1α, is capable of inducing neuronal apoptosis as well (Hesselgesser et al., 1998).

The first indication that gp120 may initiate neuronal degeneration not through direct interaction but rather indirectly, via the activation of microglia, came from a study demonstrating that removal of microglial cells from a neuronal culture protected neurons from toxic exposure to gp120 (Lipton, 1992). Supporting this mechanism that was defined *in vitro*, apoptotic neurons are often topologically associated with activated microglia in HIVE (Adle-Biassette et al., 1999). Upon stimulation with gp120, microglia release numerous neurotoxins, including arachidonic acid and proinflammatory cytokines such as tumor necrosis factor alpha (TNF-α), platelet activating factor (PAF), and interleukin-1β (IL-1β). Expression levels of these cytokines are elevated in the brains of HAD/HIVE patients. Arachidonic acid induces *N*-methyl-D-aspartate (NMDA) receptor currents in neurons, thus dysregulating this receptor (Miller et al, 1992), and increases the extracellular glutamate concentration by inhibiting glutamate uptake by glia (Barbour et al., 1989). This leads to a hyperactivation of NMDA receptors and, as a consequence, a calcium influx that may lead to lethality. Similarly, pro-apoptotic cytokines inhibit glutamate uptake and facilitate the NMDA receptor-evoked currents (Soliven and Albert, 1992) thus provoking overstimulation of the receptor. Furthemore, these cytokines were shown to increase production of arachidonic acid and in this way amplified the cascade of reactions leading to degeneration of neurons. The NMDA receptor–mediated death pathway is thought to involve mitochondrial dysfunction (Chen et al., 2002). The receptor antagonists, such as memantine, protect neurons against gp120-induced damage.

Additionally, gp120-activated macrophages/microglia produce the inducible form of nitric oxide synthase, resulting in a dramatic increase in nitric oxide detected both *in vitro* and *in vivo* (Bagetta et al., 1996). Reactive oxygen species are involved in many acute and chronic neurological diseases, including Parkinson's and Alzheimer's diseases and HAD (Simonian and Coyle, 1996; González-Scarano and Baltuch, 1999). Free radicals cause oxidative stress and cell structure damage and are able to initiate apoptotic pathways in neurons (Dawson et al., 1993). In addition to their direct role in neuronal damage, free radicals are capable of inducing the secretion of the pro-apoptotic cytokine, IL-1β, thus forming a lethal loop that is deleterious to neurons.

Another HIV protein, the transactivator of viral transcription, Tat, is released by intact, nonlysed, infected cells (Chang et al., 1997). Tat interacts with neurons, and as with gp120, this interaction may lead to dysregulation of calcium homeostasis and activation of excitatory amino acid (glutamate and NMDA) receptors. Tat-mediated potentiation of NMDA receptors is thought to be the end result of direct activation of G-protein, leading to intracellular release of calcium from endoplasmic reticulum and to activation of protein kinase C and tyrosine kinase, which mediate, perhaps synergistically, phosphorylation of NMDA receptor subunits (Haughey et al., 2001). The neurotoxic effects of Tat can be prevented by inhibition of the IP3 receptor that regulates the release of calcium from intracellular stores.

Tat is also capable of stimulating astrocytes and endothelial cells to release monocyte chemoattractant protein-1 (MCP-1), one of the chemokines most commonly associated with HAD pathogenesis (Conant et al., 1998; Toborek et al., 2003). Monocyte chemoattractant protein-1 induces influx of leukocytes into the brain (Weiss et al., 1999) and may be involved in the upregulation of adhesion molecules, further facilitating monocytic infiltration. The level of MCP-1 is markedly elevated in the brain and CSF of patients with HAD and is considered the most reliable prognostic marker for HIV-induced CNS disease (Conant et al., 1998). However, all of these scenarios presume that high levels of Tat are present extracellularly, and in many instances the concentrations required for manifestations of these *in vitro* changes are logarithmically higher than those that could ever be achieved *in vivo* given the source and physiological role of this protein.

Recently, Vpr, another important viral protein, has also been implicated in neuronotoxicity (Patel et al., 2000). Along with other toxic viral proteins, extracellular Vpr was shown to be able to induce neuronal apoptosis *in vitro*, though the *in vivo* relevance of this observation remains to be elucidated.

Besides these neurotoxic products, activated and/or infected microglia also express matrix metalloproteinases that degrade extracellular matrix integrity (Ghorpade et al., 2001). Multinucleated giant cells and the microglial nodules resulting from the infectious process in the CNS are potent sources of matrix metalloproteinases in the brains of patients with HAD. Additionally, activated resident macrophages express elevated levels of MIP-1α and MIP-1β, which are also involved in stimulation of trafficking of monocytes into the CNS and act in synergy with MCP-1 (Schmidtmayerova et al., 1996), thus providing a cellular substrate for further spread of HIV within the brain.

SUMMARY

Microglia and brain macrophages play an essential role in the pathogenesis of HIV infection of the brain. Not only are they the key cells responsible for the maintenance of brain infection, as they are the most susceptible cell type, but they are also the principal culprit in the development of neuronal pathology. Microglial cells, through their production of viral proteins and through the secretion of cytokines, mediate neuronal toxicity and apoptosis and are the clinical findings in HAD thought to be attributable to their presence and activity.

The latter function, the secretion of potentially deleterious cytokines, is not the sole province of HIV infection of the CNS: a number of other inflammatory conditions are characterized by the prominent presence of microglia and other CNS macrophages. Therefore, in diseases such as multiple sclerosis, microglia may also play a role in the neuronal and axonal degeneration that has recently been studied intensely. In fact, even in degenerative diseases such as Alzheimer's disease, the role of microglial activation and the secretion of cytokines are thought by some to be key to the pathophysiology. These findings suggest that the therapeutic modalities developed for HAD may eventually have potential uses for other diseases. At the very least, they will point the way to the development of new therapies.

ACKNOWLEDGMENTS

This work was supported by Grants NS-27405 and NS-35743 from National Institute of Health. The authors thank Dr. Ehud Lavi, of the University of Pennsylvania Department of Pathology and Laboratory Medicine, for providing Figure 40.2.

ABBREVIATIONS

AIDS	acquired immunodeficiency syndrome
HAD	HIV-associated dementia
HIV	human immunodeficiency virus
HIVE	HIV encephalitis
IL-1β	interleukin-1 beta
MCP-1	monocyte chemoattractant protein-1
MIP	macrophage inflammatory protein
MNGC	multinucleated giant cell
PAF	platelet activating factor
SAIDS	simian acquired immunodeficiency syndrome
SIV	simian immunodeficiency virus
TNF-α	tumor necrosis factor alpha

REFERENCES

Adle-Biassette, H., Chretien, F., Wingertsmann, L., Hery, C., Ereau, T., Scaravilli, F., Tardieu, M., and Gray, F. (1999) Neuronal apoptosis does not correlate with dementia in HIV infection but is related to microglial activation andaxonal damage. *Neuropathol. Appl. Neurobiol.* 25:123–133.

Albright, A.V., Shieh, J.T., Itoh, T., Lee, B., Pleasure, D., O'Connor, M.J., Doms, R.W., and Gonzalez-Scarano, F. (1999) Microglia express CCR5, CXCR4, and CCR3, but of these, CCR5 is the principal coreceptor for human immunodeficiency virus type 1 dementia isolates. *J. Virol.* 73:205–213.

Albright, A.V., Shieh, J.T., O'Connor, M.J., and Gonzalez-Scarano, F. (2000) Characterization of cultured microglia that can be infected by HIV-1. *J. Neurovirology* 6(Suppl. 1):S53–S60.

Bagetta, G., Corasaniti, M.T., Aloe, L., Berliocchi, L., Costa, N., Finazzi-Agro, A., and Nistico, G. (1996) Intracerebral injection of human immunodeficiency virus type 1 coat protein gp120 differentially affects the expression of nerve growth factor and nitric oxide synthase in the hippocampus of rat. *Proc. Natl. Acad. Sci. USA* 93:928–933.

Barbour, B., Szatkowski, M., Ingledew, N., and Attwell, D. (1989) Arachidonic acid induces a prolonged inhibition of glutamate uptake into glial cells. *Nature* 342:918–920.

Barks, J.D., Liu, X.H., Sun, R., and Silverstein, F.S. (1997) Gp120, a human immunodeficiency virus-1 coat protein, augments excitotoxic hippocampal injury in perinatal rats. *Neuroscience* 76: 397–409.

Bencherif, B. and Rottenberg, D.A. (1998) Neuroimaging of the AIDS dementia complex. *AIDS* 12:233–244.

Brenneman, D.E., Westbrook, G.L., Fitzgerald, S.P., Ennist, D.L., Elkins, K.L., Ruff, M.R., and Pert, C.B. (1988) Neuronal cell killing by the envelope protein of HIV and its prevention by vasoactive intestinal peptide. *Nature* 335:639–642.

Chang, H.C., Samaniego, F., Nair, B.C., Buonaguro, L., and Ensoli, B. (1997) HIV-1 Tat protein exits from cells via a leaderless secretory pathway and binds to extracellular matrix-associated heparan sulfate proteoglycans through its basic region. *AIDS* 11: 1421–1431.

Chen, H., Wood, C., and Petito, C.K. (2000) Comparisons of HIV-1 viral sequences in brain, choroid plexus and spleen: potential role of choroid plexus in the pathogenesis of HIV encephalitis. *J. Neurovirol.* 6:498–506.

Chen, W., Sulcove, J., Frank, I., Jaffer, S., Ozdener, H., and Kolson, D.L. (2002) Development of a human neuronal cell model for human immunodeficiency virus (HIV)-infected macrophage-induced neurotoxicity: apoptosis induced by HIV type 1 primary isolates and evidence for involvement of the Bcl-2/Bcl-xL-sensitive intrinsic apoptosis pathway. *J. Virol.* 76:9407–9419.

Clements, J.E., Babas, T., Mankowski, J.L., Suryanarayana, K., Piatak, M., Jr., Tarwater, P.M., Lifson, J.D., and Zink, M.C. (2002) The central nervous system as a reservoir for simian immunodeficiency virus (SIV): steady-state levels of SIV DNA in brain from acute through asymptomatic infection. *J. Infect. Dis.* 186: 905–913.

Conant, K., Garzino-Demo, A., Nath, A., McArthur, J.C., Halliday, W., Power, C., Gallo, R.C., and Major, E.O. (1998) Induction of monocyte chemoattractant protein-1 in HIV-1 Tat-stimulated astrocytes and elevation in AIDS dementia. *Proc. Natl. Acad. Sci. USA* 95:3117–3121.

Dawson, V.L., Dawson, T.M., Uhl, G.R., and Snyder, S.H. (1993) Human immunodeficiency virus type 1 coat protein neurotoxicity mediated by nitric oxide in primary cortical cultures. *Proc. Natl. Acad. Sci. USA* 90:3256–3259.

Ernst, T., Itti, E., Itti, L., and Chang, L. (2000) Changes in cerebral metabolism are detected prior to perfusion changes in early HIV-CMC: a coregistered (1)H MRS and SPECT study. *J. Magn. Reson. Imag.* 12:859–865.

Everall, I.P., Luthert, P.J., and Lantos, P.L. (1993) Neuronal number and volume alterations in the neocortex of HIV infected individuals. *J. Neurol. Neurosurg. Psychiatry* 56:481–486.

Flaherty, M.T., Hauer, D.A., Mankowski, J.L., Zink, M.C., and Clements, J.E. (1997) Molecular and biological characterization of a neurovirulent molecular clone of simian immunodeficiency virus. *J. Virol.* 71:5790–5798.

Ghorpade, A., Persidskaia, R., Suryadevara, R., Che, M., Liu, X.J., Persidsky, Y., and Gendelman, H.E. (2001) Mononuclear phagocyte differentiation, activation, and viral infection regulate matrix metalloproteinase expression: implications for human immunodeficiency virus type 1-associated dementia. *J. Virol.* 75: 6572–6583.

Goethe, K.E, Mitchell, J.E., Marshall, D.W., Brey, R.L., Cahill, W.T., Leger, G.D., Hoy, L.J., and Boswell, R.N. (1989) Neuropsychological and neurological function of human immunodeficiency virus seropositive asymptomatic individuals. *Arch Neurol.* 46:129–133.

Gonzalez-Scarano, F. and Baltuch, G. (1999) Microglia as mediators of inflammatory and degenerative diseases. *Annu. Rev. Neurosci.* 22:219–240.

Gorry, P.R., Taylor, J., Holm, G.H., Mehle, A., Morgan, T., Cayabyab, M., Farzan, M., Wang, H., Bell, J.E., Kunstman, K., Moore, J.P., Wolinsky, S.M., and Gabuzda, D. (2002) Increased CCR5 affinity and reduced CCR5/CD4 dependence of a neurovirulent primary human immunodeficiency virus type 1 isolate. *J. Virol.* 76:6277–6292.

Haughey, N.J., and Mattson, M.P. (2002) Calcium dysregulation and neuronal apoptosis by the HIV-1 proteins Tat and gp120. *J. Acquir. Immune. Defic. Syndr.* 31(Suppl 2):S55–S61.

Haughey, N.J., Nath, A., Mattson, M.P., Slevin, J.T., and Geiger, J.D. (2001) HIV-1 Tat through phosphorylation of NMDA receptors potentiates glutamate excitotoxicity. *J. Neurochem.* 78: 457–467.

Hesselgesser, J., Taub, D., Baskar, P., Greenberg, M., Hoxie, J., Kolson, D.L., and Horuk, R. (1998) Neuronal apoptosis induced by HIV-1 gp120 and the chemokine SDF-1 alpha is mediated by the chemokine receptor CXCR4. *Curr. Biol.* 8:595–598.

Hickey, W.F. (2001) Basic principles of immunological surveillance of the normal central nervous system. *Glia* 36:118–124.

Hughes, E.S., Bell, J.E., and Simmonds, P. (1997) Ivestigation of the dynamics of the spread of human immunodeficiency virus to brain and other tissues by evolutionary analysis of sequences from *p17gag* and *env* genes. *J. Virol.* 71:1272–1280.

Kaul, M., Garden, G.A., and Lipton, S.A. (2001) Pathways to neuronal injury and apoptosis in HIV-associated dementia. *Nature* 410:988–994.

Lassmann, H., Schmied, M., Vass, K., and Hickey, W. (1993) Bone marrow derived elements and resident microglia in brain inflammation. *Glia* 7:19–24.

Lavi, E., Strizki, J.M., Ulrich, A.M., Zhang, W., Fu, L., Wang, Q., O'Connor, M., Hoxie, J.A, and Gonzalez-Scarano, F. (1997) CXCR-4 (Fusin), a co-receptor for the type 1 human immunodeficiency virus (HIV-1), is expressed in the human brain in a variety of cell types, including microglia and neurons. *Am. J. Pathol.* 151:1035–1042.

Lipton, S.A. (1992) Requirement for macrophages in neuronal injury induced by HIV envelope protein gp120. *NeuroReport* 3:913–915.

Lui, Y., Tang, X.P., McArthur, J.C., Scott, J., and Gartner, S. (2002) Analysis of human immunodeficiency virus type 1 gp160 sequences from a patient with HIV dementia: evidence for monocyte trafficking into brain. *J. Neurovirol.* 6(Suppl. 1):S70–S81.

Mankowski, J.L., Flaherty, M.T., Spelman, J.P., Hauer, D.A., Didier, P.J., Amedee, A.M., Murphey-Corb, M., Kirstein, L.M., Munoz, A., Clements, J.E., and Zink, M.C. (1997) Pathogenesis of simian immunodeficiency virus encephalitis: viral determinants of neurovirulence. *J. Virol.* 71:6055–6060.

Martin, J., LaBranche, C.C., and González-Scarano, F. (2001) Differential CD4/CCR5 utilization, gp120 conformation, and neutralization sensitivity between envelopes from a microglia-adapted human immunodeficiency virus type 1 and its parental isolate. *J. Virol.* 75:3568–3580.

Miller, B., Sarantis, M., Traynelis, S.F., and Attwell, D. (1992) Potentiation of NMDA receptor currents by arachidonic acid. *Nature* 355:722–725.

Patel, C.A., Mukhtar, M., and Pomerantz, R.J. (2000) Human immunodeficiency virus type 1 Vpr induces apoptosis in human neuronal cells. *J. Virol.* 74:9717–9726.

Power, C., Kong, P.A., Crawford, T.O., Wesselingh, S., Glass, J.D., McArthur, J.C., and Trapp, B.D. (1993) Cerebral white matter changes in acquired immunodeficiency syndrome dementia: alterations of the blood–brain barrier. *Ann. Neurol.* 34:339–350.

Power, C., McArthur, J.C., Nath, A., Wehrly, K., Mayne, M., Nishio, J., Langelier, T., Johnson, R.T., and Chesebro, B. (1998) Neuronal death induced by brain-derived human immunodeficiency virus type 1 envelope genes differs between demented and non-demented AIDS patients. *J. Virol.* 72:9045–9053.

Puffer, B.A., Pohlmann, S., Edinger, A.L., Carlin, D., Sanchez, M.D., Reitter, J., Watry, D.D., Fox, H.S., Desrosiers, R.C., and Doms, R.W. (2002) CD4 independence of simian immunodeficiency virus Envs is associated with macrophage tropism, neutralization sensitivity, and attenuated pathogenicity. *J. Virol.* 76:2595–2605.

Ryzhova, E.V., Crino, P., Shawver, L., Westmoreland, S.V., Lackner, A.A., and González-Scarano, F. (2002) Simian immunodeficiency virus encephalitis: analysis of envelope sequences from individual brain multinucleated giant cells and tissue samples. *Virology* 297:57–67.

Sacktor, N.C., Bacellar, H., Hoover, D.R., Nance-Sproson, T.E., Selnes, O.A., Miller, E.N., Dal Pan, G.J., Kleeberger, C., Brown, A., Saah, A., and McArthur, J.C. (1996) Psychomotor slowing in HIV infection: a predictor of dementia, AIDS and death. *J. Neurovirol.* 2:404–410.

Sacktor, N.C., McDermott, M.P., Marder, K., Schifitto, G., Selnes, O.A., McArthur, J.C., Stern, Y., Albert, S., Palumbo, D., Kieburtz, K., De Marcaida, J.A., Cohen, B., and Epstein, L. (2002) HIV-associated cognitive impairment before and after the advent of combination therapy. *J. Neurovirol.* 8:136–142.

Saito, Y., Sharer, L.R., Epstein, L.G., Michaels, J., Mintz, M., Louder, M., Golding, K., Cvetkovich, T.A., and Blumberg, B.M. (1994) Overexpression of nef as a marker for restricted HIV-1 infection of astrocytes in postmortem pediatric central nervous tissues. *Neurology* 44:474–481.

Schmidtmayerova, H., Nottet, H.S., Nuovo, G., Raabe, T., Flanagan, C.R., Dubrovsky, L., Gendelman, H.E., Cerami, A., Bukrinsky, M., and Sherry, B. (1996) Human immunodeficiency virus type 1 infection alters chemokine beta peptide expression in human monocytes: implications for recruitment of leukocytes into brain and lymph nodes. *Proc. Natl. Acad. Sci. USA* 93:700–704.

Shieh, J.T., Martin, J., Baltuch, G., Malim, M.H., and Gonzalez-Scarano, F. (2000) Determinants of syncytium formation in microglia by human immunodeficiency virus type 1: role of the V1/V2 domains. *J. Virol.* 74:693–701.

Simonian, N.A. and Coyle, J.T. (1996) Oxidative stress in neurodegenerative diseases. *Annu. Rev. Pharmacol. Toxicol.* 36:83–106.

Soliven, B. and Albert, J. (1992) Tumor necrosis factor modulates Ca^{2+} currents in cultured sympathetic neurons. *J. Neurosci.* 12:2665–2671.

Strizki, J.M., Albright, A.V., Sheng, H., O'Connor, M., Perrin, L., and González-Scarano, F. (1996) Infection of primary human microglia and monocyte-derived macrophages with human immunodeficiency virus type 1 isolates: evidence of differential tropism. *J. Virol.* 70:7654–7662.

Takahashi, K., Wesselingh, S., Griffin, D.E., McArthur, J.C., Johnson, R.T., and Glass, J.D. (1996) Localization of HIV-1 in human brain using polymerase chain reaction/ in situ hybridization and immunocytochemistry. *Ann. Neurol.* 39:705–711.

Tambussi, G., Gori, A., Capiluppi, B., Balotta, C., Papagno, L., Morandini, B., Di Pietro, M., Ciuffreda, D., Saracco, A., and Lazzarin, A. (2000) Neurological symptoms during primary human immunodeficiency virus (HIV) infection correlate with high levels of HIV RNA in cerebrospinal fluid. *Clin. Infect. Dis.* 30: 962–965.

Thompson, K.A., McArthur, J.C., and Wesselingh. S.L. (2001) Correlation between neurological progression and astrocyte apoptosis in HIV-associated dementia. *Ann. Neurol.* 49:745–752.

Toborek, M., Lee, Y.W., Pu, H., Malecki, A., Flora, G., Garrido, R., Hennig, B., Bauer, H.C., and Nath, A. (2003) HIV-Tat protein induces oxidative and inflammatory pathways in brain endothelium. *J. Neurochem.* 84:169–179.

Tornatore, C., Meyers, K., Atwood, W., Conant, K., and Major, E. (1994) Temporal patterns of human immunodeficiency virus type 1 transcripts in human fetal astrocytes. *J. Virol.* 68:93–102.

van der Meer, P., Ulrich, A.M., Gonzalez-Scarano, F., and Lavi, E. (2000) Immunohistochemical analysis of CCR2, CCR3, CCR5, and CXCR4 in the human brain: potential mechanisms for HIV dementia. *Exp. Mol. Pathol.* 69:192–201.

Wang, T.H., Donaldson, W.K., Brettle, R.P., Bell, J.E., and Simmonds, P. (2001) Identification of shared population of human immunodeficiency virus type 1 infecting microglia and tissue macrophages outside the central nervous system. *J. Virol.* 75:11686–11699.

Weiss, J.M, Nath, A., Major, E.O., and Berman, J.W. (1999) HIV-1 Tat induces monocyte chemoattractant protein-1-mediated monocyte transmigration across a model of the human blood–brain barrier and up-regulates CCR5 expression on human monocytes. *J. Immunol.* 163:2953–2959.

Williams, K., Corey, S., Westmoreland, S., Pauley, D., Knight, H., deBakker, C., Alvarez, X., and Lackner, A. (2001) Perivascular microphages are the primary cell type productively infected by simian ummunodeficiency virus in the brain of macaques: implication for the neuropathogenesis of AIDS. *J. Exp. Med.* 193:905–915.

Wong, J.K., Ignacio, C.C., Torriani, F., Havlir, D., Fitch, N.J., and Richman, D.D. (1997) In vivo compartmentalization of human immunodeficiency virus: evidence from the examination of pol sequences from autopsy tissues. *J. Virol.* 71:2059–2071.

Zou Y. R., Kottmann A. H., Kuroda M., Taniuchi I., and Littman D. R. (1998) Function of the chemokine receptor CXCR4 in haematopoiesis and in cerebellar development. *Nature* 393: 595–599.

41 Focal cerebral ischemia: The multifaceted role of glial cells

ULRICH DIRNAGL AND JOSEF PRILLER

Ischemic stroke is the result of a reversible or permanent focal perfusion deficit in the territory of a brain artery. The perfusion deficit in most cases is the result of an arterio-arteriolar or cardiac embolus or the thrombotic occlusion of a brain artery. Stroke symptoms depend on the affected vascular territory and include hemiparesis, aphasia, and visual impairment. Less than a decade ago, stroke therapy was dominated by nihilism. With major breakthroughs in the understanding of stroke pathophysiology and the development of new therapeutic strategies, a worldwide campaign for the rapid recruitment and early treatment of stroke patients was initiated. Possibly as a result of these efforts, a first clinical success was achieved using recombinant tissue plasminogen activator [The National Institute for Neurological Disorders and Stroke (NINDS) and Stroke rt-PA Stroke Study Group, 1995]. Despite the recent failure of several trials using neuroprotective drugs in stroke, promising new therapeutic options are available. While the early work on stroke pathophysiology focused on blood flow and metabolism, a shift has occured toward biochemical and cellular mechanisms; recently, molecular and genetic aspects have been added. It is becoming evident that circulatory, metabolic, cellular, and molecular mechanisms have to be considered if we are to understand, treat, and possibly prevent the consequences of focal cerebral ischemia. With this shift in focus, the contribution of nonneuronal cells, and in particular glial cells, to stroke pathophysiology is becoming increasingly appreciated.

Experimental evidence suggests that a complex sequence of pathophysiological events occurs in stroke, which involves excitotoxicity, peri-infarct depolarizations, inflammation, and programmed cell death (Fig. 41.1) (Dirnagl et al., 1999). As a consequence, stroke therapy should target specific mechanisms that occur at different time points. It is apparent that drugs interfering with excitotoxicity (such as glutamate receptor antagonists) have to be administered very early after symptom onset, while drugs aiming at inflammation or apoptosis may have an extended time window (albeit a smaller overall effect). More recently, research on cerebral ischemia has begun to focus on endogenous neuroprotective mechanisms, which appear to counteract at least partially all destructive events (Fig. 41.1). According to this concept, the final infarct is the result of a "struggle" between destruction and protection. A number of such endogenous protective signaling cascades have been elaborated in more detail, and at least in animal experiments, boosting of such mechanisms protected the brain against stroke. The first clinical trials aiming at the induction of primarily endogenous neuroprotection are underway (e.g., erythropoeitin) (Ehrenreich et al., 2002).

Glial cells play important roles in the destructive as well as the protective cascades evolving in the focally ischemic or reperfused brain. Stroke results in *infarction* of brain tissue, which is defined as pannecrosis, the death of all cellular elements in a given tissue volume. Therefore, and because of the very close interaction between neuronal and nonneuronal elements in brain physiology and pathophysiology in general, we will start by looking at the principal mechanisms of ischemic damage and try to point out what we know about the specific contribution of glial cells. We will then change the perspective from affected tissue to single cells and reassess the specific contribution of the glial cell types (astroglia, microglia, oligodendrocytes) in this process.

PATHOPHYSIOLOGY OF FOCAL CEREBRAL ISCHEMIA

Early Mechanisms: Excitotoxicity, Peri-infarct Depolarizations

Energy depletion due to lack of substrate (oxygen, glucose) leads to the depolarization of neurons but also of astroglia, resulting in the release of glutamate into the extracellular space. At the same time, the energy-dependent reuptake of glutamate by astroglial cells is impeded, further increasing its extracellular concentration. As a result of receptor activation [in particular of

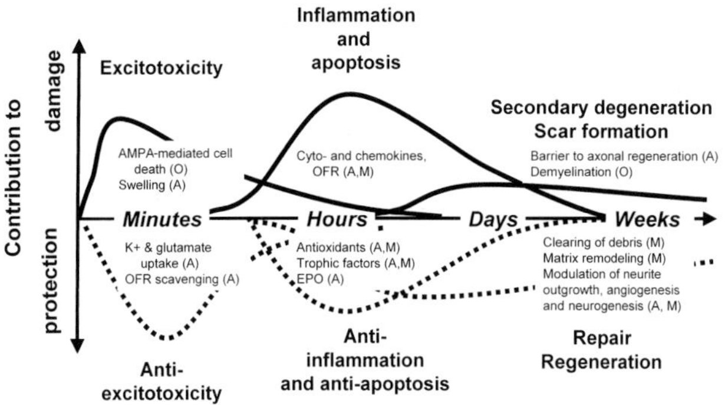

FIGURE 41.1 Putative contribution of glial cells to the temporal sequence of damage and endogenous protection following focal cerebral ischemia. A: astrocyte; EPO: erythropoietin; M: microglia; O: oligodendrocyte; OFR: oxygen free radicals.

the neuronal *N*-methyl-D-aspartate (NMDA) and AMPA receptor subtypes], intracellular calcium rises. The activation of metabotropic receptors and phospholipase C and inositol 1,4,5-triphosphate (IP3) signaling mobilizes calcium from intracellular stores, further contributing to the calcium overload. The increase in the universal second messenger, calcium, overstimulates numerous intracellular pathways and enzymes. Cell membranes are degraded (e.g., via activation of cyclooxygenase), and free radical species are produced in high concentrations in vicious circles, overwhelming endogenous scavenging mechanisms, which are mainly provided by astroglial cells. Neurons, in contrast to astroglia, depend almost exclusively on mitochondrial respiration. Neuronal mitochondrial function is impaired. In particular, the appearance of the so-called mitochondrial permeability transition (MPT) pore in the mitochondrial membrane leads to mitochondrial swelling, cessation of adenosine triphosphate (ATP) production, and possibly an oxygen free radical burst. In addition, the entry of sodium and water leads to swelling (edema) and even osmotic lysis of the cells. For review of the above mechansisms, which are generally referred to as *excitotoxicity*, see Dirnagl et al. (1999).

Due to the depolarization-induced release of neuronal and glial potassium and glutamate, repetitive depolarizations propagate and the so-called peri-infarct depolarizations may occur (Hossmann, 1996). These depolarizations are similar to spreading depressions, the putative electrophysiological correlate of the migraine aura, but since they occur in energetically compromised tissue, they may cause damage.

Glial cells appear to play an important role in these early processes. However, most of the putative functions of glial cells have been deduced from normal astrocyte biology, since little direct evidence relating to ischemia is available. As indicated above, the depolarization-induced release of excessive amounts of glutamate from neurons is a key event in triggering downstream mechanisms of tissue damage. A prominent function of astrocytes is the uptake of glutamate from the extracellular space via specialized transporters [e.g., glutamate transporter-1 (GLT-1) and glutamate/aspartate transporter-1 (GLAST-1)]. Glutamate transporter-1 knockdown exacerbates neuronal cell death and neurological deficits after experimental stroke in mice (Namura et al., 2002). In the astrocyte, glutamine synthetase converts glutamate to glutamine, which is exported to neurons for the synthesis of glutamate and gamma-aminobutyric acid (GABA) via the glutamate-glutamine shuttle. In regions of intermediate perfusion and remaining energy equivalents (the so-called penumbra), the glutamate-buffering capacity of astrocytes may be critical in limiting damage to neurons by excitotoxicity.

Astrocytes are connected with each other via gap junctions [in particular, connexin 43 (Cx43)], and thereby form a functional syncytium that is involved in ionic homeostasis and electrical coupling, K^+ buffering, and intercellular signaling. Astrocytic gap junctions remain open during ischemic conditions, and they may link ischemic astrocytes in an evolving infarct with the surroundings (Cotrina et al., 1998). Astrocytic gap junctions could have a protective function in cerebral ischemia (Nauss et al., 2001; Nakase et al., 2003). However, gap junction blockade reduces infarct volumes in rodents (Rawanduzy et al., 1997), and animals lacking Cx43 have smaller infarcts than wild-type animals (Frantseva et al., 2002). Coupling via astrocytic gap junctions has also been implicated in the propagation of spreading depression and peri-infarct depolarizations. Astrocytic Cx43 epitope masking, dephosphorylation, and cellular redistribution occur after ischemic brain injury, proceed as a temporally and spatially ordered sequence of events, and culminate in differential patterns of Cx43 modification and sequestration in the lesion center versus the periphery (Li et al., 1998). Since peri-infarct depolarizations contribute to lesion growth, inhibition of such depolarization waves may be at least partially responsible for the neuroprotection observed after astrocytic gap junction inhibition in experimental models of stroke (see above and Rawanduzy et al., 1997). For a review of the complex issue of gap junction functions in central nervous system (CNS) injury, see Perez Velazquez et al. (2003).

Astrocytes also express water channels, in particular aquaporins (AQ), which are abundant on astrocytic endfeet ensheeting capillaries (AQ4) and on cell bodies (AQ9) (Badaut et al., 2002). Aquaporin expression increases after focal cerebral ischemia (Taniguchi et al., 2000). Aquaporin-4 deletion in mice reduces brain edema after acute water intoxication and ischemic stroke (Manley et al., 2000). Astrocyte swelling, which may result from water flux across AQ channels, high glutamate and K^+, lactic acid, oxygen free radicals, and arachidonic acid, among others, is one of the earliest morphological changes detectable in focally ischemic brain tissue (Garcia et al., 1977). The high mortality that follows a large cerebral infarction is thought to be due in part to brain edema, since edema causes mass effects with raised intracranial pressure and herniation (Ayata and Ropper, 2002). Local cell swelling may also be responsible for further reducing tissue perfusion by vascular compression. Although the exact role of astrocytes in the formation of postischemic brain edema remains to be defined, the available evidence suggests that astrocytes and their increase in cell volume due to ionic and water shifts are important negative contributors to lesion growth and neurological outcome, particularly in severe cases of large artery occlusions.

Astrocytes are essential elements of the blood–brain barrier. Astrocytes lacking glial fibrillary acidic protein (GFAP) were shown to have defects in process formation, induction of the blood–brain barrier, and volume regulation. In this context, it is interesting that GFAP null mice are highly susceptible to damage by focal cerebral ischemia (Nawashiro et al., 2000).

Astrocytes are also key players in brain metabolism (Gjedde et al., 2002; Nedergaard et al., 2002). Astrocytes contain most of the glycogen in the brain (Cruz and Dienel, 2002). Wender et al. (2000) have shown that in the absence of glucose in white matter of the optic nerve, astrocytic glycogen is broken down to lactate, which is transferred to axons as an energy source. However, this transfer is unlikely to be protective in ischemia, as the presence of oxygen is required for the ATP-generating metabolism of lactate. As intrinsic anaerobes, astrocytes may be able to transiently support anaerobic metabolism and support the structural integrity of neurons in the penumbra. Along these lines, Rose et al. (1998) demonstrated that cultured spinal cord astrocytes are able to maintain a steep inwardly directed Na^+ gradient for tens of minutes during energy disruption. Another important aspect of the astrocytic contribution to early mechanisms of stroke pathophysiology is their role in the defense against oxidants. Astrocytes maintain high intracellular concentrations of certain antioxidants, contributing to their resistance to oxidative stress relative to oligodendrocytes and neurons (Wilson, 1997). The constitutive expression (e.g., glutathione peroxidase) or accumulation (e.g., ascorbate) of these antioxidants indicates that astrocytes may take part in the early detoxification of oxygen free radicals before inducible scavengers are synthesized. However, there is also evidence for a detrimental role of astrocytes in neuronal survival after focal cerebral ischemia: changes in the use of astrocytic metabolic precursors appeared to contribute significantly to neuronal death; in particular, astrocytic glutamine may contribute to glutamate excitotoxicity (Haberg et al., 2001).

Very little is known about the role of oligodendrocytes in this early phase of cerebral ischemia. Most of our knowledge is derived from work on white matter rather than gray matter, and there may be relevant differences in the pathophysiology of ischemia and the role of oligodendrocytes in both regions. Interestingly, and in contrast to previous concepts (Mabuchi et al., 2000), oligodendrocytes appear to be highly vulnerable to cerebral ischemia (McDonald et al., 1998; Lyons et al., 2000; Tekkok and Goldberg, 2001). In fact, cortical oligodendrocytes in the lesion center are lethally damaged within 3 hours after the induction of focal cerebral ischemia, thereby preceding the appearance of necrotic neurons by several hours (Pantoni, 1998). Early, non-Wallerian damage to oligodendrocytes seems to be mediated via AMPA receptors, which, in contrast to NMDA receptors, are abundant on oligodendrocytes (McDonald et al., 1998). These findings may be relevant from a clinical standpoint, as they could explain at least in part the failure of NMDA receptor antagonists in human stroke trials. When administered before or soon after the induction of focal cerebral ischemia, NMDA receptor antagonists significantly reduce infarct sizes in many stroke models. However, in contrast to AMPA receptor antagonists, they do not protect oligodendrocytes (Dewar et al., 1999; McCracken et al., 2002). Thus, while neurons may be rescued by NMDA receptor blockade, they may remain nonfunctional due to the axonal damage resulting from oligodendrocyte death.

Inflammation

A number of signals released during the early excitotoxic period are potent inducers of inflammation. Astrocytes and microglia, as well as invading leukocytes are traditionally regarded as the key cellular elements of postischemic inflammation (Stoll et al., 1998). However, while glial cells are the focus of this chapter, it should be kept in mind that endothelial cells are crucial in initiating and modulating inflammation by attracting inflammatory cells and regulating their activity.

Within minutes to hours after ischemia, the microvascular basal lamina is degraded by proteases, and selectins are expressed on endothelial cells. The induction of intercellular adhesion molecule (ICAM)-1 on endothelium parallels the mobilization of CD11b/CD18 (Mac-1) on circulating leukocytes (Zhang et al., 1995b; Lindsberg et al., 1996; Fiszer et al., 1998). Neutrophils accumulate in the cerebral microvessels of the hypoperfused region, resulting in an additional impairment of blood flow, the so-called no reflow phenomenon (del Zoppo et al., 1991). Consequently, administration of monoclonal antibodies against CD18 (Mori et al., 1992), CD11b (Chen et al., 1994), or ICAM-1 (Zhang et al., 1995a) was found to significantly reduce leukocyte accumulation and stroke severity in experimental models of cerebral ischemia. Inflammation is mediated by pro-inflammatory cytokines and chemokines, whose expression seems to be triggered initially by oxygen free radicals and oxygen free radical sensing transcription factors (O'Neill and Kaltschmidt, 1997; Iadecola et al., 1999). The two key pro-inflammatory cytokines in the setting of cerebral ischemia are interleukin (IL)-1β and tumor necrosis factor (TNF)-α, both of which are primarily produced by activated microglia and macrophages (Davies et al., 1999; Gregersen et al., 2000). The biological effects of IL-1β and TNF-α are diverse, and include the conversion of endothelium to a prothrombotic surface, the induction of leukocyte adhesion molecules, an increase in blood–brain barrier permeability, and the activation of macrophages (Priller and Dirnagl, 2002). Inhibition of either IL-1β or TNF-α activity by monoclonal antibodies or recombinant receptor antagonists after focal cerebral ischemia significantly reduced infarct sizes in rats (Yamasaki et al., 1995; Dawson et al., 1996; Relton et al., 1996). Moreover, mice expressing a dominant negative mutant of IL-1β converting enzyme developed smaller strokes (Friedlander et al., 1997). The chemokine, fractalkine, is synthesized in cortical neurons of the ischemic penumbra and in endothelial cells in the infarcted tissue, and fractalkine may attract and activate microglia and macrophages expressing the fractalkine receptor, CX_3CR1 (Tarozzo et al., 2002). Recent studies suggest that inducible nitric oxide synthase (iNOS) produced by infiltrating inflammatory cells and astrocytes also contributes to postischemic brain damage, possibly by the generation of toxic peroxynitrite and reactive oxygen species (Iadecola et al., 1997; Loihl et al., 1999). The synthesis of matrix metalloproteinases (MMPs) 2 and 9 (gelatinases A and B) in microglia and astrocytes after cerebral ischemia coincided with the breakdown of the blood–brain barrier and the neuroinflammatory response (Planas et al., 2001; Rivera et al., 2002). Interestingly, MMPs and pro-inflammtory cytokines appear to be cross-regulated after ischemic insult, since MMPs can activate IL-1β by cleavage, and IL-1β and TNF-α were found to regulate the production of MMPs in cultured microglia and astrocytes (Gottschall and Deb, 1996).

The overwhelming pro-inflammatory signaling following ischemic brain damage is counterbalanced by the production of cytokines with homeostatic and potentially neurotrophic action, such as transforming growth factor (TGF)-β1 and IL-10. Transforming growth factor-β1 suppresses the translation of cytokine mRNAs and deactivates macrophages (Tsunawaki et al., 1988; Bogdan et al., 1992). Interleukin-10 is secreted from peripheral blood mononuclear cells after ischemic stroke (Pelidou et al., 1999). Both TGF-β1 and IL-10 have been shown to protect rodents from ischemic injury (Prehn et al., 1993; Spera et al., 1998). Of all the gene transcripts upregulated in the ischemic hemisphere, metallothionein-II was identified as the one most significantly induced (Trendelenburg et al., 2002). This small, cysteine-rich molecule is synthesized almost exclusively by reactive astrocytes and has been shown to exert neuroprotective effects after cerebral ischemia (Van Lookeren Campagne et al., 1999). Purines are released on a massive scale after ischemic cell injury, and extracellular ATP was found to activate microglia and astrocytes transcriptionally *in vitro* (Priller et al., 1995, 1998). Purines may contribute to the regeneration of damaged neuronal axons by enhancing the release and activity of neurotophic factors (Rathbone et al., 1999).

Undoubtedly, microglia and macrophages are the key effector cells of the postischemic inflammatory response. Inhibition of microglial activation by tetracylines or the deficiency of tissue plasminogen activator have been shown to protect the brain against focal cerebral ischemia in rodents (Tsirka et al., 1995; Yrjänheikki et al., 1999). Microglia become activated within hours after focal cerebral ischemia (Korematsu et al., 1994; Marks et al., 2001; Ueyama et al., 2001; Tarozzo et al., 2002), characterized by the expression of major histocompatibility complex (MHC) class I and II molecules on microglia and a morphological transition from the typical ramified to an ameboid morphology. At this time after transient ischemia, neutrophils accumulate in the brain parenchyma and contribute to neuronal damage (Garcia et al., 1994). With the expression of macrophage inflammatory protein-1 in microglia and monocyte chemoattractant protein-1 in astrocytes, a switch from neutrophil to macrophage chemoattraction occurs 1–2 days after the onset of ischemia (Gourmala et al., 1997, 1999). Thereafter, activated microglia and blood-borne monocytes/macrophages predominate in the ischemic areas (Garcia et al., 1994). Since microglia and macrophages are both of mesodermal origin and share the same surface markers, it has been difficult to differentiate their roles in the setting of cerebral ischemia. Recently, we found that reconstitution of hematopoiesis with green fluorescent protein (GFP)–marked peripheral blood cell progeny in bone marrow–chimeric mice helps to discriminate the reaction of microglia from the activities of infiltrating monocytes/macrophages. Interestingly, almost a third of the blood-borne cells engrafting in the ischemic brain parenchyma differentiated into microglia within 14 days, suggesting that the early reaction of resident microglia may be supplemented by microglia recruited from the bone marrow in the course of the postischemic inflammatory response (Priller et al., 2001). Some studies have suggested that bone marrow cells may even give rise to astrocytes in the brain, and that this recruitment is enhanced after cerebral ischemia (Eglitis and Mezey, 1997; Eglitis et al., 1999). While the immune function of microglia is evident, the abilitiy of astrocytes to function as nonprofessional antigen-presenting cells in the diseased brain remains controversial (Dong and Benveniste, 2001). Nevertheless, astrocytes contribute to the production of pro-inflammatory cytokines and neuroprotective factors, such as TGF-β and metallothionein-II after cerebral ischemia.

It should be noted that in addition to the acute detrimental effects of the postischemic inflammatory response, inflammation is linked with repair and plasticity. Activated macrophages and microglia may release neurotrophic factors (Batchelor et al., 1999), and IL-1β has been shown to stimulate the synthesis of nerve growth factor (Becker et al., 1997). Mice deficient in TNF receptors had significantly larger infarcts than wild-type mice after transient ischemia and reperfusion (Bruce et al., 1996). Moreover, TNF-α has been shown to promote the remyelination of damaged axons by promoting the proliferation of oligodendrocyte progenitors during inflammation (Arnett et al., 2001).

Apoptosis

Inflammation and apoptosis in cerebral ischemia appear to have a similar temporal profile. In general, apoptosis is particularly prominent in stroke areas resulting from focal ischemia of short duration (30–60 minutes) and in the penumbral border zone, where selective neuronal degeneration may occur (see below). In addition, days and weeks after infarction, neurons in areas projecting to the infarct zone may also undergo apoptosis (e.g., in the thalamus: Soriano et al., 1996), while microglial cells in these areas become activated, either as a sign of neuronal deafferentation or of neuronophagia (Pappata et al., 2000).

Glial cells may be involved in stroke-induced apoptosis in several ways:

- By producing signals that induce apoptosis in neurons
- By dying apoptotically triggered by the same signals and in a manner similar to that of neurons (in particular oligodendrocytes: Mabuchi et al., 2000; Shibata et al., 2000)
- By self-elimination via apoptosis
- By producing factors that protect neurons against apoptosis

All of these processes are closely connected with inflammation. Inflammation produces toxins (e.g., oxygen free radicals) that induce mitochondrial and DNA damage as important upstream mediators of apoptosis in neurons and oligodendrocytes. In addition, apoptosis is a critical mechanism in limiting and terminating inflammation, although it is controversial whether inflammatory cells themselves are eliminated by apoptosis. Mabuchi et al. (2000) found macrophages expressing Bax protein and nuclear DNA fragmentation in the infarcted tissue. In contrast, no double labeling of Mac-1 and terminal deoxynucleotidyl transferase-mediated deoxyuridine triphosphate nick-end labeling (TUNEL) was recently detected in a model of mild cerebral ischemia (Katchanov et al., 2001). It is very likely that astrocytes play a major role in limiting the growth of ischemic lesions, and that antiapoptotic mechanisms are a key element of astrocyte-mediated neuroprotection after stroke. Astrocytes are a major source of growth factors that protect neurons against ischemic damage. Reactive astrocytes produce nerve growth factor, basic fibroblast growth factor, brain-derived nerve growth factor, ciliary neurotrophic factor, insulin-like growth factor-1, and transforming growth factor-β, among others (Norenberg, 1998). The trophic cytokine, erythropoietin (EPO), appears to be a highly potent endogenous neuroprotectant that is generated by astrocytes and prevents neuronal apoptosis via EPO receptor–mediated activation of Janus kinase-2 (JAK-2)/phosphoinositide-3 kinase (PI3K)–dependent pathways (Ruscher et al., 2002).

Regeneration and Repair

In most stroke survivers, functional deficits are most severe in the inital phase after the event, and neurological function recovers at least to some degree within days, weeks, or months (Jorgensen et al., 1999). While this improvement has been attributed to the reorganization of brain function toward brain areas that have survived the insult, it is increasingly appreciated that regeneration and repair contribute to recovery after stroke. Glial cells, in particular astrocytes and microglia, may play an important role in this process (see also above). The neuropathological hallmark of ischemic stroke is brain infarction, which is defined as pannecrosis, the necrotic disintegration of all cellular elements. The infarct may be surrounded by a zone of neuronal degeneration, historically termed *selective neuronal necrosis* (SNN), which is probably mechanistically more related to apoptosis (see above). Depending on the severity of the ischemic insult and the type of stroke, the ischemic infarct and selective neuronal degeneration develop over a period of hours to days. The polymorphonuclear leukocytic infiltration of the infarct area is replaced after several days by mononuclear phagocytes (which are of hematogenous origin and/or derive from microglial migration and proliferation). Tissue breakdown and phagocytosis continue, and cystic spaces filled with fluid replace the parenchyma. At the border of the lesion, which is well demarcated at that time, swollen astrocytes are abundant and astrocytes proliferate (Liu and Chen, 1994). Newly formed capillaries sprout from the marginal zone into the necrotic area. After several weeks, a glial scar surrounds the defect, which may now appear as a fluid-filled cavity.

Microglia at the infarct border and microglia/macrophages in the infarct core may produce astrocyte chemoattractants, such as osteopontin (Wang et al., 1998) and thereby organize the formation of the astroglial scar after stroke. Microglia may also contribute to tissue reorganization by secreting MMPs (in particular MMP-2: Planas et al., 2001), which lead to extracellular proteolysis and may mediate parenchymal and angiogenic recovery. Reactive astrocytes upregulate adhesion molecules and produce extracellular matrix proteins such as neural cell adhesion molecule (NCAM), laminin, tenascin, chondroitin sulfate proteoglycans, and fibronectin. Some of these products inhibit neurite outgrowth (e.g., tenascin), while others (e.g., NCAM) promote it. The role of astrogliosis after stroke remains controversial. While in the older literature a putative inhibition of axonal regeneration by glia is emphasized, recently a potentially permissive role of astrocyte proliferation and astrogliosis for axonal guidance and even neurogenesis after stroke has been stressed (Arvidsson et al., 2002). Astrocytes appear to regulate the physiological migration of neuronal precursors from the subventricular zone (Mason et al., 2001) and may even act as neural stem cells themselves (Doetsch et al., 1999). Both astrocytes and microglia/macrophages produce TGF-β1 and vascular endothelial growth factor after stroke, which are important signals for the angiogenic response (Issa et al., 1999). In addition, they may provide signals leading to the proliferation of oligodendrocytes, which can be observed around the lesion at day 5 after focal cerebral ischemia (Mandai et al., 1997).

ASSESSMENT, SUMMARY, AND CONCLUSIONS

Throughout this chapter, it has become apparent that the contributions of glial cells to stroke pathophysiology, regeneration, and repair have only recently come into focus and that our knowledge is patchy at best. Consequently, and because of the diverse nature and complex pathobiology of glial cells in general, much controversy exists and relevant aspects need to be explored in more detail. Nevertheless, it is undisputed that glial cells are major contributors to tissue damage and repair after focal cerebral ischemia. At present, the involvement of glial cells in stroke is considered to be Janus-faced (Table 41.1): while ischemia induces the production of cytotoxins in these cells, at the same time potent defense mechanisms are turned on. Since the transcription and translation of the effector proteins of inflammation and apoptosis are delayed, they represent interesting new therapeutic targets given that only a minority of stroke patients can be recruited immediately after symptom onset. In addition, if glial cells play a relevant role in tissue remodeling and repair after stroke, the modulation of their activities may open novel therapeutic avenues.

While we have focused on the contribution of glial cells to stroke pathophysiology in the temporal evolution of damage and repair, below we will synthesize and summarize our current knowledge stratified for astrocytes, microglia, and oligodendrocytes.

Astrocytes

A very thorough review of astrocytes in ischemic brain injury was presented by Norenberg (1998). Astrocytes are comparatively resistant to substrate deprivation, and are activated very early in and around a focally ischemic brain region. Reactive astrocytes are hypertrophic and hyperplastic, and can be identified by their increased expression of GFAP. Glial fibrillary acidic protein is the most important constituent of 10 nm intermediate glial filaments that accumulate as bundles. This stereotypical astrocytic response is nonspecific and

TABLE 41.1 *Janus-Faced Contribution of Glial Cells to Stroke Pathophysiology*

	Good	*Bad*
Astrocyte	Ionic and volume homeostasis Accumulation of glutamate Constitutive and inducible production of antioxidants Production of anti-apoptotic proteins (e.g., EPO) Production of trophic factors (e.g., NGF) Guidance of axons during repair Attraction and guidance of newly forming neurons	Acute swelling (vascular obstruction, herniation) Release of glutamate Production of pro-inflammatory mediators and cytotoxins (e.g., IL-1β) Astrogliosis as an impediment for axonal regeneration
Microglia	Growth and trophic factor production (e.g., TGF-β1) Oxygen free radical scavenging Phagocytosis of dead cells/debris Attraction of astrocytes involved in repair processes Degradation of extracellular matrix during remodeling	Production of pro-inflammatory mediators and cytotoxins (e.g., IL-1β, matrix metalloproteinases) Disruption of the blood–brain barrier
Oligodendrocyte	?	Secondary axonal neuronal damage by ischemia-induced apoptosis of oligodendroyctes

EPO: erythropoietin; IL-1β: interleukin-1β; NGF: nerve growth factor; TGF-β1: transforming growth factor-β1.

may occur in other conditions even in the absence of pathology, for example after spreading depression. It should be noted that the definition of the *activated state* of an astrocyte based on GFAP immunohistochemistry may be problematic given that increased staining can be caused by changes in immunological binding properties rather than increased GFAP content. In the active state, astrocytes are metabolically hyperactive, with increased numbers of mitochondria and enlarged ribosomes as well as Golgi complexes. At the molecular level, reactive astrocytes increase the production of numerous mediators, receptors, and channels that are responsible for the altered functional state of these cells in cerebral ischemia. It is not surprising that astrocyte functions that are of particular relevance to stroke include the maintenance of ionic and water homeostasis. They may help to attenuate excitotoxic conditions in the affected parenchyma by syphoning potassium (although this was proven only in the retina) and by taking up glutamate.

At the same time, and as a direct consequence, astrocytes swell, which may negatively affect the already impaired blood circulation by vascular constriction and create devastating remote effects by mass displacement and herniation. The pronounced constitutive as well as inducible antioxidant capacity of astrocytes serves to decrease the load of toxic metabolites originating from excitotoxic and inflammatory mechanisms. However, the astrocytic production of pro-inflammatory mediators may counteract this protective effect by upregulating vascular adhesion molecules, attracting hematogenous cells, and inducing microglial activation Thus, astrocytes play a key role in the induction of the inflammatory reaction to cerebral ischemia. As infarction and selective neuronal degeneration progress, astrocytes in and around the lesion (and even in remote projection areas) remain activated and even proliferate. Astrocytes are the main cellular constituent of the scar that forms around the lesion within approximately a week after the event. Astrocytes attract microglia/monocytes for the clearance of debris and the remodeling of the tissue, and they partake in angiogenesis. Very recent data indicate that they are also involved in guiding axons and newly generated neurons, which is in sharp contrast to the previously held view that glia impede axonal growth.

Microglia/macrophages

As with astrocytes, the involvement of microglia and macrophages in ischemic injury is Janus-faced. Resident microglia are rapidly activated around the ischemic lesion. They transform from a resting, ramified morphology into rod cell–shaped and ameboid phenotypes. Activated microglia proliferate and migrate to the site of injury. Their response is rather stereotypic, and the transformation of resident microglia into phagocytic cells occurs in the presence of neuronal cell death. At the same time, circulating monocytes and macrophages are recruited into the ischemic brain tissue. Activated microglia and macrophages produce pro-inflammatory cytokines, chemoattractants, and MMPs that sustain the inflammatory response. While clearing the areas of cell death, they are a source of potentially cytotoxic substances, such as nitric oxide, reactive oxygen species, proteases, and excitotoxins. Microglia and macrophages participate in the immunological reactions to cerebral ischemia by upregulating MHC and costimulatory molecules and by presenting antigens to invading lymphocytes. They also secrete factors inducing apoptosis in neurons and oligodendrocytes. On the other hand, microglia and peripheral blood mononuclear cells produce neuroprotective cytokines and trophic factors after cerebral ischemia. As outlined above, they also participate actively in tissue remodeling and angiogenesis.

Oligodendrocytes

According to recent studies, oligodendrocytes are exquisitly sensitive to hypoxia and ischemia, possibly even more so than neurons. This may have clinical consequences, since some neuroprotective strategies may fail to protect oligodendrocytes. As a consequence, neuroprotectants tested with great enthusiasm in experimental models of stroke (e.g., NMDA receptor antagonists) may have saved neurons, but not the oligodendrocytes responsible for maintaining axonal function of these neurons, which may at least partially explain the failure of these substances in clinical trials. Surprisingly little is known about the role of oligodendrocytes in regeneration and repair after stroke, although it is obvious that they must be involved in maintaining myelination or helping to remyelinate axons.

In summary, glial cells are major contributors to damage, as well as to endogenous protection and repair after stroke. The fact that the same cell types partake in damaging as well as protective signaling precludes simple therapeutic approaches aimed at blocking or inducing the activities of glial cells. Nevertheless, the recent appreciation of the high susceptibility of oligodendrocytes to AMPA-mediated cell death and the successful pilot trial on the use of EPO in stroke in humans are examples of the outstanding clinical relevance of glial mechanisms in stroke. Future studies will elucidate the interplay between glia, neurons, and other nonneuronal elements in stroke in greater detail.

ACKNOWLEDGMENTS
This work was supported by the Hermann and Lilly Schilling Foundation and the Deutsche Forschungsgemeinschaft (DFG SFB 507-A5).

REFERENCES

Arnett, H.A., Mason, J., Marino, M., Suzuki, K., Matsushima, G.K., and Ting, J.P. (2001) TNF alpha promotes proliferation of oligodendrocyte progenitors and remyelination. *Nat. Neurosci.* 4:1116–1122.

Arvidsson, A., Collin, T., Kirik, D., Kokaia, Z., and Lindvall, O. (2002) Neuronal replacement from endogenous precursors in the adult brain after stroke. *Nat. Med.* 8:963–970.

Ayata, C. and Ropper, A.H. (2002) Ischaemic brain oedema. *J. Clin. Neurosci.* 9:113–124.

Badaut, J., Lasbennes, F., Magistretti, P.J., and Regli, L. (2002) Aquaporins in brain: distribution, physiology, and pathophysiology. *J. Cereb. Blood Flow Metab.* 22:367–378.

Batchelor, P.E., Liberatore, G.T., Wong, J.Y., Porritt, M.J., Frerichs, F., Donnan, G.A., and Howells, D.W. (1999) Activated macrophages and microglia induce dopaminergic sprouting in the injured striatum and express brain-derived neurotrophic factor and glial cell line-derived neurotrophic factor. *J. Neurosci.* 19: 1708–1716.

Bogdan, C., Paik, J., Vodovotz, Y., and Nathan, C. (1992) Contrasting mechanisms for suppression of macrophage cytokine release by transforming growth factor-beta and interleukin-10. *J. Biol. Chem.* 267:23301–23308.

Bruce, A.J., Boling, W., Kindy, M.S., Peschon, J., Kraemer, P.J., Carpenter, M.K., Holtsberg, F.W., and Mattson, M.P. (1996) Altered neuronal and microglial responses to excitotoxic and ischemic brain injury in mice lacking TNF receptors. *Nat. Med.* 2:788–794.

Chen, H., Chopp, M., Zhang, R.L., Bodzin, G., Chen, Q., Rusche, J.R., and Todd, R.F., 3rd (1994) Anti-CD11b monoclonal antibody reduces ischemic cell damage after transient focal cerebral ischemia in rat. *Ann. Neurol.* 35:458–463.

Cotrina, M.L., Kang, J., Lin, J.H., Bueno, E., Hansen, T.W., He, L., Liu, Y., and Nedergaard, M. (1998) Astrocytic gap junctions remain open during ischemic conditions. *J. Neurosci.* 18:2520–2537.

Cruz, N.F. and Dienel, G.A. (2002) High glycogen levels in brains of rats with minimal environmental stimuli: implications for metabolic contributions of working astrocytes. *J. Cereb. Blood Flow Metab.* 22:1476–1489.

Davies, C.A., Loddick, S.A., Toulmond, S., Stroemer, R.P., Hunt, J., and Rothwell, N.J. (1999) The progression and topographic distribution of interleukin-1beta expression after permanent middle cerebral artery occlusion in the rat. *J. Cereb. Blood Flow Metab.* 19:87–98.

Dawson, D.A., Martin, D., and Hallenbeck, J.M. (1996) Inhibition of tumor necrosis factor-alpha reduces focal cerebral ischemic injury in the spontaneously hypertensive rat. *Neurosci. Lett.* 218: 41–44.

del Zoppo, G.J., Schmid-Schonbein, G.W., Mori, E., Copeland, B.R., and Chang, C.M. (1991) Polymorphonuclear leukocytes occlude capillaries following middle cerebral artery occlusion and reperfusion in baboons. *Stroke* 22:1276–1283.

Dewar, D., Yam, P., and McCulloch, J. (1999) Drug development for stroke: importance of protecting cerebral white matter. *Eur. J. Pharmacol.* 375:41–50.

Dirnagl, U., Iadecola, C., and Moskowitz, M.A. (1999) Pathobiology of ischaemic stroke: an integrated view. *Trends Neurosci.* 22:391–397.

Doetsch, F., Caille, I., Lim, D.A., Garcia-Verdugo, J.M., and Alvarez-Buylla, A. (1999) Subventricular zone astrocytes are neural stem cells in the adult mammalian brain. *Cell* 97:703–716.

Dong, Y. and Benveniste, E.N. (2001) Immune function of astrocytes. *Glia* 36:180–190.

Eglitis, M.A., Dawson, D., Park, K.W., and Mouradian, M.M. (1999) Targeting of marrow-derived astrocytes to the ischemic brain. *NeuroReport* 10:1289–1292.

Eglitis, M.A. and Mezey, E. (1997) Hematopoietic cells differentiate into both microglia and macroglia in the brains of adult mice. *Proc. Natl. Acad. Sci. USA* 94:4080–4085.

Ehrenreich, H., Hasselblatt, M., Dembowski, C., Cepek, L., Lewczuk, P., Stiefel, M., Rustenbeck, H.H., Breiter, N., Jacob, S., Knerlich, F., Bohn, M., Poser, W., Ruther, E., Kochen, M., Gefeller, O., Gleiter, C., Wessel, T.C., De Ryck, M., Itri, L., Prange, H., Cerami, A., Brines, M., and Siren, A.L. (2002) Erythropoietin therapy for acute stroke is both safe and beneficial. *Mol. Med.* 8:495–505.

Fiszer, U., Korczak-Kowalska, G., Palasik, W., Korlak, J., Gorski, A., and Czlonkowska, A. (1998) Increased expression of adhesion molecule CD18 (LFA-1beta) on the leukocytes of peripheral blood in patients with acute ischemic stroke. *Acta Neurol. Scand.* 97:221–224.

Frantseva, M.V., Kokarovtseva, L., and Perez Velazquez, J.L. (2002) Ischemia-induced brain damage depends on specific gap-junctional coupling. *J. Cereb. Blood Flow Metab.* 22:453–462.

Friedlander, R.M., Gagliardini, V., Hara, H., Fink, K.B., Li, W., MacDonald, G., Fishman, M.C., Greenberg, A.H., Moskowitz, M.A., and Yuan, J. (1997) Expression of a dominant negative mutant of interleukin-1 beta converting enzyme in transgenic mice prevents neuronal cell death induced by trophic factor withdrawal and ischemic brain injury. *J. Exp. Med.* 185:933–940.

Garcia, J.H., Kalimo, H., Kamijyo, Y., and Trump, B.F. (1977) Cellular events during partial cerebral ischemia. I. Electron microscopy of feline cerebral cortex after middle-cerebral-artery occlusion. *Virchows Arch. B Cell Pathol.* 25:191–206.

Garcia, J.H., Liu, K.F., Yoshida, Y., Lian, J., Chen, S., and del Zoppo, G.J. (1994) Influx of leukocytes and platelets in an evolving brain infarct (Wistar rat). *Am. J. Pathol.* 144:188–199.

Gjedde, A., Marrett, S., and Vafaee, M. (2002) Oxidative and nonoxidative metabolism of excited neurons and astrocytes. *J. Cereb. Blood Flow Metab.* 22:1–14.

Gottschall, P.E. and Deb, S. (1996) Regulation of matrix metalloproteinase expressions in astrocytes, microglia and neurons. *Neuroimmunomodulation* 3:69–75.

Gourmala, N.G., Buttini, M., Limonta, S., Sauter, A., and Boddeke, H.W. (1997) Differential and time-dependent expression of monocyte chemoattractant protein-1 mRNA by astrocytes and macrophages in rat brain: effects of ischemia and peripheral lipopolysaccharide administration. *J. Neuroimmunol.* 74: 35–44.

Gourmala, N.G., Limonta, S., Bochelen, D., Sauter, A., and Boddeke, H.W. (1999) Localization of macrophage inflammatory protein: macrophage inflammatory protein-1 expression in rat brain after peripheral administration of lipopolysaccharide and focal cerebral ischemia. *Neuroscience* 88:1255–1266.

Gregersen, R., Lambertsen, K., and Finsen, B. (2000) Microglia and macrophages are the major source of tumor necrosis factor in permanent middle cerebral artery occlusion in mice. *J. Cereb. Blood Flow Metab.* 20:53–65.

Haberg, A., Qu, H., Saether, O., Unsgard, G., Haraldseth, O., and Sonnewald, U. (2001) Differences in neurotransmitter synthesis and intermediary metabolism between glutamatergic and GABAergic neurons during 4 hours of middle cerebral artery occlusion in the rat: the role of astrocytes in neuronal survival. *J. Cereb. Blood Flow Metab.* 21:1451–1463.

Hossmann, K.A. (1996) Periinfarct depolarizations. *Cerebrovasc. Brain Metab. Rev.* 8:195–208.

Iadecola, C., Salkowski, C.A., Zhang, F., Aber, T., Nagayama, M., Vogel, S.N., and Ross, M.E. (1999) The transcription factor interferon regulatory factor 1 is expressed after cerebral ischemia and contributes to ischemic brain injury. *J. Exp. Med.* 189:719–727.

Iadecola, C., Zhang, F., Casey, R., Nagayama, M., and Ross, M.E. (1997) Delayed reduction of ischemic brain injury and neurological deficits in mice lacking the inducible nitric oxide synthase gene. *J. Neurosci.* 17:9157–9164.

Issa, R., Krupinski, J., Bujny, T., Kumar, S., Kaluza, J., and Kumar, P. (1999) Vascular endothelial growth factor and its receptor, KDR, in human brain tissue after ischemic stroke. *Lab. Invest.* 79:417–425.

Jorgensen, H.S., Nakayama, H., Raaschou, H.O., and Olsen, T.S. (1999) Stroke. Neurologic and functional recovery the Copenhagen Stroke Study. *Phys. Med. Rehabil. Clin. North Am.* 10: 887–906.

Katchanov, J., Harms, C., Gertz, K., Hauck, L., Waeber, C., Hirt, L., Priller, J., von Harsdorf, R., Brück, W., Hörtnagl, H., Dirnagl, U., Bhide, P.G., and Endres, M. (2001) Mild cerebral ischemia induces loss of cyclin-dependent kinase inhibitors and activation of cell cycle machinery before delayed neuronal cell death. *J. Neurosci.* 21:5045–5053.

Korematsu, K., Goto, S., Nagahiro, S., and Ushio, Y. (1994) Microglial response to transient focal cerebral ischemia: an immunocytochemical study on the rat cerebral cortex using anti-phosphotyrosine antibody. *J. Cereb. Blood Flow Metab.* 14:825–830.

Li, W.E., Ochalski, P.A., Hertzberg, E.L., and Nagy, J.I. (1998) Immunorecognition, ultrastructure and phosphorylation status of astrocytic gap junctions and connexin43 in rat brain after cerebral focal ischaemia. *Eur. J. Neurosci.* 10:2444–2463.

Lindsberg, P.J., Carpen, O., Paetau, A., Karjalainen-Lindsberg, M.L., and Kaste, M. (1996) Endothelial ICAM-1 expression associated with inflammatory cell response in human ischemic stroke. *Circulation* 94:939–945.

Liu, H.M. and Chen, H.H. (1994) Correlation between fibroblast growth factor expression and cell proliferation in experimental brain infarct: studied with proliferating cell nuclear antigen immunohistochemistry. *J. Neuropathol. Exp. Neurol.* 53:118–126.

Loihl, A.K., Asensio, V., Campbell, I.L., and Murphy, S. (1999) Expression of nitric oxide synthase (NOS)-2 following permanent focal ischemia and the role of nitric oxide in infarct generation in male, female and NOS-2 gene-deficient mice. *Brain Res.* 830: 155–164.

Lyons, S.A., Pastor, A., Ohlemeyer, C., Kann, O., Wiegand, F., Prass, K., Knapp, F., Kettenmann, H., and Dirnagl, U. (2000) Distinct physiologic properties of microglia and blood-borne cells in rat brain slices after permanent middle cerebral artery occlusion. *J. Cereb. Blood Flow Metab.* 20:1537–1549.

Mabuchi, T., Kitagawa, K., Ohtsuki, T., Kuwabara, K., Yagita, Y., Yanagihara, T., Hori, M., and Matsumoto, M. (2000) Contribution of microglia/macrophages to expansion of infarction and response of oligodendrocytes after focal cerebral ischemia in rats. *Stroke* 31:1735–1743.

Mandai, K., Matsumoto, M., Kitagawa, K., Matsushita, K., Ohtsuki, T., Mabuchi, T., Colman, D.R., Kamada, T., and Yanagihara, T. (1997) Ischemic damage and subsequent proliferation of oligodendrocytes in focal cerebral ischemia. *Neuroscience* 77:849–861.

Manley, G.T., Fujimura, M., Ma, T., Noshita, N., Filiz, F., Bollen, A.W., Chan, P., and Verkman, A.S. (2000) Aquaporin-4 deletion in mice reduces brain edema after acute water intoxication and ischemic stroke. *Nat. Med.* 6:159–163.

Marks, L., Carswell, H.V., Peters, E.E., Graham, D.I., Patterson, J., Dominiczak, A.F., and Macrae, I.M. (2001) Characterization of the microglial response to cerebral ischemia in the stroke-prone spontaneously hypertensive rat. *Hypertension* 38:116–122.

Mason, H.A., Ito, S., and Corfas, G. (2001) Extracellular signals that regulate the tangential migration of olfactory bulb neuronal precursors: inducers, inhibitors, and repellents. *J. Neurosci.* 21: 7654–7663.

McCracken, E., Fowler, J.H., Dewar, D., Morrison, S., and McCulloch, J. (2002) Grey matter and white matter ischemic damage is reduced by the competitive AMPA receptor antagonist, SPD 502. *J. Cereb. Blood Flow Metab.* 22:1090–1097.

McDonald, J.W., Althomsons, S.P., Hyrc, K.L., Choi, D.W., and Goldberg, M.P. (1998) Oligodendrocytes from forebrain are highly vulnerable to AMPA/kainate receptor-mediated excitotoxicity. *Nat. Med.* 4:291–297.

Mori, E., del Zoppo, G.J., Chambers, J.D., Copeland, B.R., and Arfors, K.E. (1992) Inhibition of polymorphonuclear leukocyte adherence suppresses no-reflow after focal cerebral ischemia in baboons. *Stroke* 23:712–718.

Nakase, T., Fushiki, S., and Naus, C.C. (2003) Astrocytic gap junctions composed of connexin 43 reduce apoptotic neuronal damage in cerebral ischemia. *Stroke* 34:1987–1993.

Namura, S., Maeno, H., Takami, S., Jiang, F., Kamichi, S., Wada, K., and Nagata, I. (2002) Inhibition of glial glutamate transporter GLT-1 augments brain edema after transient focal cerebral ischemia in mice. *Neurosci. Lett.* 324:117–120.

Naus, C.C., Ozog, M.A., Bechberger, J.F., and Nakase, T. (2001) A neuroprotective role for gap junctions. *Cell Commun. Adhes.* 8:325–328.

Nawashiro, H., Brenner, M., Fukui, S., Shima, K., and Hallenbeck, J.M. (2000) High susceptibility to cerebral ischemia in GFAP-null mice. *J. Cereb. Blood Flow Metab.* 20:1040–1044.

Nedergaard, M., Takano, T., and Hansen, A.J. (2002) Beyond the role of glutamate as a neurotransmitter. *Nat. Rev. Neurosci.* 3:748–755.

Norenberg, M.D. (1998) Astrocytes in ischemic injury. In: Ginsberg, M.D. and Bogousslavsky, J., eds. *Cerebrovascular Disease: Pathophysiology, Diagnosis, and Management.* Malden, MA: Blackwell Science, pp. 113–128.

O'Neill, L.A. and Kaltschmidt, C. (1997) NF-kappa B: a crucial transcription factor for glial and neuronal cell function. *Trends Neurosci.* 20:252–258.

Pantoni, L. (1998) Experimental approaches to white matter disease. *Dement. Geriatr. Cogn. Disord.* 9(Suppl 1):20-24–20-24.

Pappata, S., Levasseur, M., Gunn, R.N., Myers, R., Crouzel, C., Syrota, A., Jones, T., Kreutzberg, G.W., and Banati, R.B. (2000) Thalamic microglial activation in ischemic stroke detected in vivo by PET and [11C]PK1195. *Neurology* 55:1052–1054.

Pelidou, S.H., Kostulas, N., Matusevicius, D., Kivisakk, P., Kostulas, V., and Link, H. (1999) High levels of IL-10 secreting cells are present in blood in cerebrovascular diseases. *Eur. J. Neurol.* 6:437–442.

Perez Velazquez, J.L., Frantseva, M.V., and Naus, C.C. (2003) Gap junctions and neuronal injury: protectants or executioners? *Neuroscientist* 9:5–9.

Planas, A.M., Sole, S., and Justicia, C. (2001) Expression and activation of matrix metalloproteinase-2 and -9 in rat brain after transient focal cerebral ischemia. *Neurobiol. Dis.* 8:834–846.

Prehn, J.H., Backhauss, C., and Krieglstein, J. (1993) Transforming growth factor-beta 1 prevents glutamate neurotoxicity in rat neocortical cultures and protects mouse neocortex from ischemic injury in vivo. *J. Cereb. Blood Flow Metab.* 13:521–525.

Priller, J. and Dirnagl, U. (2002) Inflammation in stroke—a potential target for neuroprotection? *Ernst Schering Res. Found. Workshop* 39:133–157.

Priller, J., Flugel, A., Wehner, T., Boentert, M., Haas, C.A., Prinz, M., Fernandez-Klett, F., Prass, K., Bechmann, I., de Boer, B.A., Frotscher, M., Kreutzberg, G.W., Persons, D.A., and Dirnagl, U. (2001) Targeting gene-modified hematopoietic cells to the central nervous system: use of green fluorescent protein uncovers microglial engraftment. *Nat. Med.* 7:1356–1361.

Priller, J., Haas, C.A., Reddington, M., and Kreutzberg, G.W. (1995) Calcitonin gene-related peptide and ATP induce immediate early gene expression in cultured rat microglial cells. *Glia* 15:447–457.

Priller, J., Reddington, M., Haas, C.A., and Kreutzberg, G.W. (1998) Stimulation of P2Y-purinoceptors on astrocytes results in immediate early gene expression and potentiation of neuropeptide action. *Neuroscience* 85:521–525.

Rathbone, M.P., Middlemiss, P.J., Gysbers, J.W., Andrew, C., Herman, M.A., Reed, J.K., Ciccarelli, R., Di Iorio, P., and Caciagli, F. (1999) Trophic effects of purines in neurons and glial cells. *Prog. Neurobiol.* 59:663–690.

Rawanduzy, A., Hansen, A., Hansen, T.W., and Nedergaard, M. (1997) Effective reduction of infarct volume by gap junction blockade in a rodent model of stroke. *J. Neurosurg.* 87:916–920.

Relton, J.K., Martin, D., Thompson, R.C., and Russell, D.A. (1996) Peripheral administration of Interleukin-1 receptor antagonist inhibits brain damage after focal cerebral ischemia in the rat. *Exp. Neurol.* 138:206–213.

Rivera, S., Ogier, C., Jourquin, J., Timsit, S., Szklarczyk, A.W., Miller, K., Gearing, A.J., Kaczmarek, L., and Khrestchatisky, M. (2002) Gelatinase B and TIMP-1 are regulated in a cell- and time-dependent manner in association with neuronal death and glial reactivity after global forebrain ischemia. *Eur. J. Neurosci.* 15:19–32.

Rose, C.R., Waxman, S.G., and Ransom, B.R. (1998) Effects of glucose deprivation, chemical hypoxia, and simulated ischemia on Na^+ homeostasis in rat spinal cord astrocytes. *J. Neurosci.* 18:3554–3562.

Ruscher, K., Freyer, D., Karsch, M., Isaev, N., Megow, D., Sawitzki, B., Priller, J., Dirnagl, U., and Meisel, A. (2002) Erythropoietin is a paracrine mediator of ischemic tolerance in the brain: evidence from an in vitro model. *J. Neurosci.* 22:10291–10301.

Shibata, M., Hisahara, S., Hara, H., Yamawaki, T., Fukuuchi, Y., Yuan, J., Okano, H., and Miura, M. (2000) Caspases determine the vulnerability of oligodendrocytes in the ischemic brain. *J. Clin. Invest.* 106:643–653.

Spera, P.A., Ellison, J.A., Feuerstein, G.Z., and Barone, F.C. (1998) IL-10 reduces rat brain injury following focal stroke. *Neurosci. Lett.* 251:189–192.

Stoll, G., Jander, S., and Schroeter, M. (1998) Inflammation and glial responses in ischemic brain lesions. *Prog. Neurobiol.* 56:149–171.

Taniguchi, M., Yamashita, T., Kumura, E., Tamatani, M., Kobayashi, A., Yokawa, T., Maruno, M., Kato, A., Ohnishi, T., Kohmura, E., Tohyama, M., and Yoshimine, T. (2000) Induction of aquaporin-4 water channel mRNA after focal cerebral ischemia in rat. *Brain Res. Mol. Brain Res.* 78:131–137.

Tarozzo, G., Campanella, M., Ghiani, M., Bulfone, A., and Beltramo, M. (2002) Expression of fractalkine and its receptor, CX3CR1, in response to ischaemia-reperfusion brain injury in the rat. *Eur. J. Neurosci.* 15:1663–1668.

The NINDS and Stroke rt-PA Stroke Study Group (1995) Tissue plasminogen activator for acute ischemic stroke. The National Institute of Neurological Disorders and Stroke rt-PA Stroke Study Group [see comments]. *N. Engl. J. Med.* 333:1581–1587.

Trendelenburg, G., Prass, K., Priller, J., Kapinya, K., Polley, A., Muselmann, C., Ruscher, K., Kannbley, U., Schmitt, A.O., Castell, S., Wiegand, F., Meisel, A., Rosenthal, A., and Dirnagl, U. (2002) Serial analysis of gene expression identifies metallothionein-II as major neuroprotective gene in mouse focal cerebral ischemia. *J. Neurosci.* 22:5879–5888.

Tsirka, S.E., Gualandris, A., Amaral, D.G., and Strickland, S. (1995) Excitotoxin-induced neuronal degeneration and seizure are mediated by tissue plasminogen activator. *Nature* 377:340–344.

Tsunawaki, S., Sporn, M., Ding, A., and Nathan, C. (1988) Deactivation of macrophages by transforming growth factor-beta. *Nature* 334:260–262.

Ueyama, T., Ren, Y., Sakai, N., Takahashi, M., Ono, Y., Kondoh, T., Tamaki, N., and Saito, N. (2001) Generation of a constitutively active fragment of PKN in microglia/macrophages after middle cerebral artery occlusion in rats. *J. Neurochem.* 79: 903–913.

van Lookeren Campagne, M., Thibodeaux, H., van Bruggen, N., Cairns, B., Gerlai, R., Palmer, J.T., Williams, S.P., and Lowe, D.G. (1999) Evidence for a protective role of metallothionein-1 in focal cerebral ischemia. *Proc. Natl. Acad. Sci. USA* 96: 12870–12875.

Wender, R., Brown, A.M., Fern, R., Swanson, R.A., Farrell, K., and Ransom, B.R. (2000) Astrocytic glycogen influences axon function and survival during glucose deprivation in central white matter. *J. Neurosci.* 20:6804–6810.

Wilson, J.X. (1997) Antioxidant defense of the brain: a role for astrocytes. *Can. J. Physiol. Pharmacol.* 75:1149–1163.

Yamasaki, Y., Matsuura, N., Shozuhara, H., Onodera, H., Itoyama, Y., and Kogure, K. (1995) Interleukin-1 as a pathogenetic mediator of ischemic brain damage in rats. *Stroke* 26:676–680.

Yrjänheikki, J., Tikka, T., Keinanen, R., Goldsteins, G., Chan, P.H., and Koistinaho, J. (1999) A tetracycline derivative, minocycline, reduces inflammation and protects against focal cerebral ischemia with a wide therapeutic window. *Proc. Natl. Acad. Sci. USA* 96:13496–13500.

Zhang, R.L., Chopp, M., Jiang, N., Tang, W.X., Prostak, J., Manning, A.M., and Anderson, D.C. (1995a) Anti-intercellular adhesion molecule-1 antibody reduces ischemic cell damage after transient but not permanent middle cerebral artery occlusion in the Wistar rat. *Stroke* 26:1438–1442.

Zhang, R.L., Chopp, M., Zaloga, C., Zhang, Z.G., Jiang, N., Gautam, S.C., Tang, W.X., Tsang, W., Anderson, D.C., and Manning, A.M. (1995b) The temporal profiles of ICAM-1 protein and mRNA expression after transient MCA occlusion in the rat. *Brain Res.* 682:182–188.

42 Gliomas

MICHAEL WELLER

Gliomas constitute a heterogeneous group of brain tumors that are thought to derive from glial cells or their precursors. These tumors exhibit unique biological features. Their precise histogenetic origin has remained obscure. They show a highly infiltrative and invasive growth pattern in the brain but rarely metastasize outside the central nervous system. Glioma cells are paradigmatic for the ability of cancer cells to compromise cellular immune defense mechanisms. These cells are also highly resistant to the induction of apoptotic cell death, rendering futile all current approaches of cancer therapy. Gliomas have thus remained one of the most challenging types of cancer for decades.

ETIOLOGY

The cause of most gliomas remains obscure. For the vast majority of gliomas, genetic factors seem not to be predisposing factors. Similarly, no environmental factors related to glioma development have been identified except cranial irradiation, which may increase the incidence of gliomas 3- to 7-fold. In contrast, no role for cellular phones, high-tension wires, head trauma, or dietary compounds has been demonstrated. Some genetic disorders are associated with a high risk of glioma development, such as optic nerve gliomas in neurofibromatosis type I, various types of gliomas in neurofibromatosis type II and the Li-Fraumeni syndrome, subependymal giant cell astrocytoma in tuberous sclerosis, and glioblastoma in the Turcot syndrome (Kleihues and Cavenee, 2000). These associations provide interesting insights into the biochemistry of gliomagenesis and offer clues to the development of the much more common spontaneous gliomas.

Although the nomenclature of gliomas suggests a specific cell of origin, such as an oligodendrocyte or an oligodendrocyte precursor in the case of oligodendroglioma, it has not been clarified which cell population in the brain gives rise to tumors that develop several decades after birth in a tissue that is mitotically largely inactive. The new field of stem cell biology is expected to offer new hypotheses on the origin of these tumors. Thus, the combined activation of Ras and AKT in neural progenitors results in the formation of glioblastomas in mice (Holland et al., 2000), providing a novel model for gliomagenesis. Similarly autocrine stimulation by platelet-derived growth factor (PDGF) induced the formation of oligodendroglial tumors by neural progenitor cells (Dai et al., 2001). The INK4a-ARF tumor suppressor locus encodes two proteins, p16INK4a and p14ARF, which modulate the activity of the RB and p53 proteins. Although INK4a-ARF deficiency does not lead to spontaneous gliomas in rodents, it allows glioma formation from astrocytes by KRas and AKT and enhances tumor formation by neural progenitor cells (Uhrbom et al., 2002). Together, these studies support the hypothesis that brain parenchymal stem cells are the source of glioma formation in the adult mammalian brain.

HISTOPATHOLOGY

Gliomas are classified by neuropathological criteria defined by the World Health Organization (WHO) (Kleihues and Cavenee, 2000; DeAngelis, 2001). The grading of gliomas from low (I) to high (IV) malignancy is a key feature of the WHO classification and has important implications for therapy and prognosis. The most common WHO grade I tumor, pilocytic astrocytoma, is a benign lesion and mainly a tumor of childhood and early adulthood. World Health Organization grade II, III, and IV gliomas are diffusely growing, infiltrative tumors that are distinct entities histopathologically, but can be viewed as distinct stages of malignant progression among a family of related tumors, glioblastoma (WHO grade IV) being the most malignant and most common variant (Fig. 42.1*A*; Tables 42.1 and 42.2). Grade I astrocytomas are circumscribed, slowly growing tumors with low cellularity. Grade II astrocytomas are well-differentiated tumors with a diffusely infiltrative growth pattern. Grade III anaplastic astrocytomas show enhanced cellularity, nuclear atypia, and increased mitotic activity. Grade IV glioblastomas are characterized by such features plus prominent microvascular proliferation or areas of ne-

See the list of abbreviations at the end of the chapter.

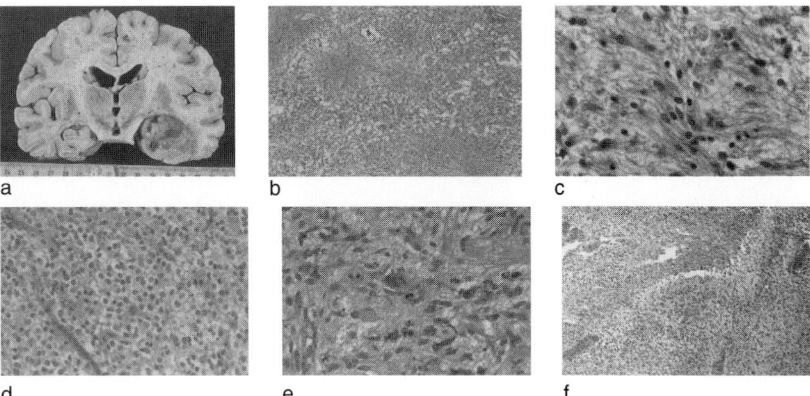

FIGURE 42.1 Macroscopic appearance of left temporal lobe glioblastoma (*a*) and histological features of common gliomas: pilocytic astrocytoma (*b*), fibrillary astrocytoma (*c*), oligodendroglioma (*d*), anaplastic astrocytoma (*e*), and glioblastoma (*f*). H&E stain. (Courtesy of R. Meyermann, Institute of Brain Research, Tübingen, Germany).

crosis (Fig. 42.1). Oligodendroglial tumors are graded as II, as III when features of anaplasia are present, or as glioblastomas without further specification if the above-mentioned criteria for glioblastoma are met. Gliomas are graded not according to the predominant grade of malignancy of the resected tissue, but according to the area of highest malignancy; for example, a tumor that for the most part corresponds to a grade II astrocytoma will still be classified as a glioblastoma should there be a single focal area meeting the criteria for glioblastoma. The diagnosis of the glial origin of a brain tumor is based on its morphological resemblance to untransformed astrocytes and the common expression of glial fibrillary acidic protein (see Chapters 2 and 6). Gliomas are often heavily infiltrated by host cells, predominantly microglial cells and macrophages, but also reactive astrocytes and fewer lymphocytes.

TABLE 42.1 *Epidemiology of Common Gliomas*

Tumor	*% of All Brain Tumors*	*Incidence per 100,000 /Year*	*Mean Age at Diagnosis*
Pilocytic astrocytoma	1.8	0.22	17
Diffuse astrocytoma	1.3	0.17	47
Anaplastic astrocytoma	4.3	0.54	50
Glioblastoma	22.6	2.94	62
Oligodendroglioma	2.6	0.32	41
Anaplastic oligodendroglioma	0.6	0.07	46
Mixed glioma	1	0.13	40
Astrocytoma, not otherwise specified	8.1	1.01	47
Malignant glioma, not otherwise specified	2.6	0.33	46

Source. Data from www.cbtrus.org/2000/table2000-2.htm (incidence rate adjusted to year 2000 U.S. standard population).

MOLECULAR GENETICS

Molecular genetic studies have provided detailed knowledge of the chromosomal and genetic changes in gliomas that include both losses and gains of genetic material (Von Deimling et al., 2000). There are clusters of alterations that are typical of, although not specific for, various types of gliomas. Molecular genetic analyses have also been instrumental in the characterization of the malignant progression from grade II to grade III and grade IV tumors. There is a high frequency of loss of heterozygosity (LOH) on chromosome 10 in glioblastoma. Other specific alterations allow the subclassification of tumors of the same histology, such as glioblastoma, by means of molecular genetic profiling (Fig. 42.2). For instance, loss of the tumor suppressor gene product, *p53*, is commonly found in grade II diffuse astrocytomas and thus also in glioblastomas (secondary glioblastoma or type I glioblastoma) progressing from these lesions (Watanabe et al., 1996). In contrast, *p53* mutations are rather uncommon in tu-

TABLE 42.2 *Relative Survival at 2 and 5 Years from the Time of Diagnosis of a Primary Brain Tumor*

	Survival at 2 years %	*Survival at 5 years %*
Pilocytic astrocytoma	91	87
Diffuse astrocytoma	67	49
Anaplastic astrocytoma	46	31
Glioblastoma	9	3
Oligodendroglioma	80	63
Anaplastic oligodendroglioma	61	38
Mixed glioma	74	59
Astrocytoma, not otherwise specified	45	35
Malignant glioma, not otherwise specified	34	27

Source. Davis et al. (1999).

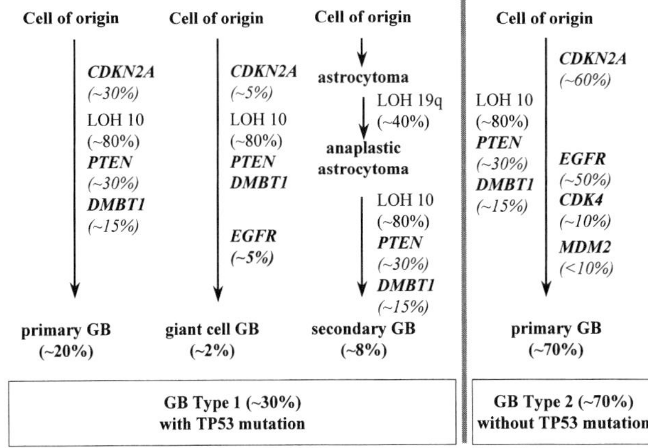

FIGURE 42.2 Molecular pathways to glioblastoma (GB) (von Deimling et al., 2000).

mors classified as glioblastoma (WHO grade IV) when diagnosed. In these tumors, it is uncertain whether there has been a clinically silent stage where the histological features of lower-grade gliomas were present. These primary (or type 2) glioblastomas, which are the most common type of glioblastoma, often exhibit enhanced expression or amplification of the epidermal growth factor receptor (EGFR) gene. Further, these tumors show alterations of the retinoblastoma (RB) protein-controlled cell cycle checkpoint. The RB protein cooperates with the cyclin-dependent kinase (CDK) inhibitor p16INK4a (encoded by the *CDKN2A* gene) to arrest the cell cycle whereas members of CDK family drive cell cycle progression. Most glioblastomas exhibit losses of both *CDKN2A* alleles, RB mutations or deletions, or *CDK4* gene amplifications, all resulting in deficient cell cycle control (Ichimura et al., 2000). Since an abnormal G0/1 transition would render cells exquisitely sensitive to *p53*-mediated apoptosis, it is not surprising that most glioblastomas also harbor abnormalities in the *p53*-controlled cell death pathway. This may involve *p53* mutation (see above), or amplification or enhanced activity of the murine double minute (MDM)-2 protein, which targets *p53* for proteasomal degradation, or loss of p14ARF, which negatively controls the action of MDM-2.

Molecular genetic studies have also assumed an important role in two areas of research on oligodendroglial tumors. First, these analyses may help to resolve the controversial issue of the mixed gliomas, the oligoastrocytomas, which are clonal in origin yet contain two morphologically distinct populations of tumor cells. Second, specific chromosomal alterations, the loss of genetic material on chromosomes 1p and 19q, have been linked to a favorable response to chemotherapy and to prolonged survival in oligodendroglial tumors (Cairncross et al., 1998; Ino et al., 2001). The identification of the gene products, which when lost confer sensitivity to chemotherapy, will represent a major step toward a better understanding of the resistance of gliomas to radiotherapy and chemotherapy.

CELL BIOLOGY

Migration, invasiveness, and induction of angiogenesis are key biological features of malignant glioma cells. The study of these biological features of brain tumor cells is currently strongly influenced by the expanding field of stem cell biology. Embryonic stem cell–derived multipotent stem cells display a broad potential and are self-renewing. They give rise to glial precursor/progenitor cells. In addition to self-renewal, all classes of these cells are characterized by extensive migration (Hatten, 1993; Sugimoto et al., 2001). Migration involves radial and tangential patterns. *Radial migration* refers to cellular locomotion along cellular processes of a specialized glial scaffold formed by the processes of radial glial cells that span the entire thickness of the developing CNS (Campbell and Götz, 2002). In contrast, *tangentially migrating* cells are thought to respond to local environmental clues to specify their ultimate fate or location. Radial migration involves interactions between neuronal and glial cells mediated by cell surface receptors and ligands. Proteins involved in tangential central nervous system (CNS) migration or axonal guidance include α_3 integrin, β_1 integrin, polysialated neural cell adhesion molecule (PSA-NCAM), semaphorin-3A, repulsive diffusible factors such as Slit, netrin, deleted in colon cancer (DCC), and ephrins. Hepatocyte growth factor (HGF)/scatter factor (SF) may also be important for the migration of interneurons in the developing CNS (Powell et al., 2001).

Some pathways involving these proteins are also essential in the migration of neoplastic astrocytes. Further key biological features of neoplastic astrocytes include invasive and angiogenic properties, resistance to multiple apoptotic stimuli, and negative immune regulatory properties. Angiogenesis is probably driven by hypoxia and mediated by the recruitment of host endothelial cells by the growing tumors. Vascular-endothelial growth factor (VEGF) is the key mediator of tumor-induced angiogenesis and has also become a major target for therapeutic intervention (see below). Migration and invasion depend on interactions of integrins expressed by glioma cells with the extracellular matrix, the activation of the urokinase-type plasminogen activator (UPA) receptor, and the expression and activity of matrix metalloproteinases (MMPs) (Mohan et al., 1999). These processes are controlled in an autocrine and paracrine fashion via the release of promigratory and proinvasive cytokines such as HGF/SF and transforming growth factor (TGF)-β. Hepatocyte growth factor/scatter factor promotes the synthesis and release of TGF-β through a signal transduction pathway involving ezrin (Wick et al., 2001). Ezrin is a member of the ezrin-radixin-moesin family proteins that cross-link actin cytoskeleton and plasma membrane. Transforming growth factor-β, in turn, promotes MMP activity.

Glioma cells have long been known to be a rich source of TGF-β, which has become one of the major targets for the experimental treatment of gliomas (see below). The synthesis, storage, and activation of TGF-β is a complex process that includes the processing of the proform of TGF-β by proprotein convertases such as furin, binding to the extracellular matrix, and activation to the mature dimeric 25 kDa TGF-β by multiple pathways (Fig. 42.3). The efficient synthesis of TGF-β requires high activity of proprotein convertases (Leitlein et al., 2001), the enzymes that also process MMP. Migration requires the survival of cells that detach from their parent cell population and inhibition of the cell death process termed *anoikis*. In that regard, enhanced expression of anti-apoptotic proteins such as B cell lymphoma (BCL)-2 or BCL-X_L supports migration and invasion *in vitro*, but it has remained controversial whether these proteins truely confer a migratory phenotype or whether their expression results in a net increase in migrated cells as a consequence of enhanced survival under unfavorable conditions.

IMMUNOLOGY

Although malignant glioma cells exhibit all characteristic features of malignant cells, these tumors appear to be essentially unable to metastasize outside the CNS. This has led to the hypothesis that the immune system mounts an effective response to glioma cells outside but not inside the CNS. Physiologically the brain is one of the body's immune-priviledged sites, that is, a site where allografts enjoy prolonged survival. While the natural milieu of the brain per se may protect a tumor from immune attack, glioma cells themselves create a locally immunosuppressed milieu, accomplished by the expression or release of immune inhibitory factors such as the cytokines, TGF-β or interleukin (IL)-10, or prostaglandins, as well as the expression of immune modulatory molecules such as CD70 or HLA-G at the cell surface (see also Chapters 11 and 22). Transforming growth factor-β again is probably a key player in the immune modulation in malignant glioma; in fact, it may be the most potent endogenous immunosuppressive molecule: it suppresses T cell activation, natural killer (NK) cell function, and the cytolytic activity of monocytes, macrophages, and microglial cells (Weller and Fontana, 1995).

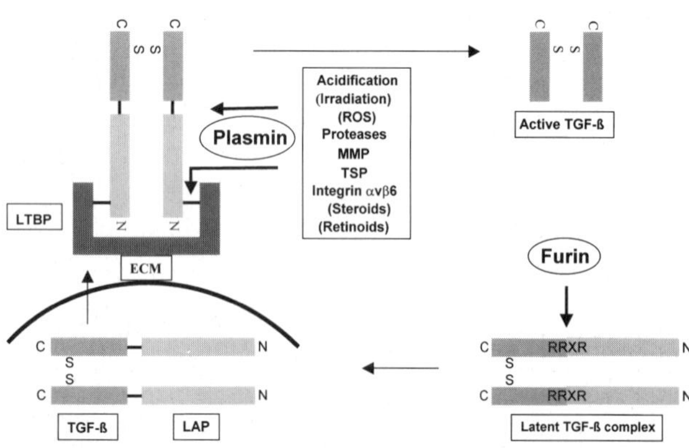

FIGURE 42.3 Synthesis and activation of transforming growth factor-β (TGF-β). The most important steps include the processing of the TGF-β precursor by furin-like proprotein convertases and the activation to the mature 25 kDa peptide by one of several stimuli. Note that modes of TGF-β activation put in brackets have remained controversial. ECM: extracellular matrix; LAP: latency-associated peptide; LTBP: laten TGF-β-binding protein; MMP: matrix metalloproteinase; ROS: reactive oxygen species; TSP: thrombospondin.

GLIOMA RESEARCH: CELL LINES AND ANIMAL MODELS

Surgically removed glioma tissue can be maintained *in vitro* and readily gives rise to polyclonal cultures and eventually long-term cell lines. Although the long-term cell lines are indispensable for molecular and cell biological studies on glioma cells, promising findings regarding the biology or experimental treatment of gliomas derived from glioma cell lines should be reconfirmed in fresh *ex vivo* polyclonal glioma cell cultures. Most animal models for gliomas suffer from their failure to mimic the infiltrative and invasive growth pattern and are not truly syngeneic. This includes the common C6 and 9L gliomas in the rat as well as the GL261 glioma in the mouse. The SMA-560 glioma in VM/Dk mice is probably the best rodent glioma for immunological studies (Serano et al., 1980). Infiltration and invasion are best mimicked by the transplantation of human glioma cell tissue into the brains of recipient nude rats (Mahesparan et al., 2003).

CLINICAL FEATURES AND DIAGNOSIS

Frequent types of clinical presentation of gliomas include seizures, personality changes, and focal neurological deficits such as hemiparesis or visual disturbances (Weller and Thomas, 2002). If clinical symptoms and signs of a brain tumor develop, the most important diagnostic step is neuroimaging, preferably magnetic resonance imaging (MRI) or cranial computed tomography (CT). Magnetic resonance imaging is superior to CT with regard to anatomical detail and the delineation of tumor tissue from edema and normal brain tissue. The uptake of the intravenous contrast agent and the formation of peritumoral edema suggest a higher grade of malignancy (Fig. 42.4). Cerebral angiography provides information on the blood supply of gliomas and may aid surgical planning. Although various neuroimaging methods are valuable tools for the diagnosis of brain tumors, for the planning of surgical procedures, and for monitoring responses to therapy, definitive diagnoses of gliomas require a surgical procedure, biopsy or gross resection, and neuropathological analysis of the tissue.

CLINICAL THERAPY

The clinical management of gliomas depends on the WHO grade of malignancy, the location of the tumor, the age of the patient, and the general condition of the patient, commonly expressed as the Karnofsky performance score. For WHO grade II, III, and IV lesions, advanced age and a low Karnofsky performance score at diagnosis are the most important predictors of a poor outcome (Weller and Thomas, 2002). The current treatment modalities used clinically include surgery, radiotherapy, and chemotherapy. Standards of care at diagnosis and at relapse are summarized in Table 42.3. Pilocytic astrocytomas are treated surgically whenever possible and may be cured by surgery alone. The management of diffuse astrocytomas has remained controversial for decades. Gross total resection is a positive prognostic factor in most retrospective series. Radiotherapy is effective in local tumor control, but the optimal time point for administering radiotherapy is much debated. Oligodendrogliomas are now more often treated with chemotherapy rather than radiotherapy as the first treatment after surgery. Anaplastic astrocytomas are commonly treated by gross total resection followed by radiotherapy, sometimes combined with chemotherapy. Chemotherapy also has modest activity at recurrence. Anaplastic oligodendrogliomas respond to chemotherapy, and are now often managed with chemotherapy up front and radiotherapy at progression. Mixed oligoastrocytomas are treated as pure oligodendrogliomas. Glioblastomas are managed by biopsy or resection followed by radiotherapy. The role of chemotherapy in the primary treatment as an adjunct to radiotherapy is uncertain. Its role at recurrence after surgery and radiotherapy is better defined.

Oncological surgery in the brain is limited. Yet, modern microsurgical and imaging techniques have led to great advances in brain tumor surgery in that the safety of the procedures has been increased and surgery-related morbidity greatly reduced.

Radiotherapy is at present the single most effective treatment for grade III and IV gliomas, although the median survival for patients with glioblastoma is prolonged for only 6 months by radiotherapy. Radiotherapy is delivered externally in a series of single fractions (fractionated radiotherapy, 2–3 Gy) or as a single dose (radiosurgery, e.g., 18–24 Gy) or interstitially by radioactive seed implantation (brachytherapy). The modes of action of radiotherapy may differ, depending on the type of tumor and the type of radiotherapy de-

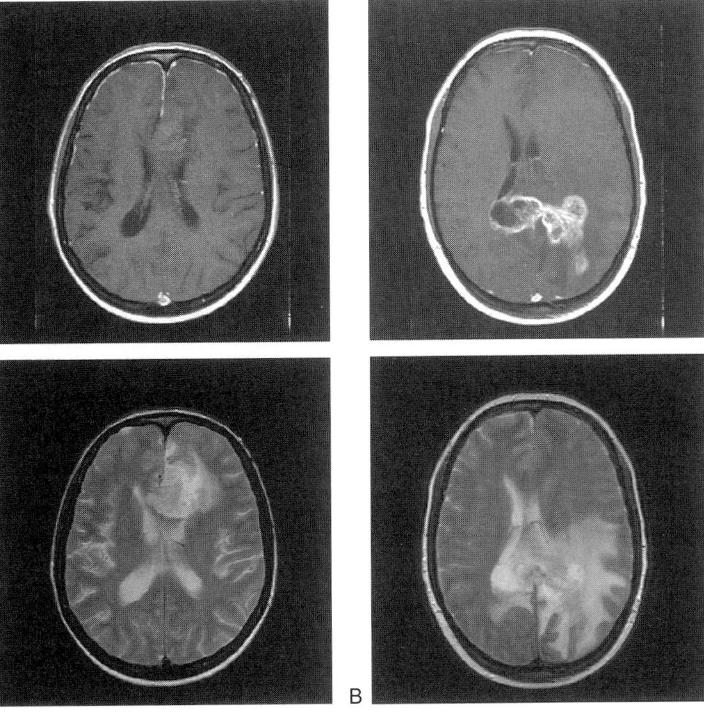

FIGURE 42.4 Magnetic resonance imaging (scan) of gliomas. *A*. Grade II oligoastrocytoma. *B*. Grade IV glioblastoma *Upper panels*: T1-weighted images after contrast enhancement. *Lower panels*: T2-weighted images. Note that the low-grade tumor in *A* is much more readily detected on T2-weighted scans, whereas contrast enhancement clearly demarcates the high-grade tumor in *B*.

TABLE 42.3 *Standards of Care for Gliomas*

	First-Line Treatment	*Treatment at Progression or Relapse*
Pilocytic astrocytoma WHO grade I	Resection	Resection, radiotherapy, or both
Diffuse astrocytoma WHO grade II	Resection/biopsy and observation *or* resection/biopsy and radiotherapy	Resection and radiotherapy (or chemotherapy)
Oligodendroglioma and oligoastrocytoma WHO grade II	Resection/biopsy and observation *or* resection/biopsy and chemotherapy or radiotherapy	Resection and chemotherapy or radiotherapy
Anaplastic astrocytoma WHO grade III	Resection/biopsy and radiotherapy ± chemotherapy	Resection and chemotherapy or radiotherapy
Anaplastic oligodendroglioma and oligoastrocytoma WHO grade III	Resection/biopsy and chemotherapy, radiotherapy, or both	Resection and chemotherapy or radiotherapy
Glioblastoma WHO grade IV	Resection/biopsy and radiotherapy ± chemotherapy	Resection and chemotherapy or radiotherapy

livered. The proliferative activity of tumor cells is the classical target of radiotherapy for cancer. It is a rather tumor-specific target in the brain since neurons never, and astrocytes rarely, divide in the normal brain. The hypothesis that radiotherapy eliminates neural stem cells in the adult human brain, and that this contributes to radiation-induced neurotoxicity, is interesting but not yet supported by experimental or clinical data. The inhibition of tumor cell proliferation is probably an important effect of radiotherapy in gliomas. In contrast, relevant cytolytic effects of radiotherapy are not achieved in most gliomas, as evidenced by the low frequency of complete responses to radiotherapy documented by CT or MRI. Further, radiotherapy is likely to compromise the vascular supply of brain tumors, notably rapidly growing tumors with heavy neovascularization such as glioblastoma. Factors that influence tumor responses and the brain's tolerance of radiotherapy are the total dose administered, the size of the fractions, the volume of brain irradiated, the age of the patient, and the type of lesion. Molecular and cell biological factors promoting resistance of glioma cells to radiotherapy include poor tumor oxygenation, preservation of DNA repair properties, and expression of antiapoptotic gene products, for example, of the BCL-2 and inhibitor-of-apoptosis (IAP) protein families.

Chemotherapy plays an overall modest role in the treatment of gliomas, with the exception of oligodendroglial tumors. The reasons for the chemoresistance of gliomas, which are similar to those discussed for radiotherapy earlier, include (*1*) poor tumor perfusion or aberrant tumor perfusion with aberrant arteriovenous shunting, limiting drug delivery to tumor cells; (*2*) hypoxia that confers resistance to most chemotherapeutic agents; (*3*) expression of membrane transport proteins such as the P-glycoprotein encoded by the multidrug resistance (*mdr*) gene or the multidrug resistance (MDR)–related protein-1 (MRP-1) gene product both by tumor cells and by cerebral endothelial cells, limiting the effects of agents such as vincristine or etoposide; and (*4*) reduced expression of proapoptotic proteins and enhanced expression of antiapoptotic proteins, for example, of the BCL-2 and IAP families. Among a wide variety of agents explored for their activity in gliomas, the nitrosoureas, nimustine, carmustine, and lomustine, and the novel agent temozolomide appear to be the most active drugs. Both are classical cancer chemotherapeutic drugs that damage DNA. The resistance to alkylating agents such as nitrosoureas is mediated in part by a DNA repair enzyme, O^6-methylguanine-DNA methyltransferase (MGMT, also referred to as O^6-alkylguanine-DNA alkyltransferase [OGAT]), which removes alkyl groups from the O^6 position of guanine, a critical target of nitrosourea-induced alkylation. The expression levels of the MGMT gene are regulated by methylation, and the determination of MGMT expression and activity may be a powerful predictor of sensitivity or resistance to alkylating agents (Esteller et al., 2000). As a corollary, the higher sensitivity of oligodendroglial tumors to chemotherapy compared with astrocytomas has been attributed to their lower MGMT expression (Silber et al., 1998; Nutt et al., 2000). The first efforts to enhance the therapeutic efficacy of nitrosoureas by inhibitors of MGMT such as O^6-benzylguanine resulted in significant hematological toxicity but not in a favorable therapeutic outcome (Quinn et al., 2002).

Suicide gene therapy is a specific approach of chemotherapy that was developed with the goal of targeting cytotoxic agents selectively to cancer cells. The concept involves the delivery by viral or liposomal gene transfer of an enzyme such as herpes simplex virus thymidine kinase (HSV-TK) to tumor cells, followed by systemic treatment with a prodrug such as ganciclovir that is converted to an active agent only in those cells that express HSV-TK. This approach has been highly successful in rodent glioma models, presumably because of the small tumor volumes and because of as yet poorly understood immunological consequences of HSV-TK gene therapy. However, there are continuing concerns regarding the safety of this procedure (Dewey et al., 1999). Further, a prospective randomized phase III trial of standard radiotherapy plus HSV-TK versus radiotherapy alone showed no effect of suicide gene therapy on progression-free or overall survival (Rainov, 2000), most likely because of a poor transduction rate of tumor cells by the retroviral vectors encoding HSV-TK.

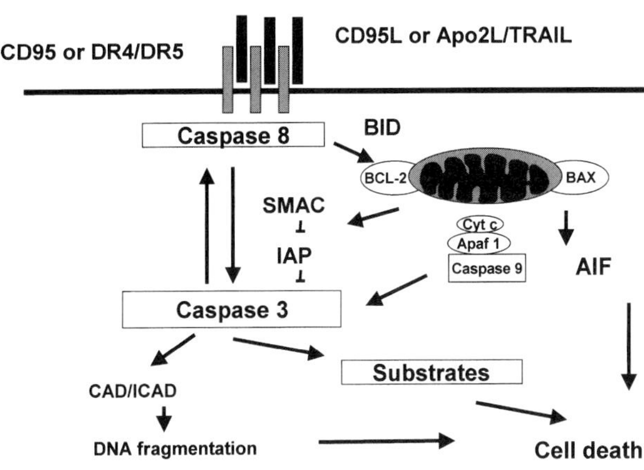

FIGURE 42.5 Molecular targets for the induction of apoptosis (for details, see text) (Fulda et al., 2002). AIF: apoptosis-inducing factor; BAX: BCL-2-associated X protein; BCL-2: B cell lymphoma; BID: BCL-2-interacting domain death agonist; CAD/ICAD: caspase 3-activated DNase/inhibitor of CAD; IAP: inhibitor-of-apoptosis protein; SMAC: second mitochondrial-derived activator of caspase.

EXPERIMENTAL THERAPY

Current experimental strategies include (*1*) cytotoxic/proapoptotic gene therapies, including suicide gene therapy, (*2*) antagonism of angiogenesis, migration, and invasion, and (*3*) various types of immunotherapy.

A better understanding of the major pathways regulating cellular sensitivity to the induction of (apoptotic) cell death has provided a whole range of molecular targets for the experimental therapy of malignant tumors, including glioblastoma. Many current articles distinguish an extrinsic and an intrinsic pathway of cell death. This distinction is artificial since the extrinsic pathway may rarely or never be triggered in the absence of a concurrent activation of the intrinsic pathway that amplifies the extrinsic pathway. The extrinsic pathway is triggered by activation of death receptors such as CD95 (Fas, APO-1) or the receptors for the tumor necrosis factor-related apoptosis-inducing ligand (TRAIL), also known as *Apo2 ligand* (Apo2L), which include the death-signaling receptors, death receptor (DR) 4/TRAIL-R1 and DR5/TRAIL-R2, as well as the non-death-inducing receptors, decoy receptors (DcR) 1/TRAIL-R3 and DcR2/TRAIL-R4 (Fig. 42.5). Trimerization of these receptors triggers the formation of a death-inducing signaling complex (DISC) containing adapter molecules such as Fas-associating protein with death domain (FADD) and consecutively the activation of a cascade of caspases, the enzymes that execute apoptosis via the cleavage of multiple protein substrates. Caspase 8 appears to be the central apical caspase in that cascade, whereas caspase 3 is thought to be the central effector caspase. Which specific protein substrates need to be cleaved by caspases to induce cell death has remained obscure. Caspase-mediated DNA degradation involves the activation of a caspase 3-activated DNase (CAD) by liberation of CAD from its inhibitor, ICAD. The intrinsic cell death pathway is initiated by the mitochondrial release of proapoptotic proteins, including cytochrome c, which mediates apoptosome formation together with apoptosis-activating factor (APAF) 1 and caspase 9, second mitochondrial-derived activator of caspase (SMAC)/direct IAP-binding protein with low pI (DIABLO), which interferes with the IAP-afforded inhibition of caspase activity, and apoptosis-inducing factor (AIF), which induces chromatin condensation and initial DNA cleavage via an unknown molecular mechanism, but in a caspase-independent manner. Caspase 3 is also considered the central executioner of the intrinsic pathway.

Control of the mitochondrial (intrinsic) cell death pathway is probably the mechanism by which BCL-2 family proteins regulate sensitivity to apoptosis. The BCL-2-interacting death-inducing protein (BID) has been proposed to mediate a death signal from death receptors and caspase 8 to the mitochondria, but this has not been confirmed in glioma cells (Glaser et al., 2001). Therapeutic approaches targeting these pathways include the upregulation of proapoptotic BCL-2 family proteins such as BCL-2-associated X protein (BAX) or natural born killer (NBK) by adenoviral gene transfer or the downregulation of antiapoptotic BCL-2 family proteins such as BCL-2 or BCL-X_L by antisense strategies, both combined with death-inducing stimuli such as radiotherapy or chemotherapy. Further, the extrinsic pathway can be triggered by recombinant or adenovirally encoded death ligands (Shinoura et al., 1998; Ambar et al., 1999), notably Apo2L/TRAIL, which appears to act rather selectively on transformed cells but spares normal brain parenchymal cells. Apo2L/TRAIL-induced glioma cell killing is potentiated in cell lines *in vitro* and in rodent glioma models *in vivo* when combined with a peptide containing the N-terminal sequence of SMAC/DIABLO that is required for the interaction with X-linked inhibitor of apoptosis (XIAP) (Fulda et al., 2002). Other approaches have targeted downstream elements of the killing pathway, for example, using adenovirally mediated overexpression of

FADD (Kondo et al., 1998) or caspases (Yu et al., 1996).

Angiogenesis, migration, and invasion are biological features that are particularly characteristic of the malignant phenotype of gliomas. Both hypoxia and acidosis stimulate the release of VEGF (Fukumura et al., 2001), the most potent inducer of angiogenesis (Plate et al., 1992). Vascular endothelial growth factor and its receptors are therefore a promising target for the prevention of angiogenesis and thus the inhibition of tumor growth (Millauer et al., 1994; Machein et al., 1999). However, anti-angiogenetic therapy alone may also have untoward side effects since efficient neutralization of the VEGF pathway, for example, using antagonistic antibodies to VEGF receptor 2, may result in enhanced tumor cell migration, presumably driven by hypoxia, and the formation of tumor satellites distant from the main tumor mass (Kunkel et al., 2001). Angiogenesis is also promoted by enhanced expression of membrane type 1 MMP (MT1-MMP) (Deruygina et al., 2002), supporting the link between migration and invasion, which also require MMP activity, and angiogenesis. Conversely, a naturally occurring fragment of MMP 2 referred to as PEX inhibits angiogenesis, migration, and invasion in human glioma xenografts (Bello et al., 2001). As indicated above, the HGF/SF pathway is also a promising target to inhibit angiogenesis, migration, and invasion (Wick et al., 2001; Abounader et al., 2002). The results of the first clinical trials targeting angiogenesis, migration, or invasion in patients with recurrent gliomas using drugs such as thalidomide (Fine et al., 2000) or marimastat (Groves et al., 2002) indicated modest activity, demonstrating the need for more innovative approaches in this field. Since migration and invasion appear to be enhanced by therapeutic irradiation (Wild-Bode et al., 2001), such agents should also be evaluated in the first-line treatment of gliomas as an adjunct to radiotherapy.

Several strategies summarized under the concept of immunotherapy are a third area of intense research into future therapies for malignant gliomas. A passive type of immunotherapy makes use of antibodies directed to proteins specifically or preferentially expressed by glioma cells, such as transferrin receptor, EGFR, or tenascin. These antibodies are radioactively labeled or linked to a toxin to induce glioma cell toxicity (Reardon et al., 2002). A related immunotoxin therapy targets the IL-4 receptor using a fusion toxin of IL-4 and pseudomonas exotoxin (Rand et al., 2000). Other strategies of immunotherapy seek to counteract the biological effects of the immunosuppressive molecules produced by glioma cells, notably TGF-β. Current strategies to inhibit TGF-β, which were successful *in vitro* or in animal models of glioma, include gene transfer of TGF-β antisense (Fakhrai et al., 1996) or the TGF-β binding protein decorin (Ständer et al., 1998) or TGF-β antibody treatment, with two clinical trials using TGF-β antisense oligonucleotides currently underway. Finally several experimental and clinical trials have evaluated active cellular immunotherapies, including the application of large quantities of lymphokine-activated killer (LAK) into the tumor cavity. None of these approaches has proven efficacy in human glioma patients. The current focus is on the development of vaccination therapies that employ fused dendritic (antigen-presenting) cells and glioma cells (Kikuchi et al., 2001; Yu et al., 2001).

Several of these innovative appoaches to glioma therapy suffer from the difficulty of delivering therapeutic molecules to glioma cells in sufficient concentrations without causing neurotoxicity. This has been particularly true of somatic suicide gene therapy (see above). The development of novel viral vectors and nonviral delivery devices such as liposomes is therefore among the key issues of current research. A second strategy involves the use of bioreactors of cells embedded in alginate that provide a local source of therapeutic molecules (Read et al., 2001). Finally, the field of stem cell biology offers new perspectives for the treatment of gliomas because stem cells may provide a novel vehicle to selectively target glioma cells within the brain parenchyma. C17.2 lacZ-expressing immortalized murine neuronal precursor cells diffusely transmigrated the whole diameter of experimental CNS-1 gliomas within 3 days when injected either into the tumor, the tail vein, or nontumorous brain tissue (Aboody et al., 2000). Further, neural progenitor cells from the cortex of C57BL6 mice have been used as vehicles to deliver therapeutic genes such as IL-4 to C6 experimental rat gliomas in Sprague-Dawley rats and to GL261 mouse gliomas in C57BL6 mice (Benedetti et al., 2000). Animals treated with progenitor cells as vehicles for IL-4 lived significantly longer than animals treated with fibroblast-derived packaging cells for the *in vivo* transfer of IL-4. The application of stem cells for the treatment of brain tumors is thus one of the most promising approaches of experimental brain tumor therapy.

SUMMARY AND PERSPECTIVES

Gliomas remain one of the most important challenges in oncology. This is because of their strong impact on the neurological function and quality of life of afflicted patients and because of the relative resistance of most of these tumors to the conventional modes of therapy of surgery, radiotherapy, and chemotherapy. The causes of gliomagenesis are largely unknown. Few patients suffer from hereditary conditions that predispose to the development of gliomas, including neurofibromatosis I and II, Li Fraumeni syndrome, and Turcot syndrome. There is no proven role for environmental factors in the development of gliomas, with the possible exception of irradiation in childhood. The possible origin of gliomas from neural or glial progenitor cells is an area of current research. Gliomas are graded by the WHO classification according to increasing malignancy from grade I to IV. The WHO grade is a strong predictor of the median survival, which is only approximately 1 year for patients with glioblastoma even with aggressive multimodality treatment consisting of surgery, radiotherapy, and chemotherapy. The difficulties in the treatment of these tumors result from the diffuse infiltrative growth pattern, which precludes radical resection, and from the apoptosis-resistant phenotype, which confers resistance to classical cancer therapies such as radiotherapy and chemotherapy.

Molecular genetic and biochemical studies indicate that the expression levels of MGMT and of still unknown gene products on chromosomes 1p and 19q determine responses to cytotoxic therapies, suggesting that the assessment of their expression may help to tailor therapy more individually in the future. Experimental treatments need to overcome the problem of delivering therapeutic molecules to the tumor cells in sufficient concentrations, but without causing neurotoxicity. Efforts to resolve this issue include the development of novel viral vectors for gene therapy and local cellular sources of therapeutic molecules (bioreactors) implanted into the postsurgical tumor cavity. Promising areas of therapeutic intervention include the activation of an apoptotic pathway at the level of death receptors, mitochondria, or caspases; the inhibition of angiogenesis, migration, and invasion; and immunotherapy targeting immunosuppressive glioma-derived molecules such as TGF-β or employing vaccination-based strategies using, for example, fusion vaccinates of dendritic and glioma cells.

ABBREVIATIONS:

AIF	apoptosis-inducing factor
APAF	apoptosis-activating factor
Apo2L	Apo2 ligand
ARF	alternative reading frame
BAX	BCL-2-associated X protein
BCL-(2, X_L)	B cell lymphoma
BID	BCL-2-interacting domain death agonist
CAD	caspase 3-activated DNase
CDK	cyclin-dependent kinase
CT	computed tomography
DcR	decoy receptor
DIABLO	direct IAP-binding protein with low pI
DISC	death-inducing signaling complex
DR	death receptor
ECM	extracellular matrix
EGFR	epidermal growth factor receptor
FADD	Fas-associating protein with death domain
HGF	hepatocyte growth factor
HSV-TK	herpes simplex virus thymidine kinase
IAP	inhibitor-of-apoptosis protein
ICAD	inhibitor of caspase 3-activated DNase
IL	interleukin
INK	inhibitor of kinase
LAK	lymphokine-activated killer
LAP	latency-associated peptide
LOH	loss of heterozygosity
LTBP	latent TGF-β-binding protein
MDM-2	murine double minute
MDR	multidrug resistance
MGMT	O^6-methylguanine-DNA methyltransferase
MMP	matrix metalloproteinase
MRI	magnetic resonance imaging
MRP	MDR-related protein
MT1-MMP	membrane type 1 MMP
NBK	natural born killer
NK	natural killer
OGAT	O^6-methylguanine-DNA alkyltransferase
PDGF	platelet-derived growth factor
PSA-NCAM	polysialated neural cell adhesion molecule
RB	retinoblastoma gene product
ROS	reactive oxygen species
SF	scatter factor
SMAC	second mitochondrial-derived activator of caspase
TGF-β	transforming growth factor-β
TRAIL	tumor necrosis factor-related apoptosis-inducing ligand
TSP	thrombospondin
UPA	urokinase-type plasminogen activator
VEGF	vascular endothelial growth factor

WHO	World Health Organization
XIAP	X-linked inhibitor of apoptosis

REFERENCES

Aboody, K.S., Brown, A., Rainov, N.G., Bower, K.A., Liu, S., Yang, W., Small, J.E., Herrlinger, U., Ourednik, V., Black, P.M., Breakefield, X.O., and Snyder, E.Y. (2000). Neural stem cells display extensive tropism for pathology in adult brain: evidence from intracranial gliomas. *Proc. Natl. Acad. Sci. USA* 97:12846–12851.

Abounader, R., Lal, B., Luddy, C., Koe, G., Davidson, B., Rosen, E.M., and Laterra, J. (2002). In vivo targeting of SF/HGF and c-met expression via U1snRNA/ribozymes inhibits glioma growth and angiogenesis and promotes apoptosis. *FASEB J.* 16:108–110.

Ambar, B.B., Frei, K., Malipiero, U., Morelli, A.E., Castro, M.G., Lowenstein, P.R., and Fontana, A. (1999). Treatment of experimental glioma by administration of adenoviral vectors expressing Fas ligand. *Hum. Gene Ther.* 10:1641–1648.

Bello, L., Lucini, V., Carrabba, G., Giussani, C., Machluf, M., Pluderi, M., Nikas, D., Zhang, J., Tomei, G., Villani, R.M., Carroll, R.S., Bikfalvi, A., and Black, P.M. (2001). Simultaneous inhibition of glioma angiogenesis, cell proliferation, and invasion by a naturally occurring fragment of human metalloproteinase-2. *Cancer Res.* 61:8730–8736.

Benedetti, S., Pirola, B., Pollo, B., Magrassi, L., Bruzzone, M.G., Rigamonti, D., Galli, R., Selleri, S., Di Meco, F., De Fraja, C., Vescovi, A., Cattaneo, E., and Finocchiaro, G. (2000). Gene therapy of experimental brain tumors using neural progenitor cells. *Nat. Med.* 6:447–450.

Cairncross, J.G., Ueki, K., Zlatescu, M.C., Lisle, D.K., Finkelstein, D.M., Hammond, R.R., Silver, J.S., Stark, P.C., Macdonald, D.R., Ino, Y., Ramsay, D.A., and Louis, D.N. (1998). Specific genetic predictors of chemotherapeutic response and survival in patients with anaplastic oligodendrogliomas. *J. Natl. Cancer Inst.* 90:1473–1479.

Campbell, K. and Götz, M. (2002). Radial glia: multipurpose cells for vertebrate brain developement. *Trends Neurosci.* 25:235–238.

Dai, C., Celestino, J.C., Okada, Y., Louis, D.N., Fuller, G.N., and Holland, E.C. (2001). PDGF autocrine stimulation dedifferentiates cultured astrocytes and induces oligodendrogliomas and oligoastrocytomas from neural progenitors and astrocytes in vivo. *Genes Dev.* 15:1913–1925.

Davis, F.G., McCarthy, B.J., Freels, S., Kupelian, V., and Bondy, M.L. (1999). The conditional probability of survival of patients with primary malignant brain tumors. Surveillance, epidemiology, and end results (SEER) data. *Cancer* 85:485–491.

DeAngelis, L.M. (2001). Brain tumors. *N. Engl. J. Med.* 344:114–122.

Deryugina, E.I., Soroceanu, L., and Strongin, A.Y. (2002). Up-regulation of vascular endothelial growth factor by membrane-type 1 matrix metalloproteinase stimulates human glioma xenograft growth and angiogenesis. *Cancer Res.* 62:580–588.

Dewey, R.A., Morrissey, G., Cowsill, C.M., Stone, D., Bolognani, F., Dodd, N.J., Southgate, T.D., Klatzmann, D., Lassmann, H., Castro, M.G., and Lowenstein, P.R. (1999). Chronic brain inflammation and persistent herpes simplex virus 1 thymidine kinase expression in survivors of syngeneic glioma treated by adenovirus-mediated gene therapy: implications for clinical trials. *Nat. Med.* 5:1256–1263.

Esteller, M., Garcia-Foncillas, J., Andion, E., Goodman, S.N., Hidalgo, O.F., Vanaclocha, V., Baylin, S.B., and Herman, J.G. (2000). Inactivation of the DNA-repair gene MGMT and the clinical response of gliomas to alkylating agents. *N. Engl. J. Med.* 343:1350–1354.

Fakhrai, H., Dorigo, O., Shawler, D.L., Lin, H., Mercola, D., Black, K..L, Royston, I., and Sobol, R.E. (1996). Eradication of established intracranial rat gliomas by transforming growth factor beta antisense gene therapy. *Proc. Natl. Acad. Sci. USA* 93:2909–2914.

Fine, H.A., Figg, W.D., Jaeckle, K., Wen, P.Y., Kyritsis, A.P., Loeffler, J.S., Levin, V.A., Black, P.M., Kaplan, R., Pluda, J.M., and Yung, W.K. (2000). Phase II trial of the antiangiogenic agent thalidomide in patients with recurrent high-grade gliomas. *J. Clin. Oncol.* 18:708–715.

Fukumura, D., Xu, L., Chen, Y., Gohongi, T., Seed, B., and Jain, R.K. (2001). Hypoxia and acidosis independently up-regulate vascular endothelial growth factor transcription in brain tumors in vivo. *Cancer Res.* 61:6020–6024.

Fulda, S., Wick, W., Weller, M., and Debatin, K.M. (2002). Smac agonists sensitize for TRAIL/Apo2L- or anticancer drug-induced apoptosis and induce regression of human glioma xenografts. *Nat. Med.* 8:808–815.

Glaser, T., Wagenknecht, B., and Weller, M. (2001). Identification of p21 as a target of cycloheximide-mediated facilitation of CD95-mediated apoptosis in human malignant glioma cells. *Oncogene* 20:4757–4767.

Groves, M.D., Puduvalli, V.K., Hess, K.R., Jaeckle, K.A., Peterson, P., Yung, W.K.A., and Levin, V.A. (2002). Phase II trial of temozolomide plus the matrix metalloproteinase inhibitor, marimastat, in recurrent and progressive glioblastoma multiforme. *J. Clin. Oncol.* 20:1383–1388.

Hatten, M.E. (1993). The role of migration in central nervous system neuronal developement. *Curr. Opin. Neurobiol.* 3:38–44.

Holland, E.C., Celestino, J., Dai, C., Schaefer, L., Sawaya, R.E., and Fuller, G.N. (2000). Combined activation of Ras and Akt in neural progenitors induces glioblastoma formation in mice. *Nat. Genet.* 25:55–57.

Ichimura, K., Bolin, M.B., Goike, H.M., Schmidt, E.E., Moshref, A., and Collins, V.P. (2000). Deregulation of the p14ARF/MDM2/p53 pathway is a prerequisite for human astrocytic gliomas with G1-S transition control gene abnormalities. *Cancer Res.* 60:417–424.

Ino, Y., Betensky, R.A., Zlatescu, M.C., Sasaki, H., Macdonald, D.R., Stemmer-Rachamimov, A.O., Ramsay, D.A., Cairncross, J.G., and Louis, D.N. (2001). Molecular subtypes of anaplastic oligodendroglioma: implications for patient management at diagnosis. *Clin. Cancer Res.* 7:839–845.

Kikuchi, T., Akasaki, Y., Irie, M., Homma, S., Abe, T., and Ohno, T. (2001). Results of a phase I clinical trial of vaccination of glioma patients with fusions of dendritic and glioma cells. *Cancer Immunol. Immunother.* 50:337–344.

Kleihues, P. and Cavenee, W.K. (2000). *World Health Organization Classification of Tumours. Pathology and Genetics. Tumours of the Nervous System.* Lyon: IARC Press.

Kondo, S., Ishizaka, Y., Okada, T., Kondo, Y., Hitomi, M., Tanaka, Y., Haqqi, T., Barnett, G.H., and Barna, B.P. (1998). FADD gene therapy for malignant gliomas in vitro and in vivo. *Hum. Gene Ther.* 9:1599–1608.

Kunkel, P., Ulbricht, U., Bohlen, P., Brockmann, M.A., Fillbrandt, R., Stavrou, D., Westphal, M., and Lamszus, K. (2001). Inhibition of glioma angiogenesis and growth in vivo by systemic treatment with a monoclonal antibody against vascular endothelial growth factor receptor-2. *Cancer Res.* 61:6624–6628.

Leitlein, J., Aulwurm, S., Waltereit, R., Naumann, U., Wagenknecht, B., Garten, W., Weller, M., and Platten, M. (2001). Processing of immunosuppressive pro-TGF-$\beta_{1,2}$ by human glioblastoma cells involves cytoplasmic and secreted furin-like proteases. *J. Immunol.* 166:7238–7243.

Machein, M.R., Risau, W., and Plate, K.H. (1999). Antiangiogenic gene therapy in a rat glioma model using a dominant-negative vascular endothelial growth factor receptor 2. *Hum. Gene Ther.* 10:1117–1128.

Mahesparan, R., Read, T.A., Lund-Johansen, M., Skaftnesmo, K.O., Bjerkvig, R., and Engebraaten, O. (2003). Expression of extracellular matrix components in a highly infiltrative in vivo glioma model. *Acta Neuropathol.* 105:49–57.

Millauer, B., Shawver, L.K., Plate, K.H., Risau, W., and Ullrich, A. (1994). Glioblastoma growth inhibited in vivo by a dominant-negative Flk-1 mutant. *Nature* 367:576–579.

Mohan, P., Chintala, S.K., and Mohanam, S. (1999). Adenovirus-mediated delivery of antisense gene to urokinase-type plasminogen activator receptor suppresses glioma invasion and tumor growth. *Cancer Res.* 59:3369–3373.

Nutt, C.L., Noble, M., Chambers, A.F., and Cairncross, J.G. (2000). Differential expression of drug resistance genes and chemosensitivity in glial cell lineages correlate with differential response of oligodendrogliomas and astrocytomas to chemotherapy. *Cancer Res.* 60:4812–4818.

Plate, K.H., Breier, G., Weich, H.A., and Risau, W. (1992). Vascular endothelial growth factor is a potential tumour angiogenesis factor in human gliomas in vivo. *Nature* 359:845–848.

Powell, E.M., Mars, W.M., and Levitt, P. (2001). Hepatocyte growth factor/scatter factor is a motogen for interneurons migrating from the ventral to the dorsal telencephalon. *Neuron* 30:79–89.

Quinn, J.A., Pluda, J., Dolan, M.E., Delaney, S., Kaplan, R., Rich, J.N., Friedman, A.H., Reardon, D.A., Sampson, J.H., Colvin, O.M., Haglund, M.M., Pegg, A.E., Moschel, R.C., McLendon, R.E., Provenzale, J.M., Gururangan, S., Tourt-Uhlig, S., Herndon, J.E., 2nd, Bigner, D.D., and Friedman, H.S. (2002). Phase II trial of carmustine plus O(6)-benzylguanine for patients with nitrosourea-resistant recurrent or progressive malignant glioma. *J. Clin. Oncol.* 20:2277–2283.

Rainov, N.G., on behalf of the GL1328 International Study Group (2000). A phase III clinical evaluation of herpes simplex virus type 1 thymidine kinase and ganciclovir gene therapy as an adjuvant to surgical resection and radiation in adults with previously untreated glioblastoma multiforme. *Hum. Gene Ther.* 11: 2389–2401.

Rand, R.W., Kreitman, R.J., Patronas, N., Varricchio, F., Pastan, I., and Puri, R.K. (2000). Intratumoral administration of recombinant circularly permuted interleukin-4-pseudomonas exotoxin in patients with high-grade glioma. *Clin. Cancer Res.* 6:2157–2165.

Read, T.A., Sorensen, D.R., Mahesparan, R., Enger, P.O., Timpl, R., Olsen, B.R., Hjelstuen, M.H., Haraldseth, O., and Bjerkvig, R. (2001). Local endostatin treatment of gliomas administered by microencapsulated producer cells. *Nat. Biotechnol.* 19:29–34.

Reardon, D.A., Akabani, G., Coleman, R.E., Friedman, A.H., Friedman, H.S., Herndon, J.E. 2nd, Cokgor, I., McLendon, R.E., Pegram, C.N., Provenzale, J.M., Quinn, J.A., Rich, J.N., Regalado, L.V., Sampson, J.H., Shafman, T.D., Wikstrand, C.J., Wong, T.Z., Zhao, X.G., Zalutsky, M.R., and Bigner, D.D. (2002). Phase II trial of murine (131)I-labeled antitenascin monoclonal antibody 81C6 administered into surgically created resection cavities of patients with newly diagnosed malignant gliomas. *J. Clin. Oncol.* 20:1389–1397.

Serano, R.D., Pegram, C.N., and Bigner, D.D. (1980) Tumorigenic cell culture lines from a spontaneous VM/Dk murine astrocytoma (SMA). *Acta Neuropathol.* 51:53–64.

Shinoura, N., Yoshida, Y., Sadata, A., Hanada, K.I., Yamamoto, S., Kirino, T., Asai, A., and Hamada, H. (1998). Apoptosis by retrovirus- and adenovirus-mediated gene transfer of Fas ligand to glioma cells: implications for gene therapy. *Hum. Gene Ther.* 9:1983–1993.

Silber, J.R., Bobola, M.S., Ghatan, S., Blank, A., Kolstoe, D.D., and Berger, M.S. (1998). O6-methylguanine-DNA methyltransferase activity in adult gliomas: relation to patient and tumor characteristics. *Cancer Res.* 58:1068–1073.

Ständer, M., Naumann, U., Dumitrescu, L., Heneka, M., Löschmann, P.A., Gulbins, E., Dichgans, J., and Weller, M. (1998). Decorin gene-transfer mediated suppression of TGF-β synthesis abrogates experimental malignant glioma growth in vivo. *Gene Ther.* 5:1187–1194.

Sugimoto, Y., Taniguchi, M., Yagi, T., Akagi, Y., Nojyo, Y., and Tamamaki, N. (2001). Guidance of glial precursor cell migration by secreted cues in the developing optic nerve. *Development* 128:3321–3330.

Uhrbom, L., Dai, C., Celestino, J.C., Rosenblum, M.K., Fuller, G.N., and Holland, E.C. (2002). Ink4a-Arf loss cooperates with KRas activation in astrocytes and neural progenitors to generate glioblastomas of various morphologies depending on activated Akt. *Cancer Res.* 62:5551–5558.

von Deimling, A., Fimmers, R., Schmidt, M.C., Bender, B., Fassbender, F., Nagel, J., Jahnke, R., Kaskel, P., Duerr, E.M., Koopmann, J., Maintz, D., Schild, S., Vogel, Y., Wick, W., Platten, M., Müller, D., Przkora, R., Waha, A., Rollbrocker, B., Wellenreuther, R., Meyer-Puttlitz, B., Schmidt, O., Mollenhauer, J., Poustka, A., Stangl, A.P., Lenartz, D., von Ammon, K., Henson, J.W., Schramm, J., Louis, D.N., and Wiestler, O.D. (2000). Comprehensive allelotype and genetic analysis of 466 human nervous system tumors. *J. Neuropathol. Exp. Neurol.* 59:544–558.

Watanabe, K., Tachibana, O., Sata, K., Yonekawa, Y., Kleihues, P., and Ohgaki H. (1996). Overexpression of the EGF receptor and p53 mutations are mutually exclusive in the evolution of primary and secondary glioblastomas. *Brain Pathol.* 6:217–223.

Weller, M. and Fontana, A. (1995). The failure of current immunotherapy for malignant glioma. Tumor-derived TGF-β, T cell apoptosis, and the immune privilege of the brain. *Brain Res. Rev.* 21:128–151.

Weller, M. and Thomas, D.G.T. (2003). *Primary tumors of the central and peripheral nervous system.* In: Brandt, T., Caplan, L.R., Dichgans, J., Diener, H.C., and Kennard, C. (Hrsg.). *Course and Treatment of Neurological Disorders.* San Diego, CA: Academic Press, pp. 827–863.

Wick, W., Grimmel, C., Wild-Bode, C., Platten, M., Arpin, M., and Weller, M. (2001). Ezrin-dependent promotion of glioma cell clonogenicity, motility and invasion mediated by BCL-2 and TGF-β_2. *J. Neurosci.* 21:3360–3368.

Wild-Bode, C., Weller, M., Rimner, A., Dichgans, J., and Wick, W. (2001). Sublethal irradiation promotes migration and invasiveness of glioma cells: implications for radiotherapy of human glioblastoma. *Cancer Res.* 61:2744–2750.

Yu, J.S., Sena-Esteves, M., Paulus, W., Breakefield, X.O., and Reeves, S.A. (1996). Retroviral delivery and tetracycline-dependent expression of IL-1beta-converting enzyme (ICE) in a rat glioma model provides controlled induction of apoptotic death in tumor cells. *Cancer Res.* 56:5423–5427.

Yu, J.S., Wheeler, C.J., Zeltzer, P.M., Ying, H., Finger, D.N., Lee, P.K., Yong, W.H., Incardona, F., Thompson, R.C, Riedinger, M.S., Zhang, W., Prins, R.M., and Black, K.L. (2001). Vaccination of malignant glioma patients with peptide-pulsed dendritic cells elicits systemic cytotoxicity and intracranial T-cell infiltration. *Cancer Res.* 61:842–847.

43 Neurological mouse mutants: a molecular-genetic analysis of myelin proteins

KLAUS-ARMIN NAVE AND UELI SUTER

FROM GENOTYPE TO PHENOTYPE

Genetics provides a powerful means to dissect basic mechanisms of development, from the function of structural or regulatory proteins to complex cellular interactions. As model organisms of mammalian brain development, mice have become the preferred genetic system due to their short gestation time (19 days) and generation cycle (3 months). A large number of defects in neural development have been associated with specific mutations in mice and have contributed to what we know about human neurological disease. Beginning in the 1950s, a number of spontaneous mutations in the mouse were shown to affect myelin formation (Sidman, 1965) and provided the first models of inherited myelin diseases in humans. Today, the ability to generate transgenic mice and rats, mouse mutations of virtually any gene, and conditional gene knockouts have resulted in a rapidly growing catalog of mutations to study myelin formation and disease.

Phenotypical differences between myelin mutants and their wild-type controls are associated, directly or indirectly, with the normal function of the studied gene. However, a specific myelin phenotype may not simply reveal that gene's function. Since mutant mice develop in the absence of that gene's function, they may respond during development with compensations that mask the full-blown phenotype or exhibit secondary changes by the time of analysis. More complex, and clinically relevant, are mutations that modify the normal function of a gene such that the gene product acquires an aberrant function and disturbs development. Specifically, a myelin protein encoded by the mutant allele may not only have lost its original function but may additionally interfere with the activity of the wild-type protein or other proteins present in the cell (*dominant-negative* effect). The chance of recognizing such dominant mutations as a genetic disease is greater than that of identifying recessive mutations in sporadic cases.

MUTATIONS AFFECTING MYELIN FORMATION

Myelination provides the electrical insulation of axons by a multilayered sheath of glial membrane and is the physical basis for rapid saltatory impulse conduction in the nervous system (see Chapter 21). This function is served by highly specialized glial cells in the central nervous system (CNS) and peripheral nervous system (PNS). The compacted myelin sheath, when assembled by oligodendrocytes and Schwann cells, uses two different but overlapping sets of myelin proteins, as shown schematically in Figure 43.1.

In rodents, most myelinating glial cells are generated late in development and differentiate after birth, when the basic wiring pattern of the nervous system has been laid down. Degeneration of oligodendrocytes and Schwann cells or their inability to assemble myelin is not immediately lethal. In fact, most mutant mice survive for several weeks or months after birth, which provides the opportunity to study the gene function *in vivo* as the animal develops a disease. Myelin-restricted phenotypes in mice include characteristic behavioral abnormalities, such as tremors, ataxia, and frequently seizures. These signs begin when normal mice assemble large amounts of myelin that then becomes a requirement for normal motor functions. We will use the term *dysmyelination* for the primary inability to assemble normal myelin; *demyelination* refers to the loss of myelin. In some mutations, both pathomechanisms overlap.

The late-onset motor phenotype of classical myelin mutants is caused by mutations in genes that are cell type–specifically expressed, such as the majority of structural myelin protein genes. The recent application of *conditional* gene targeting techniques also allows the study of the myelination-associated function of ubiquitously and very early expressed genes (Genoud et al., 2002; Feltri et al., 2002).

The following sections provide an overview of mu-

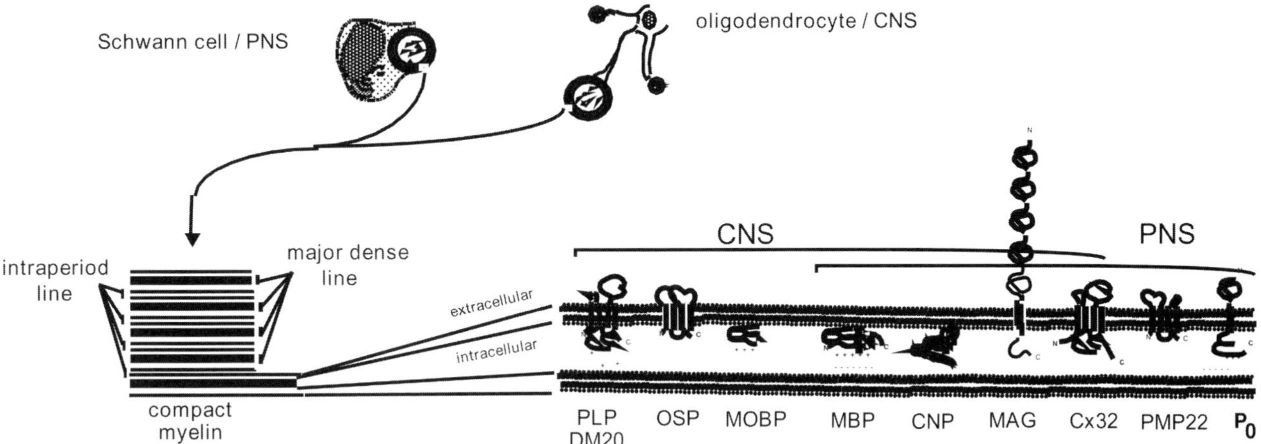

FIGURE 43.1 Schematic representation of myelin-forming glial cells in the central and peripheral nervous systems, the ultrastructure of compacted myelin, and major proteins associated with the myelin membrane. Schwann cells and oligodendrocytes incorporate an overlapping but not identical set of proteins into myelin. Indicated are only genes for which natural and engineered mouse mutants are known: PLP/DM20: proteolipid protein, OSP: oligodendrocyte-specific protein/claudin-11; MOBP: myelin-oligodendrocyte basic protein; MBP: myelin basic protein; MAG: myelin-associated glycoprotein; Cx32: connexin 32 kDa; CNP: 2′,3′-cyclic nucleotide phosphodioesterase; PMP22: peripheral myelin protein 22 kDa; and P0: protein zero. In myelin of wild-type mice, MAG is restricted to the innermost membrane facing the neuronal axon. Also, CNP and Cx32 are localized in noncompacted myelin. Not shown are protein isoforms derived by alternative RNA splicing.

tations in the mouse that have improved our understanding of structural myelin proteins. Some of this knowledge may be directly applicable to corresponding human myelin diseases.

MYELIN BASIC PROTEIN

Myelin basic protein (MBP) is a complex family of related proteins that together constitute about 30% of the protein mass in CNS myelin and about 10% in PNS myelin. The molecular weights of the major isoforms are 14, 17, 18.5, 20, and 21.5 kDa. The relationship of these structural proteins has been resolved by cloning their respective cDNAs. All MBP isoforms arise by alternative RNA splicing of a primary transcript of the *Mbp* structural gene. Inclusion of all seven exons generates the largest MBP isoform (21.5 kDa), whereas the selective exclusion of exons 2, 5, and/or 6 generates the smaller isoforms (for references to the *Mbp1* gene structure see Chapter 19). The functional difference between these proteins is not known. The *myelin-specific* transcription unit of the *Mbp1* gene (Fig. 43.2) is itself part of the considerably larger *Mbp1-Golli* gene complex (for Gene in the oligodendrocyte *l*ineage). The upstream *Golli*-specific exons encode the amino-terminal portion of MBP-like isoforms that are expressed in neurons and also outside the nervous system. Their function is unknown and most likely is unrelated to myelin.

Myelin basic proteins are positively charged, membrane-associated proteins of myelin located at the cytoplasmic surface (*major dense line*) of the glial process. The role that MBP plays in the architecture of compact myelin has been studied in the *shiverer* mouse (Chernoff, 1981). *Shiverer* mice (genetic symbol: *shi*, mouse chromosome 18) lack detectable MBP and were among the first neurological mutants successfully studied at the molecular-genetic level (Roach et al., 1983). Affected homozygotes fail to make significant amounts of myelin in the CNS and display a behavioral defect that is characteristic of most CNS myelin-deficient mice. In the second postnatal week, they develop a general body tremor that is most pronounced when the animals initiate voluntary movements. The shivering reflects a loss of proper spinal motor reflexes and is accompanied by seizures in the adult. Most *shiverer* mice die prematurely at about 6 months of age.

Biochemically, the dysmyelination is reflected in a dramatic reduction of all major myelin proteins and the complete lack of MBPs. The latter is the primary defect and is caused by a 20 kb deletion encompassing exons 3–7 of the *Mbp* gene (or exons 7–11 of the larger *Mbp-Golli* gene), as summarized in Figure 43.2. Thus, *shiverer* mice have no coding capacity for any MBP isoform (Roach et al., 1985; Molineaux et al., 1986).

Histologically, *shiverer* mice are dysmyelinated throughout the CNS, whereas peripheral myelin appears rather normal (Privat et al., 1979; Kirschner and Ganser, 1980; Rosenbluth, 1980). The ultrastructure of myelinated fibers in brain and spinal cord exhibits severe hypomyelination, and myelin-like structures—where present—appear loosely wrapped around the axon. The intracellular adhesion zone of the extended cell process (major dense line) cannot be discerned, sug-

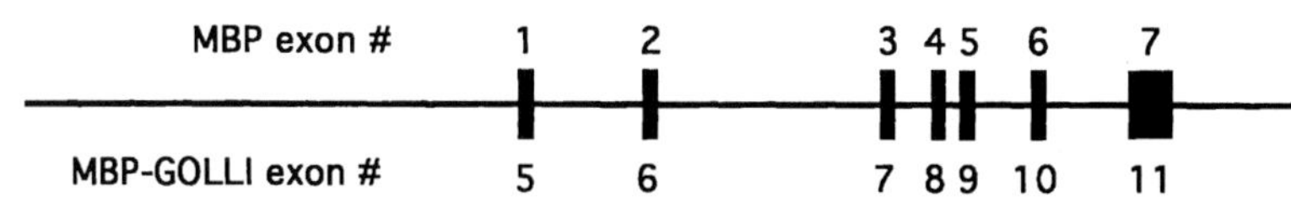

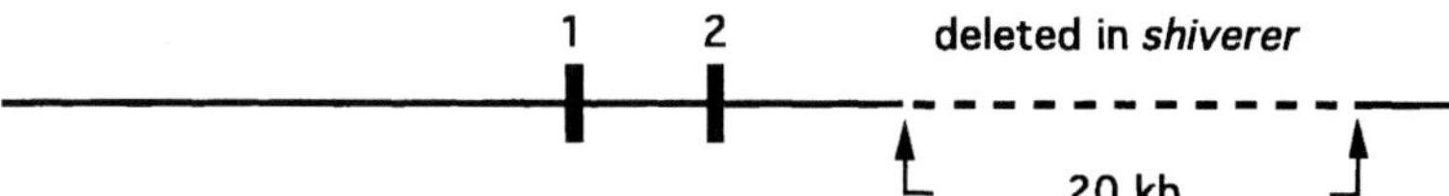

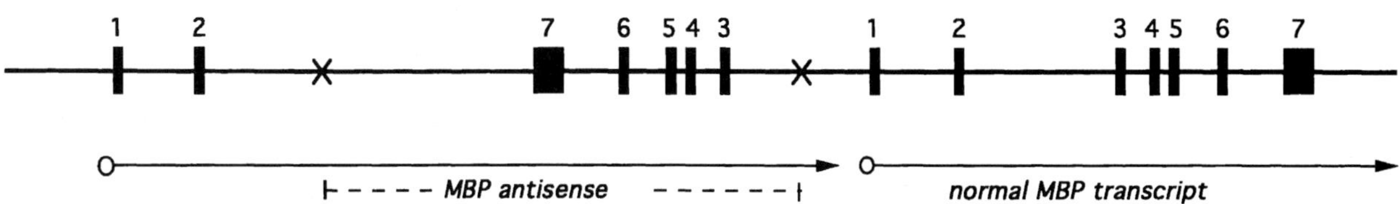

FIGURE 43.2 Genomic structure of the myelin basic protein locus, which is partially deleted in *shiverer* mice and duplicated in the *shiverer-mld* mutant. The exons of the myelin-specific *Mbp1* transcription unit (black boxes) are numbered on top, and the equivalent numbers of the larger *Mbp1-Golli* gene complex are indicated below (for further details see Chapter 19 and references). The position of a genomic deletion in *shiverer* mice is indicated by a dashed line. Normal and antisense-containing *Mbp1* transcripts are shown by horizontal arrows. An inverted segment (x——x) within the duplicated *Mbp1* gene of *shiverer-mld* mutant is labeled *MBP-antisense*. Exon sizes are not drawn to scale.

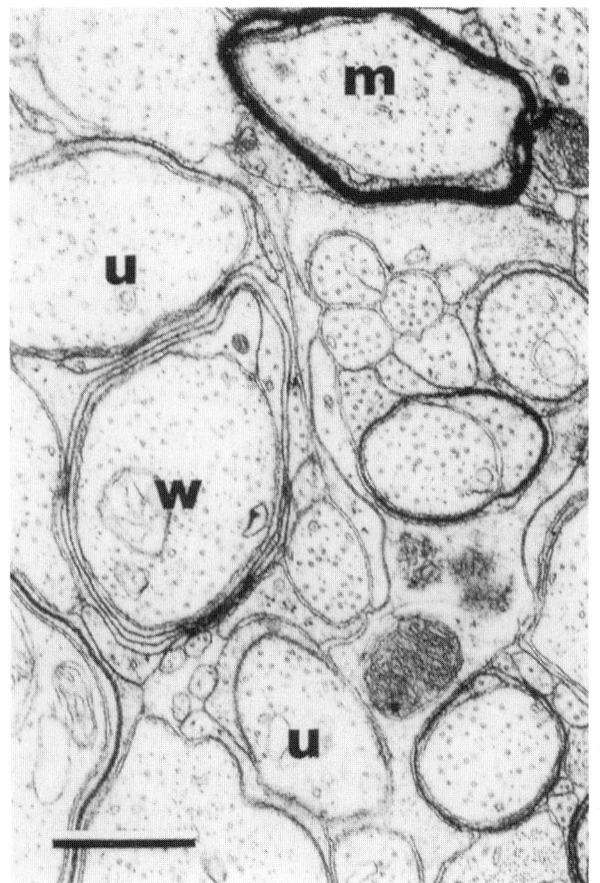

FIGURE 43.3 Electron micrograph of partially myelinated fibers in the optic nerve of *shiverer* mice (*shi/shi*) transgenic for the myelin basic protein (*Mbp1*) gene (Readhead et al., 1987). Whereas some axons remain unmyelinated (*u*) or loosely wrapped (*w*), more axons become ensheathed by compacted myelin (*m*) as the level of regained MBP expression increases in *Mbp1*-transgenic *shiverer* mice (here 12.5% of normal). Bar = 0.5 μm.

gesting that MBP itself provides a glue to membrane adhesion. However, an equally important feature is the overall lack of myelination that contrasts with assembly of myelin when other myelin proteins are absent. This suggests that MBP, unlike most myelin components, is required for myelin membrane growth.

The definitive proof that absence of MBP is solely responsible for the dysmyelinating phenotype involved the use of transgenic mice. When the entire wild-type *Mbp1* gene was reintroduced into the germline of *shiverer* mice, their tremoring phenotype disappeared as a function of regained MBP expression (up to 25% of the wild-type level) so that the mutation could be phenotypically "cured" (Readhead et al., 1987). In fact, raising MBP expression levels by increasing the transgene gene copy number in *shi/shi* and *shi/+* mice resulted in a proportional increase in myelin thickness (Popko et al., 1987; Shine et al., 1990). Thus, the amount of MBP available to oligodendrocytes is a rate-limiting step in the assembly of myelin (Fig. 43.3).

What is the functional difference among the MBP isoforms? The alternatively spliced mRNAs are individually regulated throughout brain development, suggesting isoform-specific functions. On the other hand, it has been possible to phenotypically "cure" *shiverer* mice by reintroducing transgenes that encode single MBP isoforms (Kimura et al., 1989, 1998). Thus, the major function appears common to all MBP.

A *shiverer*-like phenotype was generated in normal mice by specifically downregulating the amount of MBP mRNA available for protein synthesis (Katsuki et al., 1988). This was achieved by transgenic expression of the *Mbp1* gene in an *antisense* orientation under the control of its cognate *Mbp1* promotor (the antisense RNA hybridizes to *Mbp1* transcripts, forming RNA duplex molecules that are degraded). A similar formation of antisense *Mbp1* RNA is the presumed primary defect of the mouse mutant *myelin-deficient* (symbol: shi^{mld}), an allele of the *shiverer* mutation on chromosome 18 (Doolittle and Schweikart, 1977). Here, a tandem duplication of the entire *Mbp1* gene with the inversion of exons 3–7 created a second transcription unit immediately upstream of the intact *Mbp1* gene (Fig. 43.2) that transcribes RNA that is in part complementary to the normal *Mbp1* transcript (Popko et al., 1988). The presence of this antisense RNA most likely reduces the amount of normal MBP mRNA toward a level insufficient for myelin formation (Fremeau and Popko, 1990; Tosic et al., 1990). Morphologically, dysmyelination of shi^{mld}/shi^{mld} mice is less severe than that of *shi/shi* mice. Interestingly, the genomic inversion occurred in the same region that was deleted in *shiverer* mice, suggesting a *hot spot* of recombination in this part of the mouse *Mbp1* gene.

A puzzling observation in *shiverer* and its *mld* allele was the formation of normal myelin in the PNS that has a major dense line, despite the lack of MBP that constitutes about 10% of total peripheral myelin protein (Privat et al., 1979; Kirschner and Ganser, 1980). It was hypothesized that in *shiverer* the structural function of MBP could be compensated for by P0, the major integral myelin protein of the PNS. Specifically, the amino terminus of P0 forms a *basic* domain (Lemke and Axel, 1985) that is located at the cytoplasmic surface of the myelin membrane and may be sufficient to establish a major dense line. This hypothesis was proven experimentally several years later by the generation and ultrastructural analysis of MBP*P0 double mutant mice (Martini et al., 1995a).

Detailed morphological examinations have revealed subtle PNS abnormalities in *shiverer* that demonstrate the complexity of primary and secondary changes. For example, the number of Schmitt-Lanterman incisures in Schwann cells and their associated proteins (connexin 32 and myelin-associated glycoprotein) is about doubled in the absence of MBP (Gould et al., 1995). Does MBP counteract the formation of channel-like structures in myelin? Abnormalities of the actin cytoskeleton and its association with cyclic nucleotide phosphodiesterase were found in cultured *shiverer* oligodendrocytes (Dyer et al., 1997). Although *Mbp* is expressed only in glia, *shiverer* mice also reveal axonal abnormalities. Electron microscopy of the CNS reveals obvious defects in the maturation of the (neuronal) axonal cytoskeleton (Kirkpatrick et al., 2001). This feature is associated with reduced phosphorylation of neurofilament proteins at specific sites (Sanchez et al., 2000) and abnormal localization of the fast K^+ and Na^+ channels (Wang et al., 1995; Boiko et al., 2001). However, signs of axonal degeneration are absent.

Long-Evans *shaker* (*les*), an insertion mutation of the *Mbp* gene in rats (O'Connor et al., 1999), shows some interesting differences from *shiverer* in mice. Notably, oligodendrocytes display intracellular accumulation of vesicles and other membranous bodies (Kwiecien et al., 1998). They also fail to produce myelin beyond the first weeks of life, when the small amounts of assembled myelin are gradually lost.

MYELIN-ASSOCIATED OLIGODENDROCYTE BASIC PROTEIN

In the CNS, some homology may exist between MBP and another small basic protein (myelin-associated oligodendrocyte basic protein (MOBP). The protein is encoded by a complex transcription unit (Yamamoto et al., 1994). Myelin-associated oligodendrocyte basic protein can be immunolocalized in myelin, but also in nuclei and in the microtubular network of oligodendrocytes. Like MPB, MOBP localizes to the major dense line. Mice lacking MOBP have been generated but show no significant dysmyelination (Yamamoto et al., 1999; Sadahiro et al., 2000; Yool et al., 2002). Whether myelinated axons have a larger diameter in *Mobp* mutants than in wild-type mice and whether they display structurally abnormal radial components remains controversial. There is no obvious compensation for the lack of MOBP by MBP. Interestingly, MBP-deficient *shiverer* mice fail to incorporate the 20 kDa isoform of MOBP into myelin (Montague et al., 1999), such that the *shiverer* CNS phenotype may represent the absence of both myelin proteins. Indeed, the dysmyelination of *shiverer* is not further enhanced by the lack of MOBP in double-mutant mice (Sadahiro et al., 2000).

PROTEOLIPID PROTEIN

Proteolipid protein (PLP) is the most abundant integral membrane protein of myelin in the CNS, constituting roughly 50% of its protein mass. Two isoforms of PLP, the 30 kDa major form (PLP apoprotein or lipophilin) and the 26 kDa DM20 protein, are generated by alternative mRNA splicing (for references to the *Plp1* gene see Chapter 19). In higher vertebrates, PLP is specific to compact CNS myelin, but the *Plp1* gene is also expressed at a low levels in Schwann cells. There its function remains unclear, as little or no PLP/DM20 is detectable in PNS myelin. A remarkable feature of PLP/DM20 is its high degree of structural conservation: the primary structure (276 amino acids) is identical in mouse, rat, and humans, suggesting that PLP engages in multiple protein interactions. Chemically, PLP is a strongly hydrophobic protein with four α-helical membrane-embedded domains (Fig. 43.4) that is acylated, binds to cholesterol, and interacts with integrins. It is likely that the transmembrane domains of PLP form a tight four-helix bundle and possibly a homo-oligomeric structure. The amino and carboxyl termini are cytoplasmic and face the major dense line.

The *Plp1* gene is X-linked, and several spontaneous (X-linked recessive) mutations of the murine gene have been isolated: *jimpy* (Plp^{jp}), *myelin-synthesis deficient* (Plp^{msd}), Plp^{4J}, and *rumpshaker* (Plp^{rsh}). All of them are point mutations that alter the structure of PLP/DM20, as summarized in Figure 43.4.

Phenotypically, *jimpy*, *msd*, and *4J* mice are most severely affected, with a general body tremor and ataxia

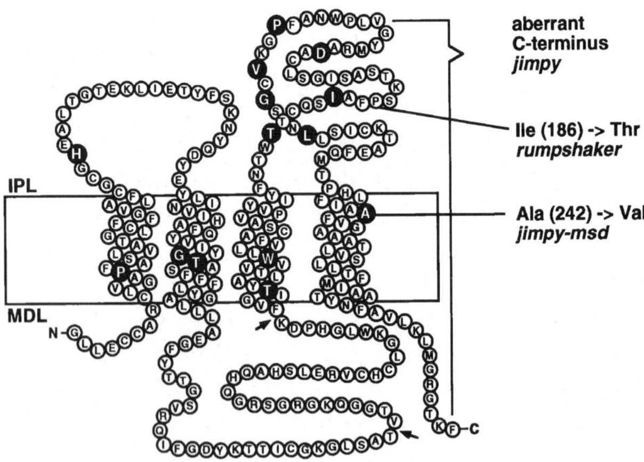

FIGURE 34.4 Topological model of myelin proteolipid protein (PLP) depicted as a four-helix bundle protein with the amino and carboxyl termini oriented to the cytoplasmic surface of the lipid bilayer (IPL: intraperiod line; MDL: major dense line). The position of residues 116–150, absent from the DM-20 isoform of PLP, is indicated by two arrows. Substitutions in spontaneous mouse mouse mutants (*jimpy*, *rumpshaker*, *jimpy-4J*, *myelin-synthesis deficient*) are shown on the right. In *jimpy*, residues 207–276 are deleted and replaced by an aberrant carboxyl terminus of 36 amino acids. Also indicated are the positions of single substitutions (black circles) underlying lethal dysmyelinations in other species including the *md* rat (Thr74 → Pro), *shaking pup* (His36 → Pro), and human patients with Pelizaeus-Merzbacher disease (Pro14 → Leu; Gly73 → Arg; Thr155 → Ile; Trp162 → Arg; Thr181 → Pro; Asp202 → His; Pro215 → Ser; Val218 → Phe; Gly220 → Cys; Leu223 → Pro). For references, see text.

beginning at 2 weeks of age. They have a reduced body weight and die with seizures and convulsions 3–4 weeks after birth. Heterozygous females that are mosaics with respect to the X-linked *Plp1* gene are behaviorally normal. *Jimpy*, the oldest of the *Plp1* mutants, is also the best-studied animal model for human Pelizaeus-Merzbacher disease (PMD).

In *jimpy* mice, the inactivation of a splice-acceptor site causes the loss of exon 5 from the *jimpy* PLP mRNA with a deletion of 74 nucleotides and a shift in the normal open reading frame (Morello et al., 1986; Nave et al., 1986; Hudson et al., 1987; Macklin et al., 1987; Nave et al., 1987). As a consequence, the encoded *jimpy* protein lacks the fourth transmembrane domain, which is replaced by an aberrant carboxyl terminus. The mutant protein is degraded in the endoplasmic reticulum, and practically no immunoreactive PLP accumulates in oligodendrocytes. Morphologically, the CNS is almost completely myelin-deficient, whereas PNS myelin appears ultrastructurally intact (Sidman et al., 1964; Herschkowitz et al., 1971). Less than 1% of the CNS axons are ensheathed. Where present, "islands" of myelin contain little more than a few layers of membrane. This myelin may be uncompacted whorles of membrane or may display a compacted but abnormal ultrastructure: here the double *intraperiod line* appears fused to a single electron-dense structure due to the absence of PLP from the intraperiod line (Duncan et al., 1989).

The major cause of dysmyelination in *jimpy*, however, is the well-documented lack of differentiated oligodendrocytes that remain immature. In fact, the proliferation of oligodendrocyte precursors is increased and is associated with an abnormally high rate of cell death (Farkas-Bargeton et al., 1972; Skoff, 1982; Knapp et al., 1986). The degeneration of *jimpy* glial cells begins when PLP becomes immunodetectable in normal mice (Skoff, 1995). Morphologically, dying oligodendrocytes in *jimpy* show the typical features of both programmed cell death (Fig. 43.5*A*) and non-apoptotic mechanisms (Thomson et al., 1999; Cerghet et al., 2001; Southwood and Gow, 2001).

The phenotype of *jimpy-msd* mice is very similar, with about twice as many glial cells escaping premature degeneration and forming visible myelin structures (Billings-Gagliardi et al., 1980). The molecular defect of *jimpy-msd* is a surprisingly conservative amino acid substitution ($Ala^{242} \rightarrow Val$) within the last transmembrane domain of PLP/DM20 (Gencic and Hudson, 1990). The spontaneous mutation *jimpy-4J* ($Plp^{jp\text{-}4J}$) has the most severe phenotype of all X-linked mutants, that is, the complete absence of CNS myelin and premature death after 24 days. Its substitution, $Ala^{38} \rightarrow Ser$, affects the first hydrophilic loop of PLP (Billings-Gagliardi et al., 1995; Pearsall et al., 1997).

Similar mutations of the *Plp1* gene have been iden-

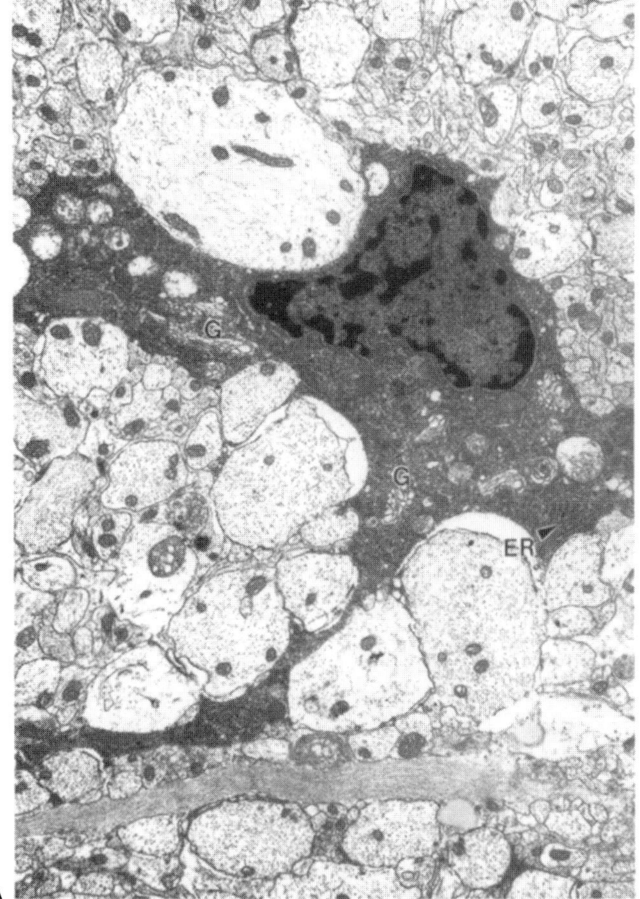

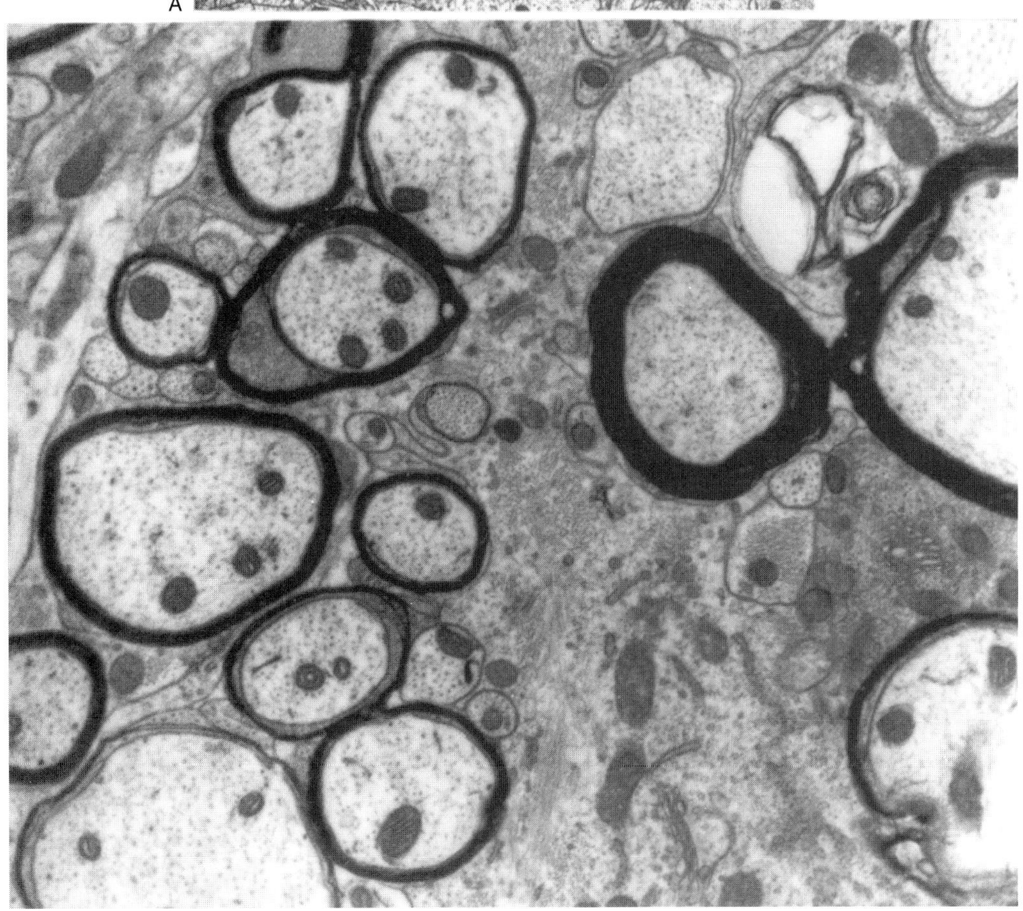

FIGURE 43.5 *A*. Electron micrograph of a dying oligodendrocyte in the spinal cord of a 3-week-old *jimpy* mouse carrying a mutation in the proteolipid protein gene. Note the chromatin condensations characteristic of apoptosis (programmed cell death) and the complete absence of myelin from surrounding axons (ER: endoplasmatic reticulum; G: Golgi apparatus. *B*. Hypomyelination in the spinal cord of *rumpshaker* mice. This mutation is allelic to *jimpy* but shows no sign of increased cell death and results in a varying degree of myelin formation. The proximity of myelinated and dysmyelinated large-caliber axons is striking and indicates abnormal oligodendrocyte differentiation rather than a structural defect of myelin assembly.

tified in other species. In a myelin-deficient strain of the rat (*md*), a point mutation induces a helix-braking change ($Thr^{74} \rightarrow Pro$) in the second transmembrane domain of PLP (Boison and Stoffel, 1989). A single base change in the canine *shaking pup* causes a helix-braking change ($His^{219} \rightarrow Pro$) close to the first transmembrane domain (Nadon et al., 1990). Ultrastructurally, the rough endoplasmic reticulum (ER) of oligodendrocytes in these mutants shows unusual vacuolar distentions, presumably caused by aberrantly folded PLP that is retained in the ER (Lipsitz et al., 1998). Using heterologous expression, Gow et al. (1994) observed the abnormal retention of mutant but not wild-type PLP/DM20 in the ER of transfected COS-7 cells. Subsequently, a genotype-phenotype correlation between intracellular retainment and disease severity was proposed (Gow and Lazzarini, 1996). The induction of several effector genes of the unfolded ER response was also demonstrated (Southwood et al., 2002).

The cause of death of PLP mutants after weeks of survival has remained a mystery. Mice do not die early as a result of CNS dysmyelination per se (Billings-Gagliardi et al., 1999). For the *md* rat, it has been shown that the toxicity of mutant PLP, which is detectable in glutamatergic neurons of the nucleus hypoglossus (not oligodendroglia), interferes with breathing control during seizure-induced hypoxia (Miller et al., 2003). Thus, it may be a neuronal dysfunction rather than the loss of myelin that causes premature death of the animals.

An interesting mutation of the *Plp1* gene is *rumpshaker* (Schneider et al., 1992), a single amino acid substitution ($Ile^{186} \rightarrow Thr$) in an extracellular loop region of PLP. PLP^{rsh} mice have more myelin than other dysmyelinated mutants, but the degree of dysmyelination varies among CNS regions. Early-myelinated (spinal cord) axons are almost normally ensheathed, whereas late-myelinated areas (optic nerve) remain severely hypomyelinated. Ultrastructurally, oligodendrocytes appear differentiated, and many escape abnormal cell death (Griffiths et al., 1990). Moreover, mutant PLP/DM20 is not degraded but is incorporated into myelin. This suggests that the specific alteration of PLP/DM20 in *rumpshaker* interferes with the oligodendrocytes' ability to initiate and complete myelination rather than with the structural function of PLP in compact myelin (Fig. 43.5*B*). On their original genetic background (C3H*101), *rumpshaker* mice are viable and have a normal life span. When backcrossed to C57 black mice, there is also substantial lethality in *rumpshaker*, suggesting a major role of modifier genes in disease expression (Al-Saktawi et al., 2003).

When the wild-type *Plp1* gene was reintroduced (as an autosomal transgene) into hemizygous *jimpy* mice in an attempt to rescue the *Plp1* mutant phenotype, the result was unexpected: the wild-type gene was normally expressed, but rescuing the *jimpy* phenotype was impossible. Apparently, in an artificially "heterozygous" situation, the X-linked *jimpy* allele is dominant over the autosomal wild-type *Plp1* transgene (Schneider et al., 1995). Presumably, normal and mutant PLP are both expressed but form aberrantly folded complexes in the ER. This is in line with the mild phenotype of *Plp1* null mutant mice (see below).

Surprisingly, PLP transgenic wild-type mice that overexpress PLP are by themselves myelin-deficient mutants with ataxia, tremors, and seizures (Kagawa et al., 1994; Readhead et al., 1994; Bradl et al., 1999). The extent of dys- and demyelination in transgenics and the survival time (a few months to 1 year) are determined by the degree of PLP/DM20 overexpression. Why *Plp1* turns into a disease gene by a duplication is not fully understood. It has been suggested that the accumulation of PLP-bound cholesterol in the lysosomal compartment of oligodendrocytes contributes to the dysmyelinated phenotype (Simons et al., 2002). *Plp1* gene duplications are also the major cause of human PMD. Several reviews have covered the various *PLP* mutations underlying PMD (Garbern et al., 1999; Woodward and Malcolm, 1999; Koeppen and Robitaille, 2002) and have drawn attention to the homology of animal models (Nave and Boespflug-Tanguy, 1996; Griffiths et al., 1998a).

Gene targeting has been used to completely inactivate the *Plp1* gene (Boison and Stoffel, 1994; Klugmann et al., 1997; Stecca et al., 2000; Sporkel et al., 2002) and has shown that PLP is not required for myelin formation. Stoffel and coworkers reported a severe perturbation of *Plp1* gene expression (close to a null mutation) resulting from the combination of a splice defect and anti-sense silencing by an inserted promoter sequence (Boison et al., 1994). Myelin lamellae were loosely wrapped, lacked the intraperiod line, and led to a profound reduction of nerve conductance velocity in the CNS. Is PLP responsible for the tight apposition of membranes in compact myelin, as suggested (Boison et al., 1995)? The PLP/DM20 null mutation studied by Klugmann et al. (1997) showed that the myelin ultrastructure at the intraperiod line was highly variable, even within a single sheath. Increased fixation artifacts are indeed an *ex vivo* sign of reduced physical stability of PLP-deficient myelin (see also Rosenbluth et al., 1996).

An unexpected observation was that myelin lacking both PLP and DM20 caused progressive, widespread CNS axonal swellings, predominantly of small-caliber axons (Griffiths et al., 1998b), probably secondary to impaired axonal transport. Such axonal degeneration profiles are not a feature of myelin mutants in general, but they demonstrate that oligodendrocytes provide axonal support, independent of myelin assembly itself (see also the section "Cyclic Nucleotide Phosphodiesterase").

What is the functional difference between PLP and DM20? Stecca et al. (2000) generated mice that express only the DM20 isoform but have the phenoytype of the PLP/DM20 null mutants. This suggests that the PLP isoform is required for maintaining axonal integrity. In contrast, Spörkel et al. (2002) independently created a DM20-only mouse but found no difference from wild-type mice, a discrepancy that cannot be explained at present. However, Griffiths et al. (1998b) noted that both PLP and DM20 cDNA transgenes are partly able to reduce the axonal pathology of null mutants, which agrees better with the findings of Spörkel et al. (2002).

The principal cellular function of PLP and DM20 is not well defined. In oligodendrocytes, the DM20-related proteolipid M6B appears to have a partially overlapping function. Mice double-deficient in PLP/DM20 and M6B mice have major developmental defects of CNS myelination, unlike either of the parental single mutants (Werner et al., in preparation).

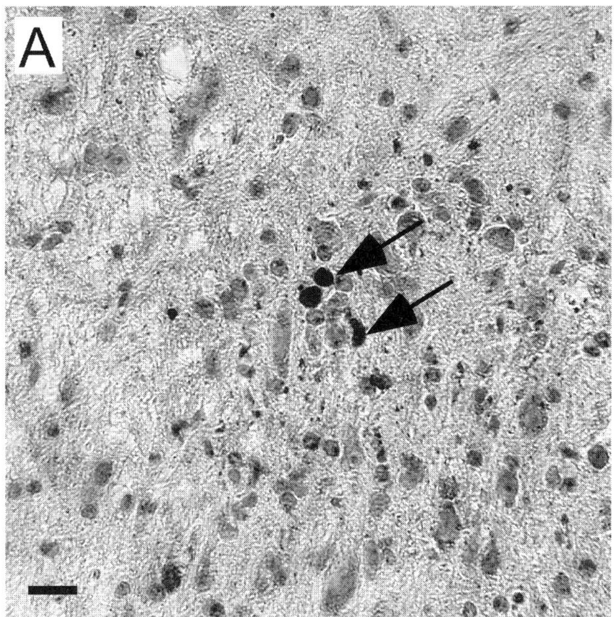

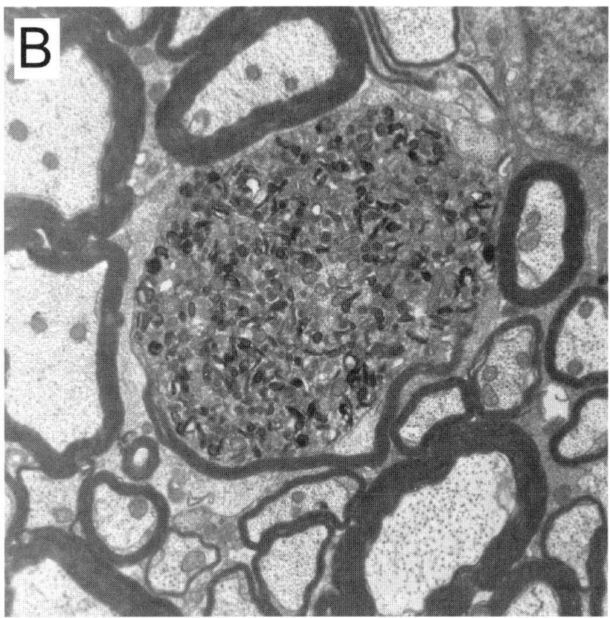

FIGURE 43.6 Axonal swellings in the central nervous system are the pathological hallmark of adult mice with a null mutation of the *Plp1* or *Cnp1* gene. As shown here for cyclic nucleotide phosphodiesterase–deficient mice, swellings are filled with axonally transported proteins and organelles, and can be visualized by immunostaining of the amyloid precursor protein (*arrows* in *A*) or by electron microscopy (in *B*). Functionally, they can be compared to a traffic jam that results in the breakdown of fast and slow axonal transport and eventually in Wallerian degeneration. (From Lappe-Siefke et al., 2003, with permission.)

CYCLIC NUCLEOTIDE PHOSPHODIESTERASE

The protein 2′,3′-cyclic nucleotide 3′-phosphodiesterase (CNP) is a widely used marker protein of oligodendrocytes and Schwann cells, but the CNP gene (the official nomenclature is *Cnp1*) is also expressed at much lower levels outside the nervous system, for example, in subsets of immune cells, photoreceptor cells, and in testis (Sprinkle, 1989).

Cnp1 mRNAs encode two protein isoforms (CNP1: 46 kDa; CNP2: 48 kDa) by alternative translation start sites. Both myelin proteins are isoprenylated at the carboxyl terminus and acylated, allowing association with cellular membranes. Cyclic nucleotide phosphodiesterase distributes within oligodendrocyte and into myelin, where it is associated with noncompacted regions (inner mesaxon, paranodal loops, and Schmidt-Lanterman incisures) but not with compact myelin (Braun et al., 1988).

The enzymatic activity of CNP remains obscure because 2′,3′-cyclic nucleotides are not present in brain. In transfection experiments, CNP overexpression caused increased outgrowth of filopodia. Moreover, overexpression of *Cnp1* in transgenic mice causes premature differentiation of oligodendrocytes, as well as specific defects in deposition of myelin basic protein and in myelin compaction (Gravel et al., 1996).

The *Cnp1* gene maps to chromosome 11 in the mouse, but natural mutations have not been reported. The targeted disruption of *Cnp1* in mice resulted in an unexpected neurodegenerative phenotype, somewhat similar to that of *Plp1* null mice (Fig. 43.6). Myelin assembly is not visibly affected and sheaths have normal stability, but the absence of CNP from oligodendrocytes causes axonal swellings, widespread neurodegeneration, and premature death before 1 year (Lappe-Siefke et al., 2003). Although this phenotype does not reveal the underlying cellular function of CNP in oligodendrocytes and in myelin, it confirms that axonal support is another principal function of oligodendrocytes, independent of myelination and the physical stability of myelin itself.

OLIGODENDROCYTE-SPECIFIC PROTEIN/CLAUDIN-11

Oligodendrocyte-specific protein (OSP) is a 22 kDa tetraspan membrane protein expressed in CNS myelin and in Sertoli cells of the testis (Bronstein et al., 1997). It belongs to the claudin family of tight junction (TJ) proteins, which play a role in cellular compartmentalization and signaling. At the ultrastructural level, OSP/claudin-11 has been localized to the interlamellar strands (radial elements) of myelin that spiral around the axon and can be considered a specialized TJ (Morita et al., 1999). A mutation of the *OSP/Claudin11* gene results in abnormal CNS myelin, with lack of radial elements and reduced nerve conduction velocity, as well as male sterility (Gow et al., 1999). Recent findings suggest that OSP can form complexes with beta-integrin and another tetraspan protein, OAP-1 (Tiwari-Woodruff et al., 2001). Whether this interaction serves a function in radial axon-glial signaling remains to be determined.

MYELIN-ASSOCIATED GLYCOPROTEIN

Another structural myelin protein of lower abundance in CNS and PNS is myelin-associated glycoprotein (MAG). The glycosylated type-I membrane protein has a molecular mass of approximately 100 kDa and belongs to the immunoglobulin superfamily of proteins. It has adhesive properties *in vitro* and when expressed in heterologous cells (Schachner and Bartsch, 2000). Due to its very restricted localization at the adaxonal surface of the myelin sheath, MAG has been a prime candidate to mediate axon-glial recognition and the first steps of myelination.

However, in MAG-deficient mice, oligodendrocytes and Schwann cells recognize axons and assemble myelin without gross abnormalities or developmental delay (Li et al., 1994; Montag et al., 1994), suggesting other functions or extensive compensatory mechanisms. Subtle myelin defects were observed at the ultrastructural level. They included multiply myelinated axons in the PNS, redundant myelin loops, and uncompacted regions at the axon-glia interface (*cytoplasmic collars*) (Montag et al., 1994). Long-term observations of *Mag* mutant mice identified onion-bulb formations in the PNS, paranodal myelin tomaculi, and degenerating axons suggestive of a mild peripheral neuropathy (Fruttiger et al., 1995; Guenard et al., 1996). In the adult optic nerve, the fraction of unmyelinated axons was higher than in wild-type controls (Bartsch et al., 1997). In aged MAG-deficient mice, a mild oligodendroglial pathology was noted, including enlarged processes with myelin-like vesicles and amorphous granular inclusions reminiscent of a "dying-back" oligodendropathy (Lassmann et al., 1997). The neural cell adhesion molecule (N-CAM) is more prominent in Schwann cells of mutant mice and was an attractive candidate to substitute for MAG function, at least in the developing PNS. However, a *Mag*Ncam* double mutant mouse could not confirm this hypothesis: peripheral myelination appeared uncompromised, even though axonal degeneration was noted months earlier than in simple MAG-deficient mice (Carenini et al., 1997).

It is now thought that the major function of MAG relates to glia-axon signaling, thereby regulating structural features of the myelinated axons, at least in the PNS (Yin et al., 1998). A principal observation was the reduced expression and phosphorylation of neurofilaments (NF-M and NF-H) in MAG-deficient mice, resulting in an increased neurofilament density and consequently a reduced diameter of myelinated PNS axons. Whether this signaling function is related to the role of MAG as an inhibitor of axonal outgrowth remains to be determined. The intracellular domain of MAG interacts with the Ser/Thr kinase fyn, and this complex may function as a receptor for axonal signals. This is indirectly suggested by the dysmyelinated phenotype of *Mag*fyn* double mutant mice that exceeds the mild phenotype of either parental single mutant (Biffiger et al., 2000).

MYELIN PROTEIN ZERO

In myelin of the PNS, the major structural component (approximately 50% of the protein mass) is P0, a glycosylated integral membrane protein with a single transmembrane domain (Lemke et al., 1988). With a molecular mass of 30 kDa and one immunoglobulin (Ig)-like extracellular domain, P0 is an ancestral member of the Ig superfamily of proteins and is found only in compact peripheral myelin. Based on these features, a role for this protein as a membrane adhesion molecule of the intraperiod line appears likely. This hypothesis was first supported by experiments in which the cloned protein was ectopically expressed in heterologous cells or incorporated into membrane vesicles and mediated homophilic binding *in vitro* (D'Urso et al., 1990; Filbin et al., 1990). The molecular basis of this interaction was elucidated by determining the three-dimensional structure of the extracellular domain of P0 (Shapiro et al., 1996). The intracellular domain of P0 contains a large number of basic residues that may interact with negatively charged phospholipids of the adjacent cytoplasmic parts of the Schwann cell membrane forming the major dense line. This hypothesis is supported by the finding in transfected fibroblasts that mutations in the intracellular domain of P0 reduce extracellular adhesion and are associated with hereditary motor and sensory neuropathies (Xu et al., 2001; see below). That P0 is required for the formation of compacted myelin was first demonstrated by the expression of *Mpz*-specific antisense RNA in cultured Schwann cells that interfered with the assembly of myelin (Owens and Boyd, 1991). Without a "spontaneous" mutation of the mouse *Mpz* (P0) gene available, precise functional *in vivo* analysis required the targeted inactivation of the gene in transgenic mice (Giese et al., 1992). As expected, myelin compaction, predominantly at the intraperiod line, was strongly affected in these mice. In addition, the abnormal myelin sheaths degenerated, as reflected in an increase of demyelinated axons in older mutants. Surprisingly, major dense lines were still abundant (see the section "Myelin Basic Protein" above). Cross-breeding of P0-deficient mice with MBP-deficient *shiverer* mice yielded P0*MBP double-deficient animals that displayed a lack of major dense lines in PNS myelin, demonstrating that P0 and MBP perform partially redundant functions in intracellular compaction (Martini et al., 1995a).

Close examination of mice with 50% reduced P0 expression revealed a late-onset but progressive demyelinating neuropathy (Martini et al., 1995b). The typical pathological features included demyelinated axons, unusually thin myelinated axons (reflecting incomplete remyelination), and supernumerary Schwann cells. These features made heterozygous mice with one functional *Mpz* gene a bona fide animal model for a human motor and sensory neuropathy caused by *Mpz* gene mutations, Charcot-Marie-Tooth disease (CMT) type 1B (Warner et al., 1996). Further analysis of the mutant mice revealed increased numbers of CD8-positive T lymphocytes and macrophages in the endoneurium. Recent findings suggest that these immune cells are actively involved in the primarily genetically mediated demyelination (reviewed by Mäurer et al., 2002).

Mice overexpressing P0 have been generated based on the rationale that other myelin components, including PLP and peripheral myelin protein-22 (see below), cause dys- and demyelination when their gene dosage is increased. P0-overexpressing mice showed various forms of hypomyelination that correlated with the level of overexpression. Pathological features ranged from thin myelin sheaths to impaired sorting of large-caliber axons (Wrabetz et al., 2000; Yin et al., 2000).

PERIPHERAL MYELIN PROTEIN-22

Peripheral myelin protein-22 is a 22 kDa integral membrane glycoprotein in compact myelin of peripheral nerves (reviewed by Naef and Suter, 1998). Peripheral myelin protein-22 and P0 have been copurified from peripheral nerve myelin, suggesting that they may form complexes in the myelin membrane (D'Urso et al., 1999). *In vitro* experiments suggest a role for PMP22 in vesicular transport, cell growth, differentiation, and apoptosis (Brancolini et al., 2000; Chies et al., 2003). Furthermore, a function as a component of TJs has been suggested (Notterpek et al., 2001).

Increased *Pmp22* gene dosage is the cause of the most frequent form of hereditary motor and sensory neuropathy (HMSN), CMT1A (reviewed by Berger et al., 2002). Decreased *Pmp22* gene dosage is responsible for hereditary neuropathy with liability to pressure palsies (HNPP), a transient neuropathy precipitated by minor injury to peripheral nerves. Point mutations in *Pmp22* lead to wide range of HMSN (reviewed by Naef and Suter, 1998).

The natural mouse mutants *Trembler* (*Tr*) and *Tr-J* are due to missense mutations in the *Pmp22* gene (Falconer, 1951; Suter et al., 1992a, 1992b). These mutations alter the primary structure of PMP22 ($G^{150} \rightarrow D$ and $L^{16} \rightarrow P$, respectively) causing intracellular protein trafficking defects, hypomyelination (Fig. 43.7), increased Schwann cell number, and aberrant Schwann cell proliferation (Henry and Sidman, 1988; Sancho et al., 2001). Grafting experiments had shown that the myelination defect in *Tr* is mainly Schwann cell autonomous (Aguayo et al., 1977). There is, however, also a strong effect of mutant Schwann cells on the axon, resulting in axonal damage (Sancho et al., 1999). This feature is not specific for *Pmp22* mutations, however, as it occurs in peripheral nerves of P0 mutant mice (reviewed by Berger et al., 2002) and is quite reminiscent of CNS axonal changes in PLP and CNP mutant mice. Secondary to axonal loss, a pronounced muscular atrophy is observed in *Pmp22* and *Mpz* mutant mice (Maier et al., 2002).

Additional *Pmp22* mutants include the in-frame deletion of exon 4 (Suh et al., 1997) and two mutagen-induced point mutations (Isaacs et al., 2000). Furthermore, *Pmp22*-overexpressing transgenic mice and rats have been generated, providing models for human CMT1A. The transgenic rat model resembles most closely the human disease (Sereda et al., 1996). These "CMT rats" carry three transgenic *Pmp22* copies and overexpress the gene about 1.6-fold (Sereda et al., 2003). The transgenic rats show reduced nerve conduction velocities (NCV) and, at the histological level, aberrant Schwann cell hypertrophy with prominent and abundant onion bulbs. Demyelination and remyelination are the main pathological features. These myelin abnormalities are more pronounced in ventral than in dorsal roots, as noted also for *Mpz* mutant mice (Martini, 1997; Wrabetz et al., 2000). The general severity of the clinical phenotype of *Pmp22* transgenic animals

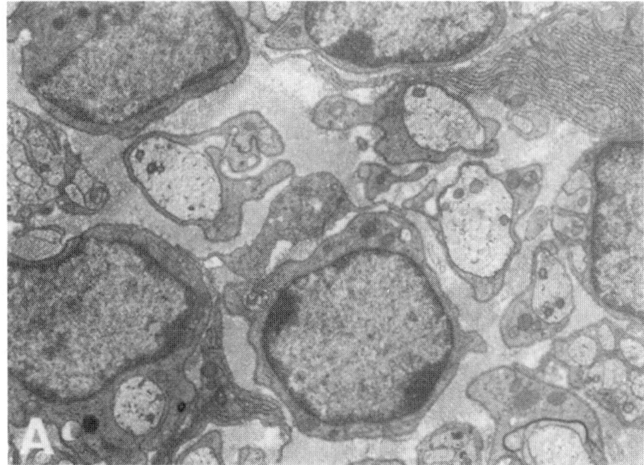

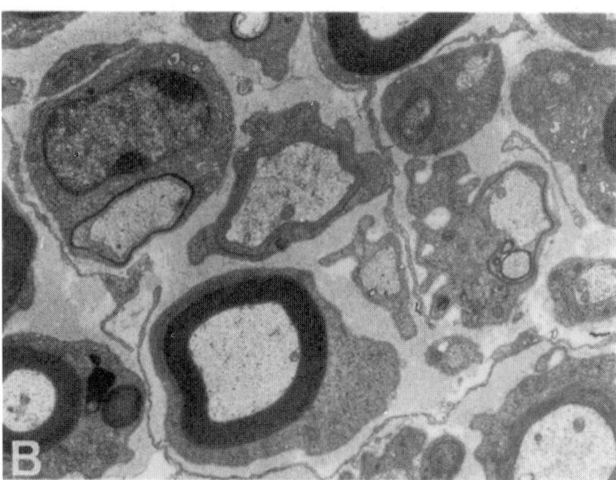

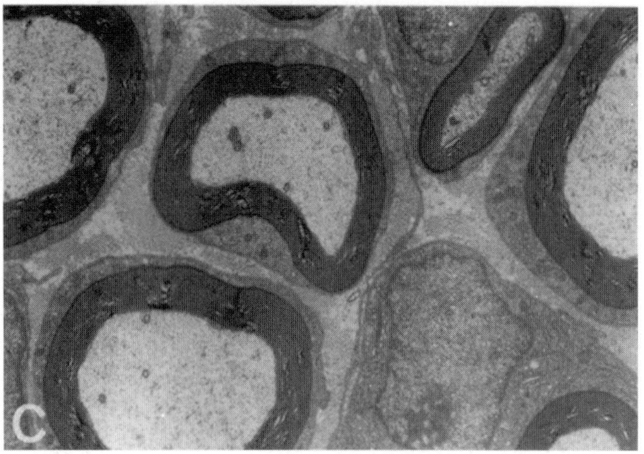

FIGURE 43.7 Transverse section of sciatic nerves from adult *trembler* mice with a point mutation in the gene encoding peripheral myelin protein-22. In homozygous animals (*Tr/Tr*), myelin is completely lacking but individual axons have been engulfed by mutant Schwann cells in a 1:1 ratio (*A*). In heterozygous trembler mice (*Tr/+*), most cells are arrested at this *promyelin* stage. Some myelin is assembled, which is abnormally thin (*arrow* in *B*) compared to the myelin of unaffected littermates (*C*). (From Henry and Sidman, 1988; with permission.)

is correlated with the degree of PMP22 overexpression (Huxley et al., 1998; Suter and Nave, 1999). Like human CMT1A patients, CMT rats develop gait abnormalities that are most likely due to secondary axonal loss and muscular atrophy rather than slowed NCV. In homozygous transgenic rats, virtually no myelin is formed in peripheral nerves, even though the program of myelin gene expression is not halted (Niemann et al., 2000). However, mice with a strongly increased *Pmp22* gene dosage exhibit defects of Schwann cell differentiation (Magyar et al., 1996).

A tetracyclin-induced *conditional* overexpression of PMP22 in adult transgenic mice also leads to rapid demyelination (Perea et al., 2001). This finding is remarkable, as it demonstrates that fully differentiated Schwann cells are also vulnerable to PMP22 overexpression and that the CMT pathology can be uncoupled from abnormal development. The authors also showed that turning off PMP22 overexpression can reverse the phenotype, which is good news for the development of a CMT1A therapy. One such approach, using the CMT rat model, is aimed at the nuclear progesterone receptor as a new pharmacological target in order to reduce pathological PMP22 overexpression (Sereda et al., 2003).

Mice with a genetic disruption of the *Pmp22* gene have been established to determine its function (Adlkofer et al., 1995). Animals lacking PMP22 are viable but show the hallmarks of severe HMSN. The onset of myelination is slightly delayed, indicating a role for PMP22 in the initial steps of myelination. Hypermyelination structures (tomacula) are abundant in peripheral nerves of young animals. They are unstable and degenerate with age, leading to a demyelination pathology that includes axonal degeneration (Sancho et al., 1999). No obvious pathological alterations have been detected outside the nervous system, possibly due to the presence of related members of the PMP22/EMP/MP20 protein family (Jetten and Suter, 2000).

Hetetrozyous mice with one functional *Pmp22* gene provide a bona fide model for HNPP and exhibit the characteristic human pathology (Adlkofer et al., 1997). This includes unstable tomacula that degenerate with age. Interestingly, older patients with HNPP may develop a chronic form of this neuropathy, which then shows similarities to CMT1.

PERIAXIN

Periaxin is a Schwann cell–specific component of the cytoskeleton that carries a PDZ (*p*ostsynaptic density protein 95, *Drosophila* *d*iscs large tumor suppressor, *z*onula occludens-1) motive (Gillespie et al., 1994). In mature nerves, periaxin interacts via dystrophin-related protein-2 (DRP2) with the dystroglycan complex (Sherman et al., 2001). In this way, laminin in the basal lamina is connected to the actin cyoskeleton of the myelinating Schwann cell. The expression of periaxin isoforms in immature cells (partially also in the nucleus) and the developmental shift in the localization of periaxin in mature Schwann cells (from an adaxonal to an abaxonal location) indicate additional functions of this protein in development (Scherer et al., 1995).

The crucial role of periaxin in myelinated peripheral nerves was elucidated by *Prx1* gene targeting (Gillespie et al., 2000). Mice lacking periaxin initially show almost normal myelin formation, but a few tomacula are present (Gillespie et al., 2000). As in PMP22-deficient mice, these structures degenerate, leading to a progressive demyelinating phenotype. Thus, the link between the basal lamina and the Schwann cell is essential for stabilizing the myelinated axon–Schwann cell unit. In contrast to most other myelin mutants, however, in which sensory nerves are largely preserved, *Prx1* mutants have a very prominent sensory neuropathy (relative to motor involvement) and develop allodynia, hyperalgesia, and neuropathic pain (Gillespie et al., 2000). In line with these findings, *Prx1* mutations have been found in human patients with CMT4F, a neuropathy with pronounced sensory abnormalities (Boerkoel et al., 2001; Guilbot et al., 2001).

CONNEXIN-32

The four-transmembrane gap junction protein connexin-32 (Cx32) is found in many cell types, but in myelinating Schwann cells it is localized in paranodes and in Schmidt-Lanterman incisures (Scherer et al., 1995). Based on this localization, it has been suggested that Cx32 is a component of reflexive gap junctions that form a direct radial pathway across the myelin sheath (Balice-Gordon et al., 1998). *Cx32* null mice have been used to test this hypothesis, but the rate of dye diffusion through myelin was not altered. Thus, other connexins such as Cx29 may perform the same function (Altevogt et al., 2002). However, the functional compensation is obviously not complete, since Cx32-deficient mice develop a demyelinating phenotype (Anzini et al., 1997) and mutations of the human *Cx32* gene are the cause of X-linked CMT1X (Bergoffen et al., 1993).

Cx32 null mice display a late-onset, progressive demyelinating peripheral neuropathy. Some features are specific to Cx32-deficient mice compared to other demyelinating mouse mutants. This includes enlarged periaxonal collars, which may reflect the consequence of disturbed communication between the outer and inner cytoplasmic aspects of myelinating Schwann cells. In addition, regenerative clusters indicative of axonal degeneration are frequent. Similar pathologies have been described for human patients with CMT1X. Interestingly, some CMT1X patients have developed CNS symptoms, but the underlying molecular mechanisms have not been identified (Kleopa et al., 2002).

A large number of different *Cx32* mutations distributed throughout the gene are associated with CMT1X. The disease mechanisms appear to be diverse but include intracellular trafficking defects and functional alterations of the mutant channels (reviewed by Abrams et al., 2000; Yum et al., 2002). It will be a challenging task to dissect these mechanisms further, in particular to determine the potential contribution of dominant-negative effects, since connexons are usually composed of six connexin subunits. Although mutant Cx32 is not coexpressed with the normal protein in the same cell (due to X chromosome inactivation), it may interact in a deleterious way with other connexins expressed by Schwann cells or oligodendrocytes. The analysis will require better knowledge of the connexin family that is expressed by myelinating cells.

BETA-1 AND BETA-4 INTEGRIN

Integrin heterodimers, including alpha-6/beta-1 and alpha-6/beta-4, link the Schwann cell surface and the basal lamina by binding to laminin (reviewed by Previtali et al., 2001). This link is crucial for the correct development of myelinated nerves, since a Cre-mediated ablation of the beta-1 gene function specifically in presumptive myelinating Schwann cells results in severe dysmyelination and impaired axonal sorting (Feltri et al., 2002).

During peripheral nerve myelination, beta-4 integrin is strongly upregulated in parallel with myelin genes (Feltri et al., 1994). However, beta-4 integrin–deficient mice, which are perinatal lethal, show normal myelin formation in organotypic dorsal root ganglion cultures, suggesting no absolute requirement for this integrin subunit in myelination (Frei et al., 1999).

TRANSCRIPTIONAL CONTROL OF MYELINATION

As shown by mice with abnormal myelin gene dosage, the expression level of myelin proteins in the PNS and CNS can have a strong effect on myelin assembly and maintainance. Thus, it is critically important for glial cells to monitor the transcriptional activity of myelin protein genes. Mutations of regulatory genes should lead to neurological deficits similar to those of mutant myelin protein genes. We therefore close this overview with a look at candidate transcription factors in myelinating glial cells.

In mice lacking the zinc finger transcription factor EGR2/Krox20, myelination is blocked at an early promyelin stage, that is, when Schwann cells begin to wrap axons (Topilko et al., 1994). Similarly, mutations of the human *EGR2/Krox20* gene lead to a wide range of demyelinating and dysmyelinating neuropathies (Warner et al., 1998). Most of these mutations are dominant and map into the highly conserved zinc finger domain required for DNA binding. They probably act by dominant-negatively inhibiting myelin gene expression. Indeed, overexpression of EGR2/Krox20 in cultured Schwann cells induces the expression of several myelin genes including *Pmp22* and *Mpz* (Nagarajan et al., 2001). In contrast, recessive mutations seem to prevent interaction of EGR2/Krox20 with the NAB corepressor, causing overactivity of the transcription factor. Here, myelination defects may be due to the overexpression of dosage-sensitive myelin genes, such as *Mpz* or *Pmp22*.

The transcription factor Sox10 is required for normal development of neural crest derivatives including Schwann cells. Cooperating with other transcription factors (SCIP/Oct-6, Pax3, and EGR2/Krox20), SOX10 regulates myelin-specific genes in Schwann cells. Null mutant mice have been generated and completely lack satellite or Schwann cells (Britsch et al., 2001), and the terminal differentiation of oligodendrocytes, including myelination, is impaired (Stolt et al., 2002).

Heterozygous mutations in the human *Sox10* gene are associated with the Waardenburg-Shah (WS4) syndrome, which is characterized by intestinal aganglionosis (Hirschsprung disease), depigmentation, and deafness (Waardenburg syndrome). These patients suffer from an aberrant development of neural crest derivatives, including enteric ganglion cells and melanocytes (hence the phenotype) but show no signs of myelin diseases. However, some WS patients with putative dominant-negative mutations in *Sox10* showed additional dysmyelination in the PNS and often in the CNS as well (reviewed by Inoue et al., 2002). Clarification of the exact nature of *Sox10* mutations that affect myelination requires further studies *in vitro* and *in vivo*.

The cyclic adenosine monophosphate (cAMP)-inducible POU protein SCIP/Oct-6 is crucially involved in the regulation of PNS myelination. SCIP/Oct-6-deficient mice show severe hypomyelination in early development, but myelinated nerves appear normal at 3 months of age (reviewed by Jaegle and Meijer, 1998). Further understanding of the exact molecular role of this and other transcription factors will require better knowledge of target genes (Bermingham et al., 2002).

CONCLUSIONS

Mouse genetics, in combination with molecular cell biology and morphology, has provided important insights into the process of myelination. For some myelin proteins, a specific function in the architecture of myelin could be demonstrated. In other cases, a more complex picture has emerged from overlapping loss-of-function and aberrant gain-of-function effects. The latter is a recurrent feature of natural point mutations with autosomal dominant (or X-linked recessive) inheritance. These mice provide helpful models for corresponding myelin diseases in humans. An important future goal is to understand how myelin proteins interact with each other, what drives the process of myelin assembly, and what is the nature of the vital axon-glia interactions in the adult nervous system.

ACKNOWLEDGMENTS

We thank Ian Griffiths and members of our laboratory for helpful discussion. For providing original electron micrographs, we are indebted to Drs. David Shine (Fig. 43.3), Robert Skoff (Fig. 43.5*A*), Ian Griffiths (Fig. 43.5*B*), and Richard Sidman (Fig. 43.7). The authors' work was supported by the Deutsche Forschungsgemeinschaft (SFB523), the Max Planck Society, the Hertie Institute of MS Research (KAN), and the Swiss National Science Foundation (US).

REFERENCES

Abrams, C.K., Oh, S., Ri, Y., and Bargiello, T.A. (2000) Mutations in connexin32: the molecular and biophysical bases for the X-linked form of Charcot-Marie-Tooth disease. *Brain Res. Brain Res. Rev.* 32:203–214.

Adlkofer, K., Frei, R., Neuberg, D.H., Zielasek, J., Toyka, K.V., and Suter, U. (1997) Heterozygous peripheral myelin protein 22–deficient mice are affected by a progressive demyelinating tomaculous neuropathy. *J. Neurosci.* 17:4662–4671.

Adlkofer, K., Martini, R., Aguzzi, A., Zielasek, J., Toyka, K.V., and Suter, U. (1995) Hypermyelination and demyelinating peripheral neuropathy in Pmp22-deficient mice. *Nat. Genet.* 11:274–280.

Aguayo, A.J., Attiwell, M., Trecarten, J., Perkins, C.S., and Bray, C.M. (1977) Abnormal myelination in transplanted *trembler* mouse Schwann cells. *Nature* 265:73–75.

Al-Saktawi, K., McLaughlin, M., Klugmann, M., Schneider, A., Barrie, J.A., McCulloch, M.C., Montague, P., Kirkham, D., Nave, K.-A., and Griffiths, I.R. (2003) Genetic background determines phenotypic severity of the Plp *rumpshaker* mutation. *J. Neurosci. Res.* 72:12–24.

Altevogt, B.M., Kleopa, K.A., Postma, F.R., Scherer, S.S., and Paul, D.L. (2002) Connexin29 is uniquely distributed within myelinating glial cells of the central and peripheral nervous systems. *J. Neurosci.* 22:6458–6470.

Anzini, P., Neuberg, D.H., Schachner, M., Nelles, E., Willecke, K., Zielasek, J., Toyka, K.V., Suter, U., and Martini, R. (1997) Structural abnormalities and deficient maintenance of peripheral nerve myelin in mice lacking the gap junction protein connexin 32. *J. Neurosci.* 17:4545–4551.

Balice-Gordon, R.J., Bone, L.J., and Scherer, S.S. (1998) Functional gap junctions in the Schwann cell myelin sheath. *J. Cell Biol.* 142:1095–1104.

Bartsch, S., Montag, D., Schachner, M., and Bartsch, U. (1997) Increased number of unmyelinated axons in optic nerves of adult mice deficient in the myelin-associated glycoprotein (MAG). *Brain Res.* 762:231–234.

Berger, P., Young, P., and Suter, U. (2002) Molecular cell biology of Charcot-Marie-Tooth disease. *Neurogenetics* 4:1–15.

Bergoffen, J., Scherer, S.S., Wang, S., Scott, M.O., Bone, L.J., Paul, D.L., Chen, K., Lensch, M.W., Chance, P.F., and Fischbeck, K.H. (1993) Connexin mutations in X-linked Charcot-Marie-Tooth disease. *Science* 262:2039–2042.

Bermingham, J.R., Jr., Shumas, S., Whisenhunt, T., Sirkowski, E.E., O'Connell, S., Scherer, S.S., and Rosenfeld, M.G. (2002) Identification of genes that are downregulated in the absence of the POU domain transcription factor pou3f1 (Oct-6, Tst-1, SCIP) in sciatic nerve. *J. Neurosci.* 22:10217–10231.

Biffiger, K., Bartsch, S., Montag, D., Aguzzi, A., Schachner, M., and Bartsch, U. (2000) Severe hypomyelination of the murine CNS in the absence of myelin-associated glycoprotein and fyn tyrosine kinase. *J. Neurosci.* 20:7430–7437.

Billings-Gagliardi, S., Adcock, L.H., and Wolf, M.K. (1980) Hypomyelinated mutant mice: description of jp^{msd} and comparison with *jp* and *qk* on their present genetic backgrounds. *Brain Res.* 194:325–338.

Billings-Gagliardi, S., Kirschner, D.A., Nadon, N.L., DiBenedetto, L.M., Karthigasan, J., Lane, P., Pearsall, G.B., and Wolf, M.K. (1995) *Jimpy 4J*: a new X-linked mouse mutation producing severe CNS hypomyelination *Dev. Neurosci.* 17:300–310

Billings-Gagliardi, S., Nunnari, J.N., Nadon, N.L., and Wolf, M.K. (1999) Evidence that CNS hypomyelination does not cause death of *jimpy-msd* mutant *Dev. Neurosci.* 21:473–482.

Boiko, T., Rasband, M.N., Levinson, S.R., Caldwell, J.H., Mandel, G., Trimmer, J.S., and Matthews, G. (2001) Compact myelin dictates the differential targeting of two sodium channel isoforms in the same axon. *Neuron* 30:91–104.

Boerkoel, C.F., Takashima, H., Stankiewicz, P., Garcia, C.A., Leber, S.M., Rhee-Morris, L., and Lupski, J.R. (2001) Periaxin mutations cause recessive Dejerine-Sottas neuropathy. *Am. J. Hum. Genet.* 68:325–333.

Boison, D., Büssow, H., D'Urso, D., Müller, H.W., and Stoffel, W. (1995) Adhesive properties of proteolipid protein are responsible for the compaction of CNS myelin sheaths. *J. Neurosci.* 15:5502–5513.

Boison, D. and Stoffel, W. (1989) Myelin-deficient rat: a point mutation in exon III (A → C, Thr75 → Pro) of the myelin proteolipid protein causes dysmyelination and oligodendrocyte death. *EMBO J.* 8:3295–3302.

Boison, D. and Stoffel, W. (1994) Disruption of the compacted myelin sheath of axons of the central nervous system in proteolipid protein-deficient mice. *Proc. Natl. Acad. Sci. USA* 91:11709–11713.

Bradl, M., Bauer, J., Inomata, T., Zielasek, J., Nave, K.A., Toyka, K., Lassmann, H., and Wekerle, H. (1999) Transgenic Lewis rats overexpressing the proteolipid protein gene: myelin degeneration and its effect on T cell-experimental autoimmune encephalomyelitis. *Acta Neuropathol. (Berl.)* 97:595–606.

Brancolini, C., Edomi, P., Marzinotto, S., and Schneider, C. (2000) Exposure at the cell surface is required for gas3/PMP22 to regulate both cell death and cell spreading: implication for the Charcot-Marie-Tooth type 1A and Dejerine-Sottas diseases. *Mol. Biol. Cell.* 11:2901–2914.

Braun, P.E., Sandillon, F., Edwards, A., Matthieu, J.M., and Privat, A. (1988) Immunocytochemical localization by electron microscopy of 2′3′-cyclic nucleotide 3′-phosphodiesterase in developing oligodendrocytes of normal and mutant brain. *J. Neurosci.* 8: 3057–3066.

Britsch, S., Goerich, D.E., Riethmacher, D., Peirano, R.I., Rossner, M., Nave, K.-A., Birchmeier, C., and Wegner, M. (2001) The transcription factor Sox10 is a key regulator of peripheral glial development. *Genes Dev.* 15:66–78.

Bronstein, J.M., Micevych, P.E., and Chen, K. (1997) Oligodendrocyte-specific protein (OSP) is a major component of CNS myelin. *J. Neurosci. Res.* 50:713–720.

Carenini, S., Montag, D., Cremer, H., Schachner, M., and Martini, R. (1997) Absence of the myelin-associated glycoprotein (MAG) and the neural cell adhesion molecule (N-CAM) interferes with the maintenance, but not with the formation of peripheral myelin. *Cell Tissue Res.* 287:3–9.

Cerghet, M., Bessert, D.A., Nave, K.-A, and Skoff, R.P. (2001) Differential expression of apoptotic markers in *jimpy* and in Plp overexpressors: evidence for different apoptotic pathways. *J. Neurocytol.* 30:841–855.

Chernoff, G.F. (1981) *Shiverer*: an autosomal recessive mutant mouse with myelin-deficiency. *J. Hered.* 72:128.

Chies, R., Nobbio, L., Edomi, P., Schenone, A., Schneider, C., and Brancolini, C. (2003) Alterations in the Arf6-regulated plasma membrane endosomal recycling pathway in cells overexpressing the tetraspan protein Gas3/PMP22. *J. Cell Sci.* 116: 987–999.

Doolittle, D.P. and Schweikart, K.M. (1977) *Myelin deficient*, a new neurological mutation in the mouse. *J. Hered.* 68:331–332.

Duncan, I.D., Hammang, J.P., Goda, S., and Quarles, R.H. (1989) Myelination in the *jimpy* mouse in the absence of proteolipid protein. *Glia* 2:148–154.

D'Urso, D., Brophy, P.J., Staugaitis, S.M., Gillespie, C.S., Frey, A.B., Stempak, J.G., and Colman, D.R. (1990) Protein zero of peripheral nerve myelin: biosynthesis, membrane insertion, and evidence for homotypic interaction. *Neuron* 4:449–460.

D'Urso, D., Ehrhardt, P., and Muller, H.W. (1999) Peripheral myelin protein 22 and protein zero: a novel association in peripheral nervous system myelin. *J. Neurosci.* 19:3396–3403.

Dyer, C.A., Phillbotte, T., Wolf, M.K., and Billings-Gagliardi, S. (1997) Regulation of cytoskeleton by myelin components: studies on *shiverer* oligodendrocytes carrying an Mbp transgene *Dev. Neurosci.* 19:395–409.

Falconer, D.S. (1951) Two new mutations, *trembler* and *reeler*, with neurological action in the house mouse. *J. Genet.* 50:192–201.

Farkas-Bargeton, E., Robain, O., and Mandel, P. (1972) Abnormal glial maturation in the white matter in *jimpy* mice. *Acta Neuropathol.* 21:272–281.

Feltri, M.L., Graus Porta, D., Previtali, S.C., Nodari, A., Migliavacca, B., Cassetti, A., Littlewood-Evans, A., Reichardt, L.F., Messing, A., Quattrini, A., Mueller, U., and Wrabetz, L. (2002) Conditional disruption of beta 1 integrin in Schwann cells impedes interactions with axons. *J. Cell Biol.* 156:199–209.

Feltri, M.L., Scherer, S.S., Nemni, R., Kamholz, J., Vogelbacker, H., Scott, M.O., Canal, N., Quaranta, V., and Wrabetz, L. (1994) Beta 4 integrin expression in myelinating Schwann cells is polarized, developmentally regulated and axonally dependent. *Development* 120:1287–1301.

Filbin, M.T., Walsh, F.S., Trapp, B.D., Pizzey, J.A., and Tennekoon, G.I. (1990) Role of myelin P0 protein as a homophilic adhesion molecule. *Nature* 344:871–872.

Frei, R., Dowling, J., Carenini, S., Fuchs, E., and Martini, R. (1999) Myelin formation by Schwann cells in the absence of beta4 integrin. *Glia* 27:269–274.

Fremeau, R.T., Jr. and Popko, B. (1990) In situ analysis of myelin basic protein gene expression in myelin-deficient oligodendrocytes: antisense hnRNA and readthrough transcription. *EMBO J.* 9:3533–3538.

Fruttiger, M., Montag, D., Schachner, M., and Martini, R. (1995) Crucial role for the myelin-associated glycoprotein in the maintenance of axon-myelin integrity. *Eur. J. Neurosci.* 7:511–515.

Garbern, J., Cambi, F., Shy, M., and Kamholz, J. (1999) The molecular pathogenesis of Pelizaeus-Merzbacher disease. *Arch. Neurol.* 56:1210–1214.

Gencic, S. and Hudson, L. (1990) Conservative amino acid substitution in the myelin proteolipid protein of *jimpy*^{msd} mice. *J. Neurosci.* 10:117–124.

Genoud, S., Lappe-Siefke, C., Goebbels, S., Radtke, F., Aguet, M., Scherer, S.S., Suter, U., Nave, K.A., and Mantei, N. (2002) Notch1 control of oligodendrocyte differentiation in the spinal cord. *J. Cell Biol.* 158:709–718.

Giese, K.P., Martini, R., Lemke, G., Soriano, P., and Schachner, M. (1992) Disruption of the P0 gene in mice leads to abnormal expression of recognition molecules, and degeneration of myelin and axons. *Cell* 71:565–576.

Gillespie, C.S., Sherman, D.L., Blair, G.E., and Brophy, P.J. (1994) Periaxin, a novel protein of myelinating Schwann cells with a possible role in axonal ensheathment. *Neuron* 12:497–508.

Gillespie, C.S., Sherman, D.L., Fleetwood-Walker, S.M., Cottrell, D.F., Tait, S., Garry, E.M., Wallace, V.C., Ure, J., Griffiths, I.R., Smith, A., and Brophy, P.J. (2000) Peripheral demyelination and neuropathic pain behavior in periaxin-deficient mice. *Neuron* 26:523–531.

Gould, R.M., Byrd, A.L., and Barbarese, E. (1995) The number of Schmidt-Lanterman incisures is more than doubled in *shiverer* PNS myelin sheaths. *J. Neurocytol.* 24:85–98.

Gow, A., Friedrich, V.L., Jr., and Lazzarini, R.A. (1994) Many naturally occurring mutations of myelin proteolipid protein impair its intracellular transport. *J. Neurosci. Res.* 37:574–583.

Gow, A. and Lazzarini, R.A. (1996) A cellular mechanism governing the severity of Pelizaeus-Merzbacher disease. *Nat. Genet.* 13:422–428.

Gow, A., Southwood, C.M., Li, J.S., Pariali, M., Riordan, G.P., Brodie, S.E., Danias, J., Bronstein, J.M., Kachar, B., and Lazzarini, R.A. (1999) CNS myelin and Sertoli cell tight junction strands are absent in Osp/claudin-11 null mice. *Cell* 99:649–659.

Gravel, M., Peterson, J., Yong, V.W., Kottis, V., Trapp, B., and Braun, P.E. (1996) Overexpression of 2′,3′-cyclic nucleotide 3′-phosphodiesterase in transgenic mice alters oligodendrocyte development and produces aberrant myelination. *Mol. Cell Neurosci.* 7:453–466.

Griffiths, I.R., Klugmann, M., Anderson, T.J., Thomson, C.E., Vouyiouklis, D.A., and Nave, K.-A. (1998a) Current concepts of PLP and its role in the nervous system. *Microsc. Res. Tech.* 41: 344–358.

Griffiths, I.R., Klugmann, M., Anderson, T., Yool, D., Thomson, C., Schwab, M.H., Schneider, A., Zimmermann, F., McCulloch, M., Nadon, N., and Nave, K.-A. (1998b) Axonal swellings and degeneration in mice lacking myelin proteolipid protein. *Science* 280:1610–1613.

Griffiths, I.R., Scott, I., McCulloch, M.C., Barrie, J.A., McPhilemy, K., and Cattanach, B.M. (1990) *Rumpshaker* mouse: a new X-linked mutation affecting myelination: evidence for a defect in PLP expression. *J. Neurocytol.* 19:273–283.

Guenard, V., Montag, D., Schachner, M., and Martini, R. (1996) Onion bulb cells in mice deficient for myelin genes share molecular properties with immature, differentiated non-myelinating, and denervated Schwann cells. *Glia* 18:27–38.

Guilbot, A., Williams, A., Ravise, N., Verny, C., Brice, A., Sherman, D.L., Brophy, P.J., LeGuern, E., Delague, V., and Bareil, C. (2001) Megarbane A mutation in periaxin is responsible for CMT4F, an autosomal recessive form of Charcot-Marie-Tooth disease. *Hum. Mol. Genet.* 10:415–421.

Henry, E.W. and Sidman, R.L. (1988) Long lives for homozygous *trembler* mutant mice despite virtual absence of peripheral nerve myelin. *Science* 241:344–346.

Herschkowitz, N., Vassella, F., and Bischoff, A. (1971) Myelin differences in the central and peripheral nervous system in the 'jimpy' mouse. *J. Neurochem.* 18:1361–1363.

Hudson, L.D., Berndt, J.A., Puckett, C., Kozak, C.A., and Lazzarini, R.A. (1987) Aberrant splicing of proteolipid protein mRNA in the dysmyelinating *jimpy* mutant mouse. *Proc. Natl. Acad. Sci. USA* 84:1454–1458.

Huxley, C., Passage, E., Robertson, A.M., Youl, B., Huston, S., Manson, A., Saberan-Djoniedi, D., Figarella-Branger, D., Pellissier, J.F., Thomas, P.K., and Fontes, M. (1998) Correlation between varying levels of *PMP22* expression and the degree of demyelination and reduction in nerve conduction velocity in transgenic mice. *Hum. Mol. Genet.* 7:449–458.

Inoue, K., Shilo, K., Boerkoel, C.F., Crowe, C., Sawady, J., Lupski, J.R., and Agamanolis, D.P. (2002) Congenital hypomyelinating neuropathy, central dysmyelination, and Waardenburg-Hirschsprung disease: phenotypes linked by SOX10 mutation. *Ann Neurol.* 52:836–842.

Isaacs, A.M., Davies, K.E., Hunter, A.J., Nolan, P.M., Vizor, L., Peters, J., Gale, D.G., Kelsell, D.P., Latham, I.D., Chase, J.M., Fisher, E.M., Bouzyk, M.M., Potter, A., Masih, M., Walsh, F.S., Sims, M.A., Doncaster, K.E., Parsons, C.A., Martin, J., Brown, S.D., Rastan, S., Spurr, N.K., and Gray, I.C. (2000) Identification of two new Pmp22 mouse mutants using large-scale mutagenesis and a novel rapid mapping strategy. *Hum. Mol. Genet.* 9:1865–1871.

Jaegle, M. and Meijer, D. (1998) Role of Oct-6 in Schwann cell differentiation *Microsc. Res. Tech.* 41:372–378.

Jetten, A.M. and Suter, U. (2000) The peripheral myelin protein 22 and epithelial membrane protein family. *Prog. Nucleic Acid Res. Mol. Biol.* 64:97–129.

Kagawa, T., Ikenaka, K., Inoue, Y., Kuriyama, S., Tsujii, T., Nakao, J., Nakajima, K., Aruga, J., Okano, H., and Mikoshiba, K. (1994) Glial cell degeneration and hypomyelination caused by overexpression of myelin proteolipid protein gene. *Neuron* 13:427–442.

Katsuki, M., Sato, M., Kimura, M., Yokoyama, M., Kobayashi, K., and Nomura, T. (1988) Conversion of normal behavior to *shiverer* by myelin basic protein antisense cDNA in transgenic mice. *Science* 241:593–595.

Kimura, M., Sato, M., Akatsuka, A., Nozawa-Kimura, S., Takahashi, R., Yokoyama, M., Nomura, T., and Katsuki, M. (1989) Restoration of myelin formation by a single type of myelin basic protein in transgenic *shiverer* mice. *Proc. Natl. Acad. Sci. USA* 86:5661–5665.

Kimura, M., Sato, M., Akatsuka, A., Saito, S., Ando, K., Yokoyama, M., and Katsuki, M. (1998) Overexpression of a minor component of myelin basic protein isoform (17.2 kDa) can restore myelinogenesis in transgenic *shiverer* mice. *Brain Res.* 785:245–252.

Kirkpatrick, L.L., Witt, A.S., Payne, H.R., Shine, H.D., and Brady, S.T. (2001) Changes in microtubule stability and density in myelin-deficient *shiverer* mouse CNS axons. *J. Neurosci.* 21: 2288–2297.

Kirschner, D.A. and Ganser, A.L. (1980) Compact myelin exists in the absence of basic protein in the *shiverer* mutant mouse. *Nature* 283:207–210.

Kleopa, K.A., Yum, S.W., and Scherer, S.S. (2002) Cellular mechanisms of connexin32 mutations associated with CNS manifestations. *J. Neurosci. Res.* 68:522–534.

Klugmann, M., Schwab, M., Pühlhofer, A., Schneider, A., Zimmermann, F., Griffiths, I.R., Nave, K.-A. (1997) Assembly of CNS myelin in the absence of proteolipid protein. *Neuron* 18:59–70.

Knapp, P.E., Skoff, R.P., and Redstone, D.W. (1986) Oligodendroglial cell death in jimpy mice: an explanation for the myelin deficit. *J. Neurosci.* 6:2813–2822.

Koeppen, A.H. and Robitaille, Y. (2002) Pelizaeus-Merzbacher disease. *J. Neuropathol. Exp. Neurol.* 61:747–759.

Kwiecien, J.M., O'Connor, L.T., Goetz, B.D., Delaney, K.H., Fletch, A.L., and Duncan, I.D. (1998) Morphological and morphometric studies of the dysmyelinating mutant, the *Long Evans shaker* rat. *J. Neurocytol.* 27:581–591.

Lappe-Siefke, C., Goebbels, S., Gravel, M., Nicksch, E., Lee, J., Braun, P.E., Griffiths, I.R., and Nave, K.-A. (2003) Disruption of the *Cnp1* gene uncouples oligodendroglial functions in axonal support and myelination. *Nat. Genet.* 33:366–374.

Lassmann, H., Bartsch, U., Montag, D., and Schachner, M. (1997) Dying-back oligodendrogliopathy: a late sequel of myelin-associated glycoprotein deficiency. *Glia* 19:104–110.

Lemke, G. and Axel, R. (1985) Isolation and sequence of a cDNA encoding the major structural protein of peripheral myelin. *Cell* 40:501–508.

Lemke, G., Lamar, E., and Patterson, J. (1988) Isolation and analysis of the gene encoding peripheral myelin protein zero. *Neuron* 1:73–83.

Li, C., Tropak, M.B., Gerlai, R., Clapoff, S., Abramow-Newerly, W., Trapp, B., Peterson, A., and Roder, J. (1994) Myelination in the absence of myelin-associated glycoprotein. *Nature* 369:747–750.

Lipsitz, D., Goetz, B.D., and Duncan, I.D. (1998) Apoptotic glial cell death and kinetics in the spinal cord of the myelin-deficient rat. *J. Neurosci. Res.* 51:497–507.

Macklin, W.B., Gardinier, M.V., King, K.D., and Kamp, K. (1987) An AG → GG transition at a splice site in the myelin proteolipid protein gene in *jimpy* mice results in the removal of an exon. *FEBS Lett.* 223:417–421.

Magyar, J.P., Martini, R., Ruelicke, T., Aguzzi, A., Adlkofer, K., Dembic, Z., Zielasek, J., Toyka, K.V., and Suter, U. (1996) Impaired differentiation of Schwann cells in transgenic mice with increased *PMP22* gene dosage. *J. Neurosci.* 16:5351–5360.

Maier, M., Berger, P., and Suter, U. (2002) Understanding Schwann cell–neurone interactions: the key to Charcot-Marie-Tooth disease? *J. Anat.* 200:357–366.

Martini, R. (1997) Animal models for inherited peripheral neuropathies. *J. Anat.* 191:321–336.

Martini, R., Mohajeri, M.H., Kasper, S., Giese, K.P., and Schachner, M. (1995a) Mice doubly deficient in the genes for P0 and myelin basic protein show that both proteins contribute to the formation of the dense line in peripheral nerve myelin. *J. Neurosci.* 15:4488–4495.

Martini, R., Zielasek, J., Toyka, K.V., Giese, K.P., and Schachner, M. (1995b) Protein zero (P0)–deficient mice show myelin degeneration in peripheral nerves characteristic of inherited human neuropathies. *Nat. Genet.* 11:281–286.

Maurer, M., Kobsar, I., Berghoff, M., Schmid, C.D., Carenini, S., and Martini, R. (2002) Role of immune cells in animal models for inherited neuropathies: facts and visions. *J. Anat.* 200:405–414.

Miller, M.J., Haxhiu, M.A., Georgiadis, P., Gudz, T.I., Kangas, C.D., and Macklin, W.B. (2003) Proteolipid protein gene mutation induces altered ventilatory response to hypoxia in the myelin-deficient rat *J. Neurosci.* 23:2265–2273.

Molineaux, S.M., Engh, H., deFerra, F., Hudson, L., and Lazzarini, R.A. (1986) Recombination within the myelin basic protein gene created the dysmyelinating *shiverer* mouse mutation. *Proc. Natl. Acad. Sci. USA* 83:7542–7546.

Montag, D., Giese, K.P., Bartsch, U., Martini, R., Lang, Y., Bluthmann, H., Karthigasan, J., Kirschner, D.A., Wintergerst, E.S., Nave, K.-A., Zielasek, J., Toyka, K.V., Lipp, H.-P., and Schachner, M. (1994) Mice deficient for the myelin-associated glycoprotein show subtle abnormalities in myelin. *Neuron* 13:229–246.

Montague, P., Kirkham, D., McCallion, A.S., Davies, R.W., Kennedy, P.G., Klugmann, M., Nave, K.-A., and Griffiths, I.R. (1999) Reduced levels of a specific myelin-associated oligodendrocytic basic protein isoform in *shiverer* myelin. *Dev. Neurosci.* 21:36–42.

Morello, D., Dautigny, A., Pham-Dinh, D., and Jollès, P. (1986) Myelin proteolipid protein (PLP and DM-20) transcripts are deleted in *jimpy* mutant mice. *EMBO J.* 5:3489–3493.

Morita, K., Sasaki, H., Fujimoto, K., Furuse, M., and Tsukita, S. (1999) Claudin-11/OSP-based tight junctions of myelin sheaths in brain and Sertoli cells in testis. *J. Cell Biol.* 145:579–588.

Nadon, N.L., Duncan, I.D., and Hudson, L.D. (1990) A point mutation in the proteolipid protein gene of the 'shaking pup' interrupts oligodendrocyte development. *Development* 110:529–537.

Naef, R. and Suter, U. (1998) Many facets of the peripheral myelin protein PMP22 in myelination and disease. *Microsc. Res. Tech.* 41:359–371.

Nagarajan, R., Svaren, J., Le, N., Araki, T., Watson, M., and Milbrandt, J. (2001) EGR2 mutations in inherited neuropathies dominant-negatively inhibit myelin gene expression. *Neuron* 30:355–368.

Nave, K.-A., Bloom, F.E., and Milner, R.J. (1987) A single nucleotide difference in the gene for myelin proteolipid protein defines the *jimpy* mutation in mouse. *J. Neurochem.* 49:1873–1877.

Nave, K.-A. and Boespflug-Tanguy, O. (1996) Developmental defects of myelin formation: from X-linked mutations to human dysmyelinating diseases. *Neuroscientist* 2:33–43.

Nave, K.-A., Lai, C., Bloom, F.E., and Milner, R.J. (1986) *Jimpy* mutant mouse: a 74–base deletion in the mRNA for myelin proteolipid protein and evidence for a primary defect in RNA splicing. *Proc. Natl. Acad. Sci. USA* 83:9264–9268.

Niemann, S., Sereda, M.W., Suter, U., Griffiths, I.R., and Nave, K.-A. (2000) Uncoupling of myelin assembly and Schwann cell differentiation by transgenic overexpression of peripheral myelin protein 22. *J. Neurosci.* 20:4120–4128.

Notterpek, L., Roux, K.J., Amici, S.A., Yazdanpour, A., Rahner, C., and Fletcher, B.S. (2001) Peripheral myelin protein 22 is a constituent of intercellular junctions in epithelia. *Proc. Natl. Acad. Sci. USA* 98:14404–14409.

O'Connor, L.T., Goetz, B.D., Kwiecien, J.M., Delaney, K.H., Fletch, A.L., and Duncan, I.D. (1999) Insertion of a retrotransposon in Mbp disrupts mRNA splicing and myelination in a new mutant rat. *J. Neurosci.* 19:3404–3413.

Owens, G.C. and Boyd, C.J. (1991) Expression of antisense P0 RNA in Schwann cells perturbs myelination. *Development* 112:639–649.

Pearsall, G.B., Nadon, N.L., Wolf, M.K., and Billings-Gagliardi, S. (1997) *Jimpy-4J* mouse has a missense mutation in exon 2 of the *Plp* gene. *Dev. Neurosci.* 19:337–341.

Perea, J., Robertson, A., Tolmachova, T., Muddle, J., King, R.H., Ponsford, S., Thomas, P.K., and Huxley, C. (2001) Induced myelination and demyelination in a conditional mouse model of Charcot-Marie-Tooth disease type 1A. *Hum. Mol. Genet.* 10:1007–1018.

Popko, B., Puckett, C., and Hood, L. (1988) A novel mutation in *myelin-deficient* mice results in unstable myelin basic protein gene transcripts. *Neuron* 1:221–225.

Popko, B., Puckett, C., Lai, E., Shine, H.D., Readhead, C., Takahashi, N., Hunt, S.W. III, Sidman, R.L., and Hood, L. (1987) *Myelin deficient* mice: expression of myelin basic protein and generation of mice with varying levels of myelin. *Cell* 48:713–721.

Previtali, S.C., Feltri, M.L., Archelos, J.J., Quattrini, A., Wrabetz, L., and Hartung, H. (2001) Role of integrins in the peripheral nervous system. *Prog. Neurobiol.* 64:35–49.

Privat, A., Jaque, C., Bourre, J.M., Dupouye, P., and Baumann, N. (1979) Absence of the major dense line in myelin of the mutant mouse *'shiverer'*. *Neurosci. Lett.* 12:107–112.

Readhead, C., Popko, B., Takahashi, N., Shine, H.D., Saavedra, R.A., Sidman, R.L., and Hood, L. (1987) Expression of a myelin basic protein gene in transgenic *shiverer* mice: correction of the dysmyelinating phenotype. *Cell* 48:703–712.

Readhead, C., Schneider, A., Griffiths, I., and Nave, K.A. (1994) Premature arrest of myelin formation in transgenic mice with increased proteolipid protein gene dosage. *Neuron* 12:583–595.

Roach, A., Boylan, K., Horvath, S., Prusiner, S.B., and Hood, L.E. (1983) Characterization of cloned cDNA representing rat myelin basic protein: absence of expression in brain of *shiverer* mutant mice. *Cell* 34:799–806.

Roach, A., Takahashi, N., Pravtcheva, D., Ruddle, F., and Hood, L. (1985) Chromosomal mapping of mouse myelin basic protein gene and structure and transcription of the partially deleted gene in *shiverer* mutant mice. *Cell* 42:149–155.

Rosenbluth, J. (1980) Central myelin in the mouse mutant *shiverer*. *J. Comp. Neurol.* 194:639–648.

Rosenbluth, J., Stoffel, W., and Schiff, R. (1996) Myelin structure in proteolipid protein (PLP)-null mouse spinal cord. *J. Comp. Neurol.* 371:336–344.

Sadahiro, S., Yoshikawa, H., Yagi, N., Yamamoto, Y., Yanagihara, T., Kimura, M., and Sakoda, S. (2000) Morphometric analysis of the myelin-associated oligodendrocytic basic protein–deficient mouse reveals a possible role for myelin-associated oligodendrocytic basic protein in regulating axonal diameter. *Neuroscience* 98:361–367.

Sanchez, I., Hassinger, L., Sihag, R.K., Cleveland, D.W., Mohan, P., and Nixon, R.A. (2000) Local control of neurofilament accumulation during radial growth of myelinating axons in vivo. Selective role of site-specific phosphorylation. *J. Cell Biol.* 151:1013–1024.

Sancho, S., Magyar, J.P., Aguzzi, A., and Suter, U. (1999) Distal axonopathy in peripheral nerves of PMP22-mutant mice. *Brain* 122:1563–1577.

Sancho, S., Young, P., and Suter, U. (2001) Regulation of Schwann cell proliferation and apoptosis in PMP22-deficient mice and mouse models of Charcot-Marie-Tooth type 1A. *Brain* 124:2177–2187.

Schachner, M. and Bartsch, U. (2000) Multiple functions of the myelin-associated glycoprotein MAG (siglec-4a) in formation and maintenance of myelin. *Glia* 29:154–165.

Scherer, S.S., Xu, Y.T., Bannerman, P.G., Sherman, D.L., and Brophy, P.J. (1995) Periaxin expression in myelinating Schwann cells: modulation by axon-glial interactions and polarized localization during development. *Development* 121:4265–4273.

Schneider, A., Montague, P., Griffiths, I.R., Fanarraga, M., Kennedy, P., Brophy, P., and Nave, K.-A. (1992) Uncoupling of hypomyelination and glial cell death by a mutation in the proteolipid protein gene. *Nature* 358:758–761.

Schneider, A.M., Griffiths, I.R., Readhead, C., and Nave, K.-A. (1995) Dominant-negative action of the *jimpy* mutation in mice complemented with an autosomal transgene for myelin proteolipid protein. *Proc. Natl. Acad. Sci. USA* 92:4447–4451.

Sereda, M.W., Griffiths, I., Puhlhofer, A., Stewart, H., Rossner, M.J., Zimmerman, F., Magyar, J.P., Schneider, A., Hund, E., Meinck, H.M., Suter, U., and Nave, K.-A. (1996) A transgenic rat model of Charcot-Marie-Tooth disease. *Neuron* 16:1049–1060.

Sereda, M.W., Meyer zu Hörste, G., Suter, U., Uzma, N., and Nave, K.-A. (2003). Therapeutic administration of anti-progesterone in a transgenic model of Charcot-Marie-Tooth disease (CMT-1A). *Nat. Med.* 9:1533–1537.

Shapiro, L., Doyle, J.P., Hensley, P., Colman, D.R., and Hendrickson, W.A. (1996) Crystal structure of the extracellular domain from P0, the major structural protein of peripheral nerve myelin. *Neuron* 17:435–449.

Sherman, D.L., Fabrizi, C., Gillespie, C.S., and Brophy, P.J. (2001) Specific disruption of a Schwann cell dystrophin–related protein complex in a demyelinating neuropathy. *Neuron* 30:677–687.

Shine, H.D., Readhead, C., Popko, B., Hood, L., and Sidman, R.L. (1990) Myelin basic protein and myelinogenesis: morphometric analysis of normal, mutant and transgenic central nervous system. *Prog. Clin. Biol. Res.* 336:81–92.

Sidman, R.L., Dickie, M.M., and Appel, S.H. (1964) Mutant mice (*quaking* and *jimpy*) with deficient myelination in the central nervous system. *Science* 144:309–311.

Sidman, R.L. (1965) *Catalog of the Neurological Mutants of the Mouse*. Cambridge, MA: Harvard University Press.

Simons, M., Kramer, E.M., Macchi, P., Rathke-Hartlieb, S., Trotter, J., Nave, K.-A., and Schulz, J.B. (2002) Overexpression of the myelin proteolipid protein leads to accumulation of cholesterol and proteolipid protein in endosomes/lysosomes: implications for Pelizaeus-Merzbacher disease. *J. Cell Biol.* 157:327–336.

Skoff, R.P. (1982) Increased proliferation of oligodendrocytes in the hypomyelinated mouse mutant-*jimpy*. *Brain Res.* 248:19–31.

Skoff, R.P. (1995) Programmed cell death in the dysmyelinating mutants. *Brain Pathol.* 5:283–288.

Southwood, C.M., Garbern, J., Jiang, W., and Gow, A. (2002) The unfolded protein response modulates disease severity in Pelizaeus-Merzbacher disease. *Neuron* 36:585–596.

Southwood C.M. and Gow, A. (2001) Molecular pathways of oligodendrocyte apoptosis revealed by mutations in the proteolipid protein gene. *Microsc. Res. Tech.* 52:700–708.

Sporkel, O., Uschkureit, T., Bussow, H., and Stoffel, W. (2002) Oligodendrocytes expressing exclusively the DM20 isoform of the proteolipid protein gene: myelination and development. *Glia* 37:19–30.

Sprinkle, T.J. (1989) 2′,3′-Cyclic nucleotide 3′-phosphodiesterase, an oligodendrocyte-Schwann cell and myelin-associated enzyme of the nervous system. *Crit. Rev. Neurobiol.* 4:235–301.

Stecca, B., Southwood, C.M., Gragerov, A., Kelley, K.A., Friedrich, V.L., and Gow, A. (2000) The evolution of lipophilin genes from invertebrates to tetrapods: DM-20 cannot replace proteolipid protein in CNS myelin. *J. Neurosci.* 20:4002–4010.

Stolt, C.C., Rehberg, S., Ader, M., Lommes, P., Riethmacher, D., Schachner, M., Bartsch, U., and Wegner, M. (2002) Terminal differentiation of myelin-forming oligodendrocytes depends on the transcription factor Sox10. *Genes Dev.* 16:165–170.

Suh, J.G., Ichihara, N., Saigoh, K., Nakabayashi, O., Yamanishi, T., Tanaka, K., Wada, K., and Kikuchi, T. (1997) An in-frame deletion in peripheral myelin protein-22 gene causes hypomyelination and cell death of the Schwann cells in the new *trembler* mutant. *Neuroscience* 79:735–744.

Suter, U., Moskow, J.J., Welcher, A.A., Snipes, G.J., Kosaras, B., Sidman, R.L., Buchberg, A.M., and Shooter, E.M. (1992b) A leucine-to-proline mutation in the putative first transmembrane domain of the 22-kDa peripheral myelin protein in the *trembler-J* mouse. *Proc. Natl. Acad. Sci. USA* 89:4382–4386.

Suter, U. and Nave, K.-A. (1999) Transgenic mouse models of CMT1A and HNPP. *Ann. N.Y. Acad. Sci.* 883:247–253.

Suter, U., Welcher, A.A., Özcelik, T., Snipes, G.J., Kosaras, B., Francke, U., Billings-Gagliardi, S., Sidman, R.L., and Shooter, E.M. (1992a) *Trembler* mouse carries a point mutation in a myelin gene. *Nature* 356:241–244.

Thomson, C.E., Anderson, T.J., McCulloch, M.C., Dickinson, P., Vouyiouklis, D.A., and Griffiths, I.R. (1999) The early phenotype associated with the *jimpy* mutation of the proteolipid protein gene. *J. Neurocytol.* 28:207–221.

Tiwari-Woodruff, S.K., Buznikov, A.G., Vu, T.Q., Micevych, P.E., Chen, K., Kornblum, H.I., and Bronstein, J.M. (2001) OSP/claudin-11 forms a complex with a novel member of the tetraspanin super family and beta1 integrin and regulates proliferation and migration of oligodendrocytes. *J. Cell Biol.* 153:295–305.

Topilko, P., Schneider-Maunoury, S., Levi, G., Baron-Van Evercooren, A., Chennoufi, A.B., Seitanidou, T., Babinet, C., and Charnay, P. (1994) Krox-20 controls myelination in the peripheral nervous system. *Nature* 371:796–799.

Tosic, M., Roach, A., de Rivaz, J.-C., Dolivo, M., and Matthieu,

J.-M. (1990) Post-transcriptional events are responsible for low expression of myelin basic protein in myelin deficient mice: role of natural antisense RNA. *EMBO J.* 9:401–406.

Wang, H., Allen, M.L., Grigg, J.J., Noebels, J.L., and Tempel, B.L. (1995) Hypomyelination alters K^+ channel expression in mouse mutants *shiverer* and *Trembler. Neuron* 15:1337–1347.

Warner, L.E., Hilz, M.J., Appel, S.H., Killian, J.M., Kolodry, E.H., Karpati, G., Carpenter, S., Watters, G.V., Wheeler, C., Witt, D., Bodell, A., Nelis, E., Van Broeckhoven, C., and Lupski, J.R. (1996) Clinical phenotypes of different MPZ (P0) mutations may include Charcot-Marie-Tooth type 1B, Dejerine-Sottas, and congenital hypomyelination. *Neuron* 17:451–460.

Warner, L.E., Mancias, P., Butler, I.J., McDonald, C.M., Keppen, L., Koob, K.G., and Lupski, J.R. (1998) Mutations in the early growth response 2 (*EGR2*) gene are associated with hereditary myelinopathies. *Nat. Genet.* 18:382–384.

Woodward, K. and Malcolm, S. (1999) Proteolipid protein gene: Pelizaeus-Merzbacher disease in humans and neurodegeneration in mice. *Trends Genet.* 15:125–128.

Wrabetz, L., Feltri, M.L., Quattrini, A., Imperiale, D., Previtali, S., D'Antonio, M., Martini, R., Yin, X., Trapp, B.D., Zhou, L., Chiu, S.Y., and Messing, A. (2000) P(0) glycoprotein overexpression causes congenital hypomyelination of peripheral nerves. *J Cell Biol.* 148:1021–1034.

Xu, W., Shy, M., Kamholz, J., Elferink, L., Xu, G., Lilien, J., and Balsamo, J. (2000) Mutations in the cytoplasmic domain of P0 reveal a role for PKC-mediated phosphorylation in adhesion and myelination. *J. Cell Biol.* 155:439–446.

Yamamoto, Y., Mizuno, R., Nishimura, T., Ogawa, Y., Yoshikawa, H., Fujimura, H., Adachi, E., Kishimoto, T., Yanagihara, T., and Sakoda, S. (1994) Cloning and expression of myelin-associated oligodendrocytic basic protein. A novel basic protein constituting the central nervous system myelin. *J. Biol. Chem.* 269:31725–31730.

Yamamoto, Y., Yoshikawa, H., Nagano, S., Kondoh, G., Sadahiro, S., Gotow, T., Yanagihara, T., and Sakoda, S. (1999) Myelin-associated oligodendrocytic basic protein is essential for normal arrangement of the radial component in central nervous system *Eur. J. Neurosci.* 11:847–855.

Yin, X., Crawford, T.O., Griffin, J.W., Tu, P., Lee, V.M., Li, C., Roder, J., and Trapp, B.D. (1998) Myelin-associated glycoprotein is a myelin signal that modulates the caliber of myelinated axons *J. Neurosci.* 18:1953–1962.

Yin, X., Kidd, G.J., Wrabetz, L., Feltri, M.L., Messing, A., and Trapp, B.D. (2000) Schwann cell myelination requires timely and precise targeting of P(0) protein. *J. Cell Biol.* 148:1009–1020.

Yool, D., Montague, P., McLaughlin, M., McCulloch, M.C., Edgar, J.M., Nave, K.-A., Davies, R.W., Griffiths, I.R., and McCallion, A.S. (2002) Phenotypic analysis of mice deficient in the major myelin protein MOBP, and evidence for a novel Mobp isoform. *Glia* 39:256–267.

Yum, S.W., Kleopa, K.A., Shumas, S., and Scherer, S.S. (2002) Diverse trafficking abnormalities of connexin32 mutants causing CMTX. *Neurobiol. Dis.* 11:43–52.

44 Astrocytic swelling in neuropathology

ALEXANDER A. MONGIN AND
HAROLD K. KIMELBERG

Brain edema is a dangerous and frequently life-threatening neurological complication. Unlike other tissues, the brain is encased within a rigid skull, and even small increases in tissue volume produce significant rises in intracranial pressure, causing compression of neural tissue and blood vessels leading to brain tissue damage mostly due to blood flow reduction. Brain edema can be broadly classified into two categories: vasogenic edema and cytotoxic (or cellular) edema (Klatzo, 1967; Kimelberg, 1995). Vasogenic edema develops upon disruption of blood–brain barrier integrity, leading to accumulation of blood components in the brain and net influx of water. In contrast, cytotoxic (or cellular) edema develops as a shift of extracellular water into intracellular compartments, without any necessary increase in total brain volume. These two types of edema are not mutually exclusive and frequently coexist in pathologies, with cellular edema typically preceding vasogenic edema. In this chapter we concentrate on the phenomenon of cellular edema, its molecular mechanisms and potential significance in several major neurological disorders. In any discussion of cellular edema, astrocytes immediately emerge into the spotlight because this cell type shows the most prominent swelling in pathological postmortem samples both in humans and in animals (Kimelberg, 1995, 2000). For example, brain trauma (Barron et al., 1988; Dietrich et al., 1994) and ischemia (Jenkins et al., 1979; Garcia et al., 1993) cause large increases in the area of astrocytic profiles, as seen in electron micrographs, with the most prominent swelling occurring in the astrocytic endfeet, which surround blood vessels and form the glia limitans. Several techniques—such as measurements of electrical impedance between two electrodes inserted in exposed brain using alternating current, measurements of extracellular tetramethyl ammonium (TMA^+) by ion-selective electrodes, and magnetic resonance imaging (MRI) measurements of the apparent diffusion coefficient (ADC) of water—allow indirect invasive or noninvasive assessments of the extracellular space *in vivo* (Van Harenveld, 1966; Sykova et al., 1994; van der Toorn et al., 1996). Although these techniques cannot determine which cell types are swollen, there is a very good correlation between the time course of extracellular space reduction, monitored as ADC changes, and astrocytic swelling, as measured in perfusion-fixed brain sections (Liu et al., 2001). We have just begun to understand why astrocytes are so prone to pathological swelling and what mechanisms underlie this phenomenon.

MOLECULAR MECHANISMS OF ASTROCYTE SWELLING

Pathological astrocytic swelling *in vivo* is likely to be a result of the interrelated actions of numerous factors, which, in turn, vary depending on the pathology. Some of these processes are universal and can be found in all cell types, such as hypoosmotic and Donnan swelling, while others are somewhat unique to astrocytes and relevant to their specialized functions in the brain, such as swelling associated with glutamate uptake. Like the majority of mammalian cells, astrocytes *in vitro* effectively regulate their volume when subjected to hypoosmotic swelling. However, under pathological conditions, cell volume regulation appears to be partially or completely suppressed. Therefore, it is important to recognize not only the factors promoting cell swelling but also those preventing effective cell volume recovery. In this section, we describe several of the most common proposed mechanisms of astrocyte swelling. Their potential significance under particular pathological conditions is discussed in the section "Astrocytic Swelling in Pathology." All the mechanisms discussed below are presented in Figure 44.1.

Changes in Osmolarity of Extracellular Fluid

A decrease in extracellular fluid osmolarity is the simplest cause of cell swelling (Fig. 44.1*A*). Although hypoosmotic media are frequently employed in *in vitro* experiments, significant osmolarity perturbations are rarely seen in the brain. Rapid hypoosmotic medium–induced

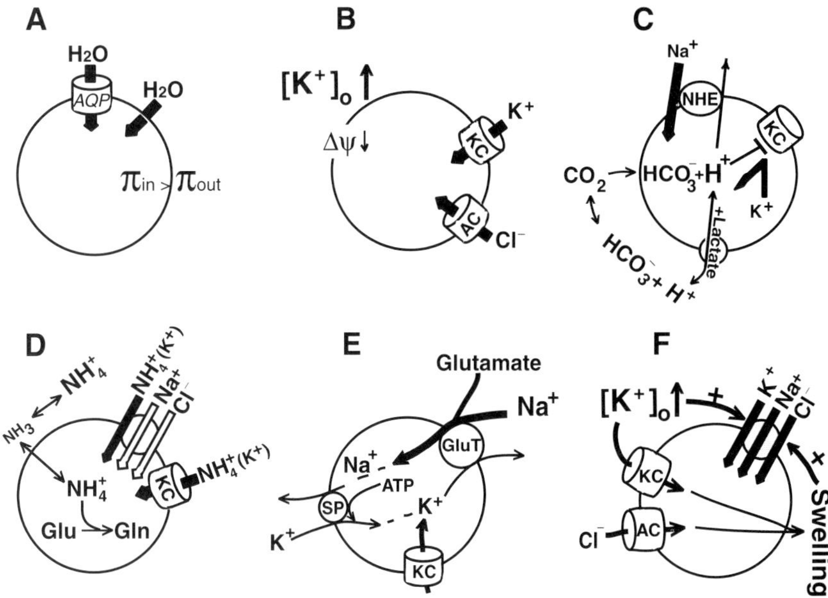

FIGURE 44.1 Molecular and cellular mechanisms of astrocyte swelling. *A.* Decrease in medium osmolarity causes cell swelling due to osmotic water influx. Water diffuses across the membrane via aquaporin water channels (*AQP*) or directly via the lipid bilayer. *B.* Elevation of the extracellular K^+ concentration causes cell swelling by a Donnan mechanism. Depolarization of cell membranes creates the inward-directed driving force for Cl^- entering the cell via anion channels (*AC*). The Cl^- influx allows for K^+ accumulation via K^+ channels (*KC*). *C.* Acidification causes swelling via several mechanisms: (*1*) Cytoplasmic acidosis activates the Na^+/H^+ exchanger (*NHE*), causing intracellular Na^+ accumulation. Combination of CO_2 diffusion and its hydration to $H^+ + HCO_3^-$ replenishes the intracellular H^+ pool and promotes osmotically significant Na^+ loading together with Cl^- accumulation due to the $Cl^-_o/HCO_3^-{}_i$ exchange (for a detailed explanation see Kimelberg and Feustel, 1998). H^+ is also shuttled across the membrane by lactate/H^+ transporters. (*2*) Cytoplasmic acidosis will also inhibit K^+ channels (*KC*), causing K^+ accumulation and preventing effective volume recovery. *D.* Ammonia enters the cell on the $Na^+,NH_4^+(K^+),2Cl^-$ cotransporter and through K^+ channels (*KC*), as well as diffusing across the membrane as nonionized NH_3. In the cell, ammonia is accumulated as glutamine (*Gln*) due to the action of glutamine synthase. Glu: glutamate. *E.* Glutamate-induced cell swelling is due to Na^+/glutamate uptake by astrocytic glutamate transporters (*GluT*). The activity of K^+ channels and of the Na^+,K^+ pump appears necessary for this type of swelling likely to replenish countertransported intracellular K^+. ATP: adenosine triphosphate; SP: Na^+,K^+ pump. *F.* The $Na^+,K^+,2Cl^-$ cotransporter may contribute to the cytoplasmic osmotic load because its activity is under positive control of extracellular K^+ and cell volume. AC: anion channels.

cell swelling is typically followed by effective cell volume regulation by a process termed *regulatory volume decrease* (RVD). In astrocytes, RVD is mediated by activation of volume-sensitive potassium and chloride/anion channels, releasing excess osmolytes from cytoplasm down their electrochemical gradients (Pasantes-Morales et al., 1994a; Vitarella et al., 1994; Lang et al., 1998). Water passively accompanies osmolyte movement across the plasma membrane during RVD. Water transport is accelerated by a class of specialized water channels called *aquaporins* (Verkman and Mitra, 2000). In the majority of mammalian cells, plasma membranes have significant water permeability; therefore, aquaporin expression is though to be rate-limiting for fast water transport such as occurs in epithelia. Astrocytes express aquaporins-4 and -9 (Venero et al., 2001). Although the physiological role of astrocytic aquaporins is not yet clear, Manley et al. (2000) have recently reported that genetic deletion of aquaporin-4 significantly reduces astrocyte swelling and brain edema in water-intoxicated animals and animals subjected to focal ischemic stroke (Fig. 44.2).

Donnan Cell Swelling

The high intracellular concentration of impermeant organic molecules (amino acids, nucleic acids, carbohydrates, high and low molecular weight proteins, etc.) generates significant osmotic force between extracellular and intracellular compartments, a process known as the *Donnan effect*. To compensate for the accumulation of water caused by the presence of organic osmolytes, cells pump out inorganic ions, predominantly Na^+ and Cl^-. Na^+ ions are extruded by the Na^+,K^+

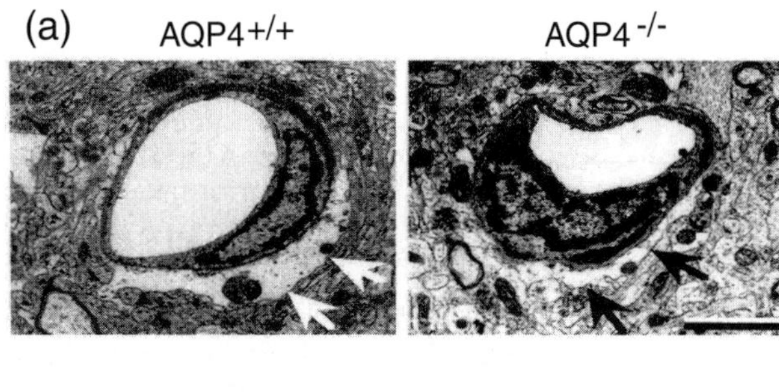

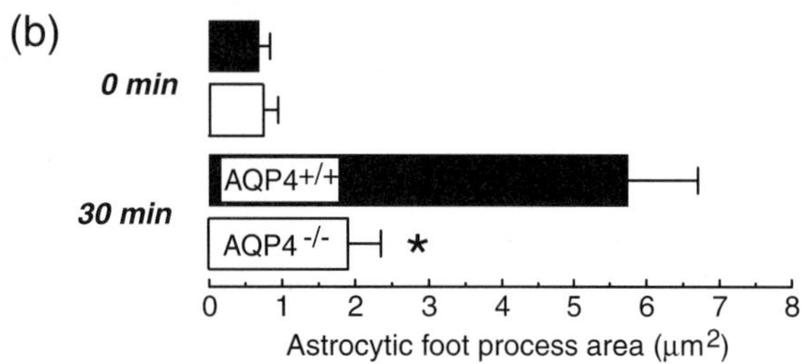

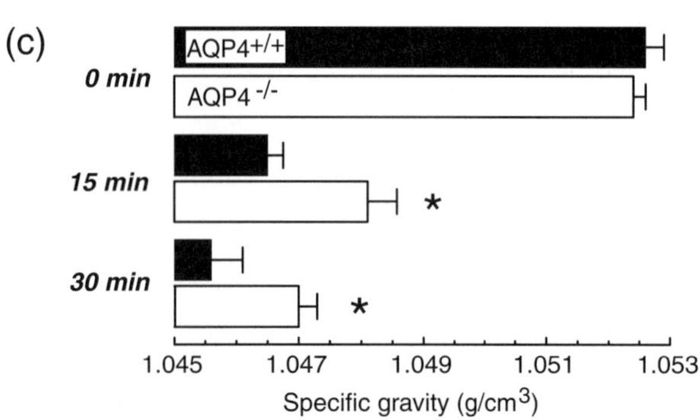

FIGURE 44.2 Contribution of aquaporin-4 (*AQP-4*) channels to perivascular astrocytic swelling in mouse brain. *a.* Electron micrograph showing profound perivascular astrocytic endfoot swelling in water-intoxicated wild-type animals (*left, white arrows*) and its reduction in animals with genetic deletion of AQP-4 (*right, black arrows*). *b.* Quantification of the perivascular astrocytic foot area before and after water intoxication in wild-type and AQP-4 knockout animals. *c.* Changes in specific gravity (a decrease represents a gain of water or brain edema) of brain tissue in wild-type and AQP-4 knockout animals subjected to water intoxication. Edema is reduced in AQP-4 knockout animals. (Data are reproduced from Manley et al., 2000, with permission of the Nature Publishing Group.)

pump (3 Na^+ out in exchange for 2 K^+ in), directly using the energy of adenosine triphosphate (ATP). The higher membrane permeability for K^+ over Na^+ results in a cytoplasmic K^+ leak and, with the electrogenic work of the Na^+,K^+ pump, creates a large negative (inside relative to outside) electric potential across the plasma membrane. This negative membrane potential passively drives Cl^- out of the cell. According to the double-Donnan hypothesis, the resulting asymmetric steady-state distribution of inorganic and organic ions, set by the Na^+,K^+ pump and the membrane potential, accommodates for the presence of impermeable anionic compounds in cytoplasm (Macknight and Leaf, 1977; Lang et al., 1998). In pathological states associated with energy depletion, inhibition of the Na^+,K^+ pump causes slow depolarization and excess Na^+ accumulation over K^+ loss inside the cell. This is accompanied by net Cl^- influx and osmotically obligated water movement, resulting in cell swelling (Macknight and Leaf, 1977). Depolarization of the astrocyte plasma membrane by high extracellular K^+ increases the inward-directed driving force for passive movement of Cl^-, accompanied by K^+ (Fig. 44.1*B*). *In vitro*, exposure of cultured astrocytes to high $[K^+]_o$ causes slow, persistent cell swelling (O'Connor et al., 1993; Rutledge et al., 1998). Since a transmembrane $[K^+]$ gradient is a prerequisite for RVD (Lang et al., 1998), cell volume regulation is suppressed under these conditions.

Acidosis and Ion Exchangers

As in most mammalian cells, regulation of intracellular pH in astrocytes involves the Na^+/H^+ and Cl^-/HCO_3^- exchangers and the electrogenic Na^+-HCO_3^- cotransporter (see Deitmer, 1995, and references therein). Activation of the Na^+/H^+ exchanger and the Na^+-HCO_3^- cotransporter causes changes in cell volume and has been linked to cell swelling in several pathologies. In ischemia/hypoxia, acidification of the cytoplasm due to proton accumulation causes astroglial cell swelling predominantly via activation of Na^+/H^+ and Cl^-/HCO_3^- exchangers (Jakubovicz et al., 1987; Kempski et al., 1988; Staub et al., 1990; Kraig and Chesler, 1990) (Fig. 44.1C). It should be stressed, however, that the Na^+/H^+ exchanger is completely inhibited at $pH_o < 6.0$, and therefore severe acidosis excludes this mechanism of cell swelling (Jakubovicz et al., 1987). Alternatively, profound extra/intracellular acidosis may cause cell swelling because of cytoplasmic solute accumulation due to inhibition of glial K^+ channels and consequent decreases in the K^+ leak (Waltz and Wuttke, 1989; Strupp et al., 1993). Intracellular acidosis potently inhibits RVD, probably due to inhibition of K^+ channels but perhaps via other unidentified mechanisms (Strupp et al., 1993; Smets et al., 2002) (Fig. 44.1C). This may contribute to persistent astrocytic swelling in ischemia and hypoxia.

Ammonia

Astrocytic swelling is a major feature of hepatic encephalopathy (Norenberg, 1977) and correlates with the plasma levels of ammonia (Swain et al., 1992). *In vitro*, ammonia induces long-lasting astrocyte swelling (Norenberg et al., 1991; Norenberg, 1995). Several *in vitro* and *in vivo* studies suggest that major causes of cell swelling are changes in glutamate metabolism and accumulation of glutamine and the product of its transamination, alanine (Swain et al., 1992; Willard-

Mack et al., 1996). Another potential reason for ammonia-induced astrocyte swelling is net NH_4^+ uptake and cytoplasm acidification followed by Na^+/H^+ exchanger activation (Nagaraja and Brookes, 1998). NH_3 freely diffuses across the plasma membrane. However, at physiological and pathological pH, practically all extracellular ammonia is in the form of NH_4^+ and it is transported into the cytosol via K^+ channels and the $Na^+,K^+(NH_4^+),2Cl^-$ cotransporter (Nagaraja and Brookes, 1998, Marcaggi and Coles, 2001) (Fig. 44.1*D*).

Glutamate Uptake

Astrocytes express two astrocyte-specific high-affinity glutamate transporters, which are termed excitatory amino acid transporter-1 (EAAT1) and EAAT2 in humans and glutamate/asparate transporter (GLAST) and glutamate transporter-1 (GLT-1), respectively, in rodents (Danbolt, 2001, and references therein). These cells represent the main sites of glutamate uptake and metabolism in brain tissue (Martinez-Hernandez et al., 1977; Danbolt, 2001). Antisense oligonucleotide knockdown experiments confirm a major role for the astrocytic GLT-1 transporter in maintaining low extracellular glutamate levels in rat brain (Rothstein et al., 1996). *In vitro*, high extracellular glutamate causes progressive astrocyte swelling (Koyama et al., 1991; O'Connor et al., 1993). This swelling depends on extracellular K^+, Na^+, and Ca^{2+} (Bender et al., 1998; Koyama et al., 2000) (Fig. 44.1*E*). It should be noted, however, that the vast majority of the published *in vitro* experiments employ very high extracellular glutamate concentrations (0.5–1 mM), exceeding those expected even under pathological conditions *in vivo*. At ≤ 100 μM, glutamate produces no or only marginal cell swelling. Therefore, it is not clear to what degree extracellular glutamate directly contributes to astrocyte swelling *in vivo*. Excitotoxic glutamate effects on neurons can be achieved at much lower concentrations. Thus, glutamate-induced astrocyte swelling *in vivo* could be indirect and mediated by glutamate effects on neuronal cells, such as increases in $[K^+]_o$ promoted by massive neuronal depolarization.

$Na^+,K^+,2Cl^-$ Cotransporter

The potential contribution of the $Na^+,K^+,2Cl^-$ cotransporter to astrocyte swelling and associated brain pathologies has only recently been evaluated. In cultured astrocytes 50–75 mM extracellular K^+ both stimulates the $Na^+,K^+,2Cl^-$ cotransporter and causes cell swelling (Su et al., 2002b). Bumetanide, a specific inhibitor of the $Na^+,K^+,2Cl^-$ cotransporter, suppresses such high K^+-induced astrocyte swelling, intracellular ($K^+ + Cl^-$) accumulation, and excitatory amino acid (EAA) release in cultured cells (Su et al., 2002b). In good agreement with the pharmacological data, genetic deletion of the NKCC1 isoform of the $Na^+,K^+,2Cl^-$ cotransporter, which is the dominant isoform in the brain, attenuates high K^+-induced cell swelling, cytoplasmic K^+ and Cl^- accumulation, and, partially, EAA release (Su et al., 2002a). Moreover, intracerebral application of bumetanide via a microdialysis probe ameliorates brain damage and reduces brain edema in rat focal ischemia (Yan et al., 2001). The astrocytic $Na^+,K^+,2Cl^-$ cotransporter is strongly stimulated by cell swelling itself (Mongin et al., 1994); therefore, $Na^+,K^+,2Cl^-$ cotransport both promotes astroglial swelling and is under positive feedback for further increases in cell volume (Fig. 44.1*F*). A combination of these two processes may represent a feedforward cycle contributing to a worsening of brain cellular edema. In hepatic encephalopathy the $Na^+,K^+,2Cl^-$ cotransporter may contribute to cell swelling via mechanisms involving NH_4^+ uptake, cytoplasm acidification, and Na^+/H^+ exchange activation by $[H^+]_i$ (Nagaraja and Brookes, 1998).

Arachidonic Acid and Its Metabolites

Several pathological states, and ischemia in particular, cause a drastic increase in tissue levels of free arachidonic acid, which can reach 0.5 mM (Rehncrona et al., 1982). When added *in vitro* to brain slices, primary astrocyte cultures, or C6 glioma cells, arachidonic acid and structurally related polyunsaturated fatty acids induce cellular edema/cell swelling in a dose-dependent manner (Chan and Fishman, 1978, 1982; Staub et al., 1994). Arachidonic acid–induced cell swelling probably involves multiple mechanisms, including inhibition of mitochondrial function and ATP synthesis, mitochondrial free radical production, and inhibition of the Na^+,K^+ pump followed by intracellular accumulation of Na^+ (Chan and Fishman, 1982; Chan et al., 1988; Staub et al., 1994; Winkler et al., 2000). Cytoplasmic acidification causes secondary activation of the Na^+/H^+ exchanger, resulting in an increased cytoplasmic Na^+ load and cell swelling (Winkler et al., 2000). Inhibition of free radical production with superoxide dismutase, the Na^+/H^+ exchanger with amiloride, or the Na^+,K^+ pump with ouabain, significantly reduces arachidonic acid–induced swelling of C6 glioma cells (Winkler et al., 2000). Importantly, arachidonic acid and other structurally similar polyunsaturated fatty acids not only promote cell swelling but also potently inhibit RVD due to the direct block of the volume-regulated anion channels (Sanchez-Olea et al., 1995).

It should be stressed, however, that in the brain the effects of arachidonic acid are not limited to glial cells or cell swelling. Arachidonic acid potently perturbs neuronal metabolism, causing $[K^+]_o$ elevation and EAA release. It also causes opening of the blood–brain barrier due to its direct effects on endothelial cells (Chan and Fishman, 1984).

ASTROCYTIC SWELLING IN PATHOLOGY

This section briefly summarizes current knowledge of astrocytic swelling and possible mechanisms of such swelling in relation to particular central nervous system (CNS) pathologies.

Ischemia

There are numerous observations at the electron microscopic (EM) level of astrocytic swelling, particularly around blood vessels, within 30 minutes of initiation of middle cerebral artery occlusion during ischemia and for up to 24 hours after reperfusion (e.g., Garcia et al., 1993, 1994). Impedance measurements (Van Harreveld, 1966) and ion-selective electrodes registering the concentration of added extracellular TMA^+ (Lundbaek and Hansen, 1992; Sykova et al., 1994) show an average reduction in the extracellular space in animal models of ischemia from 20% of the total tissue volume to 10% but as low as 4%. Methods to assess cell swelling directly and noninvasively in human subjects are still not available. However, MRI techniques using isotropic diffusion-weighted, spin-echo sequences have allowed the measurements of the ADC of water in human subjects. This gives indirect information about the amount of extracellular water, which is assumed to have a larger ADC, and hence about the volume of the extracellular space (Van der Toorn et al., 1996; Neumann-Haefelin et al., 2000; Kucinski et al., 2002). Marked decreases in ADC, which occur rapidly after initiation of ischemia, correlate very well with changes in brain tomographic density in human patients (Kucinski et al, 2002) (Fig. 44.3) and with astrocytic swelling measured by EM in perfusion-fixed brain sections in animals (Liu et al., 2001).

Clearly, multiple mechanisms contribute to cell swelling. Practically all the factors mentioned in the previous section have been linked to the development of cellular edema *in situ*. We believe that the main reasons for astrocyte swelling include intracellular accumulation of electrolytes by the Donnan mechanism and via the $Na^+,K^+,2Cl^-$ cotransporter, in combination with a potent block of volume regulatory mechanisms by arachidonic acid and acidosis (see the section "Molecular Mechanisms of Astrocytic Swelling"). Consistent with this idea, the $Na^+,K^+,2Cl^-$ cotransporter inhibitor bumetanide, and the anion channel blocker L-644,711, which blocks Cl^- channels to decrease Donnan intracellular Cl^- accumulation, attenuate cellular edema and protect against tissue damage in animal models of ischemia (Kohut et al., 1992; Yan et al., 2001). In reperfusion, activation of the Na^+/H^+ exchanger by a cytoplasmic H^+ load, production of free radicals including products of arachidonic acid oxidation, and peroxynitrite may all additionally contribute to cell swelling (see the section "Molecular Mechanisms of Astrocytic Swelling").

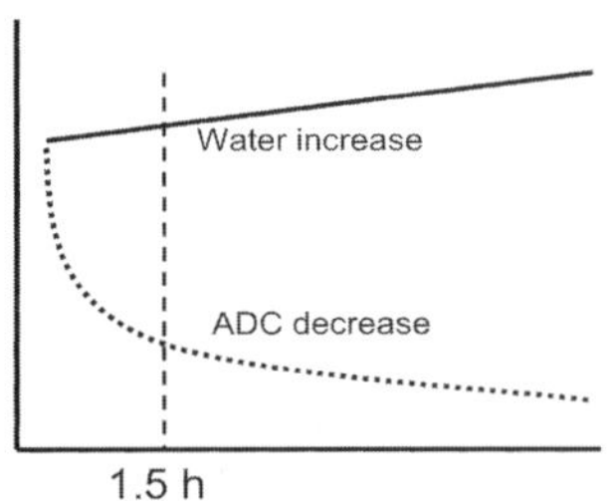

FIGURE 44.3 Schematic representation of idealized dynamic changes in the apparent diffusion coefficient (*ADC*) of water and tissue water content in human stroke. Human data before 1.5 hours are not available and are extrapolated from experimental findings in animals. Water content changes were determined based on cranial tomography and on the known linear correlation between computed tomography density and the specific gravity of tissues. (From Kucinski et al., 2002, with permission of the American Heart Association.)

A most intriguing question is, why are astrocytes so much more prone to pathological swelling than other neural cell types? Although we do not have a clear answer, studies performed over the past 10–15 years provide several important clues. Astrocytic functions in the normal brain include clearance of extracellular K^+ and glutamate, and since both substances are drastically elevated in ischemia, their uptake may cause *osmotic overload* in astrocytes and water influx into cytosol (Kimelberg, 2000). Astrocytic $Na^+,K^+,2Cl^-$ cotransporter activity is upregulated by both elevated $[K^+]_o$ and cell swelling; this phenomenon is not found in neurons (Mongin et al., 1994; Su et al., 2002a, 2002b). Astrocytes express high levels of the water channel aquaporin-4, and the genetic deletion of aquaporin-4 strongly reduces ischemia-induced brain edema, perivascular astrocytic swelling, and tissue damage in mice (Manley et al., 2000). This latter study is of particular interest. It suggests the significant contribution of aquaporin-4 to movement of water from blood vessels to the brain and from extracellular to intracellular compartments.

Traumatic Brain Injury

In a cat model of closed head injury, astrocytic swelling peaks at 30–40 minutes postinjury (Barron et al., 1988). Such swelling is also found in human head trauma, both in patients undergoing surgery and in postmortem samples, and persists for 3 hours to 3 days and probably later (Castejon, 1980; Bullock et al., 1991). A similar phenomenon has been found in humans and animals after spinal cord injury (Griffiths et al., 1978; Alessandri and Bullock, 1998). The swelling is most pronounced in perivascular astrocytic foot processes and may be a reason for compression of at least some capillaries as seen by EM (Bullock et al., 1991). Neuronal/dendritic swelling may also be seen at earlier but not later stages, preceding astrocytic edema (Mathew et al., 1996). Experimental models indicate that glutamate may be one of the key substances responsible for astrocyte swelling (Kimelberg et al., 1989; Maxwell et al., 1994). $K^+$and Cl^- uptake by the Donnan mechanism probably also contributes because chloride channels blockers prevent trauma-induced astrocytic swelling and tissue damage (Barron et al., 1988; Kimelberg et al., 1989). Typically, changes in cerebral blood flow due to brain trauma are not sufficient to induce ischemia (Mathew et al., 1996); therefore, the neuronal depolarization seen should have a nonischemic origin and may be due to spreading depression–like waves originating at the site of impact/contusion. Within hours after brain injury, changes in blood–brain barrier permeability are also seen in addition to pure cellular edema, and the damaged tissue begins to accumulate water by a vasogenic mechanism with the contribution of an inflammatory component (Mathew et al., 1994, 1996).

Hepatic Encephalopathy

Hepatic encephalopathy is a frequent neurological complication of acute or chronic liver disease (Norenberg, 1995; Blei and Larsen, 1999). Astrocytes are the only cell type showing morphological changes and are thought to play a key role in hepatic encephalopathy development (Norenberg, 1995; Haussinger et al., 2000). Acute liver failure causes brain edema and cerebral herniation, which are the main causes of the high morbidity associated with the disease. Astrocytes contribute a major portion of the cell swelling, which is proportional to the ammonia levels and in animal models can be prevented or reversed by L-methionine sulfoximine, the inhibitor of the astrocyte-specific enzyme glutamate synthetase (Blei et al., 1994; Blei and Larsen, 1999). Therefore, astrocytic swelling probably occurs due to organic osmolyte accumulation. In chronic liver failure, brain edema is absent or very mild (low-grade edema). However, astrocytic swelling also persists under chronic conditions and could contribute to the observed neurological deficits (Haussinger et al., 2000). Thus, ^{1}H-magnetic resonance spectroscopy (^{1}H-MRS) studies indicate disturbances in cell volume homeostasis and show significant changes in the content of glutamine/glutamate and the major cytoplasmic osmolyte, myo-inositol, in chronic liver dysfunction (reviewed in Haussinger et al., 2000). Interestingly, mild hypothermia (35°C) is effective in preventing brain edema and neurological deficits in animal acute liver failure despite persistent high ammonia levels (Rose et al., 2000). This finding has a good potential for clinical intervention.

Hyponatremia

Hyponatremia is defined as a pathological decrease in plasma sodium concentration, which becomes life-threatening after reaching a threshold value of approximately 120 mM. This is the condition most closely resembling hypoosmotic cell swelling *in vitro*, with the exception of its gradual development. Although hyponatremia typically originates in a misbalance in kidney electrolyte and water secretion/reuptake, the brain represents a main target organ, with brain edema being a key factor for the high morbidity. The most common causes of hyponatremia are postoperative complications (with an occurrence of about 1%), psychogenic polydipsia, congestive heart failure, complications of some pharmacological treatments, acquired immunodeficiency syndrome (AIDS), and several types of hormonal disorders including overproduction of antidiuretic hormone (ADH), glucocorticoid deficiency, and hypothyroidism (Fraser and Arieff, 1997). Theoretically, changes in extracellular osmolarity should cause cell swelling independent of cell type. However, swelling of astrocytes and neuronal dendrites is most pronounced compared to the neuronal soma (Johnson et al., 2000). The reasons for this are not completely understood and may include perivascular astrocyte localization, which is close to the source of the hyponatremic blood, combined with high aquaporin expression (Manley et al., 2000), as well as active astrocytic uptake of K^+ and neurotransmitters released by neurons (Kimelberg, 2000). Systemic hyponatremia causes an increase in aquaporin-4 immunoreactivity in perivascular astrocytic endfeet and glia limitans (Vajda et al., 2000).

Regulatory loss of electrolytes and organic osmolytes partially or completely compensates for osmotic gradients (Gullans and Verbalis, 1993; Pasantes-Morales et al., 2000). If the rate of adjustment is sufficient, patients do not show neurological deficits despite significant changes in plasma and brain osmolarity. Premenopausal women and children are at substantially higher risk of hyponatremic brain damage than either postmenopausal women or men of any age (Fraser and Arieff, 1997). This may be related to the inhibitory effects of both estrogen and progesterone on the brain's Na^+,K^+ pump (Fraser and Sarnaki, 1989; Fraser and Swanson, 1994) and on cell volume regulation (Fraser and Swanson, 1994). These data stress the significance of the Na^+,K^+ pump for slow osmoregulation and tissue adaptation to the changing osmolarity of extracellular fluid. The osmotic work of the Na^+,K^+ pump is complementary to the fast electrolyte/osmolyte loss via potassium and anion channels activated by cell swelling

(Gullans and Verbalis, 1993; Fraser and Arieff, 1997; Pasantes-Morales et al., 2000).

PATHOLOGICAL CONSEQUENCES OF ASTROCYTIC SWELLING

The previous section summarizes the substantial evidence for cellular edema of a predominantly astrocytic nature in various CNS pathologies. However the precise reasons that cell swelling is detrimental are not completely understood. Here we summarize current views on the pathological consequences of cellular (cytotoxic) edema and attempt to separate them from the detrimental effects of tissue swelling of a vasogenic etiology.

Compression of Blood Vessels

Ames et al. (1968) demonstrated some time ago that, after reversible global ischemia in rabbits, perfusion of blood vessels with carbon black resulted in incomplete filling of brain microvessels. They termed this the *no-reflow* phenomenon and considered it to be due to swelling of perivascular astrocytes constricting the vessels. No-reflow studies have been repeated for increasing times of reperfusion after focal cerebral ischemia using Evans blue to label reperfused vessels (Kuschinsky, 1997). The no-reflow phenomenon was found to depend on the duration and severity of ischemia. The issue of astrocytic swelling as the major or the only cause of the no-reflow or limited reperfusion has not been sufficiently tested. Endothelial cell swelling, thrombi formation, or vasoconstriction may also explain localized reductions in blood flow. Garcia and coworkers (1994) examined this question in a rat focal ischemia model, measuring vessel luminal diameters using injection of horseradish peroxidase just prior to sacrifice and correlating this with the increased size of astrocytic nuclei, which reflected the total astrocytic area, as measured by EM. The authors found a positive correlation between these two parameters within the first hour after occlusion, with resolution of astrocytic swelling after 48 to 72 hours.

Release of Excitatory Amino Acids

Regulatory volume decrease in astrocytes in response to swelling is predominantly due to coordinated activation of K^+ and anion channels (Pasantes-Morales et al., 1994a; Vitarella et al., 1994). Volume-regulated anion channels have relatively low selectivity and are permeable to small organic anions and uncharged molecules, including amino acids, polyols, and methylamines (Kimelberg et al., 1990, Pasantes-Morales et al., 1990, 1994b; reviewed in Kirk and Strange, 1998). In nonexcitable tissues, organic osmolyte efflux supplements Cl^- release during cell volume regulation (Kirk and Strange, 1998; Lang et al., 1998). Ironically, the same mechanism, which is designed to protect cells from swelling, probably damages brain tissue via volume-dependent release of EAAs (Kimelberg, 1995, 2000; Kimelberg and Mongin, 1998). In hypotonic media *in vitro* practically all the EAA release occurs due to activation of volume-regulated anion channels, and the time course and rate of such release mirror the time course of cell volume normalization (Vitarella et al., 1994; Rutledge et al., 1998). In contrast, application of isoosmotic high $[K^+]$ media, which resembles more closely pathological conditions *in vivo*, activates a two-phase EAA release. The first phase of the high K^+-induced EAA release occurs immediately, depends on $[K^+]_o$ and $[Na^+]_i$, and is mediated by the reversal of sodium/potassium-dependent glutamate transporters (Szatkowski and Attwell, 1994; Rutledge and Kimelberg, 1996). A second phase of the high K^+-induced EAA efflux develops more slowly and persists throughout the duration of exposure to elevated $[K^+]_o$ (Rutledge and Kimelberg, 1996; Rutledge et al., 1998). This second phase is due to the Donnan-type cell swelling and activation of the swelling-regulated anion channels. The contribution of volume-regulated anion channels to pathological EAA release *in vivo* has been recently confirmed in animal models and *in situ* preparations (Phillis et al., 1997; Basarsky et al., 1999; Seki et al., 1999) (Fig. 44.4). Although it is impossible to discriminate the cell types mediating such release *in vivo*, the evidence reviewed in this chapter strongly suggests that astrocytes are likely to be major players.

Volume-dependent EAA release may contribute to neural toxicity in all neurological disorders associated with cell swelling. Notably, several compounds that prevent astrocytic swelling and/or swelling-activated EAA release *in vitro* have been shown to provide remarkable neuroprotection in animal models of hyponatremia, brain trauma, and ischemia (Barron et al., 1988; Trachtman and Cragoe, 1989; Kohut et al., 1992; Kimelberg et al., 2000). This points to a considerable potential of anion channel blockers for clinical use. Moreover, moderate hypothermia prevents development of brain edema and neurological deficits in human ischemia, trauma, and hepatic encephalopathy and also blocks astrocytic high K^+-induced swelling and EAA release (Welsh et al., 1990; Clifton et al., 1991; Kimelberg et al., 1995; Rose et al., 2000). It should be stressed, however, that more *in vivo* studies are needed to establish a casual link between the neuroprotective effects of anion channel blockers and *in vivo* inhibition of EAA release. Two important facts should be taken into consideration when interpreting *in vivo* data. First, both volume-regulated anion chan-

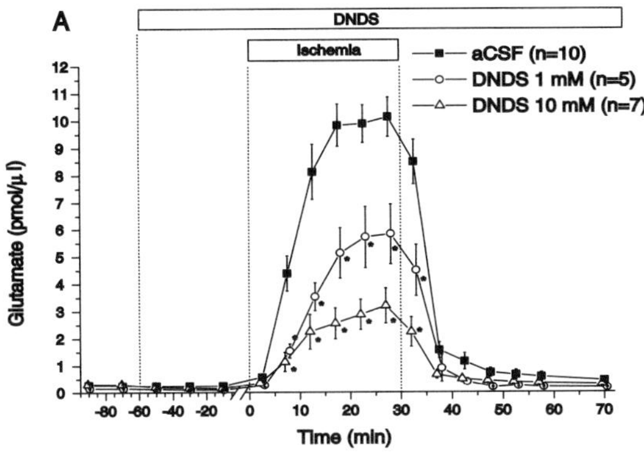

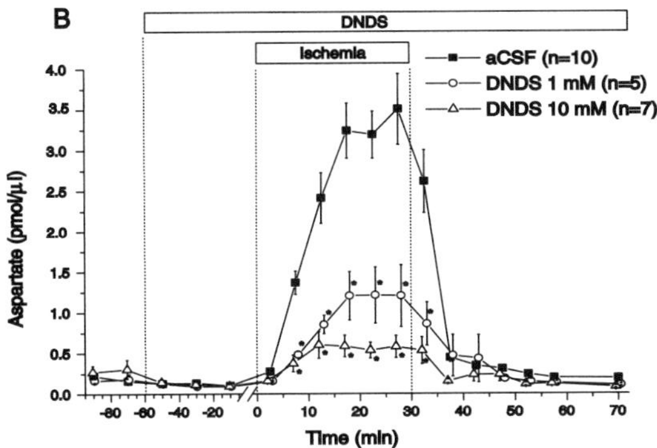

FIGURE 44.4 The anion channel blocker 4-4′-dinitrostilbene-2,2′-disulfonic acid (*DNDS*) decreases the elevation in extracellular glutamate (*A*) and aspartate (*B*) levels in the rat brain seen during ischemia. Glutamate and aspartate levels were measured in a global ischemia model with microdialysis probes placed in the striatum. One or 10 mM DNDS was perfused through the probe 60 minutes before and throughout the duration of the ischemic episode. This markedly reduced the rise in extracellular excitatory amino acid levels compared to control levels (perfusion of artificial cerebrospinal fluid, *aCSF*). Note that DNDS will be diluted outside of the probe as low as 1:10. (From Seki et al., 1999, with permission of the American Heart Association.)

nel activation and channel-mediated EAA release are strictly dependent on the intracellular ATP concentration (Jackson et al., 1994; Rutledge et al., 1999). Therefore, in the infarction core, where all intracellular ATP is depleted, the contribution of anion channels may be less or negligible. In contrast, in the ischemic penumbra, ATP levels remain as high as 50%–70% of normal tissue content; therefore, in this area, anion channels may mediate a significant portion of pathological EAA release. Another issue to be considered is the massive pathological release of neurotransmitters from depolarized and damaged neural cells. We have found that ATP, adenosine, and the nitric oxide product, peroxynitrite, greatly potentiate volume-dependent anion channels in swollen and, under some circumstances, nonswollen primary astrocyte cultures (Mongin and Kimelberg, 2002; Haskew et al., 2002) (Fig. 44.5). In pathology, such upregulation of the volume-regulated anion channels may strongly increase glutamate release from swollen, moderately swollen, or even nonswollen neural cells.

Effects of Changes in the Extracellular Milieu

The extracellular space (ECS) normally occupies 15%–25% of the brain volume and serves as a communication channel between neural cells, as described in the *volume transmission* concept (Sykova, 1997). The composition of the ECS, which includes inorganic ions, nutrients, metabolites, neurotransmitters, neuromodulators, and extracellular matrix macromolecules, dynamically changes during neuronal activity and is un-

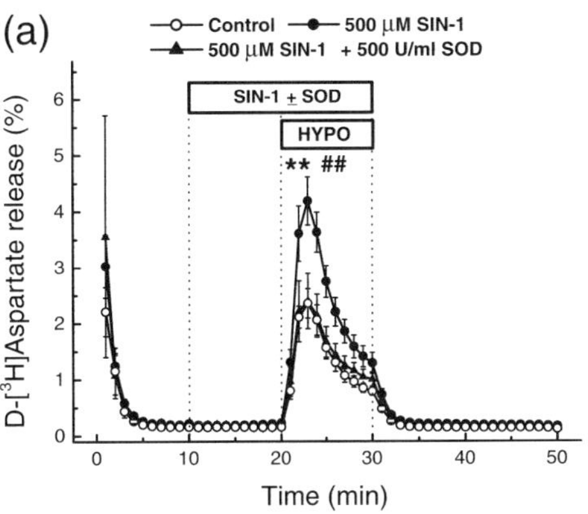

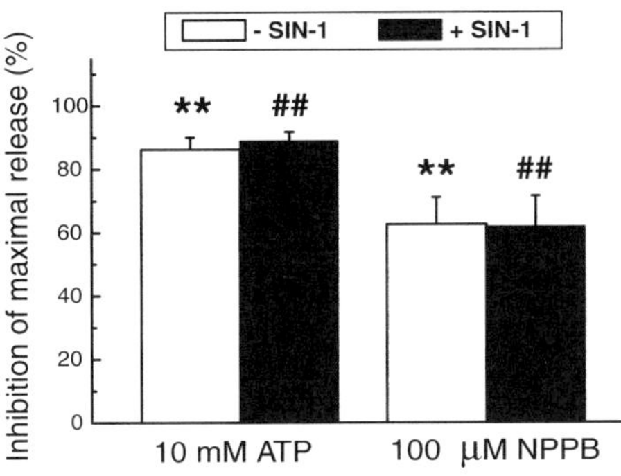

FIGURE 44.5 Peroxynitrite ($ONOO^-$) upregulates activity of volume-regulated anion channels (VRACs) in osmotically swollen astrocyte cultures. *a.* The peroxynitrite donor (SIN-1), which generates nitric oxide and superoxide anion to form $ONOO^-$, potentiated the VRAC-mediated excitatory amino acid release measured as efflux of preloaded D-[^{3}H]aspartate. This effect was abolished by the superoxide anion scavenger, superoxide dismutase (*SOD*). *b.* Hypoosmotic medium–induced D-[^{3}H]aspartate efflux was equally sensitive to the VRAC blockers extracellular adenosine triphosphate (*ATP*) and 5-nitro 2-(3-phenylpropylamine)benzoic acid (*NPPB*), both in the presence and absence of SIN-1. The inhibition was normalized to the appropriate maximum release values. These data strongly support VRAC involvement in the SIN-1-mediated excitatory amino acid release. (From Haskew et al., 2002, with permission of the International Society for Neurochemistry and Blackwell Publishing.)

der tight control of numerous homeostatic mechanisms (Sykova, 1997). Anoxia/ischemia cause dramatic changes in the ECS, reducing it in the CNS and the spinal cord from ~20% to as low as 4% (Lundbaek and Hansen, 1992; Sykova et al., 1994). The largest ECS decreases produce 5-fold increases in the extracellular concentration of K^+ and EAA, by itself sufficient for neuronal depolarization. A combination of ECS reduction with energy depletion and consequent dissipation of transmembrane ion gradients, and reversal of neurotransmitter transporters, elevates extracellular K^+ up to 80 mM and extracellular glutamate levels up to 20–50 μM (Lundbaek and Hansen, 1992; Szatkowski and Attwell, 1994; Seki et al., 1999). Other important changes include decreases in $[Na^+]_e$ to 48–59 mM, $[Cl^-]_e$ to 70–75 mM, $[Ca^{2+}]_e$ to 0.06–0.08 mM, and pH_e to 6.1–6.8 (for review see Sykova, 1997). As is evident from the previous sections (see "Astrocytic Swelling in Pathology"), increases in astrocytic volume are probably responsible for much of the ECS reduction and probably develop due to homeostatic uptake of both K^+ and neurotransmitters released by neurons (Kimelberg, 2000). Supportive of this hypothesis, onset of ECS reduction in white matter is significantly slower than in gray matter (Vorisek and Sykova, 1997).

Astrocytic Swelling and pH Control

Rapid decreases in brain pH follow ischemia and are associated with increased lactate levels (reviewed in Kimelberg and Feustel, 1998). This close association is referred to as *lactic acidosis*, often leading to the erroneous interpretation that it is the generation of lactic acid by increased glycolysis that causes the acidosis. This is wrong. The end product of glycolysis is the lactate anion, not the undissociated acid form. The protons are actually being produced from other reactions such as net hydrolysis of high-energy phosphates, principally ATP (Katsura, 1997). However, the end result is the same; increased H^+ and lactate in the tissue. A link between lactate and astrocytic swelling in pathologies, especially in ischemia, can be explained by several experimental schemes (for detailed discussion see Kimelberg and Feustel, 1998; see also the section "Molecular Mechanisms of Astrocytic Swelling" in this chapter). Cytoplasmic acidification activates the Na^+/H^+ exchanger, causing Na^+ accumulation. This process is functionally linked to Cl^-/HCO_3^- exchange, predominantly exchanging Cl^- into the cell for HCO_3^-, and is supplemented by the Na^+,HCO_3^- cotransporter. Altogether, these processes cause significant NaCl accumulation in the cytoplasm, resulting in osmotic cell swelling (Deitmer, 1995; Kimelberg and Feustel, 1998). Undissociated lactic acid and other acids in their uncharged form diffuse across membranes readily and, once inside the cell, dissociate with H^+ production. Additionally, lactate and H^+ also cross membranes on H^+ and lactate transporters. By either mechanism, but at different rates, $[H^+]$ increases in the cytoplasm and activates the Na^+/H^+ exchanger, causing osmotically relevant Na^+ uptake.

As noted in the previous sections, the responses of astrocytes to rapid swelling is to initiate RVD. Regulatory volume decrease is inhibited by decreased pH due to inhibition of either swelling-activated or already active K^+ channels. This clearly causes the swelling to persist, with continued release of EAA. Decrease in intracellular pH is most effective in inhibiting the RVD process (Smets et al., 2002). Therefore, intracellular accumulation of H^+ is more damaging than general acidosis that only increases extracellular $[H^+]$.

CONCLUSIONS AND PERSPECTIVES

In this chapter we have reviewed the evidence that cellular edema—a cell volume increase due to a shift of extracellular water to the intracellular space—is a general phenomenon occurring in numerous pathological states such as ischemia, traumatic brain injury, hepatic encephalopathy, and hyponatremia. Astrocytes are probably the major contributors to cellular edema because other cell types (oligodendrocytes and neuronal soma) are not seen to swell or show swelling only in limited regions (dendritic swelling). The reasons for such exclusive astrocytic swelling are not completely understood, but they may involve several unique features of astrocytic physiology. Such features probably include a high astrocytic capacity for K^+ and glutamate uptake (Kimelberg, 2000; Danbolt, 2001), astrocyte-specific localization of glutamate-glutamine cycle enzymes (Martinez-Hernandez et al., 1977; Danbolt, 2001), high levels of expression of aquaporin-4 (Manley et al., 2000; Venero et al., 2001), strong activation of the $Na^+,K^+,2Cl^-$ cotransporter by both cell swelling and extracellular K^+ (Mongin et al., 1994; Su et al., 2002a), and abundant expression of ion transporters and exchangers involved in pH homeostasis (Dietmer, 1995), among, no doubt, other properties. We are now beginning to understand how pathological swelling of astrocytes contributes to neural tissue damage (Fig. 44.6). Originally, swelling of perivascular astrocytic endfeet was proposed to compress microvessels and not allow for reperfusion after ischemia (the no-reflow concept; Ames et al., 1968) (Fig. 44.6*B*). Newer concepts take into account the cell swelling–related large reduction in extracellular space that significantly elevates concentrations of K^+ and neurotransmitters and limits their diffusion pathways, thereby leading to neuronal depolarization and overexcitation (Sykova, 1997) (Fig. 44.6*A*). Perhaps most importantly, astrocytic swelling leads to activation of volume-dependent anion chan-

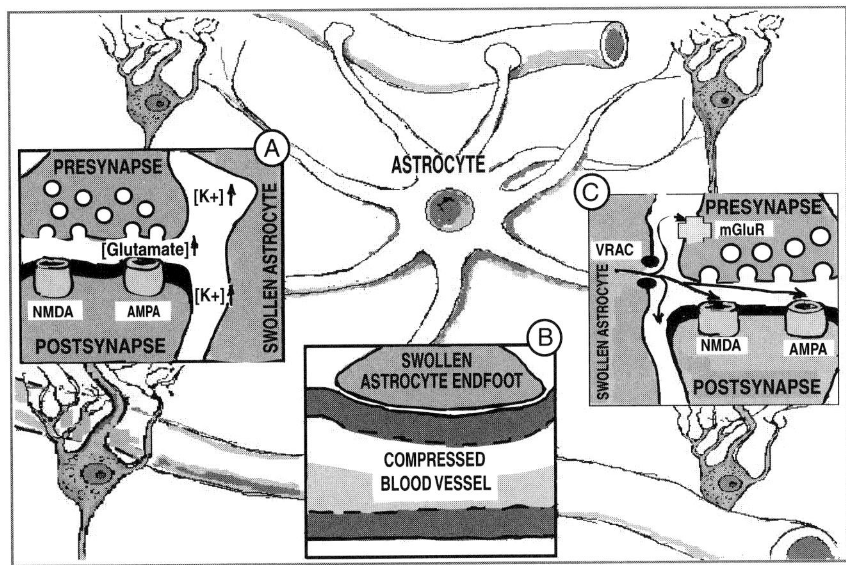

FIGURE 44.6 Major negative consequences of neuropathological astrocytic swelling. *A*. Astrocytic swelling reduces the extracellular space, causing an elevation in extracellular K^+ and glutamate concentration, both promoting neuronal depolarization and excitotoxic death. *B*. Swollen astrocytic endfeet compress microvessels, causing further reduction in blood flow. *C*. In swollen astrocytes, activation of volume-regulated anion channels (*VRACs*) causes glutamate release, which contributes to high extracellular glutamate levels and then overexcitation of pre- and postsynaptic glutamate receptors metabotropic glutamate receptors AMPA: α-amino-3-hydroxy-5-methyl-4-isoxazole propionic acid receptors; mGluR: metabotropic glutamate receptors; NMDA: *N*-methyl-D-aspartate receptors.

nels and the release of EAA, supplemented by the reversal of EAA transporters in depolarized astrocytes (reviewed in Kimelberg and Mongin, 1998; Kimelberg, 2000) (Fig. 44.6C). In animal models of ischemia and traumatic brain injury, inhibitors of anion channels decrease pathological extracellular glutamate levels, ameliorate astrocyte swelling and brain edema, and protect against tissue damage (Barron et al., 1988; Kohut et al., 1992; Phillis et al., 1997; Seki et al., 1999; Kimelberg et al., 2000, 2003). Therefore astrocytic swelling and swelling-activated EAA release may be a plausible pharmacological target in human ischemia and brain trauma, and perhaps in other neurological disorders associated with cellular edema. We clearly need more *in vivo* data to supplement and verify the wealth of basic information obtained in cell culture models. Two significant problems hamper our experimental progress: lack of the knowledge of the molecular nature of EAA-permeable, volume-activated anion channels and the absence of pharmacological tools allowing their selective inhibition (Jentsch et al., 2002). One recent report has identified the ethacrynic acid derivative 4-(2-Butyl-6,7-dichlor-2-cyclopentyl-indon-1-on-5-yl) oxybutyric acid (DCPIB) as a selective inhibitor of volume-regulated anion channels, discriminating them from cloned to-date chloride channels (Decher et al., 2001). Once commercially available, this compound, along with the progress in the molecular biology of anion channels, may strongly accelerate research in the field. Other research may explore the effects of cell swelling on astrocyte metabolism and physiology in astrocytic processes surrounding synapses and supporting synaptic transmission. Altogether, such studies will help us to understand better the role of astrocytes in normal physiology, as well as in human brain pathologies, and allow better treatment modalities.

REFERENCES

Alessandri, B. and Bullock, R. (1998) Glutamate and its receptors in the pathophysiology of brain and spinal cord injuries. *Prog. Brain Res.* 116:303–330.

Ames, A., 3rd, Wright, R.L., Kowada, M., Thurston, J.M., and Majno, G. (1968) Cerebral ischemia. II. The no-reflow phenomenon. *Am. J. Pathol.* 52:437–453.

Barron, K.D., Dentinger, M.P., Kimelberg, H.K., Nelson, L.R., Bourke, R.S., Keegan, S., Mankes, R., and Cragoe, E.J., Jr. (1988) Ultrastructural features of a brain injury model in cat. I. Vascular and neuroglial changes and the prevention of astroglial swelling by a fluorenyl (aryloxy) alkanoic acid derivative (L-644,711). *Acta Neuropathol. (Berl.)* 75:295–307.

Basarsky, T.A., Feighan, D., and MacVicar, B.A. (1999) Glutamate release through volume-activated channels during spreading depression. *J. Neurosci.* 19:6439–6445.

Bender, A.S., Schousboe, A., Reichelt, W., and Norenberg, M.D. (1998) Ionic mechanisms in glutamate-induced astrocyte swelling: role of K^+ influx. *J. Neurosci. Res.* 52:307–321.

Blei, A.T. and Larsen, F.S. (1999) Pathophysiology of cerebral edema in fulminant hepatic failure. *J. Hepatology* 31:771–776.

Blei, A.T., Olafsson, S., Therrien, G., and Butterworth, R.F. (1994) Ammonia-induced brain edema and intracranial hypertension in rats after portacaval anastomosis. *Hepatology* 19,1437–1444.

Bullock, R., Maxwell, W.L., Graham, D.I., Teasdale, G.M., and Adams, J.H. (1991) Glial swelling following human cerebral contusion: an ultrastructural study. *J. Neurol. Neurosurg. Psychiatry* 54:427–434.

Castejon, O.J. (1980) Electron microscopic study of capillary wall in human cerebral edema. *J. Neuropathol. Exp. Neurol.* 29:296–327.

Chan, P.H., Chen, S.F., and Yu, A.C. (1988) Induction of intracellular superoxide radical formation by arachidonic acid and by polyunsaturated fatty acids in primary astrocytic cultures. *J. Neurochem.* 50:1185–1193.

Chan, P.H. and Fishman, R.A. (1978) Brain edema: induction in cortical slices by polyunsaturated fatty acids. *Science* 201:358–360.

Chan, P.H. and Fishman, R.A. (1982) Alterations of membrane integrity and cellular constituents by arachidonic acid in neuroblastoma and glioma cells. *Brain Res.* 248:151–157.

Chan, P.H. and Fishman, R.A. (1984) The role of arachidonic acid in vasogenic brain edema. *Fed. Proc.* 43:210–213.

Clifton, G.L., Jiang, J.Y., Lyeth, B.G., Jenkins, L.W., Hamm, R.J., and Hayes, R.L. (1991) Marked protection by moderate hypothermia after experimental traumatic brain injury. *J. Cereb. Blood Flow Metab.* 11:114–121.

Danbolt, N.C. (2001) Glutamate uptake. *Prog. Neurobiol.* 65:1–105.

Decher, N., Lang, H.J., Nilius, B., Bruggemann, A., Busch, A.E., and Steinmeyer, K. (2001) DCPIB is a novel selective blocker of $I_{Cl,swell}$ and prevents swelling-induced shortening of guinea-pig atrial action potential duration. *Br. J. Pharmacol.* 134:1467–1479.

Deitmer, J.W. (1995) pH regulation. In: Kettenmann, H. and Ransom, B.R., eds. *Neuroglia* New York and Oxford: Oxford University Press, pp. 230–245.

Dietrich, W.D., Alonso, O., and Halley, M. (1994) Early microvascular and neuronal consequences of traumatic brain injury: a light and electron microscopic study in rats. *J. Neurotrauma* 11: 289–301.

Fraser, C.L. and Arieff, A.I. (1997) Epidemiology, pathophysiology, and management of hyponatremic encephalopathy. *Am. J. Med.* 102:67–77.

Fraser, C.L. and Sarnacki, P. (1989) Na^+-K^+-ATPase pump function in rat brain synaptosomes is different in males and females. *Am. J. Physiol.* 257:E284–E289.

Fraser, C.L. and Swanson, R.A. (1994) Female sex hormones inhibit volume regulation in rat brain astrocyte culture. *Am. J. Physiol.* 267:C909–C914.

Garcia, J.H., Liu, K.-F., Yoshida, Y., Chen, S., and Lian, J. (1994) Brain microvessels: factors altering their patency after the occlusion of a middle cerebral artery (Wistar rat). *Am. J. Pathol.* 145: 728–740.

Garcia, J.H., Yoshida, Y., Chen, H., Li, Y., Zhang, Z.G., Lian, J., Chen, S., and Chopp, M. (1993) Progression from ischemic injury to infarct following middle cerebral artery occlusion in the rat. *Am. J. Pathol.* 142:623–635.

Griffiths, I.R., Burns, N., and Crawford, A.R. (1978) Early vascular changes in the spinal gray matter following impact injury. *Acta Neuropathol. (Berl.)* 41:33–39.

Gullans, S.R. and Verbalis, J.G. (1993) Control of brain volume during hyperosmolar and hypoosmolar conditions. *Annu. Rev. Med.* 44:289–301.

Haskew, R.E., Mongin, A.A., and Kimelberg, H.K. (2002) Peroxynitrite enhances astrocytic volume-sensitive excitatory amino acid release via a src tyrosine kinase-dependent mechanism. *J. Neurochem.* 82:903–912.

Haussinger, D., Kircheis, G., Fischer, R., Schliess, F., and vom Dahl, S. (2000) Hepatic encephalopathy in chronic liver disease: a clinical manifestation of astrocyte swelling and low-grade cerebral edema? *J. Hepatol.* 32:1035–1038.

Jackson, P.S., Morrison, R., and Strange, K. (1994) The volume-sensitive organic osmolyte-anion channel VSOAC is regulated by nonhydrolytic ATP binding. *Am. J. Physiol.* 267:C1203–C1209.

Jakubovicz, D.E., Grinstein, S., and Klip, A. (1987) Cell swelling following recovery from acidification in C6 glioma cells: an in vitro model of postischemic brain edema. *Brain Res.* 435:138–146.

Jenkins, L.W., Povlishock, J.T., Becker, D.P., Miller, J.D., and Sullivan, H.G. (1979) Complete cerebral ischemia. An ultrastructural study. *Acta Neuropathol. (Berl.)* 48:113–125.

Jentsch, T.J., Stein, V., Weinreich, F., and Zdebik, A.A. (2002) Molecular structure and physiological function of chloride channels. *Physiol. Rev.* 82:503–568.

Johnson, L.J., Hanley, D.F., and Thakor, N.V. (2000) Optical light scatter imaging of cellular and sub-cellular morphology changes in stressed rat hippocampal slices. *J. Neurosci. Meth.* 98:21–31.

Katsura, K. (1997) Acidosis as a complicating factor in cerebral ischemia. In: Welch, K.M.A., Caplan, L.R., Reis, D.J., Siesjo, B.K., and WeirB., eds. *Primer on Cerebrovascular Diseases*, San Diego, CA, and London: Academic Press, pp. 159–162.

Kempski, O., Staub, F., Jansen, M., Schodel, F., and Baethmann, A. (1988) Glial swelling during extracellular acidosis in vitro. *Stroke* 19:385–392.

Kimelberg, H.K. (1995) Current concepts of brain edema. Review of laboratory investigations. *J. Neurosurg.* 83:1051–1059.

Kimelberg, H.K. (2000) Cell volume in the CNS: regulation and implications for nervous system function and pathology. *Neuroscientist* 6:14–24.

Kimelberg, H.K. and Feustel, P.J. (1998) Brain edema and pH. In: Kaila, K. and Ransom, B.R., eds. *pH and Brain Function.* New York: Wiley-Liss, pp. 651–669.

Kimelberg, H.K., Feustel, P.J., Jin, Y., Paquette, J., Boulos, A., Keller, R.W., Jr., and Tranmer, B.I. (2000) Acute treatment with tamoxifen reduces ischemic damage following middle cerebral artery occlusion. *NeuroReport* 11:2675–2679.

Kimelberg, H.K., Goderie, S.K., Higman, S., Pang, S., and Waniewski, R.A. (1990) Swelling-induced release of glutamate, aspartate, and taurine from astrocyte cultures. *J. Neurosci.* 10: 1583–1591.

Kimelberg, H.K., Jin, Y., and Feustel, P.J. (2003) Neuroprotective activity of tamoxifen in permanent focal ischemia. *J. Neurosurg.* 99:138–142.

Kimelberg, H.K. and Mongin, A.A. (1998) Swelling-activated release of excitatory amino acids in the brain: relevance for pathophysiology. *Contrib. Nephrol.* 123:240–257.

Kimelberg, H.K., Rose, J.W., Barron, K.D., Waniewski, R.A., and Cragoe, E.J. (1989) Astrocytic swelling in traumatic-hypoxic brain injury. Beneficial effects of an inhibitor of anion exchange transport and glutamate uptake in glial cells. *Mol. Chem. Neuropathol.* 11:1–31.

Kimelberg, H.K., Rutledge, E., Goderie, S., and Charniga, C. (1995) Astrocytic swelling due to hypotonic or high K^+ medium causes inhibition of glutamate and aspartate uptake and increases their release. *J. Cereb. Blood Flow Metab.* 15:409–416.

Kirk, K. and Strange, K. (1998) Functional properties and physiological roles of organic solute channels. *Annu. Rev. Physiol.* 60: 719–739.

Klatzo, I. (1967) Presidential address: neuropathological aspects of brain edema. *J. Neuropathol. Exp. Neurol.* 26:1–13.

Kohut, J.J., Bednar, M.M., Kimelberg, H.K., McAuliffe, T.L., and Gross, C.E. (1992) Reduction in ischemic brain injury in rabbits by the anion transport inhibitor L-644,711. *Stroke* 23:93–97.

Koyama, Y., Baba, A., and Iwata, H. (1991) L-Glutamate-induced swelling of cultured astrocytes is dependent on extracellular Ca^{2+}. *Neurosci. Lett.* 122:210–212.

Koyama, Y., Ishibashi, T., Okamoto, T., Matsuda, T., Hashimoto, H., and Baba, A. (2000) Transient treatments with L-glutamate and threo-beta-hydroxyaspartate induce swelling of rat cultured astrocytes. *Neurochem. Int.* 36:167–173.

Kraig, R.P. and Chesler, M. (1990) Astrocytic acidosis in hyperglycemic and complete ischemia. *J. Cereb. Blood Flow Metab.* 10:104–114.

Kucinski, T., Vaterlein, O., Glauche, V., Fiehler, J., Klotz, E., Eckert, B., Koch, C., Rother, J., and Zeumer, H. (2002) Correlation of apparent diffusion coefficient and computed tomography density in acute ischemic stroke. *Stroke* 33:1786–1791.

Kuschinsky, W. (1997) Microvascular patency in ischemia and reperfusion. In: Welch, K.M.A., Caplan, L.R., Reis, D.J., Siesjo, B.K., and Weir, B., eds. *Primer on Cerebrovascular Diseases.* San Diego, CA, and London: Academic Press, pp. 214–216.

Lang, F., Busch, G.L., Ritter, M., Volkl, H., Waldegger, S., Gulbins, E., and Haussinger, D. (1998) Functional significance of cell volume regulatory mechanisms. *Physiol. Rev.* 78:247–306.

Liu, K.F., Li, F., Tatlisumak, T., Garcia, J.H., Sotak, C.H., Fisher, M., and Fenstermacher, J.D. (2001) Regional variations in the apparent diffusion coefficient and the intracellular distribution of water in rat brain during acute focal ischemia. *Stroke* 32: 1897–1905.

Lundbaek, J.A. and Hansen, A.J. (1992) Brain interstitial volume fraction and tortuosity in anoxia. Evaluation of the ion-selective micro-electrode method. *Acta Physiol. Scand.* 146:473–484.

Macknight, A.D.C. and Leaf, A. (1977) Regulation of cellular volume. *Physiol. Rev.* 57:510–573.

Manley, G.T., Fujimura, M., Ma, T., Noshita, N., Filiz, F., Bollen, A., Chan, W.P., and Verkman, A.S. (2000) Aquaporin-4 deletion in mice reduces brain edema after acute water intoxication and ischemic stroke. *Nat. Med.* 6:159–163.

Marcaggi, P. and Coles, J.A. (2001) Ammonium in nervous tissue: transport across cell membranes, fluxes from neurons to glial cells, and role in signaling. *Prog. Neurobiol.* 64:157–183.

Martinez-Hernandez, A., Bell, K.P., and Norenberg, M.D. (1977) Glutamine synthetase: glial localization in brain. *Science* 195:1356–1358.

Mathew, P., Bullock, R., Graham, D.I., Maxwell, W.L., Teasdale, G.M., and McCulloch, J. (1996) A new experimental model of contusion in the rat. Histopathological analysis and temporal patterns of cerebral blood flow disturbances. *J. Neurosurg.* 85: 860–870.

Mathew, P., Graham, D.I., Bullock, R., Maxwell, W., McCulloch, J., and Teasdale, G. (1994) Focal brain injury: histological evidence of delayed inflammatory response in a new rodent model of focal cortical injury. *Acta Neurochir. Suppl. (Wien)* 60:428–430.

Maxwell, W.L., Bullock, R., Landholt, H., and Fujisawa, H. (1994) Massive astrocytic swelling in response to extracellular glutamate—a possible mechanism for post-traumatic brain swelling? *Acta Neurochir. Suppl. (Wien)* 60:465–467.

Mongin, A.A., Aksentsev, S.L., Orlov, S.N., Slepko, N.G., Kozlova, M.V., Maximov, G.V., and Konev, S.V. (1994) Swelling-induced K^+ influx in cultured primary astrocytes. *Brain Res.* 655:110–114.

Mongin, A.A. and Kimelberg, H.K. (2002) ATP potently modulates anion channel–mediated excitatory amino acid release from cultured astrocytes. *Am. J. Physiol.* 283:C569–C578.

Nagaraja, T.N. and Brookes, N. (1998) Intracellular acidification induced by passive and active transport of ammonium ions in astrocytes. *Am. J. Physiol.* 274:C883–C891.

Neumann-Haefelin, T., Kastrup, A., De Crespigny, A., Yenari, M.A., Ringer, T., Sun, G.H., and Moseley, M.E. (2000) Serial MRI after transient focal cerebral ischemia in rats: dynamics of tissue injury, blood-brain barrier damage, and edema formation. *Stroke* 31:1965–1972.

Norenberg, M.D. (1977) A light and electron microscopic study of experimental portal-systemic (ammonia) encephalopathy. Progression and reversal of the disorder. *Lab. Invest.* 36:618–627.

Norenberg, M.D. (1995) Hepatic encephalopathy. In: Kettenmann, H., and Ransom, B.R., eds. *Neuroglia* New York and Oxford: Oxford University Press, pp. 950–963.

Norenberg, M.D., Baker, L., Norenberg, L.O., Blicharska, J., Bruce-Gregorios, J.H., and Neary, J.T. (1991) Ammonia-induced astrocyte swelling in primary culture. *Neurochem. Res.* 16: 833–836.

O'Connor, E.R., Kimelberg, H.K., Keese, C.R., and Giaever, I. (1993) Electrical resistance method for measuring volume changes in monolayer cultures applied to primary astrocyte cultures. *Am. J. Physiol.* 264:C471–C478.

Pasantes-Morales, H., Franco, R., Torres-Marquez, M.E., Hernandez-Fonseca, K., and Ortega, A. (2000) Amino acid osmolytes in regulatory volume decrease and isovolumetric regulation in brain cells: contribution and mechanisms. *Cell Physiol. Biochem.* 10:361–370.

Pasantes-Morales, H., Moran, J., and Schousboe, A. (1990) Volume-sensitive release of taurine from cultured astrocytes: properties and mechanism. *Glia* 3:427–432.

Pasantes-Morales, H., Murray, R.A., Lilja, L., and Moran, J. (1994a) Regulatory volume decrease in cultured astrocytes. I. Potassium- and chloride-activated permeability. *Am. J. Physiol.* 266:C165–C171.

Pasantes-Morales, H. Murray, R.A., Sanchez-Olea, R., and Moran, J. (1994b) Regulatory volume decrease in cultured astrocytes. II. Permeability pathway to amino acids and polyols. *Am. J. Physiol.* 266:C172–C178.

Phillis, J.W., Song, D., and O'Regan, M.H. (1997) Inhibition by anion channel blockers of ischemia-evoked release of excitotoxic and other amino acids from rat cerebral cortex. *Brain Res.* 758:9–16.

Rehncrona, S., Westerberg, E., Akesson, B., and Siesjo, B.K. (1982) Brain cortical fatty acids and phospholipids during and following complete and severe incomplete ischemia. *J. Neurochem.* 38:84–93.

Rose, C., Michalak, A., Pannunzio, M., Chatauret, N., Rambaldi, A., and Butterworth, R.F. (2000) Mild hypothermia delays the onset of coma and prevents brain edema and extracellular brain glutamate accumulation in rats with acute liver failure. *Hepatology* 31:872–877.

Rothstein, J.D., Dykes-Hoberg, M., Pardo, C.A., Bristol, L.A., Jin, L., Kuncl, R.W., Kanai, Y., Hediger, M.A., Wang, Y., Schielke, J.P., and Welty, D.F. (1996) Knockout of glutamate transporters reveals a major role for astroglial transport in excitotoxicity and clearance of glutamate. *Neuron* 16:675–686.

Rutledge, E.M., Aschner, M., and Kimelberg, H.K. (1998) Pharmacological characterization of swelling-induced D-[^{3}H]aspartate release from primary astrocyte cultures. *Am. J. Physiol.* 274: C1511–C1520.

Rutledge, E.M. and Kimelberg, H.K. (1996) Release of [^{3}H]-D-aspartate from primary astrocyte cultures in response to raised external potassium. *J. Neurosci.* 16:7803–7811.

Rutledge, E.M., Mongin, A.A., and Kimelberg, H.K. (1999) Intracellular ATP depletion inhibits swelling-induced D-[^{3}H]aspartate release from primary astrocyte cultures. *Brain Res.* 842:39–45.

Sanchez-Olea, R., Morales-Mulia, M., Moran, J., and Pasantes-Morales, H. (1995) Inhibition by polyunsaturated fatty acids of cell volume regulation and osmolyte fluxes in astrocytes. *Am. J. Physiol.* 269:C96–C102.

Seki, Y., Feustel, P.J., Keller, R.W., Jr., Tranmer, B.I., and Kimelberg, H.K. (1999) Inhibition of ischemia-induced glutamate release in rat striatum by dihydrokinate and an anion channel blocker. *Stroke* 30:433–440.

Smets, I., Ameloot, M., Steels, P., and Van Driessche, W. (2002) Loss of cell volume regulation during metabolic inhibition in renal epithelial cells (A6): role of intracellular pH. *Am. J. Physiol.* 283: C535–C544.

Staub, F., Baethmann, A., Peters, J., Weigt, H., and Kempski, O. (1990) Effects of lactacidosis on glial cell volume and viability. *J. Cereb. Blood Flow Metab.* 10:866–876.

Staub, F., Winkler, A., Peters, J., Kempski, O., Kachel, V., and Baethmann, A. (1994) Swelling, acidosis, and irreversible damage of glial cells from exposure to arachidonic acid in vitro. *J. Cereb. Blood Flow Metab.* 14:1030–1039.

Strupp, M., Staub, F., and Grafe, P. (1993) A Ca^{2+}- and pH-dependent K^+ channel of rat C6 glioma cells and its possible role in acidosis-induced cell swelling. *Glia* 9:136–145.

Su, G., Kintner, D.B., Flagella, M., Shull, G.E., and Sun, D. (2002a) Astrocytes from Na^+-K^+-Cl^- cotransporter-null mice exhibit absence of swelling and decrease in EAA release. *Am. J. Physiol.* 282:C1147–C1160.

Su, G., Kintner, D.B., and Sun, D. (2002b) Contribution of Na^+-K^+-Cl^- cotransporter to high-$[K^+]_o$-induced swelling and EAA release in astrocytes. *Am. J. Physiol.* 282:C1136–C1146.

Swain, M., Butterworth, R.F., and Blei, A.T. (1992) Ammonia and related amino acids in the pathogenesis of brain edema in acute ischemic liver failure in rats. *Hepatology* 15:449–453.

Sykova, E. (1997) The extracellular space in the CNS: its regulation, volume and geometry in normal and pathological neuronal function. *Neuroscientist* 3:28–41.

Sykova, E., Svoboda, J., Polak, J., and Chvatal, A. (1994) Extracellular volume fraction and diffusion characteristics during progressive ischemia and terminal anoxia in the spinal cord of the rat. *J. Cereb. Blood Flow Metab.* 14:301–311.

Szatkowski, M. and Attwell, D. (1994) Triggering and execution of neuronal death in brain ischaemia: two phases of glutamate release by different mechanisms. *Trends Neurosci.* 17:359–365.

Trachtman, H. and Cragoe, E.J., Jr. (1989) Hyponatremia-induced brain edema in guinea pigs is reduced by treatment with the novel anion transport inhibitor L-644,711. *Life Sci.* 45:2141–2147.

Vajda, Z., Promeneur, D., Doczi, T., Sulyok, E., Frokiaer, J., Ottersen, O.P., and Nielsen, S. (2000) Increased aquaporin-4 immunoreactivity in rat brain in response to systemic hyponatremia. *Biochem. Biophys. Res. Commun.* 270:495–503.

van der Toorn, A., Sykova, E., Dijkhuizen, R.M., Vorisek, I., Vargova, L., Skobisova, E., van Lookeren Campagne, M., Reese, T., and Nicolay, K. (1996) Dynamic changes in water ADC, energy metabolism, extracellular space volume, and tortuosity in neonatal rat brain during global ischemia. *Magn. Reson. Med.* 36: 52–60.

Van Harreveld, A. (1966) *Brain Tissue Electrolytes.* London: Butterworths.

Venero, J.L., Vizuete, M.L., Machado, A., and Cano, J. (2001) Aquaporins in the central nervous system. *Prog. Neurobiol.* 63: 321–336.

Verkman, A.S. and Mitra, A.K. (2000) Structure and function of aquaporin water channels. *Am. J. Physiol.* 278:F13–F28.

Vitarella, D., DiRisio, D.J., Kimelberg, H.K., and Aschner, M. (1994) Potassium and taurine release are highly correlated with regulatory volume decrease in neonatal primary rat astrocyte cultures. *J. Neurochem.* 63:1143–1149.

Vorisek, I. and Sykova, E. (1997) Ischemia-induced changes in the extracellular space diffusion parameters, K^+, and pH in the developing rat cortex and corpus callosum. *J. Cereb. Blood Flow Metab.* 17:191–203.

Walz, W. and Wuttke, W.A. (1989) Resistance of astrocyte electrical membrane properties to acidosis changes in the presence of lactate. *Brain Res.* 504:82–86.

Welsh, F.A., Sims, R.E., and Harris, V.A. (1990) Mild hypothermia prevents ischemic injury in gerbil hippocampus. *J. Cereb. Blood Flow Metab.* 10:557–563.

Willard-Mack, C.L., Koehler, R.C., Hirata, T., Cork, L.C., Takahashi, H., Traystman, R.J., and Brusilow, S.W. (1996) Inhibition of glutamine synthetase reduces ammonia-induced astrocyte swelling in rat. *Neuroscience* 71:589–599.

Winkler, A.S., Baethmann, A., Peters, J., Kempski, O., and Staub, F. (2000) Mechanisms of arachidonic acid induced glial swelling. *Mol. Brain Res.* 76:419–423.

Yan, Y., Dempsey, R.J., and Sun, D. (2001) Na^+-K^+-Cl^- cotransporter in rat focal cerebral ischemia. *J. Cereb. Blood Flow Metab.* 21:711–721.

45 The activation of microglia as an early sign of disease progression in Alzheimer's disease

ROBERT VEERHUIS, JEROEN J.M. HOOZEMANS, ANNACHIARA CAGNIN, PIET EIKELENBOOM, AND RICHARD B. BANATI

Over the past decade, many studies have indicated that the number of reactive microglial cells (brain macrophages) is increased in various neurodegenerative disorders, including Parkinson's disease and Alzheimer's disease (AD). In this chapter we will focus on the role of microglia in the pathogenesis of AD.

Alzheimer's disease is characterized neuropathologically by extracellular deposits of amyloid β (Aβ) fibrils and cytoskeletal changes inside neurons. Studies in the early-onset familial forms of AD suggest that an altered metabolism of the β-amyloid precursor protein (β-APP) with progressive deposition of Aβ is the key step in the molecular pathogenesis of AD (Selkoe, 1991). These findings have led to the view that AD is an *amyloid-driven* process.

However, even though the formal diagnosis of AD includes amyloid deposition in its histopathological definition, it has long been known that the overall load of amyloid is not closely reflected in the degree of dementia. In human postmortem brain specimens, levels of fibrilllar Aβ, as found in the classical insoluble plaques, do not differ between nondemented controls and AD patients, whereas the levels of the soluble, unseen forms of Aβ seem more closely linked to the presence of dementia (Lue et al., 1999). Similarly, experimental data on the role of amyloid deposits in β-APP transgenic animal models are not unequivocal (Koistinaho et al., 2001). This seems to suggest that Aβ accumulation alone may not be sufficient to explain the disease progression and cognitive deficit.

In this context, the more recent *neuroinflammation* hypothesis posits that initial Aβ deposits and damaged neurons or neurites may elicit a localized and chronic inflammatory reaction, which, in turn, may exacerbate the pathogenetic process (Akiyama et al., 2000). Key players in this chronic inflammatory reaction are the microglia and inflammation-related proteins (including complement factors, acute-phase proteins, and proinflammatory cytokines) that normally are locally produced at low levels in the brain but the synthesis of which is upregulated in AD brain. A number of these reactants (especially cytokines and complement activation products) may attract and activate microglia.

Although the accumulation of inflammation-related proteins and microglia in AD brain may be reminiscent of an inflammatory reaction, it is not sufficient to meet the conventional definition of inflammation (McGeer and McGeer, 2001). Neutrophils are absent, and T cell subsets and immunoglobulins cannot be detected, either in the neuropil or as perivascular cuffs (Eikelenboom et al., 1994). Furthermore, expression levels of the most relevant intercellular adhesion molecules (ICAM-1, VCAM-1, E-selectin), required for leukocyte recruitment from the blood, are not increased on capillary endothelial cells in AD brains (Eikelenboom and Veerhuis, 1996). This implies that the extracellular fibrillar Aβ deposits in AD brain are associated with a locally induced, non-immune-mediated, chronic inflammatory-type response without any apparent influx of leukocytes from the blood, and that microglia are the most important immune effector cell in the brain.

In gray matter of normal brain, resting, ramified microglia are more or less evenly distributed and lack expression of major histocompatibility complex (MHC) class II proteins, whereas white matter microglia express class II molecules. In AD brain, clusters of activated microglia that have an ameboid phenotype and express MHC class II, complement receptors 3 and 4 (iC3b receptors), Fcγ receptors, and CD45 colocalize with the cerebral amyloid deposits, especially those Aβ plaques associated with neuritic changes (Rozemuller et al., 1989a; Griffin et al., 1995; Eikelenboom and Veerhuis, 1996; Akiyama et al., 2000).

In this chapter we will focus on the contribution of activated microglia to the progression of AD at various stages of the pathological cascade. Clusters of activated microglia occur only in complement-positive Aβ plaques, and effector functions of complement include the modulation of microglial activity *in vitro*. Therefore, the question of whether microglia are detrimental or beneficial in AD pathogenesis will be discussed especially in relation to the presence and modulating activities of activation products of the complement system.

SPATIAL AND TEMPORAL DISTRIBUTION OF MICROGLIAL ACTIVATION IN ALZHEIMER'S DISEASE

In the neocortex of AD brain, clusters of microglia with a rounded, phagocytic phenotype are seen only in Aβ plaques that consist of fibrillar Aβ deposits. Two types of fibrillar Aβ plaques that are associated with reactive microglia, as well as neuritic changes and reactive astrocytes, can be distinguished: (*1*) the classic neuritic plaques with a dense Aβ core that are Congo red positive and (*2*) the round, primitive plaques that lack a central core and show variable Congo red positivity. No microglial activation is seen in the nonfibrillar Aβ plaques that lack a central core, Congo red positivity, and degenerative neurites.

The number of classic congophilic amyloid deposits initially increases, but tends to decrease with disease progression from a certain stage of AD progression on. This ultimately leads to the absence of congophilic plaques and the presence of *glial nests* in severe AD cases (Brun and Englund, 1981). Amyloid β accumulation in the neuropil is the result of a dynamic balance between deposition and removal of Aβ deposits (Hyman et al., 1993). Activated microglia are closely associated with Aβ plaque-type evolution and are a relatively early pathogenetic event that precedes the process of neuropil destruction in AD patients, as shown in clinicopathological studies.

The volume densities of microglia and congophilic Aβ plaques (i.e., the volume of tissue occupied by microglia and congophilic deposits, respectively) highly correlate in AD brain at varying stages of the disease (Arends et al., 2000). When ranked in increasing order of severity of clinical dementia, the peak volume densities of activated microglia and congophilic Aβ plaques are seen in moderately affected cases, whereas Aβ and tau steadily accumulate with disease progression, suggesting that microglia clustering occurs at early stages of AD, when tau pathology is still moderate (Arends et al., 2000).

Similar results are obtained when nondemented controls, possible AD, and definite AD cases are compared (Vehmas et al., 2002). The number of human leukocyte antigen (HLA-DR)–positive microglia is increased in possible AD compared to control cases and correlates with the appearance of Aβ in the possible AD cases. Tau (Tau-2) immunoreactivity is seen in definite AD cases only, which suggests that microglial activation is an important factor in early stages of AD (Vehmas et al., 2002).

Clusters of activated microglia can be found in the majority of neuritic plaques with a dense amyloid core (Fig. 45.1) and to a limited extent in primitive Aβ plaques (Sasaki et al., 1997; Vehmas et al., 2002; Veerhuis et al., 2003).

Besides fibrillarity of the Aβ, the simultaneous presence of serum amyloid P (SAP) component and C1q, the recognition unit of the classical pathway of complement activation, seems a prerequisite for clustering of activated microglia (Veerhuis et al., 2003).

	Aß PLAQUE TYPE			
Immuno-staining	NONFIBRILLAR		FIBRILLAR (neuritic)	
Aß	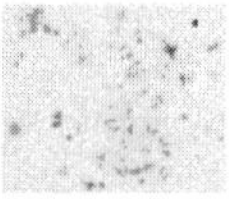 Irregularly shaped, diffuse	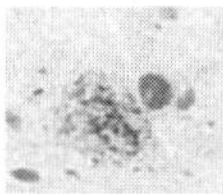 Circumscript (well demarcated)	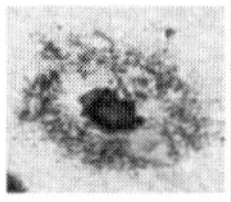 Classic with dense core	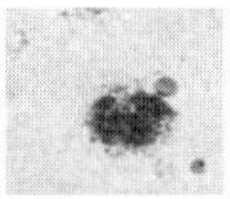 Primitive neuritic plaque
SAP	-	±	++*	+
C1q	-	±	++*	+
C4d	±	±	++*	+
C3d	±	±	++*	+
Tau (AT8)	-	-	+***	+
Clustered microglia**	-	-	++	±

FIGURE 45.1 Immunohistochemical distribution of serum amyloid P (SAP) component and complement activation products C1q, C4d, and C3d, as well as of activated microglia and hyperphosphorylated tau in morphologically distinguished cerebral Aβ plaque types. −: none; ±: maximally 50% of total; +: >75% of total; ++: all plaques.
*Much stronger immunostaining in the core than in the corona of classic plaques.
**Microglia markers KP-1 (CD68) and CR3/43 (HLA-DP/DQ/DR).
***The majority of classic amyloid β (Aβ) plaques in nondemented controls lacks tau immunoreactivity (AT8). (Adapted from Veerhuis et al., 2003.)

These findings are in line with those in Down syndrome (DS) frontal cortex specimens. Compacted Aβ plaques in all adult and old DS cases are to a large degree associated with complement factors C1q and C3 and contain activated microglia, reactive astrocytes, and dystrophic neurites. Young DS patients have predominantly diffuse-type Aβ plaques that are not detectably decorated with C1q or C3 and are devoid of microglia. Thus, the accumulation of complement activation products seems associated with the compactness of the Aβ deposits and parallels microglial activation and neurodegeneration (Stoltzner et al., 2000).

ROLE OF MICROGLIA IN ALZHEIMER'S DISEASE

Activated microglial cells may contribute to Aβ plaque formation by producing inflammatory mediators that influence APP synthesis and processing (Eikelenboom et al., 1994). Particularly in the vicinity of neuritic plaques, interleukin (IL)-1, IL-6, and tumor necrosis factor-α (TNF-α) immunoreactive microglia are found (Dickson et al., 1993; Griffin et al., 1995; Hüll et al., 1995). The functional significance of the increased cytokine expression in AD brains is still largely unknown. However, genetic studies indicate that polymorphisms of some Aβ plaque–associated pro-inflammatory cytokines (i.e., IL-1, IL-6, TNF-α) and acute-phase proteins [α1-antichymotrypsin (α1-ACT)] are genetic risks factors for AD (Kamboh et al., 1995; Nicoll et al., 2000; McCusker et al., 2001).

Interleukin-1, possibly in concert with Il-6, can regulate APP and Aβ production *in vitro* (Goldgaber et al., 1989; Rogers et al., 1999) and supposedly drives plaque evolution (Eikelenboom et al., 1994; Griffin et al., 1995). *In vivo*, a vicious circle may evolve whereby Aβ deposits stimulate further cytokine production by activated microglia, which in turn leads to even higher synthesis rates of APP and its Aβ fragments. In addition, IL-1 and IL-6 regulate acute phase protein production, some of which (α1-ACT and SAP) may control the rate of Aβ aggregation in plaques.

The role of microglial cells in the removal of plaque constituents was first suggested by Timmer, who—following up on Alzheimer's detailed account of the plaque-associated glial responses (Alzheimer, 1911)—reported that macroglia encapsulated the plaques, and that the core of senile plaques was formed by microglial cells that were mobilized to phagocytose toxic products (Timmer, 1925). Activated microglia that express HLA class II antigens, and in addition the β2-integrin α-chains CD11a, CD11b (CR3) and, more frequently, CD11c (CR4), are found in neuritic but not diffuse Aβ plaques in AD brain (Rozemuller et al., 1989b). These findings suggested that activated microglia can remove complement-opsonized Aβ fibrils or dystrophic neuronal elements in plaques through complement receptor–mediated phagocytosis.

In vitro studies have demonstrated that microglial cells can internalize Aβ aggregates (Paresce et al., 1997; Webster et al., 2001). Microglia slowly degrade Aβ. Therefore, when microglia encounter large amounts of Aβ, this leads to intracellular accumulation. Through the release of pro-inflammatory mediators and processing of the Aβ, microglia may even participate in the formation and growth of Aβ plaques (Paresce et al., 1997). Recent studies in transgenic mouse models for AD support the idea that activated microglia are involved in the removal of Aβ from the brain parenchyma. In Aβ-immunized human amyloid precursor protein (hAPP) transgenic mice, activated microglia were associated with remaining punctate Aβ deposits, suggesting that the diffuse Aβ plaques and the corona of the aggregated plaques had been cleared by the microglia (Schenk et al., 1999).

MICROGLIAL ACIVATION *IN VITRO*

Highly enriched human microglial cell cultures can be isolated from postmortem brain specimens of AD patients as well as from controls without neurological disease (Lue et al., 1996, 2001; De Groot et al., 2000). Adherent microglial cell cultures derived from human postmortem brain specimens grow as monolayer, express the leukocyte marker CD45, CD11c, CD68, and HLA-class II molecules DP, DQ, and DR, and remain viable for at least 3 weeks after isolation (De Groot et al., 2000) (Fig. 45.2). Human microglia express Fcγ receptors I and III, and to a lesser extent IIa and IIb; however, under inflammatory conditions, FcγR-IIa and -IIb expression is increased (Lue and Walker, 2002). Human microglia can secrete a variety of inflammatory mediators (Akiyama et al., 2000; Rogers et al., 2002), including complement factors, cytokines, chemokines, prostaglandins, and reactive oxygen species.

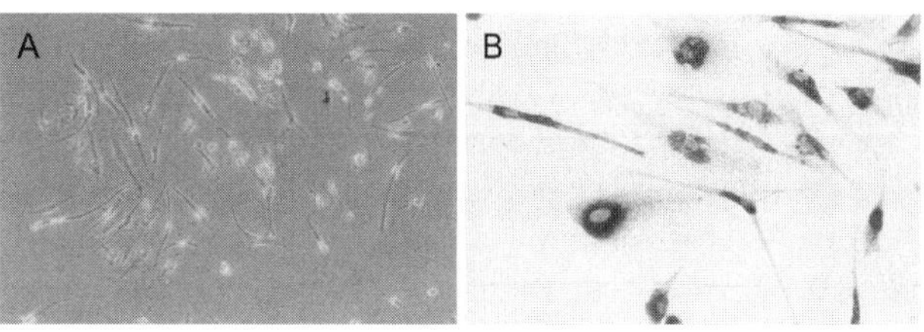

FIGURE 45.2 Human microglia isolated from subcortical white matter of postmortem adult brain. *A*. The predominant shape of isolated cells after 4 days in culture is unipolar or bipolar, with long processes. Cells exhibit bright cell bodies. Phase contrast photomicrography (10× enlargement). *B*. The adherent microglia are immunoreactive for CD68 (KP1 antibody). Hematoxylin counterstaining (40× enlargement).

The use of human microglia from adult brains offers many advantages over the use of rodent cells when research into various aspects of neurodegenerative diseases, and especially the early pathogenetic steps in AD, is performed *in vitro*. Most rodent microglial cells used in *in vitro* experiments are derived from newborn animals and mainly represent newly arrived monocytes rather than microglia.

Moreover, microglial cells in young and old rats respond differently to low doses of the pluripotent stimulator lipopolysaccharide (LPS) (Hauss-Wegrzyniak et al., 1999). Adult human microglia, when stimulated with LPS, secrete IL-6, TNF-α, and IL-10 (De Groot et al., 2001) but do not release IL-1α and IL-1β in measurable quantities, although these cytokines accumulate intracellularly (Veerhuis et al., 2003). In contrast, LPS-treated rodent microglia do not secrete TNF-α but do secrete IL-1 (Peyrin et al., 1999). Another important difference is that rodent cells secrete nitric oxide (NO) upon stimulation, whereas human cells do not (Walker et al., 2001).

Inflammation-based therapy design for AD has focused on cyclooxygenase (COX)-2–specific inhibitors to inhibit the deleterious actions of activated microglia in AD brain. *In vitro*, adult human microglia express COX-1, but not COX-2 mRNA and protein, and secrete low levels of prostaglandin E2 (PGE2) under basal conditions. Upon exposure to LPS, human microglia secrete high levels of PGE2 (De Groot et al., 2001) and have increased COX-2 mRNA and protein expression levels, whereas either the AD plaque–associated proinflammatory cytokines IL-1α, IL-1β, IL-6, TNF-α, or Aβ_{1-42} have no effect (Hoozemans et al., 2002). These findings correlate with the *in vivo* finding that microglia in AD-affected brain areas express COX-1 but not COX-2 (Yermakova et al., 1999; Hoozemans et al; 2001a) and demonstrate that human microglia *in vitro* can be used as a suitable model system to study the AD-related changes that occur *in vivo*.

Most studies report no direct stimulatory effects of Aβ on microglial cytokine release *in vitro* (Guilian, 1999), although in recent studies, preaggregated Aβ_{1-42} was shown to induce low levels of cytokine secretion by human microglia (Lue et al., 2001; Veerhuis et al., 2003).

Significant cytokine production and release of reactive oxygen species by Aβ-stimulated microglia *in vitro* requires costimulation with interferon-γ (IFN-γ), phorbol esters, or LPS (Meda et al., 1995; Van Muiswinkel et al., 1996). However, adult human microglia exposed to a mixture of Aβ_{1-42}, SAP, and C1q, a combination that is relevant to the *in vivo* situation, also secrete significantly higher levels of (pro-inflammatory) cytokines than cells treated with Aβ_{1-42} alone (Veerhuis et al., 2003). Whether this is due to increased Aβ fibrillarity or to interactions of SAP and C1q with microglial receptor sites remains elusive. Microglia are known to express receptors for C1q (Gasque et al., 2000; Webster et al., 2000).

In vitro, microglial cells secrete superoxide anion in response to C3-opsonized zymosan (Colton and Gilbert,1987; Banati et al., 1993). Pretreatment of microglia with Aβ_{1-40} (Van Muiswinkel et al., 1996) or C1q (Veerhuis et al., 2001) has a priming effect on the phorbol-myristate acetate (PMA)–induced respiratory burst and associated superoxide production. Furthermore, C1q and Aβ have synergistic effects on the oxidative burst of rat microglia (Veerhuis et al., 2001), suggesting that in the brain, complement activation products together with Aβ can stimulate microglia to produce potentially neurotoxic reactive oxygen intermediates.

In vitro, microglia can internalize fibrillar Aβ. Different types of receptors may be involved in the interaction of fibrillar Aβ with microglia, including receptors for end-glycation products receptor for advanced glycation endproducts (RAGE), Type A scavenger receptors (SR-A; Paresce et al, 1997), Fc receptors, complement receptors, and the low-density-lipoprotein receptor. Scavenger receptors-A are expressed by microglia near Aβ plaques (Christie et al., 1996) and account for a major part of Aβ uptake by microglia as judged from inhibition studies with fucoidan *in vitro* (Chung et al., 2001).

IMAGING OF MICROGLIAL ACTIVATION *IN VIVO*

Background and Rationale

The isoquinoline PK11195 is a specific ligand of the peripheral benzodiazepine binding site (PBBS), a site that is not related to the central benzodiazepine receptor associated with gamma-aminobutyric acid (GABA)–regulated channels (Gavish et al., 1999). Abundant in many peripheral organs, the PK11195-binding PBBS is minimally expressed in the normal brain *in vivo*. *In vivo* studies of conditions without blood–brain barrier damage demonstrate that the distribution pattern of increased PK11195 binding matches most closely the distribution of activated microglia rather than that of reactive astrocytes (Banati et al., 1997; Banati, 2002a). This finding is supported by high-resolution microautoradiography with [^{3}H](R)-PK11195 combined with immunohistochemical cell identification performed on the same tissue section in inflammatory diseases, such as multiple sclerosis and experimental allergic encephalomyelitis. Activated microglia, in areas where invading blood-borne cells are not a potential alternative site of binding, are thus the dominant source of binding in diseased brain tissue, including only subtly affected tissue without obvious histopathology and remote from the primary pathological focus (Banati et al., 2000).

Clinical Application

While the exact function of the PBBS has not yet been fully clarified, a clinical application for its specific ligand, PK11195, is the use as a carbon-11-labeled ligand for positron emission tomography (PET). [^{11}C](R)-PK11195 PET has been used to image active brain pathology in stroke (Banati et al., 2001), multiple sclerosis (Banati et al., 2000), herpes encephalitis (Cagnin et al., 2001a), vasculitis (Goerres et al., 2001), and AD (Cagnin et al., 2001b). The lack of significantly increased [^{11}C](R)-PK11195 binding in astrocyte-rich tissue, such as in stable epilepsy patients (low seizure frequency) with hippocampal sclerosis (Banati et al., 1999), supports the view that microglial (R)-PK11195 binding is the largest contributor to the PET signal measured *in vivo*. Also, long-established lesions identified as hypointense areas on magnetic resonance imaging (MRI) and known to be surrounded by reactive astrogliosis do not show an increased [^{11}C](R)-PK11195 PET signal (Banati et al., 2000).

Notwithstanding the final evaluation of the role of Aβ in AD, clinicopathological data confirming the strong correlation between volume densities of microglia and congophilic plaques (Arends et al., 2000) generally support the choice of using activated microglia as a target for imaging studies in AD. Recent data from [^{11}C](R)-PK11195 PET imaging demonstrated that mildly to moderately demented AD patients have a pattern of temporo-parietal signal increases, whereby the left temporal lobe appeared to be more prominently involved (Cagnin et al., 2001b) (Fig. 45.3). This may be the consequence of a selection bias since the studies focused on patients at earlier stages of the disease, in whom language, that is, left hemispheric deficits are more likely to be the first conspicuous clinical manifestations. While this is confirmation that the overall pattern of cognitive decline matches that of the anatomical distribution of the increased neuroinflammatory signal *in vivo*, a straightforward correlation of signal level with the severity of the dementia, using clinical rating scales, was not obvious. Again, this may not be too surprising, as microglial activation should reflect current disease activity rather than cumulative loss and an intellectual deficit that has been shown to be more closely correlated with the amount of Aβ deposition and neurofibrillary tangles (Arends et al., 2000). Follow-up investigations of AD patients after 1 year demonstrate that the regional increase in neuroinflammatory [^{11}C](R)-PK11195 binding, for example in the temporal lobe, to some extent anticipated the subsequent anatomical pattern of atrophy, as shown by MR-difference imaging (Cagnin et al., 2001a, 2001b). However, determining the extent to which microglial activation in patients with AD is an active promoter of neuronal damage requires more comprehensive knowledge about the particular disease state–related balance of detrimental and beneficial microglial activities.

In summary, the main clinical parameter that PET imaging of neuroinflammation is expected to provide is the rate of disease progression. Initial observations suggest that high signals can be seen in patients in whom the disease is not yet fully established (Cagnin et al., 2001b). This implies that the potentially greatest benefit of this imaging approach lies in the identification of early or possibly preclinical patients, who are also those most likely to profit from disease-slowing therapeutic intervention.

MICROGLIAL ACTIONS: GOOD OR BAD?

The local inflammatory response and microglial activation in AD has become the focuss of a therapeutic approach toward AD. However, microglia themselves,

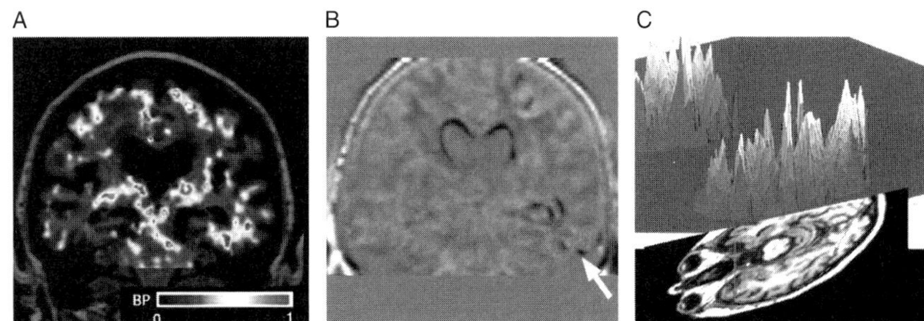

FIGURE 45.3 *A*. Alzheimer's disease patient with regionally increased [11C](R)-PK11195 signal most prominently in the left hemisphere. Bar denotes binding potential. (Cagnin et al., 2001b; Banati, 2002a.) *B*. The area of increased [11C](R)-PK11195 signal in the left temporal lobe shows progressive atrophic changes, as detected by magnetic resonance difference imaging 12 months after the [11C](R)-PK11195 scan was acquired (*arrow*; dark areas around the left ventricle and the temporal lobe indicate loss of volume). *C*. This contour plot illustrates the anterior-posterior gradient of the [11C](R)-PK11195 signal in the temporal lobe with higher values toward the posterior temporal lobe.

as well as inflammatory mediators, have neuropathic as well as neuroprotective actions.

Recent studies in transgenic mouse models (Wyss-Coray et al., 2002) illustrate well that instead of being deleterious, local complement activation and microglial activation can be beneficial through opsonization of Aβ deposits and their removal by activated microglial cells, respectively.

Transforming growth factor β (TGF-β) and hAPP double transgenic mice have high C3 levels and a reduced Aβ plaque load compared to control mice. Mice double transgenic for hAPP and sCrry (an inhibitor of C3 activation) (hAPP/sCrry mice) have two to three times more Aβ deposits than their hAPP transgenic littermates. Concomitant with the increase in Aβ deposits, the number of neurons and activated microglia decreased in the hippocampus and neocortex of hAPP/sCrry mice compared to control mice (Wyss-Coray et al., 2002).

Whether activation of microglia associated with Aβ deposits is good or bad is dependent on the time and place of activation and is complicated by intrinsic or concentration-dependent pleiotropic effects of the cytokines and other supposedly inflammatory mediators derived from activated microglia (Fig. 45.4). For instance, low-dose TNF-α and mild oxidative stress can induce the transcription of neuroprotective and/or anti-apoptotic genes, whereas excess levels of reactive oxygen species or TNF-α may cause neurotoxicity (Akiyama et al., 2000; Rozemuller and Van Muiswinkel, 2000).

Various experimental and human imaging studies based on measuring glial inflammatory responses with (R)-PK11195 appear to show evidence of both detrimental and beneficial microglial activities. In line with experimental data on the pattern of microglial activation, increased [^{11}C](R)-PK11195 PET signals are commonly observed in structurally normal-appearing regions remote from the primary lesion. For example, in stroke patients, increased [^{11}C](R)-PK11195 binding is regularly found in the ipsilateral thalamus, indicating the presence of activated microglia in the degenerating projection areas remote from the primary lesion in the cortex (Pappata et al., 2000). Similarly, patients recovering from unilateral herpes encephalitis show a distribution pattern of activated glial cells emerging over a period of months, which gradually propagates through the entire affected limbic system well beyond the initial lesion focus (Cagnin et al., 2001a). The increased [^{11}C](R)-PK11195 binding in these patients follows projecting axonal pathways, such as the large association bundles interconnecting mesocortical areas, subicular allocortices, and subcortical amygdaloid nuclei. While this can be interpreted as the result of Wallerian degeneration along the lesioned neural pathway, there is also some first evidence that peripheral denervation with long-lasting abnormal stimuli may also evoke a transsynaptic glial response beyond the first-order projection areas of the injured neural pathway. For example, increased [^{11}C](R)-PK11195 binding has been seen in the normal-appearing contralateral thalamus of patients who lost an arm 2 to 23 years ago and were suffering to various degrees from painful phantom sensations (Banati et al., 2001; Banati, 2002b). This increase in [^{11}C](R)-PK11195 binding in the thalamus but not in the somatosensory cortex indicates the presence of activated microglia, possibly as a consequence of subtle transneuronal changes. Formal histological confirmation is, however, still to come. The important implication, however, is that glial activation can occur transsynaptically and may be driven purely by altered neuronal activity. If confirmed, this would

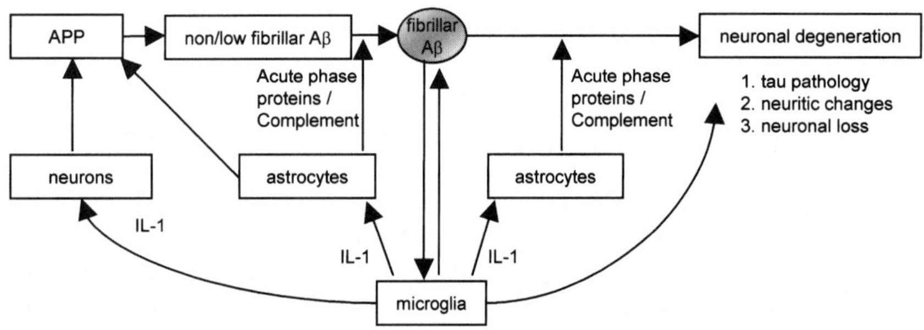

FIGURE 45.4 Key steps in the amyloid-driven cascade. Mismetabolism of the β-amyloid precursor protein (*βAPP*), spontaneously or as a result of environmental and/or genetic factors, results in enhanced production and deposition of β-amyloid (*Aβ*) in senile plaques. Activated microglia clustered In the vicinity of plaques with fibrillar Aβ deposits produce numerous factors including interleukin (IL)-1 and IL-6. These microglia derived factors may, in turn, stimulate βAPP expression, or may stimulate the synthesis of acute phase proteins that influence the conversion of nonfibrillar Aβ into fibrillar Aβ and may modulate the direct neurotoxic effects of Aβ. Other factors secreted by activated microglia (reactive oxygen species, excitotoxic amino acids) may have direct neurotoxic effects, leading to aggravation of the disease process. (Adapted from Eikelenboom et al., 2002.)

support the view that subtle activity-dependent microstructural changes in the thalamus are at least partially responsible for lasting rearrangements of the cortical representational maps (Jones, 2000) and that there is active gial participation in brain plasticity. In this specific context, microglial activation would not suggest tissue destruction but rather an adaptive process, possibly related to long-term brain plasticity.

One important factor of clinical relevance is that the presence of activated microglia per se may not equate with any damaging influence on the tissue, but may signify increased vulnerability to tissue damage (Koistinaho et al., 2002). That the latter can significantly modulate the disease course of any superimposed pathological condition, as may well be the case for age-related brain diseases, has been demonstrated in neuronal lesion models with an intact blood–brain barrier (Raivich et al., 1998; Flugel et al., 2001). Here the primary neuronal lesion triggers microglial activation and thus a state of locally increased *immune alertness* that then prepares secondarily a *site-directed* response by the peripheral immune system. This observation is important, as it points to the principal possibility that primarily neuronal pathology in the absence of overt blood–brain barrier damage can elicit secondary immune responses that themselves may contribute to further secondary disease progression.

THERAPEUTIC IMPLICATIONS

The involvement of inflammatory mechanisms in AD and the finding that a chronic inflammatory-like process takes place relatively early in the pathological cascade of the disease (Fig. 45.4), suggests the possibility of an inflammation-based approach as a therapeutic strategy aimed at preventing or retarding this chronic neurodegenerative disorder.

Because of the uncertainties about aspects of inflammation in AD, it is not surprising that two different inflammation-based therapeutic approaches have evolved: (*1*) the use of nonsteroidal anti-inflammatory drugs (NSAIDs) to reduce the inflammatory response and (*2*) vaccination to activate an inflammatory response.

Reduction of the Inflammatory Response Using Nonsteroidal Anti-Inflammatory Drugs

The idea of treating AD with anti-inflammatory drugs originated with the finding that a chronic inflammatory-like process and microglial responses occur in AD. That the neuroinflammatory response is an interesting therapeutic target for treatment with anti-inflammatory drugs was strongly supported by epidemiological studies showing that the use of classical NSAIDs can prevent or retard AD (McGeer et al., 1996; in 't Veld et al., 2001). However, recent publications on clinical trials in AD patients with anti-inflammatory drugs, such as prednisone, celecoxib (a specific COX-2 inhibitor), and hydrochloroquine, report a failure to slow the progression of dementia in AD (Aisen et al., 2000; Sainetti et al., 2000; Van Gool et al., 2001). Thus, with respect to the treatment options of AD patients with anti-inflammatory drugs, there seems to be a discrepancy between the epidemiological findings and the clinical trials with these drugs. Two major factors could determine the differences in outcome between epidemiological studies and drug trials: (*1*) the choice of drug and (*2*) the timing of the treatment. The positive epidemiological findings with NSAIDs are reported for the classical NSAIDs that are known to inhibit both COX-1 and COX-2. These, in addition, have other, non-COX-mediated, modes of action, such as activation of the nuclear receptor peroxisome proliferator-activated receptor-γ (PPARγ) and lowering of Aβ42 production (Landreth and Heneka, 2001; Weggen et al., 2001) or reduction of local C1q synthesis (Faust et al., 2002). Classic NSAIDs that were shown to reduce the risk of AD in epidemiological studies were recently studied in transgenic mice. Chronic dietary ibuprofen treatment of APPsw transgenic mice suppressed Aβ deposition and had a positive effect on behavioral changes in open field studies (Lim et al., 2001). The other explanation is the timing of anti-inflammatory treatment. Inhibition of the neuroinflammatory response at the time that clear symptoms of dementia are present might simply be too late to attenuate the detrimental effects of the inflammatory process. If that is the case, anti-inflammatory agents can be helpful in the prevention, but not the treatment, of AD.

Activation of the Immune System by Vaccination

Another inflammation-based therapeutic strategy for treatment is immunization with Aβ (Schenk et al., 1999). Antibodies against Aβ peptides could prevent Aβ from aggregating into fibrils or could stimulate the removal of Aβ by microglial cells. Amyloid β vaccination resulting in anti-Aβ antibodies in hAPP transgenic mice prevented memory loss in these animals (Morgan et al., 2000). A human Aβ vaccination trial encountered complications, however (Check, 2002). Further human studies await the outcome of investigations on whether other ways of immunization, or passive immunization rather than active immunization of a heterogeneous aging population, should be preferred.

The danger remains, however, that anti-Aβ antibodies bind to vascular amyloid and start an inflammatory reaction there, where normally no glial activation is seen (Verbeek et al., 1997).

Treatment with either anti-inflammatory drugs or immunization reflects opposite strategies in some respects. Treatment with anti-inflammatory drugs is based on reduction of the inflammatory process, whereas immunization leads to stimulation of the inflammatory process and more efficient phagocytic activity of macrophages/microglia. Since the early microglia-associated inflammatory mechanisms may have a dual role, the choice of therapy and the timing are difficult. Microglia may prevent potentially direct neurotoxic effects of Aβ through removal and breakdown. On the other hand, perhaps as a side product of the initially well-meant reaction to Aβ deposits, microglia may produce pro-inflammatory cytokines, reactive oxygen radicals, and complement factors, that either enhance the amyloid cascade or are neurotoxic.

One role may be more prominent in the earliest stages of the disease, whereas the other may be the predominant form in the end stages associated with neuronal loss. It is possible that the effects of immunization and drug therapy may act on different events in the pathological cascade. Accordingly, it will be necessary to investigate whether NSAIDs can interfere with the role of microglial cells in Aβ removal (Hoozemans et al., 2001b). On the other hand, there is the possibility that both strategies enhance each other's effects. In either case, the concept that microglia are involved in the pathogenesis of AD demands consideration in designing therapeutic strategies and warrants further investigation.

CONCLUSION

Neuroinflammatory processes (microglial activation as well as synthesis of inflammatory mediators) may have beneficial and deleterious effects with respect to the initiation and progression of AD-related neurodegenerative changes. Opposing effects, such as involvement in the production and removal of Aβ deposits, as well as neuroprotective and neurotoxic properties of microglial activation and inflammatory mediators, are described. Because it is still uncertain which mechanisms prevail, different approaches based on the knowledge that neuroinflammation is involved in AD may be pursued: (*1*) inhibition of the inflammatory reaction and thus potential slowing of the associated neurodegenerative changes, and (*2*) stimulation of a well-controlled neuroinflammatory glial response to remove Ab. Evolving new imaging approaches should enable monitoring of the effects of therapeutic compounds on microglia-mediated changes in the brain in vivo.

ACKNOWLEDGMENT

Richard B. Banati was supported by the Multiple Sclerosis Society of Great Britain and Northern Ireland, the Max-Planck-Institute of Neurobiology (Martinsried, Germany), and the Deutsche Forschungsgemeinschaft grant "The Mitochondrial Benzodiazepine Receptor as Indicator of Early CNS Pathology, Clinical Application in PET," the Medical Research Council, the European Community within the fifth framework program (QLK6-CT-1999-02004), and the International Institute for Research in Paraplegia, Zurich. Robert Verhuis and Piet Eikelenboom were supported by the European Community (BMH-4-98-6011 and QLK6-CT-1999-02004)

REFERENCES

Aisen, P.S., Davis, K.L., Berg, J.D., Schafer, K., Campbell, K., Thomas, R.G., Weiner, M.F., Farlow, M.R., Sano, M., Grundman, M., and Thal, L.J. (2000) A randomized controlled trial of prednisone in Alzheimer's disease. Alzheimer's Disease Cooperative Study. *Neurology* 54:588–593.

Akiyama, H., Barger, S., Barnum, S., Bradt, B., Bauer, J., Cole, G.M., Cooper, N.R., Eikelenboom, P., Emmerling, M., Fiebich, B.L., Finch, C.E., Frautschy, S., Griffin, W.S., Hampel, H., Hull, M., Landreth, G., Lue, L., Mrak, R., Mackenzie, I.R., McGeer, P.L., O'Banion, M.K., Pachter, J., Pasinetti, G., Plata-Salaman, C., Rogers, J., Rydel, R., Shen, Y., Streit, W., Strohmeyer, R., Tooyoma, I., Van Muiswinkel, F.L., Veerhuis, R., Walker, D., Webster, S., Wegrzyniak, B., Wenk, G., and Wyss-Coray, T. (2000) Inflammation and Alzheimer's disease. *Neurobiol. Aging* 21:383–421.

Alzheimer, A. (1911) Uber eigenartige Krankheitsfalle des späteren Alters. *Z. Gesamte Neurol. Psychiatrie*. 4:356–385. [Translation in: Banati, R.B., and Beyreuther, K. (1995) Alzheimer's disease. In: Kettenmann, H. and Ransom, B.R., eds. New York: Oxford University Press, pp. 1027–1043.]

Arends, Y.M., Duyckaerts, C., Rozemuller, J.M., Eikelenboom, P., and Hauw, J.J. (2000) Microglia, amyloid and dementia in Alzheimer's disease. A correlative study. *Neurobiol. Aging* 21:39–47.

Banati, R.B. (2002a) Visualising microglial activation in vivo. *Glia* 40:206–217.

Banati, R.B. (2002b) Brain plasticity and microglia: Is transsynaptic glial activation in the thalamus after limb denervation linked to cortical plasticity and central sensitisation? *J. Physiol. (Paris)*

Banati, R.B., Cagnin, A., Brooks, D.J., Gunn, R.N., Myers, R., Jones, T., Birch, R., and Anand, P. (2001) Long-term trans-synaptic glial responses in the human thalamus after peripheral nerve injury. *NeuroReport* 12:3439–3442.

Banati, R.B., Gehrman, J., Schubert, P., and Kreutzberg, G.W. (1993) Cytotoxicity of microglia. *Glia* 7:111–118.

Banati, R.B., Goerres, G.W., Myers, R., Gunn, R.N., Turkheimer, F.E., Kreutzberg, G.W., Brooks, D.J., Jones, T., and Duncan, J.S. (1999) [11C](R)-PK11195 positron emission tomography imaging of activated microglia in vivo in Rasmussen's encephalitis. *Neurology* 53:2199–2203.

Banati, R.B., Myers, R., and Kreutzberg, G.W. (1997) PK ("peripheral benzodiazepine")-binding sites in the CNS indicate early and discrete brain lesions: microautoradiographic detection of [3H]PK11195 binding to activated microglia. *J. Neurocytol.* 26:77–82.

Banati, R.B., Newcombe, J., Gunn, R.N., Cagnin, A., Turkheimer, F., Heppner, F., Price, G., Wegner, F., Giovannoni, G., Miller, D.H., Perkin, G.D., Smith, T., Hewson, A.K., Bydder, G., Kreutzberg, G.W., Jones, T., Cuzner, M.L., and Myers, R. (2000) The peripheral benzodiazepine binding site in the brain in multiple sclerosis: quantitative in vivo imaging of microglia as a measure of disease activity. *Brain* 123:2321–2337.

Brun, A. and Englund, E. (1981) Regional pattern of degeneration in Alzheimer's disease: neuronal loss and histopathological grading. *Histopathology* 5:549–564.

Cagnin, A., Brooks, D.J., Kennedy, A.M., Gunn, R.N., Myers, R., Turkheimer, F.E., Jones, T., and Banati, R.B. (2001a) In-vivo measurement of microglia in dementia. *Lancet* 358:461–467.

Cagnin, A., Myers, R., Gunn, R.N., Lawrence, A.D., Stevens, T., Kreutzberg, G.W., Jones, T., and Banati, R.B. (2001b) In vivo visualization of activated glia by [11C] (R)-PK11195-PET following herpes encephalitis reveals projected neuronal damage beyond the primary focal lesion. *Brain* 124:2014–2027.

Check, E. (2002) Nerve inflammation halts trial for Alzheimer's drug. *Nature* 415:426.

Christie, R.H., Freeman, M., and Hyman, B.T. (1996) Expression of the macrophage scavenger receptor, a multifunctional lipoprotein receptor, in microglia associated with senile plaques in Alzheimer's disease. *Am. J. Pathol.* 148:399–403.

Chung, H., Brazil, M.I., Irizarry, M.C., Hyman, B.T., and Maxfield, F.R. (2001) Uptake of fibrillar beta-amyloid by microglia isolated from MSR-A (type I and type II) knockout mice. *NeuroReport* 12:1151–1154.

Colton, C.A. and Gilbert, D.L. (1987) Production of superoxide anions by a CNS macrophage, the microglia. *FEBS Lett* 223: 284–288.

De Groot, C.J.A., Hulshof, S., Hoozemans, J.J.M., and Veerhuis, R. (2001) Establishment of microglial cell cultures derived from postmortem human adult brain tissue: immunophenotypical and functional characterization. *Microsc. Res. Tech.* 54:34–39.

De Groot, C.J.A., Montagne, L., Janssen, I., Ravid, R., Van der Valk, P., and Veerhuis, R. (2000) Isolation and characterization of adult microglial cells and oligodendrocytes derived from postmortem human brain tissue. *Brain Res. Protocols* 5:85–94.

Dickson, D.W., Lee, S.C., Mattiace, L.A., Yen, S.H., and Brosnan, C. (1993) Microglia and cytokines in neurological disease, with special reference to AIDS and Alzheimer's disease. *Glia* 7:75–83.

Eikelenboom, P., Bate, C., van Gool, W.A., Hoozemans, J.J.M., Rozemuller, J.M., Veerhuis, R., and Williams, A. (2002) Neuroinflammation in Alzheimer and prion disease. *Glia* 40:232–239.

Eikelenboom, P. and Veerhuis, R. (1996) The role of complement and activated microglia in pathogenesis of Alzheimer's disease. *Neurobiol. Aging* 17:673–680.

Eikelenboom, P., Zhan, S.S., van Gool, W.A., and Allsop, D. (1994) Inflammatory mechanisms in Alzheimer's disease. *Trends Pharmacol. Sci.* 15:147–150.

Faust, D., Akoglu, B., Zgouras, D., Scheuermann, E.-H., Milovic, V., and Stein, J. (2002) Anti-inflammatory drugs modulate C1q secretion in human peritoneal macrophages in vitro. *Biochem. Pharmacol.* 64:457–462.

Flugel, A., Bradl, M., Kreutzberg, G.W., and Graeber, M,B. (2001) Transformation of donor-derived bone marrow precursors into host microglia during autoimmune CNS inflammation and during the retrograde response to axotomy. *J. Neurosci. Res.* 66:74–82.

Gasque, P., Dean, Y.D., McGreal, E.P., VanBeek, J., and Morgan, B.P. (2000) Complement components of the innate immune system in health and disease in the CNS. *Immunopharmacology* 49:171–186.

Gavish, M., Bachman, I., Shoukrun, R., Katz, Y., Veenman, L., Weisinger, G., and Weizman, A. (1999) The enigma of the peripheral benzodiazepine receptor. *Pharmacol. Rev.* 51:629–650.

Goerres, G.W., Revesz, T., Duncan, J., and Banati, R.B. (2001) Imaging cerebral vasculitis in refractory epilepsy using [11C](R)-PK11195 positron emission tomography. *AJR Am. J. Roentgenol.* 176:1016–1018.

Goldgaber, D., Harris, H.W., Hla, T., Maciag, T., Donelly, R.J., Jacobsen, J.S., Vitek, M.P., and Gajdusek, D.C. (1989) Interleukin 1 regulates synthesis of amyloid beta-protein precursor mRNA in human endothelial cells. *Proc. Natl. Acad. Sci. USA* 86: 7606–7610.

Griffin, W.S.T., Sheng, J.G., Roberts, G.W., and Mrak, R.E. (1995) Interleukin-1 expression in different plaque types in Alzheimer's disease: significance in plaque evolution. *J. Neuropathol. Exp. Neurol.* 54:276–281.

Guilian, D. (1999) Microglia and the immune pathology of Alzheimer's disease. *Am. J. Hum. Genet.* 65:13–18.

Hauss-Wegrzyniak, B., Vraniak, P., and Wenk, G.L. (1999) The effects of a novel NSAID on chronic neuroinflammation are age dependent. *Neurobiol. Aging* 20:305–313.

Hoozemans, J.J.M., Rozemuller, A.J.M, Janssen, I., De Groot, C.J.A., Veerhuis, R., and Eikelenboom, P. (2001a) Cyclooxygenase expression in microglia and neurons in Alzheimer's disease and control brains. *Acta Neuropathol.* 101:2–8.

Hoozemans, J.J.M., Rozemuller, A.J.M., Veerhuis, R., and Eikelenboom, P. (2001b) Immunological aspects of Alzheimer's disease: therapeutical implications. *BioDrugs* 15:325–337.

Hoozemans, J.J.M., Veerhuis, R., Janssen, I., van Elk, E., Rozemuller, A., and Eikelenboom, P. (2002) The role of cyclo-oxygenase 1 and 2 activity in prostaglandin E(2) secretion by cultured human adult microglia: Implications for Alzheimer's disease. *Brain Res.* 951:218–226.

Hüll, M., Strauss, S., Volk, B., Berger, M., and Bauer, J. (1995) Interleukin-6 is present in early stages of plaque formation and is restricted to the brains of Alzheimer's disease patients. *Acta Neuropathol.* 89:544–551.

Hyman, B.T., Marzloff, K., and Arriagada, P.V. (1993) The lack of accumulation of senile plaques or amyloid burden in Alzheimer's disease suggests a dynamic balance between amyloid deposition and resolution. *J. Neuropathol. Exp. Neurol.* 52:594–600.

in 't Veld, B.A., Ruitenberg, A., Hofman, A., Launer, L.J., van Duijn, C.M., Stijnen, T., Breteler, M.M.B., and Stricker, B.H. (2001) Nonsteroidal antiinflammatory drugs and the risk of Alzheimer's disease. *N. Engl. J. Med.* 345:1515–1521.

Jones, E.G. (2000) Cortical and subcortical contributions to activity-dependent plasticity in primate somatosensory cortex. *Annu. Rev. Neurosci.* 23:1–37.

Kamboh, M.I., Sanghera, D.K., Ferell, R.E., and DeKosky, S.T. (1995) ApoE4-associated Alzheimer's disease risk is modified by α1-antichymotrypsin polymorphism. *Nat. Genet.* 10:468–488.

Koistinaho, M., Kettunen, M.I., Goldsteins, G., Keinanen, R., Salminen, A., Ort, M., Bures, J., Liu, D., Kauppinen, R.A., Higgins, L.S., and Koistinaho, J. (2002) Beta-amyloid precursor protein transgenic mice that harbor diffuse A beta deposits but do not form plaques show increased ischemic vulnerability: role of inflammation. *Proc. Natl. Acad. Sci USA* 99:1610–1615.

Koistinaho, M., Ort, M., Cimadevilla, J.M., Vondrous, R., Cordell, B., Koistinaho, J., Bures, J., and Higgins, L.S. (2001) Specific spatial learning deficits become severe with age in beta-amyloid precursor protein transgenic mice that harbor diffuse beta-amyloid deposits but do not form plaques. *Proc. Natl. Acad. Sci. USA* 98:14675–14680.

Landreth, G.E. and Heneka, M.T. (2001) Anti-inflammatory actions of peroxisome proliferator-activated receptor gamma agonists in Alzheimer's disease. *Neurobiol Aging* 22:937–944.

Lim, G.P., Yang, F., Chu, T., Gahtan, E., Ubeda, O., Beech, W., Overmier, J.B., Hsiao-Ashe, K., Frautschy, S.A., and Cole, G.M. (2001) Ibuprofen effects on Alzheimer pathology and open field activity in APPsw transgenic mice. *Neurobiol Aging* 22:983–991.

Lue, L.F., Brachova, L., Walker, D.G., and Rogers, J. (1996) Characterization of glial cultures from rapid autopsies of Alzheimer's and control patients. *Neurobiol. Aging* 17:421–429.

Lue, L.F., Kuo, Y.M., Roher, A.E., Brachova, L., Shen, Y., Sue, L., Beach, T., Kurth, J.H., Rydel, R.E. and Rogers, J. (1999) Soluble amyloid beta peptide concentration as a predictor of synaptic change in Alzheimer's disease. *Am. J. Pathol.* 155:853–862.

Lue, L.F., Rydel, R., Brigham, E.F., Yang, L.B., Hampel, H., Murphy, G.M.J., Brachova, L., Yan, S.D., Walker, D.G., Shen, Y., and Rogers, J. (2001) Inflammatory repertoire of Alzheimer's disease and nondemented elderly microglia in vitro. *Glia* 35:72–79.

Lue, L.F. and Walker, D.G. (2002) Modeling Alzheimer's disease immune therapy mechanisms: interactions of human postmortem microglia with antibody-opsonized amyloid beta peptide. *J. Neurosci. Res.* 70:599–610.

McCusker, S.M., Curran, M.D., Dynan, K.B., McCullagh, C.D., Urquhart, D.D., Middleton, D., Patterson, C.C., McIlroy, S.P., and Passmore, A.P. (2001) Association between polymorphism in regulatory region of gene encoding tumour necrosis factor alpha and risk of Alzheimer's disease and vascular dementia. *Lancet* 357:436–439.

McGeer, P.L. and McGeer, E.G. (2001) Inflammation, autotoxicity and Alzheimer's disease. *Neurobiol. Aging* 22:799–809.

McGeer, P.L., Schultzer, M., and McGeer, E.G. (1996) Arthritis and anti-inflammatory agents as possible protective factors for Alzheimer's disease: a review of 17 epidemiological studies. *Neurology* 47:425–432.

Meda. L., Cassatella, M.A., Szenddrei, G.I., Otvos, L.J., Baron, P., Villalba, M., Ferrari, D., and Rossi, F. (1995) Activation of microglial cells by β-amyloid protein and interferon-γ. *Nature* 374:647–650.

Morgan, D., Diamond, D.M., Gottschall, P.E., Ugen, K.E., Dickey, C., Hardy, J., Duff, K., Jantzen, P., DiCarlo, G., Wilcock, D., Connor, K., Hatcher, J., Hope, C., Gordon, M., and Arendash, G.W. (2000) A beta peptide vaccination prevents memory loss in an animal model of Alzheimer's disease. *Nature* 408:982–985.

Nicoll, J.A.R., Mrak, R.E., Graham, D.I., Stewart, J., Wilcock, G., MacGowan, S., Esiri, M.M., Murray, L.S., Dewar, D., Love, S., Moss, T., and Griffin, W.S.T. (2000) Association of interleukin-1 gene polymorphisms with Alzheimer's disease. *Ann. Neurol.* 47:365–368.

Pappata, S., Levasseur, M., Gunn, R.N., Myers, R., Crouzel, C., Syrota, A., Jones, T., Kreutzberg, G.W., and Banati, R.B. (2000) Thalamic microglial activation in ischemic stroke detected in vivo by PET and [11C] PK11195. *Neurology* 55:1052–1054.

Paresce, D.M., Chung, H., and Maxfield, F.R. (1997) Slow degradation of aggregates of aggregates of the Alzheimer's disease amyloid β-protein by microglial cells. *J. Biol. Chem.* 272:29390–29397.

Peyrin, J.M., Lasmézas, C.I., Haïk, S., Tagliavini, F., Salmona, M., Williams, A., Richie, D., DesLys, J.-P., and Dormont, D. (1999) Microglial cells respond to amyloidogenic PrP peptide by the production of inflammatory cytokines. *NeuroReport* 10:723–729.

Raivich, G., Jones, L.L., Kloss, C.U.A., Werner, A., Neumann, H., and Kreutzberg, G.W. (1998) Immune surveillance in the injured nervous system: T-lymphocytes invade the axotomized mouse facial motor nucleus and aggregate around sires of neuronal degeneration. *J. Neurosci.* 18:5804–5816.

Rogers, J., Strohmeyer, R., Kovelowski, C.J., and Li, R. (2002) Microglia and inflammatory mechanisms in the clearance of amyloid β peptide. *Glia* 40:260–269.

Rogers, J.T., Leiter, L.M., McPhee, J., Cahill, C.M., Zhan, S.S., Potter, H., and Nilsson, L.N. (1999) Translation of the Alzheimer amyloid precursor protein mRNA is upregulated by interleukin-1 through 5-untranslated region sequences. *J. Biol. Chem.* 274: 6421–6431.

Rozemuller, J.M., Eikelenboom, P., Pals, S.T., and Stam, F.C. (1989a) Microglial cells around plaques in Alzheimer's disease express leucocyte adhesion molecules of the LFA-1 family. *Neurosci. Lett.* 101:288–292.

Rozemuller, J.M., Eikelenboom, P., Stam, F.C., Beyreuther, K., and Masters, C.L. (1989b) A4 protein in Alzheimer's disease: primary and secondary cellular events in extra cellulair amyloid deposition. *J. Neuropathol. Exp. Neurol.* 48:674–691.

Rozemuller, J.M. and van Muiswinkel, F.L. (2000) Microglia and neurodegeneration. *Eur. J. Clin. Invest.* 30:469–470.

Sainetti, S.M., Ingrim, D.M., Talwalker, S., and Geis, G.S. (2000) Results of a double-blind, randomized, placebo-controlled study of celecoxib in the treatment of progression of Alzheimer's disease. In: *Proceedings of the Sixth international Stockholm/Springfield Symposium on Advances in Alzheimer Therapy*. Stockholm.

Sasaki, A., Yamaguchi, H., Ogawa, A., Sugihara, S., and Nakazato, Y. (1997) Microglial activation in early stages of amyloid β protein deposition. *Acta Neuropathol.* 94:316–322.

Schenk, D., Barbour, R., Dunn, W., Gordon, G., Grajeda, H., Guido, T., Hu, K., Huang, J., Johnson-Wood, K., Khan, K., Kholodenko, D., Lee, M., Liao, Z., Lieberburg, I., Motter, R., Mutter, L., Soriano, F., Shopp, G., Vasquez, N., Vandevert, C., Walker, S., Wogulis, M., Yednock, T., Games, D., and Seubert, P. (1999) Immunization with amyloid-attenuates Alzheimer-disease-like pathology in the PDAPP mouse. *Nature* 400:173–177.

Selkoe, D.J. (1991) The molecular pathology of Alzheimer's disease. *Neuron* 6:487–498.

Stoltzner, S.E., Grenfell, T.J., Mori, C., Wisniewski, K.E., Wisniewski, T.M., Selkoe, D.J., and Lemere, C.A. (2000) Temporal accrual of complement protein in amyloid plaques in Down's syndrome and Alzheimer's disease. *Am. J. Pathol.* 156:489–499.

Timmer, A.P. (1925) Der Anteil der Mikroglia und Makroglia am Aufbau der senilen Plaques. *Z. Neurol.* 98:43–58.

Van Gool, W.A., Weinstein, H.C., Scheltens, P.K., and Walstra, G.J. (2001) Effect of hydrochloroquine on progression of dementia in early Alzheimer's disease: an 18-month randomised, double-blind, placebo-controlled study. *Lancet* 358:455–460.

Van Muiswinkel, F.L., Veerhuis, R., and Eikelenboom, P. (1996) Amyloid β (Aβ) primes cultured rat microglial cells for an enhanced phorbol myristate-acetate induced respiratory burst activity. *J. Neurochem.* 66:2468–2476.

Veerhuis, R., Van Muiswinkel, F.L., Hack, C.E., and Eikelenboom, P. (2001) Role and regulation of early complement activation products in Alzheimer's disease. In: Rogers, J., ed. *Neuroinflammatory Mechanisms in Alzheimer's Disease: Basic and Clinical Research*. Basel, Boston, and Berlin: Birkhäuser Verlag AG, pp. 67–87.

Veerhuis, R., Van Breemen, M.J., Hoozemans, J.J.M., Morbin, M., Ouladhadj, J., Tagliavini, F., and Eikelenboom, P. (2003) Amyloid β plaque-associated proteins C1q and SAP enhance the A1–42 peptide induced cytokine secretion by adult human microglia in vitro. *Acta Neuropathol.* 105:135–144.

Vehmas, A.K., Kawas, C.H., Stewart, W.F., and Troncoso, J.C. (2002) Immune reactive cells in senile plaques and cognitive decline in Alzheimer's disease. *Neurobiol. Aging* 24:321–331.

Verbeek, M.M., Eikelenboom, P., and De Waal, R.M.W. (1997) Differences between the pathogenesis of senile plaques and congophilic angiopathy in Alzheimer's disease. *J. Neuropathol. Exp. Neurol.* 56:751—761.

Walker, D.G., Lue, L.-H., Klegeris, A., and McGeer, P.L. (2001) The involvement of glial cell-derived reactive oxygen and nitrogen species in Alzheimer's disease. In: Rogers, J., ed. *Neuroinflammatory Mechanisms in Alzheimer's Disease: Basic and Clinical Research*. Basel, Boston, and Berlin: Birkhäuser Verlag AG, pp. 173–195.

Webster, S.D., Galvan, M.D., Ferran, E., Garzon-Rodriguez, W., Glabe, C.G., and Tenner, A.J. (2001) Antibody-mediated phagocytosis of the amyloid beta-peptide in microglia is differentially modulated by C1q. *J. Immunol.* 166:7496–7503.

Webster, S.D., Park, M., Fonseca, M.I., and Tenner, A.J. (2000) Structural and functional evidence for microglial expression of C1qR(P), the C1q receptor that enhances phagocytosis. *J. Leukoc. Biol.* 67:109–116.

Weggen, S., Eriksen, J.L., Das, P., Sagi, S.A., Wang, R., Pietrzik, C.U., Findlay, K.A., Smith, T.E., Murphy, M.P., Butler, T., Kang, D.E., Marquez-Sterling, N., Golde, T.E., and Koo, E.H. (2001) A subset of NSAIDs lower amyloidogenic Abeta42 independently of cyclooxygenase activity. *Nature* 414:212–216.

Wyss-Coray, T., Yan, F.R., Lin, A.H.T., Lambris, J.D., Alexander, J.J., Quigg, R.J., and Masliah, E. (2002) Prominent neurodegeneration and increased plaque formation in complement-inhibited Alzheimer's mice. *Proc. Natl. Acad. Sci. USA* 99:10837–10842.

Yermakova, A.V., Rollins, J., Callahan, L.M., Rogers, J., and O'Banion, M.K. (1999) Cyclooxygenase-1 in human Alzheimer and control brain: quantitative analysis of expression by microglia and CA3 hippocampal neurons. *J. Neuropathol. Exp. Neurol.* 58: 1135–1146.

46 Peripheral neuropathy and the Schwann cell

RITA M. COWELL AND JAMES W. RUSSELL

THE AXON AND THE SCHWANN CELL IN NORMAL PERIPHERAL NERVE

The Schwann cell (SC) is the sole source of myelin for peripheral nerves. During axon growth in development, SC precursors proliferate and migrate to the axon, establishing a 1:1 myelinating relationship with a larger-diameter axon or ensheathing a number of smaller axons (Jessen and Mirsky, 1991; Bunge, 1993). Schwann cells are also responsible for determining the structural organization of the node of Ranvier (Arroyo and Scherer, 2000), as well as for mediating the spacing and clustering of sodium channels in the axonal membrane and the separation of sodium from potassium channels (Maier et al., 2002). At the node of Ranvier, where SC ensheathment of the axon is absent, there is a reduction in the size of the axon, and neurofilament phosphorylation is reduced. As a result, there is an increase in neurofilament density, probably due to a decreased negative charge on the neurofilament side arms and repelling of neurofilaments (Mata et al., 1992).

A correlation between axonal diameter and myelination has been observed in many species (Bunge, 1993; Elder et al., 2001), suggesting that the extent of myelination may depend on properties of the axon. In fact, axons are critically important in development of the myelin sheath (Martini, 2001). As an example, nonmyelinating SCs can be transformed into myelinating SCs after replacement of small-caliber axons with large-caliber axons (Aguayo et al., 1976). This implies that signals released from the developing axon may directly regulate myelination.

Reciprocal signaling between SCs and neuronal axons is important in development and maintenance of the peripheral nervous system (PNS) (Bunge, 1993). This chapter highlights the dependence of peripheral nerve function on SCs and presents evidence that alterations in SC protein expression and viability are responsible, in part, for diverse peripheral neuropathies.

Myelin Proteins and Hereditary Peripheral Neuropathy

Heritable peripheral neuropathies provide the most insight into the dependence of peripheral nerve on SC function. Heritable neuropathies including Charcot-Marie-Tooth (CMT) disease, hereditary neuropathy with liability to pressure palsies (HNPP), congenital hypomyelinating neuropathy (CHN), and Roussy-Lévy syndrome are caused by mutations in genes that encode myelin or SC-specific proteins (Table 46.1).

Understanding the normal regulation of intrinsic and extrinsic control of SC-axon interaction and myelination in the PNS is important in elucidating the intricate disease processes that lead to peripheral neuropathy. Myelinating SCs in the peripheral nerve express numerous cell adhesion molecules that are critical in normal SC function and SC-axon interactions (Fig. 46.1). Interestingly, heritable neuropathies often result from mutations in genes encoding one or several of these adhesion molecules, including peripheral myelin protein 22 (PMP22), myelin protein 0 (P0), and connexin 32 (Cx32) (for review see Scherer, 1997; Snipes and Orfali, 1998). Mutations in proteins that function to fasten myelin sheaths to the basal lamina, like periaxin, also can result in peripheral neuropathy. The first section of this chapter reviews PMP22, myelin P0, Cx32, and periaxin and their involvement in myelin formation and peripheral nerve function. Other, more recently discovered mutations and the corresponding proteins are listed in Table 46.1; these will not be covered in detail in this chapter.

Peripheral Myelin Protein 22

Peripheral myelin protein 22 (PMP22), a four-transmembrane domain (4-TM) myelin protein, accounts for 5% of the total myelin protein content in the PNS compact myelin and contributes to myelin stability and maintenance (for review see Muller, 2000). Duplication of or point mutations in chromosome 17p11.2–12 (PMP22) are associated with CMT IA (Thomas et al.,

TABLE 46.1 *Affected Proteins and the Associated Genetic Mutations Linked to Inherited Neuropathies*

Affected Protein	*Protein Characteristics*	*Gene Locus*	*Associated Neuropathy*
PMP22	4-TM protein; myelin stability and maintenance	17p11.2–12	CMT IA and III, Roussy-Lévy syndrome, HNPP
P0	Extracellular immunoglobulin domain; forms homotetramers; adhesion of compact myelin	1q22	CMT1B, II, and III, Roussy-Levy syndrome, and CHN
Connexin 32	4-TM protein; form pores in SC membranes for the passage of ions between layers of myelin	Xq13–22	CMT X
Periaxin	Role in SC–basal lamina associations	19q13	CMT IV
EGR2	Zinc finger transcription factor for PMP22, P0, Cx32, and periaxin genes	10q21.1–22.1	CMT III, CHN
Neurofilament light chain	Component of axonal cytoskeleton	8p21	CMT II
LITAF	Expressed in sciatic nerve; role in protein degradation pathways	16p13.1–p12.3	CMT IC
MTMR1/2	Pseudophosphatase myotubularin, peripheral nerve development	Xq28	CMT IVB1
SBF2/MTMR13	Pseudophosphatase myotubularin, phosphoinositide signaling	11p15	CMT IVB2
GDAP1	Expression in neural tissue and SCs; developmentally regulated	8q21	CMT IVA

CHN: congenital hypomyelinating neuropathy; CMT: Charcot-Marie-Tooth Disease; Cx32: connexin-32; EGR2: early growth response factor 2; GDAP1: ganglioside-induced differention-associated protein-1; HNPP: hereditary neuropathy with liability to pressure palsy; LITAF: lipopolysaccharide-induced tumor necrosis factor-a factor; MTMR: myotubularin-related gene; P0: myelin protein zero; PMP22: peripheral myelin protein 22; SBF2: SET binding factor 2; SC: Schwann cell; 4-TM: 4 transmembrane domain protein.

1997). Despite similar mutations in the majority of patients, the clinical syndrome is quite variable, ranging from subclinical disease to very severe weakness (Dyck et al., 1993). Some patients may also have additional features such as essential tremor (Roussy-Lévy syndrome) (Thomas et al., 1997), which may involve missense mutations of the *P0* gene (see below) (Plante-Bordeneuve et al., 1999).

Most patients with HNPP demonstrate a deletion of the 17p11.2–12 region containing the *PMP22* gene (Chance et al., 1993). In a minority of cases there is a loss of function point mutation in the *PMP22* gene (Lenssen et al., 1998). Patients with HNPP exhibit prominent myelin reduplication (tomaculae) consisting of redundant folds or loops of the myelin sheath. Mice with a null mutation for the *PMP22* gene exhibit similar pathological changes (Adlkofer et al., 1995); these animals have abundant tomaculae at birth and later develop demyelination and axonal loss, indicating that PMP22 is necessary for development of the peripheral nerve and maintenance of the axon and myelin sheath.

Protein 0

Protein 0 is the major protein component in peripheral myelin and is responsible for adhesion of compact myelin (Shapiro et al., 1996). Protein 0 traverses the membrane once and mediates adhesion in concentric myelin wraps. The adhesion is attributed to the extracellular immunoglobulin domain of P0 that forms a tetrameric array interlocking with a similar array in the opposing membrane (Fig. 46.1) (Shapiro et al., 1996). Protein 0 also forms a heterophilic interaction with the transmembrane protein PMP22 via the L2/HNK-1 epitopes of their glycosidic links (Griffith et al., 1992).

Several types of CMT result from mutations in the *P0* gene. A point mutation of the gene coding for myelin P0 (17p11.2–12) (Bird et al., 1997) is associated with CMT1B; pathological changes similar to those in *PMP22* mutations are observed. *Protein 0* mutations may also result in the clinical phenotype seen in CMT II, CMT III, congenital hypomyelinating neuropathy, and Roussy-Lévy syndrome (De Jonghe et al., 1999). Associated genetic defects include chromosome duplication and missense point mutations of the *P0* protein gene (Plante-Bordeneuve et al., 1999). Some patients with CMT II have a specific Thr124Met mutation of the *P0* gene (De Jonghe et al., 1999).

The P0-deficient mouse provides strong evidence that the SC is important in maintaining axonal integrity (Frei et al., 1999). Protein 0 is expressed by SC and not by motorneurons or sensory neurons, yet animals deficient in P0 develop not only severe demyelination but also a pronounced axonal pathology. When axons are ensheathed with mutant SC, their caliber is reduced and their cytoskeleton is severely damaged. It is possible that the reduction in axonal caliber is associated with reduced axonal transport resulting in distal axonal degeneration (de Waegh et al., 1992).

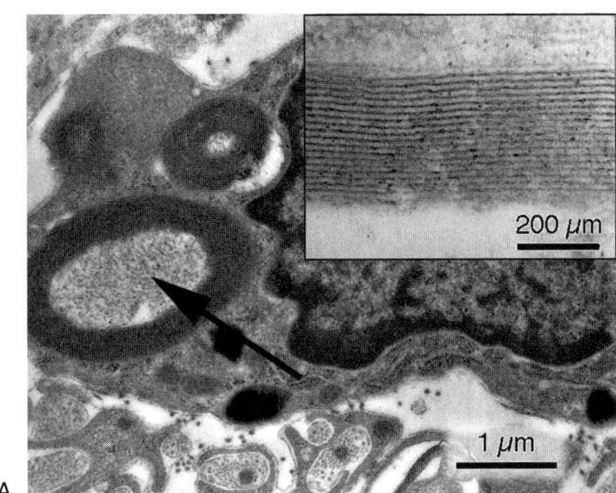

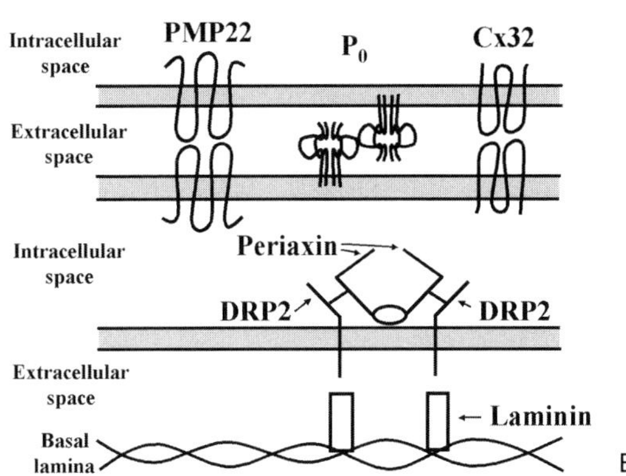

FIGURE 46.1 Myelin structure in the peripheral nerve. *A*. A large axon (*arrow*) is surrounded by concentric rings of Schwann cell (SC) cytoplasm that form the myelin sheath. The major dense lines (black: cytoplasm) and the interperiod lines (white: extracellular space) of myelin lamellae are evident in the inset. N: SC nucleus. *B*. Proteins that mediate interactions between myelin lamellae and between SCs and the basal lamina. Several proteins such as peripheral myelin protein 22kD (*PMP22*), myelin protein P0 (*P0*), and connexin 32 (*Cx 32*) mediate interactions between separate myelin laminae by binding to their structurally identical counterparts on the apposing myelin membrane. Periaxin, on the other hand, links molecules of dystrophin-related protein 2 (*DRP2*), resulting in the strong adhesion of SCs to the basal lamina. The figure was drawn with reference to Scherrer (1997) and Sherman et al. (2001).

Connexin 32

The connexins are a family of homologous 4-TM integral membrane proteins that form channels providing a low-resistance pathway for the transmission of electrical signals and the diffusion of small ions and other molecules between adjacent layers of myelin (Scherer et al., 1995). For thick myelin sheaths, the direct radial pathway through connexins can be nearly 1000 times shorter than the circumferential pathway through the SC cytoplasm (Scherer et al., 1995). Normal cellular signaling may be dependent on the pathways provided by the connexins; thus, any loss of the gap junctions could lead to demyelination and axonal loss. Mutations of connexins are associated with various other human diseases (for review see Abrams et al., 2000), and connexins are critical for normal myelination in the central nervous system (Menichella et al., 2003).

Connexin 32 is concentrated in the paranodal loops and Schmidt-Lanterman incisures of the PNS myelin. Despite its broad expression pattern (kidney, intestine, liver, spleen, stomach, pancreas, uterus, testes, brain, and peripheral nerve, peripheral neuropathy (CMT X) (Nicolson and Menter, 1995; Silander et al., 1997) is the sole clinical manifestation of Cx32 mutations. Possible mechanisms by which Cx32 mutations may disrupt cellular communication include failure of normal transcription of mRNA for Cx32 (Ionasescu et al., 1996), failure of normal translation due to a nonsense mutation or rapid degredation of RNA (Deschenes et al., 1997), failure of normal protein transport to the membrane (Deschenes et al., 1997), or failure of normal docking of hemichannels (Castro et al., 1999).

Periaxin

Periaxin is important in normal PNS myelination and exists in two isoforms due to alternate gene splicing: S-periaxin (cytoplasm) and L-periaxin (plasma membrane) (Dytrych et al., 1998). During myelination, L-periaxin is predominantly located at the adaxonal (apical) membrane, but once myelination is complete, it is localized at the abaxonal (basal) membrane (Gillespie et al., 1994), where the PDZ motif is important in organizing protein-protein interactions (Sheng, 1996). Mutations in the peraxin gene cause an inherited demyelinating neuropathy in humans (Guilbot et al., 2001); however, in periaxin-null mice, initial PNS myelination is normal, implying that periaxin is not essential for myelination to occur. Interestingly, these animals develop a late-onset demyelinating neuropathy (Gillespie et al., 2000) in which sensory deficits predominate and increases in myelin thickness are followed by phases of demyelination and remyelination.

The observed phenotype of periaxin-null mice may result from the disruption of SC–basal lamina associations. Periaxin has been shown to mediate linkage of dystrophoglycan-related protein 2 (DRP2) molecules in mature SCs (Sherman et al., 2001). Dystrophoglycan-related protein 2 binds to laminin expressed on the basal lamina, anchoring SCs to the extracellular matrix. In addition, the DRP2/periaxin complex is linked to a complex containing a short dystrophin isoform, Dp116

(Sherman et al., 2001). Splice site mutations in the human dystrophin gene also cause a demyelinating neuropathy in humans (Comi et al., 1995).

Transcription Factors Early Growth Response 2 (EGR2 or Krox-20) and Oct-6

Early growth response 2 is a zinc finger transcription factor that regulates the expression of PMP22, P0, Cx32, and periaxin (Nagarajan et al., 2001), thereby contributing to the maturation of SC and myelination of the peripheral axon (Kamholz et al., 1999). Mutated ERG2 causes hypomyelination of the PNS due to a block of SC at an early stage of differentiation. Genetic mutations in EGR2 are associated with both CHN and severe CMT I (Kamholz et al., 1999). The zinc finger mutations affect the capability of DNA binding, and the amount of residual binding directly correlates with disease severity (Warner et al., 1999). Schwann cells in mice lacking expression of EGR2 establish a 1:1 relationship with axons, but myelination does not occur (Topilko et al., 1994).

In contrast, in mice lacking expression of the POU domain transcription factor, Oct 6 [also called *suppressed cyclic AMP-inducible POU* (SCIP) and Tst 1], myelination is only delayed, not completely blocked (Bermingham et al., 1996). Thus Oct 6 is not necessarily important for the transition to myelination, but rather for its timing.

This section highlighted the evidence indicating that numerous heritable peripheral neuropathies result from genetic defects in SC and myelin proteins. In contrast to heritable peripheral neuropathies, acquired inflammatory neuropathy and diabetic neuropathy are not due to alterations in SC protein expression but rather to direct injury to SCs, myelin sheaths, and the associated axons. First, we will discuss the pathophysiology of acquired inflammatory neuropathy, with a focus on the inflammatory processes that lead to myelin destruction and axonal degeneration.

ACQUIRED INFLAMMATORY NEUROPATHY

Acquired demyelinating neuropathies include acute inflammatory demyelinating neuropathy (AIDP) and chronic inflammatory demyelinating neuropathy (CIDP). The incidence of AIDP is 1–2/100,000 per year (Schonberger et al., 1981), while the prevalence of CIDP is approximately 1–2% (Lunn et al., 1999). Clinical variants of AIDP include acute motor-sensory axonal neuropathy, acute motor axonal neuropathy, Miller Fisher syndrome, and Guillian-Barré syndrome (GBS). Each has its own characteristic set of symptoms, including a severe, progressive paralysis with sensory loss (acute motor-sensory axonal neuropathy) and the acute loss of distal sensory function with preservation of strength (GBS).

Autoantibodies and Inflammatory Neuropathy

The exact causes of inflammatory peripheral neuropathy are unknown; however, the overriding hypothesis is that peripheral nerve inflammation results from an autoimmune response leading to the direct attack on myelin or neuronal proteins by the immune system (for review see Maurer et al., 2002b). This is supported by the observation that the development of pathology, especially in AIDP, is often preceded by infection by viruses that contain oligosaccharide structures identical to those of peripheral nerve gangliosides (reviewed in Willison and Yuki, 2002). Approximately 50% of persons with AIDP have antibodies specific to gangliosides GM1 or GD1a (Takigawa et al., 2000), which are identical in structure to outer core structures of *Campylobacter jejuni* HS:19. Infected individuals, when mounting an immune response to the pathogen, inadvertently produce antibodies against their own peripheral nerve. There is some evidence that these antibodies may play a pathogenetic role in the disease (Kanda et al., 2000) by inhibiting Na^+ current conductance, leading to an abnormality of nerve conductance (Takigawa et al., 2000). In addition, autoantibodies may provide the primary stimulus for macrophage recruitment and activation via interaction with macrophage Fc receptors (Trotter et al., 1986). Demyelination may also result from the formation of antibodies to myelin proteins. Antibodies to PMP22 are associated with 52% of cases of AIDP and 35% of cases of CIDP but only 3% of other neuropathies (Gabriel et al., 2000). In animal models of inflammatory neuropathy, passive transfer of antibodies to P0 cause conduction block and demyelination in rats (Yan et al., 2001).

The T Cell Response and Macrophage Recruitment

The recognition of antigens by autoantibodies stimulates an immune response resulting in the clonal expansion of autoreactive T cells (reviewed in Maurer et al., 2002b). Normal patrolling of tissues by the autoreactive T cells brings them into proximity with their antigens and causes activation; activated T cells can release cytokines and chemokines, which recruit monocytes and macrophages to the site of the autoantigen (see below). The causal relationship between autoreactive T cell activation and the development of acquired inflammatory neuropathies has been confirmed by studies in which the transfer of T cells reactive for P0 peptides from one animal to another induced experimental autoimmune neuritis (EAN) in the acceptor animal (Olee et al., 1990).

In both AIDP and CIDP, there is evidence of mononuclear cellular infiltration and segmental demyelination (Asbury et al., 1969; Arnason and Soliven, 1993), where SCs form onion bulbs in an attempt to remyelinate the nerve segment. In active disease, macrophages penetrate the basement membrane around the fiber and displace the SC cytoplasm. The macrophage infiltration leads to focal lysis of the superficial myelin lamellae followed by penetration of the macrophage processes along interperiod lines. Macrophages then surround the denuded axon and phagocytose myelin debris. Infiltrates are observed not only in peripheral nerves, but also in cranial nerves, nerve roots, dorsal root ganglia (DRG), and autonomic ganglia (Asbury et al., 1969; Arnason and Soliven, 1993).

Currently, there is a debate as to whether macrophages are beneficial or detrimental to myelination and cell survival in neurodegenerative disease (Diemel et al., 1998; Kiefer et al., 2001). Studies with an animal model of GBS (EAN) have demonstrated that macrophage depletion inhibits development of the disease and slows disease progression (Jung et al., 1993). However, macrophages are not only required for the removal of cell debris but can release factors that promote both neuronal survival and axonal regeneration. Production of the cytokine interleukin-1 (IL-1) by infiltrating macrophages induces the expression of nerve growth factor (NGF) by SCs in injured nerve, stimulating regeneration (Lindholm et al., 1987). It is likely that macrophages play distinctly different roles, depending on the type, phase, and severity of the disease (Kiefer et al., 2001). In models of heritable neuropathies, for instance, the inhibition of T cell and macrophage infiltration reduces nerve injury (reviewed in Maurer et al., 2002a).

Cytokines and Chemokines

Many of the detrimental effects of macrophage recruitment may be due to the production of cytokines by both T cells and macrophages (reviewed in Zhu et al., 1998). Macrophages are sources of IL-1, IL-12, tumor necrosis factor-α (TNF)-α and IL-6, whereas T cells produce interferon-γ, inducing the expression of major histocompatibility complex II on macrophages, thereby increasing their efficacy as antigen-presenting cells (reviewed in Kiefer et al., 2001). While cytokines may enhance the inflammatory response, they can promote neuronal survival as well; the cytokine leukemia inhibitory factor has been shown to mediate insulin-like growth factor (IGF-I) expression after peripheral nerve injury (De Pablo et al., 2000), and a 45% increase in neuronal death after nerve transection has been observed in IL-6 knockout mice (Murphy et al., 1999).

Recent data implicate chemokines as additional mediators of inflammation within injured nerve (reviewed in Fujioka et al., 1999). Chemokines, a group of small (8–13 kDa), soluble, structurally related cytokines, regulate immune cell recruitment to sites of inflammation or injury through interactions with G-protein-coupled, membrane-bound receptors. In particular, the expression of the chemokine macrophage inflammatory protein 1α (MIP-1α/CCL3) peaks before the height of severity of symptoms in EAN, and its inhibition blocks macrophage infiltration and demyelination in the injured nerve (Zou et al., 1999). Other chemokines, such as monocyte chemoattractant protein (MCP-1), may also play key roles in macrophage recruitment. Sources of chemokines in EAN include macrophages, SCs, and endoneurial vessels (Orlikowski et al., 2003).

T Cell–Schwann Cell Interactions

The activation of autoreactive T cells is believed to play a large part in the propagation of the autoimmune response. T cell activity in inflammatory neuropathy is evidenced by an increased serum level of TNF-α in 25% of patients with CIDP; the TNF-α level correlates with severity and progression of the disease (Misawa et al., 2001). Schwann cells may contribute to T cell activation by expressing the costimulatory molecules CD80 (B7-1) and CD58 (LFA-3). CD80 expression is induced in myelinating SCs in AIDP and CIDP nerve (Kiefer et al., 2000), and both SCs and endothelial cells express CD58 in CIDP (Van Rhijn et al., 2000). Schwann cells have also been shown to act as antigen-presenting cells. These data indicate that SC may initiate and even propagate T cell activation in the inflamed peripheral nerve (Van Rhijn et al., 2000).

Complement Activation

In addition to having direct effects on axons and SCs, autoimmune antibodies can activate the complement cascade, resulting in the tagging of dead cells for removal by macrophages, chemoattraction of leukocytes, and formation of a membrane attack complex, lysing the target cell (Fig. 46.2). Immunoglobulins IgG and IgM stimulate activation of the classical complement cascade by binding complement component C1q, eventually resulting in formation of C3 and C5 convertases and the deposition of C3b and the membrane attack complex (MAC) (for review see Sahu and Lambris, 2000). Cleavage of native C3 and C5 results in the production of the potent chemoattractants C3a and C5a, which may mediate macrophage infiltration (Springer, 1994).

In EAN, depletion or inhibition of complement activation prevents the onset of axonal degeneration, suggesting that complement-mediated lysis may be involved in SC and myelin damage (Vriesendorp et al., 1998). In fact, deposition of the MAC has been ob-

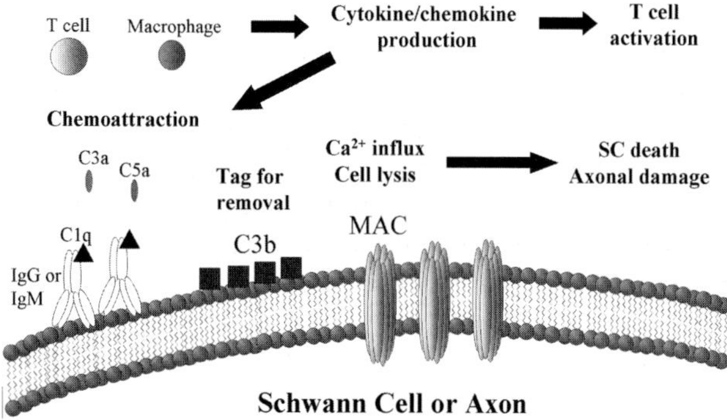

FIGURE 46.2 Inflammatory processes involved in acquired inflammatory peripheral neuropathies. In the initial phase of the disease, autoantibodies to gangliosides, myelin proteins, or neuronal proteins are deposited on Schwann cells (SCs) or axons. These antibodies may fix complement component C1q, resulting in the eventual deposition of the opsonin C3b and the membrane attack complex (*MAC*). In addition, the potent chemoattractants C3a and C5a are released, stimulating the infiltration of macrophages and T cells. Both T cells and macrophages may be sources of cytokines and chemokines, which, in addition to influencing the T cell activation state, can recruit additional macrophages and T cells. Schwann cell death and axonal damage may be mediated by MAC formation or by the toxic effects of macrophages (see text). IgG, IgM: immunoglobulins G and M.

served prior to myelin degradation and demyelination. In light of the considerable evidence that autoimmune antibodies are involved in the pathology, it is possible that fixation of antibodies to SCs and axonal membranes results in local complement activation and the initial recruitment of macrophages.

DIABETIC NEUROPATHY AND THE SCHWANN CELL

Diabetic neuropathy is the most common cause of peripheral neuropathy in the Western world and occurs in approximately 50% of diabetic patients over time (Pirart, 1978). The clinical manifestations of diabetic neuropathy are variable; however, the majority of affected patients develop a symmetrical distal and predominantly sensory neuropathy. True weakness is far less common, although a small number of patients may develop a polyradiculopathy associated with significant weakness. Diabetes is also associated with the development of mononeuropathies such as carpal tunnel syndrome and compressive ulnar neuropathy. The Diabetes Control and Complications Trial (DCCT; 1993) established a clear link between impaired glycemic control and neuropathy and showed that intensive glycemic control reduced the appearance of neuropathy by up to 70%. However, despite current optimal glycemic control diabetic patients continue to develop neuropathy, implying that other factors, possibly related to transient hyperglycemia, are implicated in the pathogenesis of diabetic neuropathy.

Schwann cells and myelin, as well as neuronal cell bodies and axons, are injured by hyperglycemia-induced dysregulation of intracellular metabolic pathways. Multiple etiologies have been proposed, including vascular insufficiency and ischemia, oxidative injury, protein glycation, and altered polyol metabolism (reviewed in Sheetz and King, 2002). Classically, many of the microvascular complications of diabetic neuropathy were thought to be due to axonal ischemia induced by impairment of neurovascular flow. Pathologically, numerous microvascular abnormalities have been described, including endothelial cell activation and proliferation, basement membrane reduplication, and monocyte and/or pericyte adhesion (Cameron et al., 2001), and reductions in these changes correlate with recovery from neuropathy. Furthermore, treatments aimed directly at improving neurovascular flow or improving metabolic regulation are important in ameliorating neuropathy (Cameron et al., 2001). However, neuropathy may develop in diabetic patients with minimal vascular ischemia (Russell and Feldman, 2001) or may not occur in patients with other evidence of ischemic complications. Thus, it is unclear if endothelial changes and impairment of neurovascular regulation are a primary cause of neuropathy or are due to the underlying destruction of SCs and peripheral axons.

Ultrastructural Abnormalities in Diabetic Neuropathy

In tissue from diabetic patients, there is evidence of mitochondrial (Mt) enlargement, SC apoptosis (programmed cell death), and marked axonal degeneration in sensory nerves (Fig. 46.3) (Vincent et al., 2002). Similar changes are observed in animal models of diabetes. The most commonly used animal model involves the injection of streptozotocin (STZ), a drug that destroys the insulin-producing cells of the pancreas.

Dramatic ultrastructural changes are evident in DRG neurons and SCs of STZ-treated rats. Prominent cytoplasmic vacuolation is present in both DRG neurons and SCs, and vacuoles are present in ballooned Mt with disrupted cristae. As evidence of apoptosis, there is condensation of chromatin and shrinkage of the nucleus and cell cytoplasm, with preservation of the cytoplasmic membrane (Sasaki et al., 1997; Russell et al., 1999; Vincent et al., 2002). Figures 46.4 and 46.5 demonstrate the appearance of apoptotic DRG neurons and SCs, respectively.

The issue of axon and ORG loss in diabetic rats is controversial (Zochodne et al., 2001). While some studies suggest that there is no loss of axons in diabetic rats (see Sharma and Thomas, 1987, for review), others have described degenerative changes and axonal loss in mixed nerves (Sharma and Thomas, 1987). Evidence of apoptosis is observed in both DRG neurons (Fig. 46.4) and SC (Fig. 46.5) *in vivo*; in addition, small re-

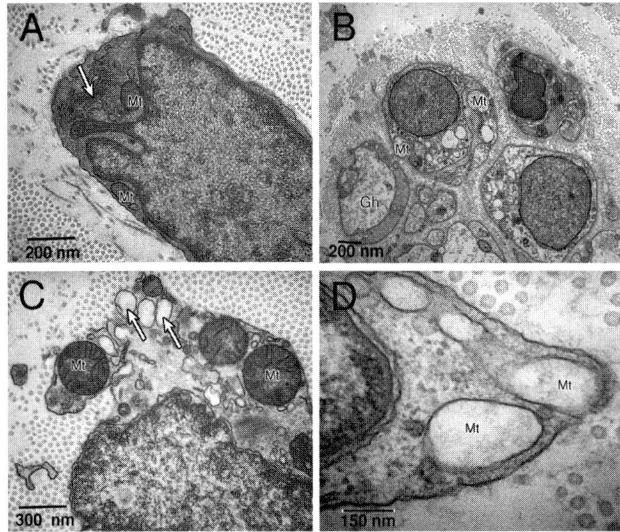

FIGURE 46.3 In human Schwann cells (SCs), there is swelling and disruption of the mitochondrium (*Mt*) and of the rough endoplasmic reticulum (RER). Schwann cell transmission electron micrographs (TEMs) were from normal human controls and patients with moderately severe diabetic neuropathy. *A*. Control SC: normal Mt and RER (*white arrow*). *B–D*. Diabetic SC: There are multiple enlarged Mt within the SC, with disruption of the normal cristae structure and formation of cytoplasmic vacuoles (*white arrows*) (Vincent et al., 2002). (Reprinted by permission from Vincent et al., 2002, Ann NY Acad Sci. copyright 2002 New York Academy of Sciences, U.S.A.)

ductions in the number of neurons, particularly the largest neurons (Kishi et al., 2002), are accompanied by loss of myelinated axons (Russell et al., 1999; Zochodne et al., 2001; Kishi et al., 2002; Vincent et al., 2004). In diabetic animals there is also evidence of myelin splitting in myelinated axons in the dorsal root.

Oxidative Injury and Diabetic Neuropathy

Evidence from several sources indicates that oxidative stress due to hyperglycemia-induced generation of reactive oxygen species (ROS) is an important mechanism leading to both the development and progression of neuropathy (Russell et al., 2002; Vincent et al., 2002, Vincent et al., 2004) and the ultrastructural changes noted above. Blocking oxidative stress using the antioxidant DL-alpha-lipoic acid in the diabetic animal prevents the development of neuropathy (Stevens et al., 2000) and restores sciatic and saphenous nerve conduction velocities in the STZ diabetic rat (Low et al., 1997).

Increased metabolic flux in the Mt due to a high glucose load causes an increase in the formation of ROS such as superoxides and highly reactive hydroxyl radicals (Fig. 46.6) (Russell et al., 2002). The reaction of superoxides with nitric oxide (formed by nitric oxide synthase) produces the toxic by-product peroxynitrite, resulting in membrane lipid peroxidation, nitration of proteins, energy depletion, degradation of DNA, and eventual apoptosis (Russell et al., 1999, 2002; Lowell et al., 2004). Concurrently, accumulation of reduced nicotine adenine dinucleotide (NADH), coupled with failure of the Mt creatine phosphate pump to regenerate adenine triphosphate (ATP) from adenine diphosphate (ADP), disrupts the Mt electron transfer chain and depletes ATP (Green and Reed, 1998).

Mitochondrial dysfunction can also lead directly to cell death by activating the caspase cascade. Caspases are a group of developmentally conserved proteases that, when activated, initiate and propagate a highly regulated series of reactions inducing apoptosis (for review, see Yuan and Yankner, 2000). Generation of

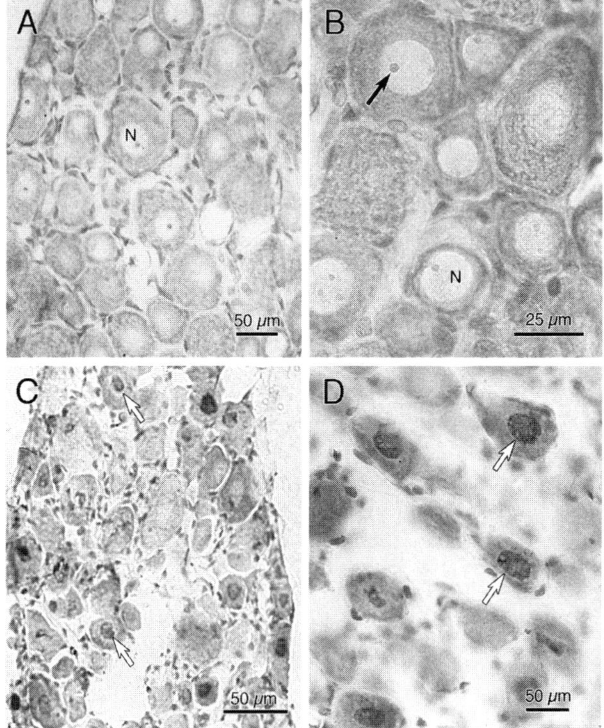

FIGURE 46.4 Hyperglycemia in streptozotocin-treated rats (*C,D*) induces apoptotic changes in dorsal root ganglion (DRG) neurons and Schwann cells compared to control animals (*A,B*). Dorsal root ganglion apoptotic nuclei were stained using the TdT-mediated dUTP-biotin nick end labeling (TUNEL) technique, and then the sections were counterstained with methyl green. *A*. Low magnification view of numerous nonapoptotic DRG neurons with normal pale nuclei (*N*). No apoptotic neurons are observed in these control sections and were rare in other control sections. *B*. Higher magnification with clear neuronal nuclei (*N*) and darker staining chromatin in the nucleolus (*arrow*). *C*. Lower magnification of DRG from diabetic animals showing numerous apoptotic neuronal nuclei (*arrows*) interspersed with nonapoptotic neurons (TUNEL staining negative) consistent with programmed cell death in single cells. *D*. Higher magnification showing nuclear chromatin condensation staining positively with the TUNEL technique (*arrows*) (Russell et al., 1999). (Reprinted from *Neurobiology of Disease*, copyright (1999), with permission from Elsevier Science.)

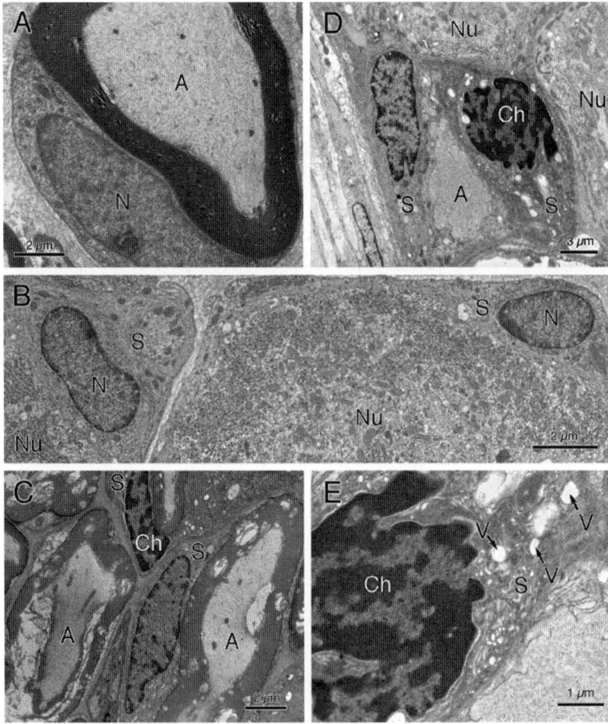

FIGURE 46.5 Electron micrograph of Schwann cells (SC) from control and streptozotocin (STZ)-treated diabetic rats. Control animals (*A,B*) and STZ-treated rats made diabetic for 1 month (*C–E*). *A*. Control SC showing normal diffuse chromatin staining in the nucleus (*N*), and a normal axon (*A*) with intact myelin lamellae showing little or no myelin splitting. *B*. Satellite cells (*S*), which are Schwann-like cells, from a control animal showing normal diffuse chromatin staining in the nucleus (*N*) and cytoplasm. The satellite cells lie adjacent to dorsal root ganglion (DRG) neurons (*Nu*) that show normal cytoplasmic components. *C*. In the dorsal root from diabetic animals, there is clumping of the chromatin (*Ch*) in the SC (*S*), atrophy of axons (*A*), and disruption of myelin surrounding the axons. *D*. In satellite cells (*S*) from a diabetic DRG, there is severe chromatin clumping (*Ch*), shrinkage of the perikaryon, and prominent vacuolation. An atrophic axon (*A*) is seen nestled between two Schwann-like satellite cells, adjacent to DRG neurons (*Nu*), which also show evidence of perikaryal vacuolation. *E*. End-stage changes in a diabetic Schwann cell (*S*). There is nuclear chromatin clumping and fragmentation (*Ch*) coupled with prominent vacuolation (*V*) resulting from ballooning of mitochondria and disruption of their cristae. Bars in each panel indicate magnification (Delaney et al., 2001). (Reproduced with permission from the *Journal of Neuropathology and Experimental Neurology*.)

ROS and the loss of Mt membrane potential ($\Delta\Psi_M$) can stimulate the release of cytochrome c into the cytosol, activating the caspase cascade. One current hypothesis is that hyperglycemia leads to SC and DRG apoptosis via the production of ROS. In support of this idea, inhibition of the glucose-induced generation of ROS with myxothiazole and thenoyltrifluoroacetone (TTFA), or prevention of $\Delta\Psi_M$ loss with bongkrekic acid, blocks induction of caspase cleavage and apoptosis (Russell et al., 2002).

Besides its roles in ROS production, glucose depletes endogenous pools of antioxidants, further potentiating ROS-mediated cellular injury. Detoxification of hydrogen peroxide (H_2O_2), generated from superoxide, occurs primarily in the Mt, where it is reduced by glutathione. Reduction of H_2O_2 by glutathione peroxidase or catalase generates oxidized glutathione disulfide, which in turn must be reduced by nicotinamide adenine dinucleotide phosphate (NADPH) to regenerate glutathione. Therefore, NADPH is required to maintain intracellular levels of glutathione. However, hyperglycemia leads to increased intracellular glucose flux through the aldose reductase (AR) pathway, depleting NADPH when reducing glucose to sorbitol. Despite promising results with AR inhibitors in experimental diabetes and small clinical studies (Greene et al., 1999), the results in large human studies of diabetic neuropathy have been less encouraging.

Diabetes is also associated with glycation of proteins called *advanced glycation end products* (AGEs). These proteins may modify a wide variety of extracellular and intracellular proteins, and AGE formation augments ROS generation by a process known as *autooxidative*

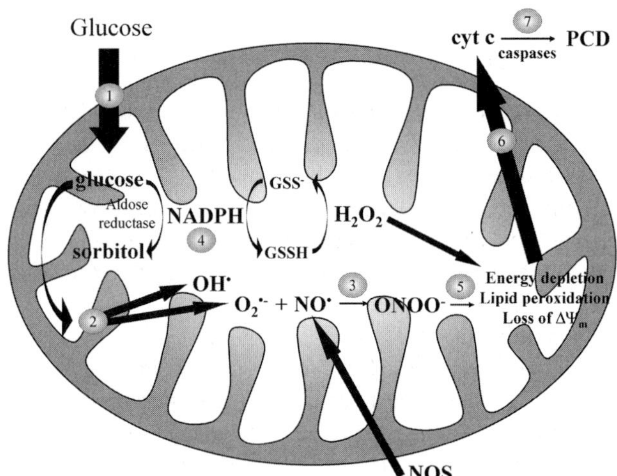

FIGURE 46.6 Oxidative stress as a stimulus for Schwann cell apoptosis in diabetic neuropathy. (*1*) The glucose supply to the mitochondrion (Mt) is increased in diabetic conditions. (*2*) A high glucose load stimulates the production of reactive oxygen species (ROS), such as the hydroxyl radical (*OH·*) and superoxides ($O_2\cdot^-$). (*3*) $O_2\cdot^-$ reacts with nitric oxide (*NO·*) produced by nitric oxide synthase (*NOS*), to form peroxynitrite (*ONOO*$^-$). (*4*) A reduction in cellular nicotinamide adenine dinucleotide phosphate (*NADPH*) levels results from activation of the aldose reductase pathway as well as from the usage of NADPH to regenerate glutathione (*GSSH*) to detoxify hydrogen peroxide (*H_2O_2*). This reduces the capacity of the Mt to neutralize ROS, favoring the production of $ONOO^-$. (*5*) $ONOO^-$ causes cellular energy depletion, DNA damage, and lipid peroxidation of Mt and other cellular proteins, resulting in a loss of Mt membrane potential ($\Delta\Psi_m$). (*7*) A loss of $\Delta\Psi_m$ stimulates the release of cytochrome c, which induces apoptosis (programmed cell death, *PCD*) by activating the caspase cascade.

glycosylation. During the normal course of aging, AGEs irreversibly modify proteins in a process called the *Maillard reaction*, leading to tissue "browning"; it is hypothesized that diabetic neuropathy may represent a form of premature aging of the nervous system.

Advanced glycation end products bind to a cell surface receptor the AGE receptor (RAGE), which activates several downstream signaling pathways, including protein kinase C (PKC) and the transcription factor NFκB. NFκB is associated with endothelial dysfunction, impaired nerve blood flow, and ischemia (Brownlee, 2001). Activation of PKC isoforms (α, β, δ, ε, ξ) is reported in some but not all tissues prone to diabetic complications (Ishii et al., 1998). Increased glycolytic pathway flux or AR pathway activity promotes *de novo* diacylglycerol (DAG) synthesis by glycerol-3-phosphate following an increase in intracellular glyceraldehyde-3-phosphate. Chronically elevated DAG, in turn, increases PKC activity. Activation of PKC promotes vasoconstriction and ischemia, increased permeability, nitric oxide dysregulation, and increased leukocyte adhesion, further inducing diabetic neuropathy. High-affinity PKC β inhibitors such as ruboxistaurin mesylate are being evaluated for treatment of human diabetic neuropathy.

Growth Factors in Normal and Diabetic Peripheral Nerve

Growth factors play an important role in myelination and maintenance of the axon, and studies are underway to determine if growth factors can promote myelination in disease states. In particular, the p75 neurotrophin receptor (p75NTR) positively regulates myelination by SCs in the PNS. Brain-derived neurotrophic factor (BDNF) probably promotes myelination by binding to p75NTR on glial cells; in contrast, neurotrophin-3 (NT3) inhibits myelination (Cosgaya et al., 2002). Expression of p75NTR is present in nonmyelinating but not myelinating glial cells and is increased in SC after nerve injury. Interestingly, neurons rather than glial cells are the major source of BDNF.

Insulin-like growth factor-I is also critical in myelination both *in vitro* and *in vivo*. Animals that overexpress IGF-I have a larger number of myelinated axons than normal littermates (Carson et al., 1993), and mice that overexpress insulin-like growth factor binding protein-1 (IGFBP-1; inhibits expression of IGF-I) have a significantly decreased number of myelinated axons in the central nervous system with thinner myelin sheaths (Ye et al., 1995). In cocultures of rat DRG and SCs, IGF-I promotes SC migration and the attachment of SC to axons (Russell et al., 2000).

Insulin-like growth factor-I may influence myelination by enhancing P0 expression. Insulin-like growth factor-I increases P0 protein expression and myelination in a dose-dependent fashion in SC-axonal cocultures (Fig. 46.7), probably by interacting with IGF-I receptors on SCs (Russell et al., 1998; Russell et al., 2000). Insulin-like growth factor-I treatment is essential for both the initiation of long-term myelination and, in part, for the determination of myelin thickness in axon-SC cocultures. In IGF-I −/− and IGF-I +/− animals axon size is reduced, and improvement in peripheral nerve conduction studies occurs with addition of IGF-I (Gao et al., 1999).

Several neurotrophic factors such as NGF, BDNF, IGF-I, and NT-3 may be reduced in diabetes, and administration of these factors may protect against diabetic neuropathy in animals (Hellweg and Hartung, 1990; Russell et al., 1999; Schmidt et al., 2001; Seyers et al., 2003; Simm et al., 2003). While normal NGF expression may prevent neuronal oxidative stress by increasing intracellular concentrations of reduced glutathione (GSH) and catalase in neurons (Sampath et al., 1994), impaired trophic support, such as the reduction in NGF expression seen in diabetic neuropathy, may cause increased peroxinitrite formation and cleavage of caspases (Park et al., 1998). Administration of NGF in experimental hyperglycemia regulates

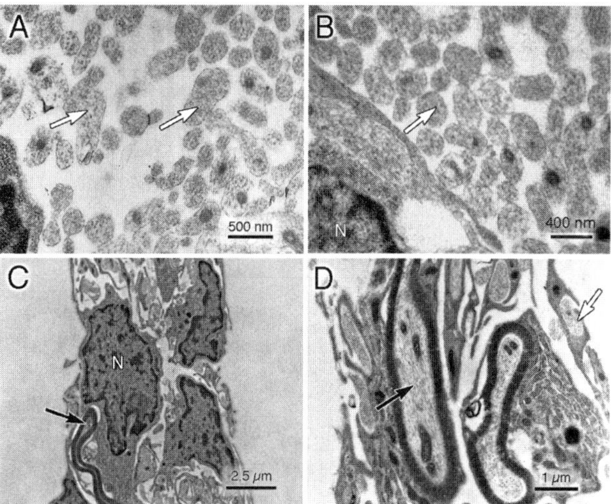

FIGURE 46.7 Transmission electron microscopy showing myelination of dorsal root ganglion (DRG) axons in vitro with insulin-like growth factor-I (IGF-I). Dissociated DRG and Schwann cells (SC) were cultured for 21 days in serum and insulin-free defined medium. *A*. Dorsal root ganglion/SC cocultures in medium alone (control) showing healthy unmyelinated axons (*white arrows*). *B*. Higher magnification shows the nucleus (*N*) of an adjacent SC. There are no SC processes extending and ensheathing the axons despite the close apposition of SC and axon. *C*. With 1 nM IGF-I there is myelination of a few individual axons (*black arrow*), although many axons remain unmyelinated. *D*. Higher magnification of *C* shows myelinated axons (*black arrow*) and, in addition, extensive attachment and ensheathment of unmyelinated axons (*white arrow*) by SC processes (Russell et al., 2000). (Reproduced with permission from the *Journal of Neuropathology and Experimental Neurology*.)

changes in the $\Delta\Psi_M$ and blocks membrane depolarization and induction of programmed cell death (PCD) in SC, probably through regulation of p75NTR (Vincent et al., 2002). Other growth factors such as BDNF may improve glycemic control, and may have a potential role in the treatment and prevention of diabetic neuropathy (Tonra et al., 1999).

Growth factors may activate several signaling proteins including PKC, p38 kinase, extracellular signal-regulated kinase (ERK), and c-jun N-terminal kinase (JNK), causing transcriptional changes and alterations in cell survival (Sheetz and King, 2002). Activation of PKC can affect the production of oxidants by activation of oxidases such as NADP(H) oxidase (Sheetz and King, 2002), and PKC may also prevent cellular injury to neurons or SCs by influencing the expression of Bcl-2-related proteins. Certain members of the Bcl-2 family, including Bcl-2, Bcl-xL, and Bag-1, act as inhibitors of cell death upstream of the caspase cascade (Reed, 1997). Protein kinase C activation upregulates Bcl-xL and Bcl-2, blocking the pro-apoptotic effect of AGEs (Giardino et al., 1996; Park et al., 1998), and both Bcl-2 and Bag-1 inhibit the generation of ROS after NGF withdrawal. While the mechanisms of action are not fully known, studies indicate that Bcl-2 stabilizes the inner Mt membrane, thus preventing the release of cytochrome c and caspase activation (Srinivasan et al., 2000).

Growth factors may also regulate other key Mt proteins to prevent induction of apoptosis. Upregulation of uncoupling protein 1 (UCP1) is mediated through increased expression of phosphoinositide-3 kinase (PI 3K) or mitogen-activated protein kinase (MAPK)/MAP-extracellular signal regulated kinase (MEK), critical signaling intermediates of both NGF and IGF-I (Valverde et al., 1997; Teruel et al., 1998). Growth factor–mediated regulation of the $\Delta\Psi_M$ by UCPs could reduce generation of ROS and prevent induction of neuronal and SC apoptosis (Vincent et al., 2002; Vincent et al., 2004).

Unfortunately, despite promising results in animal models of experimental diabetic neuropathy, growth factors have not shown significant benefit in the treatment of human diabetic neuropathy. Initial promising results in quantitative sensory tests of cold and vibration sense, and a global impression of improvement, were obtained in a phase II study in which patients randomly received either placebo or one of two doses of recombinant human NGF. Unfortunately, a larger phase III study of NGF showed no benefit (Apfel et al., 2000). In a phase II trial of human recombinant BDNF, a small improvement was observed in the cold detection threshold, but not in other quantitative sensory tests or in intra-epidermal nerve fiber measurements (Wellmer et al., 2001).

CONCLUSIONS

A normal axon-SC structural relationship is necessary for integrity of the PNS and is regulated by a variety of intrinsic structural proteins and signaling pathways. In inherited neuropathies, abnormal expression of myelin proteins causes SC dysfunction and results in demyelination and axonal loss. In acquired inflammatory neuropathies, autoimmune responses involving macrophage recruitment, complement activation, cytokine production, and T cell activation cause demyelination coupled with axonal injury. The etiology of diabetic neuropathy is complex and involves changes in vascular reactivity, metabolic pathways, oxidative stress, and regulation of a variety of signaling pathways. Many of these mechanisms are interrelated and result in injury to both the SC and the axon. From this review of peripheral neuropathies, it is clear that nerve function is dependent on SC function and myelin integrity. Future studies will focus on ways to stabilize myelin and inhibit SC apoptosis to improve outcome for the millions of people affected by these debilitating diseases.

ACKNOWLEDGMENTS

The authors would like to thank Ms. Denice Janus for secretarial assistance. The authors were supported in part by NIH Grant NS42056, The Juvenile Diabetes Research Foundation Center for the Study of Complications in Diabetes (JDRF), the Office of Research Development (Medical Research Service) and Geriatric Research Educational and Clinical Center (GRECC), Department of Veterans Affairs (JWR), and NIH Neurology Training Grant (2 T32 NS07222; RMC).

REFERENCES

Abrams, C.K., Oh, S., Ri, Y., and Bargiello, T.A. (2000) Mutations in connexin 32: the molecular and biophysical bases for the X-linked form of Charcot-Marie-Tooth disease. *Brain Res. Brain Res. Rev.* 32:203–214.

Adlkofer, K., Martini, R., Aguzzi, A., Zielasek, J., Toyka, K.V., and Suter, U. (1995) Hypermyelination and demyelinating peripheral neuropathy in *Pmp22*-deficient mice. *Nat. Genet.* 11:274–280.

Aguayo, A.J., Charron, L., and Bray, G.M. (1976) Potential of Schwann cells from unmyelinated nerves to produce myelin: a quantitative ultrastructural and radiographic study. *J. Neurocytol.* 5:565–573.

Apfel, S.C., Schwartz, S., Adornato, B.T., Freeman, R., Biton, V., Rendell, M., Vinik, A., Giuliani, M., Stevens, J.C., Barbano, R., and Dyck, P.J. (2000) Efficacy and safety of recombinant human nerve growth factor in patients with diabetic polyneuropathy: a randomized controlled trial. *JAMA* 284:2215–2221.

Arnason, B. and Soliven, B. (1993) Acute inflammatory demyelinating neuropathy. In: Dyck, P. and Thomas, P., eds. *Peripheral Neuropathy* Philadelphia: W.B. Saunders, pp. 1437–1497.

Arroyo, E.J. and Scherer, S.S. (2000) On the molecular architecture of myelinated fibers. *Histochem. Cell Biol.* 113:1–18.

Asbury, A.K., Arnason, B.G., and Adams, R.D. (1969) The inflammatory lesion in idiopathic polyneuritis: its role in pathogenesis. *Medicine* 48:173–215.

Bermingham, J.R., Jr., Scherer, S.S., O'Connell, S., Arroyo, E., Kalla, K.A., Powell, F.L., and Rosenfeld, M.G. (1996) Tst-1/oct-6/scip regulates a unique step in peripheral myelination and is required for normal respiration. *Genes Dev.* 10:1751–1762.

Bird, T.D., Kraft, G.H., Lipe, H.P., Kenney, K.L., and Sumi, S.M. (1997) Clinical and pathological phenotype of the original family with Charcot-Marie-Tooth type 1B: a 20-year study. *Ann. Neurol.* 41:463–469.

Brownlee, M. (2001) Biochemistry and molecular cell biology of diabetic complications. *Nature* 414:813–820.

Bunge, R.P. (1993) Expanding roles for the Schwann cell: ensheathment, myelination, trophism and regeneration. *Curr. Opin. Neurobiol.* 3:805–809.

Cameron, N.E., Eaton, S.E., Cotter, M.A., and Tesfaye, S. (2001) Vascular factors and metabolic interactions in the pathogenesis of diabetic neuropathy. *Diabetologia* 44:1973–1988.

Carson, M.J., Behringer, R.R., Brinster, R.L., and McMorris, F.A. (1993) Insulin-like growth factor I increases brain growth and central nervous system myelination in transgenic mice. *Neuron* 10:729–740.

Castro, C., Gomez-Hernandez, J.M., Silander, K., and Barrio, L.C. (1999) Altered formation of hemichannels and gap junction channels caused by C-terminal connexin-32 mutations. *J. Neurosci.* 19:3752–3760.

Chance, P.F., Alderson, M.K., Leppig, K.A., Lensch, M.W., Matsunami, N., Smith, B., Swanson, P.D., Odelberg, S.J., Disteche, C.M., and Bird, T.D. (1993) DNA deletion associated with hereditary neuropathy with liability to pressure palsies. *Cell* 72: 143–151.

Comi, G.P., Ciafaloni, E., de Silva, H.A., Prelle, A., Bardoni, A., Rigoletto, C., Robotti, M., Bresolin, N., Moggio, M., and Fortunato, F. (1995) A G+1 $\rightarrow$ A transversion at the 5′ splice site of intron 69 of the dystrophin gene causing the absence of peripheral nerve Dp116 and severe clinical involvement in a DMD patient. *Hum. Mol. Genet.* 4:2171–2174.

Cosgaya, J.M., Chan, J.R., and Shooter, E.M. (2002) The neurotrophin receptor p75NTR as a positive modulator of myelination. *Science* 298:1245–1248.

Cowell, R.M. and Russell, J.W. (2004) Nitrosative injury and antioxidant therapy in the management of diabetic neuropathy. *J. Investig. Med.* 52(1):33–44.

De Jonghe, P., Timmerman, V., Ceuterick, C., Nelis, E., De Vriendt, E., Lofgren, A., Vercruyssen, A., Verellen, C., Van Maldergem, L., Martin, J.J., and Van Broeckhoven, C. (1999) The Thr124Met mutation in the peripheral myelin protein zero (MPZ) gene is associated with a clinically distinct Charcot-Marie-Tooth phenotype. *Brain* 122(Pt 2):281–290.

De Pablo, F., Banner, L.R., and Patterson, P.H. (2000) IGF-I expression is decreased in LIF-deficient mice after peripheral nerve injury. *NeuroReport* 11:1365–1368.

de Waegh, S.M., Lee, V.M., and Brady, S.T. (1992) Local modulation of neurofilament phosphorylation, axonal caliber, and slow axonal transport by myelinating Schwann cells. *Cell* 68:451–463.

Delaney, C.L., Russell, J.W., Cheng, H.-L., and Feldman, E.L. (2001) Insulin-like growth factor-I and over-expression of Bcl-xL prevent glucose-mediated apoptosis in Schwann cells. *J. Neuropathol. Exp. Neurol.* 60:147–160.

Deschenes, S.M., Walcott, J.L., Wexler, T.L., Scherer, S.S., and Fischbeck, K.H. (1997) Altered trafficking of mutant connexin32. *J. Neurosci.* 17:9077–9084.

Diemel, L.T., Copelman, C.A., and Cuzner, M.L. (1998) Macrophages in CNS remyelination: friend or foe? *Neurochem. Res.* 23:341–347.

Dyck, P.J., Chance, P., Lebo, R., and Carney, J.A. (1993) Hereditary motor and sensory neuropathies. In: Dyck, P.J. and Thomas, P.K., eds. *Peripheral Neuropathy* Philadelphia: W.B. Saunders, pp. 1094–1136.

Dytrych, L., Sherman, D.L., Gillespie, C.S., and Brophy, P.J. (1998) Two PDZ domain proteins encoded by the murine periaxin gene are the result of alternative intron retention and are differentially targeted in Schwann cells. *J. Biol. Chem.* 273:5794–5800.

Elder, G.A., Friedrich, V.L., Jr., and Lazzarini, R.A. (2001) Schwann cells and oligodendrocytes read distinct signals in establishing myelin sheath thickness. *J. Neurosci. Res.* 65:493–499.

Frei, R., Motzing, S., Kinkelin, I., Schachner, M., Koltzenburg, M., and Martini, R. (1999) Loss of distal axons and sensory Merkel cells and features indicative of muscle denervation in hindlimbs of P0-deficient mice. *J. Neurosci.* 19:6058–6067.

Fujioka, T., Kolson, D.L., and Rostami, A.M. (1999) Chemokines and peripheral nerve demyelination. *J. Neurovirol.* 5:27–31.

Gabriel, C.M., Gregson, N.A., and Hughes, R.A. (2000) Anti-PMP22 antibodies in patients with inflammatory neuropathy. *J. Neuroimmunol.* 104:139–146.

Gao, W.Q., Shinsky, N., Ingle, G., Beck, K., Elias, K.A., and Powell-Braxton, L. (1999) IGF-I deficient mice show reduced peripheral nerve conduction velocities and decreased axonal diameters and respond to exogenous IGF-I treatment. *J. Neurobiol.* 39: 142–152.

Giardino, I., Edelstein, D., and Brownlee, M. (1996) BCL-2 expression or antioxidants prevent hyperglycemia-induced formation of intracellular advanced glycation endproducts in bovine endothelial cells. *J. Clin. Invest.* 97:1422–1428.

Gillespie, C.S., Sherman, D.L., Blair, G.E., and Brophy, P.J. (1994) Periaxin, a novel protein of myelinating Schwann cells with a possible role in axonal ensheathment. *Neuron* 12:497–508.

Gillespie, C.S., Sherman, D.L., Fleetwood-Walker, S.M., Cottrell, D.F., Tait, S., Garry, E.M., Wallace, V.C., Ure, J., Griffiths, I.R., Smith, A., and Brophy, P.J. (2000) Peripheral demyelination and neuropathic pain behavior in periaxin-deficient mice. *Neuron* 26:523–531.

Green, D.R. and Reed, J.C. (1998) Mitochondria and apoptosis. *Science* 281:1309–1312.

Greene, D.A., Arezzo, J.C., and Brown, M.B. (1999) Effect of aldose reductase inhibition on nerve conduction and morphometry in diabetic neuropathy. Zenarestat Study Group. *Neurology* 53: 580–591.

Griffith, L.S., Schmitz, B., and Schachner, M. (1992) L2/HNK-1 carbohydrate and protein-protein interactions mediate the homophilic binding of the neural adhesion molecule P0. *J. Neurosci.* Res 33:639–648.

Guilbot, A., Williams, A., Ravise, N., Verny, C., Brice, A., Sherman, D.L., Brophy, P.J., LeGuern, E., Delague, V., Bareil, C., Megarbane, A., and Claustres, M. (2001) A mutation in periaxin is responsible for CMT4F, an autosomal recessive form of Charcot-Marie-Tooth disease. *Hum. Mol. Genet.* 10:415–421.

Hellweg, R. and Hartung, H.-D. (1990) Endogenous levels of nerve growth factor (NGF) are altered in experimental diabetes mellitus: a possible role for NGF in the pathogenesis of diabetic neuropathy. *J. Neurosci. Res.* 26:258–267.

Ionasescu, V.V., Searby, C., Ionasescu, R., Neuhaus, I.M., and Werner, R. (1996) Mutations of the noncoding region of the connexin32 gene in X-linked dominant Charcot-Marie-Tooth neuropathy. *Neurology* 47:541–544.

Ishii, H., Koya, D., and King, G.L. (1998) Protein kinase C activation and its role in the development of vascular complication in diabetes mellitus. *J. Mol. Med.* 78:21–31.

Jessen, K.R. and Mirsky, R. (1991) Schwann cell precursors and their development. *Glia* 4:185–194.

Jung, S., Huitinga, I., Schmidt, B., Zielasek, J., Dijkstra, C.D., Toyka, K.V., and Hartung, H.P. (1993) Selective elimination of macrophages by dichlormethylene diphosphonate-containing liposomes suppresses experimental autoimmune neuritis. *J. Neurol. Sci.* 119: 195–202.

Kamholz, J., Awatramani, R., Menichella, D., Jiang, H., Xu, W., and

Shy, M. (1999) Regulation of myelin-specific gene expression. Relevance to CMT1. *Ann. NY Acad. Sci.* 883:91–108.

Kanda, T., Yamawaki, M., Iwasaki, T., and Mizusawa, H. (2000) Glycosphingolipid antibodies and blood-nerve barrier in autoimmune demyelinative neuropathy. *Neurology* 54:1459–1464.

Kiefer, R., Dangond, F., Mueller, M., Toyka, K.V., Hafler, D.A., and Hartung, H.P. (2000) Enhanced B7 costimulatory molecule expression in inflammatory human sural nerve biopsies. *J. Neurol. Neurosurg. Psychiatry* 69:362–368.

Kiefer, R., Kieseier, B.C., Stoll, G., and Hartung, H.P. (2001) The role of macrophages in immune-mediated damage to the peripheral nervous system. *Prog, Neurobiol,* 64:109–127.

Kishi, M., Tanabe, J., Schmelzer, J.D., and Low, P.A. (2002) Morphometry of dorsal root ganglion in chronic experimental diabetic neuropathy. *Diabetes* 51:819–824.

Lenssen, P.P., Gabreels-Festen, A.A., Valentijn, L.J., Jongen, P.J., van Beersum, S.E., van Engelen, B.G., van Wensen, P.J., Bolhuis, P.A., Gabreels, F.J., and Mariman, E.C. (1998) Hereditary neuropathy with liability to pressure palsies. Phenotypic differences between patients with the common deletion and a PMP22 frame shift mutation. *Brain* 121(Pt 8):1451–1458.

Lindholm, D., Heumann, R., Meyer, M., and Thoenen, H. (1987) Interleukin-1 regulates synthesis of nerve growth factor in non-neuronal cells of rat sciatic nerve. *Nature* 330:658–659.

Low, P.A., Nickander, K.K., and Tritschler, H.J. (1997) The roles of oxidative stress and antioxidant treatment in experimental diabetic neuropathy. *Diabetes* 46(Suppl 2):S38–S42.

Lunn, M.P., Manji, H., Choudhary, P.P., Hughes, R.A., and Thomas, P.K. (1999) Chronic inflammatory demyelinating polyradiculoneuropathy: a prevalence study in southeast England. *J. Neurol. Neurosurg. Psychiatry* 66:677–680.

Maier, M., Berger, P., and Suter, U. (2002) Understanding Schwann cell-neurone interactions: the key to Charcot-Marie-Tooth disease? *J. Anat.* 200:357–366.

Martini, R. (2001) The effect of myelinating Schwann cells on axons. *Muscle Nerve* 24:456–466.

Mata, M., Kupina, N., and Fink, D.J. (1992) Phosphorylation-dependent neurofilament epitopes are reduced at the node of Ranvier. *J. Neurocytol.* 21:199–210.

Maurer, M., Kobsar, I., Berghoff, M., Schmid, C.D., Carenini, S., and Martini, R. (2002a) Role of immune cells in animal models for inherited neuropathies: facts and visions. *J. Anat.* 200:405–414.

Maurer, M., Toyka, K.V., and Gold, R. (2002b) Immune mechanisms in acquired demyelinating neuropathies: lessons from animal models. *Neuromusc. Disord.* 12:405–414.

Menichella, D.M., Goodenough, D.A., Sirkowski, E., Scherer, S.S., and Paul, D.L. (2003) Connexins are critical for normal myelination in the CNS. *J. Neurosci.* 2;23(13):5963–5973.

Misawa, S., Kuwabara, S., Mori, M., Kawaguchi, N., Yoshiyama, Y., and Hattori, T. (2001) Serum levels of tumor necrosis factor-alpha in chronic inflammatory demyelinating polyneuropathy. *Neurology* 56:666–669.

Muller, H.W. (2000) Tetraspan myelin protein PMP22 and demyelinating peripheral neuropathies: new facts and hypotheses. *Glia* 29:182–185.

Murphy, P.G., Borthwick, L.S., Johnston, R.S., Kuchel, G., and Richardson, P.M. (1999) Nature of the retrograde signal from injured nerves that induces interleukin-6 mRNA in neurons. *J. Neurosci.* 19:3791–3800.

Nagarajan, R., Svaren, J., Le, N., Araki, T., Watson, M., and Milbrandt, J. (2001) *EGR2* mutations in inherited neuropathies dominant-negatively inhibit myelin gene expression. *Neuron* 30: 355–368.

Nicolson, G.L. and Menter, D.G. (1995) Trophic factors and central nervous system metastasis. *Cancer Metastasis Rev.* 14:303–321.

Olee, T., Powell, H.C., and Brostoff, S.W. (1990) New minimum length requirement for a T cell epitope for experimental allergic neuritis. *J. Neuroimmunol.* 27:187–190.

Orlikowski, D., Chazaud, B., Plonquet, A., Poron, F., Sharshar, T., Maison, P., Raphael, J.C., Gherardi, R.K., and Creange, A. (2003) Monocyte chemoattractant protein 1 and chemokine receptor CCR2 productions in Guillain-Barré syndrome and experimental autoimmune neuritis. *J. Neuroimmunol.* 134:118–127.

Park, D.S., Morris, E.J., Stefanis, L., Troy, C.M., Shelanski, M.L., Geller, H.M., and Greene, L.A. (1998) Multiple pathways of neuronal death induced by DNA-damaging agents, NGF deprivation, and oxidative stress. *J. Neurosci.* 18:830–840.

Pirart, J. (1978) Diabetes mellitus and its degenerative complications; a prospective study of 4,400 patients observed between 1947 and 1973. *Diabetes Care* 1:168–188.

Plante-Bordeneuve, V., Guiochon-Mantel, A., Lacroix, C., Lapresle, J., and Said, G. (1999) The Roussy-Levy family: from the original description to the gene. *Ann. Neurol.* 46:770–773.

Reed, J.C. (1997) Double identity for proteins of the Bcl-2 family. *Nature* 387:773–776.

Russell, J.W., Cheng, H.-L., and Golovoy, D. (2000) Insulin-like growth factor-I promotes myelination of peripheral sensory axons. *J. Neuropathol. Exp. Neurol.* 59:575–584.

Russell, J.W. and Feldman, E.L. (2001) Impaired glucose tolerance—does it cause neuropathy? *Muscle Nerve* 24:1109–1112.

Russell, J.W., Golovoy, D., Vincent, A.M., Mahendru, P., Olzmann, J.A., Mentzer, A., and Feldman, E.L. (2002) High glucose-induced oxidative stress and mitochondrial dysfunction in neurons. *FASEB J.* 16:1738–1748.

Russell, J.W., Sullivan, K.A., Windebank, A.J., Herrmann, D.N., and Feldman, E.L. (1999) Neurons undergo apoptosis in animal and cell culture models of diabetes. *Neurobiol. Dis.* 6:347–363.

Russell, J.W., Windebank, A.J., Schenone, A., and Feldman, E.L. (1998) Insulin-like growth factor-I prevents apoptosis in neurons after nerve growth factor withdrawal. *J. Neurobiol.* 36:455–467.

Sahu, A. and Lambris, J.D. (2000) Complement inhibitors: a resurgent concept in anti-inflammatory therapeutics. *Immunopharmacology* 49:133–148.

Sampath, D., Jackson, G.R., Werrbach-Perez, K., and Perez-Polo, J.R. (1994) Effects of nerve growth factor on glutathione peroxidase and catalase in PC12 cells. *J. Neurochem.* 62:2476–2479.

Sasaki, H., Schmelzer, J.D., Zollman, P.J., and Low, P.A. (1997) Neuropathology and blood flow of nerve, spinal roots and dorsal root ganglia in longstanding diabetic rats. *Acta Neuropathol.* 93:118–128.

Sayers, N.M., Beswick, L.J., Middlemas, A., Calcutt, N.A., Mizisin, A.P., Tomlinson, D.R., et al. (2003) Neurotrophin-3 prevents the proximal accumulation of neurofilament proteins in sensory neurons of streptozocin-induced diabetic rats. *Diabetes* 52(9): 2372–2380.

Scherer, S.S. (1997) Molecular genetics of demyelination: new wrinkles on an old membrane. *Neuron* 18:13–16.

Scherer, S.S., Deschenes, S.M., Xu, Y., Grinspan, J.B., Fischbeck, K.H., and Paul, D.L. (1995) Connexin32 is a myelin-related protein in the PNS and CNS. *J. Neurosci.* 15:8281–8294.

Schmidt, R.E., Dorsey, D.A., Beaudet, L.N., Parvin, C.A., and Escandon, E. (2001) Effect of NGF and neurotrophin-3 treatment on experimental diabetic autonomic neuropathy. *J. Neuropathol. Exp. Neurol.* 60:263–273.

Schonberger, L.B., Hurwitz, E.S., Katona, P., Holman, R.C., and Bregman, D.J. (1981) Guillain-Barré syndrome: its epidemiology and associations with influenza vaccination. *Ann. Neurol.* 9 (Suppl):31–38.

Shapiro, L., Doyle, J.P., Hensley, P., Colman, D.R., and Hendrickson, W.A. (1996) Crystal structure of the extracellular domain from P0, the major structural protein of peripheral nerve myelin. *Neuron* 17:435–449.

Sharma, A.K. and Thomas, P.K. (1987) Animal models: pathology and pathophysiology. In: Dyck, P.J., Thomas, P.K., Asbury, A.K., Winegrad, A.I., and Porte, D.J., eds. *Diabetic Neuropathy*. Philadelphia: W.B. Saunders, pp. 237–252.

Sheetz, M.J. and King, G.L. (2002) Molecular understanding of hyperglycemia's adverse effects for diabetic complications. *JAMA* 288:2579–2588.

Sheng, M. (1996) PDZs and receptor/channel clustering: rounding up the latest suspects. *Neuron* 17:575–578.

Sherman, D.L., Fabrizi, C., Gillespie, C.S., and Brophy, P.J. (2001) Specific disruption of a Schwann cell dystrophin-related protein complex in a demyelinating neuropathy. *Neuron* 30:677–687.

Silander, K., Meretoja, P., Pihko, H., Juvonen, V., Issakainen, J., Aula, P., and Savontaus, M.L. (1997) Screening for connexin 32 mutations in Charcot-Marie-Tooth disease families with possible X-linked inheritance. *Hum. Genet.* 100:391–397.

Sima, A.A., Li, Z.G., and Zhang, W. (2003) The insulin-like growth factor system and neurological complications in diabetes. *Exp. Diabesity Res.* 4(4):235–256.

Snipes, G.J. and Orfali, W. (1998) Common themes in peripheral neuropathy disease genes. *Cell Biol. Int.* 22:815–835.

Springer, T.A. (1994) Traffic signals for lymphocyte recirculation and leukocyte emigration: the multistep paradigm. *Cell* 76:301–314.

Srinivasan, S., Stevens, M.J., and Wiley, J.W. (2000) Diabetic peripheral neuropathy: evidence for apoptosis and associated mitochondrial dysfunction. *Diabetes* 49:1932–1938.

Stevens, M.J., Obrosova, I., Cao, X., Van Huysen, C., and Greene, D.A. (2000) Effects of DL-alpha-lipoic acid on peripheral nerve conduction, blood flow, energy metabolism, and oxidative stress in experimental diabetic neuropathy. *Diabetes* 49: 1006–1015.

Takigawa, T., Yasuda, H., Terada, M., Haneda, M., Kashiwagi, A., Saito, T., Saida, T., Kitasato, H., and Kikkawa, R. (2000) The sera from GM1 ganglioside antibody positive patients with Guillain-Barré syndrome or chronic inflammatory demyelinating polyneuropathy blocks Na^+ currents in rat single myelinated nerve fibers. *Intern. Med.* 39:123–127.

Teruel, T., Valverde, A.M., Navarro, P., Benito, M., and Lorenzo, M. (1998) Inhibition of PI 3-kinase and RAS blocks IGF-I and insulin-induced uncoupling protein 1 gene expression in brown adipocytes. *J. Cell Physiol.* 176:99–109.

The Diabetes Control and Complications Trial Research Group (1993) The effect of intensive treatment of diabetes on the development and progression of long-term complications in insulin-dependent diabetes mellitus. *N. Engl. J. Med.* 329:977–986.

Thomas, P.K., Marques, W., Jr., Davis, M.B., Sweeney, M.G., King, R.H., Bradley, J.L., Muddle, J.R., Tyson, J., Malcolm, S., and Harding, A.E. (1997) The phenotypic manifestations of chromosome 17p11.2 duplication. *Brain* 120:465–478.

Tonra, J.R., Ono, M., Liu, X., Garcia, K., Jackson, C., Yancopoulos, G.D., Wiegand, S.J., and Wong, V. (1999) Brain-derived neurotrophic factor improves blood glucose control and alleviates fasting hyperglycemia in C57BLKS-Lepr(db)/lepr(db) mice. *Diabetes* 48:588–594.

Topilko, P., Schneider-Maunoury, S., Levi, G., Baron-Van Evercooren, A., Chennoufi, A.B.Y., Seitanidou, T., Babinet, C., and Charnay, P. (1994) Krox-20 controls myelination in the peripheral nervous system. *Nature* 371:796–799.

Trotter, J., DeJong, L.J., and Smith, M.E. (1986) Opsonization with antimyelin antibody increases the uptake and intracellular metabolism of myelin in inflammatory macrophages. *J. Neurochem.* 47:779–789.

Valverde, A.M., Lorenzo, M., Navarro, P., and Benito, M. (1997) Phosphatidylinositol 3-kinase is a requirement for insulin-like growth factor I-induced differentiation, but not for mitogenesis, in fetal brown adipocytes. *Mol. Endocrinol.* 11:595–607.

Van Rhijn, I., Van den Berg, L.H., Bosboom, W.M., Otten, H.G., and Logtenberg, T. (2000) Expression of accessory molecules for T-cell activation in peripheral nerve of patients with CIDP and vasculitic neuropathy. *Brain* 123(Pt 10):2020–2029.

Vincent, A.M., Brownlee, M., and Russell, J.W. (2002) Oxidative stress and programmed cell death in diabetic neuropathy. *Ann. NY Acad. Sci.* 959:368–383.

Vincent, A.M., Olzmann, J.A., Brownlee, M., Sivitz, W.I., and Russell, J.W. (2004) Uncoupling proteins prevent glucose-induced neuronal oxidative stress and programmed cell death. *Diabetes* 53:726–734.

Vriesendorp, F.J., Flynn, R.E., Malone, M.R., and Pappolla, M.A. (1998) Systemic complement depletion reduces inflammation and demyelination in adoptive transfer experimental allergic neuritis. *Acta Neuropathol. (Berl.)* 95:297–301.

Warner, L.E., Svaren, J., Milbrandt, J., and Lupski, J.R. (1999) Functional consequences of mutations in the early growth response 2 gene (*EGR2*) correlate with severity of human myelinopathies. *Hum. Mol. Genet.* 8:1245–1251.

Wellmer, A., Misra, V.P., Sharief, M.K., Kopelman, P.G., and Anand, P. (2001) A double-blind placebo-controlled clinical trial of recombinant human brain-derived neurotrophic factor (rhBDNF) in diabetic polyneuropathy. *J. Peripher. Nerv. Syst.* 6:204–210.

Willison, H.J. and Yuki, N. (2002) Peripheral neuropathies and anti-glycolipid antibodies. *Brain* 125:2591–2625.

Yan, W.X., Archelos, J.J., Hartung, H.P., and Pollard, J.D. (2001) P0 protein is a target antigen in chronic inflammatory demyelinating polyradiculoneuropathy. *Ann. Neurol.* 50:286–292.

Ye, P., Carson, J., and D'Ercole, A.J. (1995) *In vivo* actions of insulin-like growth factor-I (IGF-I) on brain myelination: studies of IGF-I and IGF binding protein-1 (IGFBP-1) transgenic mice. *J. Neurosci.* 15:7344–7356.

Yuan, J. and Yankner, B.A. (2000) Apoptosis in the nervous system. *Nature* 407:802–809.

Zochodne, D.W., Verge, V.M., Cheng, C., Sun, H., and Johnston, J. (2001) Does diabetes target ganglion neurones? Progressive sensory neurone involvement in long-term experimental diabetes. *Brain* 124:2319–2334.

Zou, L.P., Pelidou, S.H., Abbas, N., Deretzi, G., Mix, E., Schaltzbeerg, M., Winblad, B., and Zhu, J. (1999) Dynamics of production of MIP-1alpha, MCP-1 and MIP-2 and potential role of neutralization of these chemokines in the regulation of immune responses during experimental autoimmune neuritis in Lewis rats. *J. Neuroimmunol.* 98:168–175.

Zhu, J., Mix, E., and Link, H. (1998) Cytokine production and the pathogenesis of experimental autoimmune neuritis and Guillain-Barré syndrome. *J. Neuroimmunol.* 84:40–52.

47 Reaction of glial cells in infectious disorders of the central nervous system

MARTINA DECKERT AND DIRK SCHLÜTER

Activation of resident glial cells of the central nervous system (CNS), in particular astrocytes and microglia, is a hallmark of various infectious diseases of the brain. Each cell population is characterized by a specific reaction pattern, and the temporal sequence and strength of the reaction are determined by the causative pathogen and may even be influenced by strain-specific features of the respective pathogen. The activation of both astrocytes and microglial cells is evidenced by the induction and/or upregulation of immunologically relevant cell surface molecules, cytokines, chemokines, and their receptors, thereby enabling these cell populations to interact in both an antigen-specific and an antigen-independent manner with various leukocyte populations of the immune system.

VIRAL AND PARASITIC INFECTIONS

In infections, which primarily affect the brain parenchyma, astrocytes and microglia are strongly activated. This is particularly true for infections caused by pathogens, which have the capacity to persist in the brain, such as various viruses including herpes viruses and parasites such as *Toxoplasma gondii*.

In these disorders, microglial activation may present with the formation of characteristic microglial nodules, that is, aggregates of strongly activated microglial cells. In addition, activation of astrocytes usually occurs throughout the brain, as evidenced by a strong and generalized upregulation of glial fibrillary acidic protein (GFAP) in these cells.

Depending on the infectious stimulus, resident brain cells may become activated with onset of the infection or even prior to the establishment of encephalitis. In Borna virus infection, macrophage inflammatory protein (MIP)-1α, MIP-1β, monocyte chemoattractant protein (MCP)-1, regulated on activation normal T cell expressed and secreted (RANTES), and interferon-γ (IFN-γ)-inducible protein crg-2/IP-10 were expressed prior to the formation of inflammatory infiltrates, with astrocytes being the major cellular source of crg-2/IP-10 (Lane et al., 1998; Sauder et al., 2000). It has been suggested that inflammatory protein-10 (IP-10) gene expression may be a direct response of virus-infected astrocytes, supporting the concept that local synthesis of chemokines by resident cells of the brain facilitates tracking of immune cells to areas of infection and that the pattern of chemokine expression partly determines the specific cellular composition of inflammatory infiltrates. Interestingly, the IP-10 gene was expressed more prominently than other genes in the brain of Borna virus–infected rats and mice, as well as in infections with the lymphocytic choriomeningitis virus (LCMV), mouse hepatitis virus (MHV), and mouse adenovirus type 1 infection, arguing for a specific role of this chemokine in viral infections of the CNS (Asensio et al., 1999; Charles et al., 1999). Interestingly, IP-10 is required for T cell generation and trafficking, and IP-10 possesses direct antiviral activity against herpes simplex virus (HSV)–infected neurons (Lokensgard et al., 2001; Dufour et al., 2002).

Of particular interest is the response of resident brain cells in human immunodeficiency virus (HIV) infection. In fact, microglial reactions have been characterized in great detail in this disorder. In contrast to many viruses that primarily infect neurons, such as cytomegalovirus (CMV) and herpes viruses, microglia/macrophages, but not neurons, are a major target for HIV in the brain and provide an intracerebral reservoir. Human immunodeficiency virus RNA and protein can be demonstrated in microglial cells by *in situ* hybridization and immunohistochemistry, respectively. For microglia, CCR5 together with CD4 is the major coreceptor (Albright et al., 1999; Gabuzda and Wang, 1999). Although CXCR4 and CCR3 are also expressed on microglia and can also mediate infection by certain HIV-1 isolates, this occurs at a lower efficiency than via CCR5

(He et al., 1997; Shieh et al., 1998; Vallat et al., 1998; Gabuzda and Wang, 1999). In fact, levels of CCR5 on microglia are higher than levels of CCR3 and CXCR4 (He et al., 1997; Gabuzda and Wang, 1999).

Multinucleated giant cells of the macrophage lineage and microglial nodules are a hallmark of HIV encephalitis. Interestingly, activation of microglia correlates best with clinical dementia (Si et al., 2002). Entry into and replication of HIV-1 within microglia are regulated by cytokines: interleukin-4 (IL-4) and IL-10 enhance entry of HIV-1 in microglia through upregulation of CD4 and CCR5, respectively, and IL-10-induced upregulation of CCR5 is associated with increased migration of microglia in response to MIP-1β, that is, facilitation of chemotactic microglial migration (Wang et al., 2002). Furthermore, IFN-γ-upregulates CD40 on microglia and, correspondingly, the number of CD40+ microglial cells in HIV-infected brain tissue are markedly increased (D'Aversa et al., 2002). A subsequent interaction with CD40L$^+$ cells, that is, CD4$^+$ T cells, B cells, and monocytes, induces microglial secretion of chemokines, thereby amplifying inflammatory processes.

Neuronal damage and apoptosis in HIV encephalopathy are considered to be mediated by activated microglia and macrophages, which produce neurotoxic mediators, in particular tumor necrosis factor (TNF) and nitric oxide (NO), as well as excitatory amino acids, which exert potent cytotoxic effects on neurons (Lipton et al., 1994; Kaul and Lipton, 1999). Viral coreceptors can also produce neural cell damage during HIV-1-associated dementia without simultaneously affecting viral replication. In addition, progeny of HIV-1 virions can influence neuronal signaling transduction and apoptosis; this process occurs, in part, through CXCR4, to which different gp120 isolates bind (Kaul and Lipton, 1999; Zheng et al., 1999). On the other hand, RANTES, which is produced by HIV-1-infected microglia (Si et al., 2002), and MIP-1β, the ligand for CXCR4, can protect neurons from gp120-induced apoptosis (Kaul and Lipton, 1999). In addition to microglia, astrocytes are also involved in the pathogenesis of HIV-1-associated dementia. Stromal derived factor (SDF)-1–induced activation of CXCR4 on astrocytes leads to TNF secretion, thereby contributing to neuronal apoptosis (Bezzi et al., 2001). Interference with the pathway of CXCR4-dependent signaling between astrocytes and microglia can prevent HIV-1 gp120-induced neuronal apoptosis (Bezzi et al., 2001). Conversely, TNF-α downregulates CXCR4 expression in astrocytes (Han et al., 2001). Furthermore, there is evidence that the balance between TNF-α and insulin-like growth factor I receptor (IGF-IR) signaling pathways may also control the extent of neuronal injury mediated by HIV-1-infected macrophages/microglia (Ying Wang et al., 2003).

The individual reaction patterns of microglia and astrocytes have also been studied systematically in the model of experimental murine *T. gondii* infection of the brain, a chronic encephalitis characterized by persistence of the parasite in neurons of the brain (Schluter et al., 1991). A ubiquitous, particularly strong activation of microglia and astrocytes is a hallmark of murine *Toxoplasma* encephalitis (Fig. 47.1). In this disease, astrocytes and microglial cells are characterized by a specific nonredundant reaction pattern (Schluter et al., 1997). Simultaneously with parasitic invasion of the CNS, leukocytes are recruited to the brain, resulting in

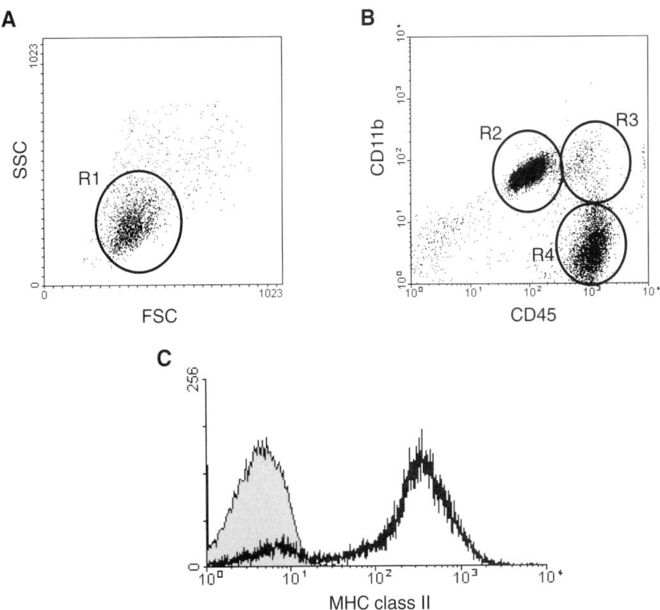

FIGURE 47.1 Analysis of microglia by flow cytometry. *A.* The granularity (SSC) and size (FSC) of leukocytes isolated from *T. gondii*-infected mouse brains (day 30 after infection) is shown. Microglia cells and most other leukocytes have low granularity and a relatively small size (R1). *B.* Leukocytes depicted in R1 (A) are further analysed by their expression of CD11b and CD45. Microglia is CD11b positive and expresses low levels of CD45 (R2). Macrophages are CD11b positive and express high levels of CD45 (R3). Other leukocytes including T and B cells are CD11b negative and express high levels of CD45 (R4). C. Microglia cells from R2 were analysed for their expression of MHC class II antigens. Most microglia cells from the *T. gondii*-infected brain express high level of MHC class II antigens (open curve). In contrast, normal microglia from uninfected mice is MHC class II negative.

the formation of *T. gondii*–associated infiltrates. At this very early stage of the infection, microglia and astrocytes are already activated. In parallel to various viral infections of the CNS, the expression of crg-2/IP-10 by astrocytes close to cerebral blood vessels and the inflamed meninges is an early event. This induction may be important for the recruitment of T lymphocytes to the *T. gondii*–infected CNS, which are required for intracerebral parasitic control (Schluter et al., 1993). In addition, major histocompatibility complex (MHC) class I and II antigens as well as the costimulatory molecules B7-1 and B7-2 are induced on microglia, (Fig. 47.1C and Fig. 47.2) persisting throughout encephalitis, thereby turning microglia into potentially antigen-presenting cells. Activation of microglia is further evidenced by upregulation of the F4/80 and CD45 antigens (Fig. 47.1B), which allow an antigen-independent interaction of microglia with lymphocytes. In addition, intercellular adhesion molecule-1 (ICAM-1) is induced on microglia, in parallel with upregulation of LFA-1, CD43, and Mac-1/CR3, all of which are ligands for ICAM-1 (Deckert-Schluter et al., 1994). In full-blown encephalitis, some microglial cells in the vicinity of parasites react with antibodies to CD11c and, thus express markers characteristic of dendritic cells. However, convincing evidence that microglia have a dendritic cell function *in vivo* in *Toxoplasma* encephalitis is still lacking. *In vivo* data demonstrating that microglia actively suppress T cell proliferation in the *T. gondii*–infected CNS argue against this assumption and, on the contrary, delineates a role for microglia in the control and regulation of T cell activity in the CNS (Schluter et al., 2002).

Whereas most of these immunologically relevant cell surface molecules were induced on microglia, astrocytes responded with an expression of MHC class I antigens to the infection. However, the expression of MHC class II antigens and ICAM-1 on single astrocytes in close proximity to parasite-associated inflammatory foci was strictly confined to the stage of maximal disease activity (Deckert-Schluter et al., 1994). This expression pattern and regulation in parallel with disease activity may reflect a further amplification loop of the neuroimmune response to ensure optimal parasite control.

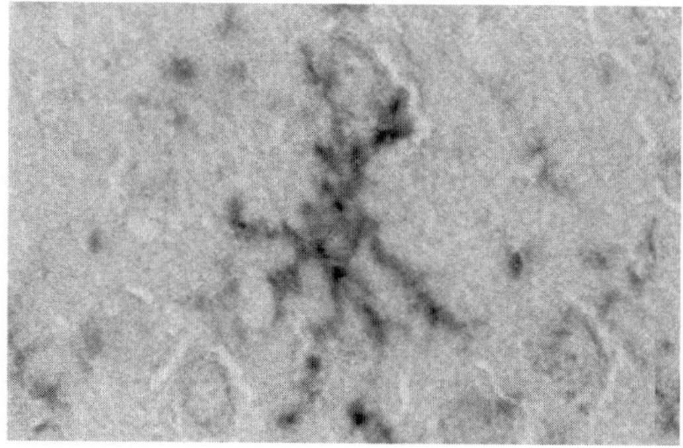

FIGURE 47.2 Histopathology of activated microglia. Early activation of microglia in murine *Toxoplasma* encephalitis at day 14 after infection. Microglial activation is characterized by the presence of prominent, short cellular processes and the induction of MHC class II antigens. I-A immunostaining, slight counterstaining with hemalum, x90.

With respect to the production of cytokines and chemokines in *Toxoplasma* encephalits, microglia and astrocytes also exhibited individual reaction patterns. Whereas astrocytes are the major cellular source for crg-2/IP-10 and MCP-1, microglia transcribes RANTES and MuMig (Strack et al., 2002). The prominent expression of crg-2 and MCP-1 may also determine the phenotype of intracerebral T cells, since these chemokines particularly attract activated T lymphocytes with an activated memory phenotype, that is, the phenotype of T cells ($CD44^{high}CD62^{low}LFA\text{-}1^{high}$) in *Toxoplasma* encephalitis. With respect to cytokines, the detailed and selective study of the cytokine profile of microglia was facilitated by the fact that microglial cells—in contrast to astrocytes—are amenable to selective isolation from the brain and can be identified by a stable genetic marker in the model of bone marrow chimeras taking advantage of CD45-congenic mouse strains. Selectively isolated microglia were found to express a panel of pro-inflammatory cytokines during *Toxoplasma* encephalitis, that is, IL-1, IL-12p35, IL-12p40, IL-15, TNF, and inducible nitric oxide synthase (iNOS), all of which have antiparasitic properties (Schluter et al., 2001). In addition, microglia expressed the potent anti-inflammatory mediator IL-10, which serves a regulatory function in *Toxoplasma* encephalitis in order to prevent an overshooting immune response with a possible subsequent immunopathology. Further studies using mouse mutants lacking either T cells or the gene for IFN-γ or the IFN-γR demonstrated that T cell–derived IFN-γ was the decisive stimulator for the induction of cell surface molecules as well as of cytokines in microglia (Deckert-Schluter et al., 1999).

Although a comprehensive pattern of cytokines produced by astrocytes in *Toxoplasma* encephalitis has not yet been delineated, topographical studies revealed that astrocytes in the vicinity of *T. gondii*–associated infiltrates expressed TNF (Schluter et al., 1997).

Taken together, these data indicate that in the various models of persistent encephalitis, microglial cells and astrocytes are characterized by a differential and individual response, the pattern, strength, and temporal profile of which are regulated by the underlying pathology and severity of the infection. The inducing pathogenic stimulus as well as the genetic background of the host determine the reaction pattern of astrocytes and microglia. This was illustrated in mouse strains, which differ genetically in their susceptibility to *T. gondii*: while microglia and astrocytes responded with the same pattern of chemokine gene expression, the onset and strength of the reaction were more prominent in susceptible mice, which developed a more severe encephalitis (Strack et al., 2002). In addition to participating in pro-inflammatory reactions, which aim at the elimination of the pathogen, microglia play a role in balancing the intracerebral immune response and controlling T cell activity, on the one hand via direct physical activity and on the other hand indirectly via production of IL-10.

Compared to microglia and astrocytes, much less is known about the immunological activity of oligodendrocytes. This is due to the difficulty of identifying oligodendrocytes *in situ* and propagating adult oligodendrocytes *in vitro*. Some experimental studies revealed MHC class I expression of oligodendrocytes in the inflamed murine brain (Evans et al., 1996; Horwitz et al., 1997; Charles et al., 1999). Oligodendrcytes do not express MHC class II antigens, although a few reports have contradicted this finding (Rodriguez et al., 1987; Horwitz et al., 1999). In humans, uncommon viral infections of oligodendrocytes may induce demyelination. Defective measles virus can cause subacute sclerosing panencephalitis (SSPE), a fatal chronic demyelinating encephalitis. In SSPE, the direct infection of oligodendrocytes results in a primary demyelination, although the accompanying T cell–mediated immune response may also contribute to oligodendrocyte death (Charles et al., 1999; Stohlman and Hinton, 2001). In immunodeficient patients, JC, a papovavirus, also infects oligodendrocytes, causing a fatal primary demyelinating disease termed *progressive multifocal leukoencephalopathy* (PML) (Stohlman and Hinton, 2001). In addition, epidemiological studies suggest a relation between the occurrence of multiple sclerosis (MS) and infections, although a particular virus has not yet been identified as being clearly associated with MS. To explore the potential mechanism(s) by which viral infections may result in oligodendrocyte damage and demyelination, two rodent models of demyelinating diseases are being studied intensely: infection with Theiler's murine encephalomyelitis virus (TMEV) and mouse hepatitis virus (MHV). Theiler's murine encephalomyelitis virus infects microglia and macrophages and induces a virus-specific intracerebral CD4 T cell response, which also causes myelin damage. Despite the absence of TMEV from oligodendrocytes, the chronic phase of this CNS infection is characterized by the induction of oligodendrocyte (proteolipid)-specific CD4 T cells (*epitope spreading*); these autoimmune CD4 T cells contribute to chronic progressive demyelination (Tompkins et al., 2002). Since oligodendrocytes do not express MHC class II antigens in TMEV infection, oligodendrocyte damage is attributed to immune mediators produced or induced by these CD4 T cells. In contrast, MHV infects numerous cell types in the murine brain, including oligodendrocytes, and induces primary demyelination. In the chronic phase, minute amounts of virus persist and, in combination with the virus-specific CD8 T cell response, may cause new foci of demyelination (Stohlman and Hinton, 2001).

BACTERIAL INFECTIONS

Most bacterial infections primarily affect the subarachnoid space and result in a rather mild glial reaction compared to infections predominantly affecting brain parenchyma, as described above for viruses and parasites.

Among meningeal infections, pneumococcal and meningococcal meningitis, as well as *Listeria (L.) monocytogenes* infection, have been studied in detail. In this regard, it is of note that in contrast to most bacteria, which induce only meningitis, *L. monocytogenes* may also cause encephalitis, abscess, or combined forms, with a striking predilection for the brain stem in both humans and mice (Schluter et al., 1996).

Once bacteria have reached the subarachnoid space, local immune reactions are usually insufficient in eliminating them and in preventing meningeal inflammation. This has been attributed to low levels of complement and the absence of antibodies from the cerebrospinal fluid (CSF). During bacterial meningitis, complement expressed locally at the infection site plays an important role because of its antipathogenic effects and its participation in the pathogenesis and killing of bacteria (Morgan and Gasque, 1996). A full complement system can be expressed by resident cells in the brain (Morgan and Gasque, 1996). The complement anaphylatoxins C5a and Ca3 are released at the site of inflammation and are powerful chemoattractants for polymorphonuclear leukocytes and macrophages, the phagocytic capacity of which is subsequently stimulated. Interestingly, expression of nerve growth factor (NGF) was induced in microglial cells in response to C3a, which can also be stimulated by IL-1β and TNF-α in this cell population (Heese et al., 1998). Release of the neuroprotective NGF appears to be involved in early processes of neuronal regeneration (Heese et al., 1998), to which microglia and astrocytes, which are major cellular sources of neurotrophic factors including NGF and neurotrophins (Goss et al., 1998), also contribute.

In general, in bacterial meningitis, the brain parenchyma adjacent to bacteria-associated inflammatory infiltrates is also involved. In the molecular layer of the adjacent cortex, activated astrocytes and activated microglial cells are evident. Concomitantly, C5aR and C3aR are expressed on these reactive astrocytes and microglial cells (Gasque et al., 1997, 1998), thereby contributing to recruitment and activation of leukocytes. In this regard, microglial induction of matrix metalloproteinase (MMP) 9 (Gottschall et al., 1995), a potent extracellular matrix–degrading enzyme, may also become functionally relevant.

Furthermore, resident brain cells may also determine the phenotypic composition of the intracerebral infiltrates in bacterial CNS infections via production of chemokines. In *Haemophilus influenzae* type b infection of the infant rat brain, MCP-1 and RANTES were induced in astrocytes and microglia, respectively, which are particularly chemoattractive for macrophages/monocytes and activated T cells (Diab et al., 1999).

With the development of ventriculitis, which may occur during bacterial meningitis and is a common feature of cerebral listeriosis, astrocytes and microglia in the periventricular brain tissue are also activated, as evidenced by an induction of cell surface molecules such as F4/80, Mac1 (CR3), MHC class I and II antigens, and ICAM-1 on microglia. While the reaction pattern, in general, does not differ from that of other infectious disorders, the activation of resident brain parenchymal cells is locally restricted to areas adjacent to bacteria, that is, the meninges and the ventricular system. Bacterial cell wall components of gram-negative bacteria bind to Toll-like receptor (tlr) 4, and cell wall components of gram-positive bacteria bind predominantly to tlr2. Activation of tlr is one of the first steps in the interaction of the host immune system with the offending pathogen and results in the rapid induction of antibacterial defense mechanisms. In pneuomococcal meningitis, tlr2 expression is upregulated, and tlr2-mediated reactions contribute to the intracerebral control of the bacteria and the reduction of intracranial complications (e.g., blood–brain barrier integrity) but do not affect the production of cytokines, chemokines, and NO. In addition, microglial cells express tlr-9 and, thus, are triggered by bacterial DNA containing motifs of unmethylated CpG dinucleotides to induce TNF-α, IL-12p40, IL-12p70, and NO, to upregulate MHC class II antigens, B7-1, B7-2, and CD40 antigens, and to enhance phagocytic activity, which may become functionally relevant with maximal disease activity (Dalpke et al., 2002). Pneumococcal cell walls induced a differential cytokine profile in microglia and astrocytes *in vitro* with induction of TNF, IL-6, IL-12, keratinocyte-derived chemokine (KC), MIP-1α, and MIP-2 in microglia and production of TNF and NO in astrocytes, respectively. While the secretion of these pro-inflammatory and antibacterial mediators is important for bacterial elimination, at least a part of these mediators may also exert detrimental effects. Among these cytokines, TNF and NO are neurotoxic. Thus, activated resident cells of the CNS may contribute to neuronal apoptosis, a complication of meningitis due to *Streptococcus pneumoniae* and *L. monocytogenes*, which was observed in the hippocampus in a segmental distribution (Nau et al., 1999; Bottcher et al., 2000; Deckert et al., 2001).

The expression pattern of cytokines and chemokines has also been investigated in a mouse model of *Staphylococcus aureus*–induced brain abscess, which has several interesting parallels with brain abscess in humans (Flaris and Mickey, 1992). In this model, MIP-2, IP-10, MIP-1α, MIP-1β, MCP-1, and T-cell activation gene-3 (TCA-3) were detected (Kielian et al., 2001). Further studies using *S. aureus*–stimulated neonatal astrocytes and microglial cell cultures identifed microglia as a major source of MIP-1α, whereas astrocytes produced RANTES under these experimental conditions (Kielian et al., 2001).

In addition to pro-inflammatory cytokines, anti-inflammatory cytokines play an important role in the regulation of intracerebral immune responses. In this regard, the potent immunosuppressive cytokine IL-10, which was found at high levels in the CSF of patients with bacterial meningitis, plays an important role: CSF obtained from patients with bacterial meningitis inhibited macrophage function, rendering macrophages even partly permissive for intracellular *L. monocytogenes* growth (Frei et al., 1993). The regulatory role of IL-10 was further illustrated in CNS listeriosis of IL-$10^{0/0}$ mice, which succumbed to a combined brain stem encephalitis, ventriculitis, and meningitis due to a hyperinflammatory syndrome (Deckert et al., 2001). While the number of intracerebral leukocytes was increased, the bacterial load was not reduced, which could be explained by the fact that there was no increased recruitment of *L. monocytogenes*–specific T cells to the brain (Deckert et al., 2001). In this mutant, the activation of microglia was more pronounced and was a generalized phenomenon compared to activation in wild-type animals, as evidenced by a stronger and ubiquitous upregulation of MHC class II antigens (Deckert et al., 2001).

Thus, these data in various models clearly demonstrate the disease-specific, individual, and finely tuned reaction pattern of astrocytes and microglia during CNS infections and their contribution to the intracerebral immune response. While both soluble mediators and the induction and/or upregulation of immunologically relevant cell surface molecules contribute to elimination of offending pathogens, microglia also serve an immunoregulatory function in order to minimize damage and destruction of vulnerable brain tissue. However, while these various components of the immune reaction serve a protective function, it is also evident that, depending on the underlying pathology, reactions of microglia and astrocytes may also be detrimental, as antibacterial effector molecules may also be neurotoxic and thereby contribute to neuronal damage, apoptosis, and, ultimately, long-term neurological sequelae.

REFERENCES

Albright, A.V., Shieh, J.T., Itoh, T., Lee, B., Pleasure, D., O'Connor, M.J., Doms, R.W., and Gonzalez-Scarano, F. (1999) Microglia express CCR5, CXCR4, and CCR3, but of these, CCR5 is the principal coreceptor for human immunodeficiency virus type 1 dementia isolates. *J. Virol.* 73:205–213.

Asensio, V.C., Kincaid, C., and Campbell, I.L. (1999) Chemokines and the inflammatory response to viral infection in the central nervous system with a focus on lymphocytic choriomeningitis virus. *J. Neurovirol.* 5:65–75.

Bezzi, P., Domercq, M., Brambilla, L., Galli, R., Schols, D., De Clercq, E., Vescovi, A., Bagetta, G., Kollias, G., Meldolesi, J., and Volterra, A. (2001) CXCR4-activated astrocyte glutamate release via TNFalpha: amplification by microglia triggers neurotoxicity. *Nat. Neurosci.* 4:702–710.

Bottcher, T., Gerber, J., Wellmer, A., Smirnov, A.V., Fakhrjanali, F., Mix, E., Pilz, J., Zettl, U.K., and Nau, R. (2000) Rifampin reduces production of reactive oxygen species of cerebrospinal fluid phagocytes and hippocampal neuronal apoptosis in experimental *Streptococcus pneumoniae* meningitis. *J. Infect. Dis.* 181:2095–2098.

Charles, P.C., Chen, X., Horwitz, M.S., and Brosnan, C.F. (1999) Differential chemokine induction by the mouse adenovirus type-1 in the central nervous system of susceptible and resistant strains of mice. *J. Neurovirol.* 5:55–64.

D'Aversa, T.G., Weidenheim, K.M., and Berman, J.W. (2002) CD40-CD40L interactions induce chemokine expression by human microglia: implications for human immunodeficiency virus encephalitis and multiple sclerosis. *Am. J. Pathol.* 160:559–567.

Dalpke, A.H., Schafer, M.K., Frey, M., Zimmermann, S., Tebbe, J., Weihe, E., and Heeg, K. (2002) Immunostimulatory CpG-DNA activates murine microglia. *J. Immunol.* 168:4854–4863.

Deckert, M., Soltek, S., Geginat, G., Lutjen, S., Montesinos-Rongen, M., Hof, H., and Schluter, D. (2001) Endogenous interleukin-10 is required for prevention of a hyperinflammatory intracerebral immune response in *Listeria monocytogenes* meningoencephalitis. *Infect. Immun.* 69:4561–4571.

Deckert-Schluter, M., Bluethmann, H., Kaefer, N., Rang, A., and Schluter, D. (1999) Interferon-gamma receptor-mediated but not tumor necrosis factor receptor type 1- or type 2-mediated signaling is crucial for the activation of cerebral blood vessel endothelial cells and microglia in murine *Toxoplasma* encephalitis. *Am. J. Pathol.* 154:1549–1561.

Deckert-Schluter, M., Schluter, D., Hof, H., Wiestler, O.D., and Lassmann, H. (1994) Differential expression of ICAM-1, VCAM-1 and their ligands LFA-1, Mac-1, CD43, VLA-4, and MHC class II antigens in murine *Toxoplasma* encephalitis: a light microscopic and ultrastructural immunohistochemical study. *J. Neuropathol. Exp. Neurol.* 53:457–468.

Diab, A., Abdalla, H., Li, H.L., Shi, F.D., Zhu, J., Hojberg, B., Lindquist, L., Wretlind, B., Bakhiet, M., and Link, H. (1999) Neutralization of macrophage inflammatory protein 2 (MIP-2) and MIP-1alpha attenuates neutrophil recruitment in the central nervous system during experimental bacterial meningitis. *Infect. Immun.* 67:2590–2601.

Dufour, J.H., Dziejman, M., Liu, M.T., Leung, J.H., Lane, T.E., and Luster, A.D. (2002) IFN-gamma-inducible protein 10 (IP-10; CXCL10)-deficient mice reveal a role for IP-10 in effector T cell generation and trafficking. *J. Immunol.* 168:3195–3204.

Evans, C.F., Horwitz, M.S., Hobbs, M.V., and Oldstone, M.B. (1996) Viral infection of transgenic mice expressing a viral protein in oligodendrocytes leads to chronic central nervous system autoimmune disease. *J. Exp. Med.* 184:2371–2384.

Flaris, N.A. and Hickey, W.F. (1992) Development and characterization of an experimental model of brain abscess in the rat. *Am. J. Pathol.* 141:1299–1307.

Frei, K., Nadal, D., Pfister, H.W., and Fontana, A. (1993) *Listeria* meningitis: identification of a cerebrospinal fluid inhibitor of macrophage listericidal function as interleukin 10. *J. Exp. Med.* 178: 1255–1261.

Gabuzda, D. and Wang, J. (1999) Chemokine receptors and virus entry in the central nervous system. *J. Neurovirol.* 5:643–658.

Gasque, P., Singhrao, S.K., Neal, J.W., Gotze, O., and Morgan, B.P. (1997) Expression of the receptor for complement C5a (CD88) is up-regulated on reactive astrocytes, microglia, and endothelial cells in the inflamed human central nervous system. *Am. J. Pathol.* 150:31–41.

Gasque, P., Singhrao, S.K., Neal, J.W., Wang, P., Sayah, S., Fontaine, M., and Morgan, B.P. (1998) The receptor for complement anaphylatoxin C3a is expressed by myeloid cells and nonmyeloid cells in inflamed human central nervous system: analysis in multiple sclerosis and bacterial meningitis. *J. Immunol.* 160:3543–3554.

Goss, J.R., O'Malley, M.E., Zou, L., Styren, S.D., Kochanek, P.M., and DeKosky, S.T. (1998) Astrocytes are the major source of nerve growth factor upregulation following traumatic brain injury in the rat. *Exp. Neurol.* 149:301–309.

Gottschall, P.E., Yu, X., and Bing, B. (1995) Increased production of gelatinase B (matrix metalloproteinase-9) and interleukin-6 by activated rat microglia in culture. *J. Neurosci. Res.* 42:335–342.

Han, Y., Wang, J., He, T., and Ransohoff, R.M. (2001) TNF-alpha down-regulates CXCR4 expression in primary murine astrocytes. *Brain Res.* 888:1–10.

He, J., Chen, Y., Farzan, M., Choe, H., Ohagen, A., Gartner, S., Busciglio, J., Yang, X., Hofmann, W., Newman, W., Mackay, C.R., Sodroski, J., and Gabuzda, D. (1997) CCR3 and CCR5 are coreceptors for HIV-1 infection of microglia. *Nature* 385:645–649.

Heese, K., Hock, C., and Otten, U. (1998) Inflammatory signals induce neurotrophin expression in human microglial cells. *J. Neurochem.* 70:699–707.

Horwitz, M.S., Evans, C.F., Klier, F.G., and Oldstone, M.B. (1999) Detailed in vivo analysis of interferon-gamma induced major histocompatibility complex expression in the the central nervous system: astrocytes fail to express major histocompatibility complex class I and II molecules. *Lab. Invest.* 79:235–242.

Horwitz, M.S., Evans, C.F., McGavern, D.B., Rodriguez, M., and Oldstone, M.B. (1997) Primary demyelination in transgenic mice expressing interferon-gamma. *Nat. Med.* 3:1037–1041.

Kaul, M. and Lipton, S.A. (1999) Chemokines and activated macrophages in HIV gp120-induced neuronal apoptosis. *Proc. Natl. Acad. Sci. USA* 96:8212–8216.

Kielian, T., Barry, B., and Hickey, W.F. (2001) CXC chemokine receptor-2 ligands are required for neutrophil-mediated host defense in experimental brain abscesses. *J. Immunol.* 166:4634–4643.

Lane, T.E., Asensio, V.C., Yu, N., Paoletti, A.D., Campbell, I.L., and Buchmeier, M.J. (1998) Dynamic regulation of alpha- and beta-chemokine expression in the central nervous system during mouse hepatitis virus–induced demyelinating disease. *J. Immunol.* 160: 970–978.

Lipton, S.A., Yeh, M., and Dreyer, E.B. (1994) Update on current models of HIV-related neuronal injury: platelet-activating factor, arachidonic acid and nitric oxide. *Adv. Neuroimmunol.* 4:181–188.

Lokensgard, J.R., Hu, S., Sheng, W., vanOijen, M., Cox, D., Cheeran, M.C., and Peterson, P.K. (2001) Robust expression of TNF-alpha, IL-1beta, RANTES, and IP-10 by human microglial cells during nonproductive infection with herpes simplex virus. *J. Neurovirol.* 7:208–219.

Morgan, B.P. and Gasque, P. (1996) Expression of complement in the brain: role in health and disease. *Immunol. Today* 17:461–466.

Nau, R., Soto, A., and Bruck, W. (1999) Apoptosis of neurons in the dentate gyrus in humans suffering from bacterial meningitis. *J. Neuropathol. Exp. Neurol.* 58:265–274.

Rodriguez, M., Pierce, M.L., and Howie, E.A. (1987) Immune response gene products (Ia antigens) on glial and endothelial cells in virus-induced demyelination. *J. Immunol.* 138:3438–3442.

Sauder, C., Hallensleben, W., Pagenstecher, A., Schneckenburger, S., Biro, L., Pertlik, D., Hausmann, J., Suter, M., and Staeheli, P. (2000) Chemokine gene expression in astrocytes of Borna disease virus–infected rats and mice in the absence of inflammation. *J. Virol.* 74:9267–9280.

Schluter, D., Chahoud, S., Lassmann, H., Schumann, A., Hof, H., and Deckert-Schluter, M. (1996) Intracerebral targets and immunomodulation of murine *Listeria monocytogenes* meningoencephalitis. *J. Neuropathol. Exp. Neurol.* 55:14–24.

Schluter, D., Deckert-Schluter, M., Schwendemann, G., Brunner, H., and Hof, H. (1993) Expression of major histocompatibility complex class II antigens and levels of interferon-gamma, tumour necrosis factor, and interleukin-6 in cerebrospinal fluid and serum in *Toxoplasma gondii*–infected SCID and immunocompetent C.B-17 mice. *Immunology* 78:430–435.

Schluter, D., Kaefer, N., Hof, H., Wiestler, O.D., and Deckert-Schluter, M. (1997) Expression pattern and cellular origin of cytokines in the normal and *Toxoplasma gondii*–infected murine brain. *Am. J. Pathol.* 150:1021–1035.

Schluter, D., Lohler, J., Deckert, M., Hof, H., and Schwendemann, G. (1991) *Toxoplasma* encephalitis of immunocompetent and nude mice: immunohistochemical characterisation of *Toxoplasma* antigen, infiltrates and major histocompatibility complex gene products. *J. Neuroimmunol.* 31:185–198.

Schluter, D., Meyer, T., Kwok, L.Y., Montesinos-Rongen, M., Lutjen, S., Strack, A., Schmitz, M.L., and Deckert, M. (2002) Phenotype and regulation of persistent intracerebral T cells in murine *Toxoplasma* encephalitis. *J. Immunol.* 169:315–322.

Schluter, D., Meyer, T., Strack, A., Reiter, S., Kretschmar, M., Wiestler, O.D., Hof, H., and Deckert, M. (2001) Regulation of microglia by CD4+ and CD8+ T cells: selective analysis in CD45-congenic normal and *Toxoplasma gondii*–infected bone marrow chimeras. *Brain Pathol.* 11:44–55.

Shieh, J.T., Albright, A.V., Sharron, M., Gartner, S., Strizki, J., Doms, R.W., and Gonzalez-Scarano, F. (1998) Chemokine receptor utilization by human immunodeficiency virus type 1 isolates that replicate in microglia. *J. Virol.* 72:4243–4249.

Si, Q., Kim, M.O., Zhao, M.L., Landau, N.R., Goldstein, H., and Lee, S. (2002) Vpr- and Nef-dependent induction of RANTES/CCL5 in microglial cells. *Virology* 301:342–353.

Stohlman, S.A. and Hinton, D.R. (2001) Viral induced demyelination. *Brain Pathol.* 11:92–106.

Strack, A., Asensio, V.C., Campbell, I.L., Schluter, D., and Deckert, M. (2002) Chemokines are differentially expressed by astrocytes, microglia and inflammatory leukocytes in *Toxoplasma* encephalitis and critically regulated by interferon-gamma. *Acta Neuropathol. (Berl.)* 103:458–468.

Strack, A., Schluter, D., Asensio, V.C., Campbell, I.L., and Deckert, M. (2002) Regulation of the kinetics of intracerebral chemokine gene expression in murine *Toxoplasma* encephalitis: Impact of host genetic factors. *Glia* 40:372–377.

Tompkins, S.M., Fuller, K.G., and Miller, S.D. (2002) Theiler's virus-mediated autoimmunity: local presentation of CNS antigens and epitope spreading. *Ann. NY Acad. Sci.* 958:26–38.

Vallat, A.V., De Girolami, U., He, J., Mhashilkar, A., Marasco, W., Shi, B., Gray, F., Bell, J., Keohane, C., Smith, T.W., and Gabuzda, D. (1998) Localization of HIV-1 co-receptors CCR5 and CXCR4 in the brain of children with AIDS. *Am. J. Pathol.* 152:167–178.

Wang, J., Crawford, K., Yuan, M., Wang, H., Gorry, P.R., and Gabuzda, D. (2002) Regulation of CC chemokine receptor 5 and CD4 expression and human immunodeficiency virus type 1 replication in human macrophages and microglia by T helper type 2 cytokines. *J. Infect. Dis.* 185:885–897.

Ying Wang, J., Peruzzi, F., Lassak, A., Del Valle, L., Radhakrishnan, S., Rappaport, J., Khalili, K., Amini, S., and Reiss, K. (2003) Neuroprotective effects of IGF-I against TNFalpha-induced neuronal damage in HIV-associated dementia. *Virology* 305:66–76.

Zheng, J., Ghorpade, A., Niemann, D., Cotter, R.L., Thylin, M.R., Epstein, L., Swartz, J.M., Shepard, R.B., Liu, X., Nukuna, A., and Gendelman, H.E. (1999) Lymphotropic virions affect chemokine receptor-mediated neural signaling and apoptosis: implications for human immunodeficiency virus type 1-associated dementia. *J. Virol.* 73:8256–8267.

Index

Page numbers followed by *f* indicate figures, page numbers followed by *t* indicate tables.